Two week loan
Benthyciad pythefnos

Please return on or before the due date to avoid overdue charges
A wnewch chi ddychwelyd ar neu cyn y dyddiad a nodir ar eich llyfr os gwelwch yn dda, er mwyn osgoi taliadau

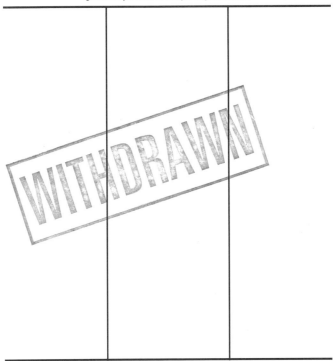

http://library.cardiff.ac.uk
http://llyfrgell.caerdydd.ac.uk

DISORDERS OF THE MOTOR UNIT

DISORDERS OF THE MOTOR UNIT

Edited by

DONALD L. SCHOTLAND, M.D.
Department of Neurology
University of Pennsylvania School of Medicine
Philadelphia, Pennsylvania

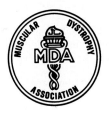

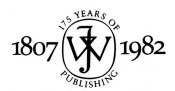

A WILEY MEDICAL PUBLICATION
JOHN WILEY & SONS
New York • Chichester • Brisbane • Toronto • Singapore

Production Editor: Rosalind Straley
Cover design: Wanda Lubelska

Library of Congress Cataloging in Publication Data:

Main entry under title:

Disorders of the motor unit.

  (A Wiley medical publication)
  Outgrowth of an international meeting in 1980
sponsored by the Muscular Dystrophy Association.
  Includes index.
  1. Neuromuscular diseases—Congresses.
2. Myoneural junction—Diseases—Congresses.
I. Schotland, Donald L.   II. Muscular Dystrophy
Association.   III. Series. [DNLM: 1. Neuromuscular
diseases—Congresses.   WE 550 D6115 1981]
RC925.D53   616.7′4   81-13119
ISBN 0-471-09507-9   AACR2

Printed in the United States of America

10 9 8 7 6 5 4 3 2 1

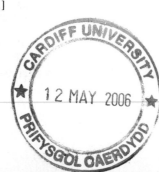

Contributors

First-Listed Authors of Each Chapter and All Panel Discussants

Albert J. Aguayo, M.D.
Department of Neurology and
  Neurosurgery
McGill University
Neurosciences Unit
Montreal General Hospital
Montreal, Canada

Edson X. Albuquerque, M.D., Ph.D.
Department of Pharmacology and
  Experimental Therapeutics
University of Maryland School of
  Medicine
Baltimore, Maryland

Wolfhard Almers, Ph.D.
Department of Physiology and
  Biophysics
University of Washington
Seattle, Washington

Stanley H. Appel, M.D.
Department of Neurology
Baylor University College of Medicine
Houston, Texas

Arthur K. Asbury, M.D.
Department of Neurology
University of Pennsylvania School of
  Medicine
Philadelphia, Pennsylvania

Valerie Askanas, M.D., Ph.D.
Medical Neurology Branch
National Institute of Neurological and
  Communicative Disorders and Stroke
National Institutes of Health
Bethesda, Maryland

Michael Bárány, M.D.
Department of Biological Chemistry
University of Illinois Medical Center
Chicago, Illinois

Robert L. Barchi, M.D., Ph.D.
Department of Neurology
University of Pennsylvania School of
  Medicine
Philadelphia, Pennsylvania

Francisco Bezanilla, Ph.D.
Department of Physiology
University of California, Los Angeles
Los Angeles, California

Eduardo Bonilla, M.D.
Department of Neurology
University of Pennsylvania School of
  Medicine
Philadelphia, Pennsylvania

Barbara I. Brown, Ph.D.
Department of Biological Chemistry
Washington University School of
  Medicine
St. Louis, Missouri

Shirley H. Bryant, Ph.D.
Department of Pharmacology
University of Cincinnati College of
  Medicine
Cincinnati, Ohio

Richard P. Bunge, M.D.
Departments of Anatomy and
  Neurobiology

Washington University School of
    Medicine
St. Louis, Missouri

Peter C. Dau, M.D.
Laboratory of Cellular Immunology
Children's Hospital of San Francisco
San Francisco, California

John R. Dedman, Ph.D.
Department of Cell Biology
Baylor University College of Medicine
Houston, Texas

Ivan Diamond, M.D., Ph.D.
Department of Neurology
University of California, San Francisco
San Francisco, California

Salvatore DiMauro, M.D.
Department of Neurology
Columbia University College of
    Physicians and Surgeons
New York, New York

Daniel B. Drachman, M.D.
Department of Neurology
Johns Hopkins University School of
    Medicine
Baltimore, Maryland

Peter J. Dyck, M.D.
Peripheral Nerve Laboratory
Mayo Medical School and Foundation
Rochester, Minnesota

Richard H. T. Edwards, M.D., Ph.D.
Departments of Human Metabolism and
    Medicine
University College Hospital
London, England

Alan E. H. Emery, M.D.
Department of Human Genetics
Western General Hospital
Edinburgh, Scotland

Andrew G. Engel, M.D.
Department Of Neurology
Mayo Clinic
Rochester, Minnesota

W. King Engel, M.D.
Medical Neurology Branch, NINCDS
National Institutes of Health
Bethesda, Maryland

Henry F. Epstein, M.D.
Department of Neurology
Baylor University College of Medicine
Houston, Texas

Douglas M. Fambrough, Ph.D.
Department of Embryology
Carnegie Institute of Washington
Baltimore, Maryland

Gerald D. Fischbach, Ph.D.
Department of Pharmacology
Harvard Medical School
Boston, Massachusetts

Sara Fuchs, Ph.D.
Department of Chemical Immunology
Weizmann Institute of Science
Rehovot, Israel

David B. P. Goodman, M.D., Ph.D.
Department of Internal Medicine
Yale University School of Medicine
New Haven, Connecticut

Paul Greengard, Ph.D.
Department of Pharmacology
Yale University School of Medicine
New Haven, Connecticut

Hanns-Dieter Gruemer, M.D.
Division of Clinical Pathology
Virginia Commonwealth University
Medical College of Virginia
Richmond, Virginia

Peter S. Harper, M.D.
Section on Medical Genetics
University Hospital of Wales
Cardiff, United Kingdom

Stephen D. Hauschka, Ph.D.
Department of Biochemistry
University of Washington
Seattle, Washington

Stephen L. Hauser, M.D.
Department of Neurosciences
Children's Hospital Medical Center
Boston, Massachusetts

Hugh E. Huxley, Ph.D.
MRC Laboratory of Molecular Biology
University Medical School
Cambridge, England

George Karpati, M.D.
Department of Neurology
Montreal Neurological Institute
Montreal, Canada

Laura Reeburgh Keller, Ph.D.
Department of Biology
University of Virginia
Charlottesville, Virginia

Peter Kornfeld, M.D.
Department of Medicine
Mt. Sinai School of Medicine
New York, New York

Gary E. Landreth, Ph.D.
Department of Anatomy
University of South Carolina
Charleston, South Carolina

Peter Libby, M.D.
Department of Medicine
Tufts University School of Medicine
Boston, Massachusetts

Jon Lindstrom, Ph.D.
Receptor Biology Laboratory
Salk Institute
La Jolla, California

Robert P. Lisak, M.D.
Department of Neurology
University of Pennsylvania School of
  Medicine
Philadelphia, Pennsylvania

Anthony N. Martonosi, M.D.
Department of Biochemistry
State University of New York
  Upstate Medical Center
Syracuse, New York

Michael Merickel, Ph.D.
Department of Neurology
Baylor University College of Medicine
Houston, Texas

John Newsom-Davis, M.D.
Department of Neurology
Royal Free Hospital
London, England

Sidney Ochs, Ph.D.
Department of Physiology
Indiana University School of Medicine
Indianapolis, Indiana

Mitsuhiro Osame, M.D.
Department of Neurology
Mayo Clinic
Rochester, Minnesota

Carl M. Pearson, M.D.
Department of Medicine
UCLA School of Medicine
Los Angeles, California

Alan Pestronk, M.D.
Department of Neurology
Johns Hopkins University School of
  Medicine
Baltimore, Maryland

Guillermo Pilar, M.D.
Physiology Section
Biological Sciences Group
University of Connecticut
Storrs, Connecticut

David Pleasure, M.D.
Department of Neurology
University of Pennsylvania School of
  Medicine
Philadelphia, Pennsylvania

Franklyn G. Prendergast, M.D., Ph.D.
Department of Pharmacology
Mayo Clinic
Rochester, Minnesota

David W. Pumplin, M.D.
Department of Anatomy
University of Maryland School of
  Medicine
Baltimore, Maryland

Michael Rasminsky, M.D., Ph.D.
McGill University
Neurosciences Unit
Montreal General Hospital
Montreal, Canada

Charles J. Rebouche, Ph.D.
Department of Neurology
Mayo Clinic
Rochester, Minnesota

Allen D. Roses, M.D.
Department of Neurology
Duke University Medical Center
Durham, North Carolina

Lee L. Rubin, Ph.D.
Rockefeller University
New York, New York

Donald B. Sanders, M.D.
Department of Neurology
University of Virginia School of
    Medicine
Charlottesville, Virginia

Henning Schmalbruch, M.D.
Institute of Neurophysiology
University of Copenhagen
Copenhagen, Denmark

Robert J. Schwartz, Ph.D.
Department of Cell Biology
Baylor University College of Medicine
Houston, Texas

Jerry W. Shay, Ph.D.
Department of Cell Biology
University of Texas Southwestern
    Medical School at Dallas
Dallas, Texas

Peter S. Spencer, Ph.D.
Institute of Neurotoxicology

Albert Einstein College of Medicine
Bronx, New York

Robert V. Storti, Ph.D.
Department of Biochemistry
University of Illinois College of
    Medicine
Chicago, Illinois

Margaret W. Thompson, M.D.
Department of Genetics
Hospital for Sick Children
Toronto, Canada

Sir John Walton, TD, MD, DSc, SRCP
Regional Neurological Center
Newcastle General Hospital
Newcastle-upon-Tyne, Great Britain

Robert H. Waterston, M.D., Ph.D.
Departments of Neurobiology and
    Anatomy
Washington University School of
    Medicine
St. Louis, Missouri

Joseph H. Willner, M.D.
Department of Neurology
Columbia University College of
    Physicians and Surgeons
New York, New York

Donald S. Wood, Ph.D.
Department of Neurology
Columbia University College of
    Physicians and Surgeons
New York, New York

David Yaffe, Ph.D.
Department of Cell Biology
Weizmann Institute of Science
Rehovot, Israel

Preface

In recent years, research in human neuromuscular disorders has accelerated at an exciting pace. For many years the Muscular Dystrophy Association (MDA) has been a major supporter of this effort, and since 1966 it has sponsored six international scientific conferences to record progress, stimulate interaction, and point to new directions of research. The international conference of 1976 focused on the pathogenesis of human muscular dystrophies. Since that time, there have been many advances in diverse fields of neuromuscular research, including biochemical genetics, membrane structure and function, cell to cell interactions, mechanism of cell death, cell culture of muscle and peripheral nerve, and metabolic disorders of muscle. In addition, new basic techniques, including the production of monoclonal antibodies, their use as specific probes, and the application of nuclear magnetic resonance to biological systems, have greatly extended our knowledge of these disorders.

Concomitant with the dramatic increase in neuromuscular research activity, MDA has expanded the focus of both its research and medical services programs to cover 40 diseases of the motor unit. It was therefore timely that MDA sponsored an international scientific conference in 1980 to analyze the advances that have occurred in research in the entire area of diseases of the motor unit. The scope of this topic has become too broad to include discussion of diseases of the motor neuron in a five-day conference. However, another international meeting to be convened by MDA in 1981 will be devoted solely to them. This book, therefore, contains a comprehensive account of neuromuscular research in peripheral nerve disease, myasthenia gravis, and disorders of muscle. The meeting from which the book is derived generated a unique excitement and a feeling of surging optimism that I believe is evident in the text of its proceedings.

This conference and much of the work that was presented would not have been possible without MDA's long-standing support as well as the special efforts of Jerry Lewis, who has served for over three decades as MDA national chairman.

MDA staff provided invaluable help in the planning of the myriad details of this meeting, whose program committee was comprised of the members of MDA's Scientific Advisory Committee from 1976 to 1980. We thank all of these people and the many others whose concerted efforts resulted in this stellar conference and the publication of this volume.

On a personal note, I should like to express my appreciation to my wife, Estherina, for her invaluable input and support throughout the preparations for the conference and this book.

D.L.S.

Contents

PART II
CELL-CELL INTERACTIONS

PART III
MYASTHENIA GRAVIS

PART IV
MEMBRANES AND MUSCULAR DYSTROPHY

SECTION A
PHYSICAL AND PHYSIOLOGICAL ASPECTS

PART V
MUSCLE AND CALCIUM

PART VI
ALTERATIONS IN METABOLIC REGULATION

PART VII
GENETIC CONTROL OF PROTEIN SYNTHESIS

PART VIII
ASPECTS OF CARRIER DETECTION

PART IX
MUSCLE IN CULTURE

DISORDERS OF
THE MOTOR UNIT

1
GUEST LECTURE: THE MECHANISM OF FORCE PRODUCTION IN MUSCLE

Hugh E. Huxley, PhD

The purpose of this review is to give a short account of some work that my colleagues and I have been doing during the past few years to try to establish, with greater certainty, the detailed molecular nature of the force-producing mechanism in muscle. This topic clearly lies some distance from most of the aspects of muscle and muscle disease that form the subject matter of this meeting. However, whatever one's own particular concern with muscle may be, I think it may be helpful to have as clear and realistic a picture as possible of what is currently believed about how muscles actually carry out their basic function of shortening and generating force.

There has been overwhelming evidence for many years that the force for muscle contraction is developed in some way by cross-bridges between actin and myosin filaments, and that their action causes the filaments to slide past each other. This general finding has been helpful in providing a reasonable picture of how muscles contract, and has also been a useful one to bear in mind when thinking about the many other forms of cell motility, especially those involving proteins closely analogous to actin and myosin in muscle.

Although the general nature of the mechanism has been well established for some time now and has been able to account for many of the physiological and biochemical properties of muscle, it has proved remarkably difficult to go the next stage further and obtain clear, convincing evidence about the details of how the cross-bridges actually function.

Thus, the application of various electron microscopic techniques enabled a great deal to be established about the general structural nature of the filaments and cross-bridges, but they did not, and still cannot, show us images of a working cross-bridge going through the various steps of its cycle of operations. Other

1

techniques, both biochemical and physiological, have given us a great deal of information about cross-bridge behavior, but the techniques involved have, by their nature, not been able to provide the structural information we need, and the basic questions that must be solved about contraction are structural ones. What is needed is a method by which we can get structural information about dynamic processes taking place on the millisecond time scale. The basic difficulties are 3-fold: the cross-bridges are very small structures, approximately 100 Å or so in length; we cannot use a chemical fixative to fix the structure in one state or another in a known way; and the changes are not only rapid, but are also cyclic, taking place continuously and asynchronously for all of the time that a muscle is active.

USE OF X-RAY DIFFRACTION

The possibility of using x-ray diffraction to study these changes had, of course, been considered ever since informative x-ray diagrams had been obtained from living muscles. However, because of the very long exposure times involved (originally many hours or even days), it was clear that major technological developments would be necessary before the data could be obtained sufficiently quickly to follow any changes that might occur during contraction. Developments have now taken place which enable us to record the x-ray diagrams in as little as 1 msec, and it is about the results that we are beginning to get with such methods that I want to write. First, however, let me explain the problem to you in a little more detail, and describe the specific pieces of information we have been trying to obtain.

SUMMARY OF THE PROBLEM

It is well established that the cross-bridges correspond, to a first approximation, to the S_1 head regions of the myosin molecules, which project out laterally from the backbones of the thick filaments so that they are in a position to interact with the actin filaments alongside. Because the adenosine triphosphate (ATP)-splitting capability of myosin is located in the head region, and because it is known from biochemical studies that the ATPase is activated by actin, there can be little doubt that the energy for contraction is being liberated at the cross-bridges by some interaction with actin, and that the sliding force from contraction is thereby being generated at the same time. What has not been established with any certainty, however, is how this force generation takes place. Of course, plausible models have been put forward.

   The so-called swinging cross-bridge model (1) envisaged that the S_1 head of myosin and the S_2 region to which it is immediately attached could hinge out sideways from the thick filament backbone (made up of the light meromyosin portions of the molecules), making use of flexible regions of the molecule at either end of the S_2 region (Fig. 1) The S_1 heads could then attach to actin and, while remaining attached, undergo some structural change that could effectively change the angle of their attachment in the appropriate direction. This would

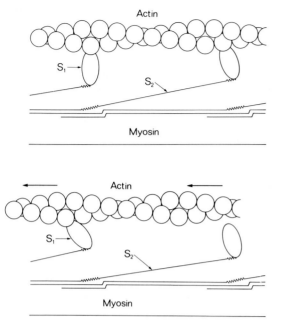

Actin

S_1

S_2

Myosin

Actin

S_1

S_2

Myosin

Fig. 1. Hypothetical scheme for cross-bridge action. Myosin heads attach to actin by swinging out laterally from backbone of thick filaments. Tension and sliding are produced by change in effective angle of attachment of cross-bridge to actin. Cross-bridge then detaches, returns to original conformation, and attaches again at another site farther along the actin filament. Adenosine triphosphate is split during each cycle. Cross-bridges all detach when muscle relaxes.

produce a sliding movement between the actin and myosin filaments. At the end of the working stroke, the cross-bridge would detach, reattach farther along the actin filament, and repeat the movement cycle. When the muscle relaxed, attachment of cross-bridges to actin would be prevented, force generation would cease, and the myosin heads would return to the thick filaments.

Now this model was all purely hypothetical. Many subsequent experiments have been interpreted very reasonably in terms of this general hypothesis, but it is essential to try to establish the hypothesis itself as firmly as possible by direct experiments. Specifically, the major points that need to be proved are the following: (*a*) Lateral movement of the cross-bridges takes place when the muscle contracts. (*b*) This movement occurs because the bridges are becoming attached to actin. (*c*) This attachment results in the generation of force in the muscle. (*d*) Longitudinal movement of bridges (e.g., axial tilting) occurs during contraction. (*e*) It is this axial movement of bridges attached to actin that generates contractile force.

TYPES OF X-RAY EVIDENCE

Evidence about these questions can be obtained by x-ray diffraction in the following way. The diagrams from muscle can be considered in two parts: the equatorial regions that provide information about the lateral organization of the muscle, and the axial regions that provide information about structures repeated along the length of the muscle. We can recognize two basic types of equatorial x-ray diagram given by vertebrate striated muscles. Each one corresponds to the pattern given by a double hexagonal lattice of filaments, with essentially the same lattice spacing of approximately 400 Å. The first type is given by resting muscle and has a strong [10] reflection (the inner reflection) and a weaker [11] reflection. The second type is given by muscle in rigor and has a weak [10] reflection and a strong [11] reflection. Fourier reconstructions show that this implies a shift of density away from the myosin filaments and toward the actin filaments. Electron micrographs of muscles in the two states show that this is indeed what has taken place, and in rigor muscles the cross-bridges can be seen attached to the actin filaments (2, 3), thereby increasing the mass near the trigonal positions of the lattice. It became possible several years ago to record the equatorial reflections from muscle during contraction by adding together the patterns given during a long series of 1- or 2-second tetani.

The equatorial x-ray diagrams from isometrically contracting muscles are quite similar to those given by muscles in rigor, with a weak [10] and a strong [11] (4), although the [11]/[10] ratio is slightly lower than it is in rigor. Whether this reflects a slightly smaller number of attached bridges or a slightly different average angle of attachment is not known. However, the most straightforward interpretation of the data is that the pattern arises in essentially the same way as in rigor, from cross-bridges attaching to actin, so the first experimental test seems to confirm the predictions of the model.

One could, nevertheless, wonder whether the change in pattern in contracting muscle could be due in whole or in part to some myosin-based control mechanism that allowed the cross-bridges to move outward on activation, so that the change did not necessarily reflect attachment to actin as such. We have investigated this possibility by recording the equatorial diagram from muscles stretched to sarcomere lengths at which thick and thin filaments no longer overlap. A strong [10] reflection is still produced by such muscles, but it does not change in intensity when the muscle is stimulated in a series of 0.5- or 1-second tetani (5). This is true even in muscles swollen in two-thirds-strength Ringer solution. Thus, the presence of actin alongside myosin is necessary for outward movement of the average center of gravity of the cross-bridges.

All the available evidence on the behavior of the control proteins on the actin filaments indicates that they operate under physiological conditions by producing changes in the binding site for myosin. These changes prevent attachment until the system is activated by calcium and are equally effective either in highly structured muscle or in muscle in solution. Therefore, it seems reasonable to deduce that the average outward movement of the cross-bridges toward actin in an activated muscle really does represent physical attachment mediated by Brownian movement. No doubt, random fluctuations of bridge position also occur in resting muscles, but in that case, the bridges that approach actin closely will not stick to it, and their average position is closer to the myosin backbone.

TIME-RESOLVED MEASUREMENTS

The next question was whether these movements are causally related to the development of force by the muscle. We can test this by finding out whether the cross-bridges become attached rapidly enough to account for the rapid onset of contractile force after stimulation. This involves measuring the changes in the equatorial x-ray diagram with a time resolution of 10 msec or so. By making use of various types of x-ray photon counters, together with high-power rotating anode x-ray tubes, we were able to begin making such time-resolved x-ray measurements some years ago, and some of the results have already been reported (5–7). The structural changes, which we interpreted as representing cross-bridge attachment to actin, occurred even faster than development of tension at the beginning of contraction, and the bridges returned to the myosin filaments as the muscles relaxed. The same changes have been seen subsequently by a number of other groups (8–10).

This result is in full agreement with what we should expect from the model, and the slight time lead of the structural change over tension may indicate a further rate process at an attached cross-bridge before it develops tension. Because it has also been shown that the characteristics of the attached pattern persist when a muscle is allowed to shorten during contraction by distances much greater than the range over which a cross-bridge would remain attached to any given site, it also follows that the attachment can be broken and re-formed during contraction, i.e., that cycling of the cross-bridges takes place. If we had found, on the other hand, that force was developed before cross-bridge movement took place or that the attached pattern disappeared if the muscle was allowed to shorten, then clearly the model would have been disproved.

AXIAL CROSS-BRIDGE MOVEMENTS

The movements with which we have been concerned so far clearly cannot themselves produce muscle shortening, because they are lateral rather than longitudinal. Thus, the crucial question we have to answer is whether there is evidence for longitudinal movement of the cross-bridges in a contracting muscle while they are attached to actin, and if so, whether we can elucidate the detailed nature and the course of that movement. The kind of longitudinal movement we are concerned with is one that will, if it occurs in an attached bridge, bring about a translation of the actin filament towards the center of the A-band. Thus, in principle, it could represent a tilting movement of the myosin head (S_1) about its attachment site to actin, with a component of the motion that tends to move the region of the myosin head to which the S_2 is attached (i.e., presumably, the opposite end of the elongated head) away from the center of the A-band; an active rotation about the S_1S_2 hinge; a change in shape of the S_1, producing essentially the same effect; a change in length of the S_2 region; or some change within the backbone of the thick filament that produces a longitudinal cross-bridge movement. There may be good reasons for thinking that one or more of these types of movement are more likely than the others, but the first step must be to examine the quality of the evidence for supposing that any significant movement at all takes place.

The structural evidence relevant to this question starts from a comparison of the axial parts of the low-angle x-ray diagram given by vertebrate striated muscle in rigor and those given by a live, resting muscle. The former gives, in place of the characteristic 430-Å myosin layer-line pattern of relaxed muscle, a pattern of layer-line reflections that can be indexed on the actin helix, with a prominent 360- to 380-Å repeat. It is apparent that a substantial proportion of the bridges have attached to actin in more or less similar orientations and are producing the characteristic "labeled actin" pattern. On the other hand, even in the earliest pictures obtained from contracting muscles, although we observed a great weakening of the myosin layer-line pattern, there was no sign of the appearance of any other layer-line pattern to replace it. This provided good initial evidence that the attached bridges (clearly present in substantial numbers because of the large change in the equatorial pattern) were attaching in a much less regular way than in rigor, i.e., that they were attached over a range of angles.

This earlier evidence, however, suffered from a number of weaknesses. The pattern was built up over a very long series of 1- or 2-second tetani, and there was no evidence (*a*) how the time course of the change in pattern during a contraction corresponded with that of the development of tension and its subsequent relaxation; (*b*) whether the change in pattern was present throughout the contraction series or developed only as the muscle fatigued; or (*c*) whether the progressive fading of the relaxed pattern that occurred during the long contraction series reflected changes in the muscle that were also making it more difficult to see evidence of a rigor pattern during contraction.

In view of the importance of the question, therefore, we have been attempting to obtain much better evidence about the behavior of the layer-line pattern during contraction, both with regard to its behavior during very short contraction series in unfatigued muscles, and also with regard to its detailed time course relative to tension. Because the layer-line patterns are weak ones, they cannot be recorded sufficiently quickly, using laboratory x-ray sources, even if electronic x-ray detectors are used, For this reason, we have carried out our experiments (11) with synchrotron radiation from the electron-positron storage ring DORIS, using the facilities provided by the European Molecular Biology Outstation at DESY, Hamburg.

USE OF SYNCHROTRON RADIATION

Storage rings were developed originally for use by physicists to investigate interactions in very high energy collisons between, for example, electrons and positrons moving in opposite directions in intersecting orbits. However, it turns out that particles confined to such orbits emit enormous quantities of radiation, much of it in the x-ray region. If one goes to enough trouble—and a great deal of effort is involved—a monochromatized beam can be produced from such a source and can be used for x-ray diffraction experiments, with the difference that the intensity can be a thousand times or more as great as that from the most powerful rotating anode x-ray tube. On this occasion, I do not want to go into the technicalities involved in generating and recording such intense x-ray beams with high time resolution. Suffice it to say that a time resolution in the millisecond range can now be achieved.

In our initial experiments we were concerned to establish whether or not the loss of layer-line intensity was a genuine effect occurring during an unfatigued contraction in a freshly dissected muscle. We used a frog sartorius muscle, maintained in an oxygenated Ringer solution and stimulated directly by platinum electrodes lying along its length on either side. Tension was measured and recorded electronically. A good-quality layer-line pattern from muscle could be recorded on an x-ray image intensifier–TV detector (12), with a total exposure time of only 1 second.

When collecting time-resolved data, only the pattern corresponding to one particular "time slot" could be recorded in a given series of experiments because of read-out time limitations with this detector. To investigate the behavior of the pattern during single twitches, we recorded the pattern during a time interval of 150 msec, and in each run of 6 to 10 twitches this time slot was set for the same time during contraction. The run was then repeated for a different time slot.

Within this limited time resolution, it could be seen that the disappearance of the layer-line pattern at the beginning of the twitch and its return during relaxation followed a time course very similar to development and decay of tension. This could be observed in quite short contraction series in which there was no doubt that the muscle was in good condition throughout and where there was none of the weakening of the resting layer-line reflections that we have observed in longer series of tetanic contractions, especially at lower temperatures; nor did we see the delayed return of off-meridional layer-line pattern after contraction that is apparent in very long contraction series (13). Thus, the experiments showed unambiguously that the loss of the layer-line pattern is a specific and reversible accompaniment of normal contraction.

USE OF FAST, POSITION-SENSITIVE DETECTORS

To compare the time course of the layer-line changes more accurately with that of tension, a different system was used. We used a position-sensitive one-dimensional proportional counter of the delay line type (14). This was positioned over the muscle pattern with its axis parallel to the meridian but displaced sideways from it so as to record the strongest parts of the set of myosin layer lines. The one-dimensional patterns were stored in 10-msec time bins synchronized electronically with the stimulation of the muscle. With the storage ring operating at 3.185 gev and 70 to 90 mA, good data could be collected from a series of approximately 100 single twitches spaced at 30-second intervals.

The most striking change in the pattern was the large decrease in all of the layer-line intensities during the time that the muscle was developing tension. The time course of the change in all of the layer lines appeared to be identical. In a typical run at 10° C the reflections began to decrease in intensity within 20 msec of stimulation, fell to a minimum by approximately 70 msec, and then returned to the resting value (or even slightly more) after 200 to 250 msec.

The relationship between change in intensity and tension could be seen much more clearly when the change in each of them was plotted as a percentage of the maximal change occurring. Both during the onset of activity and during relaxation, isometric tension and change in x-ray intensity followed a very similar time course, and this was the case in all of the records we obtained (although in one or two a very slight lag in the x-ray pattern, by approximately 20 msec or less, was noticed during relaxation). It was also seen that the change in intensity led the change in tension during the rising phase of tension by a few milliseconds at this temperature, as it does in the case of equatorial reflections (13).

We have also carried out some preliminary experiments on the behavior of the layer-line pattern in frog semitendinosus muscles stimulated at very stretched lengths, at which overlap of thin and thick filaments is either completely abolished or very greatly reduced. In all our experiments so far on stretched muscles, we have found that the decrease of the layer-line intensities during stimulation is greatly reduced compared to that seen in muscles at normal sarcomere lengths; in most of the experiments, no decrease at all in intensity was observed. We conclude provisionally that interaction with actin is necessary for helical disordering of the myosin cross-bridges to occur after stimulation. This accords with recent observations showing an absence of radial cross-bridge movement at no-overlap sarcomere lengths, as judged by the absence of change in the equatorial x-ray diagram (5) and also with recent results of Matsubara and Yagi (15).

CONCLUSIONS

The principle finding whose significance I want to consider here is the large decrease in intensity of the layer lines at resting sarcomere lengths, unaccompanied by any sign of a new layer-line pattern. It is very significant that the substantial number of attached bridges, indicated by the substantially changed equatorial x-ray diagram, gives so little helical diffraction in an axial direction. This indicates that the bridges are not all attached to actin in the same orientation, as they are in rigor. Thus, the evidence does appear to show that bridges can be attached to actin in more than one orientation, and that they move from their regular helical arrangement around the myosin filaments and occupy these different orientations, attached to actin, during contraction.

The experiments therefore provide very strong evidence that some type of longitudinal cross-bridge movement occurs during contraction. It is clear that we start off in the relaxed muscle with the cross-bridges regularly arranged in a helix around the backbone of the thick filaments and conforming to the characteristic myosin filament helical repeat of 429 Å. On stimulation, a change in the lateral position of the bridges occurs very rapidly as they attach to actin, and at the same time the helical ordering of the bridges is lost. This very rapid helical disordering that we have observed is exactly what we would expect if bridges first attached and then underwent longitudinal (tilting) movements as the muscle shortened internally against its series elastic elements, so that the population of bridges was spread over the whole range of possible attachment angles. Then, when the muscle is switched off, the bridges detach and rapidly return to their ordered resting positions.

We have attempted to get stronger positive evidence of longitudinal movement of attached cross-bridges by studying the behavior of the 143-Å meridional reflection during rapid release of the muscle. This reflection arises from the regular repeat of groups of cross-bridges along the thick filaments, and its intensity is sensitive to changes in the tilt or axial ordering of those bridges. When an isometrically contracting muscle is suddenly allowed to shorten by approximately 0.5% of its length by momentarily removing the load on it, this reflection very rapidly decreases in intensity and then recovers. This shows (given certain provisos that we have checked) that the longitudinal ordering of the cross-bridges is directly affected by changes in length of the muscle and provides strong support for the conclusion that the longitudinal filament movement is directly coupled to the change in the longitudinal position or orientation of the cross-bridges. We are still in the early stages of this work, but the important thing is that we can now make many of the x-ray diffraction observations with almost the same time resolution used in biochemical kinetic experiments (i.e., those done in stopped-flow machines) and in transient mechanical kinetic experiments. We hope this will help to establish more clearly how the cross-bridges behave when developing the sliding force between the actin and myosin filaments.

To summarize, we can now make x-ray diffraction observations on contracting muscle with sufficient time resolution to follow the changes in pattern produced by the movement of the cross-bridges. The results so far, which include experiments of increasing stringency, seem to agree very well with the predictions of the "swinging, tilting cross-bridge model," and we are now beginning to study very rapid transient responses to extend this work further.

REFERENCES

1. Huxley HE: The mechanism of muscular contraction. Science 164:1356–1366, 1969
2. Huxley HE: The double array of filaments in cross-striated muscle. J Biophys Biochem Cytol 3:631–648, 1957
3. Huxley HE: Structural differences between resting and rigor muscle. J Mol Biol 38:507–520, 1968.
4. Haselgrove JC, Huxley HE: X-ray evidence for radial cross-bridge movement and for the sliding filament model in actively contracting skeletal muscle. J Mol Biol 77:549–568, 1973
5. Huxley HE: X-ray diffraction of contracting skeletal muscle. In *Cross-Bridge Mechanism in Muscle Contraction*. Edited by Sugi H, Pollack GH, University of Tokyo Press, Tokyo, 1979, pp 391–405
6. Huxley HE: The structural basis of contraction and regulation in striated muscle. Acta Anat Nippon 50:310–325, 1975
7. Huxley HE, Haselgrove JC: The structural basis of contraction in muscle and its study by rapid x-ray diffraction methods. In *Myocardial Failure*. Edited by Riecker G, Weber A, Goodwin J. Springer-Verlag, Berlin, 1977, pp 4–15
8. Podolsky RJ, St Onge R, Yu L, et al: X-ray diffraction of actively shortening muscle. Proc Natl Acad Sci USA 73:813–817, 1976
9. Matsubara I, Yagi N: A time-resolved x-ray diffraction study of muscle during twitch. J Physiol (Lond) 278:297–307, 1978
10. Sugi H, Amemiya Y, Hashizume H: X-ray diffraction of active frog skeletal muscle before and after a slow stretch. Proc Jpn Acad 53:178–182, 1977
11. Huxley HE, Faruqi AR, Bordas J, et al: The use of synchrotron radiation in time-resolved x-ray diffraction studies of myosin layer-line reflections during muscle contraction. Nature 284:140–143, 1980
12. Reynolds GT, Milch JR, Gruner SM: A high sensitivity image intensifier–TV detector for x-ray diffraction studies. Rev Sci Instrum 49:1241–1249, 1978
13. Huxley HE: Structural changes in the actin and myosin-containing filaments during contraction. Cold Spring Harbor Symp Quant Biol 37:361–376, 1972

14. Gabriel A: Position sensitive x-ray detector. Rev Sci Instrum 48:1303–1305, 1977
15. Matsubara I, Yagi N: Myosin heads do not move on activation in highly stretched vertebrate striated muscle. Science 207:307–308, 1980

DISCUSSION

Dr. Robert Barchi: Could you comment on what you believe the role of the troponin-tropomyosin complex is? Do you think that it simply plays a permissive role by sterically blocking access to a binding site, or do you think it actually determines the nature of the interaction between the actin and the myosin headgroup?

Dr. Hugh Huxley: There is good evidence that the affinity of the myosin headgroup is greater for actin in the presence of activated tropomyosin than it is for actin that lacks the troponin-tropomyosin system. One always has fantasies about these things, but I like to think the tropomyosin moves to some position that allows the myosin head to find the right place on actin for attachment more easily than it would if presented with the actin structure alone.

Dr. Michael Bárány: Will your finding that actin is necessary for the changes in the myosin layer lines modify your swinging cross-bridge model? The original model assumed that in the resting muscle the cross-bridges are close to the backbone of the thick filaments and, on stimulation of the muscle, move toward the thin filaments. With your new finding, one may assume that the cross-bridges are near the thin filaments even in resting muscle; on stimulation of the muscle, the myosin heads will be attached to the actin molecules, and the subsequent change in the angle of attachment will cause movement.

Dr. Hugh Huxley: I would have been very happy to believe that activation did have an effect on myosin filaments and did allow the head to swing outward. But since I cannot find any evidence for such movement in the absence of actin, I see no reason to believe that this happens. There may be an activation mechanism in the myosin filament, but there is no evidence that it manifests itself in this way. Instead, I picture the myosin cross-bridges as always undergoing a certain amount of Brownian motion between the myosin and the actin filaments; when they get close to actin in an activated muscle, they stick.

Dr. Michael Bárány: My question concerns the swinging itself. Is there an absolute need for the swinging, as postulated in 1969, or would you modify the previous concept so that the swinging itself is not an absolute requirement for attachment?

Dr. Hugh Huxley: The original reason for wanting some degree of lateral movement was the rather inconvenient observation that as a muscle shortens, the filaments become farther apart. For the range of lengths within which a muscle seems to function quite well, the change in separation of the surfaces of the myosin and actin filaments may be as much as 50 Å. For a cross-bridge always to attach to actin in the same orientation in the face of this quite large difference in side spacing, one must introduce into the model some very specific feature. That was the original reason for specifying some flexibility by which the myosin head could swing out and attach to actin. That sort of outward movement does produce the expected changes in the equatorial x-ray diagram, particularly in the inner [10] reflection.

Dr. Wilfried Mommaerts: Do you keep a running catalogue of alternative explanations, and are there any that you would like to single out for comment?

Dr. Hugh Huxley: Well, in the time available I cannot deal very adequately with other suggested mechanisms, but as I tried to indicate all along, the basic sliding-filament model has a great deal of evidence in its support. Most people would probably accept that general model as a reasonable working hypothesis, and the idea that the force is developed at the cross-bridges and not by some other kind of structure would also be generally accepted. The issue becomes a bit more complicated when you start worrying about whether the cross-bridge is changing its tilt or its conformation, or whether something is going on in the S_2 portion. (This recent suggestion by Harrington is an interesting and challenging one.) However, my philosophy is that, because the enzyme is obviously located in the S_1 head, and because the S_1 head needs to be attached to actin for the site to work properly through the cycle, that is the most obvious place for the force to develop. I do not want to be dogmatic about this, but it does seem like a reasonable working hypothesis. So we do our best to design experiments that will show whether we are wrong. I would not say that it was proved that the force was developed by cross-bridge rotation, but this does seem to be a pretty reasonable hypothesis. Do you have some specific alternative model in mind?

Dr. Wilfried Mommaerts: The S_2 theory, of course, does not necessarily contradict the swinging cross-bridge model; it may just be an aspect of its mechanism.

Dr. Hugh Huxley: It would be very difficult to distinguish between the two models with regard to where the force was being generated, even if one could actually see the two models working!

Dr. Wilfried Mommaerts: Some of our unfinished work shows a diminution of circular dichroism of myosin in solution when it interacts with adenosine triphosphate, as if some conformational change in the head also continues a bit into S_2.

Dr. Hugh Huxley: There certainly are big changes in the myosin head when it interacts with actin, as evidenced by nuclear magnetic resonance (NMR) studies. If you look at S_1 on its own, it is clear that a substantial part of the molecule is in a very flexible state and gives sharp NMR spectra, which are lost when the S_1 attaches to actin. Obviously, a lot is going on in the head, but it is still quite difficult to explore the changes in detail.

Part I

PERIPHERAL NERVE DISORDERS

Overview

Arthur K. Asbury, MD

Before one can consider the disorders believed to have a primary effect on the peripheral nervous system (PNS), it is necessary to be specific about what is meant by the term "peripheral nervous system." Practically stated, the PNS is composed of all neural processes and neurons and their supporting elements that lie peripheral to the spinal root and cranial nerve entry and exit zones. This excludes the first and second cranial nerves, which are composed of central nervous system (CNS) extensions. To state the description in another way, the PNS includes the dorsal and ventral spinal roots, the dorsal root ganglia, the spinal nerves and their plexuses, the motor and sensory endings in the periphery, the cranial nerves including the sensory ganglia lying outside of the brainstem, and the bulk of the autonomic nervous system, including autonomic ganglia, postganglionic fibers, and all of the preganglionic fibers lying outside of the spinal cord and brainstem. This concept is presented in simplified fashion in Figure 1. An important corollary of this concept is that Schwann cells or their ganglionic counterparts, satellite cells, serve as the supporting and myelin-forming elements throughout all of the PNS.

Most of the neural elements with projections into the PNS, i.e., primary sensory neurons, lower motor neurons, and preganglionic autonomic neurons, also lie in part in the CNS. Therefore, these neuronal systems are vulnerable to disease processes that affect either the PNS or the CNS. In this sense, the notion that the PNS constitutes a distinct anatomic entity is an artifice, a conceptual oversimplication for ease of reference. This point should not be overlooked in thinking of disorders of peripheral nerve. The artificiality of the distinction between CNS and PNS is perhaps best brought out in the case of toxic axonopathies. With most agents known to be neurotoxic, central axons are affected in their distal parts as early and as severely as distal axons in the PNS. The degree of central involvement is often not apparent because dysfunction of peripheral motor and sensory axons masks the central effects of the neurotoxin, with the result that the clinical picture is dominated by the findings of a peripheral neuropathy. Spencer and Schaumburg (1) have recently emphasized the significance of this fact and have introduced the term "central-peripheral distal axonopathy."

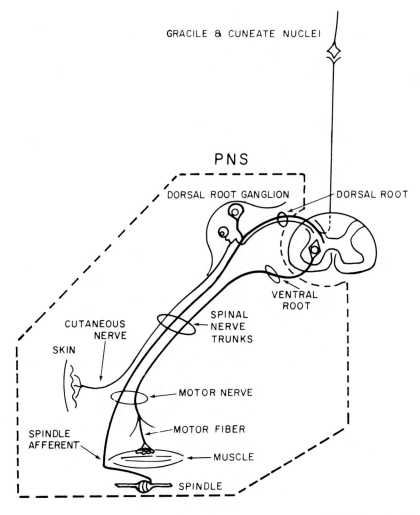

GRACILE & CUNEATE NUCLEI

PNS

DORSAL ROOT GANGLION

DORSAL ROOT

VENTRAL ROOT

CUTANEOUS NERVE

SKIN

SPINAL NERVE TRUNKS

MOTOR NERVE

MOTOR FIBER

SPINDLE AFFERENT

MUSCLE

SPINDLE

Fig. 1. Diagrammatic concept of the peripheral nervous system (PNS). (Reprinted with permission from Asbury AK, Johnson PC: *Pathology of Peripheral Nerve.* WB Saunders, Philadelphia, 1978, p 3

BASIC MECHANISMS

In our current state of knowledge, it is still useful to think in terms of the fundamental processes that affect peripheral nerve. These include wallerian degeneration, segmental demyelination, axonal degeneration, and primary lesions of nerve cell bodies. The latter three have recently been referred to as myelinopathies, axonopathies, and neuronopathies, respectively (2). All except the process of neuronopathy are illustrated diagrammatically in Figure 2.

Wallerian degeneration implies the physical interruption of an otherwise healthy axon, or interruption of an entire nerve trunk, depending on the sense and the setting in which the term is used. If a nerve trunk is severed, both axons and myelin sheath degenerate distal to the site of transection, conduction fails within 3 to 4 days as the distal nerve becomes inexcitable, chromatolysis of the nerve cell body may appear, regeneration begins early but proceeds slowly, and recovery is generally both incomplete and dysfunctional. Although physical injury to nerve trunk is the usual cause of wallerian degeneration, focal or multifocal nerve trunk ischemia may produce extensive distal degeneration. As a general rule, nerve trunk ischemia severe enough to produce focal axonal damage and distal wallerian degeneration may result from any widespread pathologic process affecting small vessels and capillaries in the vasa nervorum range (3). Multifocal nerve trunk ischemia is the usual basis for mononeuropathy multiplex encountered clinically.

Segmental demyelination implies primary damage to myelin sheath with sparing of axon. The physiologic expression of demyelination is believed to be conduction block, with the result that functional deficit may be as severe as if the axon were transected. In demyelinative neuropathies, however, recovery is often rapid, measured in days or weeks, and recovery is frequently complete. The most frequently studied models of segmental demyelination in peripheral nerve are those produced by diphtheria toxin and lead salts. With these, widening of nodal gaps, paranodal retraction and breakdown of myelin, and eventual disintegration of whole internodes of myelin are the recognized pathologic steps. But other ways in which myelin sheath may be damaged as a primary event are known. For instance, with acute nerve compression, tele-scoping of myelin at nodes of Ranvier may take place as a type of mechanical myelin injury (4). With certain agents toxic to myelin such as hexachlorophene

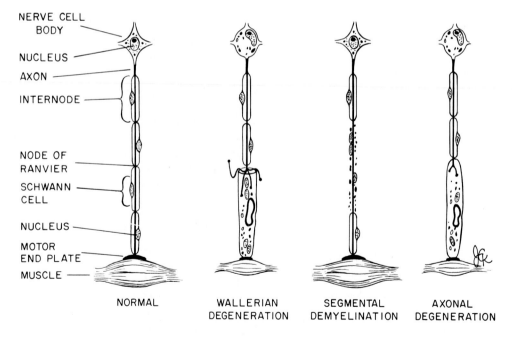

Fig. 2. Diagrammatic illustration of basic pathologic processes affecting peripheral nerve. (Reprinted with permission from Asbury AK, Johnson PC: *Pathology of Peripheral Nerve*. WB Saunders, Philadelphia, 1978, p 51

or triethyltin, striking intramyelinic edema occurs (5, 6). In other demyelinative neuropathies such as Guillain-Barré syndrome, peeling and engulfment of myelin by activated cells both at nodes of Ranvier and at other sites along the internode is the pathologic hallmark (7). In sum, there are a variety of recognizable patterns by which primary damage to peripheral nerve myelin may take place.

From their study of a number of demyelinative neuropathies, Lampert and Schochet (8) have recently made the distinction between primary Schwann cell disorders and primary myelin destruction. The distinction was made on the basis of sequential ultrastructural observations of early experimental demyelination of peripheral nerve (8). This distinction helps us most in clarifying our thinking about the pathogenesis of various demyelinative neuropathies; however, from a clinical and an electrodiagnostic standpoint, demyelination of nerve has similar features regardless of the basis of demyelination. For this reason, the term myelinopathy has clinical usefulness.

Axonal degeneration implies a widespread metabolic derangement throughout the entire neuron, which manifests itself as distal axonal breakdown. The resulting clinical picture is that of a polyneuropathy with characteristic electrodiagnostic features that allow distinction from a demyelinative process. Conventional wisdom has held that it is the longest and largest fibers that are at risk, but closer examination reveals that this rule has frequently been violated. Exogenous toxins and systemic metabolic disorders form the common bases for axonal degenerations of peripheral nerve, but the exact sequence of events culminating in axonopathy remains very much in doubt. This issue is considered further in this and subsequent chapters.

Neuronopathy implies a lesion that is manifest as destruction of the nerve cell body. It may be either motor or sensory. Examples of motor neuronopathy include poliomyelitis and motor neuron disease. Sensory neuronopathy is exemplified by the acute sensory neuronopathy syndrome (9); possibly related to an idiosyncratic effect of antimicrobial drugs; by other intoxicated states such as those produced by experimental administration of doxorubicin (10), pyridoxine hypervitaminosis (11), experimental mercurialism (12), and perhaps *cis*-platinum therapy for malignancies (13); and finally, by inflammatory disorders of dorsal root ganglia and cranial ganglia such as carcinomatous sensory neuropathy and herpes zoster. Many of these sensory neuronopathies have been recognized only recently, but they should be distinguished from axonopathies because recovery in neuronopathies is generally poor.

HISTORICAL PERSPECTIVE

In the century before 1955, interest in peripheral nerve disorders occurred in spurts during and after the major wars in response to the large number of combat-generated peripheral nerve injuries. During that century, considerable progress was made in the understanding and management of direct physical trauma to nerve trunks, but advances in understanding of nontraumatic disorders of peripheral nerve were much slower. Approximately 25 years ago, clinical and investigative interest in peripheral nerve disorders of all types began to wax and has continued to grow ever since. The reasons are manifold. Clinical interest was given impetus by the realization that fully one-third of all neurologic admissions to hospitals were neuromuscular in nature, and the great majority of these represented disorders of nerve, nerve root, and neuromuscular junction. Another major factor was technical advance, including *(a)* the redis- covery of the technique of teasing apart lengths of single nerve fibers for morphologic examination; *(b)* the introduction of new methods of microscopy, particularly ultrastructural, that were applicable to peripheral nerve; and *(c)* the rapid evolution of techniques and technologies for the electrophysiologic examination of peripheral nerve.

As the application of new methods was refined and made more rigorous and quantitative, the clinical spectrum of human neuropathies was expanded, reclassified, and subdivided. Many new entities were discovered and character- ized. Understanding of long-known entities deepened. Dozens of substances toxic to peripheral nerve were identified. The array of genetically determined neuropathies multiplied, and the diversity of their individual features became clearer. Correlative studies of clinical, morphologic, and physiologic facets of neuropathy were increasingly precise. Our neurology journals became crowded with articles on peripheral nerve and its disorders; monographs on the subject, which were once almost nonexistent, have begun to appear in the past few years.

Similarly, the fundamental neurosciences have focused a great deal of activity on peripheral nerve. Many novel approaches to the neurobiology of peripheral nerve have been developed, including axoplasmic transport and axoplasmic flow, nerve graft techniques, the characterization of neurofilamentous proteins, the advent of myelinating tissue cultures of peripheral nerve, the neurochemical dissection of myelin and determination of its immunogenicity, the cellular immunology of nerve and development of cell markers through the use of hybridomas, and the increasingly sophisticated application of biophysical tech- niques. These are only some of the areas of advance, but they give evidence of the intense interest in the biology of the PNS.

THE PRESENT AND FUTURE

Where has all of this brought us and what remains for the future? To this viewer, the progress to date, although laudable, is more apparent than real. The fundamental clinical problems remain unsolved, and for the most part, untouched. One might cite the example of pain of neuropathic origin. Despite many efforts, we are as ignorant of the basis and mechanism of neuropathic pain as ever, and our attempts to control it are, by and large, ineffective.

Another example concerns axonopathies of toxic or metabolic origin. What are the biochemical and biophysical events at a molecular level that lead to distal axonal breakdown? There is no single neuropathic disorder for which we have any knowledge of this sequence in nervous tissue. The magnitude of this question can be illustrated by the following brief review.

In distal axonopathies due to hexacarbon solvent (14–16) and carbon disulfide toxicity (17,18), striking neurofilamentous accumulation occurs within axons;

the phenomenon is somewhat less obvious in acrylamide intoxication (19). In contrast, vincristine is known to induce accumulation of neurofilaments within axons (20), but is believed to act primarily by its disruptive effect on neurotubules (21). How neurotubular disruption or neurofilamentous accumulations lead to distal axonal breakdown remains a mystery. Not all distal axonopathies manifest predominant effects on neurofibrillary structures. Other axonal organelles may bear the brunt, as for example with thallium, which induces striking mitochondrial swelling and degeneration (1). With thiamine deficiency (22) and with intoxication by organophosphates (23) and zinc pyridinethione (24), one finds axoplasmic accumulations of tubulovesicular arrays derived from smooth endoplasmic reticulum.

Taking all of these ultrastructural observations together, one might guess that there are several pathologic sequences that can lead to distal axonal degeneration. But this is as far as we can take the question at present. Do conditions that exhibit common primary effects on axonal organelles also have a common biochemical mechanism? Do conditions with different primary effects on axonal organelles eventually converge on a common biochemical pathway? Is there a single pathway or many? What degree of compromise of the axonal economy is necessary for damage to be irreversible and axonal breakdown inevitable? Efforts to address these questions, summarized by Spencer in chapter 7, are just underway.

The acquired demyelinative neuropathies, both acute and chronic, are another area of intense concern. In acute demyelinative neuropathies (Guillain-Barré syndrome), general support measures have become increasingly sophisticated and are generally successful. In more chronic demyelinative neuropathies, the judicious use of corticosteroids has proved moderately effective. The role of more potent immunosuppressants or of plasmapheresis in any of these disorders has not yet been evaluated. Of even greater concern is the lack of understanding of the pathogenesis of these myelinopathies. Although there is broad consensus that the acquired myelinopathies are immunologically mediated, the immune events that lead to demyelination are still a matter of guesswork. What host factors come into play? What immunologic circumstances must preexist? What are the antigenic stimuli in human disease? How are they introduced? What are the roles of humoral versus cellular immunopathologic events, and how do they interrelate? What role does the blood-nerve barrier play, and how is it breached? All of these questions and more must be answered before an effective level of understanding is reached in this class of myelinopathies.

Difficult as the preceding lists of questions may be to the neurologic physician, they are doubly confounded by another complexity, that of making the correct diagnosis. At present, the clinician using the means of standard examination and electrodiagnosis can usually place a particular case of neuropathic disease into a general category of myelinopathy, axonopathy, neuronopathy, or multifocal disorder. Even this degree of categorization may not be possible. One then is faced with identifying a specific underlying condition, whether it be genetic, toxic, metabolic, or immunologic, that could account for the clinical features. One must then rule out all of the other potential underlying conditions that could also account for the clinical features. This is an indirect and highly cumbersome method for establishing the correct diagnosis.

At present, approximately one-half of all cases of neuropathy are relatively readily classified by the neurologist. Of the remaining one-half, Dyck and Oviatt (25) have shown that fully 75% can be reasonably categorized and diagnosed if both the patient and the patient's relatives are studied intensively. Although this approach is effective, it is highly demanding. The future development of clear-cut diagnostic markers that can circumvent this tedious logic is a worthy goal.

REFERENCES

1. Spencer PS, Schaumburg HH: Central-peripheral distal axonopathy: the pathology of dying-back polyneuropathies. Prog Neuropathol 3:253–295, 1976

2. Schaumburg HH, Spencer PS: Toxic neuropathies. Neurology (NY) 29:429–431, 1979

3. Asbury AK: Ischemic disorders of peripheral nerve. In *Handbook of Clinical Neurology*, vol 8. Edited by Vinken PJ, Bruyn GW. North-Holland Publishing Co., Amsterdam, 1970, pp 154–165

4. Ochoa J, Fowler TJ, Gilliatt RW: Anatomical changes in peripheral nerves compressed by a pneumatic tourniquet. J Anat 113:433–455, 1972

5. Towfighi J, Gonatas NK, McCree L: Hexachlorophene neuropathy in rats. Lab Invest 29:428–436, 1973

6. Graham DI, Gonatas NK: Triethyl sulfate induced splitting of peripheral myelin in rats. Lab Invest 29:628–632, 1973

7. Prineas JW: Acute idiopathic polyneuritis: an electron microscope study. Lab Invest 26:133–147, 1972

8. Lampert PW, Schochet S: Ultrastructural changes of peripheral nerve. In *Diagnostic Electron Microscopy*, vol 2. Edited by Trump B, Jones RT. John Wiley and Sons, New York, 1979, pp 309–350

9. Sterman AB, Schaumburg HH, Asbury AK: The acute sensory neuronopathy syndrome: a distinct clinical entity. Ann Neurol 7:354–358, 1980

10. Cho E-S: Toxic effects of Adriamycin on the ganglia of the peripheral nervous system: a neuropathological study. J Neuropathol Exp Neurol 36:907–915, 1977

11. Krinke G, Schaumburg HH, Spencer PS, et al: Pyridoxine megavitaminosis produces sensory neuronopathy in the dog (abstract). Neurology (NY) 30:436, 1980

12. Jacobs JM, Carmichael N, Cavanagh JB: Ultrastructural changes in the nervous system of rabbits poisoned with methyl mercury. Toxicol Appl Pharmacol 39:249–261, 1977

13. Hemphill M, Pestronk A, Walsh T, et al: Sensory neuropathy in *cis*-platinum chemotherapy (abstract). Neurology (NY) 30:429, 1980

14. Korobkin R, Asbury AK, Sumner AJ, et al: Glue sniffing neuropathy. Arch Neurol 32:158–162, 1975

15. Saida K, Mendell JR, Weiss HS: Peripheral nerve changes induced by methyl *b*-butyl ketone and potentiation by methyl ethyl ketone. J Neuropathol Exp Neurol 35:207–225, 1976

16. Spencer PS, Schaumburg HH: Ultrastructural studies of the dying-back process. III. The evolution of experimental peripheral giant axonal degeneration. J Neuropathol Exp Neurol 36:276–299, 1977

17. Linnoila I, Haltia M, Seppalanien A-M, et al: Experimental carbon disulphide poisoning: morphological and neurophysiological studies. In *Proceedings of the VIIth International Congress on Neuropathology*. Excerpta Medica, Amsterdam, 1974, pp 383–385

18. Szendzikowski S, Stetkiewicz J, Wronska-Nofer T, et al: Pathomorphology of the experimental

lesion of the peripheral nervous system in white rats chronically exposed to carbon disulphide. In *Structure and Function of Normal and Diseased Muscle and Peripheral Nerve*. Edited by Hausmanova-Petrusewicz I, Jedrzejowski H. Polish Medical Publishers, Warsaw, 1974, pp 319–326

19. Spencer PS, Schaumburg HH: Ultrastructural studies of the dying-back process. IV. Differential vulnerability of PNS and CNS fibers in experimental central-peripheral axonopathies. J Neuropathol Exp Neurol 36:300–320, 1977

20. Wulfhekel U, Dullmann J: Ein licht- und elektronen optischer Beitrag zur Vinca-Alkaloid Polyneuropathie. Virchows Arch [Pathol Anat] 357:163–178, 1972

21. Schlaepfer WW: Vincristine-induced axonal alterations in rat peripheral nerve. J Neuropathol Exp Neurol 30:488–505, 1971

22. Takahashi K, Nakamura H: Axonal degeneration in beriberi neuropathy. Arch Neurol 33:836–841, 1976

23. Prineas JW: The pathogenesis of dying-back polyneuropathies. I. An ultrastructural study of experimental tri-ortho cresyl phosphate intoxication in the cat. J Neuropathol Exp Neurol 28:571–620, 1969

24. Sahenk Z, Mendell JR: Ultrastructural study of zinc pyridinethione-induced peripheral neuropathy. J Neuropathol Exp Neurol 38:532–550, 1979

25. Dyck PJ, Oviatt KF: When kin are evaluated, undiagnosed neuropathy commonly can be shown to be inherited. Trans Am Neurol Assoc 104:29–31, 1979

2
Does the Dystrophic Mouse Nerve Lesion Result from an Extracellular Matrix Abnormality?

Richard P. Bunge, MD

Mary B. Bunge, PhD

Ann K. Williams, BA

Lisa K. Wartels, BA

This brief chapter will be concerned primarily with an analysis of the peripheral nerve lesion in the dystrophic (dy) mouse. This lesion is now known to involve varying degrees of Schwann cell functional failure, expressed as a complete failure of Schwann cell ensheathment of certain axons in nerve root regions, with more subtle deficits (such as defects in basal lamina coverage of the axon–Schwann cell unit) in more peripheral regions of both sensory and motor nerves. In discussing these Schwann cell deficiencies we review certain recently discovered aspects of Schwann cell development, with special reference to tissue culture conditions in which normal Schwann cell behavior mimics that observed in the nerve root of the dy mouse. We also review the degree of abnormality expressed by Schwann cells in organotypic cultures of dy mouse sensory ganglia and report new tissue culture experiments showing that certain deficits expressed by dy mouse Schwann cells in culture are corrected if these cells are cocultured with normal skin fibroblasts. We develop the argument that taken together, these observations indicate that the nerve lesion in the dy mouse may be explained by an abnormality in the connective tissue components within the peripheral nerve; these extracellular matrix materials are known to be produced by both Schwann cells and fibroblasts (1).

23

NERVE LESION IN THE DY MOUSE

In Vivo Observations

In 1973, Bradley and Jenkison (2) reported a severe nerve abnormality in the dy mouse that was most apparent in certain dorsal and ventral nerve roots as they coursed from their points of contact with the spinal cord to points of egress from (or ingress to) the vertebral canal. The lesion was described as an unusual complete failure of Schwann cell function, concentrated in the midportions of the affected nerve roots. Large numbers of axons coursed through regions of the nerve root without Schwann cell ensheathment; this ensheathment failure was observed on small (normally unmyelinated) nerve fibers as well as on larger (normally myelinated) nerve fibers in both motor and sensory roots. In these regions, axons were in direct contact with one another, without intervening Schwann cell processes or endoneurial connective tissue components. Subsequent observations have established that this nerve lesion is present in each of the strains of dy mouse and that it is present in the root region of several of the cranial nerves as well [see Jaros and Bradley (3) for references]. Not only is Schwann cell ensheathment of nerve fibers deficient, but the number of Schwann cells in these regions during development is substantially reduced as a result of decreased cell proliferation (4, 5).

These initial reports stressed the severity of the nerve lesion in the root region, but subsequent systematic electron microscopic observations demonstrated more subtle abnormalities in the distal regions of the peripheral nervous system. Madrid and associates (6) demonstrated widespread deficiencies in the basal lamina that characteristically surrounds peripheral nerve Schwann cells. This observation was confirmed by Jaros and Bradley (3), who also noted abnormalities in the nodes of Ranvier and a general distortion of the form of many peripheral myelin segments (see also reference 7). Thus, it became clear that the peripheral nerve of the dy mouse is characterized by severe abnormalities in the nerve roots and by more subtle but distinct abnormalities in the more distal nerve trunks. Of the latter abnormalities, the defect in basal lamina coverage of axon–Schwann cell units was a particularly useful hallmark.

In Vitro Observations

The completeness of the Schwann cell failure in certain areas of the nerve root of the dy mouse is a unique observation. It appears to represent a failure at a very early stage of normal Schwann cell development because it involves deficiencies in Schwann cell proliferation, basic axonal ensheathment, extracellular matrix production, and myelination. It was of interest to us to determine whether the lesion present in the sensory roots of the dy mouse would be expressed in cultures prepared from dorsal root ganglia (DRG) of the dy mouse. Our observations are presented in detail elsewhere (8) and are summarized here.

Long-term cultures were established from DRG taken from the lumbar regions of embryonic or newborn mice of either a control strain of C57 BL/6J +/+ or from the dy strain C57 BL/6J dy^{2j}/dy^{2j}. The cultures were maintained for a period of 6 weeks or more so that neuronal development and Schwann cell ensheathment would be fully expressed. Morphologic analysis, undertaken by both light and electron microscopy, indicated that the substantial ensheathment failure expressed in dy nerve roots in vivo was not expressed in culture. However, many of the subtle abnormalities present in the more distal parts of the dy peripheral nerve in vivo were expressed in cultures prepared from dy mice. These included (a) discontinuities in the basal lamina surrounding both myelin-related and unmyelinating Schwann cells; (b) elongated nodes of Ranvier, occurring along otherwise well-myelinated nerve fibers; (c) relatively short myelin internodes with some increase in myelin thickness; (d) Schwann cell nuclei sometimes displaced from the midpoint along myelin segments; and (e) occasional regions of only partial ensheathment of unmyelinated nerve fibers.

We concluded from these in vitro observations that the abnormality expressed in the dy nerve in culture is one of the distal peripheral nerve rather than the nerve root. In attempting to explain the fact that the nerve root lesion was not expressed in our tissue cultures, we suggested the following hypothesis. It should be noted that in developing this hypothesis we were influenced by observations (to be discussed later) on the behavior of normal Schwann cells (under certain tissue culture conditions) that mimic the behavior of Schwann cells seen in dy nerve roots.

> The primary deficit in dy mouse peripheral nerve is in the production of an as yet unidentified component of the extracellular matrix which is required for normal Schwann cell differentiation. This component, normally manufactured by Schwann cells and/or fibroblasts, is produced in lesser amounts or in modified form in the dy mouse. The dy nerve lesion is expressed to the greatest degree in certain foci in the nerve root where endoneurial connective tissue components are greatly reduced. This paucity of components in the dy nerve root could result in part from the reduction in fibroblast number that is typical for this region normally, in contrast to the more distal nerve trunk. Also, during certain stages of development of the dy nerve root, the number of fibroblasts is exceptionally low. The paucity of fibroblasts and their products in the dy nerve root in vivo is not reproduced in culture because of the substantial fibroblast proliferation; the resulting histological picture is, therefore, that of the distal peripheral nerve rather than that of the nerve root (8).

Further tissue culture experiments yielded evidence that the basal lamina defects which characterize the dy mouse peripheral nerves can be ascribed, not to the failure of some axonal influence, but to the Schwann cell itself (9). Using preparations that make it possible to culture Schwann cells and neurons separately and to recombine these cell types, we obtained cocultures of dy Schwann cells growing in relation to normal axons and normal Schwann cells growing in relation to dy axons. The dy Schwann cells related to normal axons expressed the basal lamina defect characteristic of the Schwann cell in vivo, whereas normal Schwann cells related to dy axons did not. Because these preparations were grown without fibroblasts, the basal lamina, which is known to be deposited at least in part by the Schwann cell (1), must have been of Schwann cell origin.

In the cultures grown without fibroblasts, the Schwann cell basal lamina defect was expressed to a much greater extent than it was in cultures where fibroblasts were present. This provides some support for the view that both fibroblasts and Schwann cells may be involved in the production of the basal lamina that characteristically surrounds the axon–Schwann cell unit. The development of our hypothesis regarding the possible origin of nerve root lesions in the dy mouse, however, was primarily influenced by our observation that under certain tissue culture conditions, normal Schwann cells mimic the behavior of Schwann cells in the nerve root of the dy mouse. These conditions are explained in the next section.

CULTURED SCHWANN CELLS SOMETIMES MIMIC THOSE IN DY MICE

Culture without Collagen Contact

Under normal and well-defined conditions, it is possible to establish cultures of sensory ganglion neurons from neonatal or embryonic rodents that develop, with time, a substantial amount of normal Schwann cell ensheathment of the smaller axons and myelination of the larger axons. A dramatic abnormality of this normal Schwann cell behavior in culture can be observed if Schwann cells relate to axons that are not simultaneously in contact with the culture substratum (10, 11), which normally consists of reconstituted rat tail collagen. This exceptional situation can be observed in explant cultures of ganglia in which axons growing outward from the explant become partially detached from the tissue culture substratum after their initial growth into the more distal regions of the culture dish. Under these conditions, the proximal part of the axon may become suspended in tissue culture medium in the region immediately surrounding the explant, but the axon retains its more peripheral attachment to the substratum. In this suspended segment, where axons course through the tissue culture medium without the benefit of contact with the collagen substratum, the Schwann cells demonstrate very abnormal relationships to the axons. Here Schwann cells are restricted to the more peripheral parts of the axon bundles and do not effectively invade the bundles of neurites to separate them and provide the individual ensheathment normally observed both in these cultures and in vivo. The Schwann cells on suspended neurites produce some extracellular matrix material, but they lack the ability to align themselves with the axons. They do not substantially increase in number, and no myelination occurs in these regions.

One can demonstrate that the retarded development of these Schwann cells results from lack of contact with the tissue culture substratum by placing a narrow strip of plastic coated with reconstituted rat tail collagen over the region of the suspended fascicles, thus forcing them into contact with the collagen coat. The result is rapid reversal of the Schwann cell ensheathment. Within 24 hours the Schwann cells begin to divide and align themselves along the axons. Within several days these Schwann cells provide ensheathment for the smaller nerve fibers and myelin for the larger nerve fibers. We have interpreted this observation as demonstrating that for normal Schwann cell development, a "third element" (in addition to axon and Schwann cell) is required. In our experiments this element is provided by reconstituted rat tail collagen; presumably, it is provided within the animal by some element of the extracellular matrix. It is noteworthy, in light of the discussions regarding the dy nerve root outlined above, that the Schwann cells in this tissue culture condition display relationships to axons that are similar to those observed in the dy mouse nerve root. These observations raise the possibility that some abnormality of contact between Schwann cells and a component of the extracellular matrix may explain the abnormal Schwann cell behavior in the dy mouse nerve root.

Influence on Schwann Cell Secretion

Recent experiments in our laboratory (12, 13) using newly available defined tissue culture medium have led us to conclude that development of the normal relationship between the axon and the Schwann cell may require factors in addition to normal Schwann cells and axons and contact with a "third element." These experiments were conducted on normal rodent sensory ganglion cells grown on a substratum of reconstituted rat tail collagen. Explants were established and carried in a defined culture medium (N2) recently described by Bottenstein and Sato (14). This medium contains salts, vitamins, amino acids, and certain cofactors, with specific additions of nerve growth factor, progesterone, selenium, putrescine, insulin, and transferrin. The medium is defined in the sense that it contains only these purified protein species and lacks serum.

When sensory ganglion cells are grown (either as explants or as dissociated cells) for substantial periods of time in this culture medium, the expected axonal growth occurs. This axonal outgrowth is rapidly populated by expanding numbers of Schwann cells, demonstrating that the medium is sufficient for both growth of axons and proliferation of Schwann cells. With time, however, these cultures do not undergo the subsequent differentiation expected for normal cultures in medium containing serum and embryo extract. During the third or fourth in vitro week (when Schwann cell ensheathment of axons would normally proceed to myelination), Schwann cell differentiation appears to be arrested. The cultures do not differentiate further, even after several additional weeks in culture. Electron microscopy of these cultures reveals that large numbers of Schwann cells are generated, but the normal relationship between Schwann cell and axon does not develop. Schwann cells are in contact with the axons, but the axons are not engulfed by Schwann cell processes. The Schwann cells do not produce the basal lamina that is formed during normal development of the relationship between an axon and a Schwann cell. Thus, there is failure of Schwann cell ensheathment of the axon, as well as failure of formation of the extracellular matrix by the Schwann cell.

We have suggested elsewhere (12) that one reasonable explanation of this failure of Schwann cell function is that Schwann cells must manufacture some extracellular matrix component in order to undertake the normal ensheathment of axons. Apparently, the defined medium lacks some component necessary for this step in the differentiation of the Schwann cell. If cultures established and carried in this defined medium are subsequently shifted to medium containing serum and embryo extract, within several days the Schwann cells begin to ensheathe the axons, and basal lamina appears around the axon–Schwann cell unit. These observations raise the possibility that normal Schwann cell differentiation involves a secretory product of Schwann cells that facilitates their contact and ensheathment of axons. Schwann cells developing in N2 medium do not release this product, and normal Schwann cell–axon relationships do not develop.

CORRECTION OF DY SCHWANN CELL DEFICIT

We have argued that the abnormality observed in the dy mouse nerve may be explained by a deficit in the extracellular matrix. There is direct evidence for some abnormality in this extracellular matrix from the observation of an abnormality of the basal lamina throughout the peripheral nervous tissue of the dy mouse. The fact that this abnormality is also expressed in cultures of the same tissue further strengthens the argument that this abnormality in the dy mouse mutant is a very basic one. It is logical to suggest that if the hypothesis presented is correct, and if the extracellular matrix of peripheral nerve is the product of both Schwann cells and fibroblasts, then normal fibroblasts might be able to correct the peripheral nerve abnormality observed. It is possible to test this hypothesis in tissue cultures, and we report here the results of experiments of this type.

We first established DRG from newborn dy mice of the C57 BL/6J dy^{2j} strain as explant cultures and subjected these to intermittent treatment with antimitotic agents to remove the indigenous fibroblast population (15). This treatment suppresses Schwann cell proliferation initially, but as axons grow out of the explants in normal medium a small number of residual Schwann cells proliferate. In time, these repopulate the neuritic outgrowth with a normal complement of Schwann cells. Such cultures can be prepared from neonatal mouse tissues by using techniques similar to those described for preparing Schwann cell–neuron cultures from fetal rat DRG (15).

In separate dishes we established mouse skin fibroblasts from normal mice by removing the skin of a neonatal mouse and subjecting it to trypsin dissociation. This treatment was only moderately successful, and the dispersed cellular elements established in the culture dish grew from both small cellular aggregates and single cells. In time, these culture dishes contained small colonies of fibroblasts growing on a collagen substratum. We then transplanted the Schwann cell–neuron cultures from dy mice (prepared by the methods described) into these culture dishes in close proximity to the small explants that were generating normal skin fibroblasts. We thus obtained combination cultures containing proliferating skin fibroblasts juxtaposed with explants of DRG neurons containing a substantial indigenous Schwann cell population.

As the outgrowth from these explants formed, the neurites were populated by Schwann cells and became related to the fibroblasts provided from the skin explants (Figs. 1–4). Control cultures contained neurons and Schwann cells without fibroblasts. Light micrographs of cross sections of these two types of preparation are shown in Figures 3 and 4. In Figure 3, which shows the neuron–Schwann cell preparation in the region of the proximal outgrowth, one observes small bundles of axons and Schwann cells with none of the connective tissue elements that normally form a substantial part of the endoneurial and perineurial components of peripheral nerve. Figure 4 shows the neuron–Schwann cell preparation grown in combination with fibroblasts, which can be seen as a substantial series of layers over the fascicles of axons and Schwann cells as well as between the collagen substratum and the neurite bundles. The neurite–Schwann cell aggregates appear to be partitioned into fascicles, as would be expected in normal peripheral nerve. Electron microscopy indicates that many of the fibroblasts assume a configuration similar to that of perineurial cells in normal peripheral nerve in vivo.

Our analysis of these cultures has been primarily at the electron microscopic level, for they do not form an adequate amount of myelin to permit the extensive light microscopic analysis required to determine whether myelin internode and node of Ranvier lengths are abnormal. Electron microscopy was undertaken after 6 weeks or more in culture, at which time the cultures were considered to have developed to maturity. We systematically measured the basal lamina coverage in these cultures and compared this coverage with that seen in organotypic cultures from dy mice and in several types of control cultures prepared from C57 BL +/+ mice. The results of this extensive morphometric analysis, expressed as percentages of the Schwann cell surface covered by basal lamina, are given in Table 1.

The most crucial comparison was between cultures of dy Schwann cells and

Table 1. Basal Lamina Coverage of Axon–Schwann Cell Units in Cultures Containing Various Cell Components of Sensory Ganglia from Normal and Dystrophic Mice

Culture Component	No. of Cultures Analyzed	Days in Vitro	Basal Lamina Units Measured[a]	Basal Lamina Coverage (%)		
				Mean	Median	SEM
Culture with	1					
+/+ neurons						
+/+ Schwann cells						
+/+ fibroblasts		37	32	98.4	97.0	0.5
Culture with	3					
dy neurons		42	19	75.7	73.9	4.3
dy Schwann cells		42	5	84.2	84.6	5.0
dy fibroblasts		52	16	65.1	70.0	4.7
Culture with	2					
+/+ neurons		44	32	92.1	97.6	1.6
+/+ Schwann cells		44	17	98.1	97.6	0.5
Culture with	2					
dy neurons		44	29	71.9	77.1	3.4
dy Schwann cells		44	33	77.8	80.6	2.5
Culture with	3					
dy neurons		72	18	95.2	96.4	1.6
dy Schwann cells		72	33	96.9	97.6	1.4
+/+ fibroblasts		72	19	96.2	97.6	1.0

[a] This number indicates the number of axon–Schwann cell units analyzed from each culture. The basal lamina around the circumference of each unit was measured, including regions where defects were present. A second measurement determined the proportion of this circumference that lacked basal lamina coverage; the number given is the percentage of the entire circumference covered by basal lamina. In normal cultures with neurons, Schwann cells, and fibroblasts grown together, the mean has always been 98% to 100%. Measurements were made with a Houston Instrument Digitizer Tablet, and the data were stored and analyzed by computer.

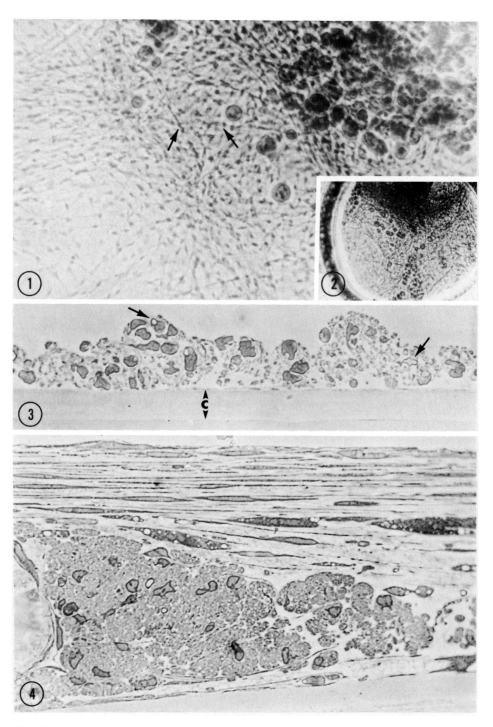

Fig. 1. Light micrograph showing the peripheral part of a sensory ganglion explant from a dy mouse. The surrounding outgrowth consists solely of nerve fibers and Schwann cells. Several individual neurons are seen at the explant margin. Myelin segments are present (arrows), but are poorly visualized at this magnification. This neuron–Schwann cell preparation lacks a fibroblast population. Electron microscopic observations were made of the proximal part of the outgrowth of this type of culture, as well as the types of culture described in Table 1. (Original magnification ×160.)

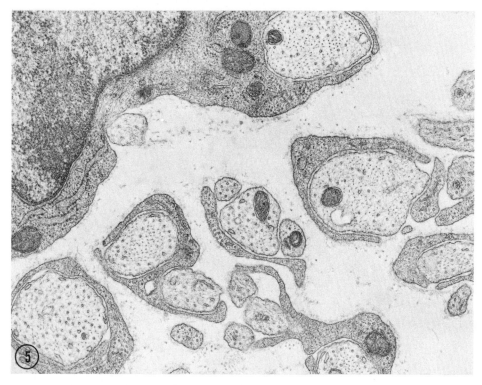

Fig. 5. Electron micrograph from the outgrowth area of a dorsal root ganglion explant taken from a dy mouse. This culture contained neurons and Schwann cells without fibroblasts. Schwann cell ensheathment is incomplete, and basal lamina coverage of the axon–Schwann cell unit is very sparse. (Original magnification ×25,000.)

neurons grown with normal fibroblasts, and preparations in which dy Schwann cells and neurons were grown in the presence of dy fibroblasts. This latter preparation was available from the work of Okada and colleagues (8) in which dy neurons, Schwann cells, and fibroblasts were grown in combination culture for 6 weeks, i.e., to maturity, without treatment with antimitotic agents. As discussed previously, the most consistent abnormality expressed in these cultures

Fig. 2. Low-power light micrograph of an explant margin in a culture that was embedded for electron microscopy; a circular score mark was made to allow selection of a specific area for sampling. This culture contained dy neurons, Schwann cells, and added normal skin fibroblasts. (An electron micrograph of this type of preparation is shown in Figure 7.) The scored circle is approximately 1 mm in diameter.

Fig. 3. Light micrograph showing cross section of an outgrowth from a culture containing only dy neurons and Schwann cells. Several myelinated fibers (arrows) are seen, as are many unmyelinated fibers with their Schwann cell ensheathment. The full thickness of the collagen substratum (**C**) is shown. (Original magnification ×950.)

Fig. 4. Light micrograph showing a cross section of an outgrowth from a culture containing dy neurons and Schwann cells grown with normal skin fibroblasts. Many layers of fibroblasts have formed over the surface of the culture, and some are admixed with the neurite fascicles. (An electron micrograph from the nerve fascicle region of this type of preparation is shown in Figure 7.) (Original magnification ×950.)

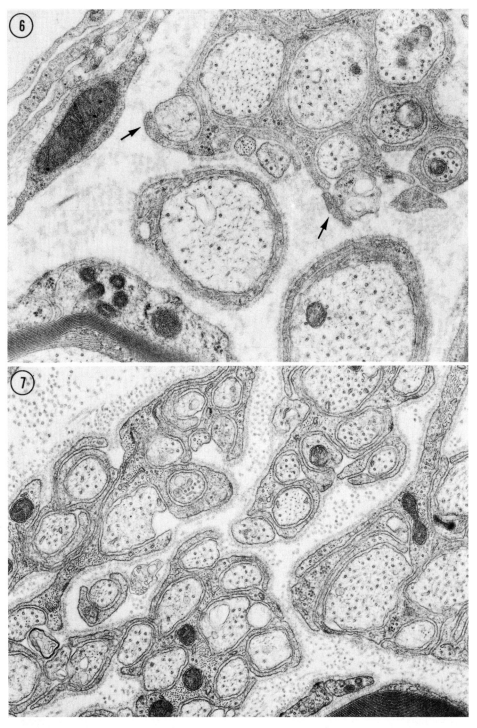

Fig. 6. Electron micrograph taken from the outgrowth area of a dorsal root ganglion explant taken from a dy mouse. This culture contained neurons, Schwann cells, and fibroblasts. Regions of the Schwann cell surface that completely lack basal lamina coverage are marked by arrows. In other regions the basal lamina shows punctate interruptions. (Original magnification ×25,000.)

32

is periodic defects in the continuity of the basal lamina surrounding the axon–Schwann cell unit. By contrast, cultures prepared with normal fibroblasts show correction of this distinctive deficit (compare Figure 5 with Figures 6 and 7; see Table 1).

We also undertook morphometric analysis of dy preparations containing dy neurons and Schwann cells only (Fig. 5). As shown in Table 1, when dy Schwann cells and neurons were grown alone, without any fibroblasts, a substantial abnormality of basal lamina formation was observed. But when dy neurons and Schwann cells were combined with normal fibroblasts, the basal lamina coverage appeared to be essentially normal. Thus, the presence of normal fibroblasts in proximity to dy neurons and Schwann cells corrects the characteristic lesion of the dy Schwann cell basal lamina, as observed by electron microscopy. By what mechanism might the fibroblast assist correction of an abnormality expressed by the Schwann cell?

It is known that Schwann cells in contact with axons produce several types of collagen (1). It is also known that the steps in collagen production involve several extracellular modifications after the release of procollagen from the cells (1). These steps involve the action of procollagen peptidases in removing terminal peptide chains from procollagen to form tropocollagen, and the action of lysyl oxidases in crosslinking tropocollagen to form collagen fibrils. Because these steps are performed extracellularly, they may be influenced by the provision of enzymes (or substrates) from cocultured cells. The formation of the complete Schwann cell basal lamina may normally involve cooperation between Schwann cell and fibroblast. In the dy nerve, both cell types may lack the necessary enzyme for a particular step in extracellular matrix processing. The provision of a normal fibroblast population could then correct this deficiency.

In general, these results agree with the observations of Peterson (16) on the expression of the dy abnormality in chimeras of dy and normal mice. His observations indicate that dy muscle in the environment of surrounding normal cells does not express characteristic dy abnormalities. In our efforts to develop additional evidence that the dy nerve lesion is corrected in an environment containing normal fibroblasts, it may be advantageous to use tissues from the 129 ReJ dy/dy mouse strain, which is known to express a more severe basal lamina abnormality than the strain used in the present study (3).

ACKNOWLEDGMENTS

We are grateful to Mr. Vincent Argiro for developing the program for the morphometric analysis of basal lamina coverage and for assistance in performing

Fig. 7. Electron micrograph taken from the outgrowth area of a dorsal root ganglion explant taken from a dy mouse and grown with skin fibroblasts from a normal mouse. The basal lamina coverage of the axon–Schwann cell units appears normal. The substantial number of collagen fibrils occupying the endoneurial space is seen only when fibroblasts are present in the culture. (Original magnification ×25,000.)

this analysis. We also thank Ms. Susan Mantia for expert secretarial aid. This work was supported by U.S. Public Health Service Grant NS 09923.

REFERENCES

1. Bunge MB, Williams AK, Wood PM, et al: Comparison of nerve cell and nerve cell plus Schwann cell cultures, with particular emphasis on basal lamina and collagen formation. J Cell Biol 84:184–202, 1980

2. Bradley WG, Jenkison M: Abnormalities of peripheral nerve in murine muscular dystrophy. J Neurol Sci 18:227–247, 1973

3. Jaros E, Bradley WG: Atypical axon–Schwann cell relationships in the common peroneal nerve of the dystrophic mouse: an ultrastructural study. Neuropathol Appl Neurobiol 5:133–147, 1979

4. Bray GM, Perkins S, Peterson AC, et al: Schwann cell multiplication deficit in the nerve roots of newborn dystrophic mice. J Neurol Sci 82:203–212, 1977

5. Jaros E, Bradley WG: Development of the amyelinated lesion in the ventral root of the dystrophic mouse: ultrastructural, quantitative and autoradiographic study. J Neurol Sci 36:317–339, 1978

6. Madrid RE, Jaros E, Cullen MJ, et al: Genetically determined defect of Schwann cell basement membrane in dystrophic mouse. Nature 257:319–321, 1975

7. Bradley WG, Jaros E, Jenkison M: The nodes of Ranvier in the nerves of mice with muscular dystrophy. J Neuropathol Exp Neurol 36:797–806, 1977

8. Okada E, Bunge RP, Bunge MB: Abnormalities expressed in long term cultures of dorsal root ganglia from the dystrophic mouse. Brain Res 194:455–470, 1980

9. Cochran M, Cornbrooks CJ, Mithen F: Persistence of basal lamina defect in cultures of dystrophic mouse Schwann cells in contact with normal mouse neurons (abstract). Soc Neurosci Abstr 5:427, 1979

10. Bunge RP, Bunge MB: Evidence that contact with connective tissue matrix is required for normal interaction between Schwann cells and nerve fibers. J Cell Biol 78:943–950, 1978

11. Bunge RP, Bunge MB, Cochran M: Some factors influencing the proliferation and differentiation of myelin-forming cells. Neurology (NY) 28:59–67, 1978

12. Moya F, Bunge RP, Bunge MB: Schwann cells proliferate but fail to differentiate in defined medium. Proc Natl Acad Sci USA (in press)

13. Bunge R, Moya F, Bunge M: Observations on the role of Schwann cell secretion in Schwann cell–axon interactions. In *Neurosecretion and Brain Peptides: Implications for Brain Function and Neurological Disease.* Edited by Martin JB. Raven Press, New York (in press)

14. Bottenstein JE, Sato GH: Growth of a rat neuroblastoma cell line in serum-free supplemented medium. Proc Natl Acad Sci USA 76:514–517, 1979

15. Wood PM: Separation of functional Schwann cells and neurons from normal peripheral nerve tissue. Brain Res 115:361–375, 1976

16. Peterson A: Mosaic analysis of dystrophic ↔ normal chimeras: an approach to mapping the site of gene expression. Ann N Y Acad Sci 317:629–648, 1979

DISCUSSION

Dr. Valarie Askanas: I just want to comment that when we used the defined (i.e., serum-free and embryo extract-free) medium, we also noticed that cultured human Schwann cells became very granulated and did not differentiate or survive as well as they did in normal medium. It could be that some ingredient of serum or embryo extract is essential for Schwann cell differentiation and survival in culture.

Dr. Walter Bradley: I would like to make the point raised by the first slide, because it is relevant to what this whole meeting is about, namely, the question of whether the Schwann cell in the root abnormality might be the basis of the muscle degeneration in the dystrophic mouse. This is obviously the first thought that comes to mind when you have a possible model of muscular dystrophy, yet you find something wrong with the nerve. One possibility is that the ephaptic transmission that Dr. Rasminsky and Dr. Kuno originally described might be the basis of overactivity of the nerve and, therefore, overactivity of the muscle, leading to muscle degeneration. But the other possibility is that these are two manifestations of a primary biochemical abnormality produced by a single gene. I do not know of any crucial evidence that can separate these two possibilities. However, we found originally that there was very little root abnormality in the thoracic region of the dystrophic mice, whereas there is muscle degeneration in the thoracic muscles. My inclination, therefore, is to suggest that the nerve and muscle changes are separate manifestations of a single biochemical abnormality of the same gene rather than one being the cause of the other.

Dr. Richard Bunge: I certainly agree. I would like to mention here that Dr. Bradley and his colleagues were responsible for the description of the basal lamina defect present throughout the peripheral nervous system. This defect was the first clue that there was something wrong with the production of extracellular matrix in these animals and was the basis for the design of much of our work.

Dr. Jarvis Seegmiller: It is fascinating that fibroblasts were able to correct the demyelinating problem of the cells in culture. Some investigators have proposed that fibroblasts from different areas of the body have different functions. Are you able to correct the defect with skin fibroblasts as well as with the ones that grow out in your explant? If so, it seems that you would have a much simpler system with which to work. Have you looked to see whether any abnormality can be found in the fibroblasts alone?

Dr. Richard Bunge: That is a very perceptive question because we have seen differences in the behavior of fibroblasts in culture. We began to take the fibroblasts from the periosteum but did use skin fibroblasts in some experiments; in fact, they are the ones that provided the correction I illustrated.

3
Cell Interactions in Nerves of Dystrophic Mice

Albert J. Aguayo, MD

C. Suzanne Perkins, BSc

Garth M. Bray, MD

In normal peripheral nerves, the relationship between axons and Schwann cells evolves through several developmental stages: the migration and growth of neurons and sheath cells, the proliferation of Schwann cells to yield a number that is appropriate to ensheathe all axons, differentiation of Schwann cells into the sheaths of myelinated and unmyelinated fibers, and finally, during maturation, an increase in the thickness of the myelin sheaths proportional to the axon (Fig. 1). This developmental sequence is altered in the peripheral nervous system of several mutant mice. In Trembler mice, Schwann cells fail to evolve beyond the stage of primary ensheathment of axons and are unable to form and sustain myelin (1, 2). In quaking mice, the initial stages of myelin formation are completed, but the maturation of the myelin sheath is impaired (3). In dystrophic mice (dystrophia muscularis), a wide spectrum of alterations affects all stages of the association between axons and Schwann cells, including ensheathment, multiplication, differentiation, and maturation. Although the precise genetic defects that cause these disorders have not been defined, much information has been obtained from physiologic (see chapter 5) and morphologic studies of neuropathies in mutant mice. The purpose of this article is 2-fold: (*a*) to summarize the main structural characteristics of the nerve disorder in dystrophic mice, and (*b*) to review the results of various experimental strategies that have been used to investigate the pathogenesis of this neuropathy.

STRUCTURE OF NERVES IN DYSTROPHIC MICE

The most striking neural abnormality in dystrophic mice is the presence of axon segments totally devoid of Schwann cells and therefore of myelin (4).

37

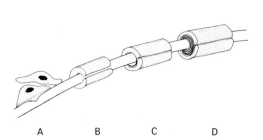

Fig. 1. Schematic representation of the development of axon–Schwann cell relationships in a myelinated peripheral nerve fiber. Multiplying Schwann cells initially contact the axon (A), which they encircle by the elaboration of cellular processes (B). After primary ensheathment, myelination commences (C) and continues until the thickness of the myelin sheath is appropriate to the size of the axon (D).

These naked axon segments are particularly prominent in the lumbosacral and cervical spinal roots (both ventral and dorsal), but are also observed in the proximal sciatic (4, 5) and cranial nerves (6). Within each affected nerve, both the longitudinal and radial distributions of the abnormally ensheathed axons are characteristic. In the affected spinal roots, the naked axons are concentrated at the mid-root level (7, 8); most axons are myelinated near the spinal cord and the exit from the spinal canal. In cross sections of nerves at the maximally affected level, the naked axon segments tend to be grouped in bundles where the plasma membranes of adjacent axons are closely apposed (Fig. 2). At the periphery of each bundle, there are usually small cells with scanty cytoplasm (Fig. 2) that contact or partially encircle the adjacent axons but do not ensheathe them normally (4, 9). These cells have been designated "uncommitted" cells by Jaros and Bradley (10). At the same cross-sectional level as the bundles of naked axons, there are also myelinated fibers in which axons are ensheathed by typical Schwann cells, although the number of such fibers is strikingly less than normal (Fig. 2). Thus, there are two populations of axon-associated cells in the spinal roots of dystrophic mice, the typical Schwann cells associated with myelinated fibers, and the "uncommitted" cells.

In many myelinated fibers in the spinal roots of dystrophic mice, the myelin is inappropriately thin (4, 7), internodal distances are short, and nodes of Ranvier may be excessively wide (11). Some axons in the dorsal roots are ensheathed by oligodendrocytes (12). No primary morphologic abnormalities have been identified in neurons or axons of dystrophic mice. The internal structure of individual axons is normal in both the unensheathed and the ensheathed axons of dystrophic mice. In addition, total numbers of anterior horn cells (13) and spinal root axons (7) are similar in dystrophic and control mice. In dystrophic spinal roots the mean diameter of the unensheathed axons is less than the mean diameter of the segments of these axons where they are ensheathed and myelinated (2). However, this observation probably reflects the dependence of axonal size on Schwann cell ensheathment (14) rather than an intrinsic abnormality of dystrophic axons.

Although the plasma membranes of adjacent unensheathed axons are directly apposed (Fig. 2) and ephaptic transmission of electrical impulses is observed (15), no special interaxonal contacts have been identified. In electron micrographs of routinely processed spinal roots, the small intercellular spaces within the bundles of naked axons may contain vesicular structures, many of which are seen in freeze-fracture electron micrographs to be axolemmal protrusions. Because these protrusions are not seen in dystrophic roots processed for freeze-fracture without chemical fixation (Bray GM, Aguayo AJ: unpublished observations), they are presumed to be aldehyde-fixation artifacts (16).

The intramembranous structure of the naked axons in dystrophic spinal roots has also been examined by freeze-fracture electron microscopy (17–19). Most regions of the unensheathed axons resemble internodal axonal membrane, but occasional patches of P-face particles (17) or E-face particles (Fig. 3) are observed that resemble the particles seen at nodes of Ranvier in myelinated fibers (20). Membrane specializations that resemble those seen at normal paranodes have also been observed in the naked axons, where they are contacted by the

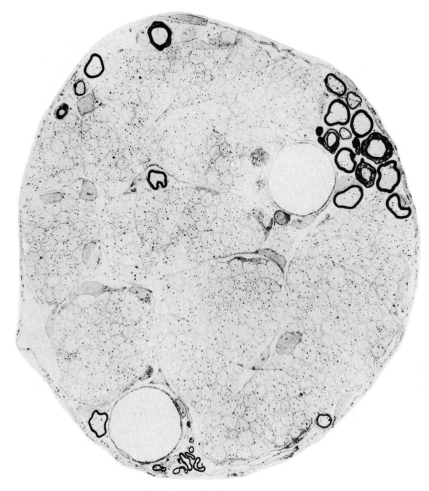

Fig. 2. Cross section at the midroot level of the fourth lumbar ventral spinal root of an adult dystrophic mouse. Most axons are naked, and only a few myelinated fibers are observed. Bundles of axons are surrounded by undifferentiated "uncommitted" Schwann cells (electron microscopic montage; bar, 10 μm). (Reprinted with permission from Bray GM, Cullen MJ, Aguayo AJ, Rasminsky M. Neurosci Lett 13:203–208, 1979.)

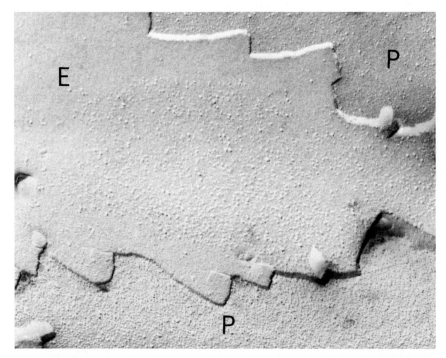

Fig. 3. Freeze-fracture replica of portions of the internal (P) and external (E) leaflets of the axolemma of naked axons in the spinal roots of dystrophic mice. The external leaflet shows a patch of relatively large particles resembling those seen at nodes of Ranvier (electron micrograph; original magnification ×64,000). (Reprinted with permission from Bray GM; Cullen MJ, Aguayo AJ, Rasminsky M. Neurosci Lett 13:203–208, 1979.)

"uncommitted" cells or differentiated Schwann cells that have ensheathed other axons (18).

In more distal parts of the peripheral nervous system, fiber diameter and myelin thickness are similar in dystrophic and control animals (11), but other abnormalities are present. The internodal lengths of large fibers are shorter than normal, nodes of Ranvier are widened (21), the Schwann cell basal lamina shows a patchy deficiency (22), and aberrant patterns of myelination are occasionally seen (5, 23, 24). In distal motor nerves, studied sequentially from birth to 72 weeks of age, axonal populations showed a progressive decrement of approximately 30% (25). The capacity of distal peripheral nerves to regenerate has also been compared in dystrophic and control animals. After crush injury, the regenerative response in terms of numbers of axons and myelin thickness was similar in dystrophic and control nerves (7), although the regeneration of motor nerve terminals may be delayed (26).

METHODS FOR STUDYING CELL INTERACTIONS IN NERVES

Because peripheral nerves are composed of complexly interwoven neuronal processes and sheath cells, it is difficult to define the exact role played by individual cellular and extracellular elements in normal and pathologic situations. Thus, in addition to the conventional techniques of quantitative and qualitative electron microscopy, radioautography, and freeze-fracture electron microscopy, several different research strategies have been used to overcome these difficulties. Two of these techniques, tissue culture and experimental nerve grafts, have been particularly useful in the study of cell interactions in dystrophic mice.

Tissue Culture

With newly developed in vitro techniques, neurites, Schwann cells, and fibroblasts have been separated and recombined to study Schwann cell multiplication, axon ensheathment, basal lamina formation, and pathogenetic mechanisms in mutant mouse neuropathies (see chapter 2).

Nerve Grafts

Experiments using radioactive, immunologic, and cytopathologic markers have established that when a segment of one nerve is grafted between the cut ends of another, Schwann cells in the donor nerves survive, multiply, and ensheath axons that regenerate from the proximal stumps of the recipient nerves. Thus, the grafted segments of such regenerated nerves represent combinations of host axons and donor sheath cells in which each may originate from a different nerve or animal or from an animal and a human nerve. To avoid graft rejection, the transplantation may be done into isogenic hosts (27) or into immune-suppressed (14, 28) or immune-deficient "nude" mice (29). Such combinations have been used to study Schwann cell differentiation (27) and multiplication (2, 30), as well as the pathogenesis of some hereditary disorders in humans (29, 31–33) and laboratory animals (14, 34, 35). Schwann cells grown in vitro may also be transplanted into peripheral nerves (14) or into the demyelinated spinal cord of mice (36).

RESULTS OF TRANSPLANTATION STUDIES

The L3 and L4 spinal roots from dystrophic and normal mice were transplanted into sciatic nerves of normal and dystrophic animals and examined by light and electron microscopy 6 to 8 weeks later. Three sets of experiments were performed.

In one group of animals, it was determined by examining the grafted nerves after regeneration that the main histologic features found in the spinal roots of dystrophic mice were not reproduced in the regenerated grafted segments. The naked axons and undifferentiated Schwann cells that characterized the dystrophic roots were not observed in any of the 4 combinations studied: dystrophic roots transplanted into normal and dystrophic sciatic nerves, or normal roots transplanted into normal and dystrophic sciatic nerves. All of the regenerated grafts contained normal-appearing myelinated and unmyelinated fibers in numerous small fascicles (2). Axon diameters and the numbers of myelin

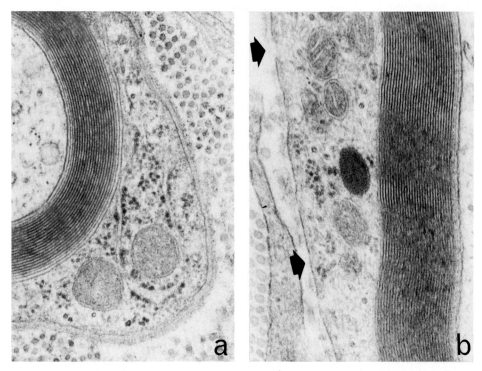

Fig. 4. (a) Electron micrograph of a Schwann cell from a normal spinal root 6 weeks after transplantation into the sciatic nerve of an adult dystrophic mouse. The basal lamina is normal. (Original magnification ×54,000.) **(b)** Electron micrograph of a Schwann cell from a dystrophic spinal root transplanted into a normal nerve. The basal lamina is thin and discontinuous (arrows). (Original magnification ×54,000).

lamellae formed around these regenerated axons were similar in normal control and dystrophic grafts. However, the generalized basal lamina deficiency that characterizes dystrophic peripheral nerves (22) was reproduced in the grafted segments that originated from dystrophic roots but not those originating from normal roots (Fig. 4).

To exclude the possibility that Schwann cells from host sciatic nerve stumps had migrated into the grafted dystrophic root segments where there were reduced numbers of Schwann cells before grafting, normal animals labeled neonatally with ^{3}H-thymidine (2), or Trembler mice whose Schwann cells could be identified by their deficient myelin formation (9), were used as hosts for dystrophic root grafts in an additional set of experiments. By both these methods, it was possible to determine that the host axons had been ensheathed by Schwann cells arising from the dystrophic spinal roots rather than the host nerves. However, these results did not permit identification of the cells of origin of the myelinated fibers in the regenerated grafts; the unensheathed cells could have originated from the differentiated typical Schwann cells in the dystrophic roots rather than from the phenotypically abnormal "uncommitted" cells. Therefore, a third set of experiments was done to investigate these cells' potential for differentiation in regenerating nerve grafts.

Because the "uncommitted" cells, rather than the typically differentiated Schwann cells of myelinated fibers, are continuously dividing in the adult dystrophic roots (Fig. 5a) (9), they were labeled cumulatively with ^{3}H-thymidine for 3 weeks before transplantation into the sciatic nerves of unlabeled host mice. After regeneration, labeled Schwann cells that had differentiated and produced myelin normally (Fig. 5b) were observed in the grafted segments (9). Thus, this experimental strategy provided proof that the "uncommitted" cells in the spinal roots were undifferentiated Schwann cells capable of differentiation after transplantation (Fig. 6). Although nerve segments would have to be grafted into dystrophic spinal roots to exclude the possibility that different environmental conditions were responsible for the differentiation of these cells in sciatic nerves, this has not been technically feasible.

The results of these nerve graft experiments suggest that the failure of axon ensheathment in the dystrophic spinal roots is caused by a block of Schwann cell differentiation rather than an intrinsic defect of these cells' ability to fulfill

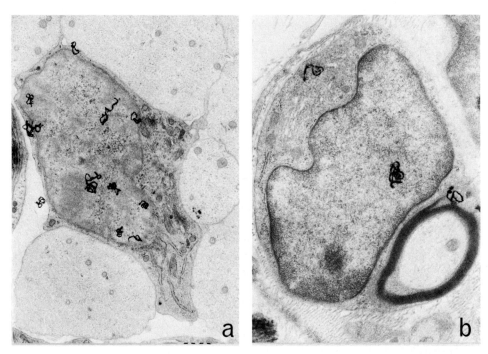

Fig. 5. **(a)** An axon-associated cell of the "uncommitted" type in the fourth lumbar ventral root of an adult dystrophic mouse labeled with ^{3}H-thymidine for 10 days before death. (Electron microscopic radioautograph; original magnification ×10,000.) (Reprinted with permission from Perkins CS, Bray GM, Aguayo AJ: Persistent multiplication of axon-associated cells in the spinal roots of dystrophic mice. Neuropathol Appl Neurobiol 6:83–91, 1980.) **(b)** A myelin-forming Schwann cell that has differentiated from a ^{3}H-thymidine-labeled "uncommitted" cell after grafting of a dystrophic spinal root into a nondystrophic peripheral nerve. (Electron microscopic radioautograph; original magnification ×13,800.) (Reprinted with permission from Perkins CS, Bray GM, Aguayo AJ: Ongoing block of Schwann cell differentiation and deployment in dystrophic mouse spinal roots. Dev Brain Res, in press.)

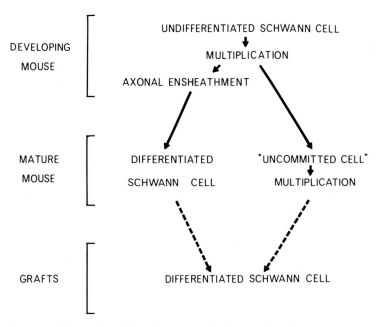

Fig. 6. Schematic illustration of Schwann cell changes in developing, mature, and transplanted spinal roots of dystrophic mice. Some dystrophic Schwann cells stop dividing and differentiate into typical Schwann cells of myelinated fibers, but other cells remain undifferentiated ("uncommitted"). After transplantation, all Schwann cells differentiate, whether the host animal is normal or dystrophic.

their ensheathing function. The basal lamina defect, on the other hand, must be related to an abnormality of the dystrophic Schwann cells, although other elements within the nerve roots that were transplanted along with the Schwann cells could be involved as well. Although these interpretations assume that, in terms of cellular interactions, regeneration reproduces the conditions of neurogenesis, it is recognized that this may not be so. The defect that initiates the spinal root abnormality in dystrophic mice may be due to conditions present only during development.

SCHWANN CELLS IN DYSTROPHIC MICE

Neonatal Proliferation

Abnormal groups of naked axons are first observed in the spinal roots of dystrophic mice shortly before birth (Perkins CS, Bray CM, Aguayo AJ: unpublished observations), and neonatal Schwann cell multiplication in these nerves is deficient in both the C57BL/dy^{2J}/dy^{2J} [37] and the 129 ReJ dy/dy animals (10). Schwann cell labeling indices, which peak on day 2 in control spinal roots, are significantly lower in dystrophic animals at this age. This deficit in neonatal Schwann cell proliferation is not generalized in dystrophic mice; labeling indices in the sciatic nerves of these animals are normal (37).

During the first 2 weeks after birth, the number of axon-associated cells in dystrophic roots is significantly lower than that in control roots, but this difference is not present in adult animals (9, 10). Although the total numbers of cells are similar for the spinal roots of both dystrophic and control animals beyond 2 weeks of age, there is an important qualitative difference: approximately one-half of the axon-associated cells in the dystrophic roots (Fig. 7) are undifferentiated Schwann cells. Thus, the population of differentiated Schwann cells in the adult dystrophic roots is markedly decreased; the failure of myelination in these nerves reflects this deficit.

Deployment and Differentiation

Early in development, nerves are composed of compact axon bundles surrounded by undifferentiated Schwann cells. In normal rodents, these cells multiply, penetrate the axon bundles, become deployed along individual axons or small groups of axons, and differentiate into the sheaths of myelinated or unmyelinated fibers (38–40). The bundles of naked axons in the spinal roots of dystrophic mice resemble the groups of unensheathed axons seen in developing nerves (4). Although normal numbers of Schwann cells eventually develop in the dystrophic spinal roots, most of them fail to migrate into the bundles or to become deployed along individual axons; rather, they remain as immature, undifferentiated cells at the margins of the axon bundles. This failure of Schwann cell differentiation is not total. Even at the most severely affected levels in the spinal roots of dystrophic mice, some Schwann cells have differentiated normally and formed myelin sheaths; other fibers showing partial, arrested, or aberrant associations between axons and Schwann cells are also occasionally observed.

Continued Multiplication

Another feature of the undifferentiated Schwann cells in the spinal roots of dystrophic mice is their continued multiplication. In contrast to normal adult animals in which Schwann cell division is uncommon in uninjured nerves, a persistence of cell division is observed in the spinal roots of dystrophic mice (9,

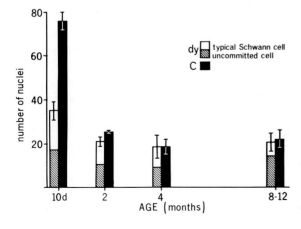

Fig. 7. Axon-associated cell nuclei in the fourth lumbar ventral roots of dystrophic and control mice studied from 10 days to 12 months of age. Total numbers per whole cross section are expressed as mean ± SEM. The proportions of typical Schwann cells and "uncommitted" cells present in dystrophic (dy) mice are compared with the total population of normal Schwann cells from control preparations (C).

10). Using cumulative labeling with ^{3}H-thymidine and electron microscopic radioautography, it was established that the cells that continue to divide in the roots of the C57BL/6J dy^{2J}/dy^{2J} animals are the undifferentiated Schwann cells (Fig. 5a) (9). Furthermore, the nerve graft experiments demonstrated that when transplanted into the sciatic nerves of other animals, these cells function as Schwann cells; they ensheathe regenerating axons, form appropiate amounts of myelin, and presumably stop dividing (Fig. 5) (9).

In their original location in the spinal roots of intact dystrophic mice, these undifferentiated Schwann cells do not proceed to ensheathe axons normally (9). This indicates that they represent a population of cells that continue to divide and fail to differentiate rather than cells that are in the process of ensheathing or reensheathing axons. Because this population of newly formed, undifferentiated Schwann cells is persistently unable to evolve into the differentiated sheath cells of myelinated and unmyelinated fibers, our observations indicate that the abnormalities in the spinal roots of dystrophic mice represent an ongoing process which, though it is first apparent during development, continues throughout the life of the animal and is not merely a failure of axon–Schwann cell relationships confined to an early stage of development.

Schwann Cell Death

Despite persistent cell division, the population of axon-associated cells (differentiated plus undifferentiated Schwann cells) remains stable in the spinal roots of dystrophic mice beyond the age of 3 weeks (9, 10). Thus, as suggested by Jaros and Bradley (10), it is probable that the proliferation of the undifferentiated Schwann cells must be balanced by an equivalent loss through cell death. A similar balancing of Schwann cell populations and multiplication may occur in other mutant mice with peripheral nerve disorders, such as the Trembler mouse (9). Perhaps continuously dividing Schwann cells in these mutants die because they prematurely exhaust a predetermined capacity for mitotic activity (41).

Basal Lamina Defects

In contrast to the focal failure of axonal ensheathment in the dystrophic spinal roots, the basal lamina defects, which are present only in Schwann cells and not in other cells of these animals (22), as well as the abnormal lengths of some nodal gaps (21, 23), are generalized and persistent abnormalities in the nerves of dystrophic mice. These generalized defects are reproduced in tissue cultures of dystrophic dorsal root ganglia (42), and the defective basal lamina is also seen in regenerated grafts of dystrophic roots transplanted into normal nerves (Fig. 4). Although these observations might suggest that the basal lamina defect is due to a primary Schwann cell abnormality, other elements that are essential for basal lamina formation may be involved as well. Axonal contact may be necessary for basal lamina formation by normal Schwann cells (43). However, in the nerve graft studies reported here as well as in tissue culture experiments (44), the basal lamina defect was reproduced when dystrophic Schwann cells became associated with normal axons, an indication that the dystrophic axons are not involved in the pathogenesis of the particular basal lamina abnormality. Fibroblasts and the extracellular matrix may also be essential for the formation of normal Schwann cell basal lamina (see chapter 2). In both the tissue culture experiments of Okada and colleagues (42) and the transplantation studies reported here, these extraneural elements as well as Schwann cells were of dystrophic origin. In addition, the basal lamina defects that develop in vitro when dystrophic Schwann cells are cocultured with normal axons in the absence of fibroblasts (44) are only partially corrected by the addition of dystrophic fibroblasts but are almost completely reversed by normal fibroblasts (see chapter 2). Thus, the basal lamina defect in vivo may be due to an aberrant interaction between the genetically abnormal Schwann cells and an abnormal component of the extracellular matrix (see chapter 2).

The relationship, if any, of the basal lamina defect to the focal failure of axonal ensheathment in the spinal roots of dystrophic mice remains to be determined (22, 45).

CONCLUSIONS

Since the initial description by Bradley and Jenkison in 1973 (4), much information has accumulated concerning various aspects of the abnormalities in the peripheral nervous system of dystrophic mice. Although the precise cause of this unique disorder has not been identified, the use of different experimental strategies has provided a greater appreciation of the dynamic processes involved in its genesis. In addition, the study of this inherited neuropathy has lead to a greater understanding of mechanisms involved in the control of cell interactions in normal peripheral nerves; in particular, the in vitro investigations of dystrophic mouse nerves have drawn attention to the importance of fibroblasts and the extracellular matrix.

On the basis of the experimental evidence reviewed in this paper, the following conclusions can be drawn concerning the peripheral nerve disorder in dystrophic mice: In focal areas of the spinal roots and cranial nerves, there is a failure of Schwann cell deployment, differentiation, control of multiplication, and survival. In these areas, many Schwann cells remain undifferentiated, divide continuously, and may die prematurely but do not evolve toward the normal ensheathment of axons.

Although the morphologic features of the dystrophic spinal roots resemble those observed in normal, immature, developing nerves, there is evidence for an ongoing process that prevents the acquisition of normal axon–Schwann cell relationships even in adult animals.

There are also other more subtle generalized abnormalities throughout the peripheral nervous system. The patchy discontinuities in the basal lamina of Schwann cells are the most striking changes in this category, but widened nodes of Ranvier and aberrant myelination also occur.

When the dystrophic spinal roots are transplanted into the peripheral nerves of normal or dystrophic mice, the failure of Schwann cells to ensheathe axons is corrected, but the basal lamina defect persists. Thus, contrary to what has been demonstrated for the neuropathies of the Trembler and quaking mutants, the major spinal root abnormality cannot be attributed solely to a primary Schwann cell disorder. Furthermore, although the basal lamina defect requires dystrophic Schwann cells for its expression, tissue culture studies suggest that even the genesis of this abnormality is more complicated and depends in part on influences arising from the extracellular matrix.

ACKNOWLEDGMENTS

The authors acknowledge the financial support of the Muscular Dystrophy Association of Canada, the Medical Research Council, and the Multiple Sclerosis Society of Canada.

REFERENCES

1. Ayers MM, Anderson RMcD: Onion bulb neuropathy in the Trembler mouse: a model of hypertrophic interstitial neuropathy (Dejerine-Sottas) in man. Acta Neuropathol 25:54–70, 1973

2. Aguayo AJ, Bray GM, Perkins CS: Axon–Schwann cell relationships in neuropathies of mutant mice. Ann NY Acad Sci 317:512–531, 1979

3. Samorajski T, Friede RL, Reimer PR: Hypomyelination in the quaking mouse: a model for the analysis of disturbed myelin formation. Neuropathol Exp Neurol 29:507–523, 1970

4. Bradley WG, Jenkison M: Abnormalities of peripheral nerves in murine muscular dystrophy. J Neurol Sci 18:227–247, 1973

5. Okada E, Mizuhira V, Nakamura H: Abnormalities of the sciatic nerves of dystrophic mice, with reference to nerve counts and mean area of axons. Bull Tokyo Med Dent Univ 22:25–43, 1975

6. Biscoe TJ, Caddy KWT, Pallot DJ, et al: Investigation of cranial and other nerves in the mouse with muscular dystrophy. J Neurol Neurosurg Psychiatry 38:391–403, 1975

7. Bray GM, Aguayo AJ: Quantitative ultrastructural studies of the axon–Schwann cell abnormality in spinal nerve roots from dystrophic mice. J Neuropathol Exp Neurol 34:517–532, 1975

8. Stirling CA: Abnormalities in Schwann cell sheaths in spinal nerve roots of dystrophic mice. J Anat 119:169–180, 1975

9. Perkins CS, Bray GM, Aguayo AJ: Persistent multiplication of axon-associated cells in the spinal roots of dystrophic mice. Neuropathol Appl Neurobiol 6:83–91, 1980

10. Jaros E, Bradley WG: Development of the amyelinated lesion in the ventral root of the dystrophic mouse. J Neurol Sci 36:317–339, 1978

11. Rasminsky M, Kearney RE, Aguayo AJ, et al: Conduction of nervous impulses in spinal roots and peripheral nerves of dystrophic mice. Brain Res 143:71–85, 1978

12. Weinberg HJ, Spencer RS, Raine CS: Aberrant PNS development in dystrophic mice. Brain Res 98:532–537, 1975

13. Papapetropoulos TA, Bradley WG: Spinal motor neurones in murine muscular dystrophy and spinal muscular atrophy: a quantitative histological study. J Neurol Neurosurg Psychiatry 35:60–65, 1972

14. Aguayo AJ, Bray GM, Perkins CS, et al: Axon–sheath cell interactions in peripheral and central nervous system transplants. Soc Neurosci Abstr 4:361–383, 1979

15. Rasminsky M: Ephaptic transmission between single nerve fibres in the spinal nerve roots of dystrophic mice. J Physiol (Lond) (in press).

16. Hasty DL, Hay ED: Freeze-fracture studies of the developing cell surface. II. Particle-free

membrane blisters on glutaraldehyde-fixed corneal fibroblasts are artifacts. J Cell Biol 78:756–768, 1978

17. Ellisman MH: Molecular specializations of the axon membrane at nodes of Ranvier are not dependent upon myelination. J Neurocytol 8:719–735, 1979

18. Rosenbluth J: Aberrant axon–Schwann cell junctions in dystrophic mouse nerves. J Neurocytol 8:655–672, 1979

19. Bray GM, Cullen MJ, Aguayo AJ, Rasminsky M. Node-like areas of intramembranous particles in the unensheathed axons of dystrophic mice. Neurosci Lett 13:203–208, 1979

20. Rosenbluth J: Intramembranous particle distribution at the node of Ranvier and adjacent axolemma in myelinated axons of the frog brain. J Neurocytol 5:731–745, 1976

21. Bradley WG, Jaros E, Jenkison M: The nodes of Ranvier in the nerves of mice with muscular dystrophy. J Neuropathol Exp Neurol 36:797–806, 1977

22. Madrid RE, Jaros E, Cullen MJ, et al: Genetically determined defect of Schwann cell basement membrane in dystrophic mouse. Nature 257:319–321, 1975

23. Jaros E, Bradley WG: Atypical axon–Schwann cell relationships in the common peroneal nerve of the dystrophic mouse: an ultrastructural study. Neuropathol Appl Neurobiol 5:133–147, 1979

24. Brown MG, Radich SJ: Polyaxonal myelination in developing dystrophic and normal mouse nerves. Muscle Nerve 2:217–222, 1979

25. Montgomery A, Swenarchuk L: Dystrophic mice show age-related muscle fibre and myelinated axon losses. Nature 267:167–169, 1977

26. Slater CR, Wolfe AFR: Abnormal reinnervation of muscles in dystrophic mice. J Physiol (Lond) 275:73P–74P, 1978

27. Aguayo AJ, Charron L, Bray GM: Potential of Schwann cells from unmyelinated nerves to produce myelin: a quantitative ultrastructural and radiographic study. J Neurocytol 5:565–573, 1976

28. Appenzeller O, Kornfeld M, Atkinson R: Pure axonal neuropathy: nerve xenografts and clinicopathological study of a family with peripheral neuropathy, hereditary ataxia, focal necrotizing encephalopathy and spongy degeneration of brain. Ann Neurol 17:251–261, 1980

29. Dyck PJ, Lais AC, Sparks MF, et al: Apportioning the role of Schwann cell and axon in the hypomyelination of HMSN-III using human sural nerve xenografts to nude mice (abstract). Neurology (NY) 29:588–589, 1979

30. Perkins CS, Aguayo AJ, Bray GM: Schwann cell multiplication in Trembler mice. Neuropathol Appl Neurobiol (in press)

31. Aguayo AJ, Kasarjian J, Skamene E, et al: Myelination of mouse axons by Schwann cells transplanted from normal and abnormal human nerves. Nature 268:753–755, 1977

32. Aguayo AJ, Perkins CS, Duncan ID, et al: Human and animal neuropathies studied in experimental nerve transplants. In *Peripheral Neuropathies*. Edited by Canal N, Pozza G. Elsevier/North-Holland Biomedical Press, Amsterdam, 1978, pp 37–48

33. Ohnishi A, Tateishi J, Matsumoto T, et al: Fabry disease: cellular expression of enzyme deficiency in nerve xenografts. Neurology (NY) 29:899–901, 1979

34. Aguayo AJ, Attiwell M, Trecarten J, et al: Abnormal myelination in transplanted Trembler mouse Schwann cells. Nature 265:73–75, 1977

35. Scaravilli F, Jacobs JM, Teixeira F: Quantitative and experimental studies on the twitcher mouse. In *Neurological Mutations Affecting Myelination*. INSERM Symposium No. 14. Edited by Bauman N. Elsevier/North-Holland Biomedical Press, Amsterdam 1980, pp 87–98

36. Duncan ID, Aguayo AJ, Bunge RP, et al: Transplantation of rat Schwann cells grown in tissue culture into the mouse spinal cord. J Neurol Sci (in press)

37. Bray GM, Perkins CS, Peterson AC, et al: Schwann cell multiplication deficit in nerve roots of newborn dystrophic mice. J Neurol Sci 32:203–212, 1977

38. Peters A, Muir AR: The relationship between axons and Schwann cells during development of peripheral nerves in the rat. Q J Exp Physiol 44:117–130, 1959

39. Webster HdeF: The geometry of peripheral myelin sheaths during their formation and growth in rat sciatic nerves. J Cell Biol 48:348–367, 1971

40. Webster HdeF, Martin JR, O'Connell MF: The relationships between interphase Schwann cells and axons before myelination: a quantitative electron microscopic study. Dev Biol 32:401–416, 1973

41. Blomquist E, Westermark B, Ponten J: Ageing of human glial cells in culture: increase in the fraction of non-dividers as demonstrated by a minicloning technique. Mech Ageing Dev 12:173–182, 1980

42. Okada E, Bunge RP, Bunge MB: Abnormalities expressed in long-term cultures of dorsal root ganglia from the dystrophic mouse. Brain Res (in press)

43. Bunge MB, Williams AK, Wood PM: Further evidence that neurons are required for the formation of basal lamina around Schwann cells. J Cell Biol (in press)

44. Cochran M, Cornbrooks CJ, Mithen E, et al: Persistence of basal lamina defect in cultures of dystrophic mouse Schwann cells in contact with normal mouse neurons. Soc Neurosci Abstr 5:427, 1979

45. Bunge RP, Bunge MB: Evidence that contact with connective tissue matrix is required for normal interaction between Schwann cells and nerve fibers. J Cell Biol 78:943–940 1978

46. Perkins CS, Bray GM, Aguayo AJ: Ongoing block of Schwann cell differentiation and deployment in dystrophic mouse spinal roots. Dev Brain Res (in press)

DISCUSSION

Dr. Richard Bunge: You showed the combinations of dystrophic and normal, but not dystrophic and dystrophic. What does the nerve root look like when the dystrophic root is put in the peripheral nerve of the dystrophic mouse?

Dr. Albert Aguayo: Normal.

Dr. Richard Bunge: Normal in terms of basal lamina coverage?

Dr. Albert Aguayo: Normal in terms of everything I mentioned.

Dr. Richard Bunge: How do you explain that?

Dr. Albert Aguayo: I have no answer for your question. Differences between what is found in vitro in the intact animal and in the regenerated transplanted nerves may depend on different experimental conditions, different requirements of the cells that are being studied, changing conditions in the neural environment, and interactions that are confined to certain growth periods only.

4
Cultured Human Schwann Cells: An Approach to Studying Peripheral Neuropathies

Valerie Askanas, MD, PhD

W. King Engel, MD

Neuropathies have been classified into two types according to their possible pathogenesis and nerve pathology: dysschwannian neuropathies are associated with segmental demyelination and slow conduction velocities, whereas dysneuronal neuropathies are associated with wallerian degeneration (1, 2). Because the Schwann cell and the neuronal axon instantly interrelate, some degree of overlap exists between the dysschwannian and dysneuronal neuropathies. Therefore, in most neuropathies, the question of whether the disease process originates in the Schwann cell or in the neuron remains to be answered.

Schwann cells can be cultured from biopsy specimens of diseased peripheral nerve. Their proliferation in a highly controlled tissue culture environment, isolated from the in vivo influence of neuronal axons and circulating serum factors, should provide important information regarding the pathogenesis of human neuropathies. If abnormalities present in the biopsied Schwann cells were reproduced in cultured Schwann cells from the same biopsy specimen, it would indicate the primary dysschwannian character of a given neuropathy. In the dysschwannian neuropathies believed to be due to circulating serum factors or to some chemical substances or toxins, the abnormalities could be induced in the cultured Schwann cells by treatment with the endogenous serum, cerebrospinal fluid, cells such as T lymphocytes, on various chemicals or toxins (Fig. 1).

We have recently described a new technique for culturing Schwann cells from biopsy specimens of adult human sural nerve (3). This several-explant reexplantation technique yields highly purified Schwann cell cultures, in which the

51

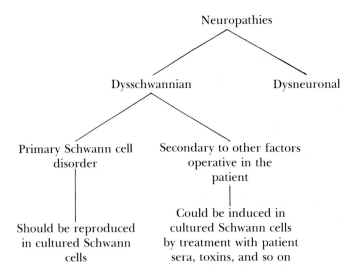

Fig. 1. Types of neuropathy.

numbers of other cells (fibroblasts, epithelial cells, endothelial cells) are greatly reduced by mechanical reexplantation rather than by cytotoxic agents. Cytotoxins are known to influence the function of Schwann cells in vivo (4). Therefore, one must attempt to avoid their potential effects on cultured Schwann cells, especially diseased ones, when one is seeking abnormalities intrinsic to the Schwann cell or abnormal responses to specific exogenous agents. Our technique provides cultures of human Schwann cells in quality suitable for a variety of histochemical, ultrastructural, cytochemical, immunologic, and biochemical studies. Our goals in culturing human Schwann cells are to study the biology of cultured human Schwann cells; to reproduce specific morphologic abnormalities; to reproduce specific biochemical abnormalities; to discover hitherto unknown morphologic or histochemical defects; to attempt myelination by cultured human Schwann cells of an "exogenous" axon.

CULTURED SCHWANN CELLS VERSUS FIBROBLAST-LIKE CELLS

Cultured human Schwann cells have a characteristic bipolar spindle shape. Under phase microscopy, their cytoplasm appears denser than the cytoplasm of fibroblast-like cells because they are more rounded transversely and have a large, elongated nucleus (Fig. 2A). The light microscopic characteristics of human Schwann cells were originally described by Murray in 1940 and 1942 (5, 6) and since then have served as a basis for distinguishing Schwann cells from other cells present in the culture system (7–9). The distinct morphologic characteristics of cultured Schwann cells enabled investigators to establish that rat neural antigen (Ran 1), defined by mouse antiserum against a chemically induced rat neural tumor, can be detected on cultured rat Schwann cells, whereas Thy 1 antigen can be detected on fibroblasts in the same culture system (10, 11), indicating different membrane properties of these cells.

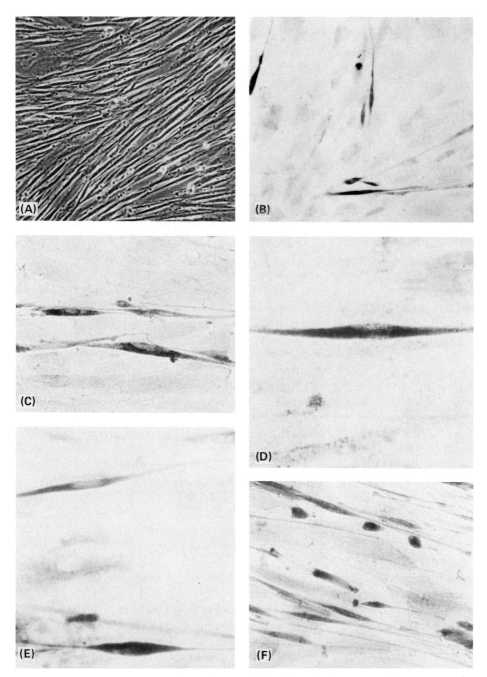

Fig. 2. Comparison of cultured Schwann cells and fibroblasts. **(A)** Nearly pure Schwann cell growth living in culture (phase contrast microscopy; original magnification ×180). **(B)** With nonspecific esterase, Schwann cells stained darkly, but fibroblasts did not stain (original magnification ×180). **(C)** With menadione-mediated α-glycerophosphate dehydrogenase, Schwann cells stained darkly, but fibroblasts did not stain (original magnification ×325). **(D)** With Sudan black, Schwann cells stained very darkly and fibroblasts were virtually unstained (original magnification ×650). **(E)** With glucose-6-phosphate dehydrogenase, Schwann cells stained darkly and fibroblasts stained very weakly (original magnification ×500). **(F)** With reduced nicotinamide adenine dinucleotide tetrazolium reductase, Schwann cells stained slightly more than fibroblasts (original magnification ×250).

53

We also demonstrated differences in membrane properties between human cultured Schwann cells and fibroblast-like cells using concanavalin A (Con A) binding to the plasmalemma of these cells. Peroxidase staining for bound Con A was performed according to a modification of the technique of Bernhard and Avrameas (12). The Con A was used at concentrations of 100, 10, 1, and 0.1 μg/ml of buffer. Elimination of Con A from the incubation medium or use of specific inhibitors of Con A binding (α-methyl-D-mannoside and α-methyl-D-glucoside) served as controls for the specificity of the reaction. At a concentration of 100 μg/ml, Con A bound uniformly strongly to the entire plasmalemma of the Schwann cells; binding to the nonSchwann cells was much weaker. When the concentration of Con A was 10 μg/ml, nonSchwann cells did not demonstrate any staining, whereas the surface of Schwann cells remained stained (Fig. 3E, F). Omitting Con A from the incubation medium or using Con A inhibitors prevented the staining.

Using Con A binding, we demonstrated similar membrane differences between cultured rat Schwann cells and fibroblast-like cells (13). To study histochemical properties of cultured human Schwann cells versus fibroblast-like cells, a battery of 18 histochemical reactions was performed, the details of which are described elsewhere (3). In summary, cultured Schwann cells stained much more strongly than did fibroblast-like cells with nonspecific esterase, glucose-6-phosphate dehydrogenase, menadione-mediated α-glycerophosphate dehydrogenase, Sudan black, and diaminobezindine peroxidase (Fig. 2B–F). They were slightly more strongly stained with reduced nicotinamide adenine dinucleotide and reduced nicotinamide adenine dinucleotide phosphate tetrazolium reductase. Succinate dehydrogenase and β-hydroxybutyrate dehydrogenase stained both types of cell approximately equally. Schwann cells were much more weakly stained than the fibroblast-like cells with alkaline phosphatase, para-aminosalicylic acid (diastase-removed material, i.e., glycogen), phosphorylase, and oil-red-O. Neither was stained with the calcium or adenosine triphosphatase reactions used in our studies.

The histochemical characteristics of cultured Schwann cells suggest the following: (a) a reliance on oxidative metabolism rather than on glycogenolysis for generation of adenosine triphosphate; (b) active peroxide production with high endogenous peroxidase; and (c) synthesis of nontriglyceride lipids as potential precursors of myelin. Recently, we have obtained biochemical evidence of the specificity of cultured Schwann cells versus cultured fibroblasts and human muscle cells. The activity of 2′,3′-cyclic nucleotide phosphohydrolase, a myelin-associated enzyme (14, 15), appeared to be approximately 20 times greater in cultured Schwann cells than in cultured fibroblasts and muscle cells (Reddy B, Askanas V, Engel WK: unpublished data).

ULTRASTRUCTURE OF CULTURED HUMAN SCHWANN CELLS

The technique for precise selection and drilling-out of individual cells from the embedded culture (16, 17) enabled ultrastructural comparison of Schwann cells versus fibroblast-like cells. Cultured Schwann cells are mononucleated. The nucleus is elongated, has 1 or 2 nucleoli, and usually has some invagination of

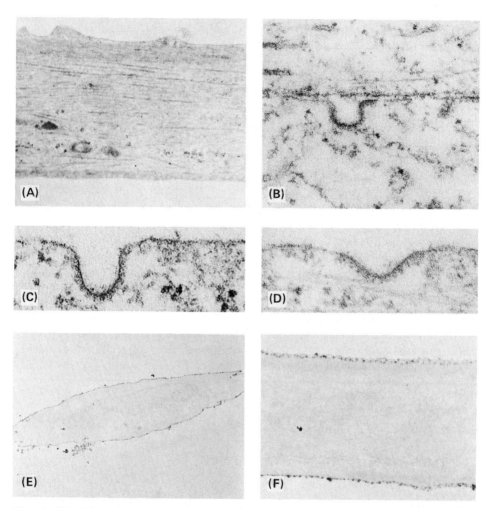

Fig. 3. (A) Polar region of Schwann cell rich in microtubules and actin-like filaments (original magnification ×12,250). **(B)** Plasmalemma of two adjacent Schwann cells showing focal invagination of thickened plasmalemma (original magnification ×60,800). **(C and D)** Higher-power electron micrograph of focal invagination of plasmalemma (original magnification ×84,000). **(E)** Low-power electron micrograph of Schwann cell with plasmalemma delineated by concanavalin A binding, without counterstain (original magnification ×4,950). **(F)** Higher-power electron micrograph showing pattern of concanavalin A binding to plasmalemma of Schwann cell, with no counterstain (original magnification ×20,600).

cytoplasm, bounded by a nuclear membrane. The cytoplasm of cultured Schwann cells is rich in ribosomes, which appear as free ribosomes, rosettes, and studding narrow endoplastic reticulum. Mitochondria are rather small and more numerous in the perinuclear area. In the perinuclear area, the Golgi apparatus is prominent. Occasional dense-core vesicles and medium-sized round, dark osmiophilic bodies are also present in the perinuclear area. Longitudinally oriented microtubules 19 nm in diameter and actin-like microfilaments 8 nm in diameter are randomly present in the perinuclear area; in the elongated ends of the Schwann cells, however, they are the most prominent structures of the cytoplasm, whereas mitochondria, ribosomes, and Golgi apparatus are very infrequent (Figs. 3A, 4, 5). Regular rounded, concentrically laminated bodies of somewhat varying periodicity and centrioles are present in some Schwann cells. Only rarely are glycogen granules evident in the Schwann cell cytoplasm.

Cultured human Schwann cells have a very well defined plasmalemma approximately 12 nm thick, but they do not have a basement membrane. A characteristic feature of the Schwann cell plasmalemma is the scattered focal invagination of a thickened membrane approximately 27 nm thick. On the cytoplasmic side of the invaginations, "fuzzy" biochemically unidentified material is present (Fig. 3B–D). The described invagination can be identified with coated pits (18).

Knowledge of the histochemical and ultrastructural properties of normal cultured human Schwann cells is important when seeking abnormalities of cultured diseased Schwann cells. In adrenomyeloneuropathy, a disease characterized by adrenal insufficiency, spastic paraparesis, and peripheral neuropathy (19, 20), we were able to demonstrate, for the first time, a biochemical defect in this disease while a patient was still alive by culturing Schwann cells and muscle cells from the patient. Cultured Schwann cells and muscle cells contained multilaminated inclusions, and they accumulated very long chain fatty acids (21). We had previously demonstrated that when excess C_{22} and C_{26} fatty acids

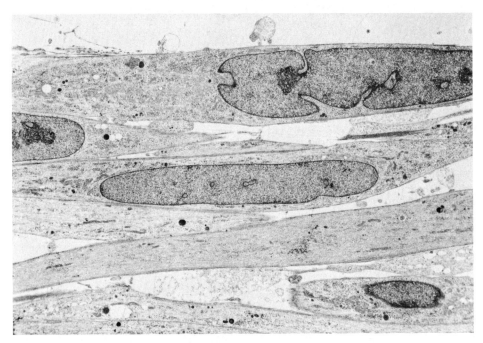

Fig. 4. Low-power electron micrograph of a field of cultured Schwann cells (original magnification $\times 3,900$).

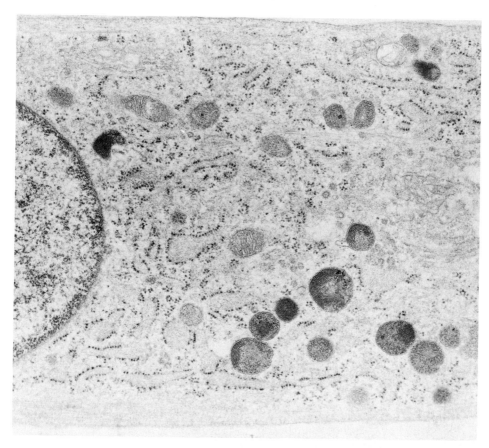

Fig. 5. Electron micrograph of perinuclear area of cultured Schwann cells, at higher magnification than Figure 4. Note abundance of ribosomes (free, rosette form, and studding the narrow endoplasmic reticulum), mitochondria, Golgi apparatus, osmiophilic bodies with concentric lamellae, and scant microtubules and microfilaments (original magnification ×34,400).

were introduced into the medium in which muscle of a patient with adreno-myeloneuropathy was cultured, the increase in these fatty acids was 6-fold greater than that of normal muscle cultured under identical conditions (21). Recently, we showed in another patient with adrenomyeloneuropathy that excess fatty acids in the culture medium intensified the ultrastructural abnormalities of cultured Schwann cells (Fig. 6A, B) (Askanas V, Moser H, Engel WK: unpublished data).

Schwann cells cultured from sural nerve biopsy specimens from a patient with continuous muscle fiber activity and peripheral neuropathy (23, 24) provided proof of dysschwannian neuropathy and a clue to the cause of neuropathy (Askanas V, Engel WK, Berginer VM, Odenwald WF, Galdi A: unpublished data). Schwann cells in the biopsy specimen of nerve contained large membrane-bound vacuoles, some of which appeared empty, and some of which contained floccular or darkly osmiophilic inclusions (Fig. 7A). The Schwann cells grew normally in culture, but vacuoles could be observed in many

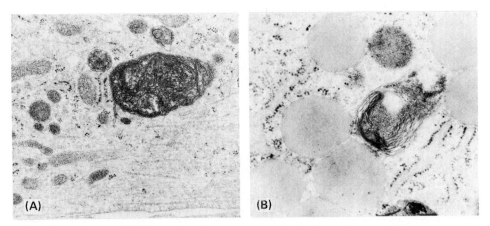

Fig. 6. Ultrastructural abnormalities in cultured Schwann cell from patient with adrenomyeloneuropathy. **(A)** No treatment with C_{26} fatty acids. Note large multilaminated inclusions (original magnification ×25,300). **(B)** After treatment with C_{26}, note multilaminated inclusion and numerous lipid droplets (original magnification ×35,100).

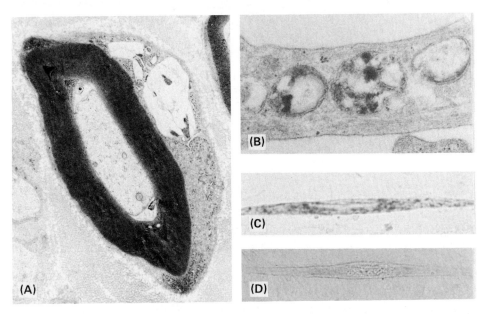

Fig. 7. (A) Large membrane-bound vacuoles containing osmiophilic inclusions in Schwann cell of biopsy specimen nerve (original magnification ×8,800). **(B)** Membrane-bound vacuoles containing osmiophilic inclusion in cultured Schwann cell (original magnification ×48,000). **(C)** Positive acid phosphatase reaction in patient's cultured Schwann cell (original magnification ×680). **(D)** Negative acid phosphatase reaction in control cultured Schwann cell (condensor lowered to visualize negatively stained Schwann cell) (original magnification ×680).

of the living Schwann cells. Ultrastructurally, vacuoles found in the cultured Schwann cells were very similar to those present in the biopsied Schwann cells. In both the biopsied and cultured Schwann cells, the vacuoles were membrane bound; some appeared empty, but some contained glycogen or floccular and darkly osmiophilic material (Fig. 7B). The patient's cultured Schwann cells stained very strongly with the reaction for acid phosphatase, whereas normal Schwann cells remained unstained (Fig. 7C, D). These studies indicate that this patient had a primary dysschwannian neuropathy because the abnormalities were reincarnated in cultured Schwann cells. The positive acid phosphatase reaction suggests that the abnormality was of lysosomal origin.

Further studies of Schwann cells cultured from abnormal human sural nerves should elucidate the pathogenesis of various neuropathies. In cultures of Schwann cells from dysschwannian neuropathies, growth abnormalities and histochemical, ultrastructural, or biochemical abnormalities caused by a metabolic defect intrinsic to the Schwann cells should be expressed, as has been demonstrated in some diseases intrinsic to the muscle cell (25–27) (see Table in *Discussion*, chapter 67).

ACKNOWLEDGMENTS

Supported in part by the Muscular Dystrophy Association of America. Excellent technical assistance in tissue culture was provided by Jane Lawrence and Linda Carter; in electron microscopy, by Ward Odenwald; in histochemistry, by Guy Cunningham; and in photography, by Gregory Zirsow.

REFERENCES

1. Engel WK: Introduction to disorders of the motor neuron, nerves and related abnormalities. In *Scientific Approaches to Clinical Neurology*. Edited by Goldensohn ES, Appel SH. Lea and Febiger, Philadelphia, 1977, pp 1250–1321

2. Engel WK: Classification of neuromuscular disorders. Birth Defects 7:18–37, 1971

3. Askanas V, Engel WK, Dalakas MC, et al: Human Schwann cells in tissue culture: histochemical and ultrastructural studies. Arch Neurol 37:329–337, 1980

4. Hall SM, Gregson NS: The effect of 5-bromodeoxyuridine on remyelination in the peripheral nervous system of the mouse. Neuropathol Appl Neurobiol 4:117–27, 1978

5. Murray MR, Stout AP: Schwann cell versus fibroblast as the origin of the specific nerve sheath tumor: observation upon normal nerve sheaths and neurinomas in vitro. Am J Pathol 16:41–60, 1940

6. Murray MR, Stout AP: Characteristics of human Schwann cell in vitro. Anat Rec 84:275–293, 1942

7. Wood PM: Separation of functional Schwann cells and neurons from normal peripheral nerve tissue. Brain Res 115:361–375, 1976

8. Wood PM, Bunge RP: Evidence that sensory axons are mitogenic for Schwann cells. Nature 256:662–664, 1975

9. Cravioto M, Lockwood R: The behavior of acoustic neuroma in tissue culture. Acta Neuropathol 12:141–157, 1969

10. Raff MC, Hornby-Smith A, Brockes JP: Cyclic AMP as a mitogenic signal for cultured rat Schwann cells. Nature 273:672–673, 1978

11. Brockes JP, Fields KL, Raff MC: Studies on cultured rat Schwann cells: establishment of purified populations from cultures of peripheral nerve. Brain Res 165:105–118, 1979

12. Bernhard W, Avremas S: Ultrastructural visualization of cellular carbohydrate components by means of concanavalin A. Exp Cell Res 64:232–236, 1974

13. Odenwald WV, Askanas V, Engel WK, et al: Ultrastructural and cytochemical characterization of Schwann cells cultured from rat peripheral nerve. Soc Neurosci Abstr 5:756, 1979

14. Sims NR, Carnegie PR: 2′,3′-cyclic nucleotide 3-phosphodiesterase. Adv Neurochem 3:1–41, 1978

15. Olafson RW, Drummond GT, Lee YF: Studies on 2′,3′-cyclic nucleotide 3′-phosphohydrolase from brain. Can J Biochem 47:961–966, 1969

16. Askanas V, Engel WK: A technique of fiber selection from human muscle tissue cultures for histochemical-electron microscopical studies. J Histochem Cytochem 22:144–151, 1975

17. Gorycki MC, Askanas V: Improved technique for electron microscopy of culture cells. Stain Technol 52:249–253, 1977

18. Goldstein JL, Anderson RGW, Brown MS: Coated pits, coated vesicles, and receptor-mediated endocytosis. Nature 279:679–685, 1979

19. Griffin JW, Goren E, Schaumburg H, et al: Adrenomyeloneuropathy: a probable variant of adrenoleucodystrophy. 1. Clinical and endocrinologic aspects. Neurology (Minneap) 27:1107–1113, 1977

20. Schaumburg HH, Powers JM, Raine CS, et al: Adrenomyeloneuropathy: a probable variant of adrenoleucodystrophy. II. General pathologic, neuropathologic and biochemical aspects. Neurology (Minneap) 27:1114–1119, 1977

21. Askanas V, McLaughlin J, Engel WK: Abnormalities in cultured muscle and peripheral nerve of a patient with adrenomyeloneuropathy. N Engl J Med 301:488–491, 1979

22. McLaughlin J, Askanas V, Engel WK: Adrenomyeloneuropathy: increased accumulation of very long chain fatty acid in cultured skeletal muscle. Biochem Biophys Res Commun 92:1202–1207, 1980

23. Issacs H: A syndrome of continuous muscle fiber activity. J Neurol Neurosurg Psychiatry 32:319–325, 1961

24. Korczyn AD, Kuritzky A, Sandbank U: Muscle hypertrophy with neuropathy. J Neurol Sci 36:399–408, 1978

25. Askanas, V, Engel WK, DiMauro S, et al: Adult-onset acid maltase deficiency: morphologic and biochemical abnormalities reproduced in cultured muscle. N Engl J Med 294:573–578, 1976

26. Askanas V, Engel WK: Normal and diseased human muscle in tissue culture. In *Handbook of Clinical Neurology*. Edited by Vinken PY, Bruyan GW. North-Holland Publishing Co., Amsterdam, 1979, pp 183–196

27. Askanas V, Engel WK, Reddy NB, et al: X-linked recessive congenital muscle fiber hypotrophy with central nuclei. Arch Neurol 36:604–609, 1979

5
Physiologic Properties of Demyelinated Nerve Fibers

Michael Rasminsky, MD, PhD

Demyelination of nerve fibers in both the peripheral and the central nervous system causes impaired ability to conduct nerve impulses, reorganization of axonal membrane, altered sensitivity to metabolic changes and pharmacologic agents, and increased excitability of nerve fibers. These consequences of demyelination are the main themes of this review.

CONDUCTION OF NERVE IMPULSES

Impaired Transmission

In both the peripheral and the central nervous system, decreased conduction velocity and conduction block are consequences of demyelination of various etiologies, including diphtheria toxin (1–4), experimental allergic neuritis (5, 6), experimental granuloma of nerve (7), and lysolecithin (8–10). Other manifestations of the impaired ability of demyelinated nerve fibers to transmit nerve impulses are an increased refractory period of transmission (2, 3), inability to transmit trains of impulses at high frequency (2, 3, 11), and posttetanic depression (5, 11). There are several recent reviews of these properties of demyelinated nerve fibers (12–16).

Structure-Function Relationships

Despite the extensive literature on conduction of nerve impulses in demyelination, we have had relatively little insight into the relationship between structure and function; for example, the minimal lesion necessary to cause conduction block has not heretofore been identified. There are a number of reasons for this. First, studies of conduction in demyelinated nerve fibers have been performed on relatively chronic lesions in which there is striking nonuniformity of involvement among various fibers in the lesion. The single-fiber technique most extensively used for studying propagation of impulses in single fibers (3, 4, 9) examines conduction in single fibers within intact rodent spinal roots; the fiber(s) studied physiologically cannot subsequently be distinguished histologically from other fibers in the same root. It has not yet been possible to perform satisfactory physiologic and morphologic studies on single identified demyelinated nerve fibers. Second, it is now clear that demyelination is followed by changes in the properties of the axonal membrane (see later). The consequences of chronic demyelination thus cannot be predicted simply as a function of fiber geometry. For example, computer simulations show that conduction velocity in myelinated fibers is relatively insensitive to nodal surface area provided that all of the exposed axonal membrane has the excitability characteristics of nodal axon (17).

The difficulties of structure-function correlation may be somewhat less in acute demyelinating lesions. Saida and colleagues (18) have injected rabbit antisera to peripheral nerve myelin or galactocerebroside (19) into the sciatic nerves of rats and have observed block of motor conduction within 2 to 5 hours. Topical application of anti-galactocerebroside serum to rat spinal roots causes blockage of conduction in single fibers after as little as 90 minutes of exposure (20); more slowly conducting, smaller-diameter fibers sustain conduction block before more rapidly conducting, larger-diameter fibers. Blockage of conduction is preceded by an increase in internodal conduction time from the normal 20 μsec to 200 μsec or more (Fig. 1). Brown and associates (21) found that during

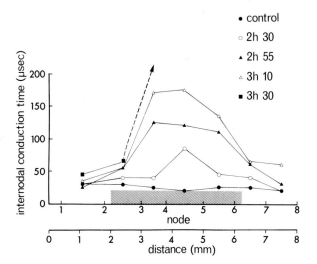

Fig. 1. Internodal conduction time for 7 successive internodes of a rat ventral root fiber before and at intervals after the root was bathed in anti-galactocerebroside serum approximately over the length indicated by the hatched bar. Zero distance is arbitrary. The positions of successive nodes of Ranvier were identified physiologically by external longitudinal current recording (3). Nodes 1 to 8 are designated in the direction of transmission of the impulses. Within the region of serum application, internodal conduction time increased from the normal control value of 20 to 25 μsec to nearly 200 μsec before conduction failure occurred at node 3 after 3.5 hours of exposure to the serum. (Rasminsky M, Sumner AJ: unpublished data.)

the first few hours of topical exposure to anti-galactocerebroside serum the major pathologic abnormality is paranodal demyelination. Thus, it appears likely that during acute demyelination, the increase in axonal surface area in the nodal region increases the nodal capacitance sufficiently to cause conduction block, the increased nodal capacitance precluding depolarization of the demyelinated node to threshold for regeneration of the action potential (Rasminsky M, Sumner A, Lafontaine S: unpublished data).

In more chronic demyelination, it is possible that paranodal demyelination has a less dramatic effect on conduction velocity. For example, in the early stages of demyelination caused by diphtheria toxin, when paranodal widening is the predominant lesion, compound action potential studies show little or no change in maximal conduction velocity (22). This finding may reflect compensation for increased nodal area by insertion of new sodium channels into the nodal axon membrane (4).

AXONAL MEMBRANE ORGANIZATION

Myelinated Nerve Fibers

Although it has been known for more than 30 years that electrical excitation is confined to nodes of Ranvier in myelinated nerve fibers (23, 24), it has only recently become clear that the axonal membrane of myelinated fibers is divided into distinct nodal and internodal domains.

The electrical excitability of axonal membrane is dependent on the presence of voltage-dependent sodium channels within the membrane. Depolarization of the membrane causes the sodium channels to open and allows current carried by sodium ions to flow inward through the membrane. The repeated regeneration of inward current at successive nodes of Ranvier is necessary for propagation of the nerve impulse. Saxitoxin binding studies have shown that the density of sodium channels in nodal axonal membrane is more than two orders of magnitude greater than that in internodal axon: the sodium channel density of rabbit nodal axonal membrane is estimated to be 10,000 to 12,000/ μm^2 in contrast to a density of less than $25/\mu m^2$ in internodal axonal membrane (25, 26) and $125 /\mu m^2$ for unmyelinated (C fiber) axonal membrane (27).

Freeze-fracture studies show a high density of particles in the external leaflet of nodal axonal membrane (E-face particles) that are present in much lower concentration in the internodal axonal membrane (28, 29). A high density of similar E-face particles is seen at the electrically excitable but not at the inexcitable nodes of the *Sternarchus* electrocyte organ (30). It is thus tempting to speculate that these E-face particles are themselves or are somehow associated with sodium channels.

Histochemical staining with ferric ion and ferrocyanate has also shown marked differences between nodal and internodal or unmyelinated axonal membrane (31, 32). The positive staining characteristic of nodes of Ranvier with this technique is also present at the excitable but not at the inexcitable nodes of the *Sternarchus* electrocyte organ (32) and at the initial segment of motor neurons (33). This stain thus appears to correlate well with the presence of excitable membrane with a high density of sodium channels.

At nodes of Ranvier of amphibian myelinated nerve fibers, there are voltage-dependent sodium and potassium channels; the potassium channels open during the latter phase of the action potential to permit outward flow of potassium current and repolarization of the membrane. Potassium channels are absent from the nodal membranes of mammalian myelinated nerve fibers (34, 35), and repolarization in these fibers is due simply to inactivation of sodium permeability. Osmotic disruption of the paranodal apparatus of mammalian nodes results in the appearance of potassium currents, indicating that potassium channels are in fact present in the ordinarily quiescent paranodal axon membrane (36). This experiment provides further evidence of partitioning of the axonal membrane into at least two distinct domains: a nodal domain characterized by a high density of sodium channels and a low density of potassium channels; and an internodal domain characterized by a low density of sodium channels and, at least in the paranodal area, an appreciable density of potassium channels.

Demyelinated Nerve Fibers

In normal myelinated nerve fibers (3, 23, 24), and probably in most rat spinal root fibers demyelinated with diphtheria toxin (3), conduction is saltatory; the sites of inward membrane current flow at nodes of Ranvier are spatially separated by the internodes, which do not participate in regeneration of the action potential. However, in some fibers demyelinated by diphtheria toxin, the spatial separation between sites of inward membrane current generation is no longer demonstrable (i.e., is at least less than 100 μm) and conduction becomes continuous over distances as long as 1.5 mm (4, 9). This implies that previously internodal axonal membrane can become electrically excitable, i.e., that bared axonal membrane can be reorganized to have a sufficient density of sodium channels to sustain continuous conduction.

Early during recovery from demyelination with lysolecithin, conduction resumes with sites of excitable membrane being separated by as little as 150 μm, in contrast to the normal internodal length of approximately 1 mm (9, 10). During the ensuing 3 weeks, the distance between sites of excitable membrane gradually increases to the approximately 300 μm characteristic of the distance between nodes of remyelinated axons (9, 10). This change in the distance between sites of excitable membrane presumably reflects an ongoing remodeling of the ion channel distribution within the axonal membrane as remyelination ensues.

Ion channel distribution within axonal membranes is one facet of the complex interaction between axons and myelin-forming glial cells (37). The details of the relationship between myelination and ion channel distribution in axonal membrane remain to be more fully elucidated. The continuous conduction observed in some diphtheria toxin–demyelinated axons (4) suggests that sodium channels distribute themselves relatively evenly throughout the bare axonal membrane in the absence of Schwann cells. On the other hand, the microsaltatory conduction observed in lysolecithin-demyelinated axons (9, 10) suggests that nodal-like aggregation of sodium channels can occur before myelination.

"Continuous" conduction has also been observed in the spinal root bare axons of dystrophic mice (38) and in regenerating nerve fibers (39), but the spatial resolution of the recording system in these experiments was not sufficient to distinguish between the truly continuous conduction characteristic of diphtheria toxin–demyelinated axons and the "microsaltatory" conduction characteristic of lysolecithin demyelination.

Node-like aggregations of intramembranous particles are seen in bare axons and at heminodes of dystrophic mouse spinal root fibers (40, 41), and Waxman and Foster (42) have observed cytochemical differentiation of axonal membrane of developing axons before formation of mature nodes of Ranvier. These observations invite the speculation (37, 41, 42) that axonal differentiation in some way directs the territory of myelination. Rosenbluth (28) has expressed the opposite view, that the interaction of myelin-forming cells with axons is responsible for constraining axonal E-face particles to nodes of Ranvier. Whatever the causal relationships between myelination and axonal differentiation ultimately prove to be, at the very least it is now clear that there is an impressive plasticity of distribution of ion channels within the axonal membrane.

SENSITIVITY TO METABOLIC CHANGES AND PHARMACOLOGIC AGENTS

The safety factor of transmission of impulses in normal myelinated fibers is high, and even relatively large changes in metabolic environment are easily tolerated without blockage of conduction. Demyelination results in a substantial reduction in the safety factor of transmission and renders conduction across demyelinated portions of nerve fibers vulnerable to factors that only marginally alter the current-generating capacity or responsiveness to stimulation of excitable membrane.

Temperature

Conduction in demyelinated fibers is reversibly blocked at temperatures within the physiologic range (43, 44). The blockage is due to the decrease with increasing temperature of *total* current generated by excitable membrane during the action potential (44, 45). Figure 2 illustrates the corresponding decrease in duration of the action potential with increased temperature. A small increase

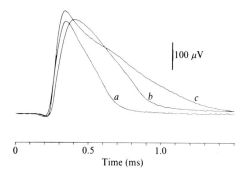

Fig. 2. Action potentials externally recorded from a rat spinal root fiber with computer averaging (**a**) at 37° C, (**b**) at 31° C, and (**c**) at 37° C after exposure to scorpion venom for 30 seconds. (Reprinted with permission from Bostock H, Sherratt RM, Sears TA: Overcoming conduction failure in demyelinated nerve by prolonging action potentials. Nature 274:385–387, 1978.)

in temperature may reduce the total current available to stimulate a critical site in a demyelinated nerve fiber from just above to just below that required to cause depolarization to threshold. In principle, a blocking temperature can be defined for each demyelinated internode (44, 46); the more severe the degree of demyelination, the lower the blocking temperature.

Calcium

Decreasing extracellular calcium lowers the threshold of excitable membrane and should thus enhance transmission in demyelinated fibers on the point of conduction block. This has been shown to be the case in computer simulations of demyelinated fibers (46), and clinical studies of patients with demyelinating disease have shown the anticipated transient reversal of neurologic deficits after maneuvers that reduce the serum calcium level (47, 48).

Pharmacologic Prolongation of the Action Potential

Blockage of Sodium Inactivation

Application of the toxin of the scorpion *Leiurus quinquestriatus* to mammalian nerve fibers results in a prolongation of the action potential (Fig. 2) due to blockage of sodium channel inactivation (49). Because the toxin affects primarily the falling phase of the action potential, it has little effect on the conduction velocity of normal fibers. However, it markedly increases the security of transmission of impulses across sites of focal demyelination as manifested by an increase of several degrees centigrade in the blocking temperature of demyelinated fibers after exposure to the toxin (49).

Blockage of Potassium Channels

In normal mammalian nerve fibers, potassium channels are not present at nodes of Ranvier (34, 35) and action potentials are not altered by the application of 4-aminopyridine (50), a drug that specifically blocks potassium channels. In demyelinated mammalian nerve fibers, as in unmyelinated mammalian fibers, application of 4-aminopyridine causes a widening of the action potential due to blockage of the component of membrane repolarization due to activation of voltage-dependent potassium channels (50). Preliminary experiments with this compound have shown an increase in blocking temperature of demyelinated fibers similar to that caused by exposure to scorpion venom (50). The compound is potentially of great therapeutic interest because of its selective effect on demyelinated fibers that appear to contain voltage-dependent potassium channels and its lack of effect on normal myelinated fibers.

INCREASED EXCITABILITY

Four patterns of increased excitability have been observed in pathologically myelinated nerve fibers: spontaneous ectopic excitation, ephaptic excitation, autoexcitation, and reflections of impulses.

Ectopic Excitation

In the lumbosacral spinal roots of dystrophic mice, many axons are bare or abnormally thinly myelinated (51). Nerve impulses arise spontaneously in mid-spinal root in these axons and are propagated both toward the spinal cord and toward the periphery (52) (Fig. 3). Sites of ectopic excitation may give rise to single impulses or bursts of impulses with instantaneous frequencies as high as 100 Hz, or they may fire continuously (52). There may be more than one site of ectopic excitation in a single pathologic fiber (53). The continuous electro-

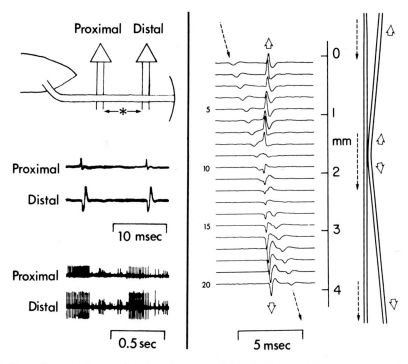

Fig. 3. Ectopic excitation and ephaptic transmission in dystrophic mouse ventral roots. *Left.* Recordings of spontaneous activity are made biphasically from pairs of wire electrodes applied to the root; upward and downward deflections reflect impulses in single fibers propagating toward and away from the spinal cord, respectively. Impulses originating in mid-root (asterisk) travel in opposite directions and propagate past the two pairs of recording electrodes (upper traces). Bursting of the single unit shown in the upper traces is shown at slower sweep speed in the lower traces. *Right.* Biphasic recordings are obtained at intervals of 200 μm along the root. From top to bottom, the recordings are progressively farther away from the spinal cord. An impulse in one fiber propagates away from the spinal cord (downward deflection in record 1 with progressively greater latency at each successive recording site) (dashed arrows). A second fiber is ephaptically excited in mid-root near recording site 9, and an impulse in this fiber (open arrows) is propagated back toward the spinal cord (upward deflections with progressively greater latencies in records 8 to 1) and toward the periphery (downward deflection with faster rise times and progressively greater latencies in records 10 to 20). (Adapted from Rasminsky (52, 53) with permission of publishers.)

myographic activity seen in the dystrophic mouse hind limb muscles can be blocked by curare (54) and is thus presumably a reflection of the ectopic activity originating in the spinal roots. This continuous muscle activity is also greatly reduced by administration of diphenylhydantoin (55), which presumably acts more directly at the site of ectopic generation of impulses.

Although a high level of spontaneous ectopic activity is not usually characteristic of experimentally demyelinated nerve fibers, such fibers have a low threshold to mechanical stimulation in both the peripheral (56) and central (57) nervous system. Spontaneous ectopic excitation of demyelinated nerve fibers can give rise to myokymia in the Guillain-Barré syndrome (58), and continuous muscle activity or myokymia of peripheral nerve origin has been reported in many patients in whom the peripheral nerve pathology is less clearly defined as demyelination (59).

Ephaptic Excitation

Cross talk between nerve fibers of dystrophic mice was first reported by Huizar and coworkers (60), and it was subsequently confirmed that ephaptic transmission occurred between spontaneously active single fibers in spinal roots of dystrophic mice (52, 53) (Fig. 3). The preferred direction of ephaptic transmission appears to be from bare axon to myelinated axon (53). Ephaptic transmission also occurs between single fibers within experimental neuromas (61), and there is preliminary evidence that it occurs in the peripheral nerves of the Trembler mouse (59), a mutant with a congenital defect of myelination. As yet there has been no persuasive experimental evidence demonstrating ephaptic transmission in experimentally demyelinated nerve fibers, although the possibility of ephaptic transmission is frequently invoked in the clinical literature of demyelinating disease (59).

Autoexcitation

Howe and associates (62) have observed after-discharges or persistent ectopic generation of impulses from chronically injured axons after cessation of tetanic stimulation of such axons. A burst of impulses arising from a site of ectopic excitation in a dystrophic mouse spinal root fiber may be provoked by a single previous impulse in the same fiber traversing the site of ectopic excitation (53). Figure 4 illustrates a diagrammatic reconstruction of a sequence of events involving ectopic excitation, autoexcitation, and ephaptic transmission in two fibers in a dystrophic mouse spinal root and shows the ability of these mechanisms to account for both temporal and lateral amplification of impulse activity generated in pathologic peripheral nerve.

Reflection of impulses

If an impulse is sufficiently delayed at a region of low safety factor in a computer-simulated axon, reexcitation and reverse propagation of the impulse may occur (63, 64). Such reflections of impulses are occasionally observed in experimentally demyelinated axons (62).

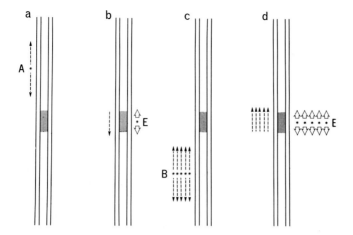

Fig. 4. Diagrammatic reconstruction of a sequence of events observed in a pair of dystrophic mouse spinal root fibers. (**a**) An impulse originates ectopically at site A in the first fiber and propagates in both directions. (**b**) This impulse ephaptically excites the second fiber at E, giving rise to a second impulse propagating in both directions; (**c**) 150 msec later, a burst of impulses arises at site B in the first fiber. (**d**) These impulses then ephaptically excite the second fiber at E. In this sequence of events, a single ectopic impulse originating in mid-root (asterisk) leads to transmission in both directions of a total of more than 10 impulses in 2 fibers. Ectopic activity is amplified both laterally by ephaptic transmission and temporally by autoexcitation. (Reprinted with permission from Rasminsky M: Ephaptic transmission between single nerve fibres in the spinal nerve roots of dystrophic mice. J Physiol (Lond), 305:151–169, 1980.)

CLINICAL IMPLICATIONS

The experimental phenomena described above lend themselves to interpretation in terms of clinical phenomena characteristic of demyelinating disease. Many of these clinical implications have been discussed in detail elsewhere (12, 14–16, 59, 65) and are summarized in Table 1.

It is useful to classify symptoms of demyelinating disease as either negative or positive in the Jacksonian sense. Negative symptoms, reflecting loss of function, are presumably due to failure of normal impulse propagation, whereas positive symptoms, reflecting excessive neural activity, presumably are due to increased excitability of nerve fibers. The pharmacologic approach to treatment of these two broad classes of symptoms should thus, in principle, be completely different. Agents tending to enhance transmission of impulses through regions of low safety factor will cause increased excitability and may thus provoke positive symptoms, whereas agents whose effectiveness against positive symptoms reflects a decrease in nerve excitability may tend to provoke negative symptoms. The clinician should be aware that any pharmacologic approach to symptomatic treatment in demyelinating disease represents a possible double-edged sword.

Table 1. Experimentally Observed Phenomena in Demyelinated Nerve Fibers and Their Clinical Correlates in Demyelinating Disease

Experimentally Observed Phenomenon	*Clinical Implications*
Conduction block, conduction slowing, inability to transmit trains of impulses, post-tetanic depression	Negative symptoms of demyelinating disease, e.g., blindness, paralysis, sensory loss, fatigability
Reorganization of axonal membrane	Recovery process in demyelination
Sensitivity to metabolic and pharmacologic agents	Transient symptomatology in central nervous system demyelination with metabolic (e.g., temperature) changes
	Possibility of pharmacologic treatment to enhance conduction through regions of low safety factor
Increased excitability of nerve fibers	Positive symptoms of demyelinating disease, e.g., tic douloureux, myokymia, visual phosphenes, Lhermitte's phenomenon

ACKNOWLEDGMENT

This research was supported by the Medical Research Council of Canada.

REFERENCES

1. McDonald WI: The effects of experimental demyelination on conduction in peripheral nerve: a histological and electrophysiological study. II. Electrophysiological observations. Brain 86:501–524, 1963
2. McDonald WI, Sears TA: The effects of experimental demyelination on conduction in the central nervous system. Brain 93:583–598, 1970
3. Rasminsky M, Sears TA: Internodal conduction in undissected demyelinated nerve fibers. J Physiol (Lond) 227:323–350, 1972
4. Bostock H, Sears TA: The internodal axon membrane: electrical excitability and continuous conduction in segmental demyelination J Physiol (Lond) 280:273–301, 1978
5. Cragg BG, Thomas PK: Changes in nerve conduction in experimental allergic neuritis. J Neurol Neurosurg Psychiatry 27:106–115, 1964
6. Hall JI: Studies on demyelinated peripheral nerves in guinea-pigs with experimental allergic neuritis: a histological and electrophysiological study. II. Electrophysiological observations. Brain 90:313–332, 1967
7. Lehmann HJ, Ule G: Electrophysiologic findings and structural changes in circumspect inflammation of peripheral nerves. Prog Brain Res 6:169–173, 1964
8. Smith KJ, Blakemore WF, McDonald WI: Central remyelination restores secure conduction. Nature 280:395–396, 1979
9. Bostock H: Conduction changes in demyelination. In *Abnormal Nerves and Muscles as Impulse Generators*. Edited by Culp W, Ochoa J. Oxford University Press, New York (in press)
10. Bostock H, Hall SM, Smith KJ: Demyelinated axons form 'nodes' prior to remyelination. J Physiol (Lond) (in press)

11. Davis FA: Impairment of repetitive impulse conduction in experimentally demyelinated and pressure injured nerves. J Neurol Neurosurg Psychiatry 35:537–544, 1972

12. McDonald WI: Pathophysiology in multiple sclerosis. Brain 97:179–196, 1974

13. Rogart RB: Ritchie JM: Pathophysiology of conduction in demyelinated nerve fibers. In *Myelin*. Edited by Morell P. Plenum Press, New York, 1977, pp 353–382

14. Rasminsky M: Physiology of conduction in demyelinated axons. In *Physiology and Pathobiology of Axons*. Edited by Waxman SG. Raven Press, New York, 1978, pp 361–376

15. Sears TA, Bostock H, Sherratt M: The pathophysiology of demyelination and its implications for the symptomatic treatment of multiple sclerosis. Neurology (NY) 28(part 2):21–26, 1978

16. Waxman SG: Conduction in myelinated, unmyelinated and demyelinated fibers. Arch Neurol 34:585–589, 1978

17. Moore JW, Joyner RW, Brill NH, et al: Simulations of conduction in uniform myelinated fibers: relative sensitivity to changes in nodal and internodal parameters. Biophys J 21:147–160, 1978

18. Saida K, Sumner AJ, Saida T, et al: Antiserum-mediated demyelination: relationship between remyelination and functional recovery. Ann Neurol 8:12–24, 1980

19. Saida K, Saida T, Brown MJ, et al: In vivo demyelination induced by intraneural injection of anti-galactocerebroside serum. Am J Pathol 95:99–110, 1979

20. Rasminsky M, Sumner A: Development of conduction block in single rat spinal root fibers locally exposed to anti-galactocerebroside serum (abstract). Neurology (NY) 30:371, 1980

21. Brown MJ, Sumner AJ, Saida T, et al: The evolution of early demyelination following topical application of anti-galactocerebroside serum in vivo (abstract). Neurology (NY) 30:371, 1980

22. Morgan-Hughes JA: Experimental diphtheric neuropathy: a pathological and electrophysiological study. J Neurol Sci 7:157–175, 1968

23. Huxley AF, Stämpfl R: Evidence for saltatory conduction in peripheral myelinated nerve fibers. J Physiol (Lond) 108:315–339, 1949

24. Tasaki I: *Nervous Transmission*. Charles C Thomas, Springfield, IL, 1953

25. Ritchie JM, Rogart RB: The density of sodium channels in mammalian myelinated nerve fibers and nature of the axonal membrane under the myelin sheath. Proc Natl Acad Sci USA 74:211–215, 1977

26. Ritchie JM: Sodium channels in muscle and nerve. In *Current Topics in Nerve and Muscle Research*. Edited by Aguayo AJ, Karpati G. Excerpta Medica, Amsterdam, 1979, pp 210–219

27. Ritchie JM, Rogart RB, Strichartz GP: A new method for labelling saxitoxin and its binding to non-myelinated fibers of the rabbit vagus, lobster walking leg and garfish olfactory nerves. J Physiol (Lond) 261:477–494, 1976

28. Rosenbluth J: Intramembranous particle distribution at the node of Ranvier and adjacent axolemma in myelinated axons of the frog brain. J Neurocytol 5:731–745, 1976

29. Kristol C, Sandri C, Akert K: Intermembranous particles at the nodes of Ranvier of the cat spinal cord: a morphometric study. Brain Res 142:391–400, 1978

30. Kristol C, Akert K, Sandri C, et al: The Ranvier nodes in the neurogenic electric organ of the knife-fish *Sternarchus*: a freeze-etching study on the distribution of membrane associated particles. Brain Res 125:197–212, 1977

31. Waxman SG, Quick DC: Cytochemical differentiation of the axon membrane in A- and C-fibres. J Neurol Neurosurg Psychiatry 40:379–386, 1977

32. Quick DC, Waxman SG: Specific staining of the axon membrane at nodes of Ranvier with ferric ion and ferrocyanide. J Neurol Sci 31:1–11, 1977

33. Waxman SG, Quick DC: Functional architecture of the initial segment. In *Physiology and Pathobiology of Axons*. Edited by Waxman SG. Raven Press, New York, 1978, pp 125–130

34. Chiu SY, Ritchie JM, Rogart RB, et al: A quantitative description of membrane currents in rabbit myelinated nerve. J Physiol (Lond) 292:149–166, 1979

35. Brismar T: Potential clamp analysis of membrane currents in rat myelinated fibers. J Physiol (Lond) 298:171–184, 1980

36. Chiu SY, Ritchie JM: Potassium channels in nodal and internodal axonal membrane of mammalian myelinated fibres. Nature 284:170–171, 1980

37. Bray GM, Rasminsky M, Aguayo AJ: Interactions between axons and their sheath cells. Annu Rev Neurosci (in press)

38. Rasminsky M, Kearney RE, Aguayo AJ, et al: Conduction of nervous impulses in spinal roots and peripheral nerves of dystrophic mice. Brain Res 143:71–85, 1978

39. Bostock H, Feasby TE, Sears TA: Continuous conduction in regenerating myelinated nerve fibres. J Physiol (Lond) 269:88P–90P, 1977

40. Bray GM, Cullen MJ, Aguayo AJ, et al: Node-like areas of intramembranous particles in the unensheathed axons of dystrophic mice. Neurosci Lett 13:203–208, 1979

41. Ellisman MH: Molecular specializations of the axon membrane at nodes of Ranvier are not dependent upon myelination. J Neurocytol 8:719–735, 1979

42. Waxman SG, Foster RE: Development of the axon membrane during differentiation of myelinated fibres in spinal nerve roots. Proc Roy Soc Lond [Biol] (in press)

43. Davis FA, Jacobson S: Altered thermal sensitivity in injured and demyelinated nerve: a possible model of temperature effects in multiple sclerosis. J Neurol Neurosurg Psychiatry 34:551–561, 1971

44. Rasminsky M: The effects of temperature on conduction in demyelinated single nerve fibers. Arch Neurol 28:287–292, 1973

45. Tasaki I, Fujita M: Action currents of single nerve fibers as modified by temperature changes. J Neurophysiol 11:311–315, 1948

46. Schauf CL, Davis FA: Impulse conduction in multiple sclerosis: a theoretical basis for modification by temperature and pharmacological agents. J Neurol Neurosurg Psychiatry 37:152–161, 1974

47. Davis FA, Becker FO, Michael JA, et al: Effect of intravenous sodium bicarbonate, disodium edetate (Na_2 EDTA), and hyperventilation on visual and oculomotor signs in multiple sclerosis. J Neurol Neurosurg Psychiatry 33:723–732, 1970

48. Becker FO, Michael JA, David FA: Acute effects of oral phosphate on visual function in multiple sclerosis. Neurology (Minneap) 24:601–607, 1974

49. Bostock H, Sherratt RM, Sears TA: Overcoming conduction failure in demyelinated nerve by prolonging action potentials. Nature 274:385–387, 1978

50. Sherratt RM, Bostock H, Sears TA: Effects of 4-aminopyridine on normal and demyelinated mammalian nerve fibers. Nature 283:570–572, 1980

51. Bradley WG, Jenkison M: Abnormalities of peripheral nerves in murine muscular dystrophy. J Neurol Sci 18:227–247, 1973

52. Rasminsky M: Ectopic generation of impulses and cross talk in spinal nerve roots of "dystrophic" mice. Ann Neurol 3:351–357, 1978

53. Rasminsky M: Ephaptic transmission between single nerve fibres in the spinal nerve roots of dystrophic mice. J Physiol (Lond) 305:151–169, 1980

54. Eberstein A, Goodgold J, Pechter BR: Effect of curare on EMG and contractile responses in the myotonic mouse. Exp Neurol 49:612–616, 1975

55. Silverman H, Atwood HL, Bloom JW: Phenytoin application in murine muscular dystrophy: behavioural improvement with no change in the abnormal intracellular Na:K ratio in skeletal muscles. Exp Neurol 62:618–627, 1978

56. Howe JF, Loeser JD, Calvin WH: Mechanosensitivity of dorsal root ganglia and chronically injured axons: a physiological basis for the radicular pain of nerve root compression. Pain 3:25–41, 1977

57. Smith KJ, McDonald WI: Spontaneous and mechanically evoked activity due to central demyelinating lesion. Nature 286:154–155, 1980

58. Wasserstrom WR, Starr A: Facial myokymia in the Guillain-Barré syndrome. Arch Neurol 34:576–577, 1977

59. Rasminsky M: Ectopic excitation, ephaptic excitation and autoexcitation in peripheral nerve

fibers of mutant mice. In *Abnormal Nerves and Muscles as Impulse Generators*. Edited by Culp W, Ochoa J. Oxford University Press, New York (in press)

60. Huizar P, Kuno M, Miyata Y: Electrophysiological properties of spinal motoneurones of normal and dystrophic mice. J Physiol (Lond) 248:231–246, 1975

61. Seltzer Z, Devor M: Ephaptic transmission in chronically damaged peripheral nerves. Neurology (NY) 29:1061–1064, 1979

62. Howe JF, Calvin WH, Loeser JD: Impulses reflected from dorsal root ganglia and from focal nerve injuries. Brain Res 16:139–144, 1976

63. Goldstein SS, Rall W: Changes of action potential shape and velocity for changing core conductor geometry. Biophys J 14:731–757, 1974

64. Ramón F, Joyner RW, Moore JW: Propagation of action potentials in inhomogeneous axon regions. Fed Proc 34:1357–1363, 1975

65. McDonald WI: Clinical consequences of conduction defects produced by demyelination. In *Abnormal Nerves and Muscles as Impulse Generators*. Edited by Culp W, Ochoa J. Oxford University Press, New York (in press)

DISCUSSION

Dr. Robert Barchi: Have you thought about, or have you carried out, any computer simulations of reentrant excitation or ephaptic transmission and the density of sodium channels you think would have to be present for those phenomena to occur? Do you think the channel density of the demyelinated areas is close to that of the node, or do you think this density is low, such as that seen on nonmyelinated fibers?

Dr. Michael Rasminsky: I really do not have any idea. Simulating ephaptic transmission is a very formidable problem, and we have been quite unsuccessful in doing it. In the dystrophic mouse spinal roots, ephaptic transmission seems, in general, to be from bare axon to myelinated axon rather than from bare axon to bare axon, but no statement can yet be made about the density of sodium channels in the dystrophic mouse axons.

Dr. Andrew Engel: How do you think antibody lyses paranodal myelin?

Dr. Michael Rasminsky: I think I would like to punt on that to one of the people in Philadelphia who has been more directly involved with the immunologic side. Dr. Sumner, do you want to respond to that?

Dr. Austin Sumner: Perhaps I could just review the background of this physiologic study, because it is the product of team effort. The germinal observations were the work of Drs. Saida, working in Dr. Silberberg's lab, the morphologic studies in Dr. Asbury's lab, and the immunologic studies of Dr. Lisak. When immune serum was injected into sciatic nerve, a rapid conduction block started in motor axons within 30 minutes and was complete within 3 hours. We were puzzled initially because there was very little preceding slowing of nerve conduction velocity and there were only subtle ultrastructural changes to account for the conduction block. A problem was posed as to whether or not this acute block was due to demyelination. When we used Dr. Rasminsky's elegant technique of recording single-fiber conduction, it became clear that conduction block is preceded by slowed conduction, but this was not observed in population studies because the fastest-conducting axons are the last to be affected. More closely timed correlative morphologic studies after topical application of anti-galactocerebroside serum to nerve roots indicate that there is early paranodal demyelination, which apparently alters the electrical properties of the nodes so as to block conduction.

Dr. Mark Brown: In answer to Dr. Engel's question, the myelin lysis reaction is complement mediated. Heated serum does not demyelinate or produce clinical paralysis, but if you add guinea pig serum as a source of complement, it does. We assume that complement is punching holes in a membrane, presumably the Schwann cell membrane, but possibly nodal axolemma as well.

Dr. Arthur Asbury: I might add that what one sees before there is myelin retraction at the paranode is either vacuolation or hyperdensity of Schwann cell cytoplasm and ballooning of Schwann cell surface membranes. Thus, Schwann cells themselves seem to be pathologically altered before the paranodal demyelinative lesion, which parallels the evolution of conduction block.

Dr. Stanley Appel: How did you rule out a direct effect of the protein on the axonal membrane as opposed to the demyelination that obviously occurs?

Dr. Michael Rasminsky: The serum is clearly not acting as a local anesthetic. With focal application of local anesthetic, conduction fails even though the nodal membrane is depolarized well beyond the threshold for generation of an action potential. With application of the anti-galactocerebroside serum, conduction fails only when depolarization at the affected nodal membrane fails to reach threshold. We also have some very preliminary data showing that the nodal capacitance is increased without a disproportionate decrease in nodal resistance. This suggests that conduction block is due simply to an increase in nodal surface area rather than holes being punched in the axonal membrane.

Dr. Andrew Engel: Following through on the question of complement-mediated lysis, have you tried to do these experiments in decomplemented animals who have been given cobra venum factor or mice that have congenital complement deficiency?

Dr. Mark Brown: Yes. The complement experiments all were done in cobra venum-treated, decomplemented animals.

Dr. Michael Rasminsky: Those experiments are in the sciatic nerve preparation, not in the spinal root preparation.

Dr. Arthur Asbury: If you decomplement the serum that is injected, there will still be a small amount of demyelination, presumably because of host complement, but if you use decomplemented animals as recipients there is no demyelination at all.

6

Axonal Atrophy Associated with Segmental Demyelination, and Axonal Degeneration in Human Neuropathy

Peter James Dyck, MD

Phillip A. Low, MD

Anthony J. Windebank, MRCP

It is commonly assumed that peripheral nerve axons respond to injury (whether physical, cellular, or chemical) in one way: by stereotyped cellular and molecular events termed wallerian degeneration. It has become increasingly evident that such a view needs to be modified. Although common pathways may be involved, cellular and molecular events may vary for different types of fiber degeneration and for different diseases.

One type of pathologic alteration, axonal atrophy, will be discussed here. This is commonly observed in human diseases in which populations of neurons (systems) degenerate. We have found evidence for this pathologic process in the distal axons of primary sensory neurons in uremic neuropathy (1) and in Friedreich's ataxia (2), but it undoubtedly occurs in many other disorders.

Evidence will be provided to show that axonal atrophy leads sequentially to myelin wrinkling, secondary segmental demyelination, and finally, axonal degeneration. If the process is chronic, remyelination may occur concomitantly with demyelination. With repair of the underlying metabolic derangement, the axon may survive. In such fibers, remyelinated segments are the hallmarks of previous segmental demyelination.

75

APPROACHES TO CLASSIFYING MYELINATED FIBER DEGENERATION

Mechanistic

Ideally, classification of the pathologic alterations of nerve cell bodies and their axons should depend on underlying cellular and molecular mechanisms. Models of axonal neuropathy, with some insights into their mechanisms, are the hexacarbon neuropathy (3, 4) discussed by Spencer (see chapter 7) and IDPN intoxication (5). An example of a model in which Schwann cells are primarily affected and in which there is emerging information on mechanisms is that of lead neuropathy (6–11). Generally, for human neuropathy, however, insufficient information is available to classify types of fiber degeneration by mechanism.

Although "fiber degeneration" refers to the static morphologic changes recognized under a microscope, it is appreciated that pathophysiologic disturbances leading to such a final event are dynamic and might have been present long before. Thus, early pathophysiologic events that lead to (or can prevent) fiber degeneration are of great interest and importance.

Nosologic

It would be helpful to the clinician if the type of fiber degeneration were specific to the disease. Such changes as the hypomyelination of hereditary motor and sensory neuropathy Type III and the giant axonal alterations and tomaculae of neuropathies with these names are characteristic, but not diagnostic, of various neuropathies. There are, of course, patterns of specific morphologic changes in addition to the type of fiber degeneration that are diagnostic of certain diseases. These include amyloidosis, leprosy, necrotizing angiopathy, sarcoidosis, metachromatic leukodystrophy, Krabbe disease, and possibly others (12). These disorders, however, may not have unique ways by which fibers degenerate, although this remains a possibility.

Descriptive

Because it is probably too early to classify fiber degeneration by mechanisms, and because fiber degeneration may not be specific by disease, we chose to classify teased fiber alterations by descriptive criteria. Based on extensive experience of teased fiber alterations in nerves (especially the sural nerve) from patients with neuropathy and from experimental neuropathies, we have proposed a descriptive classification of pathologic abnormalities of teased fibers (12).

This classification was based on aldehyde- and osmium tetroxide-fixed nerves from which fibers 6 to 10 mm long were teased in glycerin with forceps under a dissecting microscope. Teasing was always from proximal to distal ends so that the orientation of the teased fiber was known and branches would be left intact. Because the percentages of various descriptive pathologic abnormalities were to be determined, it was important that systematic approaches be used to sample fibers. An endoneurial bundle was initially split into 10 approximately equal parts, and 10 strands of fibers were teased consecutively from the extreme right-hand side of each strand irrespective of pathology.

To make the classification widely useful, we decided that it should (a) be based on the use of aldehyde- and osmium tetroxide-fixed fibers; (b) not require precise measurement; (c) not depend on organelle pathology or cytologic detail in Schwann cell or axon; (d) use criteria that were qualitative, but with defined limits; (e) need no higher magnification than that provided by a high-power dry objective.

The criteria considered for development of teased-fiber grading were: regions *without any* myelin, i.e., widened nodal gaps (paranodal demyelination) or internodal demyelination; myelin smoothness or wrinkling; thickness of myelin, especially comparison between internodes; breakdown of myelin to form ovoids or balls; focal swelling of a fiber; and reduplication of myelin into tomaculae. Measurement of internodal length and diameter, length of regions of segmental demyelination, and organelle pathology can also be used for further categorization.

A schematic drawing of the descriptive classification of pathologic abnormalities of teased fibers (evolved in our laboratory) is shown in Figure 1.

The 5 most critical and difficult judgments needed for the classification are: wrinkling (Type B), segmental demyelination (Type C), segmental remyelination (as seen in Types D and F), myelin ovoids (Type E), and degree of focal reduplication sufficient to be called tomaculae (Type G). An arbitrary definition for wrinkling is that the distance between crest and trough of the exterior edge of myelin of an internode be greater than 25% of the thickness of the fiber. During demyelination, no osmiophilic lines corresponding to myelin are seen under high-power dry objective (many early reports illustrate remyelinated lesions with existing nodes of Ranvier and describe these as demyelinative). We define a remyelinated teased fiber as one in which the myelin thickness of one or more internodes is less than one-half that of the internode with thickest myelin in the same teased fiber. We appreciate that these are arbitrary criteria. Late stages of linear rows of myeline ovoids, balls, and digestion chambers are easily missed unless a high-power objective is used. Several such deposits separated in space along an endoneurial nerve strand should be seen before identifying it as a Type E change. Finally, reduplication of myelin should at least double the diameter of the fiber before a Type G condition is identified.

We have used this classification extensively and find it sensitive in detecting and characterizing various neuropathies. In addition, it is being used increasingly by others.

To optimize results, the observer should receive special training in the use of the criteria; teased fibers at least 6 to 10 mm long should be used; grading should be done on strands containing no more than 2 or 3 fibers; and the observer should be unaware of what is being graded (identifying marks on slides should be covered, and slides from control and diseased nerves should be randomly mixed). We grade 100 fibers per nerve and calculate the percentage of fibers showing pathologic abnormality.

The frequencies of these graded pathologic abnormalities can be used in model neuropathies to find patterns characteristic of various types of fiber

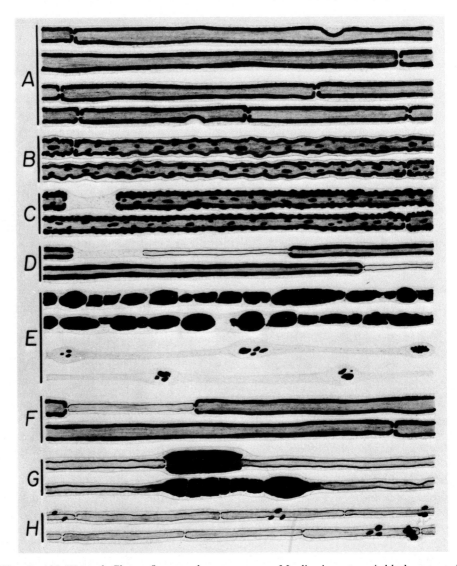

Fig. 1. **(A)** Teased fiber of normal appearance. Myelin is not wrinkled except in paranodal regions. There is no nodal separation. Variation in myelin thickness between internodes is less than 50% of the thickest internode. **(B)** Teased fiber with excessive wrinkling of myelin, otherwise like A. **(C)** Teased fiber with segmental (paranodal or internodal) demyelination (regions without recognizable myelin) with or without myelin wrinkling and variation in myelin thickness between internodes of less than 50%. **(D)** Teased fiber with segmental demyelination (as defined in **C** above) and remyelination (myelin thickness of "new" internodes is less than 50% of that of "old" internodes). **(E)** Linear rows of myelin ovoids and/or myelin balls along the entire length of the teased nerve strand. **(F)** Teased fiber without segmental demyelination but with remyelination (as defined in **D** above). **(G)** Focal reduplications of myelin to form tomaculae. A description of the other graded pathologic abnormalities can be found elsewhere (12). **CH** Small caliber fiber with thin myelin and short internodes with adjacent myelin and lipid debris typical of the regenerating fiber. (Modified, with permission, from Dyck PJ: Pathologic alterations of the peripheral nervous system of man. In *Peripheral Neuropathy.* Edited by Dyck PJ, Thomas PK, Lambert EH. WB Saunders, Philadelphia, 1975, pp 296–336.)

pathology. To illustrate, in lead neuropathy, a model of primary segmental demyelination, the frequency of Type E changes is not greater than that seen in control nerves. The earliest change is an increased frequency of Type C, followed by Type D alterations. In the permanent axotomy model, a model of axonal atrophy, the earliest alteration is a Type B change, followed later by changes of Types C, D, and F.

As we have described in earlier publications, patterns of fiber pathology are characteristic for different human neuropathies (12).

In human neuropathy, alterations of neuron cell bodies and their axons, particularly along their length, have been incompletely studied (13). Ultrastructural changes in axons include granular degeneration of microtubules and neurofilaments, accumulations of mitochondria and dense bodies, occurrence of vesicular structures and myelin figures, accumulation of glycogen, proliferation of endoplasmic reticulum, and axonal swelling as a result of focal accumulations of neurofilaments apparently displacing other organelles to one side (12, 14).

It is not known whether all of these untrastructural changes play a mechanistic role in fiber degeneration. Certainly, different patterns of pathologic alterations are seen.

SELECTIVE NEURONAL VULNERABILITY

Between Populations of Neurons

Selectivity of involvement by population of neurons is common in inherited and various metabolic neuropathies. Although complete selectivity (one population of neurons degenerating without involvement of other populations) probably never occurs, there is a surprising degree of selectivity (15). Inherited neuronal diseases can be roughly classified by the population of neurons selectively involved: spastic paraplegia involves corticospinal tract (pyramidal) neurons; progressive muscular atrophy or motor neuropathy, lower motor neurons; spinocerebellar degeneration, large-diameter primary afferent neurons; sensory neuropathy, small-diameter primary afferent neurons, and dysautonomia, autonomic neurons. Examples of how selective degeneration of populations of neurons affects symptoms, the compound action potential in vitro, and the frequency distribution of fibers according to diameter in sural nerve are described in a recent review (16).

Between Levels of Neurons

Acquired diseases of peripheral nerve may selectively affect various levels from proximal to distal ends of neurons. Polio is known to affect selectively the ventral horn region. Inflammatory demyelinating lesions may affect multiple roots (polyradiculopathy) and additionally the nerve trunks (polyradiculoneuropathy). The plexus may be selectively affected, as in brachial plexus neuropathy. Necrotizing angiopathic neuropathy may cause centrifascicular damage at watershed zones of poor perfusion, e.g., at midthigh level of the sciatic nerve.

Sarcoidosis has a predilection for certain cranial nerves. Lepromatous leprosy affects superficial nerves in acral and other regions at lower-than-core body temperature.

Particularly in inherited, metabolic, and toxic neuropathies in which populations of neurons tend to be selectively affected, there is also evidence for some selectivity by level of neuron. Before 1900, this gave rise to the distinction between an anterior horn cell of neuronal disorder and a neuritic (now neuropathic) disorder. Even then, however, there was concern that this might be too simple a separation and that in many cases the whole neuron might be affected.

HISTOLOGIC SEQUENCE OF AXONAL ATROPHY

Human Uremic Neuropathy

Studies have been published (1) on the sural nerve findings in a 24-year-old and a 44-year-old patient with mainly sensory uremic neuropathy. (a) In these patients, the density of myelinated fibers (MF) was decreased more at ankle than at midcalf level when compared to control data. (b) The histogram of myelinated fiber diameters was shifted to smaller-diameter categories at midcalf and especially at ankle level. (c) At midcalf level, 64.7% of teased fibers were excessively wrinkled (Type B), 14.8% had segmental demyelination (Type C) and remyelination (Type D), and 4% had degenerated into linear rows of myelin ovoids and balls (Type E). At ankle level, comparable percentage values were 10.6%, 25.1%, and 51.2%. Typical examples of the teased fiber abnormalities observed are shown in Figure 2. (d) Some single teased fibers had multiple regions of segmental demyelination with or without remyelination, whereas others had no segmental demyelination, an indication that segmental demyelination was clustered. (e) Regression lines relating perimeter of axon to number of myelin lamellae indicated that axis cylinders were of smaller caliber in uremic nerves than in healthy nerves (Fig. 3). (f) Thin serial sections along the length of fibers with multiple regions of segmental demyelination and remyelination provided further evidence of an underlying atrophic axis cylinder, and this was particularly apparent at "old" internodes.

These results indicated that at midcalf level, where axonal atrophy (from diameter histogram data and regression lines relating perimeter to myelin thickness) was mild, the predominant change was a Type B pathologic abnormality: fibers showed myelin irregularity (wrinkling). At ankle level, where axonal atrophy was more severe, there was an increased frequency of segmental demyelination and a greatly increased frequency of axonal degeneration. It appeared that axonal atrophy resulted in myelin wrinkling, then in paranodal and internodal demyelination, and finally, in axonal degeneration. It was clear, however, that remyelination could occur concomitantly with this process, because regions of demyelination were not infrequently covered with newly formed myelin. Although one could not be certain that the metabolic derange-

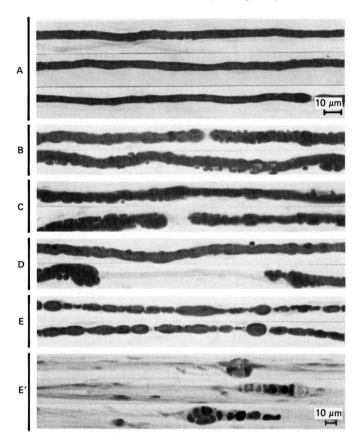

Fig. 2. Teased fibers from sural nerve of a patient with uremic neuropathy. Compare the normal teased fiber **(A)**, with the abnormalities found in uremic neuropathy: myelin wrinkling **(B)**, segmental demyelination **(C)**, segmental remyelination **(F)**, and axonal degeneration, both early **(E)** and late (E'). The stages in axonal atrophy leading to degeneration are discussed in the text. (Modified, with permission, from Dyck PJ, Johson WJ, Lambert EH, et al: Segmental demyelination secondary to axonal degeneration in uremic neuropathy. Mayo Clin Proc 46:400–431, 1971.)

ment that caused the axonal atrophy had not also caused concomitant Schwann cell disease, this seemed unlikely, especially for reason *(d)* above.

Friedreich's Ataxia

Similar findings were shown to occur in Friedreich's ataxia (2). Early in the course of Friedreich's ataxia there was a decrease in the number of large myelinated fibers. Nerves from these patients showed a greater-than-normal number of small-diameter fibers, indicating a shift to smaller-diameter categories—further evidence of atrophy. We found that large fibers selectively became atrophic; with this atrophy there was rearrangement of myelin, as

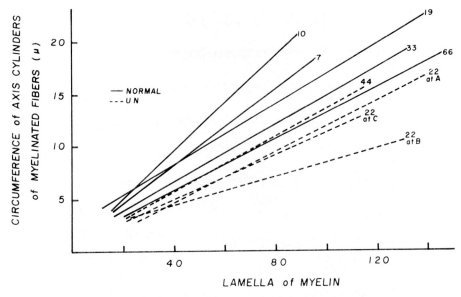

Fig. 3. Regression lines of perimeter of axis cylinders on number of myelin lamellae of myelinated fibers of control and uremic neuropathy (UN) sural nerve. Note that the regression lines, especially for distal uremic nerves, are less steep than those for control nerves, indicating axonal atrophy. (Modified, with permission, from Dyck PJ, Johnson WJ, Lambert EH, et al: Segmental demyelination secondary to axonal degeneration in uremic neuropathy. Mayo Clin Proc 46:400–431, 1971.)

described for uremia. There was a striking degree of segmental demyelination and remyelination on some fibers, whereas others had none.

Distribution of Internode Damage

An argument crucial to the view that segmental demyelination is secondary to axonal atrophy and not to concomitant interference with the metabolism of Schwann cells is the clustered distribution of segmental demyelination on certain fibers, presumably ones with axonal atrophy. Such clustered demyelination could be shown to be different from the random pattern seen in lead neuropathy (9).

MODELS OF AXONAL ATROPHY

Because of our observation of axonal atrophy and secondary segmental demyelination in uremic neuropathy and Friedreich's ataxia, we searched for an experimental model that would reproduce the morphologic changes. Initially, we attempted to damage the neuron cell body selectively, without affecting the peripheral axon or Schwann cells. We tried x-irradiation of spinal cord and ganglia, with careful shielding of the limb nerves for later study; the results were equivocal.

Various toxins used systemically to poison perikaryal protein synthesis were considered to be a problem because of the possibility that they might also affect Schwann cell protein synthesis. If segmental demyelination were seen, it would not be possible to attribute it definitely to an axonal abnormality.

We then tried the permanent axotomy model. Permanent axotomy, by hind limb amputation in kittens, was found, by morphometric evaluation 9 months after surgery, to result in failure of ventral and dorsal root myelinated fibers to attain adult calibers, despite the fact that development had continued for some time after amputation (17). Permanent axotomy in adult cats could not be shown to affect the number and size distribution of motor neuron cell bodies and spinal ganglion neuron cell bodies, but the median and peak diameters of both small and large myelinated fibers of dorsal and ventral roots were significantly smaller (approximately 30%) than those of control animals (18). This reduction in diameter was judged to be related to axonal atrophy rather than selective loss of large fibers.

We have now shown that permanent axotomy is also associated with axonal atrophy of peripheral nerve fibers. In addition, we have shown that this atrophy is initially associated with myelin irregularity (wrinkling), then with segmental demyelination, and finally, with axonal degeneration. Demyelinated segments may be remyelinated during the process. The changes are strikingly similar to those found in uremic neuropathy.

Figure 4 is a composite histogram of myelinated fiber diameters of L7 segmental nerves from the nonamputated side (above) and the amputated side (below). The median peak of diameters of all myelinated fibers and the small

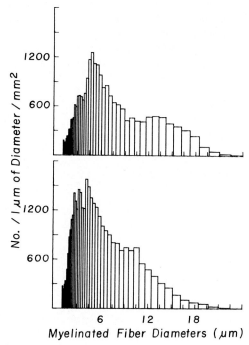

Fig. 4. Composite histograms of myelinated fiber diameters of L7 segmental nerves of cats without (above) and with (below) permanent axotomy. Note the shift of fiber diameters to smaller categories. See text for discussion. (Reprinted with permission from Dyck PJ, Lais AC, Karnes JL, et al: Permanent axotomy, a model of axonal atrophy and secondary segmental demyelination. Ann Neurol, in press.)

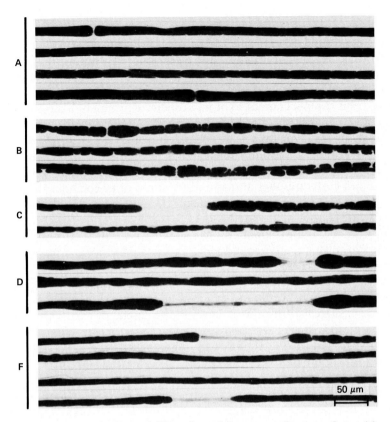

Fig. 5. Typical teased myelinated fibers from L7 segmental nerve of cat with permanent axotomy. Compared to normal fiber **(A)**, nerves from the permanent axotomy side have excessive myelin wrinkling **(B)**, segmental demyelination **(C)**, segmental remyelination **(D** and **F)**, and axonal degeneration **(E** not shown). Note the similarity of the changes encountered to those in uremic neuropathy (Fig. 2). (Reprinted with permission from Dyck PJ, Lais AC, Karnes JL, et al: Permanent axotomy: a model of axonal atrophy and secondary segmental demyelination. Ann Neurol, in press.)

Table 1. Graded Abnormalities of Teased Fibers of L7 Segmental Nerve of Cat 1 Year After Permanent Axotomy[a,b]

Cats (n = 7)	Type of Abnormality			
	A	B	C, D, F	E, H
Control	98.1	0.2	1.2	0
Axotomized	69.0	21.2	7.3	0
	$P < 0.001$	$P < 0.001$	$0.02 < P < 0.01$	$P < 0.05$

[a] Reprinted with permission from Dyck PJ, Lais AC, Karnes JL, et al: Permanent axotomy: a model of axonal atrophy and secondary segmental demyelination. Ann Neurol, in press.

[b] Data are given as percentages of the total number of abnormalities. Significance of the difference between each axotomized nerve and the opposite control nerve (no axotomy) was determined using Student's paired t test. See text and Figure 1 for descriptions of types of abnormality.

diameter peak are displaced to smaller-diameter categories, indicating fiber atrophy. Axis cylinders were affected more than myelin. Figure 5 illustrates the types of teased fiber pathologies encountered on the amputated side. The frequencies of graded teased fiber abnormalities are given in Table 1.

These experimental studies therefore mimic the findings in human neuropathy. They support the hypothesis that axonal atrophy leads initially to myelin wrinkling and later to segmental demyelination. Remyelination may occur concomitantly at sites of segmental demyelination. Ultimately, axonal degeneration occurs.

ACKNOWLEDGMENT

This work was supported in part by Peripheral Neuropathy Clinical Center Grant no. NS14304 from the National Institute of Neurological and Communicative Disorders and Stroke, by a Center Grant from the Muscular Dystrophy Association, and by Mayo, Borchard, Upton and Gallagher Funds.

REFERENCES

1. Dyck PJ, Johnson WJ, Lambert EH, et al: Segmental demyelination secondary to axonal degeneration in uremic neuropathy. Mayo Clin Proc 46:400–431, 1971

2. Dyck PJ, Lais AC: Evidence for segmental demyelination secondary to axonal degeneration in Friedreich's ataxia. In *Clinical Studies in Myology*. Edited by Kakulas BA. Excerpta Medica, Amsterdam, 1973, pp 253–263

3. Spencer PS, Schaumburg HH: Experimental neuropathy produced by 2, 5-hexanedione, a major metabolite of the neurotoxic industrial solvent methyl *n*-butyl ketone. J Neurol Neurosurg Psychiatry 38:771–775, 1975

4. Spencer PS, Schaumburg HH: Central-peripheral distal axonopathy: the pathology of dying-back polyneuropathies. In *Progress in Neuropathology*, vol 3. Edited by Zimmerman HM. Grune & Stratton, New York, 1976, pp 253–295

5. Clark AW, Griffin JW, Price DL: The axonal pathology in chronic IDPN intoxication. J Neuropathol Exp Neurol 39:42–55, 1980

6. Gombault M: Contribution a l'étude anatomique de la nevrite parenchymateuse subaigue et chronique: nevrite segmentaire peri-axile. Arch Neurol 1880–81, 1:11–38

7. Lampert PW, Schochet SS: Demyelination and remyelination in lead neuropathy. J Neuropathol Exp Neurol 27:527–544, 1968

8. Ohnishi A, Schilling K, Brimijoin WS, et al: Lead neuropathy. 1. Morphometry, nerve conduction and acetyltransferase transport: new findings of endoneurial edema associated with segmental demyelination. J Neuropathol Exp Neurol 36:499–518, 1977.

9. Dyck PJ, O'Brien PC, Ohnishi A: Lead neuropathy. 2. Random distribution of segmental demyelination among "old internodes" of myelinated fibers. J Neuropathol Exp Neurol 36:570–575, 1977

10. Low PA, Dyck PJ: Increased endoneurial fluid pressure in experimental lead neuropathy. Nature 269:427–428, 1977

11. Windebank AJ, McCall JT, Hunder HG, et al: The endoneurial content of lead related to onset and severity of segmental demyelination. J Neuropathol Exp Neurol 39:692–699, 1980

12. Dyck PJ: Pathologic alterations of the peripheral nervous system of man. In *Peripheral Neuropathy*. Edited by Dyck PJ, Thomas PK, Lambert EH. WB Saunders, Philadelphia, 1975, pp. 296–336.

13. Prineas J, Spencer PS: Pathology of the nerve cell body in disorders of the peripheral nervous system. In *Peripheral Neuropathy*. Edited by Dyck PJ, Thomas PK, Lambert EH. WB Saunders, Philadelphia, 1975, pp 253–295

14. Asbury AK, Johnson PC (eds): *Pathology of Peripheral Nerve*. WB Saunders, Philadelphia, 1978

15. Dyck PJ: Definition and basis of classification of hereditary neuropathy with neuronal atrophy and degeneration. In *Peripheral Neuropathy*. Edited by Dyck PJ, Thomas PK, Lambert EH. WB Saunders, Philadelphia 1975, pp 755–758

16. Lambert EH, Dyck PJ: Compound action potentials of sural nerve in vitro in peripheral neuropathy. In *Peripheral Neuropathy*. Edited by Dyck PJ, Thomas PK, Lambert EH. WB Saunders, Philadelphia, 1975, pp 427–441

17. Jorgensen BS, Dyck PJ: Axonal underdevelopment from axotomy in kittens. J Neuropathol Exp Neurol 38:571–578, 1979

18. Carlson J, Lais AC, Dyck PJ: Axonal atrophy from permanent peripheral axotomy in adult cat. J Neuropathol Exp Neurol 38:579–585, 1979

DISCUSSION

Dr. Alan McComas: We have looked at impulse conduction in the peripheral nerve stumps of human amputees and have found striking reductions in the amplitude of the compound action potential (typically to 10% or so of normal). Taken in conjunction with your morphologic findings, this suggests that most of the fibers you look at are perhaps no longer able to propagate nerve impulses.

Dr. Peter Dyck: That is interesting. Dr. Harper, I think, also did a physiologic study and showed a reduced conduction velocity; he postulated atrophy on that basis. Dr. McComas, did yours show reduced conduction velocity?

Dr. Alan McComas: In some fibers, conduction velocity was very close to normal. Other fibers were conducting more slowing, but even allowing for dispersion in the compound action potential, most of the fibers could not have been conducting.

Dr. Peter Dyck: How long after amputation?

Dr. Alan McComas: From 2 to 30 years.

Dr. Arthur Asbury: Did you measure the area underneath the compound action potential, or just do the amplitude?

Dr. Alan McComas: We have done both, in fact.

Dr. Ellis Stanley: We have also looked at the chronic IDPN-intoxicated rat, which has axonal atrophy and most definitely shows a slowing of conduction velocity.

Dr. Peter Dyck: That is quite a good model. The one concern is whether or not any of the IDPN could affect the protein metabolism of Schwann cells.

7
The Cellular Target Site in Distal Axonopathies

Peter S. Spencer, PhD

Michael J. Politis, PhD

Richard G. Pellegrino, MS

Herbert H. Schaumburg, MD

The usefulness of experimental toxins for exploring the etiology and pathogenesis of human axonal neuropathies has gained wide acceptance since Cavanagh (1) described the similarities between the pattern of damage in the spinocerebellar degenerations and that seen in triorthocresyl phosphate poisoning (TOCP). The presence of distal and retrograde axonal degeneration affecting long and large nerve fibers in TOCP intoxication was believed to be a consequence of dysfunction of the neuronal perikaryon and the progressive withdrawal of metabolic support from the axon (1). This hypothesis was challenged by Prineas (2, 3), who pointed out that the accumulation of tubulovesicular profiles in TOCP poisoning and of intermediate filaments in acrylamide intoxication was also compatible with a direct action of these toxins on the nerve fiber. Support for this view was subsequently provided by our experimental studies with acrylamide, n-hexane, methyl n-butyl ketone (MnBK) and 2,5-hexanedione (2,5-HD) (4–6): by following the spatial-temporal evolution of degeneration in vivo and in vitro, it was demonstrated in distal nerves that the characteristic focal swelling of the axon appeared on the proximal sides of nodes of Ranvier before the onset of distal degeneration (6, 7). Unlike the pattern predicted from dysfunction of the neuronal cell body, in which the axon was assumed to die back from its terminal region, axonal breakdown occurred in wallerian-like fashion below the position of an axonal swelling. Furthermore, some axons seemed to retain the capacity to regenerate during the period of intoxication, a property generally assumed to require a viable neuronal perikaryon. Taken together, these morphologic observations questioned the role of perikaryal dysfunction and led to the introduction of the term *distal axonopathy* as a more accurate description of the pathologic process (8).

The concept of distal axonopathy seems to have been widely accepted and has recently been applied to a number of toxin-induced axonal degenerations. Distal axonopathies that commence with multifocal pathologic changes in distal, nonterminal portions of vulnerable nerve fibers have been reported for isoniazid (9, 10), diisopropyl fluorophosphate (DFP) (11), and carbon disulfide intoxications (12).

The classic dying-back hypothesis has also been seriously challenged by experimental studies of the pattern of nerve fiber breakdown produced by methyl mercury (13), doxorubicin (14), and megavitamin levels of pyridoxine (15), compounds that do indeed appear to exert their primary effect on neuronal perikarya of dorsal root ganglia. These compounds induce a sensory neuronopathy of fairly rapid onset in which the central and peripheral axonal projections of the damaged neuron undergo a rapid, wallerian-like degeneration. The most useful agent for exploring this effect has been doxorubicin (Adriamycin) (14). After intravenous injection, anthracycline antimicrobial drugs of this type are rapidly taken up by cell nuclei (including those of sensory ganglia), intercalate between base pairs of deoxyribonucleic acid (DNA), and cause derangement and breakage of DNA strands. Cho and colleagues (14) found that pathologic changes in the nuclei of sensory neurons appear as early as 3 hours after injection of doxorubicin and, during a period of days or weeks, culminate in breakdown of neuronal perikarya. Mendell and Sahenk (16) have shown that, during this period, affected ganglia display metabolic dysfunction that may cause their distal axons to undergo anterograde degeneration. Thus, axonal degeneration accompanying metabolic failure of the perikaryon appears to follow a reverse pattern from that predicted by the dying-back hypothesis, i.e., the axon rapidly dies forward from the neuron (16, 17).

EVIDENCE FOR PRIMARY NERVE FIBER DAMAGE

Although detailed morphologic studies of distal axonopathies and sensory neuronopathies have directed attention away from the possibility that neuronal perikaryal dysfunction underlies distal axonal degeneration, and have focused on the nerve fiber itself as the possible lesion site, there is little direct evidence to support this viewpoint. The one important exception to this statement concerns the studies that Lowndes and Baker (18) conducted with DFP: when this toxin was injected into the femoral artery on one side of a cat, most of the DFP was taken up by the sciatic nerve and the animal developed a unilateral distal axonopathy on the injected side. Despite the presence of symmetric binding of DFP label in the spinal cord, no functional deficits appeared on the contralateral side. In summary, this experiment unequivocally demonstrates that the nerve itself is a major target of DFP, although it does not exclude the possibility of some minor additional toxic effect on the neuronal perikaryon.

Several investigators have tried to induce pathologic changes typical of distal axonopathy by applying the toxin directly to nerves. Zuccarello and Anzil (19) used disulfiram placed in contact with the nerve. Mendell and coworkers (20) applied a sponge soaked in MnBK to rat sciatic nerves and produced nonspecific nerve fiber breakdown. Recently, we have conducted a similar experiment with 2,5-HD, the putative primary metabolite of MnBK, and demonstrated that this compound induces giant axonal swellings filled with 10-nm neurofilaments indistinguishable from those seen in systemically intoxicated animals. This experiment, described in detail here, provides direct evidence to support the idea that distal axonopathy follows toxic attack on the nerve fiber rather than on the neuronal perikaryon.

SELECTING A TEST TOXIN

Several facets of experimental design had to be considered in choosing an appropriate toxin to test the hypothesis of direct toxic damage to the nerve fiber: (a) the compound had to be a primary neurotoxic agent, not one that might require metabolic activation to exert its effect; (b) the pathologic change induced by the compound had to be of a characteristic and readily recognizable type; and (c) a chemically related non-neurotoxic compound had to be available for use as a negative control. All of these conditions were satisfied by 2,5-HD.

Axonal Neurotoxicity of 2,5-HD

2,5-Hexanedione was first suspected to be a neurotoxic agent when DiVincenzo and colleagues (21) identified the compound as a persistent metabolite in guinea pigs intoxicated with MnBK or n-hexane. These investigators studied 6 metabolically interrelated hexacarbon compounds, all of which were subsequently found to be capable of inducing neuropathy in laboratory animals (22). By determining the rate of onset of clinical neuropathy in rats, the 6 compounds were ranked for their relative neurotoxic potency: 2,5-HD > 5-hydroxy-2-hexanol > 2,5-hexanediol > MnBK > 2-hexanol > n-hexane. This pattern correlated precisely with measurements of the relative peak serum concentrations of 2,5-HD after administration of a single dose of equimolar concentrations of each of the 6 compounds, providing strong evidence that metabolic activation to 2,5-HD was required for neurotoxic expression (22).

Additional evidence that 2,5-HD is a primary neurotoxic agent has come from studies using organotypic cord-ganglion-muscle combination cultures (7). Each of the 6 interrelated hexacarbon metabolites was able to induce a giant axonal pattern of distal axonopathy in the peripheral nerve component of these culture systems. Analysis of the nutrient fluid removed from exposed cultures revealed 2,5-HD as a common metabolite and demonstrated that this compound was among the most active in inducing the characteristic neuropathologic changes of hexacarbon neuropathy.

Characteristic Nerve Fiber Damage

2,5-Hexanedione also satisfied the criterion of producing a characteristic and readily recognizable pattern of neuropathologic damage. Rats systemically intoxicated with 0.5% 2,5-HD for a few weeks gradually developed weakness of the hindquarters and, with continued intoxication, hindlimb paralysis and forelimb weakness (23). Neuropathologic examination during stages of the disease revealed multifocal axonal swellings distally in long and large myelinated nerve fibers in limb nerves, spinal cord, cerebellum, optic nerves, and mammillary bodies (24, 25). Examination of teased peripheral nerve fibers revealed swellings first on the proximal sides of nodes of Ranvier (6), an interpretation subsequently confirmed by observing living nerve fibers undergoing the same pathologic change in tissue cultures treated with 2,5-HD (7). Individual axons of unmyelinated fibers also displayed neurofilament-filled swellings.

Giant axonal swellings contained abnormally large numbers of 10-nm intermediate filaments, often in a swirling pattern. Microtubules, smooth endoplasmic reticulum, and mitochondria were grouped together into channels that penetrated the mass of neurofilaments. Glycogen-like particles, vesicles of synaptic-vesicle proportions, dense bodies, and decorated particles were also found (6, 26). In the paranodal region of myelinated fibers, the swelling axon appeared to cause paranodal myelin to retract, so that cross sections often revealed giant axonal swellings with a thin or absent myelin sheath. Such focally demyelinated fibers were always enveloped by Schwann cell processes bordered by basal lamina. Thinly remyelinated fibers were also frequent findings in sections and teased fibers; in tissue culture, remyelination was seen to repair previously swollen and demyelinated fiber segments (7).

Schwann cells also displayed a number of changes in experimental 2,5-HD neuropathy. Spencer and Thomas (27) suggested that many of the changes observed in the adaxonal region were part of a process by which the Schwann cell sequestered and removed abnormal and effete axonal organelles. Cytoplasmic features associated with this process included Schwann cell adaxonal clusters of fine filaments, sometimes beaded, similar to those which compose Hirano bodies; Schwann cell processes invaginating the axon and surrounding abnormal axonal organelles; honeycomb structures, and dense material within the adaxonal cytoplasm. In addition to these changes in the *ad*axonal region of the Schwann cell, Powell and colleagues (26) described a number of *ab*axonal changes in Schwann cells of severely impaired animals: enlargement of the cytoplasmic compartment, increased numbers of 10-nm intermediate filaments without sidearms, many branched tubulovesicular profiles, several osmiophilic droplets, and Schwann cell inclusion bodies. Such changes were believed to lag behind development of axonal abnormalities.

Non-neurotoxic Control Compounds

The third criterion dictating the choice of a neurotoxin to test the hypothesis of local nerve fiber toxicity was the availability of a related compound free of neurotoxic properties for use as a negative control. In the case of 2,5-HD ($CH_3COCH_2CH_2COCH_3$), two compounds were commercially available: 2,4-hexanedione ($CH_3COCH_2COCH_2CH_3$), and 1,6-hexanediol ($HO(CH_2CH_2CH_2CH_2CH_2CH_2)OH$), both of which had failed to produce functional or neuropathologic evidence of neuropathy in laboratory animals (22, 28). It would also have been desirable to test the effects of local application of 2,3-hexanedione ($CH_3COCOCH_2CH_2CH_3$), another diketone that failed to induce neuropathy after systemic feeding (20, 28), but this compound became unavailable while these experiments were in progress.

Experimental Design

The sciatic nerve of male Sprague-Dawley rats was used to study the effects of local application of 2,5-HD, 2,4-hexanedione (2,4-HD), or 1,6-hexanediol (1,6-HDiol). The nerve on the opposite side of each animal was sham-operated and exposed to a saline or vehicle control. The sciatic nerve of anesthetized animals was exposed in the midthigh region and prepared by placing a piece of Parafilm between the nerve and the underlying muscle tissue. Vaseline petroleum jelly was then applied to the proximal and distal ends of the exposed portion of the nerve to form a well in which sterile cotton was placed in apposition to the nerve (Fig. 1). The test compound was then applied in 250-μl aliquots to the cotton for a period of 45 minutes. Sciatic nerves on one side of the animal were exposed to 2,5-HD (undiluted or as a 10% aqueous solution, pH 4.5), undiluted 2,4-HD, or 1,6-hexanediol (320 mg/ml of water). Saline or an aqueous solution of hydrochloric acid (pH 3.5) was applied to the nerve on the opposite side. This procedure was repeated daily for 8 days in some rats. Other animals received 0.5% 2,5-HD in their drinking water for a period of 8 days before surgery. Six hours to 16 days after surgery, the treated nerves were prepared for light and electron microscopic examination.

Nonspecific Effects of Hexacarbons

The sham-operated nerves appeared normal, except for the presence of some granulation tissue in the epineurium. Neither saline nor hydrochloric acid induced changes in nerve fascicles. Similarly, no intrafascicular changes were found in nerves exposed to 1,6-Hdiol (Fig. 2). By contrast, nerves exposed to 2,4-HD were severely damaged: the large single peroneal and tibial fascicles of the sciatic nerve displayed perimetric abnormalities consisting of nerve fiber degeneration, capillary damage, and red blood cell extravasation (Fig. 3). Nonspecific nerve fiber degeneration was also found along the perimeter of peroneal and tibial nerve fascicles exposed to 2,5-HD at 4 and 7 days after surgery. By 16 days, the perimeter contained many small, thinly myelinated regenerating nerve fibers. The smaller sural nerve component of sciatic nerves

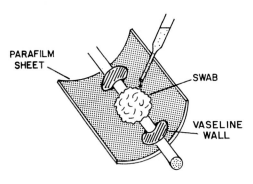

PARAFILM SHEET

SWAB

VASELINE WALL

Fig. 1. Schematic representation of the surgical preparation. The rat sciatic nerve is exposed and separated from the underlying muscle. A Parafilm sheet is slipped under the nerve, and Vaseline petroleum jelly is placed at either end of the sheet to contain the test substance. A small cotton swab is placed over the exposed nerve and is subsequently soaked with the test substance.

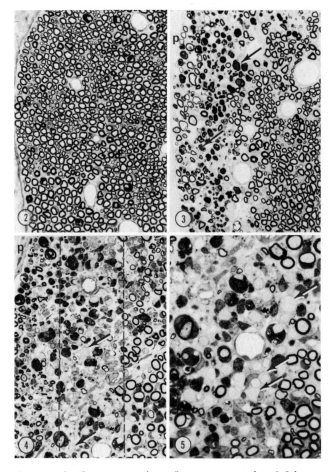

Fig. 2. Light micrograph of a cross section of nerve exposed to 1,6-hexanediol (320 mg/ml) 7 days after a single application. Nerve fibers appear normal. (A 1-μm epoxy section stained with toluidine blue; original magnification × 300.)

Fig. 3. Light micrograph of a large nerve fascicle 4 days after single application of undiluted 2,4-hexanedione. Nonspecific nerve fiber breakdown (arrows) is widespread in the endoneurium adjacent to the perineurium (p). Axons and myelin in the central part of the fascicle are preserved. (A 1-μm section stained with toluidine blue; original magnification × 300.)

Fig. 4. Light micrograph of a tibial nerve fascicle 4 days after single application of undiluted 2,5-hexanedione. Three morphologically distinct zones are seen: left area adjacent to perineurium (p) contains nonspecific breakdown of nerve fibers; central area displays swollen axons (arrows); right area shows axons of normal size and appearance. (A 1-μm section stained with toluidine blue; original magnification × 340.)

Fig. 5. Central zone of Figure 4, showing numerous swollen, demyelinated axons (arrows). (Light micrograph of 1-μm section stained with toluidine blue; original magnification × 480.)

exposed to 2,4-HD or 2,5-HD often displayed complete nerve fiber degeneration. In the light of subsequent findings with 2,5-HD such nerve fiber changes were attributed to the nonspecific effects of high concentrations of 2,4-HD and 2,5-HD.

Specific Effects of 2,5-HD

Four days after local application of 2,5-HD, cross sections of the exposed region of the nerve revealed a gradient of pathologic changes ranging from complete destruction of nerve fibers along the perimeter of the larger nerve fascicles to preservation of fibers in the central part of these fascicles (Fig. 4). This pattern was probably caused by a radial concentration gradient of the toxin, the highest levels of 2,5-HD existing beneath the perineurium, and the lowest in the center of the fascicle. Between the outer necrotic perimeter and the central zone of largely intact fibers, the most prominent structures were swollen myelinated and demyelinated axons. On light microscopic examination of 1-μm sections stained with toluidine blue, many swollen axons had a waxy appearance similar to the giant axonal swellings found in systemic hexacarbon neuropathy (Figs. 4 and 5.) Untrastructural examination of these fibers revealed giant axons uniformly filled with 10-nm neurofilaments (Fig. 6) and neurotubules scattered in small clusters or surrounding mitochondria. Myelin sheaths in cross section were thin or absent. By 16 days, many swollen and unswollen fibers in this zone had thin myelin sheaths and were surrounded by supernumerary Schwann cells or reduplicated basal lamina, features indicative of remyelination. Swollen, neurofilament-filled axons were more numerous under the position of 2,5-HD application in nerves removed from animals that had also received 2,5-HD orally before surgery. Comparable changes were not seen in nerves treated with 2,4-HD.

These findings demonstrate that the specific hallmarks of hexacarbon neuropathy develop in peripheral nerves at sites of 2,5-HD application, and strongly suggest that systemic 2,5-HD distal axonopathy is induced by direct toxic damage of the nerve fiber. There is no evidence from this experiment to indicate that the neuronal perikaryon participated in the development of nerve fiber damage: any 2,5-HD that escaped into the systemic circulation would have had equal access to neuronal perikarya supplying right and left sciatic nerves, but damage was restricted to the region locally exposed to 2,5-HD, even in systemically 2,5-HD-intoxicated animals.

The Role of Axonal Transport

The significance of a focal and selective axonal accumulation of 10-nm intermediate filaments after the application of 2,5-HD is of considerable interest in relation to the mechanism of distal axonal degeneration. Neurofilaments are associated with 3 major polypeptides that behave in a constitutive fashion as they move down the axon in a slow wave of axonal transport moving at 1 to 2 mm/day (29). Griffin and colleagues (30) have demonstrated that axonal transport of neurofilaments can be stopped focally by systemic intoxication with β,β′-iminodipropionitrile, the pathologic correlate being the development

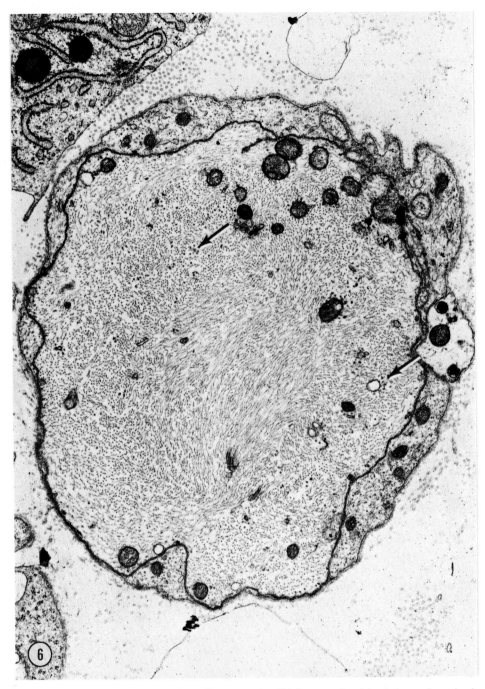

Fig. 6. Electron micrograph of swollen axon in tibial nerve fascicle 4 days after single application of undiluted 2,5-hexanedione. The axoplasm is uniformly packed with 10-nm neurofilaments. Small groups of microtubules (arrows) are scattered in the axoplasm. A thin layer of myelin is present. (Thin epoxy section stained with uranyl acetate and lead citrate; original magnification × 15,000.)

of giant axons containing masses of neurofilaments in proximal axons. From these observations, it seems likely that local or systemic application of 2,5-HD to peripheral nerves also results in a focal blockade of neurofilament transport, but in a distal distribution.

Savolainen (31) has suggested that neurotoxic hexacarbons, and other compounds that cause neurofilaments to accumulate, might bind to neurofilaments and affect their normal function. D.G. Graham (personal communication) has further proposed that 2,5-DH reacts with ε-amino groups of neurofilaments to form a conjugated imine. These ideas raise the possibility that 2,5-HD slowly denatures the neurofilament proteins during their movement along the axon, so that eventually they are unable to be transported further. Neurofilaments exposed to the toxin for the longest period of time, i.e., those sited distally in long fibers, would be the first ones affected in this way. Thus, denatured neurofilament proteins unable to traverse the nodal axon would collect on the proximal side, where they would form paranodal swellings. With time, neurofilaments in more proximal regions would become similarly affected, whereupon axonal swellings would develop in more proximal paranodes.

The neurofilament-filled giant axons produced by neurotoxic hexacarbons are also associated with focal abnormalities of fast transport. Griffin and colleagues (32) demonstrated in animals intoxicated with 2,5-HDiol that fast anterogradely transported material selectively accumulated in the swollen, filamentous regions, suggesting that it was held up in these areas during passage along the axon. These observations are consistent with the temporal slowing in the rate of fast anterograde axonal transport reported (20) in animals intoxicated with MnBK, because the number and proximal ascent of swellings are direct functions of the duration of intoxication. The dependence of fast axonal transport on the normal functioning of glycolysis (33) led Sabri and Spencer (34) to examine the effects of MnBK and 2,5-HD on glycolytic enzymes. The selective inhibition of glyceraldehyde-3-phosphate dehydrogenase (GAPDH) and phosphofructokinase in vitro and in vivo (Sabri MI: published data) led these investigators to suggest that an impairment of energy metabolism might underlie the reported abnormalities in fast axonal transport (20, 31).

Uses of the New Model

The 2,5-HD axonal mononeuropathy described in this paper provides an opportunity to explore further the mechanisms underlying axonal degeneration in distal axonopathies. For example, the behavior of anterogradely and retrogradely transported materials could be examined with conventional techniques, and the locally applied marker described by Gainer and colleagues (35) could be used to determine the fate of slowly transported materials.

We have also used the model to examine the behavior of GAPDH and lactic dehydrogenase (LDH) after a single application of 2,5-HD or 2,4-HD to the hindlimb nerves of rats. Left sciatic nerves were exposed to the diketones and right sciatic nerves, to saline. After 1, 2, 4, and 7 days, nerves were assayed for GAPDH and LDH activity. Two days postoperatively, before the appearance of axonal swellings, there was a significant (approximately 50%) reduction in

GAPDH activity in nerves exposed to 2,5-HD. The GAPDH activity in 2,4-HD-treated nerves and the LDH activity in 2,5-HD-treated nerves were comparable to the saline control activities. With time, GAPDH activity at sites of 2,5-HD application returned to control values. These data suggest that 2,5-HD might reversibly inhibit energy-dependent axonal transport systems at the site of toxin application.

Effects of 2,4-HD and 2,5-HD on Schwann Cells

Schwann cell changes are also seen in the local nerve lesion produced by hexacarbon compounds. The central portions of larger nerve fascicles of sciatic nerves exposed to 2,4-HD or 2,5-HD consistently contained myelinated nerve fibers with hypertrophied cytoplasm and an eccentric Schwann cell nucleus. The response in these fibers appeared to be primary and probably nonspecific, because it was not associated with axonal degeneration or demyelination. The enlarged cytoplasm contained several vacuoles, numerous mitochondria, prominent Golgi apparatus, and abundant rough endoplasmic reticulum (Fig. 7).

Occasional Schwann cells associated with demyelinated axons in areas of 2,5-HD-treated nerves displayed an increased number of cytoplasmic intermediate

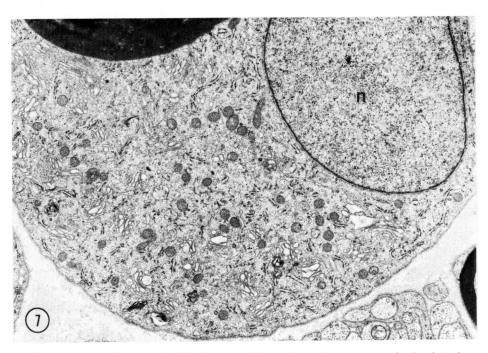

Fig. 7. Electron micrograph of Schwann cell cytoplasm from nerve obtained 4 days after application of 2,5-hexanedione. An abundance of rough endoplasmic reticulum and Golgi apparatus is present. The nucleus (n) is large and eccentrically located. These Schwann cell abnormalities, which were also seen in fascicles exposed to 2,4-hexanedione, occurred in the central portion of the endoneurium in association with normal-appearing myelin and axoplasm. (Thin epoxy section stained with uranyl acetate and lead citrate; original magnification × 10,000.)

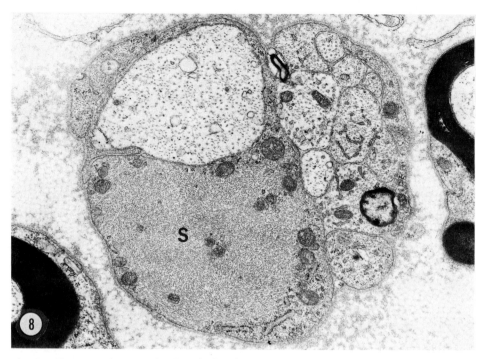

Fig. 8. Electron micrograph of an isolated example of excessive intermediate filaments in the Schwann cell cytoplasm (S) of a nerve fiber 4 days after exposure to 2,5-hexanedione. The axon displays no abnormalities. (Thin epoxy section stained with uranyl acetate and lead citrate; original magnification × 14,500.)

filaments, mitochondria, and small vesicles. Although these changes may be reactive, on one occasion, an extraordinary number of intermediate filaments was found (Fig. 8). The latter is pertinent to the suggestion that neurotoxic hexacarbons may induce a generalized cellular proliferation of intermediate filaments similar to that reported in the childhood disorder of giant axonal neuropathy (36). Comparable changes have been found in animals with advanced 2,5-HD neuropathy. Because they seem to postdate the appearance of axonal abnormality (26), it is not known whether they are primary or secondary. The answer to this question probably awaits an analysis of the structure and function of Schwann cells along long lengths of single teased nerve fibers displaying distal axonal abnormalities. Changes affecting all cells would point to a primary effect of 2,5-HD on the Schwann cell, whereas abnormalities restricted to distal regions of affected nerve fibers would indicate that the Schwann cell changes accompany axonal damage (37).

SUMMARY

This report has provided direct evidence in support of the idea that the causation of axonal degeneration in central-peripheral distal axonopathies should be sought in the nerve fiber rather than in the neuronal perikaryon.

There is increasing evidence to suggest that abnormalities of slow and fast axonal transport are responsible for the fine structural changes that precede nerve fiber breakdown. It seems probable that axonal neurotoxins such as 2,5-HD will continue to play an important role in the elucidation of these diseases, as well as in the expansion of our understanding of the biochemical mechanisms underlying axonal transport.

ACKNOWLEDGMENTS

Monica Bischoff and Kathy Ederle provided expert technical assistance. We would also like to thank Laurell Edwards for typing the manuscript. This work was supported by National Science Foundation grant PFR 78-12701, by National Institutes of Occupational Safety and Health grants OH 00535 and OH 00851, by National Institute of Environmental Health Sciences grant ES 02168, by National Research Service Award Training Grant NS 07098, and by National Institutes of Health Training Grant 5T 32 GM 7288 from the National Institute of General Medical Sciences.

REFERENCES

1. Cavanagh, JB: The significance of the "dying-back" process in experimental and human neurological disease. Int Rev Exp Pathol 3:219–267, 1964

2. Prineas JB: The pathogenesis of dying-back polyneuropathies. I. An ultrastructural study of experimental tri*ortho*cresyl phosphate intoxication in the cat. J Neuropathol Exp Neurol 28:571–597, 1969

3. Prineas JB: The pathogenesis of dying-back polyneuropathies. II. An ultrastructural study of experimental acrylamide intoxication in the cat. J Neuropathol Exp Neurol 28:598–621, 1969

4. Schaumburg HH, Wiśniewski HM, Spencer PS: Ultrastructural studies of the dying-back process. I. Peripheral nerve terminal and axon degeneration in systemic acrylamide intoxication. J Neuropathol Exp Neurol 33:260–284, 1974

5. Spencer PS, Schaumburg HH: A review of acrylamide neurotoxicity. II. Experimental animal neurotoxicity and pathologic mechanisms, Can J Neurol Sci 1:151–169, 1974

6. Spencer PS, Schaumburg HH: Ultrastructural studies of the dying-back process. III. The evolution of experimental peripheral giant axonal degeneration. J Neuropathol Exp Neurol 36:279–299, 1977

7. Veronesi B, Peterson ER, Spencer PS: Reproduction and analysis of methyl *n*-butyl ketone neuropathy in organotypic tissue culture. In *Experimental and Clinical Neurotoxicology*. Edited by Spencer PS, Schaumburg HH. Williams & Wilkins, Baltimore, 1980, pp 863–873

8. Spencer PS, Schaumburg HH: Central-peripheral distal axonopathy: the pathology of dying-back polyneuropathies. In *Progress in Neuropathology*, vol III. Edited by Zimmerman H. Grune & Stratton, New York, 1976, pp 253–295

9. Jacobs JM, Miller RH, Whittle A, Cavanagh JB: Studies on the early changes in acute isoniazid neuropathy in the rat. Acta Neuropathol 47:85–92, 1979

10. Jacobs JM, Miller RH, Cavanagh JB: The distribution of degenerative changes in INH neuropathy: further evidence for focal axonal lesions. Acta Neuropathol 48:1–10, 1979

11. Bouldin TW, Cavanagh, JB: Organophosphorus neuropathy. I. A teased-fiber study of the spatio-temporal spread of axonal degeneration. Am J Pathol 94:241–252, 1979

12. Seppalainen AM, Haltia M: Carbon disulfide. In *Experimental and Clinical Neurotoxicology*. Edited by Spencer PS, Schaumburg HH. Williams & Wilkins, Baltimore, 1980, pp 356–373

13. Jacobs JM: Vascular permeability and neural injury. In *Experimental and Clinical Neurotoxicology*. Edited by Spencer PS, Schaumburg HH. Williams & Wilkins, Baltimore, 1980, pp 102–117

14. Cho E-S, Spencer PS, Jortner BS, et al: A single intravenous injection of doxorubicin (Adriamycin®) induces sensory neuronopathy in rats. Neurotoxicology 1:583–592, 1980

15. Krinke G, Schaumburg HH, Spencer PS, et al: Pyridoxine megavitaminosis produces degeneration of peripheral sensory neurons (sensory neuronopathy) in the dog. Neurotoxicology (in press)

16. Mendell JR, Sahenk Z: Interference of neuronal processing and axoplasmic transport by toxic chemicals. In *Experimental and Clinical Neurotoxicology*. Edited by Spencer PS, Schaumburg HH. Williams & Wilkins, Baltimore, 1980, pp 139–160

17. Spencer PS, Schaumburg HH: Pathobiology of neurotoxic axonal degeneration. In *Physiology and Pathobiology of Axons*. Edited by Waxman S. Raven Press, New York, 1978, pp 265–282

18. Lowndes HE, Baker T: Toxic site of action in distal axonopathies. In *Experimental and Clinical Neurotoxicology*. Edited by Spencer PS, Schaumburg HH. Williams & Wilkins, Baltimore, 1980, pp 193–205

19. Zuccarello M, Anzil AP: A localized model of experimental neuropathy by topical application of disulfiram. Exp Neurol 64:699–703, 1979

20. Mendell JR, Sahenk Z, Saida K, et al: Alterations of fast axoplasmic transport in experimental methyl *n*-butyl ketone neuropathy. Brain Res 133:107–118, 1977

21. DiVincenzo GD, Kaplan CJ, Dedinas J: Characterization of the metabolites of methyl *n*-butyl ketone, methyl iso-butyl ketone and methyl ethyl ketone in guinea pig serum and their clearance. Toxicol Appl Pharmacol 36:511–522, 1976

22. O'Donoghue JL, Krasavage WJ: Identification and characterization of methyl *n*-butyl ketone neurotoxicity in laboratory animals. In *Experimental and Clinical Neurotoxicology*. Edited by Spencer PS, Schaumburg HH. Williams & Wilkins, Baltimore, 1980, pp 856–862

23. Spencer PS, Schaumburg HH: Experimental neuropathy produced by 2,5-hexanedione, a major metabolite of the neurotoxic industrial solvent methyl *n*-butyl ketone. J Neurol Neurosurg Psychiatry 8:771–775, 1975

24. Spencer PS, Schaumburg HH: Ultrastructural studies of the dying-back process. IV. Differential vulnerability of PNS and CNS fibers in experimental central-peripheral distal axonopathies. J Neuropathol Exp Neurol 36:300–320, 1977

25. Schaumburg HH, Spencer PS: Environmental hydrocarbons produce degeneration in cat hypothalamus and optic tract. Science 199:199–200, 1978

26. Powell HC, Koch T, Garrett R, et al: Schwann cell abnormalities in 2,5-hexanedione neuropathy. J Neurocytol 7:517–528, 1978

27. Spencer PS, Thomas PK: Ultrastructural studies of the dying-back process. II. The sequestration and removal by Schwann cells and oligodendrocytes of organelles from normal and diseased axons. J Neurocytol 3:763–783, 1974

28. Spencer PS, Bischoff MB, Schaumburg HH: On the specific molecular configuration of neurotoxic aliphatic hexacarbon compounds causing central-peripheral distal axonopathy. Toxicol Appl Pharmacol 44:17–28, 1978

29. Hoffman PN, Lasek RJ: The slow component of axonal transport: identification of major structural polypeptides of the axon and their generality among mammalian neurons. J Cell Biol 66:351–366, 1975

30. Griffin JW, Hoffman PN, Clark AW, et al: Slow axonal transport of neurofilament proteins: impairment by β,β'-iminodipropionitrile. Science 202:633–635, 1978

31. Savolainen H: Some aspects of the mechanisms by which industrial solvents produce neurotoxic effects. Chem Biol Interact 18:1–10, 1977

32. Griffin JW, Price DL, Spencer PS: Fast axonal transport through giant axonal swellings in hexacarbon neuropathy (abstract). J Neuropathol Exp Neurol 36:603, 1977

33. Sabri MI, Ochs S: Relationship of ATP and creatine phosphate to fast axoplasmic transport in mammalian nerve. J Neurochem 19:2821–2828, 1972

34. Sabri, MI, Spencer, PS: Toxic distal axonopathy: biochemical studies and hypothetical mech-

anisms. In *Experimental and Clinical Neurotoxicology*. Edited by Spencer PS, Schaumburg HH. Williams & Wilkins, Baltimore, 1980, pp 206–210

35. Fink DH, Gainer H: Retrograde axonal transport of endogenous proteins in sciatic nerve demonstrated by covalent labeling in vivo. Science 208:303–305, 1980

36. Prineas JW, Ouvrier RA, Wright RG, et al: Giant axonal neuropathy, a generalized disorder of microfilament formation. J Neuropathol Exp Neurol 35:458–470, 1976

37. Politis MJ, Pellegrino RG, Spencer PS: Ultrastructural studies of the dying-back process. V. Axonal neurofilaments accumulate at sites of 2,5-hexanedione application: evidence for nerve fiber dysfunction in experimental hexacarbon neuropathy. J Neurocytol 9:505–516, 1980

DISCUSSION

Dr. Michael Rasminsky: You show very elegantly that 2,5-HD acts on the axon. However, I still do not understand why the pathology should, in general, first appear distally. What is your current explanation for this?

Dr. Peter Spencer: The explanation is in a constant state of flux and reappraisal. We have suggested that 2,5-HD may inhibit certain glycolytic enzymes within the axon on which the transport mechanism(s) depend. There is evidence to show that 2,5-HD inhibits glyceraldehyde phosphate dehydrogenase and phosphofructokinase both in vitro and in vivo, but we do not know whether this phenomenon is causally related to the onset of axonal abnormalities. The idea here is that glycolytic enzymes, manufactured in and exported from the neuronal perikaryon, become progressively inhibited during passage along the axon, so that insufficient levels of enzymes reach distal regions, causing transport difficulties and degeneration. This hypothesis is now being tested. Another idea is that neurofilaments exported down the axon slowly undergo molecular deformation after contact with 2,5-HD (Graham DE: personal communication). Eventually, when the neurofilament proteins reach the distal portion of the axon, they cannot be transported further, and they accumulate in giant axonal swellings. These then are two current ideas: the first addresses the origin of the fast axonal transport abnormality; the second considers the causation of the putative slow axonal transport problem, which is believed to result in neurofilament accumulation.

Dr. Peter Dyck: I would like to address the question of nomenclature. It is a very old concept that, in some diseases, the whole neuron is diseased, whereas in other diseases the distal axon and other parts are affected. I am a little concerned that we use words too loosely. For example, in the axotomy model, clearly the disease process begins distally but has a proximal effect.

Dr. Peter Spencer: I fully agree with you. I think this terminology will be useful for a few years and then will be replaced by another, more illuminating nosology. This terminology was specifically developed in relation to the toxic models of experimental neuropathy in an attempt to try to understand some of the patterns found in human neuropathy.

Dr. Peter Dyck: I want to amplify this point. For example, in terms of myelinopathy, we really do not know whether the lesion lies in the myelin sheath or in the Schwann cell. I think we should not use those "buzz" words; they imply that we know when we do not.

Dr. Peter Spencer: I think that one can justifiably use the word "toxin" or even "axonal toxin" in the case of nerve fibers treated with 2,5-HD. With regard to myelinopathies, this is merely a category that indicates the possibility of a direct effect on the myelin sheath, the Schwann cell perikaryon, or the myelinating cell transport systems between the perikaryon and the myelin sheath, which of course, no one has been able to address at the present time.

Dr. Arthur Asbury: Before I call on Dr. Ochs, I am going to respond to Dr. Dyck, with whom I frequently disagree. It seems to me that there are clinical and electrodiagnostic features that allow one clearly to categorize various types of neuropathy. Just to be arbitrary, I think these divisions are easily recognized, such as the one in which there is a predominantly demyelinative component, therefore referred to as "myelinopathy." This does not imply anything about whether the Schwann cell or the enclosed myelin sheath is the primary target. But, for these purposes, I do not think that it matters. The main thing is to distinguish a demyelinative process from an axonal process, and for that reason, perhaps these terms have a categorizing usefulness.

Dr. Peter Dyck: But that is exactly my point. You cannot distinguish, by those criteria, a primary from a secondary process.

Dr. Arthur Asbury: I do not think we need to at this stage. It is better to use these terms than to refer to all cases as "neuropathy," nonspecifically.

Dr. Peter Dyck: But why not use descriptive criteria and not attach precise terms? I am very much in favor of categorization, but consider, for example, anterior horn cell versus distal motor neuropathy. We are not at the stage where we understand the similarities and differences; there are in-between forms. Let's not be so black and white.

Dr. Arthur Asbury: Thank you Dr. Dyck. We reversed our roles for once.

Dr. Sidney Ochs: Dr. Dyck, could you calculate from the dying-back phenomenon, to see whether it matches the presumed slow rates of transport? Do they have any correlation at all?

Dr. Peter Spencer: We do not know, because the rate of onset of the abnormality depends on the rate of the intoxication, which is a function of both the amount of toxin administered and the frequency of application. Relating back to the discourse between Dr. Asbury and Dr. Dyck, it is entirely possible, that distal axonopathy is not a specific entity. Perhaps one could "flood" the nerve with amounts of 2,5-HD sufficient to arrest axonally transported material in the intermediate portion of the axon or even proximally. Then, of course, the whole nomenclature would have to be rethought.

Part II

CELL—CELL
INTERACTIONS

Overview

Daniel B. Drachman, MD

Nerve cells and the target cells they innervate function in a highly interdependent manner. Firing a neuron excites (or inhibits) the innervated target cell, and may precipitate a cascade of downstream events. Conversely, changes in the target cell's activity may be reflected by alterations in the activity of the innervating cell.

These intimate functional relationships presuppose that nerve cells and their targets are appropriately connected, are maintained in a state of readiness for function, and are properly adapted for the specialized jobs they perform. By using mechanisms that have been the subject of intensive investigation, nerve cells and target cells manage to attain such functionally appropriate arrangements in development, and to maintain them thereafter. These nerve cell–target cell interactions comprise the subject of this session. The term "trophic" has been applied to such relationships, and it is here defined as *relatively long-term interactions between nerve cells and target cells in which the structure or function of either member of the pair is influenced.*

This definition does not presuppose or exclude any particular mechanism of long-term interaction. Specifically, although it is not meant to describe the individual events of neurotransmission, it does not exclude the cumulative effects of repeated transmission if they have a long-term influence on the cells involved.

In this session, our interests turn not only to motor nerves and skeletal muscle—the theme of this conference—but also to other neural systems, for the lessons that can be learned from them. The speakers will discuss: *(a)* mechanisms by which motor nerves regulate certain key properties of skeletal muscle; *(b)* factors that influence sprouting and regeneration of motor nerves; *(c)* formation of neuromuscular junctions; *(d)* The role of basement membrane in retaining and directing junctional specialization in vivo; *(e)* The reverse influence of the peripheral field on the innervating cells; and *(f)* the mechanisms by which nerve growth factor enters and affects sympathetic neurons.

8
Neurotrophic Interactions Between Nerves and Muscles: Role of Acetylcholine

Daniel B. Drachman, MD

Alan Pestronk, MD

Elis F. Stanley, PhD

Motor innervation plays an important role in the trophic regulation of many properties of skeletal muscle. Elimination of the influence of the nerve by surgical denervation results in a variety of changes in the physiologic, biochemical, and structural properties of muscle fibers (1). The question of how the nerves normally prevent these denervation changes has been the subject of continuing controversy. The hypothesis that acetylcholine (ACh) may serve as a mediator of neurotrophic influences has been considered (2) almost since its discovery as the natural neuromuscular transmitter. However, it has been suggested that unrelated factors, e.g., materials carried by axonal transport, may participate as well (3–5). It now appears that ACh transmission may have a key role in the regulation of at least some properties of skeletal muscle, including extrajunctional ACh receptors and the resting membrane potential. On the other hand, the older concept of a unitary trophic factor that influences *all* muscle properties is no longer tenable. The purpose of this presentation is to summarize the available evidence, and to add new observations concerning the role of ACh transmission and the muscle usage it produces in the regulation of skeletal muscle properties.

ACh TRANSMISSION

By way of background, the following summary of present concepts about ACh transmission is included.

Acetylcholine is synthesized chiefly in motor nerve terminals (6) and is believed

107

to be stored in vesicles (quanta) containing approximately 10^4 molecules (7), and possibly in the cytoplasm as well (8). Spontaneous release of ACh occurs in both quantal (9) and nonquantal (10, 11) forms. The release of one or a few quanta gives rise to depolarizations of small amplitude (miniature endplate potentials, or mepps) that remain localized to the region of the endplate. Spontaneous nonquantal release of ACh is believed to occur continuously, in much larger amounts than quantal release, without producing discrete depolarization potentials (9–11).

Conducted nerve impulses release large numbers of ACh quanta (approximately 150 to 200 per impulse), giving rise to endplate potentials of relatively large amplitude (epps). These epps trigger a complex sequence of events, including propagated muscle action potentials, excitation-contraction coupling, and muscle contraction, relaxation, and energy utilization, which may collectively be called "usage" or "activity" of muscle. Any of these electrochemical or mechanical events might theoretically be involved in trophic interactions, but it must be remembered that the nerve's only means of initiating them is via release of ACh. Thus, trophic influences due to ACh transmission might in theory result from the effects of spontaneously released ACh, and/or from the usage triggered by ACh.

NEUROTROPHIC ROLE OF ACh: EARLY STUDIES

The first experimental studies suggesting that ACh plays a role as a mediator of neurotrophic influences used botulinum toxin to interfere with neuromuscular ACh transmission (12). Purified botulinum toxin is a crystallizable protein (13) that acts presynaptically to prevent the release of ACh (14). It appears to block the nerve terminals' specialized ACh release sites (15), through which most quantal ACh release takes place. This produces a marked decrease in both spontaneous and impulse-directed quantal ACh release, resulting in muscle paralysis (disuse) and a reduction of the frequency of mepps to approximately 5% to 10% of normal (16, 17).

The effects of prolonged treatment with botulinum toxin resemble those produced by denervation in many respects. The denervation-like changes include skeletal muscle atrophy (18), fibrillations (19), supersensitivity to ACh and increased extrajunctional ACh receptor (AChR) density (12, 17), reduction of muscle acetylcholinesterase (20), slowing of isometric muscle contraction and relaxation (21), decreased histochemical differentiation (22), and susceptibility to innervation by foreign nerves (23).

THE ROLE OF MUSCLE USAGE

These denervation-like effects of botulinum treatment were unequivocal, yet their interpretation raised further questions about the role of ACh as a mediator of trophic influences. Because botulinum toxin blocks impulse-triggered (as well as spontaneously released) ACh (24), it produces muscle paralysis; one may ask what part the muscle disuse per se plays in the development of denervation changes. Conversely, what part does neurally triggered usage of muscle contribute to the normal regulation of these muscle properties?

The idea that contractile activity has a trophic influence on skeletal muscle is an old one (25, 26); in recent years it has been reexamined by several new experimental approaches that permit more precise definition of its role in the regulation of muscle properties. In these investigations, a given property of muscle known to be under neural control is selected for study and is measured quantitatively under conditions of experimentally altered muscle activity.

Stimulation of Skeletal Muscle

In this approach, a denervated muscle is directly stimulated electrically in an effort to replace the missing influence of the nerve. Several reports have documented the effectiveness of electrical stimulation in preventing or reversing denervation changes (27–29). However, to evaluate the normal biologic contribution of usage, it is essential to mimic the nerve's natural pattern of impulse activity. Using the rat diaphragm, we were able to estimate the amount of stimulation normally provided by the phrenic nerve, because respiration occurs in a regular, rhythmic pattern. Stimulation of the denervated hemidiaphragms of rats in imitation of the normal phrenic nerve pattern prevented the denervation-induced increase of extrajunctional ACh sensitivity largely, but not completely (27). Thus suggested an important, but partial regulatory role of muscle activity. If the amount and frequency of stimulation are increased, extrajunctional ACh sensitivity and other denervation effects can be completely prevented or reversed (30).

Disuse

A more accurate method of assessing the biologic contribution of nerve-induced muscle usage is to block all nerve impulse conduction while leaving the neuromuscular system otherwise intact, and compare the effects quantitatively with those of denervation. Earlier attempts to produce disuse resulted in only partial inactivity (26, 31) or caused damage to axons (32). We and others have recently devised an experimental method of producing pure disuse, based on the local application of tetrodotoxin (TTX) to the sciatic nerves of rats (33–35). By repeated injection of TTX into the nerve at 48-hour intervals, complete blockade of nerve conduction can be maintained for long periods of time (33). The TTX interrupts action potential conduction at the site of application by blocking sodium channels (36), but has no other effect on the nerves. It does not interfere with axonal transport, produce morphologic changes in nerves, or prevent spontaneous release of ACh from nerve terminals (33).

We have studied the effects of TTX-induced disuse on two neurally regulated properties of rat skeletal muscles, extrajunctional AChRs (33) and the resting membrane potential (RMP) (37), and have compared them with the effects of surgical denervation. The AChRs were measured by a method that uses binding of ^{125}I-labeled α-bungarotoxin (α-BuTx) (38). Normally, AChRs are virtually confined to the region of the neuromuscular junction, with very few receptors located extrajunctionally. After denervation, there is a striking increase in the number of extrajunctional AChRs, eventually reaching a level many thousand times higher than that of the innervated muscle (39, 40).

The TTX-induced disuse produced a denervation-like increase of extrajunctional AChRs in the rat soleus muscle, but the effect was only approximately half as great as that of denervation at the two time points studied (33). Similarly, disuse resulted in a delayed fall of the RMP indicative of an incomplete denervation effect (35, 37). The normal RMP of the rate soleus is approximately -80 mV when recorded in vivo. After surgical section of the nerve, the RMP begins to fall approximately 18 hours later, reaching a minimum value of -65 mV at 48 hours (41). The TTX-induced disuse resulted in a much slower fall in the RMP that began at 36 to 48 hours and finally reached -65 mV at 7 days.

These findings show that impulse-dependent ACh release and the muscle usage it produces have only a partial effect in regulating extrajunctional AChRs and the RMP of skeletal muscles.

Nerve Stump Length

Nerve stump experiments have been used to determine whether some factors contained in the stump of a severed motor nerve left attached to the muscle is capable of delaying the onset of a denervation change. Luco and Eyzaguirre (42) first demonstrated that the onset of fibrillations occurred later in muscles with long stumps attached compared to those with nerves sectioned close to the muscle. Other experiments have since confirmed the effect of long nerve stumps in delaying the onset of a variety of denervation changes (43, 44). Similarly, we have found that the RMP recorded in vivo begins to fall approximately 3 hours later in rat soleus muscles with 40-mm stumps than in those with 2-mm stumps, giving a delay of approximately 45 minutes per cm of nerve (41).

These findings indicate that some factor other than activity must account for the difference in timing, because all of the denervated muscles were inactive, regardless of the stump length. Luco and Eyzaguirre (42) originally suggested that the delay might be related to more prolonged spontaneous ACh release in the longer nerve stumps. This hypothesis is consistent with the finding that the persistence of mepps is also proportional to the length of the stump (45), although nothing is yet known about the effect of nerve stump length on nonquantal release of ACh.

WHAT IS THE REMAINING NEUROTROPHIC FACTOR?

Because impulse-dependent ACh release (and muscle activity) were shown to account for only part of the nerve's regulation of skeletal muscle properties, some other influence exhibited by the nerve must surely contribute the remainder. The likely candidates included a "trophic substance" delivered to the muscle, perhaps by axonal transport (5), or alternatively, ACh released spontaneously by quantal and/or nonquantal mechanisms. Several clues led us to suspect spontaneous ACh release. Quantitative comparison of the increase of extrajunctional AChRs occurring with botulinum toxin treatment (17) and

TTX-induced disuse (33) showed that the effect of botulinum was significantly greater, although it was not equivalent to the effect of surgical denervation. Because botulinum toxin is known to block a substantial fraction of the spontaneous release of ACh in addition to its effect on impulse-directed ACh release, this suggested that the spontaneous ACh release might be important. Furthermore, other studies showed that postsynaptic ACh-blocking agents given alone (46) or in addition to botulinum toxin (47) produced rather large denervation-like effects.

To resolve the question of the remaining neural influence, we undertook to block ACh transmission as thoroughly as possible, to determine whether its denervation-like effects are quantitatively equivalent to those of surgical nerve section. For this purpose, we used α-BuTx because of its postsynaptic site of action, great potency, and specificity (48, 49). Previous studies had shown that intramuscular injection of α-BuTx results in a limited period of complete neuromuscular blockade (46, 50) despite the presumed irreversibility of its binding to AChRs. To produce prolonged blockade, we developed a method of local infusion into the soleus muscles of rats, using implantable osmotic pumps. With this method, we have been able to achieve virtually complete blockade of ACh transmission for as long as 7 days (51).

We again elected to study extrajunctional AChRs and the muscle RMP as parameters of the denervation-like effects. By using the same two muscle properties as in our previous disuse experiments, we were able to make quantitative comparisons of the effects of α-BuTx treatment and those of TTX-induced disuse and surgical denervation. Our results showed that α-BuTx infusion produced an increase in the number of extrajunctional AChRs equivalent to that produced by surgical denervation, with the same time course at 4 and 7 days. Details of these experimental findings are reported elsewhere (51). Similarly, the effect of α-BuTx treatment on the muscle RMP was identical to that of surgical section of the soleus nerve at its point of attachment to the muscle. In both the denervated and α-BuTx-treated animals, the fall in RMP began at 18 to 24 hours and reached a maximum change of 15 mV at 36 to 42 hours, as measured in vivo (52).

These findings now demonstrate that the effects of cholinergic blockade are quantitatively equivalent to those of surgical denervation, with respect to the two neurally regulated properties of muscle studied. Our results are in general agreement with those of earlier studies, but the previous reports did not establish the quantitative completeness of the effects. In some studies, the use of intermittent injections of the pharmacologic agents produced incomplete ACh blockade and resulted in partial denervation-like effects (47, 53). In one report, systemic administration of postsynaptic blocking agents resulted in high levels of extrajunctional AChRs and a fall in the RMP, but the data presented were conflicting and were not sufficient to permit quantitative conclusions regarding the completeness of the effects (46). In our investigations, the method of direct infusion produced continuous local blockade of ACh transmission; its simplicity permitted the use of relatively large numbers of animals; and the reproducibility of the methods of measurement of AChRs and RMPs allowed quantitative comparison with the effects of surgical denervation.

The simplest interpretation of our findings is that the observed denervation-like changes in the extrajunctional AChRs and the RMP are attributable to the only known action of α-BuTx: the highly specific blockade of AChRs (48). Control studies have not revealed any other effects of α-BuTx on the function or structure of motor nerves. In particular, α-BuTx neither interferes with fast axonal transport (Drachman DB, Griffin JW, Pestronk A, et al: unpublished data) or decreases ACh release (54). Moreover, prolonged treatment with α-BuTx does not alter motor nerve terminal morphology, as shown by light (50) and electron microscopy (Drachman DB, Griffin JW, Pestronk A, et al: unpublished data). These findings make it highly improbable that α-BuTx interferes with some other aspect of nerve–muscle interaction. Indeed, because the effects of specific blockade of ACh transmission have now been shown to equal those of surgical denervation, there seems no need to postulate other neural factors in the regulation of extrajunctional AChRs and the muscle RMP.

ROLE OF SPONTANEOUS ACh TRANSMISSION

The separate contribution of spontaneously released ACh to the neural regulation of these muscle properties cannot be directly measured because there is, at present, no means of blocking spontaneous ACh release alone. However, the evidence summarized above allows us to draw the conclusion that both spontaneous and impulse-dependent ACh contribute to the neurotrophic influences. Because elimination of the impulse-dependent release of ACh (disuse) produced only a partial denervation-like effect, whereas blockade of all ACh transmission (by α-BuTx) resulted in a complete effect, the difference is attributable to the spontaneously released ACh.

Similar reasoning suggests that both the quantal and the nonquantal forms of spontaneous ACh release may contribute to the regulation of muscle properties. Thus, treatment with botulinum toxin, which blocks nearly all quantal release of ACh, resulted in an increase in the number of AChRs that was significantly less than that produced by α-BuTx or denervation. The greater effect of α-BuTx appears to be due to its ability to block all ACh because of its postsynaptic site of action and high affinity for AChRs. Thus, it must interfere with nonquantal, as well as quantal, ACh transmission. We are led to conclude that the influence of the motor nerve in regulating the RMP and extrajunctional AChRs is due to the combination of these forms of ACh transmission (Fig. 1).

ARE ALL MUSCLE PROPERTIES REGULATED BY ACh TRANSMISSION?

Extrajunctional AChRs and the RMP are only two of the many properties of skeletal muscle that are under neurotrophic influence. It is worth emphasizing that the rules that govern neural regulation of these two parameters cannot a priori be assumed to apply to other muscle properties. Previous studies of the effects of botulinum toxin suggest that many muscle properties are partly or wholly regulated by ACh transmission as noted above (12, 17–23). On the other hand, there is evidence that blockade of ACh transmission does not interfere with other neurotrophic influences, such as the formation of neuromuscular

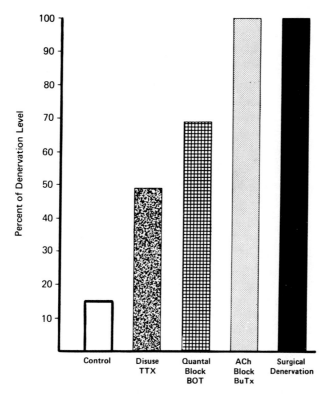

Fig. 1. Relative increase at 4 days of soleus muscle extrajunctional acetylcholine receptors (AChRs) is produced by different treatments. In each case the treatment was maintained for 7 days. Note that the effect of α-bungarotoxin (BuTx) treatment was equivalent to that of denervation. Botulinum toxin (BOT) treatment resulted in a less pronounced increase of AChRs. The effect of tetrodotoxin (TTX)-induced disuse was smaller, but still highly significant.

junctions and the localization of subsynaptic AChRs (55–58). Thus, the factors involved in the neural regulation of each muscle property must be evaluated individually. Finally, many trophic relationships have been described in a variety of systems other than skeletal muscle (1). Clearly, the neural factors involved in the regulation of these systems cannot be assumed to correspond to those in the muscle system, and must be separately evaluated.

In conclusion, the findings described here have demonstrated the importance of ACh transmission in the neurotrophic regulation of two key properties of skeletal muscle. Future study will be necessary to identify the mechanism at the level of the muscle cell by which ACh transmission is linked to control of cellular properties.

ACKNOWLEDGMENTS

Supported by National Institutes of Health grants RO1 HD04817 and PO1 NS10820, and by a grant from the Muscular Dystrophy Association. We are grateful to Dr. J Griffin and Dr. D Price for their contributions to parts of the studies quoted and for their continued help and advice; to CF Barlow for help in preparing the manuscript; and to RN Adams and MJ Peper for expert technical assistance.

REFERENCES

1. Drachman DB (ed): Trophic functions of the neuron. Ann NY Acad Sci 228:1–423, 1974

2. Cannon WB, Rosenblueth A: *The Supersensitivity of Denervated Structures*. MacMillan, New York, 1949

3. Albuquerque EX, Warnick JE, Tasse JR, et al: Effects of vinblastine and colchicine on neural regulation of the fast and slow skeletal muscles of the rat. Exp Neurol 37:607–634, 1972

4. Fernandez HL, Ramirez BU: Muscle fibrillation induced by blockade of axoplasmic transport in motor nerves. Brain Res 79:385–395, 1974

5. Ochs S: Systems of material transport in nerve fibers (axoplasmic transport) related to nerve function and trophic control. Ann NY Acad Sci 228:202–223, 1974

6. Hebb CO, Krnjević K, Silver A: Acetylcholine and choline acetyltransferase in the diaphragm of the rat. J Physiol (Lond) 171:504–513, 1964

7. Hartzell HC, Kuffler SW, Yoshikami D: The number of acetylcholine molecules in a quantum and the interaction between quanta at the subsynaptic membrane of the skeletal neuromuscular synapse. Cold Spring Harbor Symp Quant Biol 40:175–186, 1976

8. Tauc L: Are vesicles necessary for release of acetylcholine at cholinergic synapses? Biochem Pharmacol 27:3493–3498, 1979

9. Fatt P, Katz B: Spontaneous subthreshold activity at motor nerve endings. J Physiol (Lond) 117:109–128, 1952

10. Potter LT: Synthesis, storage and release of ^{14}C-acetylcholine in isolated rat diaphragm muscles. J Physiol (Lond) 206:145–166, 1970

11. Katz B, Miledi R: Transmitter leakage from motor nerve endings. Proc Roy Soc Lond [Biol] 196:159–172, 1977

12. Thesleff S: Supersensitivity of skeletal muscle produced by botulinum toxin. J Physiol (Lond) 151:598–607, 1960

13. Duff JT, Wright GG, Klerer J, et al: Studies on immunity to toxins of *Clostridium botulinum*. I. A simplified procedure for isolation of type A toxin. J Bacteriol 73:42–47, 1957

14. Brooks V: An intracellular study of the action of repetitive nerve volleys and of botulinum toxin on miniature end-plate potentials. J Physiol (Lond) 134:264–277, 1956

15. Kao I, Drachman DB, Price DL: Botulinum toxin: mechanism of presynaptic blockade. Science 193:1256–1258, 1976

16. Boroff DA, del Castillo J, Evoy WH, et al: Observations on the action of type A botulinum toxin on frog neuromuscular junctions. J Physiol (Lond) 20:227–253, 1974

17. Pestronk A, Drachman DB, Griffin JW: Effect of botulinum toxin on trophic regulation of acetylcholine receptors. Nature 264:787–789, 1976

18. Drachman DB: Is acetylcholine the trophic neuromuscular transmitter? Arch Neurol 17:206–218, 1967

19. Josefson JO, Thesleff S: Electromyographic findings in experimental botulinum intoxication. Acta Physiol Scand 51:163–168, 1961

20. Drachman DB: Neurotrophic regulation of muscle cholinesterase: effects of botulinum toxin and denervation. J Physiol (Lond) 226:619–627, 1972

21. Drachman DB, Johnston DM: Neurotrophic regulation of dynamic properties of skeletal muscle: effects of botulinum toxin and denervation. J Physiol (Lond) 234:29–42, 1973

22. Drachman DB, Romanul FCA: Effect of neuromuscular blockade on enzymatic activities of muscles. Arch Neurol 23:85–89, 1970

23. Hoffman WW, Thesleff S, Zelena J: Innervation of botulinum poisoned skeletal muscles by accessory nerves. J Physiol (Lond) 171:27P–28P, 1964

24. Thesleff S, Lundh H: Mode of action of botulinum toxin and the effect of drug antagonists. Adv Cytopharmacol 3:35–43, 1979

25. Brown-Sequard E: *Experimental Researches Applied to Physiology and Pathology.* H. Bailliere, New York, 1853

26. Tower S: Trophic control of non-nervous tissues and quiescent region of the spinal cord. J Comp Neurol 67:241–267, 1937

27. Drachman DB, Witzke F: Trophic regulation of acetylcholine sensitivity of muscle: effect of electrical stimulation. Science 176:514–516, 1972

28. Lømo T, Rosenthal J: Control of ACh sensitivity by muscle activity in the rat. J Physiol (Lond) 221:493–513, 1972

29. Purves D, Sakmann B: The effect of contractile activity on fibrillation and extrajunctional acetylcholine-sensitivity in rat muscle maintained in organ culture. J Physiol (Lond) 237:157–182, 1974

30. Lømo T, Westgaard RH: Control of ACh sensitivity in rat muscle fibers. Cold Spring Harbor Symp Quant Biol 40:263–274, 1975

31. Fischbach GD, Robbins N: Changes in contractile properties of disused soleus muscles. J Physiol (Lond) 201:305–320, 1969

32. Robert ED, Oester YT: Nerve impulse and trophic effect. Arch Neurol 22:57–63, 1970

33. Pestronk A, Drachman DB, Griffin J: Disuse of muscle: effect on extrajunctional acetylcholine receptors. Nature 260:352–358, 1976

34. Lavoie P-A, Collier B, Tenenhouse A: Comparison of α-bungarotoxin binding to skeletal muscles after inactivity or denervation. Nature 260:349–350, 1976

35. Mills RG, Bray JJ, Hubbard JI: Effects of inactivity on membrane potentials in rat muscle. Brain Res 150:607–610, 1978

36. Evans MH: Tetrodotoxin, saxitoxin, and related substances: their applications in neurobiology. Int Rev Neurobiol 15:83–166, 1972

37. Stanley EF, Drachman DB: Effect of disuse on the resting membrane potential of skeletal muscle. Exp. Neurol 64:231–234, 1979

38. Fambrough DM: Acetylcholine receptors: revised estimates of extrajunctional receptor density in denervated rat diaphragm. J Gen Physiol 64:468–472, 1974

39. Fambrough DM: Control of acetylcholine receptors in skeletal muscle. Physiol Rev 59:165–227, 1979

40. Edwards C: The effects of innervation on the properties of acetylcholine receptors in muscle. Neuroscience 4:565–584, 1979

41. Stanley EF, Drachman DB: Denervation and the time course of resting membrane potential changes in skeletal muscle in vivo. Exp Neurol 69:253–259, 1980

42. Luco JV, Eyzaguirre C: Fibrillation and hypersensitivity to ACh in denervated muscle: effect of length of degenerating nerve fibers. J Neurophysiol 18:65–73, 1955

43. Harris JB, Thesleff S: Nerve stump length and membrane changes in denervated skeletal muscle. Nature 236:60–61, 1972

44. Uchitel O, Robbins N: On the appearance of acetylcholine receptors in denervated rat diaphragm, and its dependence on nerve stump length. Brain Res 153:539–548, 1978

45. Miledi R, Slater CR: On the degeneration of rat neuromuscular junctions after nerve section. J Physiol (Lond) 207:507–528, 1970

46. Berg DK, Hall ZW: Increased extrajunctional sensitivity produced by chronic post-synaptic neuromuscular blockade. J Physiol (Lond) 244:659–676, 1975

47. Mathers DA, Thesleff S: Studies on neurotrophic regulation of murine skeletal muscle. J Physiol 282:105–114, 1978

48. Lee CY: Chemistry and pharmacology of polypeptide toxins in snake venoms. Annu Rev Pharmacol 12:265–286, 1972

49. Miledi R, Potter LT: Acetylcholine receptors in muscle fibers. Nature 233:599–603, 1971

50. Pestronk A, Drachman DB: Motor nerve sprouting and acetylcholine receptors. Science 199:1223–1225, 1978

51. Pestronk A, Drachman DB, Stanley EF, et al: Cholinergic transmission regulates extrajunctional acetylcholine receptors. Exp Neurol (in press)

52. Stanley EF, Drachman DB, Pestronk A, et al: The role of ACh transmission in the neural regulation of muscle resting membrane potential (abstract). Soc Neurosci Abstr 6:384, 1980

53. Chang CC, Chuang S-T, Huang MC: Effects of chronic treatment with various neuromuscular blocking agents on the number and distribution of acetylcholine receptors in the rat diaphragm. J Physiol (Lond) 250:161–173, 1975

54. Miledi R, Molenaar PC, Polak RL: α-Bungarotoxin enhances transmitter "released" at the neuromuscular junction. Nature 272:641–642, 1978

55. Steinbach JH, Harris AJ, Patrick J, et al: Nerve-muscle interactions in vitro. J Gen Physiol 62:255–270, 1968

56. Crain SM, Peterson ER: Development of neural connection in culture. Ann NY Acad Sci 228:6–33, 1974

57. Freeman SS, Engel AG, Drachman DB: Experimental acetylcholine blockade of the neuro-muscular junction: effects on end-plate and muscle fiber ultrastructure. Ann NY Acad Sci 274:46–59, 1976

58. Giacobini-Robecchi MB, Giacobini G, Filogmao G, et al: Effects of the type A toxin from *Clostridium botulinum* on the development of skeletal muscles and of their innervation in chick embryo. Brain Res 83:107–121, 1975

DISCUSSION

Dr. Stephen Thesleff: You have described two factors, muscle activity and the release of acetylcholine. Would you care to speculate how these two factors might govern the synthesis of muscle proteins that govern resting potential and receptors?

Dr. Daniel Drachman: Your question really asks what the response is at the level of the muscle. Up to now, we have been studying the nature of the nerve's signal, i.e., how the nerve "talks to the muscle." Now we have to find out how the muscle "listens," i.e., the mechanism of transduction of the neural signal that leads to changes in protein synthesis. That is the next step, and a crucial one. We think our studies show that the nerve communicates with the muscle by means of cholinergic transmission, at least with respect to the control of resting membrane potential and extrajunctional ACh receptors.

Dr. Henry Epstein: Understanding your qualifications, I want to ask for your comments on the growth of nerves toward specific targets during normal development, which you did not discuss specifically. Would you comment on both that concept and the alternative paradigms of normal development versus postdevelopmental changes?

Dr. Daniel Drachman: I have not commented on factors regulating the growth of nerves to target cells because the latter part of the program is devoted specifically to that subject. Dr. Pestronk and Dr. McMahan will be talking about nerve outgrowth and formation of junctions. That aspect of cell-to-cell inter-action is a different side of the nerve-muscle relationship. I am glad that you have brought it up, because it allows me to emphasize that there are many different kinds of regulatory functions. We would certainly not suggest that cholinergic transmission regulates cell outgrowth or formation of junctions, about which we will hear much more later.

Dr. Richard Almon: Not to be heretical in a trophic factor conference, but with regard to the increase in cholinergic receptors, we have recently shown that if you castrate male animals you get a slight increase in cholinergic receptors. There are also data in the literature showing that treatment with glucocorticoids produces a depolarization similar to that produced by denervation. Our tentative hypothesis was simply that if you disturb the balanced functioning of the muscle, you generate this response. Glucocorticoids will, of course, cause the atrophy types of effect (depolarization and perhaps extrajunctional receptors). These effects may simply represent a response of the muscle to disturbance of its balance of function, rather than having to do with the nerve or anything else.

Dr. Daniel Drachman: If I understand you correctly, androgenic hormones have functions similar to those which we attribute to the neurotrophic effect. A great many factors affect the resting membrane potential and, for that matter, many other properties of skeletal muscle, such as the distribution of extrajunctional receptors. Not all such regulatory factors are "neurotrophic." Our goal is to try to determine what the nerve is actually doing. The literature on this subject has been cluttered with reports that confuse those two issues. I am not saying that you do not separate them, but the literature is replete with reports of various factors that apparently have nothing to do with the nerve, whereas what we are trying to define as precisely as possible is what the nerve itself is doing, i.e., how the nerve talks to the muscle.

9
Neuromuscular Interdependence During Development

Guillermo Pilar, MD

Jeremy B. Tuttle, PhD

Lynn T. Landmesser, PhD

TARGET INFLUENCE ON NEURONAL DEVELOPMENT

At some point in normal development, neurons make contact with their peripheral targets, whether these are muscle cells or other neurons. Although most neurons that have been studied show a period of relatively autonomous development (1–4), they begin to show an obvious dependence on their targets at about the time they would normally form peripheral contacts. In most vertebrate systems studied, neurons that are prevented from establishing peripheral contacts die (1–3, 5–7). In some systems, such neurons may show other indications of failure to proceed along a normal course of differentiation, even before cell death. For example, the normal elaboration or rough endoplasmic reticulum fails to occur in peripherally deprived avain ciliary ganglion cells (8), and the sprouting of collateral axons fails to occur in the ciliary and trochlear ganglia (7, 8).

If at some later time the communication between neuron and target is interrupted either by axotomy (9, 10) or application of colchicine (9, 11), a number of changes ensue. Synaptic transmission onto the cells in question is depressed (9–12), there may be a reduction in the postsynaptic sensitivity to transmitter (13, 14), and the presynaptic terminals may physically retract from the neurons (10, 11). The neurons may also show changes in excitability (12) and in the activity of various enzymes (15, 16). Finally, axotomy may also result in cell death (17).

It is clear, then, that the peripheral target is essential for survival and for normal phenotypic differentiation of neurons. What is lacking is an understand-

119

ing of the detailed cellular mechanisms by which the target structure exerts its influence. In general, several possibilities exist. It is possible that the target may supply the neurons with essential trophic factor(s). For instance, nerve growth factor (NGF) has been shown to prevent a number of axotomy-induced alterations (18) in sympathetic neurons. Furthermore, it is retrogradely transported (19), and NGF obtained via retrograde transport has been shown to allow survival of sympathetic neurons in culture (20).

The role that synapse formation may play in the retrograde transport of trophic factors in normal development has not yet been clearly defined. It is also possible that the neuron could detect some alteration in the axonal endings associated with synapse formation per se. This could then exert influence on the cell independent of target-derived trophic factors. Finally, contact with the target and synapse formation may be necessary for normal functional activity. Some event associated with functional activation might directly affect different aspects of neuronal differentiation.

It is important to emphasize that each or all of these potential modes of interaction with the target may occur during neuronal development, and that different aspects of neuronal differentiation may be dependent on different types of interaction. These interactions have been best studied in somatic and autonomic motoneurons. This paper will focus on one of the most completely studied systems, the avian ciliary ganglion. We review what has been determined about the nature of these interactions from normal or manipulated in vivo development, and we show how these interactions can be further dissected by controlled experiments in cell culture.

Neuronal Survival

The chick ciliary ganglion is a parasympathetic autonomic structure composed of approximately 3,500 neurons that innervate the striated iris and ciliary muscles (ciliary cells) and the smooth choroidal muscles (choroid cells) within the eye (2, 21). The ciliary cells send their axons out 3 main ciliary nerve branches, each of which innervates a characteristic part of the target (22) (Fig. 1). Both ganglionic and peripheral synapses are cholinergic.

After early ablation of the peripheral target, ganglion cells differentiated normally up to a point, sending out axons and receiving functional connections from preganglionic fibers (2). However, most cells later died between developmental stages (St) 34 and 40 (day 8 to 14 of a 21-day incubation period). During normal development, approximately half of the original complement of 6,200 cells also died during the same stages (2, 3). Some ultrastructural differences were observed in comparisons of normal cell death with that induced by peripheral target removal (8). Nonetheless, these results were taken to indicate that interaction with the peripheral target is required for neuronal survival, and that neurons are normally produced in excess and compete for some aspect of their target. Those that lose the competition die (8).

If this hypothesis is valid, it should be possible to rescue neurons by increasing the amount of available peripheral target. Indeed, this procedure has been shown to rescue at least some of the neurons normally destined to die in the chick spinal cord (23). Similar results were achieved in the ciliary ganglion by

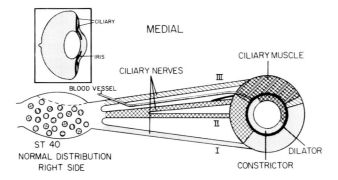

Fig. 1. Schematic diagram of the peripheral innervation pattern of the ciliary population of the avian ciliary ganglion. Each of the main ciliary nerve branches emanating from the ganglion innervates different parts of the target: branch I (stippled) innervates the iris constrictor and the lateral portion of the ciliary muscle; branch II (cross-hatched) innervates intermediate areas of the ciliary muscle as well as the iris constrictor; branch III (hatched) innervates only the medial portion of the ciliary muscle. A small branch (solid) emerging from branch II innervates the iris dilator. The cell bodies that project from each of these nerves are not localized, but are distributed throughout the ciliary portion of the ganglion. *Inset*: Sagittal section bisecting the lens of the eye, showing the position of the intrinsic eye muscles. (Reprinted with permission from Pilar G, Landmesser L, Burstein L: Competition for survival among developing ciliary ganglion cells. J Neurophysiol 43:233–253, 1980.)

keeping the peripheral target constant, but reducing the number of competing ganglion cells (22). By axotomizing 2 of the 3 ciliary nerve branches between St 32 and 34 (7- to 8-day incubation), the cells projecting out these branches were caused to die. This reduced the ciliary cell population from a mean ± SD of 1,523 ± 339 to 529 ± 117 cells. We then determined whether any of the cells projecting out the intact branch (branch III in Figure 1) could be saved by this procedure.

It was observed that the number of cells projecting out branch III was normally reduced from 948 ± 131 to 302 ± 66 cells during the cell death period. However, in the experimental series, the number of cells was reduced to only 549 ± 97. It was therefore possible to rescue approximately 40% of the cells that normally would have died.

These results were interpreted as showing that neurons normally compete with each other for survival. Competition was also implicated in slowing the rate of neuronal maturation because axons from such reduced populations of ganglion cells became larger and were myelinated sooner than were contralateral control ganglion cells (22). It was assumed that the neurons were probably competing for some aspect of their peripheral target, but it was not possible to define exactly what this was. It was also not possible to define why certain neurons survived, whereas others died. Why did some neurons appear fit? Finally, why were we not able to rescue all of the neurons? It seemed that many of these questions would be difficult to answer in a convincing manner in the relatively complicated in vivo system, where it was difficult to assess the behavior of individual neurons. Dissociated ciliary cells in culture were therefore studied in an effort to learn more about the factors affecting neuronal survival (24) and to facilitate study of neuromuscular interdependence.

Neuronal Survival Protein

Parasympathetic ciliary neurons had resisted successful long-term culture, presumably because a "growth factor" similar to NGF had not been isolated (25). Our discovery of methods that allowed long-term culture of the neurons (24, 26, 27) led to an effort to isolate the factors responsible, an effort that was also conducted in several other laboratories (28–30). All of these efforts have focused on the peripheral target as a source of the appropriate trophic agent: the usual muscle target (28), other muscle tissues (29), culture medium conditioned by muscle (25, 30), or whole embryo (24). However, most investigators have not studied long-term survival, relying instead on short-term (1- to 4-day) assays of trophic activity. Because of these and other methodologic differences, and because of the state of rapid flux of this research, the question of the role of specific trophic agents transferred from the periphery during development cannot now be answered. However, several salient observations are available.

In contrast to the situation in vivo, all of the neurons of the ciliary ganglion can survive for 1 month in culture (24, 31) when they are dissected and dissociated before to the normal cell death period. In our hands, long-term survival depends on a relatively small protein termed (neuronal survival protein (NSP) of molecular weight $\simeq$ 12,000) daltons. This protein can be purified from a saline extract of 8- to 10-day embryos (Tuttle JB, Pilar G, Greene C, Lucas-Lenard J: unpublished observations). The presence of striated muscle in coculture will also support survival (32). Thus, in cell culture, all of the neurons ordinarily destined to die can be rescued either by an appropriate target tissue or by the inclusion of NSP in the culture medium. It is reasonable to adopt as a working hypothesis that the target dependence for neuronal survival in vivo derives from the ability of the target to supply a protein similar or identical to NSP. Furthermore, the neurons that normally die in vivo do not do so as the result of some fatal defect, but rather, the lack of appropriate trophic support. However, as our other studies (see later) have shown, survival alone does not ensure normal and complete development.

Maturation of Neuromuscular Junctions

There have been many studies of the embryologic development of the neuromuscular system (33–35). Nonetheless, a definitive correlation in the same system between the maturation of acetylcholine (ACh) machinery and the functional and structural changes during development has not been made. Our investigations of the avian iris neuromuscular junction in vivo demonstrated a striking temporal correlation between synaptic reliability, the response of ACh synthesis to demand, and the morphologic transformation of multiple undifferentiated endings to a large nerve terminal (Vaca K, Pilar G, Tuttle J: unpublished observations).

These changes are illustrated in Figures 2 and 3, which include information from the time of formation of initial junctions until synaptic maturation was reached. Figure 2 shows the time course of the several parameters of neuro-muscular development studied, and Figure 3 illustrates the prodigious ultra-structural alterations of the iris synaptic region.

The activities of choline acetyltransferase (CAT) and acetylcholinesterase (AChE) (Fig. 2A) were measured in the iris, and their developmental courses were compared with physiologic and morphologic findings at the same synapses (Figs. 2B, C). These enzymes are involved in the metabolism of ACh, the transmitter in the peripheral neuromuscular junctions formed by the ciliary nerve terminal on the iris muscle.

Because CAT is transported from the soma to the terminals, the presence of CAT was used as an index of the enzyme activity in the ganglion cell. Virtually all CAT activity measured in the iris preparation was localized to the ciliary nerve endings, whereas AChE is primarily postsynaptic (36). Before the formation of neuromuscular junctions (St 26, or 5 days of incubation), low but measurable CAT activity was assayed in the iris terminal, an indication that ganglion cells were biochemically differentiated as cholinergic neurons at this time.

When neuromuscular junctions started to form (St 34, or 8 days of incubation) there was a 200-fold specific increase in CAT, a reflection of an increased synthesis of the enzyme in the ganglion cell somas (36). Consequently, it was hypothesized that the synapse formation triggers CAT synthesis, the implication being that the neurons respond to a signal ascending the axon from the terminal. In other words, the target organ, iris muscle, instructs the neuron into its secretory state. The nerve terminals also formed multiple small contacts between the axons and the target myoepithelial cells, and these early contacts had sparse synaptic specialization (Fig. 3A). Later (St 41), synaptic vesicles were more conspicuous; they were usually heterogeneous in shape, and several endings commonly abutted the postsynaptic membrane (Fig. 3B).

There also occurred a 2-fold increase in AChE at St 34; a more marked increase was observed later, after junctions were established (St 38 to 40) (Fig. 2A). The developmental sequence of largely postsynaptic AChE activity probably reflects AChE induction in the subneural region, and may suggest that the specific induction of AChE in the postjunctional cells is due to an influence of the prejunctional neuronal element.

The graph of Figure 2 also illustrates later changes that took place during the maturation of the neuromuscular apparatus. The CAT activity (Fig. 2A) continuously increased over time, coinciding with the initially slow growth of the nerve terminals (St 40 to 1 day after hatching). At St 41 the endings began to have the morphologic appearance of mature terminals containing an increas-ing number of synaptic vesicles (Fig. 3B) (Vaca K, Pilar G, Tuttle J: unpublished observations). By 2 days after hatching, CAT activity again increased more rapidly, coinciding with the enlargement of the nerve terminals (Fig. 3C). At this point, endings as long as 30 μm were not uncommon. The latest inflection of the AChE activity curve (Fig. 2C, 1 day) apparently once again followed the pattern of growth of muscle fibers, as evidenced by the increase of the amount of protein measured in the iris (Fig. 2B).

The ability to synthesize ACh was also studied over the same developmental period. The precursor for ACh, choline (Ch^+), is taken up via a Na^+-dependent

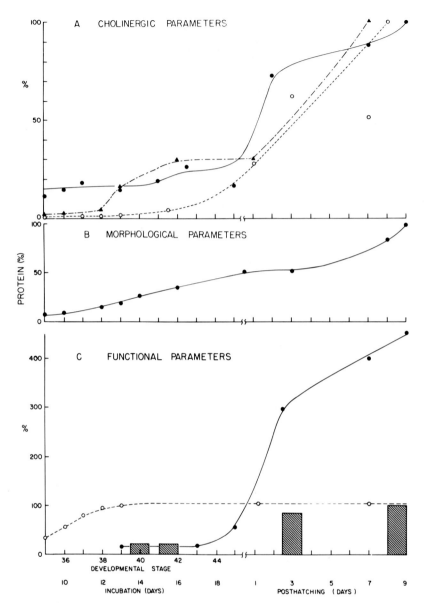

Fig. 2. Biochemical, morphologic, and functional parameters of the maturation of the avian iris neuromuscular junctions during development. To observe the correlation in the time course of the different parameters, all original data were plotted as percentages of the mature values (10 days after hatching). (**A**) Choline acetyltransferase activity (●) is given as a percentage of acetylcholine (ACH) synthesized/8 min/iris. Data are from Chiappinelli and colleagues (36). Acetylcholinesterase (▲) is given as a percentage of ACh hydrolized/hr/iris. Sodium-dependent ACh synthesis/iris (○) is given as a percentage of total ACh synthesis; results are unpublished data of Vaca, Pilar, and Tuttle. (**B**) Morphologic parameters. Development pattern of total protein content of the iris muscle. This graph from Chiappinelli and associates (36) should be consulted with the ultra-structural samples of the neuromuscular contacts illustrated in Figure 3, at their different stages of development. (**C**) Functional parameters. Neuromuscular transmission (○) is

124

high-affinity transport system that is primarily localized to the nerve terminals (37). This uptake mechanism is closely associated with ACh synthesis: after AChE inhibition, more than 96% of the Ch^+ taken up via the high-affinity pathway is acetylated (38). Because nearly all ACh formed in the nerve terminals is dependent on the presence of extracellular Na^+, the time of appearance of the high-affinity carrier was studied by measuring the level of Na^+-dependent ACh synthesis (Fig. 2A). The process is detectable when neuromuscular junctions are first formed, and remains essentially unchanged until hatching time, when a substantial increase in transport is clearly observable. Of course, CAT activity also increases during the same time period (Fig. 2A).

Two physiologic landmarks punctuate the developmental course of the iris neuromuscular apparatus. One is the first appearance of neuromuscular transmission at St 34. There occurs at that time a concurrent increase in CAT activity as well as augmented Na^+-dependent ACh synthesis (36, and Vaca K, Pilar G, Tuttle J: unpublished observations). The second physiologic landmark takes place around hatching time, when pupillary reflex activity becomes necessary and a sustained contraction is required for accommodation. Contraction can be maintained because the neuromuscular transmission is highly efficient.

This was examined by studying synaptic transmission in isolated iris preparations during periods of prolonged stimulation. Postsynaptic electrical activity remained unchanged during repetitive ciliary nerve stimulation (Fig. 2C). This is in marked contrast to the readily fatigued synapses observed in the embryonic tissue under similar conditions of nerve stimulation. The small hatched bars at St 40 and 42 show the decrease in amplitude of the postsynaptic response after 30 seconds of the initiation of electrical stimulation. This transmission block is presynaptic in origin, for even after prolonged indirect stimulation, the iris responds to direct electrical stimuli with contraction (36, and Vaca K, Pilar G, Tuttle J: unpublished observations).

The strikingly high safety factor for synaptic transmission in the mature iris would seem to require an efficient synaptic capacity to synthesize ACh, and this was indeed observed (Fig. 2A). But most remarkable was the response of ACh synthesis to a conditioning depolarization (Fig. 2C). The Na^+-dependent ACh synthesis at hatching increased 5-fold after challenge with a high extracellular K^+ concentration, $[K^+]_o$. It was of interest to observe that large endings virtually filled with synaptic vesicles had developed at this time (Fig. 3C).

---

shown as a percentage of transmission through iris neuromuscular junctions, from the data of Chiappinelli and colleagues (36), determined by comparing iris aperture elicited by tetanic nerve stimulation and contraction stimulated by high extracellular K^+ concentration ($[K^+]_o$). The ACh synthesis on demand (●) is shown as Na^+-dependent ACh synthesis in response to high $[K^+]_o$ conditioning depolarization; these are unpublished data of Vaca, Pilar, and Tuttle. Bars indicate efficacy of neuromuscular transmission, measured as the area under the extracellular recordings of electrical activity of the iris muscle elicited by 20-Hz repetitive stimulation. Each bar is the ratio of the initial response to the area of the response 30 seconds after the initiation of the electrical pulses. Thus, the ratio represents an index of the ability of the synapses to withstand fatigue.

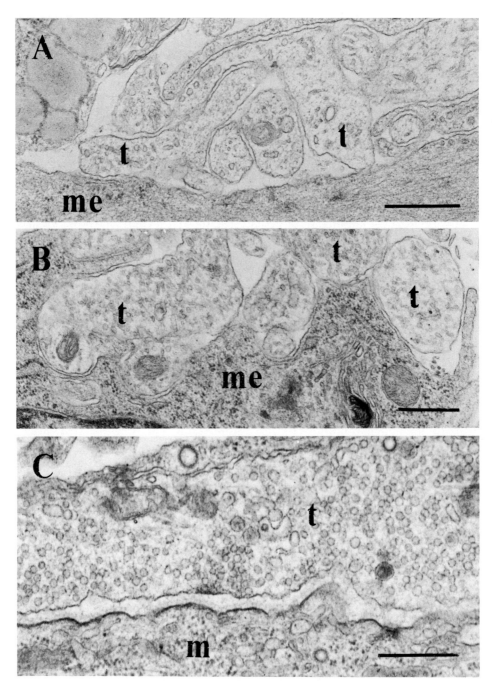

Fig. 3. Nerve-muscle contacts between ciliary endings and iris. Electron micrographs of isolated avian iris fixed in 2% glutaraldehyde, postfixed in 1% osmium tetroxide, embedded in Epon, and sectioned along the longitudinal axis of the muscle fibers. Thin sections were stained with uranyl acetate and lead citrate. Bar represents 0.5 μm; m, muscle; me, myoepithelial cell; t, nerve terminal. (**A**) The St 39 group of axons and nerve terminals in possible synaptic contact with a myoepithelial cell, characterized by a packed filamentous structure that confers to the cell an electron-dense appearance.

Synthesis in the embryonic terminals was unresponsive to such stimuli, which explains the easy fatigability of the embryonic synapses.

Several conclusions can be drawn from the temporal correlation of functional, biochemical, and morphologic alterations during the formation and maturation of the iris neuromuscular junctions. The initial synaptic contacts require only a minimum of specialization to assure transmission across the iris junctions. Only after functional demands occur around hatching is there a rapid development of the system to the mature form. Thus, activity may modulate the terminal maturation of the synapse.

The transformation of the iris neuromuscular system during development apparently involves several steps. Some reflect an autonomous growth of the embryonic tissues, and others depend on a more complex interaction between the neurons and their peripheral targets. Our studies in vivo provided some clues as to when these interactions took place, but little about the mechanisms or signals involved. In the complex milieu of the intact embryo, it would be an awesome task to characterize these phenomena. Thus, study of nerve terminal maturation and its dependence on target interaction was continued in primary cell culture, where the homogeneity of this population of parasympathetic motoneurons offers a unique opportunity.

Differentiation In Vitro

The dissociation of neurons for cell culture has been termed a "catastrophic intervention" (39). One necessarily axotomizes, usually denervates, and completely disrupts all of the other normal interrelationships that exist between developing neurons and other associated tissues. Therefore, when a novel cell type is developed as a cultured preparation, it is wise to examine the developmental course in cell culture and compare it when possible to that which occurs normally during embryogenesis. However, the caveat that arises from this interruption must never be forgotten. In one sense, all neuronal development in cell culture exemplifies phenomena of regeneration, rather than embryogenesis, in a vastly altered environment.

Ciliary ganglion neurons apparently adapt quite well to cell culture (24) (Fig. 4A). In fact, it was surprising to find that even more neurons survived in vitro than normally did in vivo; more survived than could be rescued by reduced interneuronal competition (22). Therefore, in addition to isolation of the factor

---

Notice the scarcity of organelles in the terminals, the small size of the appositions, and the multiterminal contacts. (Reprinted with permission from Pilar G, Landmesser L, Burstein L: Competition for survival among developing ciliary ganglion cells. J Neurophysiol 43:233–253, 1980 (**B**) At St 41 several nerve terminals abut onto a myoepithelial cell. No basement membrane is interposed at the contact site, and, as in A, the cleft is approximately 30 to 40 nm, certainly narrower than in the mature stage (C), approximately 100 nm. Synaptic vesicles are heterogeneous in shape and of small dimensions when compared to those present in the mature synapses. (**C**) At 2 days the neuromuscular junction is well developed. This is a portion of an 18-μm nerve terminal filled with round synaptic vesicles; some are aggregated near a presynaptic membrane density, probably a releasing site. The postsynaptic membrane also showed areas of electron density that might represent regions of ACh receptor accumulation.

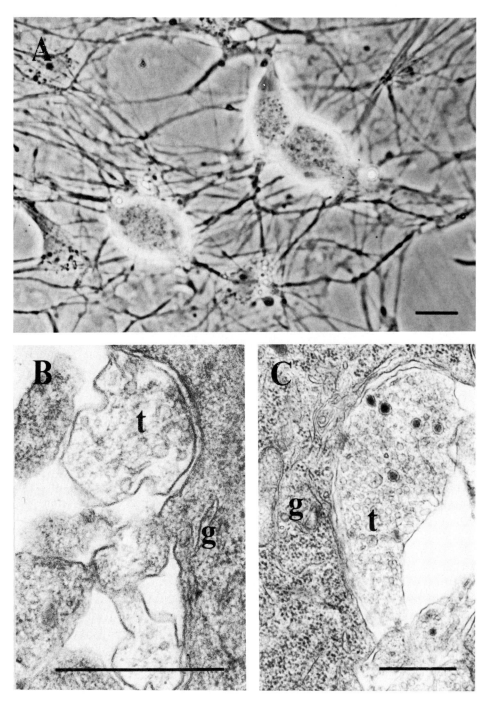

Fig. 4. Ciliary ganglion neurons in dissociated cell culture. (**A**) Phase contrast photograph of neurons after 5 days of culture. Note the extensive network of neurites. Bar represents 10 μm. (**B** and **C**) Electron micrographs of interneuronal synapses formed between cultured neurons. At 8 days in vitro, cultures were fixed in glutaraldehyde, postfixed in osmium tetroxide, dehydrated, embedded in Epon, stained with uranyl acetate and lead citrate, and sectioned for viewing. Cultured neurons readily formed normal-appearing terminals (t) on ganglion cell bodies (g) as well as axons (not shown). Synaptic specializations included varied vesicle population (C) and membrane densities. Vesicle aggregations at points of increased membrane electron opacity were also common. Bar represents 0.5 μm.

128

critical to survival (NSP), examination of the developmental course of the neurons in culture became important.

Intracellular recordings could readily be obtained from the ciliary ganglion neurons as soon as 3 hours after dissociation. In all cases, action potentials could be elicited by direct stimulation through the recording electrode. A survey of the active and passive membrane electrical properties of the cultured neurons showed that they were quite similar to those of neurons in vivo, with only the duration and waveform of the action potential from freshly isolated cells an unexplained variant (24). Similar variations have been observed for dorsal root ganglion neurons in culture (40). At no time was there any evidence of synaptic interaction between the neurons during the initial 3 weeks of culture (41). This was surprising, because an ultrastructural survey of some cultured neurons revealed typical synaptic contacts on the cell bodies and en passant between axons (Figs. 4B, C) (41). Both of these findings were pursued.

An exhaustive search for interneuronal synaptic interaction was conducted. Recordings were obtained in growth medium, normal saline, and high-Ca^{++} saline and included records from cell pairs with direct intracellular stimulation of each in turn and single-cell recordings with extracellular stimulation of other cells and processes. Because the cultures were observed under Nomarski optics at $350 \times$ during these experiments, any apparent contact could be tested under direct visual guidance. Despite this effort, no spontaneous or elicited synaptic activity was ever detected in recordings from more than 150 neurons in more than 10 different culture sets. Sister cultures, however, continued to show typical interneuronal synapses when examined under the electron microscope.

Obviously, ciliary ganglion neurons in culture share many similarities with those in vivo, yet respond to the new situation with some novel properties. Ganglion cells in vivo do not form functional or other synapses among themselves, despite ample opportunity to do so (21, 42, 43). Rather, axons extend directly to the periphery. In culture alone, with no periphery available, interneuronal synapses are formed, but they appear to be nonfunctional. The basis for this synaptic silence was examined.

Cholinergic synaptic transmission depends on 3 factors. (a) The formation of adequate supplies of transmitter (ACh), and thus the ability to take up and acetylate Ch^+ in vivo, demands a high-affinity Ch^+ uptake system and the enzyme CAT (44). Normally, these capabilities are restricted to the synaptic terminal region (45). (b) Sufficient ACh must be released in response to adequate threshold stimuli. (c) There must be postsynaptic sensitivity to the transmitter, usually mediated by specific ACh receptors capable of altering the membrane conductance of the postsynaptic cell.

The transmitter metabolism of the cultured neurons that we examined appeared to be fairly normal (24, 45, 46) (Table 1). The cultures developed quite respectable CAT activity (24) with a time course similar to that seen in vivo. The CAT levels in the cultures, however, tended to plateau after approximately 2 weeks of culture; in vivo, the ganglion and its terminals in the iris continued to accumulate increasing levels of the enzyme up to and beyond the time of hatching. At 1 week in culture, the neurons accumulated ^3H-Ch^+, and 25% to 35% of the total was taken up via the Na^+-dependent pathway. Furthermore, ^3H-Ch^+ accumulated via this process was the predominant source

Table 1. Cholinergic Development of Ciliary Ganglion Neurons in the Presence and Absence of Target Myotubes[a]

Variable	Neurons	Myotubes and Neurons
Basal ACh synthesis (pmol/10^4 cells/30 min)	5.30 ± 1.74	13.00 ± 2.67
Depolarization-stimulated ACh Synthesis (pmol/10^4 cells/30 min)	6.28 ± 1.33	20.92 ± 1.96
% Increase in ACh synthesis (stimulated/basal)	18	61
Ca^{++}-dependent ACh release (pmol/10^4 cells/5 min)	1.10 ± 0.20	5.70 ± 0.60
CAT activity (pmol/cell/60 min)	0.23 ± 0.03	0.46 ± 0.07
% Neurons responsive to iontophoretic ACh	21	100

Abbreviations: ACh, acetylcholine; CAT, choline acetyltransferase.

[a] Pectoral myoblasts (11 days in ovo) were grown to fusion and treated with 10^{-5} M cytosine arabinoside for 48 hours; they subsequently received a plating of ganglion cell dissociate in fresh medium. Control cultures of neurons were plated at the same time onto collagen-coated surfaces. All tests were performed 1 week after the neurons were plated. For the measurements of stimulated synthesis and release of ACh, depolarization was induced with 55 mM K^+; details of the method will be published elsewhere. Values are expressed as the mean $\pm$ SEM for at least 5 cultures.

of Ch^+ for ACh synthesis. Conversion of 50% of the ^3H-Ch^+ transported was typical. Thus, the cultured neurons possessed adequate machinery for transmitter synthesis. When challenged by depolarization in high-K^+ medium, a significant proportion of the ^3H-ACh synthesized was released into the incubation medium (Table 1). However, only slightly more than half of the ACh release required extracellular Ca^{++}; depolarization in nominally Ca^{++}-free saline also caused some transmitter release.

The final requisite for synaptic function, postsynaptic sensitivity, was tested by the iontophoretic application of ACh from high-resistance (47) micropipettes. Soon after (3 to 48 hours) the neurons were dissociated and plated, sensitivity to ACh was easily demonstrated (Table 1). Transmission through the ciliary ganglion is established at the time of dissection, so one would expect freshly dissociated neurons to retain at least a portion of the receptors already active in vivo. However, neurons tested in older cultures, especially during the second week, generally lacked any demonstrable sensitivity to ACh. The combination of large frequency of insensitive neurons, restricted "spots" of sensitivity in those that do respond, and a lack of matching between sites of contact and membrane sensitivity probably accounts for the observed dearth of synaptic interaction. Alterations in receptor dynamics (48), transmitter sensitivity (13), and receptor binding (14) after axotomy have been reported, so the changes we observed in the ACh sensitivity of cultured ciliary ganglion neurons may be related directly to the trauma of dissociation.

The cultures studied above contained only ganglion cells, with no other target available to the developing neurons. Does the availability of a suitable target tissue (striated muscle) alter any of the development so far described? Cultures of pectoral muscle myoblasts were allowed to grow to fusion, and ciliary ganglion neurons were then plated onto the preformed myotubes. One week later, the cultures were tested for their ability to synthesize ACh, release the transmitter in response to depolarization, and respond to iontophoretically applied ACh. In all cases, the results were dramatic (Table 1). The neurons in coculture had a relatively uniform high sensitivity to ACh; none failed to respond. The presence of the muscle tissue prevented the loss of active receptors for the transmitter.

Synthesis of ACh by the cultures was also markedly affected; resting levels of synthesis per cell in the cocultures were 2.5 times higher than those in cultures of ganglion cells alone, and CAT levels were also increased (49) (Table 1). Most striking, though, was the increase in synthesis in response to a conditioning depolarization. The neurons plated alone increased ACh synthesis by only a small amount (18%), whereas those growing on the myotubes more than doubled synthesis of the transmitter (Table 1). Thus, after 1 week in culture with myotubes, the neurons were able to acetylate Ch^+ at a rate comparable to that of mature parasympathetic neurons. It should be noted that in vivo, the ability to respond to the conditioning depolarization with accelerated synthesis does not appear until just before hatching (~21 days), whereas the 8-day ganglion cells plated onto muscle for 7 additional days (total, 15 days) already responded briskly. Thus, their development in this regard was considerably accelerated.

Investigation of these phenomena in culture will continue for some time before definitive statements concerning their relevance to normal development can be advanced. Nonetheless, it is obvious that appropriate target tissues can profoundly influence neurodevelopment both in vivo and in vitro. Synapse formation per se does not seem to be sufficient for normal development. Ciliary ganglion neurons formed ultrastructurally normal interneuronal synapses, yet these nonfunctional contacts were not as trophically effective as the presence of striated muscle, even though the muscle was derived from an alien source (pectoral as opposed to iris muscle). It is also apparent that a specific survival-promoting protein (NSP) does not ensure full neuronal expression of developmental capability in culture, because its presence in the medium does not duplicate the trophic influence of target tissue. In preliminary tests, culture medium conditioned by striated muscle also seems incapable of promoting the development of ciliary ganglion neurons (Vaca K, Tuttle J, Pilar G: unpublished observations). Thus, appropriate synapses with the target tissue may indeed provide an essentially unique influence on neuronal development, whether through the transfer of specific substances or more efficient acquisition of whatever signals are involved. Our continuing work with neurons manipulated both in vitro and in vivo may allow some of these principles of interaction and regulation to be revealed. As the next section will suggest, neuron-target interaction flows in both directions, with each tissue responding to the presence of the other, a symbiosis of development.

NEURONAL INFLUENCE ON MUSCLE DEVELOPMENT

Several influences of nerve on muscle are well documented in a variety of systems both in vivo and in vitro. One example is the dependence of the myosin adenosine triphosphatase on the innervation of striated muscle (50). Another is the influence of nerve on localization of muscle AChE (51). These latter observations are now being extended to in vitro studies (52). Finally, the distribution of ACh receptors in muscle is also regulated to a large extent by motor neurons (53). Iris muscle also displays a striking dependence on neural innervation. The muscle fibers of the iris undergo considerable transformation during embryogenesis. An initial more radial organization of the contractile proteins (similar to that found in smooth muscle) of the precursor myoepithelial cells gradually changes to the regular sarcomeric organization characteristic of the mature iris. This conversion is under nerve influence (22).

We have also discovered during a study of the nature of the ACh receptor in the iris muscle membrane that the receptor changed from the muscarinic to the nicotinic type during the period of innervation. As early as St 36 (10 days of incubation), it was possible to record muscular activity from the iris muscle elicited by electrical stimulation of the ciliary nerves or by application of ACh to the bath. The form of the mechanical response as well as the kind of synaptic receptor involved in the response steadily altered with age. Initially, contraction of the iris is mediated exclusively by muscarinic receptors, but at the time of hatching, transmission is primarily nicotinic (54). The receptor type was determined pharmacologically in iris preparations using quinuclidinyl benzilate (muscarinic receptors) and α-bungarotoxin (nicotinic receptors) (55). To determine whether this alteration of receptor type was due to the presence of nerve activity or was temporally specified, the role played by the ciliary neurons was investigated. Preganglionic and postganglionic denervations were performed on chicks after hatching, when the iris response is almost entirely mediated by nicotinic receptors. After section of the ciliary nerves, but not after preganglionic denervation, the nicotinic component of the response was reduced, yielding a partially muscarinic response. This suggests that the presence of the nerve rather than the activity of the nerve affects receptor expression. The discovery of a "naturally occurring" muscle receptor transformation mediated by the innervating nerve is a novel finding in neuron-muscle interaction; it may help to increase our understanding of this relationship.

In summary, an examination of the development of the avian ciliary ganglion–iris system has provided further insight into the nature of the symbiotic relationship that exists between nerve and muscle (see reference 56 for a review of some other aspects). Continued inquiry into the many unsolved questions raised in this short synopsis should reveal further the intricacies of neuroembryogenesis.

ACKNOWLEDGMENTS

We gratefully acknowledge the participation of Dr. Ken Vaca, Dr. Ramon Núñez (a Muscular Dystrophy Association Fellow), and Christopher Greene in some aspects of this work and for useful discussion. We also thank B Wolmer and P Vaillancourt for help in preparing the manuscript. This work was supported by National Institutes of Health Research Grants NS10338, NS10666, and NS05382, and by the University of Connecticut Research Foundation. JB

Tuttle is a recipient of a fellowship from the National Spinal Cord Injury Foundation.

REFERENCES

1. Prestige MC: The control of cell number in the lumbar ventral horns during the development of *Xenopus laevis* tadpoles. J Embryol Exp Morphol 18:359–387, 1967

2. Landmesser L, Pilar G: Synapse formation during embryogenesis on ganglion cells lacking a periphery. J Physiol (Lond) 241:715–736, 1974

3. Landmesser L, Pilar G: Fate of ganglionic synapses and ganglion cell axons during normal and induced cell death. J Cell Biol 68:357–374, 1976

4. Oppenheim RW, Chu-Wong IW, Maderdrut JL: Cell death of motoneurons in the chick embryo spinal cord. III. The differentiation of motoneurons prior to their induced degeneration following limbbud removal. J Comp Neurol 177:87–112, 1978

5. Hamburger V: Regression versus peripheral control of differentiation in motor hypoplasia. Am J Anat 102:365–410, 1958

6. Chu-Wong IW, Oppenheim RW: Cell death of motoneurons in the check embryo spinal cord. II. A quantitative and qualitative analysis of degeneration in the ventral root including evidence for axon outgrowth and limb innervation prior to cell death. J Comp Neurol 177:59–86, 1978

7. Sohal GS, Weidman TA, Stoney SD: Development of the trochlear nerve: effects of early removal of periphery. Exp Neurol 59:331–341, 1978

8. Pilar G, Landmesser L: Ultrastructural difference during embryonic cell death in normal and peripherally deprived ciliary ganglia. J Cell Biol 68:339–356, 1976

9. Pilar G, Landmesser L: Axotomy mimicked by localized colchicine application. Science 177:1116–1118, 1972

10. Purves D: Functional and structural changes in mammalian sympathetic neurons following interruption of their axons. J Physiol (Lond) 252:429–463, 1975

11. Purves D: Functional and structural changes in mammalian sympathetic neurons following colchicine application to post-ganglionic nerves. J Physiol (Lond) 259:159–175, 1976

12. Kuno M, Llinás R: Alterations of synaptic action in chromatolyzed motoneurons of the cat. J Physiol (Lond) 210:823–838, 1970

13. Brenner HR, Martin AR: Reduction in acetylcholine sensitivity of axotomized ciliary ganglion cells. J Physiol (Lond) 260:159–175, 1976

14. Fumagálli L, de Renzis G, Miani N: α-Bungarotoxin-acetylcholine receptors in the chick ciliary ganglion: effects of deafferentation and axotomy. Brain Res 153:87–98, 1978

15. Cheah TB, Geffen LB: Effects of axonal injury on norepinephrine, tyrosine hydroxylase and monoamine oxidase levels in sympathetic ganglia. J Neurobiol 4:443–452, 1973

16. Reis DJ, Ross RA: Dynamic changes in brain dopamine β-hydroxylase activity during antero-grade and retrograde reactions to injury of central noradrenergic axons. Brain Res 57:307–326, 1973

17. Lieberman AR: The axon reaction. Int Rev Neurobiol 14:49–124, 1971

18. Purves D, Nja A: The effects of nerve growth factor and its antiserum on synapses in the superior cervical ganglion of the guinea pig. J Physiol (Lond) 277:53–75, 1978

19. Hendry IA, Stoeckel K, Thoenen H, et al: Retrograde axonal transport of nerve growth factor. Brain Res 68:103–121, 1974

20. Campenot RB: Local control of neurite development by nerve growth factor. Proc Natl Acad Sci USA 74:4516–4519, 1977

21. Marwitt R, Pilar G, Weakley JN: Characterization of two cell populations in the avain ciliary ganglion. Brain Res 25:317–334, 1971

22. Pilar G, Landmesser L, Burstein L: Competition for survival among developing ciliary ganglion cells. J Neurophysiol 43:233–253, 1980

23. Hollyday M, Hamburger V: Reduction of the naturally occurring motor neuron loss by enlargement of the periphery. J Comp Neurol 170:311–320, 1976

24. Tuttle JB, Suszkiw J, Ard M: Long term survival and development of dissociated parasympathetic neurons in culture. Brain Res 183:161–180, 1980

25. Helfand SL, Smith GA, Wessels NK: Survival and development in culture of dissociated parasympathetic neurons from ciliary ganglia. Dev Biol 50:541–547, 1976

26. Tuttle JB: Dissociated cell culture of chick ciliary ganglion survival and development with and without target tissues (abstract). Soc Neurosci Abstr 3:1529, 1977

27. Tuttle JB, Suszkiw J, Ard M: Neuronal survival and CAT activity in dissociated cell cultures of ciliary ganglion (abstract). Soc Neurosci Abstr 4:596, 1978

28. Varon S, Manthorpe M, Adler R: Cholinergic neuronotrophic factors. 1. Survival, neurite outgrowth and choline acetyltransferase activity in monolayer cultures from chick embryo ciliary ganglia. Brain Res 173:29–45, 1979

29. McLennan I, Hendry I: Parasympathetic neuronal survival induced by factors from muscle. Neurosci Lett 10:269–273, 1978

30. Collins F: Axon initiation by ciliary neurons in culture. Dev Biol 65:50–57, 1978

31. Nishi R, Berg D: Survival and development of ciliary ganglion neurons grown alone in cell culture. Nature 277:232–234, 1979

32. Nishi R, Berg D: Dissociated ciliary ganglion neurons in vitro: survival and synapse formation. Proc Natl Acad Sci USA 74:5171–5175, 1977

33. Filogamo G, Gabella G: The development of neuromuscular correlations in vertebrates. Arch Biol (Liege) 78:9–60, 1967

34. Bennett MR, Pettigrew: The formation of synapses in striated muscle during development. J Physiol (Lond) 241:515–545, 1974

35. Kullberg RW, Lentz TL, Cohen MW: Development of the myotomal neuromuscular junction in *Xenopus laevis*: an electrophysiological and fine structural study. Dev Biol 60:101–129, 1977

36. Chiappinelli V, Giacobini E, Pilar G, et al: Induction of cholinergic enzymes in chick ciliary ganglion and iris muscle cells during synapse formation. J Physiol (Lond) 257:749–766, 1976

37. Suszkiw JB, Pilar G: Selective localization of a high affinity choline uptake system and its role in ACh formation in cholinergic nerve terminals. J Neurochem 26:1133–1138, 1976

38. Beach RL, Vaca K, Pilar G: Ionic and metabolic requirements for high-affinity choline uptake and acetylcholine synthesis in nerve terminals at a neuromuscular junction. J Neurochem 34:1387–1398, 1980

39. Fischbach GD, Nelson PG: Cell culture in neurobiology. In *Handbook of Physiology*, Sec 1, The Nervous System, vol 1, Cellular Biology of Neurons, part 2. Edited by Kandel ER. American Physiological Society, Bethesda, MD, 1977, pp 719–774.

40. Scott BS, Edwards BAV: Electric membrane properties of adult mouse DRG neurons and the effect of culture duration. J Neurobiol 11:291–301, 1980

41. Pilar G, Tuttle JB: Ciliary ganglion neurons form ineffective synapses in dissociated cell culture (abstract). Soc Neurosci Abstr 4:1092, 1978

42. Terzuolo C: Richerche sul ganglio ciliari degli ucelli: connessionie mutamenti in relazione all'eta'e dopo recisione delle fibre pregangliari. Z Zellforsch 36:255–267, 1951

43. Cantino D, Mugnaini E: The structural basis for electronic coupling in the avian ciliary ganglion: a study with thin sectioning and freeze-fracturing. J Neurocytol 4:505–536, 1975

44. Pilar G, Vaca K: Regulation of acetylcholine synthesis in cholinergic nerve terminals. Prog Brain Res 49:97–106, 1979

45. Vaca K, Tuttle JB, Pilar G: Trophic effects of nerve on muscle I. Acetylcholine synthesis (abstract). Soc Neurosci Abstr 5:771, 1979

46. Pilar G, Tuttle JB, Vaca K: Trophic effects of nerve on muscle. II. Acetylcholine sensitivity and release (abstract). Soc Neurosci Abstr 5:770, 1979

47. Dreyer F, Peper K: Iontophoretic application of acetylcholine: advantages of high resistance pipettes in connection with an electronic current pump. Pfluegers Arch 348:263–272, 1974

48. Carbonetto S, Fambrough D: Synthesis, insertion into the plasma membrane and turnover of α-bungarotoxin receptors in chick sympathetic neurons. J Cell Biol 81:555–569, 1979

49. Schrier BK: Surface culture of fetal mammalian brain cells: effect of subculture on morphology and choline acetyltransferase activity. J Neurobiol 4:117–124, 1973

50. Bárány M, Close RI: The transformation of myosin in cross-innervated rat muscle. J Physiol (Lond) 213:455–474, 1971

51. Guth L: Trophic influences of nerve on muscle. Physiol Rev 48:645–687, 1968

52. Fischbach GD, Frank E, Jessell TM, et al: Accumulation of acetylcholine receptors and acetylcholinesterase at newly formed nerve-muscle synapses. Pharmacol Rev 30:411–428, 1979

53. Harris AJ: Inductive functions of the nervous system. Annu Rev Physiol 36:251–305, 1974

54. Nunez R, Pilar G, Vaca K: Muscarinic-nicotinic changes in the cholinergic receptors involved in iris activation during development (abstract). Soc Neurosci Abstr 6:99, 1980

55. Vaca K, Nunez R, Pilar G: Neural control of acetylcholine receptor and contraction in avian iris (abstract). Soc Neurosci Abstr 6:99, 1980

56. Gutmann F: Neurotrophic relations. Annu Rev Physiol 38:177–216, 1976

DISCUSSION

Dr. Richard Bunge: If the neurons are growing with muscle and simultaneously make synaptic contact with one another, do those synaptic contacts then have physiologic activity? Is that known?

Dr. Lynn Landmesser: I have to refer you to Dr. Pilar; this work was carried out in his lab.

Dr. Guillermo Pilar: Yes, synaptic activity was seen under coculture conditions. I might add that morphologically, these interneuronal synaptic contacts are more numerous than are the neuron-muscle contacts. We were a bit surprised at this. Because the muscle is the natural target of these ganglion cells, we expected that the interneuronal synapses would be transitory and would be present in smaller numbers or absent altogether.

Dr. Stephen Thesleff: Have you tried to culture your neurons with higher-than-normal concentrations of extracellular calcium? There are indications that the intracellular level of calcium may govern the synthesis of cholinergic receptors. One of the common things between transmitter effect and usage is the influx of calcium ions. In addition, some tissue culture work by Dr. Shainberg shows that you can increase the number of receptors by affecting the intracellular calcium concentration, either by changing the extracellular calcium concentration or by drugs that release intracellular calcium.

Dr. Lynn Landmesser: We have not tried that.

Dr. Stephen Hauschka: In your coculture experiment, have you done a control in which the neurons were cultured with muscle connective tissue cells and in which no muscle cells were present? The idea here would be to control for nonspecific effects of presumably non-innervated cells on the survival of the ciliary neurons and, consequently, the persistence of ACh receptors.

Dr. Guillermo Pilar: We cultured the ganglon cells with fibroblasts; under these conditions, there was no effect comparable to the effect of muscle.

Dr. Allen Roses: What is the evidence that the synapses between these cells are cholinergic?

Dr. Lynn Landmesser: Are you asking about the synapses that form in culture between these cells?

Dr. Allen Roses: Correct.

Dr. Lynn Landmesser: I guess I can only say that it is circumstantial. The cells are obviously cholinergic in that they release ACh. You saw the evidence that I presented of the whole cultures doing that. Since we did not actually detect cholinergic transmission between them without coculture with muscle, I could not really say that any of the individual ultrastructural contacts that I showed you were indeed cholinergic synapses. However, there is no reason to suspect otherwise.

Dr. Allen Roses: No binding studies of α-bungarotoxin?

Dr. Lynn Landmesser: I do not know of any.

Dr. Guillermo Pilar: As you know, binding studies with α-bungarotoxin have been done in ciliary ganglion cells, and they show 2 fractions of bungarotoxin with different binding affinities for the receptor sites. The original bungarotoxin fraction, the α_2 fraction, which has been isolated by Dr. D. Berg, did not functionally block the receptors of the autonomic ganglion cells. The recently isolated α_1 fraction did block the cholinergic responses in these ganglion cells. We have not yet done the experiments because the bungarotoxin that we have is the one that is ineffective in blocking synaptic transmission in these ganglion cells.

Dr. Daniel Drachman: Some years ago you did a very interesting experiment in which you were able to innervate skeletal muscle with vagus nerves; that situation is similar to the kind of thing you are talking about here. Would you comment on the efficiency and the "trophic" effects, so to speak, of that kind of inappropriate innervation in skeletal muscle?

Dr. Lynn Landmesser: That is a little difficult, because the influences are in the opposite direction.

Dr. Daniel Drachman: Yes, exactly.

Dr. Lynn Landmesser: My feeling is that these inappropriate synaptic contacts were able to maintain muscle fiber properties, to a certain degree, under normal conditions.

Dr. Daniel Drachman: To a certain degree?

Dr. Lynn Landmesser: To a certain degree, although there were some differences from normal. The differences in that situation were less than those in the present situation.

10

Induction of High Acetylcholine Receptor Density at Nerve-Muscle Synapses In Vitro

Gerald D. Fischbach, PhD

Acetylcholine receptors (AChRs) are integral membrane proteins that are packed in the tips of postjunctional folds of adult vertebrate motor endplates at a density in excess of $20,000/mm^2$. Immediately outside of the postsynaptic "gutter" the receptor density is less than $10/mm^2$. We have been investigating how this remarkable clustering of receptors comes about during nerve-muscle synapse formation in vitro. Many of the experiments outlined below have been summarized recently (1).

Chick myotubes can be innervated in culture with dissociated spinal cord neurons, with neurites that grow out of thin slices cut from 4-day, 7-day, or 14-day embryonic cords (explants), or with ciliary ganglion neurons. In nearly all of the studies cited here spinal cord explants were used. Mononucleated muscle precursor cells dissociated from 11-day embryonic pectoral muscles fuse with one another during a 2- to 4-day period after they are plated at a density of 10^3 cells/cm^2 on a collagen-coated substrate. After fusion is nearly complete, proliferating fibroblasts can be eliminated by adding 10^{-5} M cytosine to the medium for 24 to 48 hours. The myotubes that remain are not as firmly attached to the substrate as are those that grow on top of and within a fibroblast bed, and many of them detach after 10 to 14 days. They are electrically excitable, however, and, most important for our experiments, they are sensitive to ACh over their entire surface.

Synapses form rapidly in vitro. We have evoked synaptic potentials by stimulating cholinergic growth cones within 2 hours after they contacted a myotube. We have not yet tested the distribution of AChRs at these very young functional contacts, but after 2 to 3 days of coculture, sharp peaks of ACh sensitivity are present at sites of transmitter release. In every case examined to date, transmitter release, detected by focal extracellular recording or by focal depolarization in the presence of tetrodotoxin (TTX), was restricted to short (5 to 10 μm) segments along the length of motor axon–myotube contacts. Motor axons may course along individual myotubes for several hundred micrometers, so this restricted distribution of active release sites is quite striking.

The finding that AChR clusters are more or less restricted to sites of transmitter release suggests that they are induced in some way by the motor nerve. However, an interesting alternative explanation was evident from the first experiments in which the distribution of AChRs on uninnervated myotubes was mapped in detail. Sharp relative peaks of ACh sensitivity and clusters of α-bungarotoxin (α-BuTx) binding sites similar to those found at synapses can be found on myotubes that have never been exposed to neurons in vitro. Thus, it seemed possible that AChR clusters were present at synapses not because they were induced, but because exploring motor nerves sought out and synapsed on preexisting hot spots.

To decide between these alternatives, Eric Frank and I mapped the distribution of ACh sensitivity over the surface of individual myotubes before and then again after they were contacted and innervated by spinal cord neurites. The answer was clear. Motor axons can induce hot spots; they need not seek out preexisting clusters. We watched several growth cones pass within a few micromotors of hot spots, but none formed synapses at these sites. Altogether we observed 22 new hot spots appear beneath cholinergic neurites. Hot spots on uninnervated myotubes are remarkably stable with time, so the appearance of new clusters at sites of transmitter release cannot be due to chance.

Synapse formation is a rare event in spinal cord explant-myotube cocultures. Only a few of the emergent neurites innervate most of the surrounding myotubes, and sites of transmitter release are difficult to locate. Thus, we do not know whether synapse formation is more likely at preexisting hot spots. We can conclude, however, that such receptor clusters are not necessary for synapse formation.

Anderson and coworkers (2, 3) used α-BuTx coupled with tetramethyl rhodamine (TMR) to study the distribution of AChRs on *Xenopus* myocytes that were dissociated from somites of developmental stage 21 embryos. They noted discrete patches of fluorescence on uninnervated cells, but they also concluded that ingrowing neurites induce new AChR clusters. Their conclusion was based on the observation that distinctive long streaks of fluorescence were found along neurite-myocyte contacts. Uninnervated clusters were ovoid in shape. Because subneurite streaks of fluorescence were observed even when myocyte AChRs were labeled with TMR-α-BuTx before addition of neural tube cells, Anderson and colleagues suggested that clusters form by migration of receptors within the plane of the membrane lipid bilayer.

The fact that AChRs can migrate does not exclude the additional possibility of local insertion of newly synthesized receptors at functional contacts. There is a relatively large number of coated vesicles in the myoplasm at established chick nerve-muscle synapses, and many of these vesicles contain α-BuTx binding sites (4, 5). Specific intracellular binding sites were visualized in saponin-permeabilized cells with horseradish peroxidase (HRP)-α-BuTx conjugates.

Only a few (15%) of coated vesicles could be filled with unconjugated HRP added to the bathing medium, so it is likely that most of them were en route to the cell surface rather than involved in endocytosis.

One coated vesicle-worth of receptor may represent a minimal building block of postsynaptic membrane. The appearance of small fluorescent specks over the surface of *Xenopus* myocytes and chick myotubes exposed to TMR-α-BuTx is consistent with this notion, as are the small islands of intramembranous particles observed in freeze-fracture replicas of cultured muscle cells (6–8).

Quantitative estimates are needed to decide which mechanism (migration or local insertion) is most important at different stages of synapse formation. It may be that receptor migration makes an important contribution to the initial formation of subsynaptic clusters, but that after a few hours the high postsynaptic receptor density is maintained by insertion of newly synthesized receptors.

How do motor nerves induce hot spots? The AChR clusters appear at synapses that form in the presence of α-BuTx or TTX, so it is unlikely that nerve or muscle activity is an important factor. Some indirect evidence for mediation by a water-soluble neuronal factor has been obtained. Saline extracts of embryonic rat brain increase the number of ^{125}I-α-BuTx binding sites and induce receptor clusters on rat L6 myotubes (9). The density of binding sites is quite low in these cells compared to primary rate myotubes, and the distribution of sites ordinarily is quite uniform. Extracts of a neuroblastoma cell line increase the number of receptor clusters on mouse myotubes, but in this system the total number of receptors is apparently unchanged (10). We found that saline extracts of chick spinal cord or brain produce a 4- to 5-fold increase in receptor number and a 40-fold increase in the number of receptor clusters in chick myotubes (11). This effect is not due to a general increase in protein synthesis and it is apparently unique to extracts prepared from neuronal tissue.

In our first experiments we found that nearly all of the activity migrated with material of low molecular weight (less than approximately 2,000 daltons) on Biogel P150 and P4 columns. The activity was soluble in acidified acetone, and it was not destroyed by boiling for 5 minutes. It was, however, destroyed by brief exposure to trypsin. Therefore, we have proceeded on the assumption that one or more small peptides are capable of increasing the rate of AChR synthesis and of altering the distribution of AChRs.

Most recently we have followed procedures for extraction of peptides described by Bennett and associates (12, 13). After extraction in 1% triflou-roacetic acid (TFA), amino acids and salts are removed by passing the material over an octadecylsilica (C_{18}) column. At pH 2.5, peptides are retained and can be eluted with an organic solvent. The eluate is then applied to an analytical C_{18} column and eluted with a 0% to 60% acetonitrile gradient applied under high pressure. Receptor-inducing activity is consistently eluted at 30% to 40% acetonitrile.

In the immediate future we plan to complete the purification and determine the amino acid sequence of active molecules. Specific antisera raised against completely pure or partially purified material will be extremely useful in attempts to decide whether or not material purified from brain homogenates is present in and released from cholinergic motor nerve terminals.

REFERENCES

1. Fischbach GD, Frank E, Jessell TM, et al: Accumulation of acetylcholine receptors and acetylcholinesterase at newly formed nerve-muscle synapses. Pharmacol Rev 30:411–428, 1979
2. Anderson MJ, Cohen MW: Nerve-induced and spontaneous redistribution of acetylcholine receptors on cultured muscle cells. J Physiol (Lond) 268:757–773, 1977
3. Anderson MJ, Cohen MW, Zorychta E: Effects of innervation on the distribution of acetylcholine receptors on cultured muscle cells. J Physiol (Lond) 268:731–756, 1977
4. Bursztajn S, Fischbach GD: Coated vesicles in cultured myotubes contain acetylcholine receptors (abstract). Soc Neurosci Abstr 5:477, 1979
5. Bursztajn S, Fischbach GD: Accumulation of coated vesicles bearing α-BTX binding sites in brain treated myotubes (abstract). Neurosci Soc Abstr 6:358, 1980
6. Yee A, Karnovsky MJ, Fischbach GD: Clusters of intramembranous particles on cultured myotubes at sites that are highly sensitive to acetylcholine. Proc Natl Acad Sci USA 75:3004–3008, 1978
7. Peng B, Nakajima Y: Membrane particle aggregates in innervated and non-innervated cultures of *Xenopus* embryonic muscle cells. Proc Natl Acad Sci USA 75:500–504, 1978
8. Cohen SA, Pumplin DW: Clusters of intramembranous particles associated with binding sites for α-bungarotoxin in cultured chick myotubes. J Cell Biol 82:494–516, 1979
9. Podleski TR, Axelrod D, Ravdin P, et al: Nerve extract induces increase and redistribution of acetylcholine receptors on cloned muscle cells. Proc Natl Acad Sci USA 75:2035–2039, 1978
10. Christian CN, Daniels MO, Sigiyama H, et al: A factor from neurons that increases the number of acetylcholine receptor aggregates on cultured muscle cells. Proc Natl Acad Sci USA 75:4011–4015, 1978
11. Jessell T, Siegel R, Fischbach GD: Spinal cord and brain extracts increase acetylcholine receptor number on cultured chick myotubes. Soc Neurosci Abstr 4:369, 1978
12. Bennett HPJ, Hudson AM, McMartin C, Purdon GE: Use of octadecasilyl-silica for the extraction and purification of peptides in biological studies. Biochem J 168:9–13, 1977
13. Bennett HPJ, Hudson AM, Kelly L, et al: A rapid method, using octadecasilyl-silica, for the extraction of certain peptides from tissues. Biochem J 175:1139–1141, 1978

DISCUSSION

Dr. Donald Fischman: Dr. Fischbach, this very beautiful presentation still leaves us with the question of why all contacts between nerve and muscle do not form functional junctions; presumably, there are unique regions on the myotube that promote the interaction. Can you suggest what properties or what unique inhomogeneities of the muscle cell surface provide that information?

Dr. Gerald Fischbach: I do not know why hot spots are restricted to only a few micrometers along the length of motor axons in the chick cultures. As you suggest, either there is something uniquely receptive about the muscle, or receptor-aggregating material is only released at certain sites and exerts a local action. There are inhomogeneities in the muscle. For example, we have tried to locate the intracellular pool of AChRs that Drs. Fambrough and Devreotes (1975) defined. It appears that Golgi membranes and coated vesicles are concentrated in the myoplasm at synapses. If this is the route of receptor synthesis and insertion into the surface membrane, then it may explain why subneural hot spots are focal.

Dr. Alan Horwitz: Gerry, can you innervate myoballs, and do the myoballs show hot spots?

Dr. Gerald Fischbach: It is possible to grow muscle cells as spheres (myoballs) instead of elongated cylinders. We have not tried to innervate spherical cells. Experiments I have done with ACh iontophoresis indicate some inhomogeneity on spheres, but I have never seen hot spots as striking as those formed on elongated myotubes.

Dr. Richard Strohman: The lag period before the increase in the number of receptors looks a little bit like the TTX effect that Changeaux reported. Do you know anything about your factor in terms of what it might do to relax the fibers and bring on that kind of a response in terms of receptor?

Dr. Gerald Fischbach: I want to make the point that we may be dealing with something different from extrajunctional receptors. Everyone is now well aware that activity plays an important role in regulating the number of extrajunctional receptors. The clustering of receptors at synapses that I have described occurs in the presence of TTX or α-BuTx, so activity probably does not play a role in the formation of synaptic receptor clusters. Brain extracts produce the same effect in the presence of TTX, so the effect is not simply due to inactivity. The latency is a puzzle. I am encouraged that recent experiments suggest that we may be able to reduce the latency by allowing muscle cells to grow for a longer time in vitro before adding the extracts.

inhibitor complex. The characterization of a 22,000-dalton species that has the chemical and kinetic properties of a βNGF precursor and is cleaved by the γ subunit to produce βNGF (38, 39) offers direct evidence for this model. The further finding that epidermal growth factor (EGF) is released from its precursor, proEGF, only by the trypsin-like enzyme (EGF-binding protein) with which it is associated in the gland in its specific HMW complex (HMW-EGF) suggests that the specificity of precursor cleavage implied by the model holds (40).

Aside from its biosynthesis in the mouse submaxillary gland, little is known about specific sites of synthesis in other animals, although there are indications that they are widespread. Many normal or transformed cells secrete an NGF-like material in culture (41–43), but whether effector organs have the capacity to synthesize NGF in vitro, as the retrograde trophic function implies, remains to be proved. The recent finding of significant levels of NGF in the prostate glands of the guinea pig and bull (44, 45) are of considerable interest for exploring further the biosynthetic mechanisms of NGF.

MECHANISM OF ACTION OF NGF

The in vitro studies aimed at elucidating the mechanisms whereby NGF exerts its several roles have used whole sympathetic or sensory ganglia or single-cell dissociates of the ganglia. More recently, several NGF-responsive cell lines have been established from a transplantable rat pheochromocytoma (18, 19, 46). One of these, the PC12 clone, has been extensively used. In medium containing serum, PC12 cells retain many of the properties of the pheochromocytoma, but when exposed to NGF, the cells acquire a number of the properties of sympathetic neurons, including generation of neurites (19, 47). The first step in the modulation of neuronal response by NGF is its interaction with specific NGF receptors on the surface of the responsive cells. The characteristics of this interaction are discussed at some length later. Some of the consequences of this interaction are described first.

Synthetic Events

In an important study, Burstein and Greene (48) reported that NGF-induced regeneration of neurites from PC12 cells does not require ribonucleic acid (RNA) synthesis if the time interval between divesting cells of their original neurites and inducing regeneration is not too long. This led to the suggestion (49) that neurite outgrowth requires both the NGF-induced synthesis of certain gene products as well as the binding of NGF to its receptor to initiate other transcription-independent events. Primed PC12 cells that have once grown neurites require only the latter step to regenerate neurites. The turnover of the NGF-induced gene products means, however, that primed cells revert in time to naive cells. In contrast, the survival function of NGF as expressed in naive PC12 cells does not require transcription of RNA (50).

The induction of tyrosine hydroxylase for the regulation of norepinephrine synthesis by retrogradely transported NGF is also not blocked in vivo by inhibitors of RNA synthesis, although it is in vitro (51–53). This raises the possibility that enzyme induction, like neurite outgrowth, requires both transcriptional and nontranscriptional events. It should also be noted that the transcription events necessary for neurite outgrowth in naive PC12 cells give rise to changes in only a very few proteins in the cell (54).

Linking Mechanisms

With respect to possible linking mechanisms or second messengers, which are brought into play after the NGF-receptor interaction, the role of cyclic adenosine monophosphate (cAMP) is perhaps the most interesting. There is evidence both for (55) and against (56) changes in cAMP induced by NGF. However, cAMP or its analogues induce neurite outgrowth from PC12 cells (55) and modulate the synthesis of the same set of proteins as NGF (57). In contrast, cAMP does not apparently alter the synthesis of the set of glycoproteins in PC12 cells, as does NGF (Burstein DE, Greene LA: unpublished data). The interrelationships among the mechanisms of action of cAMP and NGF need to be explored further.

There is good evidence that the uptake of small molecules is rather rapidly affected by NGF (58), perhaps as a consequence of NGF-induced alterations in Na^+ pump activity. The role of Ca^{++} fluxes is more controversial (55, 59). The cell surface of PC12 cells also changes dramatically and rapidly in the presence of NGF (60). It will be of considerable interest to continue attempts to link all these phenomena to the several mechanisms of action of NGF. One of the keys is an understanding of the NGF-NGF receptor interactions.

NGF Receptors

Sensory and Sympathetic Neurons
Early work from several laboratories identified specific NGF receptors on the plasma membrane of sensory and sympathetic neurons. Most recently, Sutter and colleagues (61) studied single-cell dissociates from 8-day-old chick embryos and provided evidence from both steady-state and kinetic data for 2 distinct saturable receptor sites with dissociation constants of approximately 10^{-11} and 10^{-9} M, respectively. The number of low-affinity receptors is approximately 10 to 20 times the number of high-affinity receptors. The binding of the labeled βNGF is specific for both receptors. The difference in affinities of the 2 receptors arises from differences in the rate at which ^{125}I-βNGF dissociates from the receptors, being about 100-fold faster for the low-affinity site (half-time, ~6 seconds) than for the high-affinity site (half-time, 10 minutes). These 2 different rates of dissociation are observed with cells in which the 2 receptors are loaded with ^{125}I-βNGF to different extents. In addition, the ratio of the ^{125}I-βNGF released with either of the 2 dissociation rate constants depends solely on the occupancy of the 2 sites before dissociation is started. These facts suggest that the receptors act apparently independently.

The same results are obtained when a large excess of unlabeled βNGF is added to initiate dissociation, eliminating the possibility that the low-affinity receptors are generated from high-affinity receptors by negative cooperativity. If negative cooperativity were involved, the addition of unlabeled βNGF would convert all of the receptors rapidly to the low-affinity state and only one rate of dissociation, the fast one, would be observed. Furthermore, although the rate of dissociation is accelerated when unlabeled βNGF is added to increase receptor occupancy, a property previously believed to denote negative cooperativity, it is also increased when the cells are added to a dilute solution of βNGF to decrease receptor occupancy (61). This suggests that in the absence of added βNGF, the dissociation of ^{125}I-βNGF is hindered by its interactions with membrane components other than the receptor. In line with this, vigorous stirring of membrane fractions during the dissociation accelerates the release of ^{125}I-βNGF by disturbing the inhibiting diffusion barrier, bringing the rate close to that obtained with added βNGF (62). Although it is not possible to carry out the same experiment with whole cells, because they rupture during stirring, the experiments with the membrane fractions offer an explanation for the acceleration of dissociation by unlabeled βNGF without invoking negative cooperativity.

These results raise the question of the role of the 2 βNGF receptors and their possible interrelationship. Are the 2 receptors different molecules subserving different functions for NGF, or despite the evidence against conversion of high- to low-affinity receptors, are they simply different states of the same molecular receptor? The question of whether the 2 receptors are related has been approached by studying the biologic and binding activities of βNGF after oxidation of 1 of the 3 tryptophan residues in each of its chains with N-bromosuccinimide (29). This derivative retains approximately 3% to 5% of the biologic activity of βNGF. (Cytotoxicity assays show that this is not due to residual unmodified βNGF).

The decrease in biologic activity is paralleled by a similar decrease in binding; significantly, specific binding to both receptors is decreased to 2.5% of that of βNGF. This result can be interpreted as evidence for the same ligand binding site on the 2 receptors. It should be noted that, at least with sensory neurons, the high-affinity receptors do not arise from internalization of low-affinity receptors together with their labeled βNGF, because similar biphasic steady-state and kinetic data are obtained at 2° C and at 37° C (61). Internalization processes are inhibited at this lower temperature. Sympathetic neurons from chick embryo (11 to 15 days of age) also display the same 2 receptor types in approximately the same numbers and proportions (63).

PC12 Cells

The differences in the dissociation rates of ^{125}I-βNGF from high- and low-affinity receptors provides a method for measuring binding to high- and low-affinity receptors independently. The dissociation curves for ^{125}I-βNGF bound to PC12 cells (64) are similar to those seen with sensory neurons (61). The ^{125}I-βNGF is released rapidly from the low-affinity receptors but more slowly from the high-affinity receptors at 37° C (Fig. 1). Release from high-affinity receptors is almost completely inhibited at 0° C (Fig. 1). Washing PC12 cells with medium containing unlabeled βNGF at 0° C therefore quantitatively releases ^{125}I-βNGF

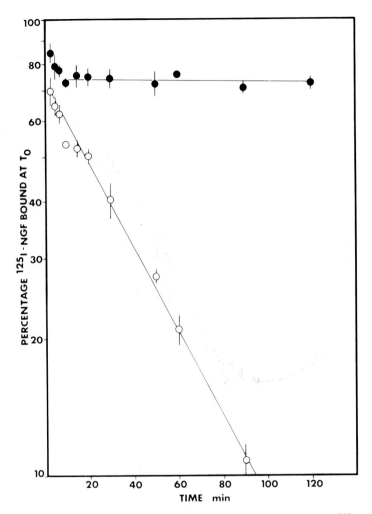

Fig. 1. Kinetics of dissociation of ^{125}I-labeled β-nerve growth factor (^{125}I-NGF) from PC12 cells. The PC12 cells were incubated with 16 pM ^{125}I-NGF for 30 minutes at 37° C. At time zero (T_0), the dissociation reaction was initiated by addition of unlabeled NGF to a final concentration of 85 nM. The dissociation reaction was carried out at 37° C with 1 aliquot of cells (○). A second aliquot was cooled to 0.5° C before the dissociation was initiated, and the incubation was carried out at that temperature (●). Each point represents the mean ±SD of 3 samples. (Reprinted with permission from Landreth GE, Shooter EM: Nerve growth factor receptors on PC12 cells: ligand induced conversion from low to high affinity states. Proc Natl Acad Sci USA 77:4751–4754, 1980.)

bound to low-affinity receptors, but not that bound to high-affinity receptors. Using this method, it is possible to follow the binding to both types of receptor as a function of time, as shown in Figure 2.

High-affinity binding follows the same general time course as total or low-affinity binding (Fig. 2A), but there are important differences. During the first 30 seconds, only low-affinity binding is observed (Fig. 2B). After this lag, high-affinity binding appears, but with a slower time course than that of low-affinity binding (Figs. 2B, C). Thus, ^{125}I-βNGF binds first to low-affinity receptors, suggesting that the high-affinity receptor is generated by a ligand-induced change in the low-affinity receptor. This idea is strengthened by the observation that high-affinity binding continues even when there is no ^{125}I-βNGF in the external medium.

In the experiment shown in Figure 3, binding of ^{125}I-βNGF was interrupted after 2 minutes, and the cells were collected and washed in a βNGF-free medium; this procedure removes the free ^{125}I-βNGF but does not release significant amounts of ^{125}I-βNGF from either low- or high-affinity receptors. When these cells were resuspended in βNGF-free medium, high-affinity binding increased with time and a similar number of low-affinity receptors were lost. Because there was no free ^{125}I-βNGF, the high-affinity receptors must have been derived from the low-affinity receptors.

The high-affinity receptors produced on the PC12 cells are trypsin resistant at 0° C, and the appearance of the trypsin-resistant pool of ^{125}I-βNGF parallels the time course of the appearance of high-affinity receptors. Despite this, a major fraction of the ^{125}I-βNGF bound to the high-affinity receptors can be recovered by adding medium containing unlabeled βNGF, provided that the binding time is of the order of 20 to 30 minutes (see Fig. 1). Thus, the conversion and the appearance of trypsin resistance are phenomena that largely occur on the cell surface.

Sensory neurons from 8-day-old chick embryos show no lag in the appearance of high-affinity binding (Sutter A: unpublished data), suggesting either that once formed, the high-affinity receptors remain stable, even after release of bound βNGF, or that the conversion of low- to high-affinity receptors is much

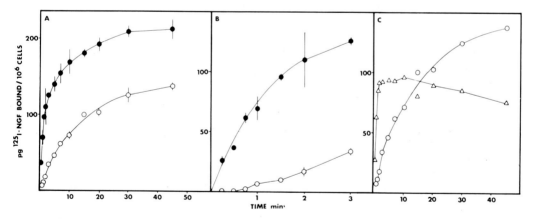

Fig. 2. Kinetics of association of ^{125}I-labeled β-nerve growth factor (^{125}I-NGF) to PC12 cells. The association of ^{125}I-NGF to PC12 cells was initiated by addition of 14 pM ^{125}I-NGF; total binding and high-affinity binding were measured at the indicated times. (**A** and **B**) Time course of association for total binding (●) and high-affinity binding (○). (**C**) Low-affinity binding (△), determined by subtracting high-affinity binding from total binding. Each point represents the mean ±SD of 3 determinations. (Reprinted with permission from Landreth GE, Shooter EM: Nerve growth factor receptors on PC12 cells: ligand induced conversion from low to high affinity states. Proc Natl Acad Sci USA 77:4751–4754, 1980.)

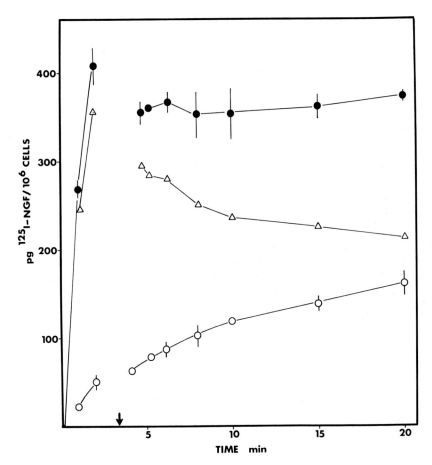

Fig. 3. Effect on nerve growth factor (NGF) binding of removing ^{125}I-NGF from the medium. The PC12 cells were incubated with 35 pM ^{125}I-NGF at 37° C for 2 minutes. The cells were centrifuged for 1 minute at 1,000 g, the medium containing ^{125}I-NGF was aspirated, and the cells were resuspended in the same volume of fresh medium (arrow). Total binding (●), high-affinity binding (○), and low-affinity binding (△) were determined as described in the text. Each point represents the mean ±SD of 3 determinations. (Reprinted with permission from Proc Natl Acad Sci USA 77:4751–4755, 1980.)

more rapid on sensory neurons than on PC12 cells. The actual mechanism of the conversion to the high-affinity state is not yet known, but the data are compatible with the 2-step ligand-receptor interaction put forward in the mobile receptor hypothesis of Boeynaems and Dumont (65) and Jacobs and Cuatrecasas (66). According to this hypothesis, receptors in the plane of the membrane change the apparent affinity with which they bind hormone when they interact with other effector molecules in the membrane.

Events After Binding. The PC12 cell handles the receptor-bound ^{125}I-βNGF in two ways. (*a*) It can internalize the ^{125}I-βNGF and its receptor and degrade them in the lysosomes, subsequently releasing ^{125}I-tyrosine into the medium.

(b) It can internalize the ^{125}I-βNGF receptor complex and translocate it to the nucleus (67). The internalization and degradation of the bound ^{125}I-βNGF is the first major event that occurs after binding of ^{125}I-βNGF to PC12 cells on plates (Layer P: unpublished observations). Under conditions in which the cytoskeleton of the cell is less organized, e.g., cells in suspension, the degradative phase is less pronounced. Probably as a consequence, the lag before ^{125}I-βNGF appears in the nucleus is quite short (67). The translocation of ^{125}I-βNGF from the surface of the cell to the nucleus is temperature sensitive, supporting the notion that it is mediated by vesicular bound ^{125}I-βNGF.

The nuclear receptors for NGF are located on the inner nuclear matrix and not on the chromatin of the PC12 cell. Although the high-affinity nuclear receptor has the same dissociation constant as its plasma membrane counterpart, it differs from the latter in its resistance to solubilization by Triton X-100. When PC12 cells are exposed to ^{125}I-βNGF, the cells and the nuclei enlarge, and the amount of ^{125}I-βNGF translocated to the nucleus is roughly equal to the increase in the number of receptors on the nucleus, suggesting that the ^{125}I-βNGF receptor complex may be inserted as a unit into the nuclear membrane.

The degradative phase for PC12 cells on a substratum lasts for approximately 3 to 5 hours, and no translocation to the nucleus occurs during this time. Thereafter, ^{125}I-βNGF appears in the nucleus and the amount steadily increases during the next 5 to 6 days in culture to reach approximately 10% to 15% of the total ^{125}I-βNGF bound to the cell. Neurite outgrowth is apparent after an even longer lag, typically becoming visible after approximately 24 hours. In long-term experiments, there is a rough correlation between the amount of nuclear bound ^{125}I-βNGF and the number of cells that possess neurites. The ^{125}I-βNGF that is translocated to the nucleus remains intact, as judged by electrophoresis on polyacrylamide gels in the presence of sodium dodecyl sulfate of ^{125}I-βNGF from isolated and highly purified nuclei.

Physiologic Relevance of Nuclear Translocation. Which of the two fates of the internalized NGF produces the signal for neurite outgrowth: its degradation in the lysosomes, or its translocation to the nucleus? Evidence in favor of the latter has now been obtained by interfering with binding and internalization in a specific manner using anti-βNGF antibody. A rapidly responding variant of the PC12 cell, the PCR cell, was used in these experiments. The cells were continuously incubated with ^{125}I-βNGF in monolayer and anti-βNGF antibody was added at increasing time intervals after the addition of label. The subsequent appearance of ^{125}I-βNGF in the nucleus was determined at 24 hours. Addition of antibody at any time up to 4 hours prevented translocation to the nucleus. With longer pulses, increasing amounts of ^{125}I-βNGF appeared on the nucleus. When the cells were examined at 24 hours for neurite outgrowth before the nuclei were isolated, the commitment to neurite outgrowth closely paralleled the curve for nuclear binding. No neurite outgrowth occurred when antibody was added within the first 4 hours, but increasing numbers of cells generated neurites as the nuclear binding increased. It appears, therefore, that translocation to the nucleus is a prerequisite for the generation of a neurite.

The nuclear binding that is measured in these time course experiments is high-affinity binding, which raises the interesting possibility that it is the ^{125}I-βNGF internalized on high-affinity, but not low-affinity, receptors that is translocated to the nucleus. One can then ask, is lysosomal degradation restricted to ^{125}I-βNGF internalized on low-affinity receptors? If so, this would suggest that vesicles carrying high- and low-affinity receptors travel through the cell on entirely separate pathways. Alternatively, if vesicles containing high-affinity receptors are also transported to lysosomes and degraded, then nuclear translocation results from a fraction of the internalized ^{125}I-βNGF that bypasses the lysosomal pathway after the major degradative phase of the cell's reaction to ligand binding has occurred.

CONCLUSION

Evidence that the translocation of intact NGF to the nucleus of PC12 cells is crucial to initiation of neurite outgrowth emphasizes the role of this translocation in one of the long-term effects of NGF. The question then remains as to whether any of the short-term effects of NGF, such as changes in membrane permeability or rapid fluxes in cAMP content, link into and are part of the neurite outgrowth mechanism or subserve entirely different roles for NGF. The availability of the PC12 clonal cell line makes it possible to seek answers for these questions.

ACKNOWLEDGMENTS

This work was supported by grants from the National Institute of Neurological and Communicative Diseases and Stroke (NS-04270) and the American Cancer Society (BC-325). GE Landreth was supported by a National Institutes of Health (NIH) National Research Service Award; BA Yankner, by the Medical Scientist Training Program (NIH Training Grant GM 07635); and P Layer, by Fellowships from the Deutscheforschungsgemeinshaft and NATO.

REFERENCES

1. Levi-Montalcini R: The nerve growth factor: its mode of action on sensory and sympathetic nerve cells. Harvey Lect 60:217–259, 1966
2. Levi-Montalcini R, Angeletti PU: Nerve growth factor. Physiol Rev 48:534–569, 1968
3. Levi-Montalcini R, Booker B: Destruction of the sympathetic ganglia in mammals by an antiserum to the nerve growth protein. Proc Natl Acad Sci USA 46:384–391, 1960
4. Levi-Montalcini R, Angeletti PU: Immunosympathectomy. Pharmacol Rev 18:619–628, 1966
5. Dolkart-Gorin P, Johnson EM: Experimental auto-immune model of nerve growth factor deprivation: effects on developing peripheral sympathetic and sensory neurons. Proc Natl Acad Sci USA 76:5382–5386, 1979
6. Hendry IA: The effects of axotomy on the development of the rat superior cervical ganglion. Brain Res 90:235–244, 1975
7. Hendry IA: The response of adrenergic neurons to axotomy and nerve growth factor. Brain Res 94:87–97, 1975

8. Stöckel K, Thoenen H: Retrograde axonal transport of nerve growth factor (NGF): specificity and biological importance. Brain Res 85:337–341, 1975

9. Thoenen H, Otten U, Schwab M: Orthograde and retrograde signals for the regulation of gene expression: the peripheral sympathetic nervous system as a model. In *The Neurosciences Fourth Study Program*. Edited by Schmitt FO, Worden FE. MIT Press, Cambridge, MA, 1979, pp 911–928

10. Hendry IA, Stöckel K, Thoenen H, et al: The retrograde axonal transport of nerve growth factor. Brain Res 68:103–121, 1974

11. Paravicini U, Stöckel K, Thoenen H: Biological importance of retrograde axonal transport of nerve growth factor in adrenergic neurons. Brain Res 84:279–291, 1975

12. Levi-Montalcini R: The nerve growth factor: its role in growth, differentiation and function of the sympathetic adrenergic neuron. Prog Brain Res 45:235–256, 1976

13. Gundersen RW, Barrett JN: Neuronal chemotaxis: chick dorsal root axons turn toward high concentrations of nerve growth factor. Science 206:1079–1080, 1979

14. Bjerre B, Bjorklund A, Stenevi U: Stimulation of growth of new axonal sprouts from lesioned monoamine neurones in adult rat brain by nerve growth factor. Brain Res 60:161–176, 1973

15. Szutowicz A, Frazier WA, Bradshaw RA: Subcellular localization of nerve growth factor receptors: thirteen-day chick embryo brain. J Biol Chem 251:1516–1523, 1976

16. Szutowicz A, Frazier WA, Bradshaw RA: Subcellular localization of nerve growth factor receptors: developmental correlations in chick embryo brain. J Biol Chem 251:1524–1528, 1976

17. Zimmermann A, Sutter A, Samuelson J, et al: Serological assay for the detection of cell surface receptors of nerve growth factor. J Supramolec Struct 9:351–361, 1978

18. Tischler AS, Greene LA: Nerve growth factor-induced process formation by cultured rat pheochromocytoma cell. Nature 258:341–342, 1975

19. Greene LA, Tischler AS: Establishment of a noradrenergic clonal line of rat adrenal pheochromocytoma cells which respond to nerve growth factor. Proc Natl Acad Sci USA 73:2424–2428, 1976

20. Unsicker K, Chamley JH: Growth characteristics of postnatal rat adrenal medulla in culture. Cell Tissue Res 177:247–268, 1977

21. Aloe L, Levi-Montalcini R: Nerve growth factor-induced transformation of immature chromaffin cells in vivo into sympathetic neurons: effect of antiserum to nerve growth factor. Proc Natl Acad Sci USA 76:1246–1250, 1979

22. Server AC, Shooter EM: Nerve growth factor. Adv Protein Chem 31:339–409, 1977

23. Angeletti RH, Bradshaw RA: Nerve growth factor from mouse submaxillary gland: amino acid sequence. Proc Natl Acad Sci USA 68:2417–2420, 1971

24. Frazier WA, Angeletti RH, Bradshaw RA: Nerve growth factor and insulin. Science 176:482–488, 1972

25. Schwabe C, McDonald JK: Relaxin: a disulfide homolog of insulin. Science 197:914–915, 1977

26. Rinderknecht E, Humbel RE: The amino acid sequence of human insulin-like growth factor I and its structural homology with proinsulin. J Biol Chem 253:2769–2776, 1978

27. Rinderknecht E, Humbel RE: Primary structure of human insulin-like growth factor II. FEBS Lett 89:283–286, 1978

28. Mobley WC, Schenker A, Shooter EM: Characterization and isolation of proteolytically modified nerve growth factor. Biochemistry 15:5543–5551, 1976

29. Cohen P, Sutter A, Landreth G, et al: Identification of tryptophan-21 as essential for the biological activity of mouse nerve growth factor. J Biol Chem 255:2949–2954, 1980

30. Varon S, Nomura J, Shooter EM: The isolation of the mouse nerve growth factor protein in a high molecular weight form. Biochemistry 6:2202–2209, 1967

31. Varon S, Nomura J, Shooter EM: Reversible dissociation of the mouse nerve growth factor protein into different subunits. Biochemistry 7:1296–1303, 1968

32. Burton LE, Wilson WH, Shooter EM: Nerve growth factor in mouse saliva: rapid isolation

procedures for and characterization of 7S nerve growth factor. J Biol Chem 253:7807–7812, 1978

33. Pattison SE, Dunn MF: On the relationship of zinc ion to the structure and function of the 7S nerve growth factor protein. Biochemistry 14:2733–2739, 1975

34. Bothwell MA, Shooter EM: Thermodynamics of the interaction of the subunits of 7S nerve growth factor. J Biol Chem 253:8458–8464, 1978

35. Stach RW, Shooter EM: The biological activity of cross-linked 7S nerve growth factor. J Neurochem 34:1499–1505, 1980

36. Bradshaw RA: Nerve growth factor. Annu Rev Biochem 47:191–216, 1978

37. Young M, Saide JD, Murphy RA, et al: Nerve growth factor: multiple dissociation products in homogenates of the mouse submandibular gland. Purification and molecular properties of the intact undissociated form of the protein. Biochemistry 17:1490–1498, 1978

38. Berger EA, Shooter EM: Evidence for pro-βNGF, a biosynthetic precursor to β nerve growth factor. Proc Natl Acad Sci USA 74:3647–3651, 1977

39. Berger EA, Shooter EM: The biosynthesis of β nerve growth factor on mouse submaxillary gland. J Biol Chem 243:804–810, 1978

40. Frey P, Forand R, Maciag T, et al: The biosynthesis precursor of epidermal growth factor and the mechanism of its processing. Proc Natl Acad Sci USA 76:6294–6298, 1979

41. Longo AM: Synthesis of nerve growth factor in rat glioma cells. Dev Biol 65:260–270, 1978

42. Pantazis NJ, Blanchard MH, Arnason BGW, et al: Molecular properties of the nerve growth factor secreted by L cells. Proc Natl Acad Sci USA 74:1492–1496, 1977

43. Murphy RA, Singer RH, Saide JD, et al: Synthesis and secretion of a high molecular weight form of nerve growth factor by skeletal muscle cells in culture. Proc Natl Acad Sci USA 74:4496–4500, 1977

44. Harper GP, Barde YA, Burnstock G, et al: Guinea pig prostate is a rich source of nerve growth factor. Nature 279:160–162, 1979

45. Harper GP, Thoenen H: Nerve growth factor: biological significance, measurement and distribution. J Neurochem 34:5–16, 1980

46. Goodman R, Herschman HR: Nerve growth factor mediated induction of tyrosine-hydroxylase in a clonal pheochromocytoma cell line. Proc Natl Acad Sci USA 75:4587–4590, 1978

47. Tischler AS, Greene LA: Morphologic and cytochemical properties of a clonal line of rat adrenal pheochromocytoma cells which respond to nerve growth factor. Lab Invest 39:77–89, 1978

48. Burstein DE, Greene LA: Evidence for RNA synthesis-dependent and synthesis-independent pathways in stimulation of neurite outgrowth by nerve growth factor. Proc Natl Acad Sci USA 75:6059–6063, 1978

49. Greene LA, Burstein DE, McGuire JC, et al: Cell culture studies on mechanism of action of nerve growth factor. In *Aspects of Developmental Neurobiology*. Edited by Ferrendelli J. Society for Neuroscience, Bethesda, MD, 1979, pp 153–171

50. Greene LA: Nerve growth factor prevents the death and stimulates neuronal differentiation of clonal PC12 pheochromocytoma cells in serum-free medium. J Cell Biol 78:747–755, 1978

51. Rohrer H, Otten U, Thoenen H: Role of RNA synthesis in selective induction of tyrosine hydroxylase by nerve growth factor. Brain Res 159:436–439, 1978

52. Stockel K, Paravicini U, Thoenen H: Specificity of the retrograde axonal transport of nerve growth factor. Brain Res 76:413–421, 1974

53. Macdonnell PC, Tolson N, Guroff G: Selective de novo synthesis of tyrosine hydroxylase in organ cultures of rat superior cervical ganglia after in vivo administration of nerve growth factor. J Biol Chem 252:5859–5863, 1977

54. McGuire JC, Greene LA, Furano AV: NGF stimulates incorporation of glucose or glucosamine into an external glycoprotein in cultured rat PC12 pheochromocytoma cells. Cell 15:357–365, 1978

55. Schubert D, LaCorbiere M, Whitlock C, et al: Alterations in the surface properties of cells responsive to nerve growth factor. Nature 273:718–723, 1978

56. Otten U, Hatanaka H, Thoenen H: Role of cyclic nucleotides in NGF-mediated induction of tyrosine hydroxylase in rat sympathetic ganglia and adrenal medulla. Brain Res 140:385–389, 1978

57. Garrels JI, Schubert D: Modulation of protein synthesis by nerve growth factor. J Biol Chem 254:7978–7985, 1979

58. Skaper SD, Varon S: Nerve growth factor action on 2-deoxy-D-glucose transport in dorsal root ganglionic dissociates from chick embryo. Brain Res 163:89–100, 1979

59. Landreth GE, Cohen P, Shooter EM: Calcium transmembrane fluxes and NGF action on a clonal cell line of rat pheochromocytoma (PC12). Nature 286:202–204, 1980

60. Connolly JL, Greene LA, Viscarello RR, et al: Rapid sequential changes in surface morphology of PC12 pheochromocytoma cells in response to nerve growth factor. J Cell Biol 82:820–827, 1979

61. Sutter A, Riopelle RJ, Harris-Warrick RM: Nerve growth factor receptors: characterization of two distinct classes of binding sites on chick embryo sensory ganglia cells. J Biol Chem 254:5972–5982, 1979

62. Riopelle RJ, Klearman M, Sutter A: Nerve growth factor receptors: analysis of the interaction of nerve growth factor with membranes of chick embryo dorsal root ganglion. Brain Res 199:63–77, 1980

63. Godfrey EW, Shooter EM: Nerve growth factor receptors on chick sympathetic ganglion cells (abstract). Soc Neurosci Abstr 5:767, 1979

64. Landreth GE, Shooter EM: Nerve growth factor receptors on PC12 cells: ligand-induced conversion from low- to high-affinity states. Proc Natl Acad Sci USA 77:4751–4755, 1980

65. Boeynaems JM, Dumont JE: Quantitative analysis of the binding of ligands to their receptors. J Cyclic Nucleotide Res 1:123–142, 1975

66. Jacobs S, Cuatrecasas P: The mobile receptor hypothesis and cooperativity of hormone binding. Biochim Biophys Acta 433:482–495, 1976

67. Yankner BA, Shooter EM: Nerve growth factor in the nucleus: interaction with receptors on the nuclear membrane. Proc Natl Acad Sci USA 76:1269–1273, 1979

DISCUSSION

Dr. John Bird: Would you care to elaborate on the translocation of the nerve growth factor (NGF) and receptor to the nucleus? Do you have any ideas about how these vesicles that are internalized bypass the lysosomal apparatus?

Dr. Eric Shooter: Not yet. This part of the study has yet to be done in detail. That NGF is carried in internalized vesicles can be fairly readily shown by sucrose gradient analyses of cellular organelles at appropriate times after ^{125}I-NGF binding. However, the time course of transport of the vesicles to various internal organelles such as the nucleus or the lysosome remains to be determined. I described one scheme in which vesicles containing low- and high-affinity receptors travel in the cell by different pathways. An alternative model would be one in which both types of vesicle are initially directed to the lysosomes for degradation; not until all lysosomes were completely filled would vesicles containing high-affinity receptors be allowed to bypass that pathway and go to the nucleus. The use of agents that inhibit fusion of vesicles and lysosomes or inhibit the lysosomal enzymes themselves should allow us to answer this question.

Dr. James Florini: Your initial slide suggested that DNA replication was involved in the mechanism of NGF action. I was under the impression that NGF is usually referred to as not being mitogenic.

Dr. Eric Shooter: Yes, that is correct. The slide included a signal directed at DNA replication only for the PC12 cells. In this regard, there is increasing evidence in a variety of mammalian cells that the control of DNA replication in the replisome occurs on the inner nuclear membrane, the exact location to which NGF (and possibly its receptor) is translocated.

Dr. Richard Bunge: I am a little concerned about the extrapolation from PC12 cells to the superior cervical ganglion adenergic neuron in vivo. Is there not, in fact, evidence of an NGF-independent initial neuritic outgrowth of adrenergic autonomic neurons in the early development of the rat? I am referring to the evidence from Dr. Ira Black's lab. Is there really any evidence that NGF is necessary for the initiation of a neurite in the adrenergic autonomic neuron, which is not a PC12 cell?

Dr. Eric Shooter: The experiments reported by Dr. Black and his colleagues showing that superior cervical sympathetic ganglia from 13- to 15-day-old embryonic mice initiate neuritic outgrowth in the absence of NGF, and indeed in the presence of anti-NGF antibody, are of great interest. It is possible to explain this phenomenon on the basis of the prior exposure of these ganglia to NGF. If this has occurred, the sympathetic neurons might have accumulated enough nuclear-bound NGF to allow for neurite initiation even in the absence of added NGF in vitro. The alternative explanation, as Dr. Black has emphasized, is that the sympathetic neurons in the newly formed ganglion are dependent on another factor before their dependence on NGF.

Dr. Richard Bunge: But there's the paradox. The neuron has not really put out the neurite. You have to speculate that it sees NGF in its immediate environment, not from the target; how can it get NGF from the target until it initiates a neurite that reaches the target? I would like to have you speculate on that.

Dr. Eric Shooter: That is one of the missing links in the whole NGF story. We do not know where NGF is produced in the developing embryo. Where do these embryonic sensory and sympathetic nerve cells get NGF if not from the target? It should be pointed out, however, that neurons do not need neurites to be able to sense and respond to NGF. The cell bodies of primary sympathetic sensory neurons as well as nerve PC12 cells possess specific NGF receptors.

12
Calcium and the Mechanism of Axoplasmic Transport

Sidney Ochs, PhD

Axoplasmic transport, the movement of materials in nerve fibers and dendrites, is recognized as basic to a full understanding of neuronal form and function. The processes of excitability and conduction of the nerve impulse, neurotransmission, neurotransduction, the maintenance of form of the axon and satellite cells, and the trophic effect of neurons on other cells are all dependent on axoplasmic transport and the supply of components needed to maintain those various functions. It remains a valid working hypothesis that some defect in the supply of a trophic meterial or related component carried down to the nerve terminals is responsible for some forms of dystrophy.

Although the general outlines of the phenomenon of axoplasmic transport are well recognized (1–5), the mechanism has not been identified. Two fundamental findings were used to construct a model of the transport mechanism, the transport filament hypothesis (6, 7): *(a)* a wide variety of material, from small molecules to organelles, are transported at the same fast rate; *(b)* metabolic energy is required to maintain transport. Recently, we found that Ca^{2+} is also an essential part of the transport mechanism, and this is the basis for the modification of the original transport filament model described in this paper.

THE BASIC TRANSPORT FILAMENT MODEL

Fast Transport Properties

Using ^3H-leucine injected into the L7 dorsal root ganglion or into the L7 motor neuron region of the cat spinal cord, a consistent and regular rate of fast axoplasmic transport was shown by a crest of labeled incorporated proteins and polypeptides moving down the sciatic nerves at a rate of 410 mm/day (7, 8). Differential centrifugation and gel filtration of portions of the nerve containing the radioactivity in the crest and plateau regions showed that both the crest and

157

the plateau contained a wide range of labeled soluble proteins, smaller polypeptides, and relatively large particles.

Among the latter was a well-defined organelle, the dense-core vesicle (DCV) of adrenergic nerve fibers containing norepinephrine (NE) and dopamine β-hydroxylase (DBH). Using NE and DBH as markers, the DCV has been shown to move at a rate close to 410 mm/day (9, 10). The enzyme acetylcholinesterase (AChE), which was present in a particulate fraction, also moved at this fast rate (11). Even the mitochondrion, a much larger structure, can for a short time move at rates approaching these fast rates (12–14).

Fast transport is not restricted to vesicular or particulate structures. Soluble proteins also can have this fast rate. A particularly interesting example is tyrosine hydroxylase (TH), which was shown by Brimijoin and Wiermaa (9) to have both a fast and slow rate of transport. The list of components that undergo fast transport is now a long one, and small amounts of other substances previously considered to be transported only slowly are now known to undergo fast transport as well (15).

Requirement for ATP

Axoplasmic transport requires a constant supply of adenosine triphosphate (ATP) derived from oxidative phosphorylation (16). This was inferred from in vitro studies in which the usual pattern of axoplasmic transport was maintained when oxygen was supplied (8). Nitrogen anoxia or the administration of cyanide, dinitrophenol, or azide blocks oxidative phosphorylation and ATP formation and, in turn, blocks transport within 15 to 20 minutes (16, 17).

Iodoacetic acid (IAA) was used to block glycolysis and caused a characteristic decrement of ATP with a block of transport 1.5 to 2 hours later (18). The level of organic phosphate (∼P), the combined amounts of ATP and creatine phosphate (CP), fell from a control level of 1.0 to 1.2 μmol/g to approximately half that amount in nerves made anoxic (19) at the same time that axoplasmic transport and excitability were blocked. Similarly, a decrease in ∼P to that level was seen 1.5 to 2 hours after glycolysis was blocked with IAA at the time that fast transport was also blocked. The correlation between the block of fast axoplasmic transport and the decrease in ∼P indicated that ATP is required to maintain the transport mechanism (16).

The Original Transport Filament Model

To account for the variety of components transported and the need for ATP, the transport filament hypothesis was advanced (6, 7). The various species transported are bound to a common carrier, a "transport filament" that is moved along the microtubules by side arms; the energy required for their movement is supplied by ATP (Fig. 1).

In the transport filament model, the Ca^{2+},Mg^{2+}–adenosine triphosphatase (Ca,Mg-ATPase) found in mammalian nerve (20) was considered to be located on the side arms along the microtubules. The side arms would bind to the transport filaments and, in the presence of ATP, change their conformation to pull the filaments and the components bound to them axially in the fiber. We

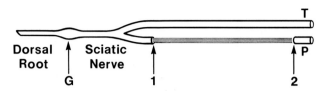

Fig. 1. Schematic diagram of desheathed and sheathed branches of sciatic nerve, showing the dorsal root ganglion (G) and the tibial (T) and peroneal (P) branches. The latter is desheathed from point 1, approximately 35 mm distal to the ganglion, to point 2, approximately 135 mm from the ganglion.

had expected transport to be sensitive to a lack of Ca^{2+} or Mg^{2+} in the in vitro incubation medium. However, until recently, except for some isolated suggestive findings (21), it was generally considered that axoplasmic transport in the nerve fiber did not depend on Ca^{2+}. Fast axoplasmic transport in vitro was maintained as usual in a Ca^{2+}-depleted medium with or without ethyleneglycol tetra-acetic acid (EGTA) added (7, 22–25). The apparent lack of influence of a variation of Ca^{2+} on transport was eventually traced to the low permeability of the perineural sheath to Ca^{2+} (26), as described in the following section.

EFFECT OF IONS

Calcium

Desheathed Nerve Preparation

To show the effect of a depletion of Ca^{2+}, a sufficiently long length of nerve must be desheathed. The preparation that proved satisfactory was made using the peroneal branch of the cat sciatic nerve. The tibial and peroneal branches of the sciatic nerve are readily separated by dividing the epineurium up to a point approximately 30 mm below the L7 dorsal root ganglion. Above this point, the nerve fibers from the L7 dorsal root ganglion cross over to enter their two nerve branches. At a point 35 mm below the ganglion, the sheath was slit down the length of the peroneal branch, which was cut circumferentially at the proximal end and peeled down from the nerve to about 135 mm distal to the ganglion. This left a relatively long length of uniformly desheathed nerve for study of in vitro transport in medium in which the concentrations of Ca^{2+} and other ions could be varied (Fig. 1).

The typical procedure was to inject the L7 dorsal root ganglion of the cat with the precursor ^{3}H-leucine, and allow 2 hours for flow of radioactively labeled proteins down into the fibers of the two nerve branches. Within 2 hours this reaches 2×17 mm/hr = 34 mm. The nerves were then removed, and the peroneal branch was desheathed just below the front of the transported radioactivity, starting at 35 mm below the ganglion. The nerve preparation was then placed in an Erlenmeyer flask containing a given ionic medium for in vitro transport at 38° C and was well oxygenated for the determined time of incubation.

Lack of Calcium

Axoplasmic transport was well maintained in vitro in both the sheathed tibial nerve branch and the desheathed peroneal nerve branch when these preparations were placed in a Ringer solution (Fig. 2).

The overall mean ± SD rates of transport were 17.43 ± 1.53 mm/hr for the desheathed peroneal branch and 17.64 ± 1.54 mm/hr for the sheathed tibial branch. These values were not significantly different from those previously found for fast transport in mammalian nerve (17 mm/hr ≃ 410 mm/day) determined both in vitro and in vivo (21, 27).

In medium containing only isotonic NaCl, in vitro axoplasmic transport was characteristically blocked in the desheathed peroneal nerves (Fig. 3). The decrease in labeled activity began within 30 minutes after exposure to the Ca^{2+}-free medium. The slope fell to the baseline, indicating complete block, 2.6 hours after exposure to the Ca^{2+}-free NaCl medium. In contrast, transport at the usual rate with its usual form was maintained in the sheathed tibial nerve branch. This result is consistent with a large number of earlier observations showing a normal axoplasmic transport in sheathed nerves in vitro in Ca^{2+}-free medium.

A similar block of transport was seen in the desheathed peroneal nerve incubated in a Ca^{2+}-free buffered isotonic sucrose medium, and also when a concentration of 4 mM EGTA was added to a Ringer solution to chelate the Ca^{2+} present (28). Hammershlag and coworkers (22), using a smaller length of

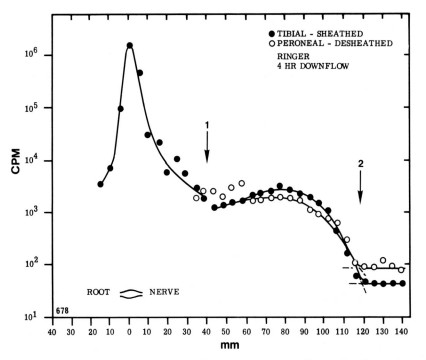

Fig. 2. Four-hour downflow with Ringer in vitro. Arrow 1 shows the time when the nerve was placed in the in vitro Ringer medium. Arrow 2 shows the expected transport distance, calculated from a flow of 17 mm/hr.

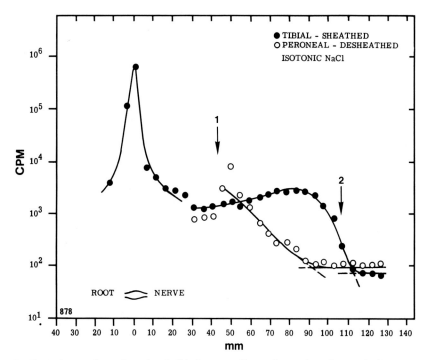

Fig. 3. Four-hour downflow in Ca^{2+}-free medium (isotonic saline solution). Arrow 1 shows the time when the nerve was placed in the isotonic NaCl medium; arrow 2 shows the calculated transport distance.

desheathed frog nerve, confirmed that transport was blocked when Ca^{2+} was deleted from the in vitro medium.

Excess Calcium

When 5 mM Ca^{2+} was added to a buffered isotonic NaCl medium, transport in the desheathed peroneal nerve was maintained at the normal form and rate. The rate of axoplasmic transport was 17 mm/hr. Addition of 5 mM Ca^{2+} to a buffered isotonic sucrose solution produced similar results. Thus, Ca^{2+} appears to be essential for the maintenance of transport. However, a Ca^{2+} concentration of 5 mM is higher than that usually present in tissues or Ringer solution. When 1.5 mM Ca^{2+} (a normal level) was added to isotonic NaCl or sucrose, there was some tendency for the crest of outflow in the desheathed branch to be less prominent and for the front to have a somewhat shallower slope than that normally seen. This indicated that Ca^{2+} could maintain transport by itself at somewhat higher levels, but some other component was needed to maintain the normal pattern of outflow at normal concentrations of Ca^{2+}. The component required was K^+.

When 4 mM K^+ (a level of K^+ usually found in extracellular fluid) was added to incubation medium containing 1.5 mM Ca^{2+}, the outflow pattern of axoplasmic transport was normal (Fig. 4). The rate of axoplasmic transport was the same as that of the sheathed nerves, and the crest and slope of the front were normal. Even with a Ca^{2+} concentration as low as 0.75 mM, the normal

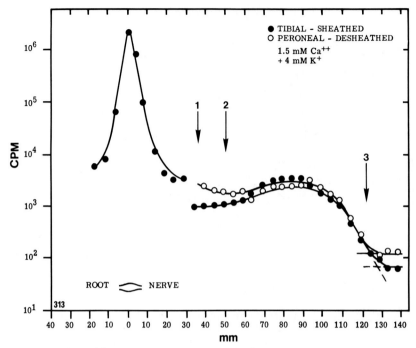

Fig. 4. Downflow in Ca^{2+} medium with 4 mM K^+ added. Arrow 1 shows the time when the nerve was placed in the isotonic NaCl medium; arrow 2, the time when the preparation was placed in isotonic NaCl solution containing 1.5 mM Ca^{2+} and 4 mM K^+. Arrow 3 shows the calculated transport distance.

rate and shape of outflow in the desheathed nerves were maintained. At a Ca^{2+} concentration of 0.5 mM or less, however, transport was impaired and then blocked (28).

Potassium

When 4 mM K^+ alone was added to Ca^{2+}-free NaCl medium, transport was blocked, as in desheathed nerves in isotonic NaCl or sucrose. This indicates that K^+ cannot substitute for Ca^{2+}, but can facilitate the action of Ca^{2+} at the levels normally present in the tissues.

Full transport was maintained when much higher levels of K^+ were present in the incubation medium. Axoplasmic transport appeared to be normal when 75 to 100 mM K^+ replaced Na^+ in the medium, even when no Ca^{2+} was present (28). Presumably, this level of K^+ can cause retention of Ca^{2+} in the fibers.

One can infer from the maintenance of transport in the presence of such high levels of K^+ that depolarization of the membrane does not affect transport. The lack of a close relationship between membrane excitability and axoplasmic transport had earlier been shown by the action of tetrodotoxin or procaine in amounts adequate to block excitability without effect on axoplasmic transport (17); similar results with lidocaine were reported by Fink and associates (29).

Magnesium

To assess the ability of Mg^{2+} to sustain axoplasmic transport, 3 to 5 mM Mg^{2+} was added to an isotonic NaCl medium. Axoplasmic transport was partially maintained, as shown by the somewhat later time at which a block occurred compared to that seen in a Mg^{2+}-free NaCl medium (28, 30): the average time to block of transport in 5 mM Mg^{2+} was approximately 3.3 hours, compared to 2.6 hours in Mg^{2+}-free NaCl or sucrose medium. The addition of 4 mM KCl to the 5 mM Mg^{2+} medium did not significantly further increase the time to block.

The difference between Mg^{2+} and Ca^{2+} in maintaining transport was enhanced when lower concentrations of the two cations were compared. Transport was well maintained in NaCl medium containing 0.75 mM Ca^{2+} and 4 mM KCl, but was blocked in medium containing 0.75 mM Mg^{2+} (28). In addition, Mg^{2+} acted synergistically with Ca^{2+}. Addition of 1.5 mM Mg^{2+} to a solution containing 0.25 mM Ca^{2+}, a concentration of Ca^{2+} too low to support transport by itself, produced a normal pattern and rate of axoplasmic transport. It is possible that Mg^{2+} acts at the same site as Ca^{2+} within the fiber, but it is more likely that Mg^{2+} reduces the efflux of Ca^{2+} from nerves incubated in a low-Ca^{2+} medium and thus maintains the level of free Ca^{2+} within the fibers needed to sustain transport (see *Role of Calcium in Nerve*).

Sodium

With Ca^{2+} in the medium, transport is maintained whether or not Na^+ is present. This indicates that transport is unaffected by external Na^+. However, there is some evidence to suggest that an increased intraaxonal concentration of Na^+ does affect transport. The level of Na^+ in axons can be increased by blocking the Na^+ pump with ouabain (31, 32), and ouabain blocks axoplasmic transport (7, 33). Recent studies using the desheathed nerve preparation have shown that the block obtained with ouabain was more pronounced in an isotonic NaCl medium than a sucrose medium without Na^+ (Ochs S: unpublished observations).

Changes in the Na^+ level of the medium do not affect the intraaxonal level because of the low permeability of the membrane to Na^+. An agent that increases the content of axonal Na^+ by altering membrane permeability is batrachotoxin (BTX) (34). In our earlier studies (35), we found that micromolar concentrations of BTX block axoplasmic transport. The possibility that BTX could increase the Na^+ content in the axons was discounted at that time because a similar block was seen in nerves incubated in isotonic sucrose as well as medium containing Na^+ (35). However, those experiments were carried out using sheathed nerves. Using the desheathed nerve preparation, we recently found that lower concentrations of BTX (18 to 180 nM) blocked transport when nerves were placed in an isotonic Na^+ medium, but not when they were placed in an isotonic sucrose medium lacking Na^+ (28, and Worth RM, Ochs S: unpublished observations).

In our earlier studies, higher levels of BTX produced a more rapid block of transport. This and other findings suggested that BTX might also act directly on the transport mechanism. Such an action was recently shown to follow the intraneuronal injection of BTX, which blocked transport without affecting membrane potentials (36). Thus, both an intraaxonal increase in Na^+ and an internal action of BTX may account for the block of transport. Boegman and Albuquerque (37) have recently shown that the block of axoplasmic transport produced by subarachnoid injection of BTX into the spinal cord can be short lasting, with recovery occurring after 1 day. This result probably depends on the concentration of BTX achieved at axons somewhere along there trajectory from the motoneuron cell bodies to their entry into the peripheral nerve trunk.

ROLE OF CALCIUM IN NERVE

Reversibility of Block

If the cause of block is depletion of Ca^{2+} from the fibers to below some critical level, then axoplasmic transport should be restored in desheathed nerves exposed to Ca^{2+}-free medium when the preparation is returned to medium containing a normal concentration of Ca^{2+}. Nerves placed in a Ca^{2+}-free medium for 3 hours and then returned to medium containing Ca^{2+} for an additional 3 to 5 hours of downflow in vitro showed transport beyond the point of block expected in a Ca^{2+}-free medium (Fig. 5). Block of transport in the

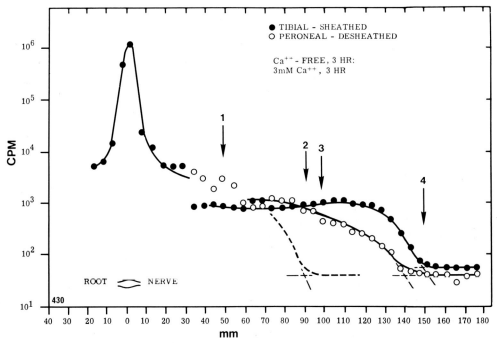

Fig. 5. Reversibility of block in Ca^{2+}-free medium with Ca^{2+}. Arrow 1 shows when the nerve preparation was placed in isotonic NaCl medium. Arrow 2 shows the expected transport distance in Ca^{2+}-free medium (dashed line). Arrow 3 shows when the nerve was placed in NaCl medium containing 3 mM Ca^{2+}. Arrow 4 shows the calculated normal transport distance.

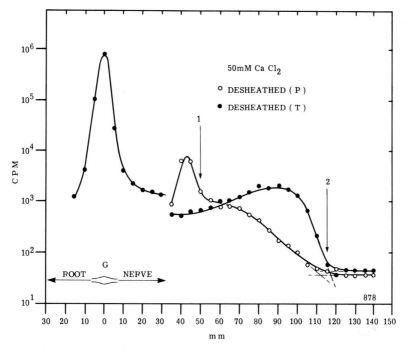

Fig. 6. Downflow in high-Ca^{2+} medium. Arrow 1 shows when the nerve was placed in NaCl medium containing 50 mM Ca^{2+}. Arrow 2 shows the calculated transport distance.

Ca^{2+}-free medium could be reversed quickly (within 30 minutes after exposure to medium containing Ca^{2+}).

Concentrations of Ca^{2+} as high as 20 to 35 mM might have little effect on transport in the desheathed nerve preparation if the exposure were not prolonged. Desheathed nerves exposed to Ca^{2+} levels higher than 50 to 60 mM showed evidence of block of transport (Fig. 6). It should be noted that even with an isotonic concentration of Ca^{2+} in the medium, axoplasmic transport in the sheathed tibial nerve was unaffected, an example of the low permeability of the perineurial sheath to Ca^{2+}.

The block of transport seen in the desheathed nerve when higher levels of Ca^{2+} were present suggests that the regulatory mechanism in the fibers was overloaded. At lower Ca^{2+} levels, regulatory mechanisms appear to be effective. This conclusion was supported by additional evidence: after exposure to Ca^{2+} concentrations as high as 60 mM for 3 hours (with consequent transport block), nerves were returned to Ringer solution containing little or no Ca^{2+}; transport continued well beyond the time at which it would normally fail in nerves exposed to such high concentrations of Ca^{2+} (28). Longer exposure to such high Ca^{2+} levels leads to irreversible loss of function with visible signs of damage. Electron microscopy (EM) reveals loss of neurofilaments and microtubules, and changes in mitochondria and endoplasmic reticulum (ER). Entry of enough Ca^{2+} to overload the Ca^{2+}-regulatory mechanisms would result in high levels of free Ca^{2+}, leading to activation of proteolytic enzymes and other processes that cause axonal damage.

Regulatory Mechanisms for Calcium

The experiments described indicate that regulatory mechanisms in the nerve fibers act to maintain the level of Ca^{2+} that is optimal for axoplasmic transport. For a complete analysis of Ca^{2+} regulation we must know the level of free Ca^{2+} in mammalian nerves as well as the total level of Ca^{2+} present. As yet, the free Ca^{2+} level is unknown.

The best information we have comes from studies of the giant axons, where a concentration of approximately 10^{-7} M has been determined (32, 38). The total concentration of Ca^{2+} is much higher (approximately 0.4 mM), with most of the Ca^{2+} in bound or sequestered form. Most of it is in the mitochondria, which are known to sequester Ca^{2+} (39–41). The sequestration of Ca^{2+} in mitochondria is seen in giant axons and in mammalian axons using oxalate or pyroantimonate, as well as in the ER (42–45). In addition, Ca^{2+} is bound in the axoplasm, probably to a Ca^{2+}-binding protein (CaBP) found in mammalian nerve (46, 47).

Changes in the sequestration of Ca^{2+} in the mitochondria and ER could be seen in EM studies using pyroantimonate to chelate Ca^{2+} in nerves exposed to high concentrations of Ca^{2+} in the incubation medium (48). The densely staining granules in EM sections were identified as containing Ca^{2+}, much of it in nerves incubated in a 40 mM Ca^{2+} solution compared to Ringer medium. The accumulation of Ca^{2+} was fairly rapid. The time course of augmentation and depletion of Ca^{2+} levels in nerves incubated in high- and low-Ca^{2+} medium was more recently examined using ^{45}Ca efflux. Placing nerves in a Ca^{2+}-free medium caused an early and maintained increase in Ca^{2+} efflux (Chan SY, Ochs S: unpublished observations), as would be expected from the studies showing an early block of transport when Ca^{2+} was deleted from the medium.

The changes in internal Na^+, suggested previously to affect transport, might act through an effect on Ca^{2+}-regulatory mechanisms, probably on the mitochondria that regulate Ca^{2+} (32, 41). Metabolic agents may also act indirectly through an effect on mitochondria and their regulation of Ca^{2+} (49). Some indication of an involvement of the mitochondria in nerves exposed to a low Ca^{2+} medium was suggested by small decreases in ATP and CP levels, changes not great enough in themselves to block transport (see *Requirement for ATP*.)

Eventually, the Ca^{2+} that enters the nerve fibers passively as a result of its electrochemical gradient and the increased permeability to Ca^{2+} during membrane activation is removed from the fiber by a Na^+-Ca^{2+} exchange mechanism in the membrane (32, 38, 50) or a Ca^{2+} pump that requires ATP (32, 51, 52). If high Ca^{2+} results by any means, its pathologic actions probably come about by its activation of proteolytic enzymes (53). The low permeability of the axolemmal membrane permits normal function to persist for a time in the face of a high Ca^{2+} concentration in the medium, but if this concentration is too high, enough Ca^{2+} enters to overcome the Ca^{2+}-regulatory mechanisms, causing pathologic effects inimical to transport.

THE NEW TRANSPORT FILAMENT MODEL

The various Ca^{2+}-regulatory mechanisms present in the axons and the requirement for Ca^{2+} to maintain transport are taken into account in the new transport filament model shown in Figure 7. As in the basic transport filament model presented earlier, ATP is required. It is assumed that an optimal level of Ca^{2+} in the axoplasm is required for the action of Ca,Mg-ATPase, pictured as being present on the side arms of the microtubules. The K_m for Ca,Mg-ATPase previously assessed (20, 54), however, was higher than the 10^{-7} M concentration of free Ca^{2+} likely to be present in the axoplasm. The Ca,Mg-ATPase could be activated to respond to this low level of Ca^{2+} by calmodulin (55, 56). Our recent studies have shown that the CaBP we had previously found in nerve (46) is very similar if not identical to the calmodulin also obtained from nerve (47). In the presence of micromolar concentrations of Ca^{2+}, calmodulin activates the Ca,Mg-ATPase obtained from nerve (57).

In a further step toward relating the Ca,Mg-ATPase activity to the side arms of the microtubules, we have obtained a preparation of purified tubulin with Ca,Mg-ATPase remaining present as part of its microtubular-associated protein. This was done by several cycles of disassembly-assembly of microtubules at low and high temperatures and centrifugation. The Ca,Mg-ATPase associated with the tubulin was found to require Ca^{2+} in submicromolar concentrations for maximal activity and to be activated by calmodulin (58). As evidence for that, triflouperazine (TFP) was found to inhibit the Ca,Mg-ATPase activity: the TFP bound to calmodulin and inactivated it. Further support for a calmodulin requirement related to transport was that TFP could also block axoplasmic transport (Fig. 8).

Thus, calmodulin is related to the transport process itself. We can thereby account for the sensitivity of transport to the small changes in free axoplasmic Ca^{2+} resulting from exposure of the desheathed nerve to a low-Ca^{2+} medium; this treatment reduces the level of Ca^{2+} below that required for calmodulin activation of Ca,Mg-ATPase and utilization of ATP.

Two possibilities remain to account for how transport comes about. (a) The

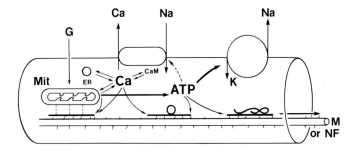

Fig. 7. Transport filament model. The mitochondrion (Mit) supplies adenosine triphosphate (ATP) to the pump that controls NA^+ and K^+ levels in the fiber and to the side arms that move the transport filaments along microtubules (M). Transport filaments are shown with various components bound to them and carried down the fiber. In addition, Ca^{2+} is shown in the fiber, where it participates in movement of transport filaments, possibly by permitting calmodulin (CaM) carried on the transport filaments to activate locally the Ca^{2+}, Mg^{2+}-adenosine triphosphatase (Ca,Mg-ATPase) on the side arms. The Ca^{2+} concentration is regulated by its sequestration in the mitochondria and endoplasmic reticulum (ER), and by binding to Ca^{2+}-binding protein (CaM). A Ca^{2+}-Na^+ exchange or Ca^{2+} pump is shown in the membrane as part of the Ca^{2+}-regulatory mechanisms acting to eject excess Ca^{2+}. NF = neurofilament; G = glucose.

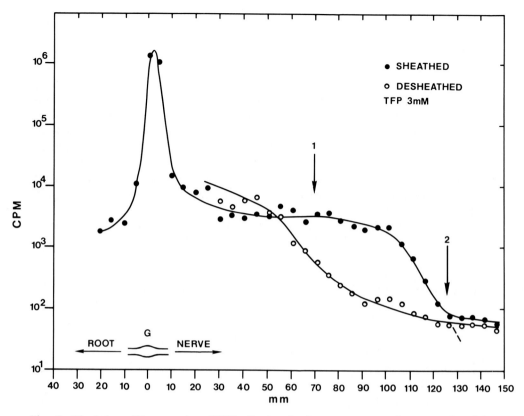

Fig. 8. Block by trifluoperazine (TFP). Desheathed nerve preparation was placed in medium containing 3 mM TFP at arrow 1. Arrow 2 shows expected transport distance.

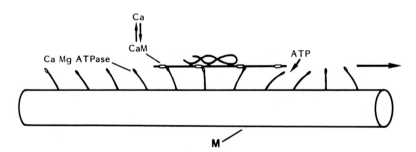

Fig. 9. Hypothesis of calmodulin Ca-Mg-ATPase interaction. Calmodulin (CaM) is shown on the transport filaments, which, as they move down the axon, contact the Ca^{2+},Mg^{2+}-adenosine triphosphatase (Ca,Mg-ATPase) to activate it and thus ultilize adenosine triphosphate (ATP) when micromolar levels of Ca^{2+} are present in the axoplasm. An alternative hypothesis is that calmodulin and Ca,Mg-ATPase are both on the side arms and a modulator bound to the transport filament moves to contact the side arm, permitting calmodulin to activate the Ca,MG-ATPase and thereby produce conformational changes that move the transport filaments foward. M = microtubule.

168

transport filaments could contain calmodulin, so that as the filaments are moved forward, the calmodulin activates the side arm Ca,Mg-ATPase to use ATP for movement of the transport filaments. This would allow ATP to be used just at the site at which a micromovement of the side arm is required to pull the transport filament forward. The advantage of such localized use of energy at the point of need is apparent (Fig. 9).

We have obtained evidence for the fast transport of some small amount of calmodulin (59). *(b)* Alternatively, calmodulin could be associated with the Ca,Mg-ATPase of the side arm; some additional component on the transport filament, when that component joins it, could allow calmodulin to activate the Ca,Mg-ATPase of the side arms. Further study is required to determine just how calmodulin and the Ca,Mg-ATPase of the microtubular side arms interact to bring about transport filament movement.

REFERENCES

1. Livett BG: Axonal transport and neuronal dynamics: contributions to the study of neuronal connectivity. Int Rev Physiol 10:37–124, 1976

2. Ochs S, Worth RM: Axoplasmic transport in normal and pathological systems. In *Physiology and Pathobiology of Axons.* Edited by Waxman SG. Raven Press, New York, 1978, pp 251–264

3. Wilson DL, Stone GC: Axoplasmic transport of proteins. Annu Rev Biophys 8:27–45, 1979

4. Schwartz JH: Axonal transport: components, mechanisms, and specificity. Annu Rev Neurosci 2:467–504, 1979

5. Grafstein B, Forman DS: Intracellular transport in neurons. Physiol Rev 60:1167–1283, 1980

6. Ochs S: Local supply of energy to the fast axoplasmic transport mechanism. Proc Natl Acad Sci USA 68:1279–1282, 1971

7. Ochs S: Fast transport of materials in mammalian nerve fibers. Science 176:252–260, 1972

8. Ochs S, Sabri MI, Johnson J: Fast transport system of materials in mammalian nerve fibers. Science 163:686–687, 1969

9. Brimijoin S, Wiermaa MJ: Rapid axonal transport of tyrosine hydroxylase in rabbit sciatic nerves. Brain Res 120:77–96, 1977

10. Ben-Jonathan N, Maxson RE, Ochs S: Fast axoplasmic transport of noradrenaline and dopamine in mammalian peripheral nerve. J Physiol (Lond) 281:315–324, 1978

11. Ranish N, Ochs S: Fast axoplasmic transport of acetylcholinesterase in mammalian nerve fibres. J Neurochem 19:2641–2649, 1972

12. Kirkpatrick JB, Bray JJ, Palmer SM: Visualization of axoplasmic flow in vitro by Nomarski microscopy: comparison to rapid flow of radioactive proteins. Brain Res 43:1–10, 1972

13. Cooper RD, Smith RS: The movement of optically detectable organelles in myelinated axons of *Xenopus laevis.* J Physiol (Lond) 242:77–97, 1974

14. Forman DS, Padjen AL: Siggins GR: Axonal transport of organelles visualized by light microscopy: cinemicrographic and computer analysis. Brain Res 136:197–213, 1977

15. Stromska DP, Igbal Z, Ochs S: Fast axoplasmic transport of tubulin and triad proteins (abstract). Soc Neurosci Abstr 5:63, 1979

16. Ochs S: Energy metabolism and supply of ~P to the fast axoplasmic transport mechanism in nerve. Fed Proc 33:1049–1058, 1974

17. Ochs S, Hollingsworth D: Dependence of fast axoplasmic transport in nerve on oxidative metabolism. J Neurochem 18:107–114, 1971

18. Ochs S, Smith CB: Fast axoplasmic transport in mammalian nerve in vitro after block of glycolysis with iodoacetic acid. J Neurochem 18:833–843, 1971

19. Sabri MI, Ochs S: Relation of ATP and creatine phosphate to fast axoplasmic transport in mammalian nerve. J Neurochem 19:2821–2828, 1972

20. Khan MA, Ochs S: Mg^{2+}-Ca^{2+} activated ATPase in mammalian nerves: relation to fast axoplasmic transport and block with colchicine (abstract). Abstr Am Soc Neurochem 3:93, 1972

21. Ochs S: Rate of fast axoplasmic transport in mammalian nerve fibers. J. Physiol (Lond) 227:627–645, 1972

22. Hammerschlag R, Dravid AR, Chiu AY: Mechanisms of axonal transport: proposed role for calcium ions. Science 188:273–275, 1975

23. Edstrom A: Effects of Ca^{2+} and Mg^{2+} on rapid axonal transport of proteins in vitro in frog sciatic nerves. J Cell Biol 61:812–818, 1974

24. Banks P, Mayor D, Mraz P: Metabolic aspects of the synthesis and intra-axonal transport of noradrenaline storage vesicles. J Physiol (Lond) 229:383–394, 1973

25. Abe T, Haga T, Kurokawa M: Rapid transport of phosphatidylcholine occurring simultaneously with protein transport in the frog sciatic nerve. Biochem J 136:731–740, 1973

26. Ochs S, Worth RM, Chan SY: Calcium requirement for axoplasmic transport in the desheathed peroneal nerve. Nature 270:748–750, 1977

27. Ochs S, Smith C: Low temperature slowing and cold-block of fast axoplasmic transport in mammalian nerves in vitro. J Neurobiol 6: 85–102, 1975

28. Chan SY, Ochs S, Worth RM: The requirement of Ca^{2+} and the effect of other ions on axoplasmic transport in mammalian nerve. J Physiol (Lond) 301:477–504, 1980

29. Fink BR, Kennedy RD, Hendrickson AE, Middaugh ME: Lidocaine inhibition of rapid axonal transport. Anesthesiology 36:422–432, 1972

30. Ochs S: Calcium requirement for axoplasmic transport and the role of the perineurial sheath. In *Nerve Repair and Regeneration: Its Clinical and Experimental Basis*. Edited by Jewett DL, McCarroll HR. CV Mosby Company, St. Louis, 1980, pp 77–88

31. Baker PF, Blaustein MP, Hodgkin AL, Steinhardt RA: The influence of calcium on sodium efflux in squid axons. J Physiol (Lond) 200:431–458, 1969

32. Baker PF: Transport and metabolism of calcium ions in nerve. Prog Biophys Molec Biol 24:177–223, 1972

33. Partlow LM, Ross CD, Motwani R, McDougal DB Jr: Transport of axonal enzymes in surviving segments of frog sciatic nerve. J Gen Physiol 60:388–405, 1972

34. Narahashi T, Albuquerque EX, Deguchi T: Effects of batrachotoxin on membrane potential and conductance of squid giant axons. J Gen Physiol 58:54–70, 1971

35. Ochs S, Worth R: Batrachotoxin block of fast axoplasmic transport in mammalian nerve fibers. Science 187:1087–1089, 1975

36. Kumara-Siri MH: Batrachotoxin inhibits axonal transport without affecting membrane potential in single neurons of *Aplysia california*. J Neurobiol 10:509–512, 1979

37. Boegman RJ, Albuquerque EX: Axonal transport in rats rendered paraplegic following a single subarachnoid injection of either batrachotoxin or 6-aminonicotinamide into the spinal cord. J Physiol (Lond) 11:283–290, 1980

38. Blaustein MP: The interrelationship between sodium and calcium fluxes across cell membranes. Rev Physiol Biochem Pharmacol 70:33–82, 1974

39. Lehninger AL, Carafoli E, Rossi CS: Energy-linked ion movements in mitochondrial systems. Adv Enzymol 29:259–320, 1967

40. Bygrave FL: Mitochondria and the control of intracellular calcium. Biol Rev 53:43–79, 1978

41. Carafoli E, Crompton M: The regulation of intracellular calcium. In *Current Topics in Membranes and Transport*, vol 10, Membrane Properties: Mechanical Aspects, Receptors, Energetics and Calcium Dependence on Transport. Edited by Bronner F, Kleinzeller A. Academic Press, New York, 1978, pp 151–216

42. Theron JJ, Meyer BJ, Boekkooi S, Loots JM: Ultrastructural localization of calcium in peripheral nerves of the rat. S Afr Med J 48:1795–1798, 1975

43. Hinderlang-Gertner C, Stoeckel ME, Porte A, Stutinsky F: Colchicine effects on neurosescretory

neurons and other hypothalamic and hypophysical cells, with special reference to changes in the cytoplasmic membranes. Cell Tissue Res 170:17–41, 1976

44. Duce IR, Keen P: Can neuronal smooth endoplasmic reticulum function as a calcium reservoir? Neuroscience 3:837–848, 1978

45. Henkart MP, Reese TS, Brinley FJ Jr: Endoplasmic reticulum sequesters calcium in the squid giant axon. Science 202:1300–1303, 1978

46. Igbal Z, Ochs S: Fast axoplasmic transport of a calcium-binding protein in mammalian nerve. J Neurochem 31:409–418, 1978

47. Igbal Z, Garg BP, Ochs S: Calmodulin activation of brain and nerve Ca^{2+}-Mg^{2+}-ATPase (abstract). Soc Neurosci Abstr 5:60, 1979

48. Chan SY, Jersild R, Ochs S: Calcium localization in mammalian nerve fibers in relation to its regulation and axoplasmic transport (abstract). Soc Neurosci Abstr 5:59, 1979

49. Blaustein MP, Hodgkin AL: The effect of cyanide on the efflux of calcium from squid axons. J Physiol (Lond) 200:497–527, 1969

50. Brinley FJ: Calcium and magnesium metabolism in cephalopod axons. Fed Proc 35:2572–2573, 1976

51. Baker PF, Glitsch HG: Does metabolic energy participate directly in the Na^+-dependent extrusion of Ca^{2+} ions from squid giant axons? J Physiol (Lond) 233:33P–46P, 1973

52. DiPolo R: Ca pump driven by ATP in squid axons. Nature 274:390–392, 1978

53. Schlaepfer WW: Calcium-induced degeneration of axoplasm in isolated segments of rat peripheral nerve. Brain Res 69:203–215, 1974

54. Sheckert GN, Lasek RJ: Neurofilament-associated Mg^{2+}-Ca^{2+}-ATPase from squid giant axon. Trans Am Soc Neurochem 8:179, 1977

55. Cheung WY: Calmodulin plays a pivotal role in cellular regulation. Science 207:19–27, 1980

56. Means AR, Dedman JR: Calmodulin: an intracellular calcium receptor. Nature 285:73–77, 1980

57. Igbal Z, Ochs S: CDR protein in mammalian nerve (abstract). Fed Proc 38:849, 1979

58. Ochs S, Igbal Z: Calmodulin and calcium activation of tubulin associated Ca-ATPase (abstract). Soc Neurosci Abstr 6:501, 1980

59. Igbal Z, Ochs S. Calmodulin in mammalian nerve. J Neurobiol 11:311–318, 1980

DISCUSSION

Dr. Michael Bárány: We did a lot of work with trifluoperazine (TFP) and found that its solubility is very low, so we now use chlorpromazine instead. I believe that, even with as much as 3 mM TFP, you would not get reversal of the reaction; such reversibility is necessary to prove the underlying mechanism. If you used chlorpromazine, you could work with a concentration at least 5 times lower than that of TFP and the reaction might be reversible.

Dr. Sidney Ochs: There have been several reports that chlorpromazine blocks transport, but no known mechanism was reported. In our particular system I think we are at the limit of solubility of TFP.

Dr. Michael Bárány: I believe that microtubular systems contain protein kinase.

Dr. Sidney Ochs: Yes, but we are not sure whether the protein kinase is the one that calmodulin actually works on. Calmodulin works on perhaps 14 different enzymes, and the number is growing every day. Whether kinase is definitely involved we really do not know. There is a Ca,Mg-ATPase in red cell membranes that is controlled by calmodulin, so there are many enzymes that are not kinases.

Dr. Anthony Means: Dr. Ochs, which procedure do you use to prepare your microtubules, the one of Borisy or the one of Shelanski, because they are different.

Dr. Sidney Ochs: For a number of reasons, we have concentrated on the Borisy procedure. As you know, this is not the best procedure for dissociating calmodulin, because it does not use EGTA. Early on, we had a little difficulty with the Shelanski procedure, so we have used a 3-cycle Borisy procedure. We get a dome-shaped activation curve with a pCa at about 7, but we are now returning to the Shelanski procedure because it yields cleaner bands.

Dr. Anthony Means: The Borisy procedure uses no glycerol.

Dr. Sidney Ochs: Yes, that is true.

Dr. Anthony Means: Under those conditions, neurofilament proteins are also copurified with the tubulin. It has been demonstrated that some of the protein kinases and phosphodiesterases and possibly one of the ATPases are neurofilament proteins, not microtubular proteins. We have also found that in both axons and dendrites of peripheral nerves one finds calmodulin associated with mitochondrial inner and outer membranes, and also with neurofilaments. When one localizes one enzyme known to be stimulated by calmodulin, the myosin light chain kinase, by immunocytochemical procedures, one also finds an association with the neurofilaments of the nerve processes. These data suggest that calmodulin may be involved in force generation in nerves as well as in non-neuronal cells.

Dr. Sidney Ochs: I should mention that your work on the microtubules in mitotic dividing cells is another example of the importance of calmodulin in terms of regulating disassembly of microtubules. There are a number of reasons for us to try very hard to purify the Ca-ATPase of microtubules; it is imperative if this model is to stand up. We are hoping that the Shelanski method or some modification of it will give us that kind of preparation.

13
Sprouting and Regeneration of Motor Nerves

Alan Pestronk, MD

Daniel B. Drachman, MD

Motor nerves are known to sprout under a variety of normal, pathologic, and experimental conditions (1). Sprouting appears to be essential for the mainte-nance and restoration of nerve-muscle connections. At normal neuromuscular junctions, nerve terminal sprouting allows continued renewal of motor nerve endings (2, 3). During development, axons sprout to reach and innervate appropriate target tissues such as muscle. In the mature animal, in which connections between nerves and target tissues have previously been established, partial denervation from any cause can elicit collateral sprouting (4). Finally, regeneration of nerves occurs after accidental or experimental nerve injury. Clinically, the various forms of nerve sprouting occur in denervating diseases such as the spinal muscular atrophies, poliomyelitis, or peripheral neuropathies, and in some of the "myopathies" including Duchenne muscular dystrophy, myotonic dystrophy, and myasthenia gravis (5, 6). In this paper we will discuss several aspects of motor nerve sprouting.

MORPHOLOGY OF THE NEUROMUSCULAR JUNCTION

Using light microscopic techniques, the region of the neuromuscular junction, or endplate, is defined as a localized area of cholinesterase staining on the muscle fiber. Motor axons normally terminate within this area, forming an arborization on the skeletal muscle fibers (Figs. 1, 2). In most adult mammalian muscle the nerve terminal arborization lies entirely within the region of the endplate, and it is rare to find branches of axon terminals extending beyond this cholinesterase-stained zone. Exceptions to this rule occur in the extraocular muscles and on intrafusal muscle fibers.

The morphologic features of the terminal axonal branches differ according to the histologic technique used to demonstrate them. Intravital methylene blue

NORMAL

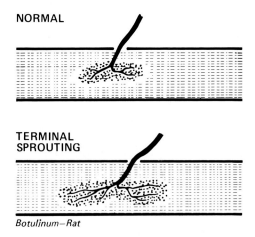

**TERMINAL
SPROUTING**

Botulinum—Rat

Fig. 1. Diagrammatic representation of combined cholinesterase-silver-strained endplates from the soleus muscle of a 2-month-old rat (original magnification ×600). *Above:* Normal endplate is short and the axon has 3 terminal branch points. *Below:* Terminal sprouting at an endplate 7 days after treatment with botulinum toxin. Endplate length has increased and the axon terminal has 5 branch points.

or zinc iodide–osmium tetroxide stains demonstrate terminal branches as "swollen" structures (5, 7). Silver stains usually impart a fine, tapered appearance to the terminals (Fig. 2).

For our studies we have developed a combined cholinesterase-silver stain that displays the cholinesterase-containing endplate as a well-demarcated blue zone against which the black silver-stained nerve terminals stand out clearly (8). The silver stain reproducibly demonstrates the preterminal axon, its terminal arborization, and any terminal or ultraterminal outgrowth (see later). The simultaneous cholinesterase stain allows the reliable identification and measurement of the endplate zone and the nerve terminal arborization within this area. The stain is effective in frozen longitudinal sections of muscle in all species tested, including mouse, rat, and human. The neuromuscular junctions can be

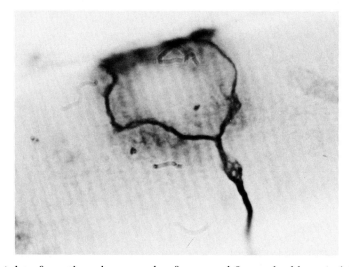

Fig. 2. Endplate from the soleus muscle of a normal 2-month-old rat (original magnification ×1,000). Black silver-stained nerve terminals end within gray cholinesterase zone.

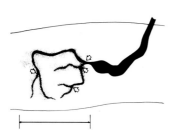

Fig. 3. Diagram showing morphometry of neuromuscular junction. The endplate length, outlined by the cholinesterase stain (dotted area), is measured parallel to the length of the muscle fiber (interval marker). The nerve terminal branch points are indicated by the open arrows. (Reprinted with permission from Pestronk A, Drachman DB: Motor nerve sprouting and acetylcholine receptors. Science 199:1223, 1978. Copyright 1978 by the American Association for the Advancement of Science.)

evaluated quantitatively (Fig. 3) by (*a*) counting the number of nerve terminal branch points within each endplate area, and (*b*) measuring the length of each endplate as outlined by the cholinesterase stain (8).

FORMS OF MOTOR NERVE OUTGROWTH

There may be several distinct forms of motor nerve outgrowth.

1. *Nerve terminal sprouting,* also called endplate proliferation, is the enlargement of an endplate on a muscle fiber. Using the combined cholinesterase-silver stain, this form of sprouting appears as an elongation of the area of endplate cholinesterase staining and the increased branching of nerve terminals within this area (Fig. 1). In mammals, terminal sprouting occurs continuously as a normal process (2). In amphibians, it varies seasonally (3). It probably serves to replace terminals as they are damaged or lost, and thus maintains the integrity of neuromuscular junctions.

2. We use the term *ultraterminal sprouting* to define outgrowth originating from a nerve terminal arborization and extending beyond the cholinesterase-stained endplate zone (Figs. 4, 5). When ultraterminal sprouts reinnervate a neighboring denervated muscle fiber, they may be a form of collateral sprouting (see later) (Fig. 4).

3. *Collateral sprouting* is the growth of an intact axon beyond its original endplate area to innervate a neighboring muscle fiber (Fig. 4). These axonal branches

COLLATERAL SPROUTING

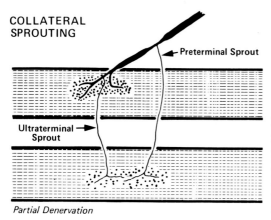

Partial Denervation

Fig. 4. Collateral sprouting from an intact axon (above) to reinnervate a nearby denervated muscle fiber (below). Branches originate from a node of Ranvier (preterminal sprout) and from the terminal arborization (ultraterminal sprout).

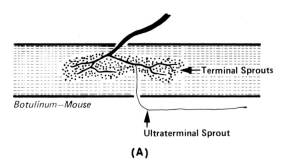

(A)

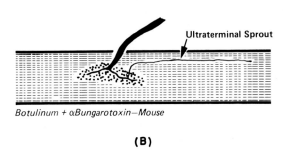

(B)

Fig. 5. Sprouting at endplates from mouse soleus 7 days after treatment with botulinum toxin. (**A**) Note the presence of both terminal and ultraterminal sprouts. (**B** This muscle has been treated daily with α-bungarotoxin, in addition to the botulinum toxin. Note that terminal sprouting is inhibited, although ultraterminal sprouts still occur.

may originate from nodes of Ranvier (preterminal sprouts) or from nerve terminals within the endplate area (ultraterminal sprouts). Collateral sprouts are most commonly seen in partially denervated muscle, where they reinnervate neighboring muscle fibers that have lost their nerve supply.

4. The term *axonal regeneration* will be used here in a restricted sense to define a fourth type of sprouting: nerve outgrowth that is elicited by interruption of or damage to an axon. This form of sprouting differs from the others; the axon appears to have an inherent capacity to regenerate after injury, without requiring an external stimulus. However, external factors may influence the speed and direction of axonal regeneration.

CONTROL OF NERVE TERMINAL SPROUTING

Denervation Changes in Muscle

There is much evidence that skeletal muscle plays an important role in controlling nerve terminal sprouting. In particular, denervation changes in muscle seem to elicit nerve terminal sprouting (7, 9).

Nerve terminal sprouting is seen in situations where reduced neuromuscular transmission results in denervation-like changes in muscle. For example, Duchen and Strich (10) originally observed nerve terminal sprouting after presynaptic blockade produced by botulinum toxin. In the rat soleus muscle, treatment with botulinum toxin produces only nerve terminal sprouting (Fig. 1). The cholinesterase-stained endplate zone elongates, and nerve terminal branching increases within this area. No nerve terminal branches extend beyond the cholinesterase-stained endplate area during the first 2 weeks after treatment.

To study the relationship between muscle denervation and motor nerve sprouting, we produced denervation changes in muscle by 3 different means and measured their effects on nerve terminal sprouting (9). Functional denervation of muscle was brought about by (a) presynaptic blockade of acetylcholine (ACh) transmission, produced by botulinum toxin (11–13); (b) muscle disuse due to tetrodotoxin (TTX) blockade of nerve impulse conduction (14, 15); and (c) postsynaptic blockade of neuromuscular transmission, produced by α-bungarotoxin (α-BuTx) (16). As an indicator of denervation changes produced in the muscles by each of these procedures, we measured the extrajunctional acetylcholine receptors (AChRs) by means of ^{125}I-α-BuTx binding.

There were two main findings. First, there was a close correlation between the degree of sprouting and the measured levels of extrajunctional AChRs, except in the postsynaptic blockade experiments. Second, when α-BuTx was used to produce postsynaptic blockade, there was no significant sprouting compared with the control preparations.

Mean endplate length increased by 22 μm and nerve terminal branching increased by 56% over control values 7 days after treatment with botulinum toxin. This high degree of sprouting was correlated with a high level of extrajunctional AChRs (308 AChRs/μm^2 compared with a normal value of 22 AChRs/μm^2).

Disuse alone, induced by TTX blockade of nerve conduction, resulted in a less marked sprouting response. Mean endplate length increased by 11 μm and nerve terminal branching increased by 46% after 7 days of disuse. Correspondingly, disuse produced a smaller increase of extrajunctional AChRs than did botulinum treatment (106 AChRs/μm^2). In individual muscles, there was a strong correlation between the degree of terminal sprouting and extrajunctional AChR density (r = 0.9; $P \ll 0.001$).

In contrast to these results, no significant sprouting occurred after injections of α-BuTx, despite high levels of extrajunctional AChRs (251 AChR/μm^2). Nerve terminal branching and endplate length in α-BuTx-treated muscles were not different from those in control muscles.

There are at least two possible explanations for the failure of α-BuTx-induced postsynaptic blockade to elicit terminal sprouting: (a) the resulting denervation changes may not be sufficient or appropriate to evoke nerve terminal sprouting; (b) α-BuTx itself might interfere with terminal sprouting.

To resolve this problem, we tested the ability of α-BuTx to inhibit terminal sprouting by applying it in a situation where a pronounced sprouting response otherwise occurs, i.e., after administration of botulinum toxin. Our results showed virtually complete inhibition of sprouting in muscles injected with α-BuTx in addition to botulinum toxin, whereas other muscles treated with botulinum toxin showed a marked sprouting response. In contrast, the combined botulinum toxin–α-BuTx treatment resulted in markedly increased levels of extrajunctional AChRs slightly greater than those in muscles treated with botulinum toxin alone. Thus, α-BuTx appears to inhibit nerve terminal sprouting without reducing the denervation changes in muscle.

Most other studies have found similar effects of α-BuTx on terminal sprouting. For example, α-BuTx also inhibits terminal sprouting during development. There is a reduction in endplate size and in the complexity of nerve terminal branching when α-BuTx (17) or another α-neurotoxin (18) is administered to developing chicken embryos.

Holland and Brown (19) have disputed the finding that α-BuTx inhibits nerve terminal sprouting. They examined the effect of α-BuTx on nerve outgrowth occurring in the mouse soleus muscle after the application of botulinum toxin. They noted that nerve outgrowth continued to occur despite treatment with α-BuTx, and erroneously interpreted this as a failure of α-BuTx to inhibit terminal sprouting. We repeated these experiments and found that the disparity in results was due to the fact that these authors did not distinguish between nerve terminal sprouting and other forms of nerve outgrowth.

Using both the zinc iodide–osmium tetroxide and cholinesterase-silver staining techniques, we found that, in the mouse soleus, application of botulinum toxin results in both nerve terminal and ultraterminal sprouting (Fig. 5A). In contrast, only nerve terminal sprouting occurs in the rat soleus (Fig. 1). As in our previous study, we found that α-BuTx inhibits botulin-induced nerve terminal sprouting (i.e., endplate elongation and terminal branching within the endplate area) in the mouse. However, the botulin-induced ultraterminal sprouting that occurs in the mouse (but not the rat) is not affected by α-BuTx treatment (Fig. 5B). The different effect of α-BuTx on terminal and ultraterminal sprouting suggests that these types of outgrowth are controlled by different mechanisms. To avoid confusion and misinterpretation, future studies should clearly define the type of nerve outgrowth under investigation.

The inhibitory effect of α-BuTx on terminal sprouting is not due to a general interference with the ability of the nerve to grow, because other types of sprouting are not affected. As noted previously, when α-BuTx is injected into the botulin-treated mouse soleus, nerve terminal sprouting is inhibited, whereas ultraterminal sprouts from the same nerve terminals grow normally (Fig. 5B). In addition, α-BuTx has no effect on collateral preterminal or ultraterminal sprouting (Pestronk A, Drachman DB: unpublished observations) or axonal regeneration (9).

It seems most likely that the specific inhibition of nerve terminal sprouting produced by α-BuTx results from its only known action, a highly specific and irreversible blockade of AChRs (16). The mechanism by which AChR blockade might inhibit terminal sprouting is not known. The evidence that newly synthesized AChRs, which appear in functionally denervated muscle, may play a role in motor nerve terminal sprouting is summarized here: (a) As noted previously, functional denervation produced by botulinum toxin or by TTX-induced disuse results in nerve terminal sprouting. The degree of sprouting correlates closely with the level of extrajunctional AChRs. (b) Procedures that reduce the number of extrajunctional AChRs inhibit the tendency to sprout. Implantation of the normal nerve into botulin-treated muscle decreases both extrajunctional AChRs and terminal sprouting (20). Direct electrical stimulation of botulin-treated muscle decreases extrajunctional AChRs and terminal sprouting (7). (c) Specific pharmacologic blockade of AChRs with α-BuTx inhibits terminal sprouting. Possible mechanisms for this effect include α-BuTx blockade of the AChR recognition site, steric hindrance of a nearby site, or some as yet undefined secondary consequence of AChR blockade.

Effects of AChRs on Nerve Terminals

If an interaction between nerve terminals and AChRs plays an important role in terminal sprouting, then one would predict that AChRs might have a direct effect on motor nerve terminal morphology. We recently tested this idea by isolating AChRs from the torpedo electric organ and then injecting the solubilized receptors directly into the soleus muscles of the rat. Light microscopic examination of muscle, after 7 days of AChR injection, showed that nerve terminals had abnormal nodular thickenings (Fig. 6) and an increased number of branch points. Nodular thickenings in nerve terminals were found at 35% of neuromuscular junctions in muscles injected with AChRs compared to less than 5% of those in control muscles. This appeared to be a specific effect of the AChRs, because injection of solubilized AChRs whose receptor site was blocked with α-BuTx produced significantly fewer changes, with nodular swellings at only 15% of nerve terminals. Injections of other materials, such as albumin, did not produce any significant morphologic changes. (Pestronk A, Drachman DB: unpublished observations.)

The relationship of the changes induced by injection of solubilized AChRs to the terminal sprouting evoked by denervation changes in muscle needs further clarification. In particular, the nodular changes in nerve terminals produced by injection of AChRs do not occur in the sprouting response evoked by denervation changes in muscle. However, the presence of morphologic changes induced by AChRs suggests that nerve terminals may interact directly with the soluble AChRs.

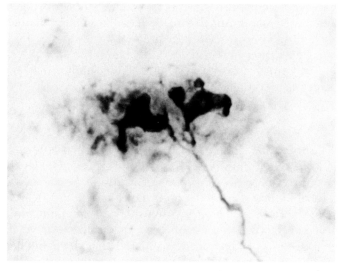

Fig. 6. Cholinesterase-silver-stained endplate (original magnification ×1,000) from a rat soleus muscle injected for 7 days with solubilized acetylcholine receptors. Nerve terminal branches are swollen and nodular.

It is tempting to speculate that in the intact animal a similar process of local interaction of nerve terminals with AChRs in muscle membrane takes place. In this way the new appearance of "extrajunctional" AChRs within and immediately adjoining the endplate could induce nerve terminal branching and enlargement of the endplate. The mechanism by which nerve terminals interact with AChRs in muscle membrane and the role of this interaction in nerve terminal sprouting must be defined by future studies.

Terminal Sprouting at Old Synaptic Sites

Recent evidence suggests that nerve terminal sprouting, a single type of nerve outgrowth, can be induced by several different mechanisms. For example, in some situations nerve terminal sprouting can occur in the absence of AChRs. In the frog, regenerating axons reinnervate denervated muscle fibers at the original synaptic sites. These axons undergo terminal sprouting, i.e., branching, and an increase in the area of synaptic contact until much of the old synaptic site is reoccupied. It appears that muscle AChRs are not involved in this process, because the terminal sprouting continues to occur on basal lamina even though the muscle beneath it has been removed (21).

In the rat, terminal sprouting of regenerating axons not only reinnervates the original synaptic sites but also extends beyond this area. The resulting reinnervated endplates (cholinesterase zones) are larger than the original ones. When regeneration occurs in the presence of AChR blockade, the terminal sprouting reinnervates the original endplate area as before, but the expansion of the endplate due to formation of new areas of neuromuscular contact is inhibited (Pestronk A, Drachman DB: unpublished observations).

These results suggest that terminal sprouting may be elicited by two mechanisms. The AChRs play an important role when nerve terminal sprouting occurs into areas without prior synaptic contact, such as during development, after treatment with botulinum toxin, or in enlargement of the endplate by regenerating axons. However, AChRs are not necessary to initiate terminal sprouting in regenerating nerves if the basal lamina from a prior synaptic site is present. The characteristics of "synaptic" basal lamina that evoke terminal sprouting from regenerating nerves are not known.

"Trophic" Factors

The role of "trophic" or chemical factors in evoking nerve terminal sprouting is not well defined. At this time there is no clear evidence that any such substances are involved in nerve terminal sprouting where local factors such as AChRs and basal lamina seem to be important.

On the other hand, diffusible factors may play a role in initiating or directing other types of outgrowth, such as collateral sprouting, because these must be evoked over a distance. It has been postulated that denervated tissues either release sprout-eliciting factors or cease manufacturing a growth-inhibiting agent. An alternative suggestion has been that products of nerve damage or degeneration may stimulate nerve outgrowth (1). However, these speculations, in general, apply to collateral sprouting, and results regarding one type of outgrowth cannot be generalized to another without sufficient evidence linking the two.

INTRINSIC MECHANISMS OF NERVE OUTGROWTH: EFFECTS OF AGING

The tendency of a nerve to sprout depends on intrinsic characteristics of the axon, as well as on extrinsic factors such as denervation changes in the target tissue. For example, after treatment with botulinum toxin, sprouting occurs earlier and is more profuse in slow muscle than in fast muscle (22), although the degree of denervation changes in the muscles is similar (14). In the central nervous system adrenergic neurons seem to have a particular ability to undergo collateral sprouting in response to denervation of nearby neurons (23).

One factor that plays an important role in the ability of axons to grow is aging (24, 25). We have found that in the rat both nerve terminal sprouting and axonal regeneration after injury are most active in young animals, decline with advancing age, and are markedly impaired in senescence (26).

Nerve Terminal Sprouting

To examine the effect of aging on nerve terminal sprouting, we measured nerve terminal sprouting after treatment with botulinum toxin in rats of different ages (26). In 2-month-old (young adult) animals there was a large degree of terminal sprouting in the soleus muscle 7 days after treatment with botulin. Endplate length increased by 30% and terminal branch points, by 52%. In 10- and 18-month-old (mature adult) animals there was less terminal sprouting, with increases of 25% in endplate length and 15% in terminal branch points. In senescent 28-month-old rats there was no significant terminal sprouting 7 days after treatment with botulinum toxin. Thus, with increasing age, terminal sprouting progressively declined.

One possible explanation for the changes in terminal sprouting might be age-dependent differences in the stimulus to sprout. Because levels of extra-junctional AChRs are indicative of denervation changes in muscle and may play a role in terminal sprouting, we measured AChRs in the botulinum toxin–treated muscles. Rats of all ages showed similar increases in the number of extrajunctional AChRs. Thus, the impairment of terminal sprouting in the older animals could not be attributed to lower levels of extrajunctional AChRs or to failure of botulinum toxin to produce denervation changes in muscle.

These results suggest that the decreasing amount of nerve terminal sprouting is attributable to some age-dependent change in the axon that impairs its inherent ability to grow. This defect could, in turn, lead to the denervation and reinnervation changes seen in muscles of aging rats. As nerve terminals are lost by a normal turnover process (2, 27–29), they may fail to be replaced because of impaired terminal outgrowth. Some muscle fibers would become atrophic, and others might be reinnervated by a process of collateral sprouting of neighboring nerves. This sequence of events at the level of the distal motor axon might explain the observed denervation atrophy, type grouping, and loss of muscle fibers in aging, with no loss of proximal motor axons (30, 31).

Axonal Regeneration

To learn whether the failure of sprouting was limited to nerve terminals or whether it involved other types of nerve outgrowth as well, we studied the effect of aging on axonal regeneration (26). We used a focal crush injury to elicit regeneration. The extent of axonal regeneration in peripheral motor and sensory axons was measured using radiolabeled proteins carried by axonal transport. These proteins are known to accumulate in the growth cones of regenerating axons. Thus, the pattern of radioactivity gives information about the distribution of sprout tips.

Our results in both motor and sensory axons showed that in young animals the rate of regeneration of most axons was close to that of the fastest-growing ones, resulting in relatively synchronized outgrowth at approximately 4.5 mm/day. In older rats, the rate of axonal regeneration was retarded in an increasing proportion of axons, leading to a less synchronized and slower average rate of outgrowth. In the oldest rats studied (28-month-old animals) outgrowth was most markedly impaired. However, in all age groups, at least some axons continued to regenerate at a rapid rate.

It thus appears that at least two types of neuronal outgrowth, nerve terminal sprouting and axonal regeneration, are impaired with increasing age. This provides further evidence that, with aging, changes occur within the axon that impair its ability to grow. The cellular mechanisms that progressively impair outgrowth in many axons with increasing age are not known.

CONCLUSION

It appears that there are at least 4 different kinds of nerve outgrowth. Recent results suggest that several different factors may regulate even a single type of outgrowth. For example, AChRs, intrinsic axonal factors, and "synaptic basal lamina" can play an important role in nerve terminal sprouting. Future study of the control of terminal sprouting and other forms of nerve outgrowth must take into account the multifactorial nature of the sprouting process.

It should also be noted that each type of motor nerve outgrowth should be analyzed separately to determine the factors controlling them. Results regarding one type of nerve outgrowth cannot be generalized to another without sufficient evidence linking the two. For example, in the mouse soleus, α-BuTx inhibits the nerve terminal sprouting that normally appears after treatment with botulinum toxin, whereas ultraterminal sprouting from the same axons is unaffected. Future studies should clearly define the type of nerve outgrowth under investigation to avoid misinterpretation. Examination of each type of outgrowth and the analogies between them should contribute to our general understanding of neuronal growth and plasticity in both the peripheral and the central nervous system.

ACKNOWLEDGMENTS

We wish to thank Robert Adams, Julie Tomasloff, Linda Mickley, Kenneth Fahnestock, and Marilyn Peper for their technical assistance. CF Barlow and

MJ Klein provided expert assistance with the manuscript. The original research carried out in the authors' laboratories was supported in part by National Institutes of Health (NIH) grants 5 PO1 NS10920 and 5 RO1 HD04817, and grants from the Muscular Dystrophy Association. Dr. Pestronk was supported by a Teacher-Investigator Award from the NIH.

REFERENCES

1. Diamond J, Cooper E, Turner C, et al: Trophic regulation of nerve sprouting. Science 193:371–377, 1976

2. Barker D, Ip MC: Sprouting and degeneration of mammalian motor axons in normal and deafferented skeletal muscle. Proc R Soc [Biol] 163:538–554, 1966

3. Wernig A, Pécot-Dechavassine M, Stöver, H: Sprouting and regression of the nerve at frog neuromuscular junction in normal conditions and after prolonged paralysis with curare. J Neurocytol 9:277–303, 1980

4. Hoffman H: Local reinnervation in partially denervated muscle: a histophysiological study. Aust J Exp Biol 28:383–397, 1950

5. Coërs C. Telerman-Toppet N, Gerard J: Terminal denervation ratio in neuromuscular disease. Arch Neurol 29:210–222, 1973

6. Bickerstaff ER, Woolf AL: The intramuscular nerve endings in myasthenia gravis. Brain 83:10–23, 1960

7. Brown MC, Ironton R: Motor nerve sprouting induced by prolonged tetrodotoxin block of nerve action potentials. Nature 265:459–461, 1977

8. Pestronk A, Drachman DB: A new stain for quantitative measurement of sprouting at neuromuscular junctions. Muscle Nerve 1:70–74, 1978

9. Pestronk A, Drachman DB: Motor nerve sprouting and acetylcholine receptors. Science 199:1223–1225, 1978

10. Duchen LW, Strich SJ: The effects of botulinum toxin on the pattern of innervation of skeletal muscle in the mouse. Q J Exp Physiol 53:84–89, 1968

11. Brooks VB: The action of botulinum toxin on motor-nerve filaments, J Physiol (Lond) 123:501–515, 1954

12. Tonge DA: Chronic effects of botulinum toxin on neuromuscular transmission and sensitivity to acetylcholine in slow and fast skeletal muscle of the mouse. J Physiol (Lond) 241:127–139, 1974

13. Pestronk A, Drachman DB: Effect of botulinum toxin on trophic regulation of acetylcholine receptors. Nature 264:787–789, 1976

14. Pestronk A, Drachman DB, Griffin JW: Effect of muscle disuse on acetylcholine receptors. Nature 260:352–353, 1976

15. Lavoie PA, Collier G, Tenehouse A: Comparison of α-bungarotoxin binding to skeletal muscle after inactivity or denervation. Nature 260:349–350, 1976

16. Berg DK, Kelly RB, Sargent PB, et al: Binding of bungarotoxin to acetylcholine receptors in mammalian muscle. Proc Natl Acad Sci USA 69:147–151, 1972

17. Freeman SS, Engel AG, Drachman DB: Experimental acetylcholine blockade of the neuromuscular junction: effects on endplate and muscle fiber ultrastructure. Ann NY Acad Sci 274:46–59, 1976

18. Giacobini G, Filogamo G, Weber M, et al: Effects of a snake α-neurotoxin on the development of innervated skeletal muscles in chick embryo. Proc Natl Acad Sci USA 70:1708–1712, 1973

19. Holland RL, Brown MC: Postsynaptic transmission block can cause terminal sprouting of a motor nerve. Science 207:649–651, 1980

20. Duchen LW, Tonge DA: The effects of implantation of an extra nerve on axonal sprouting usually induced by botulinum toxin in skeletal muscle of the mouse. J Anat 124:205–215, 1977

21. Marshall LM, Sanes JR, McMahan UJ: Reinnervation of original synaptic sites on muscle fiber basement membrane after disruption of the muscle cells. Proc Natl Acad Sci USA 74:3073–3077, 1977

22. Bowden REM, Duchen LW: The anatomy and pathology of the neuromuscular junction. In *Neuromuscular Junction*. Edited by Zaimis E. Springer-Verlag, Berlin, 1976, pp 23–97

23. Moore RY, Bjorklund A, Stenevi U: Growth and plasticity of adrenergic neurons. In *The Neurosciences Third Study Program*. Edited by Schmitt FO, Worden FG. MIT Press, Cambridge, MA, 1974, pp 961–977

24. Gutmann E, Gutmann L, Medawar PB, et al: The rate of regeneration of nerve. J Exp Biol 19:14–44, 1942

25. Black MM, Lasek RJ: Slowing of the rate of axonal regeneration during growth and maturation. Exp Neurol 63:108–119, 1979

26. Pestronk A, Drachman DB, Griffin JW: Effects of aging on sprouting and regeneration. Exp Neurol 70:62–85, 1980

27. Tuffery AR: Growth and degeneration of motor endplates in normal cat hind limb muscles. J Anat 110:221–247, 1971

28. Fujisawa K: Some observations on the skeletal muscle of aged rats. III. Abnormalities of terminal axons found in motor endplates. Exp Gerontol 11:43–47, 1976

29. Ruffolo RR Jr, Eisenbarth GS, Thompson JM, et al: Synapse turnover: a mechanism for acquiring synapse specificity. Proc Natl Acad Sci USA 75:2281–2285, 1978

30. Birren JE, Wall PD: Age changes in conduction velocity, refractory period, number of fibers, connective tissue space and blood vessels in sciatic nerve of rats. J Comp Neurol 104:1–16, 1956

31. Gutmann E, Hanzlikova V: Motor unit in old age. Nature 209:921–922, 1966

DISCUSSION

Dr. Andrew Engel: One comment: destruction of the junctional folds, by whatever mechanisms, seems to turn on local sprouting. One question: have you looked at the ultrastructure of the sprouts that seems to appear after local injection of the AChR? Could the swelling of the nerve terminals be caused by Triton-X, which contaminates the receptor preparation?

Dr. Alan Pestronk: With regard to your comment, the sprouting that occurs after disruption of the junctional folds is complicated and is seen over a long period of time. Over a short period of time, in the experimental autoimmune myasthenia gravis (EAMG) model, the disease actually inhibits the amount of sprouting that can occur during a defined period of time. In answer to your question, we have not looked at the ultrastructure.

Dr. Daniel Drachman: One point worth making is that the bungarotoxin-blocked receptor did not elicit the same kinds of change as did receptor alone and, of course, both preparations contained the Triton X.

Dr. Andrew Engel: I would like to follow through on the previous question. We also looked at the endplate in rats with EAMG. In chronic EAMG there is sprouting with "elongation" of the end-plate as judged by methylene blue and cholinesterase preparations and by electron microscopy. This is seen about 50 to 60 days after the induction of the disease.

Dr. Alan Pestronk: There is no question that there is sprouting in that model. However, the speed at which those terminals can sprout is much slower than normal. For instance, if we administer botulinum toxin to normal animals and EAMG animals, sprouting occurs more slowly in the EAMG animals. It does occur over a long period of time, but antibody does not totally block the receptor and does not totally inhibit the denervation changes.

Dr. Andrew Engel: If I understand your argument that extrajunctional AChRs induce nerve terminal sprouting, you are saying that there is much less sprouting after bungarotoxin than after botulinum toxin. Another interpretation is that the botulinum toxin acts directly on the nerve terminal to induce sprouting.

Dr. Alan Pestronk: Bungarotoxin actually inhibits the sprouting seen after botulinum toxin. In addition, most of the evidence suggests that botulinum toxin can elicit sprouting only by inducing denervation changes in muscle. If one eliminates the denervation changes in muscle without reducing the botulinum toxin-induced blockade, one reduces the amount of nerve terminal sprouting.

Dr. Henning Schmalbruch: Do you have an explanation for why axons do not sprout in partially denervated muscles in newborn rats? This might be important for our understanding of the development of Werdnig-Hoffmann's disease.

Dr. Alan Pestronk: No. The stimuli that evoke collateral sprouting are very poorly defined.

14

Regeneration of the Neuromuscular Junction: Steps Toward Defining the Molecular Basis of the Interaction Between Nerve and Muscle

Lee L. Rubin, PhD

U. J. McMahan, PhD

Less than 0.1% of a muscle fiber's surface is occupied by presynaptic nerve terminals, yet this relatively tiny region is highly specialized in its molecular composition. For example, the concentration of acetylcholine receptors (AChRs) in the portion of the myofiber plasma membrane that lies opposite the nerve terminals is at least 500 times greater than elsewhere on the muscle cell (1–4), and when one stains for acetylcholinesterase (AChE) on the surface of myofibers it is seen only at the neuromuscular junction (5, 6). Moreover, specific components of the myofiber surface at the junction play an important role in reestablishing neuromuscular function after trauma; damaged axons and myofibers regenerate to reform neuromuscular junctions precisely at original synaptic sites within a muscle (7–9).

Our laboratory has undertaken a series of experiments to identify structures at the muscle fiber synaptic site that influence restoration of the neuromuscular junction after damage and to determine what information these structures provide. Findings to date demonstrate that factors which direct the growth and differentiation of regenerating axons and the differentiation of the postsynaptic membrane of regenerating myofibers are tightly bound to the myofiber's extracellular matrix and are maintained for days in the absence of myofibers and axons. At least some of the factors are associated with the portion of the myofiber's basal lamina sheath that is situated in the narrow space between the nerve terminal and the myofiber. Documentation of these findings is presented elsewhere (10–14). Here we review evidence that supports some of the major conclusions and present a brief account of our initial attempts to define the molecular nature of the components of the extracellular matrix that influence regeneration.

BASAL LAMINA DIRECTS SYNAPTIC DIFFERENTIATION

Each vertebrate skeletal muscle cell is ensheathed by basal lamina (Fig. 1), a felt-like material containing collagen (11, 15–17). The basal lamina sheath is approximately 15 nm thick and is separated from the lipid-rich plasma membrane of the muscle cell by a narrow electron-lucent gap. Delicate strands of material run from the surface of the plasma membrane to the basal lamina (18). At the neuromuscular junction the myofiber basal lamina extends through the synaptic cleft. The postsynaptic membrane at vertebrate neuromuscular junctions is depressed at regular intervals, forming junctional folds that can be as much as 1 μm deep. Projections of the myofiber's basal lamina sheath extend into the folds.

Molecules associated with the synaptic portion of the myofiber basal lamina distinguish it from other portions of the basal lamina. For example, much of the junctional AChE is attached to or is a part of the basal lamina (19–21). Moreover, Sanes and Hall (17) have made antibodies that bind selectively to the synaptic portion of the myofiber basal lamina.

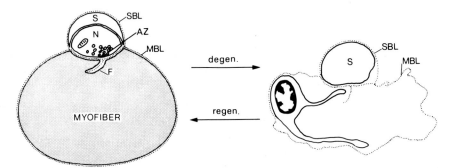

Fig. 1. Degeneration and regeneration of myofibers and axon terminals. Myofibers are normally ensheathed by basal lamina (MBL), which passes between the nerve terminal (N) and myofiber at the neuromuscular junction. Basal lamina also projects into junctional folds. Seven days after damage to nerve and muscle, myofibers and nerve terminals degenerate and are phagocytized. The basal lamina sheaths remain intact and contain mononucleated cells. The portion of basal lamina that extended into junctional folds also persists. Schwann cell processes (S) occupy the position of the nerve terminal on the presynaptic side of the myofiber basal lamina. By 2 weeks after damage to the nerve and muscle, new myofibers form within the basal lamina sheaths of the original myofibers and axons regrow to establish neuromuscular junctions at original synaptic sites on the sheaths. The new nerve terminals have active zones (AZ), and the myofibers have junctional folds as do the original ones. SBL, Schwann cell basal lamina.

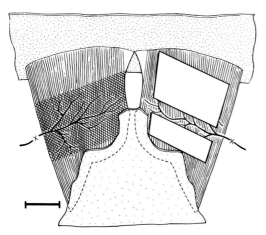

Fig. 2. The cutaneous pectoralis muscles. Slabs have been cut from the right muscle, leaving a narrow band of damaged muscle fiber segments in the region of innervation. The shaded area in the left muscle is the portion of the muscle that was frozen to kill all cells at the neuromuscular junctions. Points of nerve damage are marked with an X. Bar, 3 mm.

The presence of factors associated with basal lamina that influence regeneration of motor axons and myofibers was demonstrated in the following way. Experiments were done using the thin, paired cutaneous pectoralis muscles (Fig. 2) of the frog, which are situated just beneath the skin of the chest. The frog neuromuscular junction has the same general features as mammalian neuromuscular junctions (22, 23). Each myofiber is innervated by one myelinated motor axon that terminates in an arborization of unmyelinated branches. Each terminal branch is capped by a Schwann cell and is situated in a shallow gutter in the myofiber surface. The Schwann cell also has a basal lamina; it fuses with that of the myofiber at the edge of the junction. Each terminal branch has thousands of synaptic vesicles that contain the transmitter, acetylcholine. The vesicles are situated mainly in the half of the terminal that faces the muscle fiber, and some are focused on patches of osmiophilic material that line the cytoplasmic surface of the presynaptic membrane. The patches of osmiophilic material and their vesicle clusters occur at approximately 1-μm intervals along each terminal branch; it is at these sites, called "active zones" (24), that vesicles fuse with presynaptic membrane during synaptic transmission (24, 25). Junctional folds in the myofiber plasma membrane occur just opposite the active zones; accordingly, they also are distributed at 1-μm intervals along the synaptic gutter.

The cutaneous pectoralis muscles in anesthetized frogs were denervated, and at the same time slabs of muscle on each side of the region of innervation were removed, leaving behind a narrow band of cut muscle fiber segments (Fig. 2) (10). Within 1 week, the damaged myofiber segments degenerated and were phagocytized, as were the nerve terminals, but the basal lamina tubes of the myofiber segments remained intact (Fig. 1). Original synaptic sites were identified, even on these empty tubes, by the accumulation of AChE. The basal lamina tubes contained mononucleated cells that included macrophages and myoblasts. The myoblasts divided and fused to form new myofibers within the basal lamina sheaths of the original myofibers, and damaged axons grew to reinnervate precisely the original synaptic sites on the sheaths; by 2 weeks after damage, the new neuromuscular junctions looked and performed much like the original ones (10) (Fig. 1).

To study reinnervation of the basal lamina sheaths in the absence of myofibers, the frogs were x-irradiated near the time of the operation, preventing mitosis of the myoblasts and hence the formation of myofibers for at least 1 month (11). In muscles that had been damaged, denervated, and x-irradiated, axons returned precisely to original synaptic sites on the basal lamina sheaths even though their target cells, the myofibers, were absent (11). The terminals accumulated synaptic vesicles, most of which were in the half of the terminal that faced the myofiber basal lamina as at normal neuromuscular junctions. In addition, active zones, including both vesicle clusters and patches of osmiophilic material, were situated on the nerve terminal plasma membrane. The active zones occurred at intervals and were opposite basal lamina that had projected into the junctional folds of the original myofibers; thus, they were situated at the same spots as the active zones of the original nerve terminals.

These findings lead to the conclusion that factors which direct the morphogenesis of regenerating nerve terminals are associated with the synaptic portion of the myofiber basal lamina and that they are concentrated at discrete intervals. Because the myofibers were prevented from regenerating and nerves did not reach the synaptic basal lamina for more than a week after damage, these factors must be maintained for several days in the absence of presynaptic and postsynaptic cells.

To determine whether or not the presence of the nerve is required for the accumulation of AChRs and the formation of folds in regenerating myofibers, damaged muscles were permitted to regenerate (i.e., animals were not x-irradiated) and the damaged nerve was prevented from reinnervating them (12). The distribution of AChRs on the regenerating myofibers were examined by labeling the receptors with ^{125}I-α-bungarotoxin and then observing autoradiographs of cross sections of the muscles by light microscopy.

We found that AChR clusters of nearly normal density were located precisely at the original synaptic sites on the basal lamina as marked by AChE staining. Nearly all of the original synaptic sites had clusters of AChRs and nearly all clusters of comparable size and density were situated at original synaptic sites. Folds similar to junctional folds developed in the myofiber surface and they were also selectively localized to the original synaptic sites in the basal lamina.

To remove from synaptic sites Schwann cells that might have released the factors that organized the AChRs, and thus to demonstrate that the basal lamina contains such factors, additional experiments were done to kill the Schwann cells as well as the axon terminals and original myofibers (13). The muscles were frozen in the region of innervation, resulting in degeneration and phagocytosis of all cellular components in that area. Large portions of the basal lamina sheaths remained intact, and new myofibers regenerated within them. Even in the absence of Schwann cells (and nerve terminals), AChRs accumulated and folds developed at the original synaptic sites on the basal lamina sheaths.

Altogether these results demonstrate that formation of the active zones in regenerating nerve terminals and the postsynaptic apparatus in regenerating myofibers is directed by factors associated with the myofiber basal lamina sheath, a morphologically well-defined component of the muscle's extracellular matrix. Knowledge of where molecules involved in regeneration of the neuromuscular junction are situated is an important step toward identifying them and learning how they are regulated.

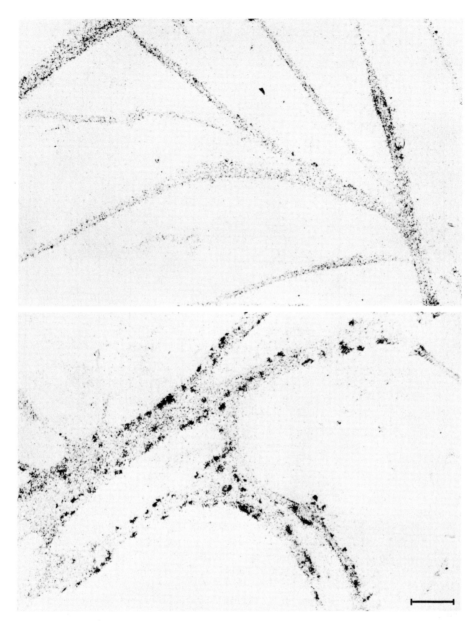

Fig. 3. The extracellular matrix fraction from the *Torpedo* electric organ induces clusters of acetylcholine receptors (AChRs) on cultured chick muscle cells. In 6-day chick muscle cultures, AChRs were labeled by incubating the cultures with 5 nM ^{125}I-α-bungarotoxin for 60 minutes at 37° C. The unbound toxin was washed away by rinsing in medium lacking toxin for 45 minutes. Experimental cultures then received 375 μg of the extracellular matrix fraction, and all cultures were incubated at 37° C for 8 hours. The cultures were fixed, coated with Kodak NTB2 emulsion, and exposed for 5 days. *Top:* Autoradiograph of myofibers from a control culture. *Bottom:* Autoradiograph of myofibers from a culture treated with the extracellular matrix fraction. In the culture treated with the extracellular matrix fraction, grains produced by ^{125}I-α-bungarotoxin are arranged in numerous dense patches, indicating that the extracellular matrix particles organized AChRs of the myofibers into clusters. Bar, 60 μm.

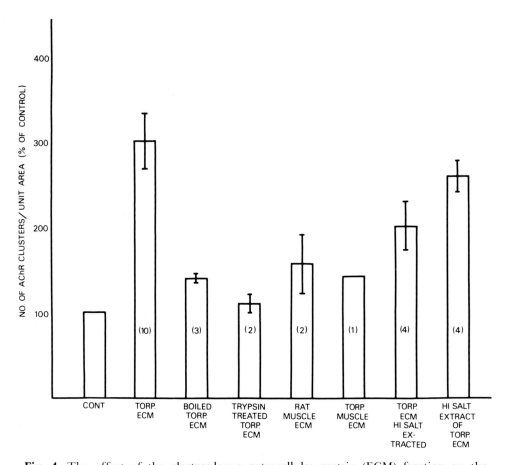

Fig. 4. The effect of the electroplaque extracellular matrix (ECM) fraction on the organization of acetylcholine receptors (AChRs) can be altered by a variety of treatments to the matrix; active molecules can be extracted from the matrix by high salt concentration, and ECM fractions from rat and *Torpedo* muscle have less influence on the organization of myofiber AChRs than does matrix from electroplaque. Cultures were processed as described in the legend to Figure 3. The number of AChR clusters/unit surface area of myofiber for each culture was determined by counting the number of autoradiographic grain clusters in 12 fields at a magnification of 160×. In each experiment on an ECM fraction, 2 to 4 cultures were analyzed, and the density of AChR clusters was expressed as a percentage of the density of clusters in control cultures that had been run in parallel. The number of experiments for each fraction is indicated in its column. Error bars give standard error of the mean except when only 2 experiments were conducted, in which case the range is indicated. The mean ± SEM density of clusters in control cultures was 22.3 ± 1.7 (n = 26). Measurements of the number and size of myofibers showed the average for 12 fields to be virtually the same from preparation to preparation. For the method of preparation, of control and *Torpedo* ECM, see legend to Figure 3. For boiled *Torpedo* ECM, the matrix fraction was boiled for 20 minutes, then resuspended by passage through a 25-gauge needle. For trypsin-treated ECM, the matrix fraction was treated with trypsin (1 mg/ml) in 150 mM NaCl in 10 mM Tris buffer at pH 7.5 for 60 minutes and then with soybean trypsin inhibitor (1 mg/ml) in the same buffer for 15 minutes. The particulate fraction was pelleted in a microfuge, washed, and resuspended. Rat and *Torpedo* muscle ECM were prepared according to the

EXTRACELLULAR MATRIX FRACTIONS THAT ORGANIZE AChRs

A step toward identifying the molecules involved in neuromuscular regeneration is to dissect chemically the extracellular components of synapses and then examine the influence of specific molecular constituents on the differentiation of nerve terminals and of the postsynaptic apparatus. Accordingly, we carried out a series of studies to develop an in vitro preparation in which extracellular matrix, nerve terminals, and muscle cells could be easily manipulated. We used the electric organ of *Torpedo californica* as the source of extracellular material.

The electric cells of the *Torpedo* are innervated by cholinergic axons, and at least 100 times more of their surface area than that of myofibers is covered by nerve terminals. For this reason, they should yield far more synaptic basal lamina per gram of tissue than should muscle. The principal aims of the experiments described here were to determine whether fractions containing extracellular matrix are rich in molecules that organize AChRs on myotubes and, if so, to reveal some of the characteristics of these molecules.

Fractions containing electric organ extracellular matrix were obtained by procedures similar to those of Meezan and colleagues (26), who isolated basal lamina from kidney and blood vessels. Our extracellular matrix fractions consisted of insoluble particles that ranged in size from less than 1 μm to 30 μm in their greatest dimension. Electron microscopy showed that the particles consisted of collagen fibrils, found only in extracellular matrix, and fine filamentous and granular material. The particles also stained intensely for AChE, an enzyme associated with basal lamina at the neuromuscular junction.

When particles of extracellular matrix were added to cultures of chick myotubes whose surface AChRs had been irreversibly labeled with ^{125}I-α-bungarotoxin, autoradiographs showed that within 2 hours there was an increase in the number of AChR clusters per unit surface area of myofiber. By 8 hours the particles had induced a 3-fold increase in clusters (Figs. 3, 4). Thus, the particles, of extracellular matrix had a marked effect on the distribution of AChRs. Because the AChRs were labeled before the addition of particles to the cultures, clusters induced by the particles must have been formed by the lateral migration of receptor molecules. Patches of AChRs opposite nerve terminals at nerve-muscle synapses developing in culture also form by lateral migration of the receptor molecules (28).

Further experiments on the extracellular matrix fractions revealed the following:

1. Boiled or trypsin-treated extracellular matrix particles produced only a small increase (30% to 50% at 8 hours) in clusters (Fig. 4); thus, production of

---

same procedures used for making electric organ ECM. For high-salt extracted *Torpedo* ECM, ECM was twice suspended in 2 M MgCl$_2$ in 10 mM Tris pH 7.5 for 60 minutes at 0° C, centrifuged, washed in NaCl-Tris buffer, and resuspended. For high-salt extraction of ECM, the ECM was treated with high salt as above and the high salt soluble material was dialyzed against NaCl-Tris buffer. Insoluble material was removed by centrifugation, and 10 to 20 μg of soluble protein were added to the culture. Protein concentration was measured by the method of Bradford (27). Aliquots of particulate fractions were dissolved in 1 N NaOH and heated to 35° C for several hours before they were assayed.

most AChR clusters is dependent on a heat-labile component of the extracellular matrix, which is probably proteinaceous.

2. The extracellular matrix particles had little, if any, effect on the number and size of myofibers; thus, the action of the matrix particles on the myotubes appears to be selective.

3. Extracellular matrix fractions from rat and *Torpedo* muscles produced an effect similar to that of boiled or trypsin-treated matrix fractions from the electric organ (Fig. 4); thus, the extracellular matrix fraction of *Torpedo* electric organ is rich in molecules that direct the organization of AChRs in comparison to similar fractions from muscle.

Studies of AChE have demonstrated that this enzyme can be dissociated from *Torpedo* electroplaque homogenates with high salt concentration (29). We therefore examined high-salt extracts from the extracellular matrix fraction to determine whether molecules that direct the organization of AChRs also can be removed by this procedure. As shown in Figure 4, after high-salt extraction, the influence of the particles on the formation of AChR clusters was markedly reduced, whereas material extracted by high salt concentration had a profound influence on the organization of AChRs. The apparent specific activity of the extracted material was 10 to 20 times that of unextracted extracellular matrix. Thus, molecules that are active in aggregating AChRs on cultured myotubes can be removed from the extracellular matrix fraction by a relatively simple and gentle procedure.

Factors that organize AChRs on cultured myofibers have been extracted from embryonic spinal cord by Podleski and colleagues (30), from neuron-conditioned medium by Christian and associates (31), and from chick central nervous system and Jessell and coworkers (32). The active molecules extracted by Podleski and colleagues and Christian and associates had a molecular weight of more than 15,000 daltons. Jessell and coworkers found active components with molecular weights much less than 15,000 daltons. We do not yet know the molecular weight of the factors extracted from *Torpedo* extracellular matrix. The factors are retained by an ultrafiltration membrane that has a molecular weight cut-off at 50,000 daltons, so the active molecules may have a molecular weight greater than this.

There may be several different molecules that can organize AChRs when applied to myofibers, but only one may be localized to the neuromuscular junction. To determine whether the material we have extracted from electroplaque extracellular matrix is similar to factors in myofiber basal lamina that influence the organization of AChRs in regenerating muscle cells and to examine its mode of action, we plan further experiments aimed at purifying the active molecules and making histologic markers for them.

REFERENCES

1. Fambrough DM, Hartzell HC: Acetylcholine receptors: number and distribution at neuromuscular junctions in rat diaphragm. Science 176:189–191, 1972

2. Kuffler SW, Yoshikami D: The distribution of acetylcholine sensitivity at the postsynaptic membrane of vertebrate skeletal twitch muscles: iontophoretic mapping in the micron range. J Physiol (Lond) 244:703–730, 1975

3. Burden S: Development of the neuromuscular junction in the chick embryo: the number, distribution, and stability of acetylcholine receptors. Dev Biol 57:317–329, 1977

4. Matthews-Bellinger J, Salpeter MM: Distribution of acetylcholine receptors at frog neuromuscular junctions with a discussion of some physiological implications. J Physiol (Lond) 279:197–213, 1978

5. Couteaux R: Localization of cholinesterase at neuromuscular junctions. Int Rev Cytol 4:335–375, 1955

6. McMahan UJ, Spitzer NC, Peper K: Visual identification of nerve terminals in living isolated skeletal muscle. Proc R Soc [B] 181:421–430, 1972

7. Tello F: Degeneration et regeneration des plaques motrices après la section des nerfs. Trav Lab Rèch Biol Univ Madrid 5:117–149, 1907

8. Gutmann E, Young JZ: The re-innervation of muscle after various periods of atrophy. J Anat 78:15–43, 1944

9. Letinsky MS, Fischbeck KH, McMahan UJ: Precision of reinnervation of original postsynaptic sites in frog muscle after a nerve crush. J Neurocytol 5:691–718, 1976

10. Marshall LM, Sanes JR, McMahan UJ: Reinnervation of original synaptic sites on muscle fiber basement membrane after disruption of the muscle cells. Proc Natl Acad Sci USA 74:3073–3077, 1977

11. Sanes JR, Marshall LM, McMahan UJ: Reinnervation of muscle fiber basal lamina after removal of muscle fibers. J Cell Biol 78:176–198, 1978

12. Burden SJ, Sargent PB, McMahan UJ: Acetylcholine receptors in regenerating muscle accumulate at original synaptic sites in the absence of the nerve. J Cell Biol 82:412–425, 1979

13. McMahan UJ, Sargent PB, Rubin LL, Burden SJ: Factors that influence the organization of acetylcholine receptors in regenerating muscle are associated with the basal lamina at the neuromuscular junction. In *Ontogenesis and Functional Mechanisms of Peripheral Synapses.* Edited by Taxi J. Elsevier/North-Holland Biomedical Press, Amsterdam, 1980, pp 345–354

14. McMahan UJ, Edgington DR, Kuffler DP: Factors that influence regeneration of the neuromuscular junction. J Exp Biol (in press)

15. Uehara Y, Campbell GR, Burnstock G: Muscle and its innervation. Arnold, London, 1976

16. Carlson EC, Brendel K, Hjelle JT, Meezan E: Ultrastructural and biochemical analyses of isolated basement membranes from kidney glomeruli and tubules and brain and retinal microvessels. J Ultrastruct Res 62:26–53, 1978

17. Sanes JR, Hall ZW: Antibodies that bind specifically to synaptic sites on muscle fiber basal lamina. J Cell Biol 83:357–370, 1979

18. Heuser J: 3-D visualization of membrane and cytoplasmic specializations at the frog neuromuscular junction. In *Ontogenesis and Functional Mechanisms of Peripheral Synapses.* Edited by Taxi J. Elsevier/North Holland Biomedical Press, Amsterdam, 1980, pp 139–155

19. Hall ZW, Kelly RB: Enzymatic detachment of endplate acetylcholinesterase from muscle. Nature 232:62–63, 1971

20. Betz W, Sakmann BJ: Effects of proteolytic enzymes on function and structure of frog neuromuscular junctions. J Physiol (Lond) 230:673–688, 1973

21. McMahan UJ, Sanes JR, Marshall LM: Cholinesterase is associated with the basal lamina at the neuromuscular junction. Nature 271:172–174, 1978

22. Birks R, Huxley HE, Katz B: The fine structure of the neuromuscular junction of the frog. J Physiol (Lond) 150:134–144, 1960

23. Zacks SI: *The Motor Endplate.* RE Krieger Publishing Co, Huntington, 1973, pp 52–70

24. Couteaux R, Pécot-Dechavássine M: Vésicules synaptiques et poches au niveau des 'zones actives' de la jonction neuromusculaire. C R Acad Sci [D] (Paris) 271:2346–2349, 1970

25. Heuser JE, Reese TS, Dennis MJ, Jan Y, Jan L, Evans L: Synaptic vesicle exocytosis captured by quick freezing and correlated with quantal transmitter release. J Cell Biol 81:275–300, 1979

26. Meezan E, Hjelle JJ, Brendel K, Carlson EC: A simple versatile, nondisruptive method for the isolation of morphologically and chemically pure basement membranes from several tissues. Life Sci 17:1721–1732, 1975

27. Bradford MM: A rapid and sensitive method for the quantitation of microgram quantities of protein utilizing the principle of protein-dye binding. Anal Biochem 72:248–254, 1976

28. Anderson MJ, Cohen MW: Nerve-induced and spontaneous redistribution of acetylcholine receptors on cultured muscle cells. J Physiol (Lond) 268:757–773, 1977

29. Lwebuga-Mukasa JS, Lappi S, Taylor P: Molecular forms of acetylcholinesterase from *Torpedo californica:* their relationship to synaptic membranes. Biochemistry 15:1425–1434, 1976

30. Podleski TR, Axelrod D, Ravdin P, Greenberg I, Johnson MM, Salpeter MM: Nerve extract induces increase and redistribution of acetylcholine receptors on cloned muscle cells. Proc Natl Acad Sci USA 75:2035–2039, 1978

31. Christian CN, Daniels MP, Sugiyama H, Vogel Z, Jacques L, Nelson PG: A factor from neurons increases the number of acetylcholine receptor aggregates on cultured muscle cells. Proc Natl Acad Sci USA 75:4011–4015, 1978

32. Jessell TM, Siegel RE, Fischbach GD: Induction of acetylcholine receptors on cultured skeletal muscle by a factor extracted from brain and spinal cord. Proc Natl Acad Sci USA 76:5397–5401, 1979

DISCUSSION

Dr. Robert Barchi: It is possible that these nerve terminals may be growing back down a gradient of ACh. This could occur if the growing nerve were releasing very low concentrations of ACh that formed a diffusion gradient in all directions. The AChE left in the muscle basal lamina would locally lower the ACh concentration, and the nerve tip could be growing down this negative concentration gradient. Have you ever tried adding irreversible organophosphate inhibitors or something like that to the basal lamina to block AChE before you reinnervate?

Dr. Jackson McMahan: Yes, we have used diisopropyl fluorophosphate to block all of the AChE that we can detect by staining. We cannot rule out the possibility that some molecules of AChE do not get inhibited. In any event, the regenerating axons still grow precisely to original synaptic spots on myofiber basal lamina sheaths in the absence of the myofibers.

Dr. Richard Almon: As you and, I think, Dr. Fischbach pointed out, extrajunctional and junctional receptors are not identical. With respect to both your and the previous talk, is it possible that extrajunctional hot spots are, in fact, junctional receptors and that the extrajunctional receptors that one sees outside the hot spots are true extrajunctional receptors? Conceivably, on denervation, the extrajunctional hot spots occur and are, in fact, the true denervation signal, rather than the diffuse extrajunctional receptors.

Dr. Jackson McMahan: Dr. Fischbach, would you like to answer that question?

Dr. Gerald Fischbach: Most studies suggest that the receptors that appear clustered on uninnervated fibers are more like extrajunctional than junctional receptors, but the issue becomes a bit semantic: the difference depends on how you define one rather than the other. In terms of metabolic half-life and mean channel open time, they seem to be more like extrajunctional receptors even though they are clustered.

15
Cell Surface and Secretory Proteins of Skeletal Muscle

Douglas M. Fambrough, PhD

Richard Rotundo, PhD

John M. Gardner, PhD

Ellen K. Bayne, PhD

Eric Wakshull, PhD

M. John Anderson, PhD

A focus of research in our laboratory has been the metabolism of acetylcholine receptors (AChRs) in skeletal muscle (1). Recently, we have extended these studies to the acetylcholinesterases (AChEs), which include both membrane-associated and secreted forms (2). Many of the major features of their metabolism are shared by these glycoproteins. In carrying out such comparative studies, we have been motivated in part by our interest in the involvement of both of these molecules in neuromuscular transmission and in part by curiosity about the basic cellular mechanisms for handling membrane and secretory proteins. A couple of comparative experiments are described here to illustrate first some aspects of membrane biogenesis and secretion, and then some aspects of membrane protein turnover. These comparisons allow us to generate working hypotheses about cell surface and secretory proteins in skeletal muscle. Later we describe some of our efforts to use monoclonal antibody technology (3) to study these proteins further.

ACETYLCHOLINE RECEPTORS AND ACETYLCHOLINESTERASE

Biosynthesis and Transport

Metabolic labeling with isotopically heavy amino acids has provided direct evidence for the rapid translation of AChR messenger ribonucleic acids and

197

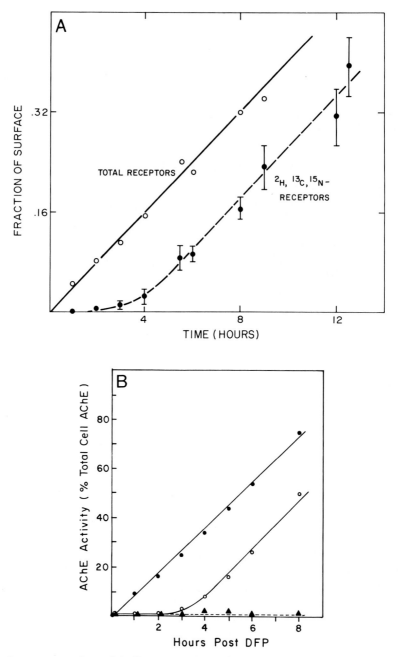

Fig. 1. Appearance of acetylcholine receptors (AChRs) and secretory acetylcholinesterase (AChE) at the cell surface. (**A**) Kinetics of appearance of AChRs at the cell surface after block of preexisting cell surface AChRs with unlabeled α-bungarotoxin. At time zero, the muscle cultures were switched to a medium containing ^2H, ^{13}C, ^{15}N-labeled amino acids and the appearance of total (○) and of dense-labeled (●) AChRs was measured. (Reprinted with permission from Devreotes PN, Gardner JM, Fambrough DM: Kinetics of acetylcholine receptor biosynthesis and subsequent incorporation into plasma membrane of cultured chick skeletal muscle. Cell 10:365:373, 1977.) (**B**) Kinetics of secretion

198

assembly of newly synthesized polypeptide chains into full-sized AChR units (4). Binding studies and electron microscopic (EM) autoradiography have identified the Golgi apparatus as the major intracellular residence of newly synthesized AChR molecules (5). Kinetic studies with both heavy amino acid labeling and with EM techniques have established that the intracellular residence time for the newly made AChRs is approximately 3 hours, after which the receptors become incorporated into the plasma membrane.

Figure 1A illustrates the time course of appearance of new cell surface AChRs in cultured skeletal muscle after the preexisting receptors had been blocked with α-bungarotoxin (α-BuTx). New sites begin appearing immediately, indicating a continuous replenishment of surface receptors. If the cells are switched to fresh medium containing dense amino acids at this time, it is possible to examine directly the kinetics of appearance of dense labeled AChRs on the surface. The dense AChRs begin to appear several hours after the switch. The lag before appearance of dense AChRs on the surface has been shown to reflect the intracellular biosynthesis-transit time for AChRs. Approximately 2 hours of this time is required for the transport of newly synthesized AChR molecules through the Golgi apparatus.

Figure 1B illustrates the kinetics of secretion of AChE into the culture medium by myogenic cells. When the cells are placed in esterase-free culture medium, there is a linear accumulation of enzyme in the medium during the next several hours. If diisopropyl fluorophosphate (DFP) is used to inactivate both cell surface and intracellular AChE molecules, there is a delay of several hours before the secretion of functional AChE molecules resumes. During this period the myotubes replenish their intracellular pool of AChE. Only then does the secretion of active enzyme resume. The graphs in Figure 1 illustrate that the incorporation of AChRs into the plasma membrane and the secretion of AChE into the culture medium follow similar kinetics. In fact, partial inhibition of these processes with various reagents results in quantitatively similar decreases in the appearance of both molecules. No strategy that we have used has yet succeeded in separating the two processes.

The simplest explanation for the coupling of membrane biogenesis and secretion is that membrane and secretory glycoproteins follow a similar pathway through intracellular organelles during biosynthesis and posttranslational modification. Our experiments suggest that such a pathway might also include a common vehicle of transport from Golgi apparatus to the cell surface, leading both to the exteriorization of AChRs and the liberation of AChE. One

---

of AChE from chick muscle cultures. At time zero, some cultures were treated with diisopropyl fluorophosphate (DFP) to inactivate both cell surface and internal AChE molecules (○). The secretion of AChE was then followed by measuring the accumulation of AChE in the culture medium. Untreated cultures served as positive controls (●). Experiments A and B are designed to show, respectively, that AChRs and AChE are synthesized several hours before their appearance at the cell surface. The cycloheximide control (▲) shows that new protein synthesis is required for appearance of secretory AChE after a DFP block. (Reprinted with permission from Rotundo RL, Fambrough DM: Synthesis, transport and fate of acetylcholinesterase in cultured chick embryo muscle cells. Cell 22:583–594, 1980.)

experimental test of this hypothesis would be to demonstrate the occurrence of AChRs and AChE (both newly synthesized) in post-Golgi transport vesicles. Another potential approach would be to determine whether the kinetics of biosynthesis and secretion, or incorporation into plasma membrane, apply generally to all plasma membrane and secretory proteins. This will require the identification of other secretory and membrane proteins, as well as examination of their production and exteriorization by developing muscle cells.

Thus, some of our current research goals are: (a) to identify other plasma membrane proteins and secretory proteins produced by skeletal muscle fibers; (b) to determine whether or not these substances follow more than one kinetic path from biosynthesis to exteriorization; and (c) to determine more directly whether membrane proteins and secretory proteins (or some subset of the two) are cotransported from Golgi apparatus to plasma membrane.

Turnover

The cell surface AChR and surface-bound AChE constitute a pair of membrane proteins whose turnover rates can be measured simultaneously on the same myotubes. For example, AChR turnover rate can be estimated by determining the kinetics of degradation of iodinated α-BuTx bound to AChRs (1). The turnover rate thus obtained is only slightly slower than that determined by direct labeling (6). If anything, it slightly overestimates the lifespan of AChR molecules. Likewise, cell-surface AChE can be labeled covalently with radioactive DFP to study its fate. Figure 2 illustrates results of such a comparative study of AChR and AChE turnover in cultured chick muscle. Less direct experiments, such as measuring the survival of the populations of AChRs and AChE after blockade of biosynthesis of new functional molecules with the inhibitor tunicamycin, led to the same conclusion: the AChR and the membrane-bound AChE turn over at very different rates.

At present it is not known what cellular mechanisms are responsible for these remarkably different turnover rates, nor even whether it is reasonable to expect any consistency in turnover rate among other membrane proteins. In fact, one long-standing problem has been the paucity of well-characterized membrane proteins to study. A similar problem exists for secretory proteins. Secretion has been studied mostly in the context of exocrine and endocrine glands. In such cases the secretory components may be stored for release on demand. This is a specialized form of secretion that does not seem to be coupled tightly to renewal of plasma membrane components. In the case of skeletal muscle, the secretory products are not well characterized. Presumably, a major function of the secretory proteins of skeletal muscle is to provide building material for renewal or expansion of extracellular matrix, including the prominent basement membrane that surrounds each muscle fiber. Few matrix components have been characterized even crudely, and the cellular sources of this material have been a matter of speculation.

To understand what regulates the synthesis, transport, and turnover of both membrane and secretory proteins, it is thus essential to identify additional components for study. For this purpose, our laboratory has begun to apply recently developed techniques for the generation of monoclonal antibodies.

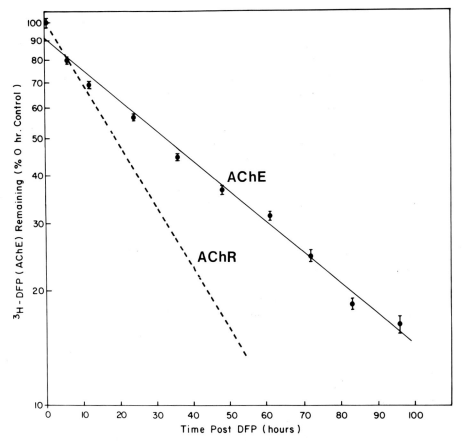

Fig. 2. Kinetics of turnover of cell surface–associated acetylcholinesterase (AChE) and acetylcholine receptors (AChRs) on cultured chick myotubes. Cell surface AChE was tagged selectively with [3]-labeled diisopropyl fluorophosphate (DFP) by treating cultures with unlabeled DFP in the presence of a water-soluble AChE inhibitor, BW 284c51, which protected the cell surface AChE from DFP blockade. The unbound DFP was then removed, and the cell surface AChE was labeled with ^{3}H-DFP in the absence of the BW compound. Subsequently, the amount of radioactivity remaining bound to AChE was measured as a function of time (○). The turnover of AChRs was measured on cells from the same set, treated in the same manner with DFP and then with ^{125}I-labeled α-bungarotoxin to label the AChRs. Receptor turnover was then estimated as the rate of loss of radioactivity from the cultures (dashed line).

STUDIES USING MONOCLONAL ANTIBODIES

Monoclonal antibodies are products of clonally derived immunoglobulin-secreting cells. Each monoclonal antibody is a single molecular species and has a simple target specificity. Köhler and Milstein (3) have developed methods that allow the investigator to generate continuous tissue culture cell lines which produce antibodies of preselected target specificity. We have used these techniques to generate monoclonal antibodies whose targets are various muscle membrane and secretory proteins. Each monoclonal antibody has specificity for a target antigen that is potentially as unique as is α-BuTx for the AChR.

With monoclonal antibody technology two major experimental difficulties can be overcome. One is the problem of identifying plasma membrane proteins unambiguously. The other is the problem of determining the type of cell on which a particular membrane protein is located.

A particularly useful property of proteinaceous probes such as monoclonal antibodies is that they do not cross cell membranes. Thus, if it can be shown that a monoclonal antibody binds to living cells, its binding signifies a set of exterior sites. Furthermore, when the antibodies are labeled with tracers detectable by fluorescence microscopy or autoradiography, then the distribution of the binding sites can be determined. Figure 3 illustrates cases in which various monoclonal antibodies from our collection show cell type–specific binding for neurons, myoblasts, and myotubes in culture.

We envision monoclonal antibodies being of great utility at four steps in our research program:

1. Identification and localization of antigenic sites on cells. As described previously, the antibodies can be used to define cell surface components and distinguish which cell type bears the antigen.

2. Quantification of antigenic sites. Using directly labeled monoclonal antibody, the number of antigenic sites can be determined.

3. Purification of antigen. The antibodies are valuable in assays for antigen during purification, and in some cases, for detection of antigen after separations such as electrophoresis and isoelectric focusing.

4. Determination of antigen function. A useful property of multivalent anti-

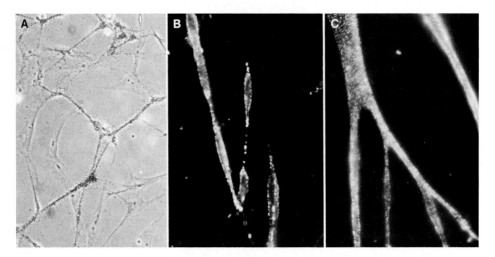

Fig. 3. Distribution of target antigen for hybridoma 24 IgG on nerve and myogenic cell cultures. (**A**) Autoradiograph showing silver grains over neuronal cell bodies and processes in chick spinal cord tissue culture exposed to no. 24 antibody and then to iodinated rabbit anti-mouse antibody. (**B** and **C**). Immunofluorescence staining of myoblasts (**B**) and myotubes (**C**) with no. 24 IgG followed by fluoresceinated rabbit anti-mouse antibody.

bodies is that they can trigger rapid turnover of cell-surface antigens. This is a feature of the disease myasthenia gravis, wherein antibodies against AChRs cause accelerated turnover of the receptors. If we search for deficits in membrane function after chronic exposure of muscle cells to monoclonal antibodies that interact with membrane proteins, we may discover the functions of some of the target antigens. In this way we hope to identify some interesting ion channels and transport molecules.

Producing the Antibodies

We have used various immunogens to generate clones of antibody-producing cells, henceforth called hybridomas. Most of the hybridomas were produced from Balb/c mice, which we immunized with a crude muscle membrane preparation. Leg muscle from 14-day chick embryos was homogenized in a dilute salt solution. Membranes were sedimented at 20,000 g for 15 minutes, washed several times to remove soluble proteins, and used together with Freund's complete adjuvant as immunogen. After the initial immunization and a boost with antigen 1 month later, spleen cells were isolated (3 days after the boost) and fused with myeloma cells (SP2/0 nonsecreting cells). The fusion protocol was essentially that of Kennett and associates (7) and used polyethylene glycol (PEG 1000) as fusagen. Hybridoma cells were selected by their ability to grow in hypoxanthine-aminopterin-thymidine (HAT) medium. Medium from culture wells that contained rapidly growing hybrid cells was tested for the presence of antibodies directed against chick skeletal muscle. The first test consisted of determining whether any antibody in the culture medium would bind to exposed antigens on primary cultures of chick muscle. An iodinated second antibody directed against the Fab portion of mouse antibodies was used to estimate the amount of bound mouse immunoglobulin (see legend to Fig. 3).

Other screening tests have included (*a*) indirect fluorescent antibody staining, both of cultured muscle and of frozen sections of adult tissues, and (*b*) antibody binding to antigens that had been adsorbed to microtiter wells. The fluorescent antibody assays have been particularly useful in identifying extracellular matrix antigens, whereas the microtiter well assay has been valuable both in purifying solubilized antigens and in screening for hybridomas that secrete monoclonal antibodies against easily purified material such as collagen and coated vesicles.

Hybridomas judged useful in the screening tests were cloned in soft agar as many as 3 times. At this stage we routinely overlayed the agar clones with rabbit anti-mouse IgM or rabbit anti-mouse IgG serum. Under these conditions secreting clones become centers of precipitin rings and the isotype of the secreted antibody can be determined. High secretor IgG and IgM clones were rescreened and then grown as ascites tumors in the peritoneal cavity of mice. The ascites fluid was fractionated by ammonium sulfate precipitation, and the antibody was purified by gel filtration on Ultragel 22 (LKB) and/or by ion exchange chromatography on diethylaminoethyl-52 Sephadex (Pharmacia). In this manner, as much as 250 mg of antibody (at least 80% pure) was obtained. In many experiments, such purified antibody was derivatized and used in direct immunoassays. For example, iodinated antibody was used to measure the on and off rates for binding to antigen.

Cell Specificity

Several of our monoclonal antibodies have interesting specificities for cells of myogenic or neurogenic origin. Two of these antibodies recognize different antigens on myoblasts that disappear or decrease drastically in amount after muscle cell fusion. One of these antigens is shared by fibroblasts. The other is absent from fibroblasts but occurs on Schwann cells as a prominent antigen. Still other antibodies recognize both neurons and muscle fibers but do not bind to various nonexcitable cells (Fig. 3). Reagents such as these should prove useful in studies of myogenesis and analysis of cell-surface proteins of muscle and nerve. However, two technical problems must be solved in our laboratory before full utility of these antibodies can be achieved. First, the antigens must be identified (as polypeptides or other molecular species) so that biochemical experiments can proceed. Second, the functions of the antigens must be determined if the antibodies are to be of major use in physiologic experiments. It has been our judgment that most rapid progress could be made by studying antigens that are among the secretory proteins. For these antigens the problem of biochemical identity is simplified. As our proficiency in the use of monoclonal antibodies increases, the approach to the membrane antigens will become easier.

"Deep Six" Procedure

A problem in studying secretion from skeletal muscle is the presence of cells other than muscle fibers. In culture this problem is often fought by treatment with antimitotic drugs, which affect surviving myotubes as well as killing or halting the growth of other cell types. Monoclonal antibodies have provided us with another solution. Among our collection of hybridomas is one that secretes an IgM that, together with guinea pig complement, will kill all dividing cells, leaving a population consisting of almost pure myotubes (at least 97% of nuclei in multinucleated syncytia and another fraction in differentiated mononucleated muscle elements). After this treatment (which we affectionately refer to as "the deep six" procedure, because the hybridoma was arbitrarily numbered 6), the secretory proteins of the myotubes can be labeled with radioactive amino acids and analyzed by standard techniques. An example of a "deep-sixed" culture is shown in Figure 4.

Muscle Secretory Proteins

The secretory proteins of muscle fibers in tissue culture are a complex mixture. After reduction, denaturation, and electrophoresis on polyacrylamide gels in the presence of sodium dodecyl sulfate (Fig. 5), the pattern of radioactively labeled polypeptides includes species ranging in molecular weight (MW) from more than 300,000 daltons to less than 40,000 daltons. Some of these peptides are proline rich, as determined by metabolic labeling with ^{3}H-proline. A subset of these are probably collagenous, because they have MWs similar to those of procollagen subunits (160,000 to 200,000 daltons) and are selectively destroyed by purified bacterial collagenase. One of our monoclonal antibodies appears to recognize a subset of these molecules. Another pair of proline-labeled peptides (MW, approximately 230,000 daltons) appear to be subunits of fibronectin. We have prepared hybridomas from mice immunized with purified fibronectin and have demonstrated that IgG from one hybridoma binds to these components.

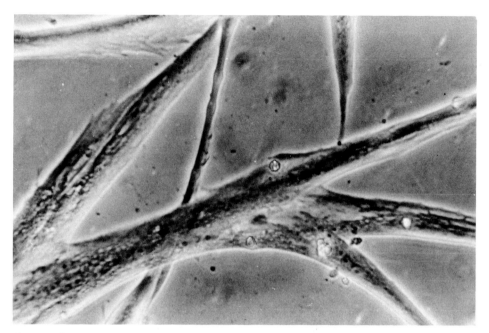

Fig. 4. Phase micrograph of chick muscle culture after "deep six" procedure, which eliminates fibroblasts and myoblasts by complement-mediated lysis. Hybridoma no. 6 IgM in a concentration of 1 µg/ml and 20% guinea pig complement were used in complete medium for 1 hour at 37° C to eliminate mononucleated cells.

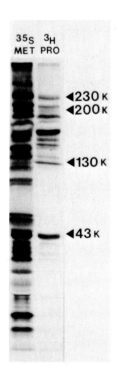

Fig. 5. Sodium dodecyl sulfate polyacrylamide gel electrophoretic patterns of chick skeletal muscle fiber secretory proteins metabolically labeled with ^{35}S-methionine and ^{3}H-proline. The proline-rich components include a fibronectin doublet with apparent molecular weights of approximately 230,000 daltons and several collagenous peptides in the molecular weight range 160,000 to 200,000 daltons. Some approximate molecular weights, based on the electrophoretic migration of standards, are indicated at right.

One of the first questions we asked about the secretory products of cultured muscle cells is whether they display a single schedule of biosynthesis and secretion. In a series of pulse and pulse-chase labeling experiments, using purified muscle cultures, we found that virtually all of the major secretory components appeared in the culture medium after a delay of approximately 2 hours. Thus, the kinetics are similar to those determined for secretion of AChE, suggesting that a single carrier mechanism may deliver all of these components to the cell surface. The lag between biosynthesis and secretion also provides a strong argument against the appearance of any of these components in the medium due to cell lysis or leakage of cytoplasmic proteins from the cells.

Extracellular Matrix Components

A group of monoclonal antibodies in our collection defines several of the components of the extracellular matrix of skeletal muscle. The uniqueness of the antigens is proved by obvious differences in their abundance and in location. Some striking examples are illustrated in Figure 6. Cross sections of adult chicken skeletal muscle were fluorescently stained with various hybridoma antibodies. These micrographs illustrate several morphologic classes of binding sites that can be distinguished by light microscopy: the continuous rings of

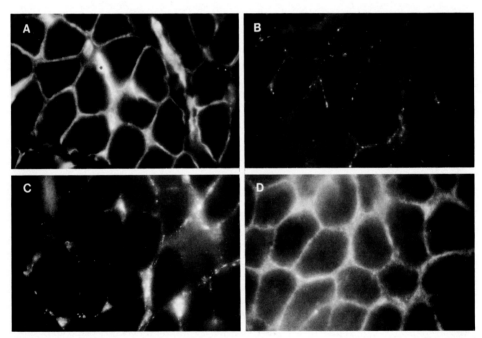

Fig. 6. Immunofluorescent staining of adult chicken skeletal muscle cross sections with monoclonal antibodies to various components of the extracellular matrix. This series demonstrates the different arrangements of some of these antigens. (**A**) Staining of a presumed basal lamina component with hybridoma 33 IgG. (**B**) Punctate distribution of hybridoma 3 antibody staining between muscle fibers. (**C**) Staining of fibronectin with hybridoma B3 IgG. (**D**) Staining of the extracellular matrix with hybridoma 15 IgG. An intensely stained neuromuscular junction (*) is indicated in panel A.

basement membrane around each muscle fiber (A); small punctate accumulations of antigen between adjacent fibers (B); fibronectin-containing elements that run between fibers (C); and an antigen that is diffusely distributed throughout the endomysium (D). At present we are using ultrastructural techniques to determine more exactly the distribution of each of these antigens.

In the study of extracellular matrix, the combined use of monoclonal antibodies and tissue culture techniques seems very powerful. As it turns out, each of the antigens we identified within the extracellular matrix of adult muscle also appears to be synthesized by embryonic muscle in tissue culture. Furthermore, each of the components interacts with sites in the culture environment, resulting in the attachment of the antigen to substrate and cells. The substrate binding (Fig. 7) suggests that antigens may exist as soluble secretory components. Thus, it should be possible to identify soluble secretory components corresponding to each matrix antigen. The matrix itself is highly cross linked by covalent interactions in vivo and has proved intractable to conventional biochemical analysis (8). Analysis of the soluble products before covalent cross linking is an obvious route around the problem.

Our present efforts therefore include identification of the secretory proteins that become components of the extracellular matrix, and analysis of their biosynthesis, secretion, and assembly. It is clear already that the assembly will

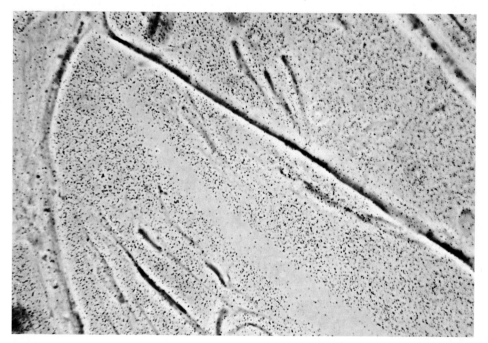

Fig. 7. Autoradiograph of chick muscle culture after exposure to hybridoma B1 antibody and then to iodinated rabbit anti-mouse IgG. Silver grains are distributed preferentially over the culture dish where no cells are located. The area relatively free of silver grains was formerly occupied by a myotube that pulled loose from the dish but is still visible in this photograph.

be a most interesting aspect to study. Assembly of such an orderly extracellular structure must involve specific interactions between individual matrix components. It also must involve interaction between secretory components and elements of the plasma membrane. One such interaction, between the muscle fiber membrane and a basal lamina component, has become a matter of keen interest to us, for it may relate to the problem of synaptogenesis and membrane organization (see chapter 14 and references 9 and 10).

In Figure 6A, an area of bright fluorescence is marked by an asterisk, indicating that this area was not only rich in binding sites for the antibody but also was an endplate region, as determined by fluorescent α-BuTx binding in the same section. This correspondence in location of AChRs and the antigen is better illustrated in Figure 8, where a grazing longitudinal section through a 3-week-old chicken anterior latissimus dorsi muscle is stained with tetramethylrhodamine-labeled α-BuTx and fluoresceinated antibody (double-antibody method). The antibody binding sites are located all along the muscle fiber surface as well as at the neuromuscular junction. At the junction there is close correspondence in the distribution of AChRs and accumulations of the antigen. (Unlike the AChRs, this antigen is not solubilized by non-ionic detergents.)

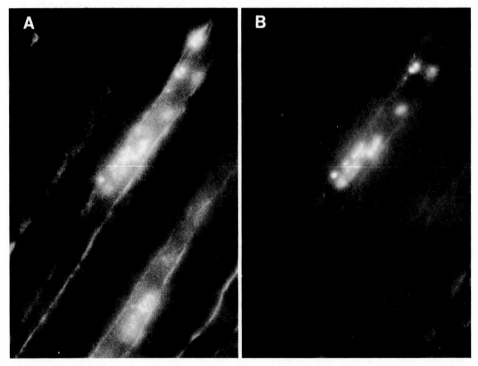

Fig. 8. Distribution of "33 antigen" and acetylcholine receptors in adult chicken skeletal muscle. Muscle was first exposed to rhodamine labeled α-bungarotoxin, then frozen and sectioned longitudinally. Sections were treated with monoclonal antibody (1 μg/ml) from hybridoma number 33 and fluorescein-labeled rabbit anti-mouse IgG. (**A**) Fluorescein fluorescence showing the high concentration of 33 antigen at a neuromuscular junction as well as labeling along muscle surface. (**B**) Binding of rhodamine-labeled α-bungarotoxin to the same neuromuscular junction.

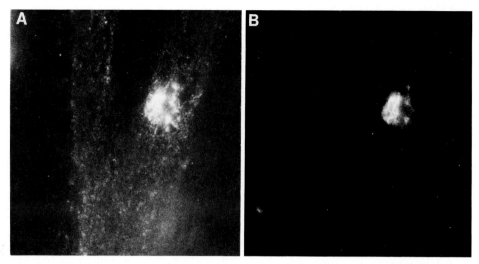

Fig. 9. Colocalization of "33 antigen" and acetylcholine receptors (AChRs) in tissue culture of chick skeletal muscle. Live cultures were exposed to rhodamine-labeled α-bungarotoxin, then to IgG (1 μg/ml) from hybridoma 33, and finally to fluorescein-labeled rabbit anti-mouse IgG. (**A**) Fluorescein fluorescence showing distribution of 33 antigen along myotube, with high concentration of antigen in a complex patch. (**B**) Rhodamine fluorescence showing clustered AChRs to which α-bungarotoxin had bound.

Accumulation of the same antigen was also examined in skeletal muscle cultures. Our original autoradiographs showed antibody binding reminiscent of the distribution of AChRs in cultured muscle except that some specific dish-associated binding also occurred. More recent studies using indirect immuno-fluorescence techniques demonstrate that the binding sites consist of a complex extracellular web and structured patches on myotubes. Double fluorescent labeling with tetramethylrhodamine-labeled α-BuTx and fluoresceinated anti-body has shown that virtually all AChR clusters on the myotubes are associated with patches of antigen (Fig. 9). However, some antigen patches occur where there is no clustering of AChRs. This is most evident in young cultures, where AChR clustering is less marked, suggesting that receptors may aggregate in response to accumulations of the antigen or in response to events that led to antigen accumulation. The colocalization of AChRs and this antigen in aneural muscle cultures suggests that a complex set of interactions, involving biosynthetic products of the muscle itself, can result in the formation of discrete sites of chemical specialization on the muscle surface. The organization at such regions mirrors, at least in part, the organization of elements of the neuromuscular junction. That such interactions, involving only the muscle, occur in tissue culture brightens the prospect that the underlying molecular mechanisms may soon yield to experimental analysis.

ACKNOWLEDGMENTS

We wish to thank Delores Somerville for her excellent technical assistance. We also thank Dr. Barbara Migeon, Dr. Patricia Gearhart, Dr. John Cebra, Dr.

Hillary Koprowski, Dr. David Gottlieb, and Dr. Cesar Milstein for technical advice and generous gifts of cell lines and reagents. This research was supported by a grant from the Muscular Dystrophy Association. Dr. Rotundo and Dr. Wakshull were supported by Muscular Dystrophy Association postdoctoral fellowships.

REFERENCES

1. Fambrough DM: Control of acetylcholine receptors in skeletal muscle. Physiol Rev 59:165–227, 1979

2. Rotundo R, Fambrough DM: Molecular forms of chicken embryo acetylcholinesterase in vitro and in vivo: isolation and characterization. J Biol Chem 254:4790–4799, 1979

3. Köhler G, Milstein C: Continuous cultures of fused cells secreting antibody of predefined specificity. Nature 256:495–497, 1975

4. Devreotes PN, Gardner JM, Fambrough DM: Kinetics of acetylcholine receptor biosynthesis and subsequent incorporation into plasma membrane of cultured chick skeletal muscle. Cell 10:365–373, 1977

5. Fambrough DM, Devreotes PN: Newly synthesized acetylcholine receptors are located in the Golgi apparatus. J Cell Biol 76: 237–244, 1978

6. Gardner JM, Fambrough DM: Acetylcholine receptor degradation measured by density labeling: effects of cholinergic ligands and evidence against recycling. Cell 16:661–674, 1979

7. Kennett RH, Denis KA, Tung AS, Klinman NR: Hybrid plasmacytoma production: fusions with adult spleen cells, monoclonal spleen fragments, neonatal spleen cells and human spleen cells. In *Lymphocyte Hybridomas*. Edited by Melchers F, Potter M, Warner NL. Curr Top Microbiol Immunol 81:77–91, 1978

8. Kefalides NA, Alper R, Clark CC: Biochemistry and metabolism of basement membranes. Int Rev Cytol 61:167–228, 1979

9. Sanes JR, Marshall LM, McMahan UJ: Reinnervation of muscle fiber basal lamina after removal of myofibers: differentiation of regenerating axons at original synaptic sites. J Cell Biol 78:176–198, 1978

10. Burden SJ, Sargent PB, McMahan UJ: Acetylcholine receptors in regenerating muscle accumulate at original synaptic sites in the absence of the nerve. J Cell Biol 82:412–435, 1979

11. Rotundo RL, Fambrough DM: Synthesis, transport and fate of acetylcholinesterase in cultured chick embryo muscle cells. Cell 22:583–594, 1980

DISCUSSION

Dr. Daniel Drachman: There are some obvious parallels between your findings and those of Drs. McMahan, Pestronk, and Fischbach. In each case, basal lamina structures might be correlated with the aggregation of receptors and/or with sites for nerve attachment. Can you comment on the similarity or differences, and perhaps say something about what you think some of these basal lamina factors are?

Dr. Douglas Fambrough: I guess the big question is whether or not there is a lot more in the extracellular matrix than we know so far. Have I tagged most of the components of extracellular matrix or just a little bit of what is there? Has Dr. McMahan defined something that is made by muscle, something that is contributed by nerve, or something that is modified either by nerve or by some product of muscle? There is no way to tell at the moment, but we are going to find out in the next few years, especially with so many good investigators entering this area. The view that one gets of extracellular matrix (the basal lamina in particular) from reviews of the literature is that it is not very complicated. Only three things are defined in it: a type of protocollagen and a couple of ill-defined glycoproteins. One problem is that all of these components of basal lamina are covalently cross linked. Dr. Bunge mentioned this morning the hydroxylation of lysines and cross linking with transaminases and so on that occur in the extracellular space. You wind up with a matrix that you can only begin to analyze after pepsin digestion and separation of fragments. However, in the culture system, you have a handle on all the molecules as they come out of the cell, before all those extracellular modifications occur. I think that cultures are going to contribute centrally to analysis of what is made in the first place. Unraveling the modifications that result during intercellular interactions to produce the final "stigma" on the cells is going to require more clever approaches.

Dr. Richard Strohman: I am a stranger to all this, but when the nerve grows back to the empty muscle and localizes itself specifically at that place, where else could it go? Doesn't it grow back along a very well-defined and restricted pathway anyway?

Dr. Alan Pestronk: Yes. In some experiments we have ripped out the original nerve all the way back to the spinal cord and then implanted a foreign nerve far away and asked whether the axons grow back to these spots in the empty basal lamina sheaths. They do so just as precisely as if it had been the original nerve. We forced them to grow over nonsynaptic basal lamina to reach these spots.

Dr. Richard Strohman: In the reverse case, where the muscle grows back, are there receptor clusters anywhere else except at that particular place?

Dr. Alan Pestronk: About 90% of the receptor clusters on the muscle fiber are at the original synaptic spots, and about 90% of the original spots have receptor clusters.

Dr. Barry Wilson: How many monoclonal antibodies do you have to sort out?

Dr. Douglas Fambrough: Thirty that we bothered to clone grow as ascites forms, and we are able to purify at least 100 mg of antibody. Once you get things going, you can make more hybridomas than you can handle. You have to define your priorities after a while; many things are possible and they all take a lot of work. It is a long way from defining an antigen by antibody binding to saying what you have functionally.

Dr. Donald Fischman: I was struck by your discussion of individual monoclonal antibodies recognizing several peptides. Most of us working with these antibodies are beginning to recognize the naiveté of assuming that monoclonal antibodies would be the direct path for "plucking out" specific proteins from complex mixtures. It is clear now that the monoclonal antibodies recognize specific determinants, but these may be shared. Perhaps this fact tells us something about secreted or integral membrane proteins that share common determinants. Would you comment on the possible functional implications of what I think is a very important observation?

Dr. Douglas Fambrough: There are a lot of levels of answer to that. I will make it really short. In the case that we documented well, all of the antigenic determinants were collagenous-type molecules. We do not have anything that looks like an anti-sugar, for instance, that would be a part of a spectrum of different proteins. I also ought to point out that, on a couple of occasions, we independently cloned from a fusion hybridomas making antibody to the same determinants. Cloning cells from different culture wells does not ensure that each resultant ligand is unique. I should also point out that many of the originally cloned hybrids are low secreters; if you plate them in agar and look at how well individual subclones secrete, it varies all over the place. A large number of subclones do not secrete at all. Something we routinely do now is select among subclones of a cloned line and then isolate antibody from high secreters.

Dr. Guillermo Pilar: Do you think this kind of recognition by the basal membrane in regenerating muscle also operates in the developing muscle at the time of synapse formation?

Dr. Alan Pestronk: The basal lamina forms at about the time the neuromuscular junction is forming. However, this has not been studied very intensively. What we can get from the literature is that about the first place the basal lamina appears on a muscle cell is at the neuromuscular junction. Perhaps it serves to stabilize elements at the synaptic site that are involved in the differentiation of pre- and postsynaptic membrane. That would be one way to look at what is going on.

Part III

MYASTHENIA GRAVIS

16
Mechanisms of Acetylcholine Receptor Loss in Myasthenia Gravis

Daniel B. Drachman, MD

Alan Pestronk, MD

Elis F. Stanley, PhD

Robert N. Adams, MA

The neuromuscular junction was first implicated as the site of the abnormality in myasthenia gravis (MG) because of the similarity between MG and curare poisoning (1) and the remarkable response of many patients to anticholinesterase drugs (2, 3). Further confirmation of a defect in neuromuscular transmission came from physiologic studies demonstrating a decremental response to repetitive nerve stimulation in MG, like that seen with pharmacologic blockade of the junction (4). However, the exact site and nature of the defect remained elusive until the development and application of a new set of tools, neurotoxins from snake venoms (5), which permitted the specific identification of the acetylcholine receptor (AChR) abnormality in 1973 (6). Since that time, it has become clear that the basic defect in MG is a decrease in the number of available AChRs at neuromuscular junctions, brought about by an antibody-mediated autoimmune attack. Our understanding of the pathogenesis of the receptor defect in MG has advanced with remarkable rapidity and has begun to serve as a rational basis for the design of treatment. The purpose of this paper is to summarize current concepts of the mechanisms of AChR loss in MG.

REDUCTION OF AChRs IN MG

In 1964, Elmqvist and colleagues (7) applied microelectrode techniques to the investigation of intercostal muscles from myasthenic patients and made the important observation that the amplitude of miniature endplate potentials (mepps) was reduced to approximately 20% of normal. They suggested that the reduction of mepp amplitudes might be due to a decrease in the number of ACh molecules per quantum, resulting from an abnormality of the motor nerve terminals in MG. This concept of a presynaptic defect, although incorrect, was widely accepted for many years; evidence from physiologic, pharmacologic, and morphologic studies did not further define the precise site of the defect (8). However, it seemed theoretically possible that a decrease in the number of available postsynaptic AChRs could account for the electrophysiologic and clinical features of MG.

To test the receptor hypothesis, we obtained "motor point" biopsies from groups of patients with MG and from control subjects (6). The strips of muscle containing endplates were incubated with ^{125}I-α-bungarotoxin (^{125}I-α-BuTx) to saturate the AChRs, and the number of available AChRs was determined from the amount of bound radioactivity. The neuromuscular junctions of myasthenic patients bound only 11% to 30% as much radioactivity as those of normal subjects, indicating that they had a markedly reduced number of available AChRs. These observations have now been confirmed in several laboratories by a variety of techniques using α-BuTx binding (9–12) or electrophysiologic measurements (13, 14) (Table 1). Indeed, recent data from our laboratory suggest that the radiometric measurement of junctional AChRs in muscle biopsies may be clinically valuable as one of the most sensitive diagnostic tests for MG (Pestronk A, Drachman DB: unpublished observations).

Role of AChR Deficit in MG

These observations raised the question of whether the decrease in number of available AChRs per se could account for the physiologic abnormalities in MG,

Table 1. Evidence for Reduction of Acetylcholine Receptors in Muscle of Myasthenic Patients

Method	Result		Reference No.
	Normal	*MG*	
^{125}I-α-BuTx binding			
Scintillation counting (no. AChR sites/ NMJ)	3.7×10^7	0.54×10^7	6
Autoradiography (arbitrary units)	3.75/4	1.54/4	6
γ = Counting (AchR sites/NMJ)	1.54×10^7	0.49×10^7	11
γ = Counting (mol AChR/g muscle)	28.6×10^{-14}	10.3×10^{-14}	10
Peroxidase α-BuTx			
Electron microscopy (AChR surface/ presynaptic membrane surface)	3.06	0.98	12
ACh iontophoresis			
ACh sensitivity (mV/nC)	2,302	675	13

Abbreviations: MG, myasthenia gravis; BuTx, bungarotoxin; AChR, acetylcholine receptor; NMJ, neuromuscular junction; nC, nanocoulomb.

or whether it represented a secondary effect. To resolve this issue, we developed an experimental animal model in which the number of available AChRs in rats was reduced by specific pharmacologic blockade with α-cobratoxin (15). The receptor-blocked animals showed all the features of human MG: they were weak and had decremental responses on repetitive nerve stimulation that were typical of the pattern in MG. The decremental responses were exaggerated by small doses of D-tubocurarine and were markedly improved by administration of anticholinesterase agents. Posttetanic responses, believed to be particularly characteristic of MG (16), were also reproduced by the AChR-blockade model. Furthermore, α-cobratoxin has been shown to reduce the amplitude of mepps (17). The cobratoxin model strongly supported the hypothesis that a decreased number of available AChRs is sufficient to account for the clinical and physiologic defects of human MG.

Morphologic studies of neuromuscular junctions of myasthenic patients have provided another line of evidence consistent with a postsynaptic defect (18–21). The postsynaptic membranes showed sparse, shallow folds with markedly simplified geometric patterns. The motor nerve terminals contained the normal complement of structurally intact ACh vesicles, although the presynaptic nerve endings were often elongated and reduced in diameter (19, 20). These studies did not distinguish whether the pre- or postsynaptic abnormalities were primary, but it now seems clear that the changes in the postsynaptic membrane are the important ones and reflect the underlying AChR deficit.

The physiologic abnormalities in neuromuscular transmission appear to be accounted for by the AChR deficit alone. No additional disorders of pre- or postsynaptic function have been found that might further impair neuromuscular transmission in MG. Release of ACh from myasthenic neuromuscular junctions, both at rest and after stimulation, has been reported to be normal, or possibly even increased (7, 12, 22, 23). Furthermore, no functional abnormality of the AChRs remaining at myasthenic neuromuscular junctions (in terms of open times and current flow) has been found (14). Thus, a postsynaptic deficit of AChRs appears to be the underlying abnormality in MG.

ANTI-AChR ANTIBODIES IN MG

The autoimmune nature of MG was first suspected on the basis of indirect evidence, including its association with other autoimmune diseases (24) and the high incidence of thymic abnormalities in patients with MG (25). Moreover, antibodies against skeletal muscle were found in a majority of myasthenic patients (26), and complement levels were reduced in some cases (27). A further clue came from an experimental animal model of MG (EAMG) produced by immunization with purified AChRs from the electric organs of eels or rays (28). Animals injected with these substances manifest certain features of MG, consistent with the concept of an autoimmune response directed against the receptors (29–33).

Based on the knowledge of a receptor deficit in MG, and the analogy to the experimental animal model, the search for antibodies directed against AChRs in myasthenic patients was soon begun. Antireceptor antibodies were identified by a variety of techniques, all of which depend on α-BuTx for their specificity (34–38). With the most sensitive radioimmunoassay, circulating antibodies against AChR have been detected in nearly 90% of myasthenic patients (38), although the titer bears only an approximate relationship to the patient's clinical condition.

The question of whether the circulating antibodies are pathogenic, or merely represent a secondary response to AChR damage caused by some other agent, is critical in understanding the disease mechanisms in MG. To test the pathogenicity of the antibodies, we injected myasthenic patients' immunoglobulins into laboratory mice daily so as to maintain physiologic levels of the human IgG for 1 to 14 days (39, 40). Some of the recipient mice became weak within a few days and showed decremental responses to repetitive nerve stimulation. The most reliable tests were the measurement of mepp amplitudes and the determination of the number of AChRs per neuromuscular junction. Passive transfer of immunoglobulin from more than 90% of myasthenic patients resulted in decreased mepp amplitudes, reduced numbers of junctional AChRs, or both, usually within a few days of treatment (40). Immunoglobulin G was identified as the active immunoglobulin fraction by purification and absorption studies. The recipient animal's complement enhanced the effect of the myasthenic IgG, but a substantial abnormality was present in complement-depleted mice. Thus, the passive transfer experiments clearly demonstrated the pathogenicity of IgG from myasthenic patients.

Further confirmation of the role of antibodies in MG has come from studies of the ultrastructure of myasthenic neuromuscular junctions. By means of high-resolution electron microscopy, Rash and colleagues (41) found material resembling IgG in configuration and dimensions in the region of junctional AChRs. Engel and associates (42) identified IgG at postsynaptic membranes of human myasthenic junctions, using an immunoperoxidase technique.

EFFECTS OF MYASTHENIC ANTIBODIES ON AChRs

Theoretically, myasthenic patients' antibodies might reduce the number of available AChRs by several possible mechanisms: *(a)* by altering the turnover of AChRs through an increase in the rate of degradation or a decrease in the rate of synthesis; *(b)* by blocking the active site of the receptor; *(c)* by damaging the AChRs, possibly in conjunction with complement and/or cellular elements.

The evidence now available suggests that accelerated degradation of AChRs, blockade, and damage may all be involved, but the relative role of each mechanism has yet to be determined.

Accelerated Degradation of AChRs

Receptor degradation has been measured in a rat skeletal muscle tissue culture system, using a modification of the method of Devreotes and Fambrough (43). ^{125}I-α-BuTx is used to label the AChRs of cultured rat myotubes. As the labeled receptors undergo degradation, the attached ^{125}I-α-BuTx is broken down to ^{125}I-tyrosine, which appears in the culture medium. The rate of degradation can be calculated from the rate of release of radioactivity into the medium, and is normally approximately 4% per hour for rat skeletal muscle.

The addition of immunoglobulin from myasthenic patients to the cultures resulted in a 2- to 3-fold increase in the rate of AChR degradation (44, 45). The acceleration of degradation was triggered by IgG alone, without requiring other humoral or cellular components of the immune system. The addition of complement did not alter the rate of degradation (Table 2). Both the normal AChR degradation process and the acceleration produced by myasthenic immunoglobulin are temperature dependent and can be partially inhibited by dinitrophenol (44, 45), suggesting that they involve energy-dependent processes. Similar results have also been reported using immunoglobulin preparations from animals with EAMG (46).

Selectivity of Degradation

Theoretically, the myasthenic IgG might increase AChR degradation by accelerating the muscle cell's overall receptor-degrading mechanism or by altering only AChRs to which IgG is bound, so that these receptors are selectively degraded at a more rapid rate.

To distinguish between these possibilities, we prepared cultures in which one set of AChRs was directly exposed to myasthenic patients' IgG for 2 hours; a second set of AChRs was synthesized and inserted by the muscle cells after the IgG exposure (47) (Fig. 1). Each set of receptors was separately labeled with ^{125}I-α-BuTx, and the degradation rate for each was independently followed. Only the set of AChRs directly exposed to myasthenic IgG (and presumably having IgG bound to the receptors) was degraded at a rate 2 to 3 times normal. By contrast, the second set of receptors (in cultures treated identically, but

Table 2. Effects of Protease Inhibitors on Loss and Degradation of Acetylcholine Receptors[a]

Preparation	Apparent Degradation Rate (%/hr)	^{125}I-α-BuTx Bound (cpm/dish)
Pooled control IgG		
No inhibitor	3.81 ± 0.24	20,472 ± 1,936
Antipain (100 μg/ml)	1.38 ± 0.25	21,136 ± 856
Leupeptin (100 μg/ml)	1.02 ± 0.35	21,265 ± 4,751
Myasthenic patient's IgG		
No inhibitor	8.57 ± 0.11	7,789 ± 761
Antipain (100 μg/ml)	4.05 ± 0.48	7,526 ± 400
Leupeptin (100 μg/ml)	2.39 ± 0.51	5,368 ± 150

[a] Sets of 30 cultures were treated with control immunoglobulin or a myasthenic patient's immunoglobulin. Inhibitors of lysosomal enzymes were added to sets of 5 cultures each. Mean ± SD degradation rates are given as percentages of acetylcholine receptors (AChRs) degraded per hour. Note that both leupeptin and antipain inhibited degradation in control cultures and in cultures treated with myasthenic immunoglobulin. Eight hours after addition of control or myasthenic immunoglobulin, sets of 5 cultures each were labeled with ^{125}I-α-bungarotoxin (^{125}I-α-BuTx) to measure the remaining surface AChRs. Note that the protease inhibitors did not prevent the accelerated loss of AChRs from cultures treated with myasthenic IgG, despite their effects on lysosomal degradation of AChRs.

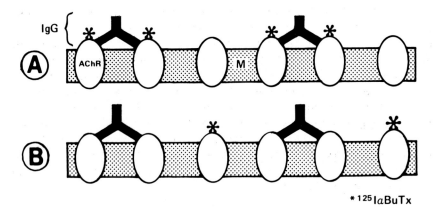

Fig. 1. Muscle (M) cultures in set A were first labeled with ^{125}I-α-bungarotoxin (^{125}I-α-BuTx), then treated for 2 hours with myasthenic IgG. The ^{125}I-BuTx-labeled (*) acetylcholine receptors (AChRs) have bound IgG. The M cultures in set B were first treated with myasthenic IgG. All existing AChRs were then blocked with unlabeled α-BuTx. After 6 hours of incubation to allow for synthesis and incorporation of additional AChRs, the new AChRs were labeled with ^{125}I-α-BuTx (*). Thus, the labeled AChRs do not have bound IgG, although other receptors in the same cultures do. The degradation rate of labeled AChRs in set A (with bound IgG) was accelerated, whereas that of labeled AChRs in set B (without bound IgG) was not accelerated. (Reprinted by permission from Drachman DB, Adams RN, Stanley EF, et al: Mechanisms of acetylcholine receptor loss in myasthenia gravis. J Neurol Neurosurg Psychiatry 43:601–610, 1980.)

without bound IgG) was degraded at the control rate. This suggested that the binding of IgG altered the receptors in some way that caused them to be preferentially selected for degradation. Our findings are not consistent with an overall acceleration of the muscle cell's receptor-degrading mechanism.

Cross-linking of AChRs
Immunoglobulin G molecules are known to be Y shaped, with 2 arms capable of binding to identical antigenic sites, thereby linking them together. Certain actions of IgG, such as the induction of "capping" of lymphocytes are known to require cross-linking (47). We have recently found that the ability of myasthenic patients' immunoglobulin to induce accelerated degradation of AChRs depends on its capacity to cross link the receptors (48). To test the effect of cross-linking, we prepared pure IgG, divalent F(ab′)$_2$ fragments, and monovalent Fab fragments from myasthenic and control sera by standard purification and enzymatic cleavage methods. When added to muscle cultures, the divalent preparations, IgG and F(ab′)$_2$, produced equally accelerated rates of AChR degradation (Fig. 2A, B). By contrast, the monovalent Fab fragments failed to accelerate the degradation rate, although they bound to AChRs of cultured skeletal muscle (Fig. 2C). When a second "piggyback" antibody directed against Fab fragments was added, it caused accelerated degradation of the Fab-AChR complexes, presumably as a result of cross-linking them (Fig. 2D). To determine whether direct contact of an antibody with the AChR is necessary for accelerated degradation, another method of cross-linking was also tested.

In this experiment, only α-BuTx was directly attached to the AChRs in cultured muscle. Antibodies prepared against α-BuTx were used to cross link the α-BuTx-AChR complexes (Fig. 2E), again resulting in 2- to 3-fold acceleration of the rate of degradation of AChRs. These findings clearly demonstrate that cross-linking of AChRs by antibodies from myasthenic patients is the factor that triggers their rapid degradation, and they have now been confirmed by

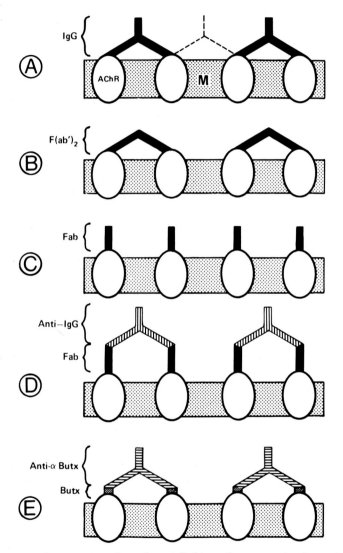

Fig. 2. Diagrammatic representation of cross-linking of receptors by the various antibody fragments. M denotes muscle membrane; AChR, acetylcholine receptor; α-BuTx, α-bungarotoxin. Acceleration of degradation was observed in the experimental conditions shown in panels A, B, D, and E. As shown in panel C, Fab alone failed to accelerate AChR degradation. (Reprinted by permission from the *New England Journal of Medicine* from Drachman DB, Angus DW, Adams RN, et al: Myasthenic antibodies cross-link acetylcholine receptors to accelerate degradation. N Engl J Med 298:1116–1122, 1978.)

studies in other laboratories using antibody fragments derived from sera of EAMG animals (50).

Endocytosis of AChRs

The normal process of AChR degradation begins with endocytosis, or "internalization" of the receptors, which are then broken down within the muscle cell by lysosomal enzymes (51, 52). The antibody-dependent mechanism of accelerated degradation is also believed to involve endocytosis and enzymatic lysis. There is increasing evidence that endocytosis, rather than lysosomal degradation, may be the step that determines the rate of loss of surface AChRs: (a) Morphologic studies suggest that the antibody-induced acceleration of AChR degradation begins with redistribution of the receptors within the muscle membrane, which then leads to their rapid endocytosis. Autoradiography and fluorescence microscopy of cultured skeletal muscle have shown that the addition of anti-AChR serum causes AChRs to aggregate in patches (53, 54). Freeze-fracture electron microscopy gives a picture of the molecular events that take place after the addition of myasthenic IgG to cultured skeletal muscle (chapter 23 of this volume, and Pumplin DW, Drachman DB: unpublished data) because it permits visualization of the AChRs as particles within the muscle membrane (55). The AChRs are first redistributed in clusters and aggregates. "Coated pits" then form in the regions of AChR aggregates, and apparently serve as vehicles to transport the AChRs within the muscle cell. (b) The role of lysosomal enzymes in the degradation process has been explored by the use of the enzyme inhibitors leupeptin and antipain. When added to normal or antibody-treated skeletal muscle cultures, these agents retard the release of degradation products into the medium (52, 56). However, the enzyme inhibitors do not slow the rapid loss of AChRs from the surface membranes of muscle treated with myasthenic IgG (Table 2).

Taken together, this evidence supports the concept that the endocytotic step is the critical one for the degradation of both normal and antibody-treated AChRs; the lysosomal enzyme system is capable of disposing of all the AChRs presented to it, unless it is specifically inhibited.

Effect of Myasthenic Immunoglobulin on AChRs

There are important differences between AChRs at neuromuscular junctions and those at extrajunctional sites of cultured or denervated muscle. Junctional receptors have far slow turnover rates (half-life of approximately 10 days compared to 18 hours for extrajunctional receptors), different immunologic reactivity, and different physical and pharmacologic properties (57). These differences raised questions about the applicability of the results of tissue culture experiments to intact neuromuscular junctions. Because junctional AChRs can be labeled with ^{125}I-α-BuTx in vivo and their degradation rates can be determined from the loss of bound reactivity (58, 59), the effect of myasthenic immunoglobulin on ACh turnover can be tested in the intact animal.

Stanley and Drachman (60) showed that treatment of mice with immunoglobulin from myasthenic patients accelerated the rate of degradation of labeled AChRs from the intact diaphragm approximately 3-fold, as in the tissue culture system. The loss of bound radioactivity was due almost entirely to degradation; chromatographic analysis revealed that the radioactive material released from diaphragms treated with myasthenic immunoglobulin consisted of ^{125}I-tyrosine, a breakdown product of ^{125}I-α-BuTx. Similar findings have been reported from other laboratories, using EAMG sera in vitro (61, 62). These results suggest that accelerated degradation may play a role in bringing about the reduction of AChRs at neuromuscular junctions of patients with MG.

Synthesis and Incorporation of AChRs

In contrast to its pronounced effect on AChR degradation, myasthenic immunoglobulin does not alter the rate of synthesis and incorporation of AChRs in muscle cultures (47). To measure new receptor synthesis, sets of rat skeletal muscle cultures were first treated overnight with immunoglobulin from myasthenic or control patients. Immediately after removal of the immunoglobulin, surface AChRs were blocked with cold α-BuTx; the cultures were then incubated for an additional period of 6 or 8 hours to allow the synthesis and incorporation of new AChRs to take place. At the end of this interval, the cultures were saturated with ^{125}I-α-BuTx, to measure the number of new surface AChRs. The results showed that treatment with myasthenic IgG did not alter the rate of synthesis and incorporation of new AChRs.

A recent report (63) of an apparent decrease in AChR synthesis of muscle cells treated with myasthenic serum illustrates one of the pitfalls in interpretation of AChR turnover experiments. The authors attempted to measure AChR synthesis in muscle cultures during exposure to myasthenic IgG (rather than afterwards, as above). At the end of the test period of synthesis and incorporation, they found fewer AChRs than expected, and attributed the apparent deficit to reduced AChR synthesis. However, their method of estimating AChR synthesis entails the erroneous assumption that newly inserted AChRs are degraded at the same rate as receptors of average age. We have found that new AChRs are lost approximately 30% to 50% faster than average AChRs, and that myasthenic Ig causes a proportionately greater increase in the AChR degradation rate (47, and Drachman DB, Adams RN: unpublished observations), thus fully accounting for the apparent receptor deficit. Although there is no evidence that myasthenic immunoglobulin alters the rate of AChR synthesis acutely, the possibility that a compensatory change may occur during long-term exposure has yet to be tested.

Blockade of AChRs

The hypothesis that a curare-like substance might be present in the serum of myasthenic patients was proposed as early as 1938 (64), yet the role of blockade of AChRs in the pathogenesis of MG is still controversial. One would like to know whether antibodies from myasthenic patients can interfere with ACh transmission by occupying the active site of the AChR itself, or by binding nearby and thus interfering with the ability of ACh to interact with this site. Present evidence indicates that many myasthenic patients have antibodies capable of blocking the active sites of AChRs, but the relative importance of this mechanism in impairing ACh transmission is not yet clear.

Several studies have shown that the addition of sera from myasthenic patients to AChR preparations may interfere with the binding of α-BuTx in a proportion of cases varying from 7% to 68% (34, 36, 38). These striking differences in results must be due to variations in the AChR preparations used, in the biologic activity of individual patients' sera, and in specific details of the experimental conditions.

We have recently developed a method that optimizes the blockade of the active site of AChRs by myasthenic immunoglobulin, using the rat skeletal muscle culture system. The cultures are cooled to 4° C to eliminate degradation and to minimize possible dissociation of antibody. They are treated overnight in the cold with immunoglobulin prepared from myasthenic patients' sera, and are then saturated with ^{125}I-α-BuTx in the cold. The decrease of α-BuTx binding sites in the cultures treated with myasthenic immunoglobulin is attributable to AChR blockade by the antibodies. Our findings indicate that serum immunoglobulins from approximately 80% of myasthenic patients produced significant blockade of ^{125}I-α-BuTx binding (Drachman DB, Adams RN: unpublished observations). It is not certain whether this represents binding of the antibody directly at, or near, the active site of the AChR. In the latter instance, steric hindrance could account for the blocking effect.

Although these studies demonstrate the potential ability of the antibody to block access to the active site of the AChR, the significance of this effect in neuromuscular transmission is not at all clear. The antibodies' ability to block α-BuTx binding may not necessarily parallel their ability to interfere with ACh binding by receptors at the neuromuscular junction. Although α-BuTx undoubtedly binds at or very near the active site of the receptor (65), there are important differences between α-BuTx and ACh. α-Bungarotoxin is much larger (molecular weight, 8,000 daltons) than ACh (molecular weight, 182 daltons) and therefore could be excluded from a site only partially blocked by the antibody, which might be accessible to the smaller ACh molecule. On the other hand, the affinity of α-BuTx for the receptors is much higher than that of ACh. Therefore α-BuTx might displace blocking antibody and bind to the receptor under circumstances in which ACh binding would be impaired. These considerations make it difficult to translate findings based on α-BuTx binding studies into definite conclusions about ACh transmission.

Inhibition of Neuromuscular Transmission

Sera from some patients may have a reversible inhibitory effect on neuromuscular transmission suggestive of receptor blockade. The addition of myasthenic sera to marginally affected EAMG animals in vivo (66) or to neuromuscular junctions in vitro (67) has been reported to interfere with ACh transmission, although another in vitro study failed to show an effect (68).

Plasmapheresis has been reported to produce very rapid clinical improvement within hours to days in occasional cases, suggesting removal of a blocking antibody (69). Similarly, thoracic duct drainage of lymph from myasthenic patients produced clinical improvement within 48 hours, whereas reinfusion of the lymph increased myasthenic weakness within hours (70). The rapidity and reversibility of these changes have suggested that at least one action of the antibody might be functional blockade of AChRs, but such circumstantial evidence does not rule out other possible explanations.

Antibodies Binding to AChR but Not Blocking

The large majority of MG patients have a significant proportion of antibodies that bind to the AChR at loci other than the active site. In the commonly used radioimmunoassay, the active site of the AChR is already occupied by ^{125}I-α-BuTx, so that one can measure only antibodies directed against other determinants (35, 37). This indicates that nonsite-directed antibodies are present in myasthenic patients and undoubtedly contribute to the pathogenesis of MG by the other mechanisms outlined in this paper. However, the existence of such antibodies cannot be used as evidence against the possibility of an antibody population capable of blocking the receptor's active site.

On balance, the evidence now available suggests that at least some myasthenic patients have antibodies capable of blocking AChRs under appropriate conditions. However, the relative role of receptor blockade in producing clinically significant impairment of neuromuscular transmission is as yet unresolved, and is likely to differ in individual patients.

Structural Damage to Neuromuscular Junctions

Light and electron microscopic studies of neuromuscular junctions have revealed a variety of morphologic abnormalities that may contribute to the impairment of neuromuscular transmission. The junctional folds are sparse and shallow, with a decreased area of contact with the nerve terminals (18–21). These structural changes result from the interaction of antibodies with AChRs. The antibodies, perhaps in collaboration with complement, may produce the fragmentation and shedding of postsynaptic membrane into the synaptic space that has been seen by electron microscopy (41, 42). An alternative hypothesis, not yet tested, is that a sufficient amount of postsynaptic membrane may be endocytosed concomitantly with the increased endocytosis of AChRs to result in the simplification of junctional folds. The altered geometry of the neuromuscular junction not only reflects the loss of AChRs, but may itself impair neuromuscular transmission because of the reduced contact between nerve and muscle membranes.

A possible role of complement in the pathogenesis of MG was first suggested by the observation that complement levels are decreased in myasthenic patients, especially during clinical exacerbations (27). To test the effect of complement on antibody-dependent loss of AChRs, we used the mouse passive transfer model (40). The mice were depleted of the C3 component of complement by the use of "cobra venom factor," a purified fraction derived from the venom of the Indian cobra *Naja naja*. The C3-depleted mice and nondepleted control mice were treated with immunoglobulin from 7 different patients. In each case, C3 depletion reduced, but did not eliminate, the effect of myasthenic immunoglobulin on mepp amplitudes and number of AChRs per neuromuscular junction. The participation of the early part of the complement system up to and including C3 in this reaction implies that it enhances, but is not essential for, the effect of myasthenic antibody on AChRs.

The role of complement has received further support from morphologic studies demonstrating C3 and C9 at neuromuscular junctions of myasthenic patients (42) and from studies of complement fixation by anti-AChR antibodies from myasthenic patients (71).

As noted above, and in Table 1, we have found that complement does not contribute in vitro to the antibody-induced loss of AChRs in rat skeletal muscle cultures. It thus appears unlikely that complement acts by enhancing accelerated degradation or blockade induced by myasthenic antibody.

Cell-mediated Immunity

This discussion has focused on antibody-mediated mechanisms in the pathogenesis of MG. However, several recent studies have suggested an important role for lymphocytes in the autoimmune responses.

B lymphocytes represent the "final common path" in the production of antibody. Lymphocytes from the peripheral blood and from thymuses of myasthenic patients have been shown to produce anti-AChR antibodies when cultured in vitro (72). Furthermore, it has been suggested that some abnormality of the regulatory functions of lymphocytes may be involved in the development of the autoimmune response in at least some myasthenic patients (73, 74). The concurrence of other autoimmune diseases in some myasthenic patients implies a loss of immunoregulatory control mechanisms. Detailed studies of subsets of lymphocytes have produced a bewildering variety of results concerning suppressor cells and responses to mitogens that are beyond the scope of this paper. It has recently been shown that peripheral blood lymphocytes from myasthenic patients are stimulated to undergo increased cell division ("blast transformation") when incubated in the presence of AChRs from electric eels or rays (75–77). However, the relationship between lymphocyte responsiveness and the clinical status of MG patients is as yet unclear. In general, stimulation of lymphocytes in response to a specific antigen indicates that the cells have previously been sensitized to that antigen. However, it is not yet known whether the positive responses in MG are derived from T cells or B cells, nor what role the responding cells play in the immunopathogenesis of the disease.

The implications of these observations are by no means clear at present. The interactions between T lymphocytes and B lymphocytes are highly complex, and both classes of cell may be involved in humoral as well as cellular immune reactions (78). At present, there is little evidence for a cell-mediated effector mechanism in MG, but it seems likely that defects of immune regulation may exist in at least some myasthenic patients.

CONCLUSIONS

The fundamental abnormality affecting the neuromuscular junctions of myasthenic patients is a decrease in the number of available AChRs due to an autoimmune attack directed against the receptors. Antibodies to AChR are present in most patients, and there is evidence that they have a predominant pathogenic role in the disease. The mechanisms of antibody action involve acceleration of the rate of degradation of AChRs that requires cross-linking of the receptors. In addition, antibodies may block AChRs and may participate in producing destructive changes, perhaps in conjunction with complement. Although the target of the autoimmune attack in myasthenic patients is probably always the AChRs, it is not yet clear which of these immune mechanisms are most important. It is likely that the relative role of each mechanism varies from patient to patient. This may account for our inability thus far to find correlations between the titer or properties of the antibodies and the patient's clinical condition. One of the goals of future research will be to identify the relative importance of each of these mechanisms in individual patients. Based on this kind of detailed knowledge, it should be possible to tailor specific immuno-therapeutic measures to the abnormalities found.

ACKNOWLEDGMENTS

We are deeply indebted to the many colleagues who participated in the studies described here. CF Barlow provided expert assistance with the manuscript. The original research carried out in the authors' laboratories was supported in part by National Institutes of Health (NIH) grants 5 PO1 NS10920 and 5 RO1 HD04817, and grants from the Muscular Dystrophy Association and the Myasthenia Gravis Foundation. A. Pestronk was supported by a Teacher-Investigator Award from the NIH.

REFERENCES

1. Oppenheim H: *Zur Myasthenische Paralyse*. S. Karger, Berlin, 1901
2. Remen L: Zur pathogenese und therapie der myasthenia gravis pseudoparalytica. Dtsch Z Nervenheilk 128:66–78, 1932
3. Walker MB: Treatment of myasthenia gravis with physostigmine. Lancet 1:1200–1201, 1934
4. Harvey AM, Masland RL: The electromyogram in myasthenia gravis. Bull Johns Hopkins Hosp 69:1–13, 1941
5. Lee CY: Chemistry and pharmacology of polypeptide toxins in snake venoms. Annu Rev Pharmacol 12:265–286, 1972
6. Fambrough DM, Drachman DB, Satyamurti S: Neuromuscular junction in myasthenia gravis: decreased acetylcholine receptors. Science 182:293–295, 1973
7. Elmqvist D, Hoffmann WW, Kugelberg J, et al: An electrophysiological investigation of neuromuscular transmission in myasthenia gravis. J Physiol (Lond) 174:417–434, 1964
8. Fields WS: Myasthenia gravis. Ann NY Acad Sci 183:1–386, 1971
9. Drachman DB, Kao I, Pestronk A, et al: Myasthenia gravis as a receptor disorder. Ann NY Acad Sci 273:226–234, 1976
10. Engel AG, Lindstrom JM, Lambert EH, et al: Ultrastructural localization of the acetylcholine receptor in myasthenia gravis and in its experimental autoimmune model. Neurology (Minneap) 27:307–315, 1977
11. Ito Y, Miledi R, Vincent A, et al: Acetylcholine receptors and endplate electrophysiology in myasthenia gravis. Brain 101:345–368, 1978
12. Lindstrom JM, Lambert EH: Content of acetylcholine receptor and antibodies bound to receptor in myasthenia gravis, experimental autoimmune myasthenia gravis, and Eaton-Lambert syndrome. Neurology (NY) 28:130–138, 1978
13. Albuquerque EX, Rash JE, Mayer RF, et al: An electrophysiological and morphological study of the neuromuscular junctions in patients with myasthenia gravis. Exp Neurol 51:536–563, 1976

14. Cull-Candy SC, Miledi R, Trautman A: End-plate currents at normal and myasthenic human end-plates. J Physiol (Lond) 287:247–265, 1979

15. Satyamurti S, Drachman DB, Slone F: Blockade of acetylcholine receptors: a model of myasthenia gravis. Science 187:955–957, 1975

16. Desmedt JE: The neuromuscular disorder in myasthenia gravis. In *New Developments in EMG and Clinical Neurophysiology*. Edited by Desmedt JE. S Karger, Basel, 1973, pp 241–304

17. Chang CC, Lee CY: Electrophysiological study of neuromuscular blocking action of cobra neurotoxin. Br J Pharmacol Chemother 28:172–181, 1966

18. Zachs SI, Bauer WC, Blumberg JM: The fine structure of the myasthenic neuromuscular junction. J Neuropathol Exp Neurol 21:335–347, 1962

19. Woolf AL: Morphology of the myasthenic neuromuscular junction. Ann NY Acad Sci 135:35–58, 1966

20. Engel AG, Santa T: Histometric analysis of the ultrastructure of the neuromuscular junction in myasthenia gravis and in the myasthenic syndrome. Ann NY Acad Sci 183:46–63, 1971

21. Bergman RA, Johns RJ, Afifi AK: Ultrastructural alterations in muscle from patients with myasthenia gravis and Eaton-Lambert syndrome. Ann NY Acad Sci 183:88–122, 1971

22. Molenaar PC, Polak RL, Miledi R, et al: The cholinergic synapse. Prog Brain Res 49:449–458, 1979

23. Cull-Candy SG, Miledi R, Trautman A, et al: On the release of transmitter at normal, myasthenia gravis and myasthenic syndrome affected human endplates. J Physiol (Lond) 299:621–638, 1980

24. Simpson JA: Myasthenia gravis: a new hypothesis. Scott Med J 4:419–436, 1960

25. Castleman B: The pathology of the thymus gland in myasthenia gravis. Ann NY Acad Sci 135:496–503, 1966

26. Strauss AJL, Segal BC, Hsu KC, et al: Immunofluorescence demonstration of a muscle binding complement-fixing serum globulin fraction in myasthenia gravis. Proc Soc Exp Biol Med 105:184–191, 1960

27. Nastuk WL, Plescia OJ, Osserman KE: Changes in serum complement activity in patients with myasthenia gravis. Proc Soc Exp Biol Med 105:177–184, 1960

28. Patrick J, Lindstrom J: Autoimmune response to acetylcholine receptor. Science 180:871–872, 1973

29. Green DPL, Miledi R, de la Mora MP, et al: Acetylcholine receptors. Philos Trans R Soc Lond [Biol] 270:551–559, 1975

30. Granato DA, Fulpius BW, Moody JF: Experimental myasthenia in Balb/C mice immunized with rat acetylcholine receptor from rat denervated muscle. Proc Natl Acad Sci USA 73:2872–2876, 1976

31. Heilbronn E, Mattson C, Thornell L-E, et al: Experimental myasthenia in rabbits: biochemical, immunological, electrophysiolo_ ᵎ-al and morphological aspects. Ann NY Acad Sci 274:337–353, 1976

32. Lambert EH, Lindstrom JM, Lennon VA: Endplate potentials in experimental autoimmune myasthenia gravis in rats. Ann NY Acad Sci 274:300–318, 1976

33. Sanders DB, Schleifer LS, Eldefrawi ME, et al: An immunologically induced defect of neuromuscular transmission in rats and rabbits. Ann NY Acad Sci 274:319–336, 1976

34. Almon RR, Andrew CG, Appel SH: Serum globulin in myasthenia gravis: inhibition of α-bungarotoxin binding to acetylcholine receptors. Science 186:55–57, 1974

35. Appel SH, Almon RR, Levy N: Acetylcholine receptor antibodies in myasthenia gravis. N Engl J Med 293:760–761, 1975

36. Bender AN, Engel WK, Ringel SP, et al: Myasthenia gravis: a serum factor blocking acetylcholine receptors of the human neuromuscular junction. Lancet 1:607–608, 1975

37. Lindstrom JM, Seybold ME, Lennon VA, et al: Antibody to acetylcholine receptor in myasthenia gravis: prevalence, clinical correlates, and diagnostic value. Neurology (Minneap) 26:1054–1059, 1976

38. Mittag T, Kornfeld P, Tormay A, et al: Detection of antiacetylcholine receptor factors in serum and thymus from patients with myasthenia gravis. N Engl J Med 294:691–694, 1976

39. Toyka KV, Drachman DB, Pestronk A, et al: Myasthenia gravis: passive transfer from man to mouse. Science 190:397–399, 1975

40. Toyka KV, Drachman DB, Griffin DE, et al: Myasthenia gravis: study of humoral immune mechanisms by passive transfer to mice. N Engl N Med 296:125–131, 1977

41. Rash JE, Albuquerque EX, Hudson CS, et al: Studies on human myasthenia gravis: electrophysiological and ultrastructural evidence compatible with antibody labeling of the acetylcholine receptor complex. Proc Natl Acad Sci USA 73:4584–4588, 1976

42. Engel AG, Sahashi K, Lambert EH, et al: The ultrastructural localization of the acetylcholine receptor, immunoglobulin G and the third and ninth complement components at the motor endplate and their implications for the pathogenesis of myasthenia gravis. In *Current Topics in Nerve and Muscle Research*. Edited by Aguayo AJ, Karpati G. Excerpta Medica, Amsterdam, 1979, pp 111–122.

43. Devreotes PN, Fambrough DM: Acetylcholine receptor turnover in membrane of developing muscle fibers. J Cell Biol 65:335–358, 1975

44. Kao I, Drachman DB: Myasthenic immunoglobulin accelerates acetylcholine receptor degradation. Science 196:527–529, 1977

45. Appel SH, Anwyl R, McAdams MW, et al: Accelerated degradation acetylcholine receptor from cultured rat myotubes with myasthenia gravis sera and globulins. Proc Natl Acad Sci USA 74:2130–2134, 1977

46. Heinemann S, Bevan S, Kullberg R, et al: Modulation of acetylcholine receptor by antibody against the receptor. Proc Natl Acad Sci USA 74:3090–3094, 1977

47. Drachman DB, Angus CW, Adams RN, et al: Effect of myasthenic patients' immunoglobulin on acetylcholine receptor turnover: selectivity of degradation process. Proc Natl Acad Sci USA 75:3422–3426, 1978

48. Taylor RB, Duffus WPH, Raff MC, et al: Redistribution and pinocytosis of lymphocyte surface immunoglobulin antibody. Nature [New Biol] 233:225–229, 1971

49. Drachman DB, Angus CW, Adams RN, et al: Myasthenic antibodies cross-link acetylcholine receptors to accelerate degradation. N Engl J Med 298:1116–1122, 1978

50. Tarrab-Hazdai R, Yaffe D, Prives Y, et al: Effects of macrophages and antibodies from myasthenic animals on muscle cells in culture. In *Plasmapheresis and the Immunobiology of Myasthenia Gravis*. Edited by Dau PC. Houghton Mifflin Professional Publishers, Boston, 1979, pp 32–40

51. Devreotes PN, Fambrough DM: Turnover of acetylcholine receptors in skeletal muscle. Cold Spring Harbor Symp Quant Biol 40:237–251, 1976

52. Libby P, Bursztajn S, Goldberg AJ: Degradation of the acetylcholine receptor in cultured muscle cells: selective inhibitors and the fate of undegraded receptors. Cell 9:481–491, 1980

53. Tarrab-Hazdai R, Yaffe D, Prives Y, et al: Effects of macrophages and antibodies from myasthenic animals on muscle cells in culture. In *Plasmapheresis and the Immunobiology of Myasthenia Gravis*. Edited by Dau PC. Houghton Mifflin Professional Publishers, Boston, 1979, pp 32–40.

54. Lennon VA: Immunofluorescence analysis of surface acetylcholine receptors on muscle: modulation by auto-antibodies. In *Cholinergic Mechanisms and Psychopharmacology*. Edited by Jenden DJ. Plenum Press, New York 1978, pp 77–92

55. Cohen SA, Pumplin DW: Clusters of intramembrane particles associated with binding sites for α-bungarotoxin in cultured chick myotubes. J Cell Biol 82:494–516, 1979

56. Drachman DB, Adams RN, Stanley EF, et al: Mechanisms of acetylcholine receptor loss in myasthenia gravis. J Neurol Neurosurg Psychiatry 43:601–610, 1980

57. Brockes JP, Berg DK, Hall ZW: The biochemical properties and regulation of acetylcholine receptors in normal and denervated muscle. Cold Spring Harbor Symp Quant Biol 30:253–262, 1976

58. Berg DK, Hall ZW: Loss of bungarotoxin from junctional and extrajunctional receptors in rat diaphragm muscle in vivo and in organ culture. J Physiol (Lond) 252:771–789, 1975

59. Chang CC, Huang MD: Turnover of junctional and extrajunctional acetylcholine receptors of the rat diaphragm. Nature 253:643–644, 1975

60. Stanley EF, Drachman DB: Effect of myasthenic immunoglobulin on acetylcholine receptors of intact mammalian neuromuscular junctions. Science 200:1285–1287, 1978

61. Reiness CW, Weinberg CB, Hall ZW: Antibody to acetylcholine receptor increases degradation of junctional and extrajunctional receptors in adult muscle. Nature 274:68–70, 1978

62. Merlie JP, Heinemann S, Lindstrom JM: Acetylcholine receptor degradation in adult rat diaphragms in organ culture and the effect of anti-acetylcholine receptor antibodies. J Biol Chem 254:6300–6327, 1979

63. Appel SH, Elias SB, Chauvin P: The role of acetylcholine receptor antibodies in myasthenia gravis. Fed Proc 38:2385–2391, 1979

64. Walker MB: Myasthenia gravis: Case in which fatigue of forearm muscles could induce paralysis of extraocular muscle. Proc R Soc Med 31:722, 1938

65. Heidmann T, Changeux J-P: Structural and functional properties of the acetylcholine receptor protein in its purified and membrane bound state. Annu Rev Biochem 47:315–357, 1978

66. Heilbronn E, Hammarstrom L, Lefvert AK, et al: Effects of acetylcholine receptor antibodies in mice and rabbits. In *Plasmapheresis and the Immunobiology of Myasthenia Gravis*. Edited by Dau PC. Houghton Mifflin Professional Publishers, Boston, 1979, pp 92–96

67. Shibuya N, Mori K, Nakazawa Y: Serum factor blocks neuromuscular transmission in myasthenia gravis: electrophysiological study with intracellular microelectrodes. Neurology (NY) 28:804–811, 1978

68. Albuquerque EX, Lebeda FJ, Appel SH, et al: Effects of normal and myasthenic serum factors on innervated and chronically denervated mammalian muscle. Ann NY Acad Sci 274:475–492, 1976

69. Dau PC, Lindstrom JM, Cassel CK, et al: Plasmapheresis and immunosuppressive drug therapy in myasthenia gravis. N Engl J Med 297:1134–1140, 1977

70. Matell G, Bergstrom K, Franksson C: Effects of some immunosuppressive procedures on myasthenia gravis. Ann NY Acad Sci 274:659–676, 1976

71. Tarrab-Hazdai R, Abramsky O, Fuchs S, et al: Humoral antibodies to acetylcholine receptor in patients with myasthenia gravis. Lancet 2:340–342, 1975

72. Vincent A, Scadding GK, Clarke C, et al: Anti-acetylcholine receptor antibody synthesis in culture. In *Plasmapheresis and the Immunobiology of Myasthenia Gravis*. Edited by Dau PC. Houghton Mifflin Professional Publishers, Boston, 1979, pp 59–71.

73. Penn AS: Immunological features of myasthenia gravis. In *Current Topics in Nerve and Muscle Research*. Edited by Aguayo AJ, Karpati G. Excerpta Medica, Amsterdam, 1979, pp 123–132

74. Shore A, Limatibul S, Dosch H-M, et al: Identification of two serum components regulating the expression of T-lymphocyte function in childhood myasthenia gravis. N Engl J Med 301:625–629, 1979

75. Abramsky O, Aharonov A, Webb C, et al: Cellular immune response to acetylcholine receptor-rich fraction in patients with myasthenia gravis. Clin Exp Immunol 19:11–16, 1975

76. Richman DP, Patrick J, Arnason BGW, et al: Cellular immunity in myasthenia gravis. N Engl J Med 294:694–698, 1976

77. Conti-Tronconi B, Morgutti M, Sghirlanzoni A, et al: Cellular immune response against acetylcholine receptor in myasthenia gravis. Neurology (NY) 29:496–501, 1979

78. Greaves MF, Owen JJT, Raff MC: *T and B Lymphocytes: Origins, Properties and Roles in Immune Responses*. American Elsevier Publishing Co., New York, Amsterdam 1974

DISCUSSION

Dr. Richard Almon: I have two questions. First, accelerated degradation is not necessarily a mechanism for reduced number of receptors. It is quite possible that there could be a compensatory increase in synthesis, leading to a new steady state with no net change in the number receptors. Have you looked at this? My second question is related to the fact that your turnover mechanisms were all directed at extrajunctional receptors in tissue culture. As you know, in our original papers we observed quite distinct antigenic differences, at least in the rat, between junctional and extrajunctional receptors, which have been followed up very elegantly by Dr. Zach Hall.

Dr. Daniel Drachman: Let me answer your second question first. Dr. Elis Stanley and I have done a detailed study and have shown that junctional receptors are degraded at an accelerated rate. Using our passive transfer model, both in vivo and in vitro, we have found accelerated degradation of AChRs. You also asked what happens to synthesis. In our culture system, at a time when degradation is proceeding rapidly, there is no change in synthesis. However, I do not exclude the possibility that there may be a chronic compensatory increase in synthesis and insertion of receptors, because we have not measured that.

Dr. Stanley Appel: I just want to comment that our data support an alteration in AChR synthesis. There is a technical problem in interpreting the difference in our data, since our studies were done with antibodies present and your studies were carried out in the absence of antibodies.

Dr. Henry Epstein: With respect to your passive transfer experiments, have you ever compared monovalent versus bivalent antibodies?

Dr. Daniel Drachman: Yes we have. We have used monovalent Fab antibody fragments and have shown that they do not cause accelerated degradation of receptors.

Dr. Angela Vicent: With regard to synthesis of receptors during passive transfer of myasthenic IgG to mice: Dr. Steve Wilson, Dr. John Newsom-Davis, and I have found that there does seem to be an increased compensatory synthesis of AChRs during passive transfer over a period of 7 days.

Dr. Daniel Drachman: Your experiment suggests that there may be compensatory increase in AChR synthesis over the long term.

Dr. Andrew Engel: I would like to comment on your comment that there is "possibly" a role of complement in the destruction of the junctional folds. We have observed and published excellent correlation between the localization of C9 and sites where destruction of junctional folds occurs. In fact, there is a one-to-one correspondence, and the evidence is unambiguous.

Dr. Daniel Drachman: I would be very happy to amend my comment. There is a role for complement in loss of AChRs, as our passive transfer experiments and your immunoelectron microscopic studies have shown.

17
Molecular Studies of Acetylcholine Receptors and Myasthenia Gravis

Jon Lindstrom, PhD

Socrates Tzartos, PhD

Bianca Conti-Tronconi, MD

Bill Gullick, PhD

In 1960, John Simpson proposed that myasthenia gravis (MG) was caused by an autoimmune response to acetylcholine receptor (AChR) (1). He proposed that the anti-AChR antibodies acted as curare-like antagonists of muscle AChR. He was correct in proposing that anti-AChR antibodies were the primary pathologic effector in MG, but the pathologic mechanisms by which they act proved to be quite complex (reviewed in 2–4). The hypothesis that antibodies to AChR might be involved in MG could not be tested until 13 years later, when techniques for quantifying AChRs using ^{125}I-labeled α-bungarotoxin (^{125}I-BuTx) were available.

In 1972, Lindstrom and Patrick (5) purified AChR from the electric organs of *Electrophorus electricus*, and in 1973 they reported that rabbits immunized with this AChR weakened and died (6). Methods were developed for measuring antibodies to AChR in these rabbits (7), and it was proposed that these antibodies were responsible for impairing neuromuscular transmission in the rabbits. This animal model was termed experimental autoimmune myasthenia gravis (EAMG). The same basic assay procedure for measuring antibodies used in EAMG was modified for use in MG by substituting human muscle AChR as antigen and was later used to detect anti-AChR antibodies in patients with MG (8, 9). The reason for immunizing the rabbits was not to test whether AChR could provoke MG. Instead, we wanted antibodies to test whether the newly purified protein was, in fact, AChR by whether or not those antibodies could block the function of AChR in electric organ cells. They could (7, 10). This indirect test was devised because at that time we had no direct techniques for reconstituting our detergent-solubilized purified cholinergic ligand-binding protein back into membranes to test whether binding of an agonist to the protein caused opening of a cation-specific channel across the membrane. In fact, only in the last year or so have methods been developed for solubilizing AChRs without denaturing their channels, purifying them, and then reconstituting them into membranes (11, 12).

This brief history was presented to give a perspective on the importance of developing critical techniques in one area before it becomes possible to make advances in a related area. The observation of EAMG in rabbits immunized with AChR from the electric organs of electric eels in 1973 (6) suggested that there must be some similarity in structure between AChR from fish electric organs and AChR from mammalian muscle, but only now is it starting to become clear just what the subunit structure of electric organ AChR is (13–15) and how detailed is its similarity to that of muscle AChR (16–19).

We have been developing new techniques that we hope will be valuable both for the study of the AChR molecule and for its role in MG and EAMG. We have been using the methods of Köhler and Milstein (20) to prepare hybridomas secreting monoclonal antibodies (mAbs) to AChR (21–26). Spleen cells from an immunized animal are fused with myeloma cells to produce hybrid cells that produce antibodies characteristic of the spleen cell and have the immortality characteristic of the myeloma. The mAbs produced by cloned hybridomas provide monospecific probes for specific sites on the surface of the AChR molecule. These probes are very important, because although many ligands for the ACh binding site are known, the cation channel and most of the rest of this complex macromolecule remain unexplored.

We are developing techniques for mapping the binding specificities of mAbs to AChR (18, 21–26). These same techniques are applicable in many cases to mapping the specificities of antibodies from patients with MG and animals with EAMG (26). This is important for two reasons. First, the population of antibody specificities in a patient with MG is something of a "fossil record" of what the stimulating antigen was. The identity of the stimulating antigen is important to ascertain, because although we are gaining a modest understanding of the mechanisms by which antibodies can act in MG (reviewed in 2–4), we have no idea what triggers and sustains their formation. We do not know whether a uniquely immunogenic AChR antigen is involved (but see 27), or whether the lesion is entirely a deficit of immunoregulation. Second, although there is good evidence that impairment of neuromuscular transmission in EAMG and MG occurs by humoral rather than cellular immune effectors, there is not a strict correlation between total anti-AChR titer and severity of weakness (8). No doubt this is due, in part, to the complexity of the pathologic mechanisms involved, but it also suggests that some antibody specificities are more effective at impairing transmission than others.

The following sections will first briefly review the structure of the AChR molecule and the pathologic mechanisms of EAMG, and then review some of our recent findings from studies of AChRs using mAbs. We hope that these studies with mAbs will provide the beginning of an understanding not only of the molecular biology of the AChR molecule, but also the molecular biology of MG.

STRUCTURE OF THE AChR MOLECULE

Because it is available in the largest amounts, AChR from the electric organs of the marine ray *Torpedo californica* is the AChR whose structure is best understood. Torpedo AChR contains 4 kinds of subunit designated α, β, γ, and δ whose apparent molecular weights (MWs) are, respectively, approximately 38,000, 50,000, 57,000, and 64,000 daltons (15, 28–32). Karlin and coworkers (13, 14) proposed that each AChR monomer contained 2 α subunits and one subunit each of β, γ, and δ on the basis of several observations: *(a)* the apparent MWs of the subunits; *(b)* the apparent MW of torpedo AChR monomers (250,000 daltons); *(c)* 1 mol of ^{125}I-α-BuTx is bound per 125,000 g of protein; *(d)* all toxin binding can be blocked by cholinergic ligands; *(e)* the affinity labeling reagent 4-(*N*-maleimido)benzyltrimethylammonium iodide (MBTA) labels α subunits, and the binding of MBTA is prevented by both cholinergic ligands and toxin. Direct measurement of the subunit amounts supported this ratio (15). Affinity labeling with MBTA (14) and other agents (31, 32) showed that α subunits composed at least part of the ACh binding site. Only one of the two toxin binding sites is blocked by MBTA (14). Toxin specifically bound to AChR can be covalently cross-linked to not only α subunits, but also to the other subunits (33–35), showing that parts of all of the subunits are under or near the area occupied by the nearly 40-Å diameter (36) toxin molecules.

In the past, AChR was usually solubilized in the detergents Triton X-100 or sodium cholate. Although AChR solubilized in this way retains its ability to bind toxin, the cation channel whose opening is regulated by ACh binding is irreversibly denatured (11). If AChR is solubilized in cholate-lipid mixtures, the channel is not denatured, and removal of the cholate by dialysis results in formation of vesicles that exhibit carbamylcholine-induced influx of ^{22}Na$^+$ (37). The AChR can be solubilized in cholate-lipid mixtures and subsequently purified to homogeneity by affinity chromatography (11, 12). Because monomers are fully active (38), it is clear that the cation channel is a component of the α$_2$βγδ structure of the monomer.

By negative staining, the extracellular surface of torpedo AChR appears in electron micrographs as a doughnut of 90- to 100-Å diameter with a negatively stained center (39–44). X-ray crystallography of AChR-rich membrane fragments (41) and electron microscopy (44, 45) suggest that the AChR molecule may be a 100-Å tall asymmetric mushroom-shaped structure with most of its mass on the extracellular surface of the membrane and only its stem traversing the membrane. Some evidence suggests (46) that a pit runs the length of the molecule, and this might correspond to the channel. Each subunit contains carbohydrate (15, 47), and part of each subunit is exposed on the extracellular surface (16), but it is not known which subunits cross the membrane.

For several years there has been controversy about the subunit structure of AChR, because several laboratories observed only α subunits in torpedo (48) and muscle AChR (49), and because AChR from *E. electricus* appeared to have subunits corresponding to only 3 of the 4 seen in torpedo AChR (17). It now seems likely that these differences in subunit structure are apparent rather than real, and result from selective proteolytic nicking of the β, γ, and δ subunits during purification (18, 50). After intentional proteolysis, the nicked subunits of torpedo AChR remain associated and can still bind toxin and function in reconstituted vesicles (50, 51). By including in the initial homogenate a sulfhydryl alkylating agent (iodoacetamide) that may act by inhibiting a protease, AChR containing 4 kinds of subunit can be purified from *Electrophorus*. These subunits correspond by apparent MWs and cross reaction with anti-subunit antibodies to the 4 subunits of torpedo AChR (18). Antigenic determinants corresponding to these 4 subunits can be found in AChRs from human (16) and bovine (17) muscle. The AChR purified from rat muscle by Nathanson and Hall (19) contains subunits that correspond by affinity labeling and apparent MWs to the 4 subunits of torpedo AChR.

Thus, it is gradually becoming apparent that the AChR monomers of fish electric organs and mammalian muscle are very similar macromolecules with similarly complex subunit structures. These molecules contain both the ACh binding sites and the cation-specific channel whose opening they regulate.

EXPERIMENTAL AUTOIMMUNE MYASTHENIA GRAVIS

As a consequence of the similarity between the structure of AChRs from fish electric organ and mammalian muscle, immunization of mammals, or frogs for that matter, with purified fish AChR in adjuvant causes the formation of antibodies to the fish AChR that cross-react with muscle AChR (reviewed in 2–4). Torpedo AChR is a potent immunogen (52), and muscle AChR is a very potent inducer of EAMG (53, 54). Because most antibodies are directed at conformationally dependent determinants, denatured AChR subunits are much less effective at inducing EAMG (16, 17).

EAMG differs fundamentally from MG in that it is triggered and sustained by intentional immunization with exogenous AChR in adjuvant and does not depend absolutely on any preexisting defect in the immune system of the immunized animal. However, the pathologic mechanisms by which the antibody-mediated immune response to AChR impairs neuromuscular transmission in chronic EAMG appear identical to those involved in MG. There is also an acute form of EAMG observed in rats shortly after immunization, but only if they are given special adjuvants. The acute phase does not seem to have a human counterpart. Because we have recently reviewed MG and EAMG in detail (2–4), here EAMG will be reviewed only very briefly to emphasize certain fundamental points.

Acute EAMG occurs 8 to 11 days after immunization of rats with AChR in complete Freund's adjuvant, only if they are also injected with the additional adjuvant, pertussis vaccine (55). A very similar acute response occurs in normal rats injected with anti-AChR antibodies from animals with chronic EAMG. Acute and passively transferred EAMG are characterized by extensive phago-cytic invasion of the endplates, which destroys the postsynaptic membrane

(56–58). Only a small fraction of muscle AChRs have antibodies bound (56). The phagocytic attack is triggered by complement activation secondary to the binding of antibody (58). If it is not fatal, the phagocytic response terminates after 2 or 3 days.

The weakness characteristic of chronic EAMG occurs approximately 30 days after immunization, whether or not an acute phase has occurred (59). Phagocytes are not observed (60–63). Chronic EAMG is characterized by a simplified postsynaptic membrane (60–63) bound with antibodies (53, 63) and complement (63), whose ACh sensitivity is reduced (64) as a consequence of loss of active AChR (53, 60). Most of the AChRs that remain have antibodies bound (53). The primary lesion impairing neuromuscular transmission appears to be loss of AChR, but disruption of sites of ACh release and AChR localization is probably also important. Antibodies bound to AChR can impair their function, but the effects in general are small (58, 65). Complement-mediated focal lysis probably accounts for much of the observed simplification of the folded structure of the postsynaptic membrane and for some AChR loss. The primary cause of AChR loss in EAMG, as in MG, is probably antigenic modulation (52, 65–69). Antigenic modulation is an antibody-induced increase in the rate of AChR destruction (65–69). It is triggered by antibody cross-linking of AChR (52, 69), involves aggregation of AChRs (70) and probably is rate limited by facilitated endocytosis (52). Thereafter, antigenic modulation seems to resemble normal AChR turnover as described by Fambrough and coworkers (71), including lysozomal destruction of the internalized AChR. Antigenic modulation has been demonstrated both with muscle cells in tissue and organ culture (52, 65, 67–69) and with muscle removed from animals with EAMG (66).

MONOCLONAL ANTIBODIES

Several groups have reported passive transfer of EAMG by injection of mAbs that cross react with mammalian muscle (21, 72, 73). Lennon and Lambert (72) have also reported that EAMG can be actively transferred by hybridoma cells producing cross-reacting mAbs in vivo. EAMG was transferred by mAbs that were not directed at the ACh binding site of AChR (21, 72). This is consistent with many other results (reviewed in 2–4) indicating that it is not necessary for antibody molecules to behave as AChR antagonists to cause EAMG.

It is clear that some specificities of anti-AChR antibodies could not cause EAMG or MG. The mAbs that do not cross react with muscle AChR (72) are a trivial and uninteresting example. Antibodies that could bind only to the intracellular surface of AChR would be a trivial but interesting example. We have not identified such a mAb yet, but we have found one that cannot bind to AChR in membranes (22).

More interesting are mAbs that can bind to AChR in muscle, but differ more subtly in their functional effects. We have found that the α subunit is highly immunogenic (17, 21), so that many of the antibodies to AChR are directed at this subunit. Most antibodies to the α subunit can be shown to cross-link the two α subunits within an AChR monomer (23). These could not cross-link AChR and, like monovalent F(ab) (52, 69) would not be expected to cause antigenic modulation. When cross-reacting mAbs of this type that fix complement can be developed, they should permit us to look at the effects of complement on neuromuscular transmission independent of the effects of antigenic modulation. Some mAbs to α are directed at determinants so that the mAbs cross-link the AChR (23). We have studied a mAb of this type that cross reacts with muscle AChR and have shown that it can cause antigenic modulation in vitro. The mAbs of this specificity, a subclass of mAbs that do not fix complement, and complement-fixing mAb converted to $F(ab)_2$ should permit study of the effects of antigenic modulation on neuromuscular transmission independent of the effects of complement. The most important kind of mAbs for future studies of the AChR molecule itself will be those which directly impair AChR cation channel function (26).

A prerequisite for using mAbs to study AChR is to map the binding specificity of the mAbs. A first step is to test for cross reaction with AChR from species other than the immunogen (21). In our studies we have used several different immunogens to obtain mAbs of different specificities (21–26). As immunogens we have used Triton-solubilized AChR purified from *Torpedo*, *Electrophorus*, and bovine muscle, as well as the purified subunits of *Torpedo* AChR. We have mapped the subunit specificity of many of the mAbs (21) using techniques we had developed for studying anti-subunit sera (17, 18). The method consists of using a mixture of purified ^{125}I-labeled AChR subunits (17) or sodium dodecyl sulfate (SDS)–dissociated ^{125}I-AChR as antigen (18). The mAb and bound ^{125}I-subunit are precipitated with anti-Ig coupled to agarose beads. Then the bound ^{125}I subunit is dissociated with SDS and identified by electrophoresis. Cross-reaction can be quantified using immunoprecipitation of purified ^{125}I-labeled subunits (21).

For finer scale mapping of mAb binding specificity, we have used ^{125}I-labeled proteolytic fragments of purified AChR subunits as antigen (22). As the subunits are sequenced, this should permit precise localization of the mAb binding sites. Antibodies to native AChR are directed primarily at conformationally dependent determinants (16, 17); thus, cross-reaction with SDS-denatured ^{125}I-labeled subunits is often limited or nonexistent. A technique was developed for mapping mAbs that do not react detectably with denatured subunits (21, 24). The AChR is coupled to agarose and then it is saturated with a mAb of known specificity or with anti-subunit serum. This "protecting" antibody is covalently bound to the AChR with glutaraldehyde. Then other mAbs are tested for their ability to bind to the agarose-AChR-protecting antibody complex. With this method, mapped mAbs can be used to localize unmapped mAbs. We have also studied competitive binding of mAbs to solubilized AChR by studying the size of the complexes by ultracentrifugation (23). Conclusions of the two methods agree. Our mapping techniques can discern at least 6 antigenic determinants on the α subunits of *T. californica* (23).

Using these mapping methods we are beginning to characterize our growing library of mAbs (59 to date) and thereby to characterize the structure of AChR. We are also undertaking studies of the effect of these mAbs on the function of AChR reconstituted into model membranes and on neuromuscular transmission in vivo.

As an example of the approach we are taking, consider only mAbs no. 6 and no. 35 (21–24). Monoclonal antibody no. 6 is a 7S rat immunoglobulin (23) that reacts with an antigenic determinant on the torpedo α subunit (21). Binding is highly dependent on the native conformation of AChR, but some cross-reaction with denatured α is detectable (21). A similar antigenic determinant was detected by cross reaction with all other AChR tested (21), but although its affinity for torpedo AChR is very high, its affinity for AChR from other species is much lower. Monoclonal antibody 6 binds on the extracellular surface of AChR outside the area occupied by bound α-BuTx (21), but to the same peptide fragments which contain both the MBTA binding site and the site(s) where carbohydrate is bound (22). Binding of mAb 6 to AChR has no detectable effect on its function (26). This antibody can passively transfer EAMG (21), indicating that muscle AChR has a similar determinant to which mAb 6 can bind in vivo and cause the fixation of complement. The antigenic determinant for mAb 6 is highly immunogenic, and approximately half of the antibodies in an antiserum to native AChR are bound at this site, or close enough to be inhibited by bound mAb 6 (21).

By analogy with other proteins (74, 75), we expect that the antigenic determinant for mAb 6 is probably formed by a continuous sequence of 5 or 6 amino acids located on a fold or end of the α polypeptide chain. In the native molecule the antigenic determinant for mAb 6 on each α subunit is oriented so that the determinants on two adjacent molecules can be crosslinked by a single mAb 6 molecule (23). Because there are 2 α subunits per monomer, a maximum of 2 mAb 6 molecules can bind per monomer (23).

Monoclonal antibody no. 35 is a 7S rat antibody to *Electrophorus* AChR that cross-reacts competitively with the same determinant recognized by mAb (23, 24). Monoclonal antibody no. 35 cross-reacts with AChR from other species with higher affinity than does mAb 6 (24). Thus, it can be used not only to crosslink electric organ and muscle AChR in solution, but also to crosslink muscle cell AChR within the plane of the membrane. This causes antigenic modulation, and is consistent with the idea that muscle AChRs, like electric organ AChRs, have two α subunits per monomer (23).

The amount of information available from the partial characterization of these two mAbs should give some idea of the large amount of information that should become available with the further characterization of these and many other mAbs. The results, we believe, will contribute significantly both to the elucidation of the structure and function of the AChR molecule, and to the understanding of the molecular biology of MG.

ACKNOWLEDGMENTS

The research reported here was supported by grants to J Lindstrom from the Muscular Dystrophy Association, the National Institutes of Health (grant no. NS11323), and the Los Angeles Chapter of the Myasthenia Gravis Foundation. S Tzartos is supported by a postdoctoral fellowship from the Muscular Dystrophy Association.

REFERENCES

1. Simpson J: Myasthenia gravis: a new hypothesis. Scott Med J 5:419–436, 1960

2. Lindstrom J: Autoimmune response to acetylcholine receptors in myasthenia gravis and its animal model. Adv Immunol 27:1–50, 1979

3. Lindstrom J, Dau P: The biology of myasthenia gravis. Annu Rev Pharmacol Toxicol 20:337–362, 1980

4. Lindstrom J, Engel A: Myasthenia gravis and the nicotinic cholinergic receptor. In *Receptor Regulation*, edited by Lefkowitz R, in the series *Receptors and Recognition*, edited by Cuatracasas P, Greaves M. Chapman and Hall, London (in press)

5. Lindstrom J, Patrick J: Purification of the acetylcholine receptor by affinity chromatography. In *Synaptic Transmission and Neuronal Interaction*. Edited by Bennett MVL. Raven Press, New York, 1974, pp 191–216

6. Patrick J, Lindstrom J: Autoimmune response to acetylcholine receptor. Science 180:871–872, 1973

7. Patrick J, Lindstrom J, Culp B, McMillan J: Studies on purified eel acetylcholine receptor and anti-acetylcholine receptor antibody. Proc Natl Acad Sci USA 70:3334–3338, 1973

8. Lindstrom JM, Seybold ME, Lennon VA, et al: Antibody to acetylcholine receptor in myasthenia gravis: prevalence, clinical correlates and diagnostic value. Neurology (Minneap) 26:1054–1059, 1976

9. Lindstrom J: An assay for antibodies to human acetylcholine receptor in serum from patients with myasthenia gravis. J Clin Immunol Immunopathol 7:36–43, 1977

10. Lindstrom J, Einarson B, Francy M: Acetylcholine receptors and myasthenia gravis: the effect of antibodies to eel acetylcholine receptors in electric organ cells. In *Cellular Neurobiology*. Edited by Hall Z, Kelley R. A R Liss, New York, 1977, pp 119–130

11. Lindstrom J, Anholt R, Einarson B, et al: Purification of acetylcholine receptors with functional cation channels and reconstitution into lipid vesicles. J Biol Chem 255:8340–8350, 1980

12. Huganir R, Schell M, Racker E: Reconstitution of the purified acetylcholine receptor from *Torpedo californica*. FEBS Lett 108:155–160, 1979

13. Reynolds JA, Karlin A: Molecular weight in detergent solution of acetylcholine receptor from *Torpedo californica*. Biochemistry 17:2035–2038, 1978

14. Damle V, Karlin A: Affinity labeling of one of two α-neurotoxin binding sites in acetylcholine receptor from *Torpedo californica*. Biochemistry 17:2039–2045, 1978

15. Lindstrom J, Merlie J, Yogeeswaran G: Biochemical properties of acetylcholine receptor subunits from *Torpedo californica*. Biochemistry 18:4465–4470, 1979

16. Lindstrom J, Einarson B, Merlie J: Immunization of rats with polypeptide chains from *Torpedo* acetylcholine receptor causes an autoimmune response to receptors in rat muscle. Proc Natl Acad Sci USA 75:769–773, 1978

17. Lindstrom J, Walter B, Einarson B: Immunochemical similarities between subunits of acetylcholine receptors from *Torpedo*, *Electrophorus*, and mammalian muscle. Biochemistry 18:4470–4480, 1979

18. Lindstrom J, Cooper J, Tzartos S: Acetylcholine receptors from *Torpedo* and *Electrophorus* have similar subunit structures. Biochemistry 19:1454–1458, 1980

19. Nathanson N, Hall Z: Subunit structure and peptide mapping of junctional and extrajunctional acetylcholine receptors from rat muscle. Biochemistry 18:3392–3401, 1979

20. Köhler G, Milstein C: Continuous cultures of fused cells secreting antibody of predefined specificity. Nature 256:495–497, 1975

21. Tzartos S, Lindstrom J: Monoclonal antibodies used to probe acetylcholine receptor structure: localization of the main immunogenic region and detection of similarities between subunits. Proc Natl Acad Sci USA 77:755–759, 1980

22. Gullick W, Tzartos S, Lindstrom J: Monoclonal antibodies as probes of acetylcholine receptor structure. I. Peptide mapping. Biochemistry (in press)

23. Conti-Tronconi B, Tzartos S, Lindstrom J: Monoclonal antibodies as probes of acetylcholine receptor structure. II. Binding to native receptor. Biochemistry (in press)

24. Tzartos S, Lindstrom J: Production and characterization of monoclonal antibodies for use as probes of the acetylcholine receptor. In *Monoclonal Antibodies in Endocrine Research*. Edited by Fellows R, Eisenbarth G. Raven Press, New York (in press)

25. Lindstrom J, Einarson B, Tzartos S: Production and assay of antibodies to acetylcholine receptors. In *Methods in Enzymology: Immunochemical Techniques*. Edited by Van Vunahio H, Langone JJ. Academic Press, New York (in press)

26. Lindstrom J, Tzartos S, Gullick W: Structure and function of the acetylcholine receptor molecule studied using monoclonal antibodies. Ann NY Acad Sci (in press)

27. Weinberg C, Hall Z: Antibodies from patients with myasthenia gravis recognize determinants unique to extrajunctional acetylcholine receptors. Proc Natl Acad Sci USA 76:504–508, 1979

28. Weill C, McNamee MG, Karlin A: Affinity labeling of purified acetylcholine receptor from *Torpedo californica*. Biochem Biophys Res Commun 61:997–1003, 1974

29. Raftery MA, Vandlen RL, Reed KL, et al: Characterization of *Torpedo californica* acetylcholine receptor: its subunit composition and ligand binding properties. Cold Spring Harbor Symp Quant Biol 40:193–202, 1975

30. Hucho F, Bandini G, Suarez-Isla B: The acetylcholine receptor as part of a protein complex in receptor-enriched membrane fragments from *Torpedo californica* electric tissue. Eur J Biochem 83:335–340, 1978

31. Damle V, McLaughlin M, Karlin A: Bromoacetylcholine as an affinity label of the acetylcholine receptor from *Torpedo californica*. Biochem Biophys Res Commun 84:845–851, 1978

32. Witzemann V, Raftery M: Selective photoaffinity labeling of acetylcholine receptor using a cholinergic analogue. Biochemistry 16:5862–5868, 1977

33. Witzemann V, Raftery M: Affinity directed crosslinking of acetylcholine receptor polypeptide components in post-synaptic membranes. Biochem Biophys Res Commun 85:623–631, 1978

34. Nathanson N, Hall Z: In situ labeling of *Torpedo* and rat muscle acetylcholine receptor by a photoaffinity derivative of an α-bungarotoxin. J Biol Chem 255:1698–1703, 1980

35. Hamilton SL, McLaughlin M, Karlin A: Crosslinking of the acetylcholine receptor from *Torpedo* electric tissue (abstract). Fed Proc 37:529, 1978

36. Kimball M, Sato A, Richardson J, et al: Molecular conformation of erabutoxin β: atomic coordinates at 2.5 Å resolution. Biochem Biophys Res Commun 88:950–959, 1979

37. Epstein M, Racker E: Reconstitution of carbamylcholine-dependent sodium ion flux and desensitization of the acetylcholine receptor from *Torpedo californica*. J Biol Chem 253:6660–6662, 1978

38. Anholt R, Lindstrom J, Montal M: Functional equivalence of monomeric and dimeric forms of purified acetylcholine receptor from *Torpedo californica* in reconstituted lipid vesicles. Eur J Biochem 109:481–487, 1980

39. Cartaud J, Benedetti LL, Cohen JB, et al: Presence of a lattice structure in membrane fragments rich in nicotinic receptor protein from the electric organ of *Torpedo marmorata*. FEBS Lett 33:109–113, 1973

40. Nickel E, Potter LT: Ultrastructure of isolated membranes of *Torpedo* electric tissue. Brain Res 57:508–517, 1973

41. Ross MJ, Klymkowsky MW, Agard DA, et al: Structural studies of a membrane-bound acetylcholine receptor from *Torpedo californica*. J Mol Biol 116:635–659, 1977

42. Allen T, Potter LT: Postsynaptic membranes in the electric tissue of *Narcine*: isolation and characterization. Tissue Cell 9:609–622, 1977

43. Cartaud J, Benedetti E, Sobel A, Changeux JP: A morphological study of the cholinergic receptor protein from *Torpedo marmorata* in its membrane environment and in its detergent extracted purified form. J Cell Sci 29:313–337, 1978

44. Zingsheim H, Neugebauer D, Barrantes F, et al: Structural details of membrane bound acetylcholine receptor from *Torpedo marmorata*. Proc Natl Acad Sci USA 77:952–956, 1980

45. Klymkowsky M, Stroud R: Immunospecific identification and three-dimensional structure of a membrane-bound acetylcholine receptor from *Torpedo californica*. J Mol Biol 128:319–334, 1979

46. Potter LT, Smith DS: Postsynaptic membranes in the electric tissue of *Narcine*. Tissue Cell 9:585–644, 1977

47. Vandlen R, Wilson C, Eisenach J, et al: Studies of the composition of purified *Torpedo californica* acetylcholine receptor and its subunits. Biochemistry 18:1845–1854, 1979

48. Sobel A, Weber M, Changeux JP: Large-scale purification of the acetylcholine receptor protein in its membrane-bound and detergent-extracted forms from *Torpedo marmorata* electric organ. Eur J Biochem 80:215–224, 1977

49. Shorr RG, Dolly O, Barnard E: Composition of acetylcholine receptor protein from skeletal muscle. Nature 274:283–284, 1978

50. Lindstrom J, Gullick W, Conti-Tronconi B, Ellisman M: Preteolytic nicking of the acetylcholine receptor. Biochemistry 19:4791–4795, 1980

51. Huganir R, Racker E: Endogenous and exogenous proteolysis of the acetylcholine receptor from *Torpedo californica*. J Supramolec Struct (in press)

52. Lindstrom J, Einarson B: Antigenic modulation and receptor loss in EAMG. Muscle Nerve 2:173–179, 1979

53. Lindstrom JM, Einarson B, Lennon VA, et al: Pathological mechanisms in EAMG. I. Immunogenicity of syngeneic muscle acetylcholine receptor and quantitative extraction of receptor and antibody: receptor complexes from muscles of rats with experimental autoimmune myasthenia gravis. J Exp Med 144:726–738, 1976

54. Granato D, Fulpius BW, Moody J: Experimental myasthenia in Balb/c mice immunized with rat acetylcholine receptor from rat denervated muscle. Proc Natl Acad Sci USA 73:2872–2876, 1976

55. Lennon VA, Lindstrom JM, Seybold ME: Experimental autoimmune myasthenia: a model of myasthenia gravis in rats and guinea pigs. J Exp Med 141:1365–1375, 1975

56. Lindstrom JM, Engel AG, Seybold ME, et al: Pathological mechanisms in EAMG. II. Passive transfer of experimental autoimmune myasthenia gravis in rats with anti-acetylcholine receptor antibodies. J Exp Med 144:739–753, 1976

57. Engel A, Sakakibara H, Sahashi K, et al: Passively transferred experimental autoimmune myasthenia gravis. Neurology (NY) 29:179–188, 1978

58. Lennon VA, Seybold ME, Lindstrom J, et al: Role of complement in pathogenesis of experimental autoimmune myasthenia gravis. J Exp Med 147:973–983, 1977

59. Lindstrom J, Lennon V, Seybold M, et al: Experimental autoimmune myasthenia gravis and myasthenia gravis: biochemical and immunochemical aspects. Ann NY Acad Sci 274:254–274, 1976

60. Engel AG, Lindstrom JM, Lambert EH, et al: Ultra-structural localization of the acetylcholine receptor in myasthenia gravis and in its experimental autoimmune model. Neurology (NY) 27:307–315, 1977

61. Engel A, Tsujihata M, Lambert E, et al: Experimental autoimmune myasthenia gravis: a sequential and quantitative study of the neuromuscular junction ultrastructure and electrophysiologic correlation. J Neuropathol Exp Neurol 35:569–587, 1976

62. Engel A, Tsujihata M, Lindstrom J, et al: End-plate fine structure in myasthenia gravis and in experimental autoimmune myasthenia gravis. Ann NY Acad Sci 274:60–79, 1976

63. Sahashi K, Engel AG, Lindstrom J, et al: Ultrastructural localization of immune complexes (IgG and C3) at the end-plate in experimental autoimmune myasthenia gravis. J Neuropathol Exp Neurol 37:212–223, 1978

64. Lambert EH, Lindstrom JM, Lennon VA: End-plate potentials in experimental autoimmune myasthenia gravis in rats. Ann NY Acad Sci 274:300–318, 1976

65. Heinemann S, Bevan S, Kullberg R, et al: Modulation of the acetylcholine receptor by anti-receptor antibody. Proc Natl Acad Sci USA 74:3090–3094, 1977

66. Merlie J, Heinemann S, Einarson B, et al: Degradation of acetylcholine receptor in diaphragms of rats with experimental autoimmune myasthenia gravis. J Biol Chem 254:6328–6332, 1979

67. Merlie JP, Heinemann SJ, Lindstrom J: Acetylcholine receptor degradation in adult rat diaphragms in organ culture and the effect of anti-acetylcholine receptor antibodies. J Biol Chem 254:6320–6327, 1979

68. Kao I, Drachman DB: Myasthenic immunoglobulin accelerates acetylcholine receptor degradation. Science 196:527–529, 1977

69. Drachman DB, Angus CW, Adams RN, et al: Myasthenic antibodies cross-link acetylcholine receptors to accelerate degradation. N Engl J Med 298:1116–1122, 1978

70. Prives J, Hoffman L, Tarrab-Hazdai R, et al: Ligand induced changes in stability and distribution of acetylcholine receptors on surface membranes of muscle cells. Life Sci 24:1713–1718, 1979

71. Fambrough D: Control of acetylcholine receptors in skeletal muscle. Physiol Rev 59:165–227, 1979

72. Lennon V, Lambert E: Myasthenia gravis induced by monoclonal antibodies to acetylcholine receptors. Nature 285:238–240, 1980

73. Gomez C, Richman D, Wollmann R, et al: Passive transfer of experimental autoimmune myasthenia gravis using monoclonal anti-receptor antibodies. Nature 286:738–739, 1980

74. Atassi MZ: Antigenic structure of myoglobin: the complete immunochemical anatomy of a protein and conclusions relating to antigenic structures of proteins. Immunochemistry 12:423–438, 1975.

75. Atassi MZ: Precise determination of the entire antigenic structure of lysozyme. Immunochemistry 15:909–936, 1978

DISCUSSION

Dr. Andrew Engel: I would like to correct the impression you have that modulation alone is responsible for loss of the receptor. In fact, the diagram of the myasthenic endplate (which is based on electron micrographs) indicates marked simplification of the junctional folds. We should not ignore the morphologic and immunoelectron microscopic evidence that some receptor loss is due to complement-mediated lysis of the junctional folds.

Dr. Jon Lindstrom: I agree.

Dr. Edson X. Albuquerque: I would like to introduce a slight modification on your model of the AChR: it would be appropriate to extend the channel component to cross the entire membrane and go inside the cell. We recently showed that a number of channel-reactive agents react with active sites outside as well as inside the cell. We demonstrated this by using agents such as quaternary phencyclidine, quaternary piperocaine, and quaternary histrionicotoxin. Other quaternary agents, including tetraethylammonium and atropine methylsulfate, had no effect on the ionic channel of the AChR when applied inside the cell. Thus, it is clear that the ionic channel of the AChR has binding sites located outside as well as inside the cell.

Dr. Jon Lindstrom: Actually, the model of structure I showed did not depict the cation channel as extending through the center of the molecule from the exterior to the interior of the cell. The gating mechanism could be anywhere along such a channel. It would not be surprising to find that some agents could affect the channel if introduced from within the cell. It is not known whether quaternary agents act at the same sites when applied from outside the cell and inside the cell.

Dr. Michael Garlepp: Are many antibodies in human MG directed at carbohydrate?

Dr. Jon Lindstrom: I do not know what fraction of the antibodies in human MG are directed against carbohydrate, but we have tried to get at the problem in a couple of ways in animals. I was especially worried that the anti-subunit sera might be directed against carbohydrate, because these antisera are very efficient in their cross-reaction with native receptor. If you were to ask what sort of determinant would survive denaturation in SDS and react perfectly well with native receptors, carbohydrate would be a good answer. Then anti-subunit sera would be directed against just the carbohydrate-rich parts of the subunits. But it turns out that peptide maps of the subunits show that the antibodies are directed at all parts of the receptor subunit, not just the carbohydrate-rich parts.

Dr. Ivan Diamond: Do any of the antibodies you have raised against specific subunits either affect Na^+ flux in your reconstituted preparation or perhaps affect the desensitization of that response?

Dr. Jon Lindstrom: Of the 60 monoclonal antibodies we have sitting in the freezer, we have tested only a few. We have found two that do affect the Na^+ flux. These are not directed at the ACh binding site, which has us very excited. Unfortunately, these two antibodies have quite low affinity for the AChR; they are difficult to map and difficult to deal with. The bulk of these monoclonal antibodies, like mAb 6, are very nice magic bullets; you can add them in very low concentrations and they bind stoichiometrically. You can use them as you might use a toxin. In summary, I cannot tell you yet which subunit is the channel.

18
Molecular Approaches to Myasthenia Gravis

Sara Fuchs, PhD

Carmela Feingold, MSc

Daniel Bartfeld, MSc

Daria Mochly-Rosen, MSc

Ilana Schmidt-Hopfeld, MSc

Rebeca Tarrab-Hazdai, PhD

Special interest in the immunologic properties of the nicotinic acetylcholine receptor (AChR) arises from the involvement of an autoimmune response against this receptor in myasthenia gravis (MG) (1, 2). It has been known since 1973 that immunization of animals with AChR isolated and purified from electric organs of electric fish leads to the development of an experimental autoimmune myasthenia gravis (EAMG) that mimics many of the manifestations of MG (2, 3). Research in our group deals mainly with EAMG and with structural analysis of the AChR, which is involved as an autoantigen in both the human and the experimental disease. We report here some recent studies from our laboratory on the structure and function of AChR, monoclonal antibodies, attempts to regulate EAMG by anti-idiotypes, and a surface antigen on thymic lymphocytes that cross reacts with AChR. These studies were aimed at elucidating the molecular origin and immunologic nature of MG and possibly at developing approaches to regulate MG.

STRUCTURE AND FUNCTION OF AChR

In attempts to elucidate the molecular requirements for the cholinergic and/or myasthenic activities of the AChR, we have studied the pharmacologic and immunologic features of various modifications and derivatives of the AChR molecule. By this approach we hope to identify, characterize, and isolate minimal fragments of AChR that are responsible for its biologic activities, to

245

map the active sites, and to find out whether the cholinergic and myasthenic active sites overlap. Such analyses may also lead to the preparation and characterization of derivatives or fragments of the receptor molecule with the potential to regulate the immune response to AChR and the autoimmune disease resulting from it. The various AChR preparations that have been investigated in our laboratory and their biologic activities are summarized in Table 1.

Denatured AChR

We have shown previously that irreversible denaturation of AChR, which destroys the secondary and tertiary structure of the protein, abolishes both the pharmacologic and myasthenic activities of the receptor. Thus, a reduced carboxymethylated receptor preparation (RCM-AChR) does not bind α-neu-rotoxins or other cholinergic ligands and does not lead to any myasthenic symptoms when used to immunize of rabbits (4, 5). However, the RCM-AChR is immunogenic in rabbits and cross reacts with intact AChR via nonstructural antigenic determinants, which are common to the native and denatured receptor preparations. Other conformational antigenic determinants in AChR are abolished by denaturation.

The RCM-AChR itself is not myasthenic, but has an immunosuppressive effect on EAMG by either preventing the onset of the disease or reversing the clinical symptoms in myasthenic rabbits. The preventive and therapeutic effects of RCM-AChR are accompanied by a change in the specificity of the immune response toward the characteristic specificity of RCM-AChR (5). The cross reactivity between AChR and RCM-AChR and the nonpathogenicity of the latter appear to be crucial in governing the immunosuppressive effect of denatured AChR on EAMG.

Like denatured AChR, the isolated individual subunits of the receptor do not induce any myasthenic symptoms. They bind very effectively to anti-RCM-AChR and, on reacting with anti-AChR, they bind only to the antibody fraction that is directed against nonstructural antigenic determinants in AChR.

Table 1. Structure and Function of the Acetylcholine Receptor

Derivative	Modification	Bind Cholinergic Ligands	Induce EAMG
RCM-AChR	Denaturation by reduction and alkylation in 6 M guanidine (4, 5)	No	No
T-AChR	Trypsinization (6)	Yes	Yes
PA-AChR	Polyalanylation of lysines (free amino groups) with DL-alanine carboxyanhydride (7)	Yes	No
Ni-AChR	Nitration of tyrosines with tetranitromethane (Mochly-Rosen D, Fuchs S: unpublished data)	No	No

Abbreviations: RCM-AChR, reduced carboxymethylated acetylcholine receptor (AChR); T-AChR, trypsinated AChR; PA-AChR, polyalanylated AChR; Ni-AChR, nitrated AChR; EAMG, experimental autoimmune myasthenia gravis.

Trypsinated AChR

Another modification of the AChR that we have studied in detail is obtained by trypsinization of AChR, which cleaves and "shaves" the nonstructural portions of the receptor that are susceptible to proteolytic degradation. This treatment yields a simpler and smaller AChR molecule that retains both the cholinergic binding site and the myasthenic activity of AChR (6). After additional steps of repurification, trypsinated AChR (T-AChR) has a sedimentation coefficient of 8.0S and on sodium dodecyl sulfate acrylamide gel electrophoresis shows one major band with a molecular weight of approximately 27,000 daltons. This 27,000-dalton subunit appears to originate from the 40,000-dalton subunit of the receptor and represents an active AChR molecule with lower structural complexity than that of the intact detergent-purified receptor. The availability of T-AChR thus facilitates analysis of the molecular origin of the biologic activities of AChR.

Polyalanylated AChR

Modifying the lysine residues in the AChR by attaching poly-DL-alanine side chains to free amino groups in the protein resulted in a derivative that retained the cholinergic specificity of the receptor but lost the myasthenic activity (7). Polyalanylated AChR (PA-AChR) is the only AChR derivative we have studied that exhibits dissociation of the myasthenic and cholinergic activities of the receptor (7). These studies suggest that the receptor site for myasthenic activity is not necessarily identical to the site for pharmacologic activity. The finding that polyalanylation of lysines does not interfere with the binding properties of AChR to various cholinergic ligands may imply either that lysine residues (or other amino groups) do not participate in the cholinergic binding site or that these particular residues in the active site were not susceptible to the modification.

Nitrated AChR

We have recently shown that reacting tyrosine residues in the AChR with tetranitromethane abolishes both cholinergic and myasthenic activities of the receptor, as was observed after denaturation. Like denatured AChR, nitrated AChR (Ni-AChR) may also have a suppressive effect on EAMG (Mochly-Rosen D, Fuchs S: unpublished data).

Further modifications of the AChR and development of additional derivatives will add information on the structural features of the biologically active sites of the molecule and will contribute to the design of additional specific immunosuppressive preparations for EAMG.

MONOCLONAL ANTIBODIES

As immunochemical analyses and various antibody fractionations show, the AChR is a complex antigen expressing many antigenic determinants, only some of which may be involved in the pathogenesis of MG (5, 8, 9). To obtain antibodies of defined, restricted specificity, we used somatic cell hybridization to prepare monoclonal antibodies (10, 11).

To establish monoclonal antibodies with anti-AChR activity, spleen cells from myasthenic mice immunized with purified *Torpedo* AChR were fused with NSl nonsecreting myeloma cells (11). Hybrids with anti-AChR antibody activity were selected, and positive hybridomas were cloned and propagated in vivo as ascitic fluids. The various clones were characterized for their antigenic specificity by measuring their binding to various preparations and derivatives of AChR representing different antigenic determinants. The anti-AChR sera bound to all of the antigens derived from AChR, but the individual clones possessed defined, restricted specificities. Some clones were directed selectively against structural (conformational) antigenic determinants of AChR and thus bound T-AChR but not RCM-AChR. Other clones were directed against nonstructural antigenic determinants represented by RCM-AChR. All our monoclonal antibodies bound to membranous AChR, indicating that they were directed against antigenic determinants exposed also on the membrane-bound receptor. Only part of the monoclonal antibodies reacted with mouse muscle AChR.

One monoclonal antibody, designated A.F.5.5, appears to be of special interest in being directed against the cholinergic site of the receptor. This specificity has not been detected in AChR-immunized animals (12, 13), although it might be of biologic importance. The ability to select for a particular antibody specificity, even one that is extremely minor, is one of the advantages offered by the lymphocyte hybridization method. We have demonstrated that α-bungarotoxin and other cholinergic agonists and antagonists inhibit the binding of AChR to the antibody clone A.F.5.5 in a pharmacologic manner. The ligand concentrations required for 50% inhibition of the binding of ^{125}I-AChR to A.F.5.5 are similar to the concentrations required for 50% inhibition of the binding of ^{125}I-α-bungarotoxin to AChR (Table 2).

Some of our preliminary experiments showed that A.F.5.5 inhibits the carbamylcholine-induced sodium influx into AChR-enriched membrane vesicles. Passive transfer of these antibodies leads to myasthenic symptoms. How-

Table 2. Inhibition of the Binding of A.F.5.5 and α-Bungarotoxin to the Acetylcholine Receptor (AChR) by Cholinergic Ligands

	Ligand Concentration (M) at 50% inhibition of Binding to AChR	
Ligand	Inhibition of A.F.5.5 Binding	Inhibition of α-Bungarotoxin Binding
α-Bungarotoxin	3.0×10^{-10}	1.5×10^{-10}
Naja naja siamensis toxin	1.3×10^{-8}	1.0×10^{-9}
D-Tubocurarine	6.2×10^{-6}	9.0×10^{-6}
Hexamethonium	1.6×10^{-3}	5.6×10^{-4}
Decamethonium	3.3×10^{-4}	5.0×10^{-5}
Carbamylcholine	0.5×10^{-4}	1.7×10^{-4}
Acetylcholine	6.1×10^{-4}	1.0×10^{-5}
Atropine	$> 10^{-2}$	1.2×10^{-2}

ever, we still do not know whether this particular specificity has a unique role in EAMG and human MG. In other recent reports, myasthenic symptoms have been transferred by monoclonal antibodies not directed to the cholinergic binding site (14, 15).

It is of interest that the monoclonal antibody (A.F.5.5) directed against the cholinergic active site of AChR binds weakly to both the 40,000- and the 65,000-dalton subunit of the receptor (α and δ subunits, respectively), which suggests the possibility of some structural homology between these two subunits.

The applications of monoclonal antibodies in general are manifold. The potential of the particular clone against the biologically active site of AChR is even broader, both in structure analysis of this site and in screening for nicotinic receptors in a wide range of tissues and species.

REGULATION OF EAMG BY ANTI-IDIOTYPES

According to the network theory of Jerne (16), anti-idiotypes might normally be involved in modulating the degree and duration of immune responses. Thus, anti-idiotypes may have a regulatory role in autoimmune diseases or other immunologic disorders, and it has been suggested that remissions in autoimmune diseases might be associated with an increase of specific anti-idiotypic activity (17). Immunization with a person's antibodies or lymphocytes carrying the same idiotypes may furnish an efficient way to produce specific anti-idiotypic antibodies. Alternatively, active autoimmunization with a person's own idiotypes might result in an enhanced specific anti-idiotypic reactivity that could suppress or block the effect of the idiotype.

The application of anti-idiotypic antibodies provides a possible approach for specific regulation of the immune response to AChR and of MG. Anti-idiotypic serum specific for anti-AChR idiotypes has previously been prepared in C57BL/ 6 mice by repeated injection of anti-AChR antibodies produced in and purified from syngeneic mice or, alternatively, by immunization with syngeneic spleen cells educated in vitro with AChR (18). The anti-idiotypic serum reacted specifically with anti-AChR antibodies of several mouse strains and of other species. It also inhibited the binding of AChR to anti-AChR antibodies, suggesting that idiotypic determinant(s) against which the sera are directed are associated with the antigen combining site.

We recently elicited in rabbits anti-idiotypic antibodies against anti-AChR antibodies and tested their effect in regulating EAMG (19). The anti-idiotypes were prepared by repeated immunizations with purified anti-AChR antibodies. When the idiotypes (antibodies) originated from other rabbits, we induced immunologic tolerance against the normal immunoglobulins of the donor rabbits before immunization with purified antibodies (Fig. 1). This step was necessary to avoid the production of anti–normal immunoglobulins, because our rabbits were not genetically identical. The anti-idiotypic response was assayed by the direct binding of the idiotype to the anti-idiotypic serum in a solid-phase radioimmunoassay.

The anti-idiotypic sera against a certain rabbit's idiotypes cross reacted with anti-AChR antibodies produced in other rabbits, as had previously been

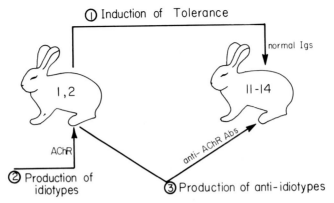

Fig. 1. Induction of anti-idiotypes in rabbits: ① Tolerance was induced in rabbits 11–14 against the normal immunoglobulins of rabbits 1 and 2 by intravenous injection of 10 mg of immunoglobulins. ② Anti–acetylcholine receptor (AChR) antibodies (idiotypes) were raised in rabbits 1 and 2 by one injection of 20 μg of *Torpedo californica* AChR in complete Freund's adjuvant (CFA). ③ Anti-anti-AChR (anti-idiotypes) were induced in rabbits 11–14 by repeated intradermal injections of 100 μg of purified anti-AChR antibodies (elicited in rabbits 1 and 2) in CFA.

reported in mice (18). After 5 immunizations with anti-AChR antibodies, the rabbits were injected with 100 μg of purified *Torpedo* AChR to test for the effect on EAMG of the specific anti-idiotypic response. Two control rabbits were similarly immunized with normal immunoglobulins (Nig) before injection of AChR, and 2 other control rabbits were injected with AChR only (Fig. 2). As shown in Figure 2, EAMG was suppressed in the rabbits producing anti-idiotypes (rabbits 11–14). In 2 rabbits (rabbits 12 and 14) there was a delay in the onset of the disease, and 2 immunizations with AChR were required. In 2 other rabbits (rabbits 11 and 13) there was complete protection against the disease for at least several months.

In another experiment, EAMG was also suppressed in rabbits immunized against their own anti-AChR antibodies. The rabbits were first injected once with subclinical doses of AChR (20 μg per rabbit). Anti-AChR antibodies were purified from the serum of these rabbits on an AChR-Sepharose adsorbent, and the purified antibodies (in complete Freund's adjuvant) were administered repeatedly to the same rabbits to elicit an anti-idiotypic response. When these rabbits were then challenged as many as 3 times with myasthenic doses of AChR (100 μg for each challenge), protection against EAMG was observed. Such experiments, together with the possible cross reactivity between anti-AChR idiotypes from various sources, may render the approach of anti-idiotypes valuable for regulating EAMG and human MG.

AChR AND THE THYMUS

The role of the thymus in MG has been widely investigated but is still not thoroughly understood. We have previously reported on an immunologic cross reactivity, both humoral and cellular, between a thymic component and the AChR (20). This cross reactivity could provide a molecular explanation for involvement of the thymus in MG. Studies from other laboratories have suggested that the cross reactivity between the AChR and the thymus could stem from myoid cells in the thymus (21, 22) and/or from epithelial cells of the thymus that contain nicotinic AChR (23). Using immunofluorescence and radioimmunologic techniques, we recently demonstrated that thymic lympho-

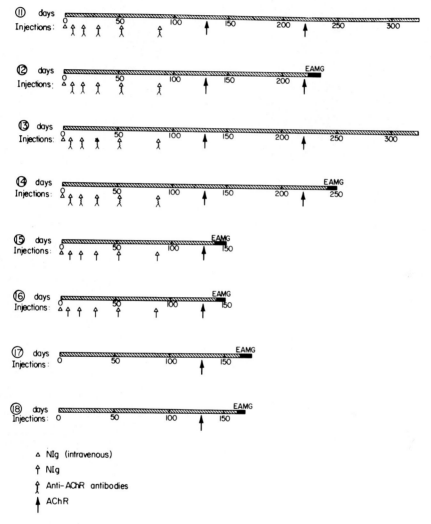

Fig. 2. Effect of anti-idiotypic response on experimental autoimmune myasthenia gravis (EAMG). Anti-idiotypes were induced in rabbits 11–14 as described in Figure 1. Control rabbits 15 and 16 were injected on the same days as rabbits 11–14 with the normal immunoglobulins (NIg) of rabbits 1 and 2 (Figure 1). After 120 days from the beginning of these experiments, rabbits 11–16 plus control rabbits 17 and 18 (not pretreatment) were injected once or twice with 100 μg of AChR in CFA, and development of EAMG was tested.

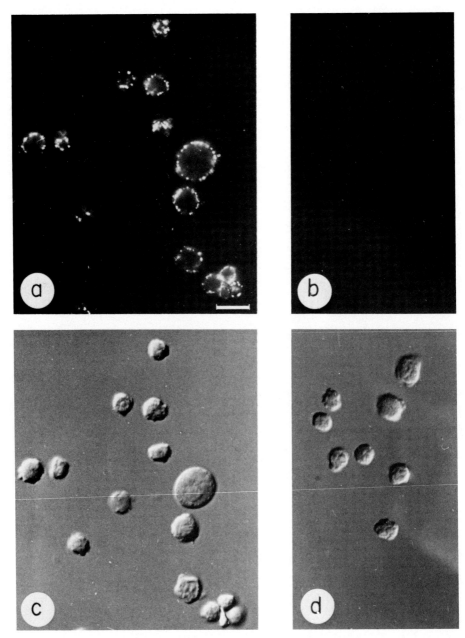

Fig. 3. Immunofluorescence staining of C57BL/6 thymocytes with anti–acetylcholine receptor (AChR) antibodies. **(a)** Epifluoresecence of cells incubated with rabbit anti-AChR IgG followed by rhodamine-goat anti-rabbit IgG, compared to **(b)** control cells incubated with rabbit anti-ovalbumin immunoglobulin instead of anti-AChR. Parts **c** and **d** show the same fields as **a** and **b**, respectively, but were photographed with Nomarski optics (differential interference contrast). Bar indicates 10 μm.

cytes bear a surface antigen that binds specifically to antibodies against nicotinic AChR, and we defined this antigen as "AChR-like" (24).

Thymocytes of normal mice were fluorescently labeled by treatment with rabbit anti–*Torpedo* AChR immunoglobulins, followed by fluorescein or rhodamine conjugated goat anti-rabbit immunoglobulins (Fig. 3). The fluorescence was evenly distributed on the cell surface in minute patches (Fig. 3a), and capping of the patches was observed after removal of sodium azide and further incubation at 37° C (24). Control immunoglobulins from normal rabbit serum or from rabbit anti-ovalbumin serum did not result in any staining (Fig. 3b, d).

The microscopic findings were verified by quantitative analysis in the fluorescence-activated cell sorter. Specific fluorescence peaks were obtained after labeling with rabbit anti-AChR serum, immunoglobulins, or purified antibodies. Increasing the amounts of the specific immunoglobulins or antibodies added resulted in a shift of the fluorescence peak toward higher intensity (Fig. 4). The labeled cells were shown to be of the size of lymphocytes by light scattering. Specific binding to mouse thymocytes was demonstrated with anti–*Torpedo* AChR sera, immunoglobulins, or antibodies elicited in monkeys, rats, and even syngeneic mice. These results were observed by both immunofluorescence experiments and radioimmunoassay (Table 3) (24).

The presence of an "AChR-like" antigen on mouse thymocytes is not associated with susceptibility to EAMG. Thymocytes of either a susceptible mouse strain (C57BL/6) (25) or a nonsusceptible one (SJL) bind anti-AChR antibodies similarly (Table 3).

It should be pointed out that we did not succeed in demonstrating significant receptor activity, measured by toxin binding experiments, in thymocytes or thymic extracts. This fact and the finding that antibodies against a pharmacologically inactive, denatured AChR preparation (RCM-AChR) (4) cross react

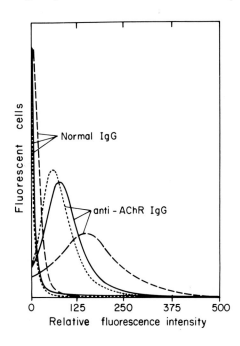

Fig. 4. Immunofluorescence profile monitored in the fluorescence-activated cell sorter of C57BL/6 thymocytes labeled with rabbit anti–acetylcholine receptor (AChR) immunoglobulins and with normal rabbit immunoglobulins. Dotted line, application of 200 μg of IgG; solid line, 300 μg of IgG; dashed line, 600 μg of IgG. Fluorescein-conjugated goat anti-IgG was used for staining.

Table 3. Binding of Anti-Acetylcholine Receptor (AChR) to Mouse Thymocytes[a]

Thymocytes	Sample	Binding (cpm)	
Sera (dilution)		(1/2)	(1/4)
C57BL/6	Rabbit anti-AChR	46,420	37,310
	Rabbit anti-RCM-AChR	49,140	47,420
	Rabbit anti-ovalbumin	15,750	10,700
C57BL/6	Monkey anti-AChR	75,210	68,420
	Monkey normal serum	20,210	19,460
C57BL/6	Mouse (C57BL/6) anti-AChR	46,320	22,470
	Mouse (C57BL/6) normal serum	19,200	9,720
Purified antibodies (μg)		(24)	(18)
C57BL/6	Rabbit anti-AChR	10,510	4,950
	Rabbit anti-RCM-AChR	ND[b]	4,610
	Rabbit anti-ovalbumin	1,950	40
SJL	Rabbit anti-AChR	8,720	2,920
	Rabbit anti-ovalbumin	1,130	230

[a] Thymocytes (10^5 to 10^6 suspended in 50 μl phosphate-buffered saline containing 2% bovine serum albumin and 0.02% sodium azide as diluent) were added to 100-μl aliquots of the tested antibodies in wells of microtiter plates. Quantification of the specifically bound antibodies was determined as described by Fuchs and coworkers (24). For definitions of abbreviations, see Table 1.
[b] Not done.

with the thymus suggest that the immunologically cross-reactive material on thymocytes is not an active nicotinic receptor. Nevertheless, an immunologic cross reactivity by itself could explain the association between the thymus and the neuromuscular junction in MG: the thymus or a modified form of it could be the primary antigen in the spontaneous disease or could be damaged by a cross-reactive autoimmune attack by anti-AChR antibodies. We are trying now to isolate this "AChR-like" antigen to study its structure, its relationship to AChR, and its possible role in the pathogenesis of MG.

ACKNOWLEDGMENTS

This work was supported by grants from the Muscular Dystrophy Association of America, the United States–Israel Binational Science Foundation (BSF), and the Los Angeles Chapter of the Myasthenia Gravis Foundation.

REFERENCES

1. Drachman DB: Myasthenia gravis. N Engl J Med 298:136–142, 1978
2. Fuchs S: Immunology of the nicotinic acetylcholine receptor. Curr Top Microbiol Immunol 85:1–29, 1979
3. Patrick J, Lindstrom J: Autoimmune response to acetylcholine receptor. Science 180:871–872, 1973

4. Bartfeld D, Fuchs S: Immunological characterization of an irreversibly denatured acetylcholine receptor. FEBS Lett 77:214–218, 1977

5. Bartfeld D, Fuchs S: Specific immunosuppression of experimental autoimmune myasthenia gravis by denatured acetylcholine receptor. Proc Natl Acad Sci USA 75:4006–4010, 1978

6. Bartfeld D, Fuchs S: Active acetylcholine receptor fragment obtained by tryptic digestion of acetylcholine receptor from *Torpedo californica*. Biochem Biophys Res Commun 89:512–519, 1979

7. Tarrab-Hazdai R, Schmidt-Sole Y, Mochly-Rosen D, et al: Modification of acetylcholine receptor: chemical and immunological characterization of polyalanyl acetylcholine receptor. FEBS Lett 118:35–38, 1980

8. Bartfeld D, Fuchs S: Fractionation of antibodies to acetylcholine receptor according to antigenic specificity. FEBS Lett 105:303–306, 1979

9. Fuchs S, Bartfeld D, Eshhar Z, et al: Immune regulation of experimental myasthenia. J Neurol Neurosurg Psychol 43:634–643, 1980

10. Köhler G, Milstein C: Continuous cultures of fused cells secreting antibody of predefined specificity. Nature 256:495–497, 1975

11. Mochly-Rosen D, Fuchs S, Eshhar Z: Monoclonal antibodies against defined determinants of acetylcholine receptor. FEBS Lett 106:389–392, 1979

12. Aharonov A, Tarrab-Hazdai R, Silman I: Immunochemical studies on acetylcholine receptor from *Torpedo californica*. Immunochemistry 14:129–137, 1977

13. Lindstrom J: Immunological studies of acetylcholine receptors. J Supramolec Struct 4:389–403, 1976

14. Lennon VA, Lambert EH: Myasthenia gravis induced by monoclonal antibodies to acetylcholine receptors. Nature 285:238–240, 1980

15. Richman DP, Gomez CM, Berman PW, et al: Monoclonal anti-acetylcholine receptor antibodies can cause experimental myasthenia. Nature 286:738–739, 1980

16. Jerne NK: The immune system. Sci Am 229:52–60, 1973

17. Carnegie PR, Mackay IR: Vulnerability of cell surface receptors to autoimmune reactions. Lancet 2:684–686, 1975

18. Schwartz M, Novick D, Givol D, et al: Induction of anti-idiotypic antibodies by immunization with syngeneic spleen cells educated with acetylcholine receptor. Nature 273:543–545, 1978

19. Feingold C, Fuchs S: Regulation of experimental autoimmune myasthenia gravis in rabbits by anti-idiotypes. Israel J Med Sci (in press)

20. Aharonov A, Tarrab-Hazdai R, Abramsky O, et al: Immunological relationship between acetylcholine receptor and thymus: a possible significance in myasthenia gravis. Proc Natl Acad Sci USA 72:1456–1459, 1975

21. Wekerle H, Paterson B, Ketelsen UP, et al: Striated muscle fibers differentiate in monolayer cultures of adult thymus reticulum. Nature 256:493–494, 1975

22. Kao I, Drachman DB: Thymic muscle cells bear acetylcholine receptors: possible relation to myasthenia gravis. Science 195:74–75, 1977

23. Engel WK, Trotter JL, McFarlin DE, et al: Thymic epithelial cell contains acetylcholine receptor. Lancet 1:1310–1311, 1977

24. Fuchs S, Schmidt-Hopfeld I, Tridente G, et al: Thymic lymphocytes bear a surface antigen which cross reacts with acetylcholine receptor. Nature 287:162–164, 1980

25. Fuchs S, Nevo D, Tarrab-Hazdai R, et al: Strain differences in the autoimmune response of mice to acetylcholine receptors. Nature 263:329–330, 1976

DISCUSSION

Dr. David Richman: I would just like to mention a bit of the monoclonal antibody work that one of our students, M. Gomez, and Drs. Berman, Arnason, Fitch and I have been doing. We have raised hybridoma clones making monoclonal anti-receptor antibody against *Torpedo* receptor. We have about 11 clones, a number of which cross react with mammalian receptor and have various pharmacologic activities. One clone is completely blocked by α-bungarotoxin (α-BuTx) but not by any of the other cholinergic ligands, and another set of clones is partially blocked by various cholinergic ligands. In another clone the titers are increased in the presence of some ligands. When antibodies from the last 2 groups are passively transferred to syngeneic rats, they produce experimental autoimmune myasthenia gravis (EAMG) identical to that produced by passive transfer of myasthenic serum. In electron micrographs of the neuromuscular junction from one of these animals 3 days after injection, one can see macrophages invading the muscle fiber, and apparently separating the endplate from the rest of the fiber. The antibodies used were only partially affected by ligands. Interestingly, the antibody that was completely blocked by α-BuTx did not passively transfer the disease. These results demonstrated that a single antibody, binding to a single determinant and having a single set of effector functions, can produce EAMG. Therefore, loss of regulation of a single immunocyte clone can result in an autoimmune disease.

Dr. Sara Fuchs: I am familiar with this work. I also think that the two clones that Dr. Lennon has been able to transfer the disease with are not directed against the cholinergic binding site. We will probably find that not all clones that can transfer the disease are directed against the cholinergic binding site. I believe that the clone directed against this binding site has some unique activity, but this remains to be shown.

Dr. Edson Albuquerque: Dr. Fuchs, have you studied the effect of agents that react with the AChR ionic channel during the activation process produced by the agonist? We have noticed that heterologous serum did not affect channel lifetime at the endplate region of the myasthenic muscle, but the homologous serum accelerated the decay time constant of the endplate current, miniature endplate current, and channel lifetime of the microiontophoretically evoked noise. This means that we will have to clarify a possible allosteric interaction of the homologous serum of the patient on the AChR channel properties.

Dr. Sara Fuchs: We have not done any experiments concerning this line, but plan to. We would like very much to find an antibody clone that might be specific against the channel. Perhaps we should start our fusion with cells from animals that have been immunized with AChR-rich membrane fragments, which have a higher chance of resulting in monoclonal antibodies against the channel.

Dr. Angela Vincent: To turn to anti-idiotypes, I think it is of considerable interest and importance to know whether the idiotype of spontaneously produced anti-AChR antibodies in the human disease are similar to those produced by immunization in the experimental disease. Do rabbit anti-idiotype antibodies bind to human anti-AChR antibodies? You showed a couple of years ago that they bound to experimentally produced anti-AChR from several species.

Dr. Sara Fuchs: I did not have time to go through the cross reactivity between idiotypes, which we had observed previously. I do not think we have shown it with human antibodies.

19
Abnormalities of Immunologic Control Mechanisms and Autoimmunity in Myasthenia Gravis

Robert P. Lisak, MD

Arnold I. Levinson, MD

Burton Zweiman, MD

Myasthenia gravis (MG) is an immunopathologically mediated disease of unknown etiology. Most of the available studies in humans support the concept of a humoral immune response, specifically, Type II of Coombs and Gell (1), or Type II or V of Roitt (2), directed against components of the postsynaptic acetylcholine receptor (AChR) (3–6). Current controversies concerning these antibodies include: (*a*) the nature of the antigenic components of the receptor (7–9); (*b*) the relationship between antibodies to various antigenic sites and production of clinical-pathologic disease (9–11); (*c*) the relative importance of the various classes of immunoglobulins and subclasses of antibodies that comprise the heterogeneous population of AChR antibodies (12–16); (*d*) the relationship between amounts and biologic properties of antibodies to clinical severity, including the relationship to therapy. The possible role of a cell-mediated cell-determined (T-cell) immunopathologic reaction (Type IV) directed against receptor in humans is not clear (17–19). Although immune complexes may (20, 21) or may not (22) be found to circulate in the serum of patients with MG, tissue damage due to complex deposition, as in serum sickness (Type III), is unlikely.

The use of experimental and natural animal models of MG has been instrumental in increasing our understanding of disease pathogenesis. These models include experimental autoimmune MG (23, 24), neonatal autoimmune MG (25), passive transfer of MG to mice or other species with immunoglobulin from myasthenics (26, 27), experimental heteroantisera (28) and mouse monoclonal antibodies to receptor (9, 29), and congenital and acquired canine MG (30).

The fundamental etiology of MG is not known, as is the case for other putative immunopathologically mediated diseases such as systemic lupus erythematosus, rheumatoid arthritis, and polymyositis and dermatomyositis. We would like now to review investigations by our group and by others who are attempting to grapple with this question in MG.

The occurrence of an autoimmune disease in a patient not actively immunized with material containing a putative tissue antigen implies a change in the normal immune response. When autoimmunity develops in some subjects but not others after sensitization with tissue antigens, it is likely that an aberrant (in type or degree) immune response has also occurred. The reasons for the development of these immunopathologically mediated responses are not known, although several hypotheses have been put forth. Such hypotheses have evolved over the years as we have gained increased insight into the normal, highly complex immune system.

It was once held that the appearance of a group (clone) of cells that recognized self would not be tolerated, and that such cells were ordinarily eliminated. In autoimmune states, especially Type II and Type IV hypersensitivity reactions, persistence of these forbidden clones was believed to lead to autoimmunity. Recent immunologic studies have clearly indicated that autoreactive cells exist in normal persons, implying that autoimmunity is a failure to control or regulate, rather than to eliminate these cells (31, 32). Other explanations for immunologic reactions to self antigens have included sensitization to an antigen to which the immune system has not been exposed during development. This failure of recognition by the immune system that this "hidden antigen" is, indeed, self results in an immune response to the antigen. It has become clear that certain potential autoantigens, most notably thyroglobulin (33), are not hidden antigens, thereby negating this theory as the sole or even likely explanation for autoimmunity.

It was postulated that the failure to eliminate forbidden clones or to prevent clinical disease due to emergence of normally present autoreactive cells was due to defective immune surveillance or immunodeficiency (34, 35). There have been many studies addressing the question of immunodeficiency in MG in which humoral (36–41) and cell-mediated (42–49) immunologic parameters were investigated using the in vivo and in vitro techniques then in vogue. In summary, some groups found evidence for immune deficiency in some patients with MG, but overall, a consistent abnormality was not demonstrated.

With increasing recognition of the roles of T and B lymphocytes and monocytes in human immune responses, techniques using markers for such cells were applied to the study of MG. Several published studies either did or did not show a decrease in the percentage of T lymphocytes in the blood and thymus of patients with MG (46, 50–59). The next phase of enumeration of cells with immunoregulatory function brings us to suppressor and helper T cells and markers to identify such cells in humans. We (60) and others (61) reported an increase in myasthenic patients in the percentage of peripheral blood T cells bearing receptor for the Fc portion of IgG, called T_γ or T_G cells.

These cells were shown to have suppressor and cytotoxic properties in vitro (62). The T cells with receptor for the Fc portion of IgM are called T_μ or T_M and have helper or suppressor functions in certain in vitro assays. Our group also demonstrated that there was an increase in both T_γ and T_μ cells in the thymus of some patients with MG. In normal subjects the vast majority ($\geq 95\%$) of thymic T cells do not bear either marker (T null cells).

Recently, allogeneic sera, heteroantisera, and monoclonal antibodies have been produced that are reported to be capable of identifying various populations and subpopulations of blood and thymic T cells (63–65). The T-cell nature of T_γ cells has also been called into question (66) using these newer reagents. Some of these markers allow the selection of cells or elimination of cells with various functions including in vitro suppressor, cytotoxic, and helper activity. These monoclonal antibodies, as well as others being produced in other laboratories, will undoubtedly be used to enumerate T-cell subpopulations in the blood (and thymus) of patients with MG and other autoimmune diseases. They will also be important in studying the functions of lymphocyte subpopulations in autoimmunity. However, an exchange of reagents between various laboratories will be necessary to interpret data from different groups.

In addition to assays enumerating subsets of lymphocytes there have been in vitro studies of lymphocyte function looking for evidence for changes in suppressor function. Mischak and colleagues (67) measured the in vitro suppressive effect of lymphocytes treated with a mitogen, concanavalin A (Con A) on the proliferative response of other lymphocytes (67); depression of normal suppressor activity was found. Other groups found a decrease (68) or an increase in in vitro suppressor activity (54) with two other assays.

It should be pointed out that (a) some of the Con A assays measure a suppressive effect on a nonspecific mitogen proliferative response, the physiologic correlates of which are not known, and (b) the assays measure T-cell suppression of a T-cell property that may have little relevance to MG. In MG, the large number of autoantibodies, including anti-AChR antibodies, suggests that T-B cell interrelationships are likely to be of greater importance.

Shore and coworkers (69) have recently demonstrated an in vitro defect in T-cell suppression of B-cell function in patients with juvenile MG using ovalbumin as the antigen in their assay. We have recently adapted a reverse hemolytic plaque assay that enables us to look at the spontaneous and pokeweed mitogen (PWM)-driven polyclonal Ig-secreting cell response (70). This assay allows us to examine levels of Ig-secreting cells circulating in the blood and to examine polyclonal T–B cell interrelationships, albeit in vitro. We have begun to study the cells of patients with MG. The details of our early data will be published elsewhere (71). To date, we have found that, overall, patients with MG have greater levels of circulating Ig-secreting cells than do control subjects. There is a tendency for the higher levels to be found in patients with more severe disease. Lymphocytes from patients with MG, as a group, did not respond differently from those of normal subjects when cultured with PWM, although several patients had very high levels of Ig-secreting cells in this assay. We would anticipate that these functional assays will be expanded to study the PWM-driven IgG, IgM, and IgA responses, because the majority of autoantibodies found in patients with MG are of the IgG class. Moreover, we ultimately hope to analyze T–B cell interactions in relation to production of anti-AChR antibodies.

The very frequent occurrence of thymic germinal center follicular hyperplasia or tumor in MG and the sometimes dramatic improvement in the neuromuscular manifestations following thymectomy have prompted speculation that thymic abnormalities may play a role in disordered immunoregulation. Possible support for this concept includes: (*a*) increased numbers of surface immunoglobulin-positive (50, 55, 58) cells in the thymus of patients with MG; (*b*) increased in vitro secretion of immunoglobulin by thymic cells from some myasthenic patients in response to PWM stimulation (72); (*c*) in vitro secretion of anti-AChR antibodies by thymic lymphocytes (73); (*d*) evidence previously reported by us (50, 51) and others (18, 58) that thymocytes may be autoreactive with blood lymphocytes in MG; (*e*) reports of cross-reactivity between AChR and an antigenic determinant in the myoepithelial component of the thymus (74). The pathogenic and etiologic significance of these findings remain to be clarified.

A third consideration in the control of immune regulation is the role of serum factors. A host of serum factors are reported to have a role in immunoregulation. Among the most interesting are antilymphocyte antibodies. Shore and colleagues (69) reported an IgG class antibody in the serum of juvenile myasthenic patients that is directed against theophylline-sensitive T-suppressor cells. Interestingly, a deficit of these suppressor cells was found in the same patients. We (75) and others (68, 76, 77) have reported an increase in cold-reactive (IgM) antilymphocyte antibodies in the serum of myasthenic patients. We did not find a correlation between the presence of such antibodies and a decrease in blood T-cell levels. However, we did not enumerate subpopulations of T cells, as measured by any of the current markers, or study the unfractionated blood cells for in vitro suppressor and helper activity. In systemic lupus erythematosus the presence of these antibodies is believed to be corrected with clinical disease (78) and to play a role in perturbing the normal regulatory state of the immune system in these patients (79). A complicating but intriguing feature of antilymphocyte antibodies in MG is related to the probable presence of the AChR on some lymphocytes in laboratory animals and humans (80, 81). Serum antibodies against such receptors on lymphocyte surfaces could profoundly affect T-cell regulatory activity in myasthenic patients, particularly if the receptors were preferentially concentrated on suppressor T cells (81, 82). Whether such changes are a cause or a result of disease activity is not known. Ideally, one should: (*a*) find increased serum antibodies just before and during the early stages of increased disease activity; (*b*) show that these antibodies preferentially react with a subpopulation of T cells believed to have suppressor activity using cells obtained from normal subjects and cells obtained from myasthenic patients themselves during periods of relative quiescence; (*c*) show a change in the proportion of suppressor and helper cells and an accompanying loss of functional suppressor activity from unfractionated blood cells; (*d*) show that the interaction of these antibodies and lymphocytes results in a loss of normal T–B cell interrelationships in cells from normal persons and perhaps results in antigen-specific abnormalities when cells from stable myasthenic patients are used; (*e*) find a relative return toward the normal state of all parameters during periods of relative quiescence. Serial studies of individual patients will probably be required to determine whether this sequence of events actually occurs.

There are other potential immunoregulatory mechanisms in addition to nonspecific suppressor lymphocytes, including monocyte-macrophages, antigen bridging, and idiotype networks (82–84). In this latter system, the antigen-binding region of each immunoglobulin (antibody) itself acts as an antigen to which another antibody is directed. This immunoglobulin likewise elicits another immunoglobulin specific for its antigen binding site.

The postulated changes in nonspecific or broad-based suppressor-helper T-cell balance results in different immunopathologic diseases and autoantibodies or at least a relatively limited range of antibodies in most patients. This suggests that the changes in the suppressor-helper balance discussed earlier are permissive and may be required for disease induction and changes in disease activity. The changes do not explain the actual specificity of which autoantibodies and which diseases appear. Changes in the normal idiotype network could be the second part of disease or antibody induction (85, 86). If only a restricted anti-idiotype fails to appear, only certain clones might be likely to show increased reactivity during periods of decreased control. Whether heredity plays a role in this second signal for disease specificity is not known, however.

In this talk we have attempted to outline what has been done, some present courses of research, and future approaches to elucidate the factors responsible for the development and disease activity in MG. With newer markers for cell subpopulations, functional studies of cell populations and subpopulations, and exploration of serum factors in conjunction with clinical correlations, one can anticipate continued progress in the search for the cause of MG.

REFERENCES

1. Coombs RRA, Gell PGH: Classification of allergic reactions responsible for clinical hypersensitivity. In *Clinical Aspects of Immunity*. Edited by Gell PGH, Coombs RRA. FA Davis, Philadelphia, 1975, pp 575–596

2. Roitt I (ed): *Essential Immunology*. Blackwell Scientific Publications, London, 1977, pp 151–187

3. Almon RR, Andrew CG, Appel SH: Serum globulin in myasthenia gravis: inhibition of α bungarotoxin binding of acetylcholine receptors. Science 186:55–57, 1974

4. Bender AN, Ringel SP, Engel WK, et al: Myasthenia gravis: a serum factor blocking acetylcholine receptors of the human neuromuscular junction. Lancet 1:607–609, 1975

5. Aharonov A, Abramsky O, Tarrab-Hazdai R, Fuchs S: Humoral antibodies to acetylcholine receptor in patients with myasthenia gravis. Lancet 2:340–342, 1975

6. Lennon VA: Immunology of the acetylcholine receptor. Immunol Commun 5:323–344, 1975

7. Lindstrom JM, Campbell M, Nave B: Specificities of antibodies to acetylcholine receptors. Muscle Nerve, 1:140–145, 1978

8. Lindstrom J, Einarison B, Merle J: Immunization of rats with polypeptide chains from *Torpedo* acetylcholine receptor causes an autoimmune response to receptors in rat muscle. Proc Natl Acad Sci USA 75:769–773, 1978

9. Tzartos SJ, Lindstrom JM: Monoclonal antibodies used to probe acetylcholine receptor structure: localization of the main immunogenic region and detection of similarities between subunits. Proc Natl Acad Sci USA 77:755–759, 1980

10. Lindstrom JM, Seybold ME, Lennon VA, et al: Antibody to acetylcholine receptor in myasthenia gravis: prevalence, clinical correlates, and diagnostic value. Neurology (Minneap) 26:1054–1059, 1976

11. Dwyer DS, Bradley RJ, Oh SJ, Kemp GE: A modified assay for antibody against the nicotinic acetylcholine receptor in myasthenia gravis. Clin Exp Immunol 37:448–451, 1979

12. Zurn AD, Fulpus BW: Accessibility to antibodies of acetylcholine receptors in the neuromuscular junction. Clin Exp Immunol 24:9–17, 1976

13. Lefvert AK, Bergstrom K: Immunoglobulin in myasthenia gravis: effect of human lymph IgG3 and F(ab')₂ fragments on a cholinergic receptor preparation from *Torpedo marmorata*, Eur J Clin Invest 7:115–119, 1977

14. Brenner T, Abramsky O, Lisak RP, et al: Antibody to acetylcholine receptor in myasthenia gravis: radioimmunoassay. Israel J Med Sci 14:986–989, 1978

15. Lefvert AK, Bergstrom K, Matell G, et al: Determination of acetylcholine receptor antibody in myasthenia gravis: clinical usefulness and pathogenic implications. J Neurol Neurosurg Psychiatry 41:394–403, 1978

16. Newsom-Davis J: Antiacetylcholine receptor antibody in myasthenia gravis. In *Clinical Neuroimmunology*. Edited by Rose FC, Blackwell Scientific Publications, London, 1979, pp 128–136

17. Abramsky O, Aharonov A, Webb C, Fuchs S: Cellular immune response to acetylcholine receptor-rich fraction in patients with myasthenia gravis. Clin Exp Immunol 19:11–16, 1975

18. Richmond DP, Patrick J, Arnason BGW: Cellular immunity in myasthenia gravis. N Engl J Med 294:694–698, 1976

19. Conti-Tronconi BM, Dipadova F, Morgutti M, et al: Stimulation of lymphocytes by cholinergic receptor in myasthenia gravis. J Neuropathol Exp Neurol 36:157–162, 1977

20. Casali P, Bargini P, Zanussi C: Immune complexes in myasthenia gravis. Lancet 1:378, 1976

21. Behan WMH, Behan PO: Immune complexes in myasthenia gravis. J Neurol Neurosurg Psychiatry 42:595–599, 1979

22. Tachovsky T, Koprowski H, Lisak RP, et al: Circulating immune complexes in multiple sclerosis and other neurological diseases. Lancet 2:997–999, 1976

23. Patrick J, Lindstrom J: Autoimmune response to acetylcholine receptor. Science 180:871–872, 1973

24. Tarrab-Hazdai R, Aharonov A, Silman I, et al: Experimental autoimmune myasthenia induced in monkeys by purified acetylcholine receptor. Nature 256:128–130, 1975

25. Sanders DB, Cobbs EE, Winfield JB: Neonatal experimental autoimmune myasthenia gravis. Muscle Nerve 1:145–160, 1978

26. Toyka KV, Drachman DB, Pestronk A, Kao I: Myasthenia gravis: passive transfer from man to mouse. Science 190:397–399, 1975

27. Heilbronn E, Hammarstrom L, Lefvert AK, et al: Effect of acetylcholine receptor antibodies in mice and rabbits. In *Plasmapheresis and the Immunobiology of Myasthenia Gravis*. Edited by Dau PC. Houghton Mifflin Professional Publishers, Boston, 1979, pp 92–96

28. Lindstrom JM, Engel Am, Seybold ME, et al: Pathological mechanisms in experimental autoimmune myasthenia gravis. II. Passive transfer of experimental autoimmune myasthenia gravis in rats with antiacetylcholine receptor antibodies. J Exp Med 144:739–753, 1976

29. Gomez CM, Richmond DP, Wollman RL, et al: Passive transfer of experimental autoimmune myasthenia gravis using monoclonal antiacetylcholine receptor antibodies (abstract). Neurology (Minneap) 30:388, 1970

30. Lennon VA, Palmer AC, Pflugfelder C, Indrieri RJ: Myasthenia gravis in dogs: acetylcholine receptor deficiency with and without autoantibodies, In *Genetic Control of Autoimmune Disease*. Edited by Rose NL, Bigazzi PE, Warner NL, Elsevier/North Holland Biomedical Press, Amsterdam, 1978, pp 295–306

31. Allison AC: Autoimmune diseases: concepts of pathogenesis and control. In *Autoimmunity*. Edited by Talal N. Academic Press, New York, 1977, pp 92–140

32. Gershon RK: Suppressor T-cell dysfunction as a possible cause of autoimmunity. In *Autoimmunity*. Edited by Talal N. Academic Press, New York, 1977, pp 171–183

33. Torrigiani G, Doniach D, Roitt IM: Serum thyroglobulin levels in healthy subjects and in patients with thyroid disease. J Clin Endocrinol Metab 29:305–314, 1969

34. Fudenberg HH: Are autoimmune diseases immunologic deficiency states? In *Immunology*. Edited by Good RA, Fisher DW. Sinauer Associates, Stamford, 1971, pp 175–183

35. Weigle WO: Recent observations and concepts in immunological unresponsiveness and autoimmunity. Clin Exp Immunol 9:437–447, 1971

36. Adner MM, Sherman JD, Ise C, et al: An immunologic survey of forty-eight patients with myasthenia gravis. N Engl J Med 271:1327–1333, 1964

37. Kornfeld P, Siegal S, Weiner LB, Osserman KE: Studies in myasthenia gravis: immunologic response in thymectomized and non-thymectomized patients. Ann Intern Med 63:416–428, 1965

38. Bundey S, Doniach D, Soothill JF: Immunological studies in patients with juvenile-onset myasthenia gravis and their relatives. Clin Exp Immunol 11:321–332, 1972

39. Behan PO, Simpson JA, Behan WMH: Decreased serum-IgA in myasthenia gravis. Lancet 1:593–594, 1976

40. Lisak RP, Zweiman B: Serum immunoglobulin levels in myasthenia gravis, polymyositis and dermatomyositis. J Neurol Neurosurg Psychiatry 39:34–37, 1976

41. Dawkins RL, O'Reilly C, Grimsley G, Zilko PJ: Myasthenia gravis: the role of immunologic deficiency. Ann NY Acad Sci 274:461–467, 1976

42. Hausley J, Oppenheim JJ: Lymphocyte transformation in thymectomized and non-thymectomized patients with myasthenia gravis. Br Med J 2:679–681, 1967

43. Behan WMH, Behan PO, Simpson JA: Absence of cellular hypersensitivity to muscle and thymic antigens in myasthenia gravis. J Neurol Neurosurg Psychiatry 38:1039–1047, 1975

44. Lisak RP, Zweiman B: Mitogen and muscle extract induced in vitro proliferative responses in myasthenia gravis, dermatomyositis, and polymyositis. J Neurol Neurosurg Psychiatry 38:521–524, 1975

45. Simpson JA, Behan PO, Dick HM: Studies on the nature of autoimmunity in myasthenia gravis. Evidence for an immunodeficiency type. Ann NY Acad Sci 274:382–389, 1976

46. Huang S-W, Rose JW, Mayer RF: Assessment of cellular and humoral immunity of myasthenics. N Neurol Neurosurg Psychiatry 40:1053–1089, 1977

47. Gross WL, Kruger J, Groschel-Stewart U, et al: Studies on HLA antigens and cellular and humoral autoimmune phenomena in patients with myasthenia gravis. Clin Exp Immunol 27:48–54, 1977

48. Fukawa M, Torisu M, Miyakara T, et al: Immunologic studies on myasthenia gravis: operative indication and cell-mediated immunity. Surgery 83:293–302, 1978

49. Kawanami S, Kanaide A, Itoyama Y, Kuroiva Y: Lymphocyte function in myasthenia gravis. J Neurol Neurosurg Psychiatry 42:734–740, 1979

50. Abdou NI, Lisak, RP, Zweiman B, et al: The thymus in myasthenia gravis: evidence for altered cell populations. N Engl J Med 291:1271–1275, 1974

51. Lisak RP, Abdou NI, Zweiman B, et al: Aspects of lymphocyte function in myasthenia gravis. Ann NY Acad Sci 274:402–410, 1976

52. Koziner B, Block KJ, Perlo VP: Distribution of peripheral blood latex injesting cells, T-cells and B-cells in patients with myasthenia gravis. Ann NY Acad Sci 274:411–420, 1976

53. Namba T, Nakata Y, Grob D: The role of humoral and cellular immune factors in neuromuscular block in myasthenia gravis. Ann NY Acad Sci 274:493–515, 1976

54. Birnbaum G, Tsairis P: Suppressor lymphocytes in myasthenia gravis and effect of adult thymectomy. Ann NY Acad Sci 274:527–535, 1976

55. Shirai T, Miyata M, Nakase A, Itoh T: Lymphocyte subpopulations in neoplastic and non-neoplastic thymus and in blood of patients with myasthenia gravis. Clin Exp Immunol 26:118–123, 1976

56. Birnbaum G, Tsairis P: Thymic lymphocytes in myasthenia gravis. Ann Neurol 1:331–333, 1977

57. Lisak RP, Zweiman B, Phillips SM: Thymic and peripheral blood T and B-cell levels in myasthenia gravis. Neurology (NY) 28:1298–1301, 1978

58. Opelz G, Keesey J, Glovsky M, Gale RP: Autoreactivity between lymphocytes and thymus cells in myasthenia gravis. Arch Neurol 35:413–415, 1978

59. Aarli JA, Hermann P, Matre R, et al: Lymphocyte populations in thymus and blood from patients with myasthenia gravis. J Neurol Neurosurg Psychiatry 42:29–34, 1979

60. Lisak RP, Smiley R, Schotland DL, et al: Abnormalities of T-cell subpopulations in blood and thymus of patients with myasthenia gravis. J Neurol Sci 44:69–76, 1979

61. Piantelli M, Lauriola L, Carbone A, et al: Subpopulations of T lymphocytes in myasthenia gravis patients. Clin Exp Immunol 36:85–89, 1979

62. Moretta L, Ferrarini L, Cooper MD: Characteristics of human T-cell subpopulations as defined by specific receptors for immunoglobulins. Contemp Top Immunobiol 8:19–53, 1978

63. Kung PC, Goldstein G, Reinherz EL, Schlossman SF: Monoclonal antibodies defining distinctive human T-cell surface antigens. Science 206:347–349, 1979

64. Reinherz EL, Kung PC, Goldstein G, Schlossman SF: Separation of functional subsets of human T-cells by a monoclonal antibody. Proc Natl Acad Sci USA 76:4061–4065, 1979

65. Reinherz EL, Kung PC, Goldstein G, et al: Discrete stages of human intrathymic differentiation: analysis of normal thymocytes and leukemic lymphoblasts of T-cell lineage. Proc Natl Acad Sci USA 77:1588–1592, 1980

66. Reinherz EL, Moretta L, Kung PC, et al: Human T lymphocyte subpopulations defined by Fc receptors and monoclonal antibodies: a comparison. J Exp Med 151:969–974, 1980

67. Mischak RP, Dau PC, Gonzalez RL, Spitler LE: In vitro testing of suppressor cell activity in myasthenia gravis. In *Plasmapheresis and Immunobiology of Myasthenia Gravis*. Edited by Dau PC. Houghton Mifflin Professional Publishers, Boston, 1979, pp 72–78

68. Zilko PJ, Dawkins RL, Holmes K, Witt C: Genetic control of suppressor lymphocyte function in myasthenia gravis: relationship of impaired suppressor function to HLA B8/DRW3 and cold reactive lymphocytotoxic antibodies. Clin Immunol Immunopathol 14:222–230, 1979

69. Shore A, Limatibul S, Dosch H-M, Gelfand EW: Identification of two serum components regulating the expression of T-lymphocyte function in childhood myasthenia gravis. N Engl J Med 301:625–629, 1979

70. Levinson AI, Dziarski A, Pincus T, et al: Heterogeneity of polyclonal B cell activity in systemic lupus erythematosus. J C Lab Clin Immunol (in press)

71. Levinson AI, Dziarski A, Lisak RP, et al: Analysis of polyclonal B-cell activity in myasthenia gravis. Neurology (NY), (in press)

72. Smiley JD, Bradley J, Daly D, Ziff M: Immunoglobulin synthesis in vitro by human thymus: comparison of myasthenia gravis and normal thymus. Clin Exp Immunol 4:387–399, 1969

73. Vincent A, Scadding GK, Thomas HC, Newsom-Davis J: In vitro synthesis of antiacetylcholine receptor antibody by thymic lymphocytes in myasthenia gravis. Lancet 1:305–307, 1978

74. Aharanov A, Tarrab-Hazdai R, Abramsky O, Fuchs S: Immunologic relationships between acetylcholine receptor and thymus: a possible significance in myasthenia gravis. Proc Natl Acad Sci USA 72:1456–1459, 1975

75. Lisak RP, Guerro F, Zweiman B: Cold reactive antilymphocyte antibodies in neurologic diseases. J Neurol Neurosurg Psychiatry 42:1054–1057, 1979

76. Kreisler MJ, Naito S, Terrasaki PI: Cytotoxins in disease. V. Various diseases. Transplant Proc 3:112–114, 1971

77. Knapp W, Pateisky K: Lymphotoxins in myasthenia gravis. Z Immunitaetsforsch Immunobiol 144:329–339, 1972

78. Butler WT, Sharp JT, Rossen RD, et al: Relationship of the clinical course of systemic lupus erythematosus to the presence of circulating lymphocytotoxins antibodies. Arthritis Rheum 15:231–237, 1972

79. Messner RP: Naturally occurring antilymphocyte antibodies. In *Lymphocytes and Their Interactions*. Edited by Williams RC Jr. Raven Press, New York, 1975, pp 169–181

80. Strom TB, Carpenter CB, Garovoy MR, et al: The modulating influence of cyclic nucleotides upon lymphocyte-mediated cytotoxicity. J Exp Med 138:381–393, 1973

81. Tridente G, Andrighetto G, Beltrame S, et al: The thymus in myasthenia gravis: identification of lymphocyte subsets in thymus and thymoma by cell separation analysis, T and B-cell markers, and response to adrenergic and cholinergic agents. In *Developments in Clinical Immunology*. Edited by Ricci M, Fauci AS, Arcangel P, Torzuoli P. Academic Press, New York, 1978, pp 81–103

82. Richmond DP, Arnason BGW: Nicotinic acetylcholine receptor: evidence for a functionally distinct receptor on human lymphocytes. Proc Natl Acad Sci USA 76:4632–4635, 1979

83. Jerne NK: Towards a network theory of the immune system. Ann Immunol (Paris) 125C:375–389, 1974

84. Binz H, Wigzell H: Specific transplantation tolerance induced by autoimmunization against the individuals own, naturally occurring idiotypic, antigen-binding receptors. J Exp Med 144:1438–1457, 1976

85. Talal N: Autoimmunity and the immunologic network. Arthritis Rheum 21:853–861, 1978

86. Bona C, Paul WE: Cellular basis of regulation of expression of idiotype. I. T-suppressor cells specific for MOPC460 idiotype regulate the expression of cells secreting anti-TNP antibodies bearing 460 idiotype. J Exp Med 149:592–600, 1979

DISCUSSION

Dr. John Newsom-Davis   I have a comment in relation to the increased B-cell content you found in hyperplastic thymuses. We have studied 35 patients undergoing thymectomy, and in most patients whose thymus showed hyperplasia, lymphocytes isolated from the thymus made anti-AChR antibody in culture. In general, the rates of antibody production correlated with the duration of the disease. However, even in those whose thymus cells showed the highest rates of antibody production, it appeared that the thymus as a whole made only a very small proportion of the total amount of antibody required per day, probably less than 1%. On the other hand, it does seem that the thymus, if not a major site of anti-AChR antibody production, can assist other cells in making antibody. When thymus cells subjected to irradiation, which abolishes antibody production and perhaps suppressor activity, are cocultured with peripheral blood lymphocytes, they can cause these cells to produce antibody; when cultured alone, these lymphocytes produce at best very small amounts. Thus, the thymus may contain either helper cells or antigen or possibly both and these may assist anti-AChR antibody production by peripheral blood lymphocytes.

Dr. Robert Lisak: The work that Dr. Newsom-Davis has just described is very interesting. It would also be interesting to see in various patients with MG whether the same thymic cells would have the ability to help or would fail to suppress lymphocyte production of some of other autoantibodies, such as anti-thyroglobulin and antinuclear antibodies, or whether the thymic helper cell is specific only for the pathogenic anti-AChR.

Dr. Carl Pearson: Have you studied any patients with rheumatoid arthritis who developed MG who were on D-penicillamine? Even if you have not, could you speculate about the various mechanisms that you have discussed as to where you think D-penicillamine might be operating, especially because the MG disappears when D-penicillamine is discontinued.

Dr. Robert Lisak: That is an interesting question. Actually, there is a very nice discussion of that situation in a review article by Dr. Talal, which is cited in our presentation. He postulates that the antibodies and disease may occur in a subject who has the appropriate immunologic immunogenetic tendency. The incidence of penicillamine-induced MG, although it occurs in Wilson's disease, seems to be greater in rheumatoid arthritis. Rheumatoid arthritis itself occurs more frequently with MG than one would expect by chance. Somehow, because of genetic or other factors, the drug bypasses temporarily the immune regulatory circuit. When you stop the drug, however, the circuit goes back to normal. In the patient with idiopathic MG, the regulatory circuit is more or less permanently bypassed by a mechanism that we do not understand. I think it is a perfectly reasonable explanation in view of the current thought of suppressor-helper cell interactions and idiotypic control.

Dr. Michael Garlepp: Are any of your suppressor cell function assays or your enumeration of T_γ cells or any other types of suppressor cells related at all to anti-AChR titers?

Dr. Robert Lisak: We have not looked at T_γ or T_μ cells and antibodies simultaneously in enough patients to answer that question. We have looked at antibodies to receptor simultaneously with Dr. Levinson's assay, and increased plaque-forming cells did not correlate with total anti-AChR antibodies as measured by Drs. Brenner and Abramsky. We have not looked at the correlation as yet with other markers for T-cell subsets. We are trying to get the system going with some of the newer markers of Dr. Kung to see whether there is a correlation. It would be nice if there were, in view of some of Dr. Richman's work on the possibility of an AChR on T-suppressor cells.

Dr. Douglas Fambrough: I thought this was a most appropriate place for me to put in my two cents on the question of sharing monoclonal antibodies among laboratories. The great thing about monoclonal antibodies, besides their power to define special parts of molecules, is that you can make more than you can possibly use of any single one, plus you can generate many more different ones than you could ever use, once you get the hang of it. Yet, I have encountered several cases in which people who have even published on their monoclonal antibodies have been unwilling to share the antibody or the cell line. I think that is crazy. The other great thing about monoclonal antibody technology is that it provides the possibility of one laboratory reproducing another laboratory's data. I have some ideas about rules for sharing that I would like to give you in a few seconds. First, I think it is reasonable that a laboratory which makes a cell line be given an opportunity to publish a refereed paper on it before distributing it. Second, I think that since graduate students' and postdoctoral fellows' careers are often tied up with certain projects involving monoclonal antibodies, it is reasonable for a laboratory to define those problems and request respect for that person's efforts when they give out monoclonal antibodies. Other laboratories should not outcompete the generous laboratory on those projects. Otherwise, it seems to me that there should be a free sharing of at least as much antibody as people need to do experiments. The question about cell lines is complicated by the free enterprise system, and I do not have that all worked out. Personally, I would not want to patent the monoclonal antibody technology, none of which the inventors patented! Probably, in the long run, what we should all do is give our cell lines to a center that would raise them and give them out. In the meantime, I think we should all be happy to give out either purified antibody or cell lines, whichever is more convenient to the recipient. Just one other comment: it seems to me that, having produced a cell line, you are not entitled to be an author on every future paper involving that line.

Dr. Robert Lisak: This has been a problem related to the T-cell markers, as those of you who do cell immunology may know. Obtaining these markers for human and even some of the murine markers has been a big problem for people trying to confirm some of the reported changes.

20
Summary: Myasthenia Gravis

Stanley H. Appel, MD

Stanton B. Elias, MD

Our role in this morning's session on myasthenia gravis (MG) is to summarize in brief fashion the past accomplishments and future directions in the field. Since the last international scientific conference sponsored by The Muscular Dystrophy Association 4 years ago, our knowledge and understanding of MG have progressed dramatically.

Myasthenia gravis is now well accepted as an autoimmune disease, whereas only several years ago data supporting this concept were entirely circumstantial and primarily related to the involvement of the thymus. More than 70% of patients with MG have thymic hyperplasia, and 15% of patients have thymomas (1). In addition, a small percentage of cases of MG are associated with other autoimmune disease, and more than 10% of patients with MG may also exhibit thyroid dysfunction (2).

The present evidence supporting MG as an autoimmune disease is based on availability of animal models such as experimental autoimmune myasthenia gravis (EAMG), which can be induced by the injection of purified acetylcholine receptor (AChR) (3). Although the acute phase of this disease has many differences from MG, the chronic phase closely resembles the human disorder physiologically, pharmacologically, immunologically (4), and morphologically (5). The presence of circulating antibodies to AChR in as many as 85% of patients with MG (6, 7) and the ability to transfer the disease to mice passively with immunoglobulin from affected patients (8) have provided further evidence for an autoimmune pathogenesis. In addition, immune complexes containing immunoglobulin and several components of complement have been localized to the neuromuscular junctions of human myasthenic intercostal endplates (9).

The site of this immune attack is postsynaptic, as evidenced by the simplification and atrophy of the muscle postsynaptic membrane (10) and the decreased number of postjunctional AChRs (11). The remaining receptors appear to have a slightly altered configuration as assessed by toxin binding in detergent extracts of intercostal muscles from patients with MG (12). The diminution in bungarotoxin binding to AChRs correlates with the decreased amplitude of miniature endplate potentials, and thereby helps explain the altered safety margin of the myasthenic neuromuscular junction. Furthermore, the sensitivity of the post-synaptic muscle surface to iontophoretically applied ACh is reduced (13).

The mechanisms by which anti-AChR antibodies reduce the number of AChRs have been explored both in vivo and in vitro. In myotube cultures in vitro, myasthenic antibodies accelerate endocytosis of the AChR in a manner similar to antigenic modulation in lymphocytes (14–16). This reaction is independent of complement. Similar enhanced degradation can be demonstrated with myasthenic anti-AChR antibodies in model systems in innervated muscles in vivo (17).

An additional important mechanism is complement-dependent membrane lysis and extrusion of fragments containing AChR into the intersynaptic cleft (9). By electron microscopy, the debris in the cleft appears to possess immune complexes, and this reaction may help to explain not only the loss of AChRs but also the loss of postjunctional membrane, with resulting atrophy. In tissue culture myotubes, the antibodies not only accelerate degradation but also impair insertion and synthesis of AChRs (18). Although a high percentage of sera from myasthenic patients contain antibodies that block bungarotoxin binding (19), these blocking antibodies have not been demonstrated to play a significant role in the disturbance of neuromuscular function (16, 20). However, it is possible that such receptor-antibody interactions might also affect the ACh-induced ion channel or the affinity of ACh for its receptor. Although both of these mechanisms are theoretically possible, neither has received experimental support (21).

It is now clear that anti-AChR antibodies are the key determinants of the altered physiology in MG. However, there are numerous examples of cases in which high titers of anti-AChR antibodies are associated with minimal clinical dysfunction; conversely, low titers of anti-AChR antibodies may be associated with severe clinical disease. The major point to be emphasized is that many factors may influence the ability of the anti-AChR antibody to decrease the number of AChRs. Hormonal factors are among the most likely candidates, primarily through their influence on general muscle metabolism, but also through effects specifically related to AChR metabolism.

In our own laboratories, Dr. Blosser has been able to demonstrate an increase in the number of AChRs on chick myotubes in the presence of agents that increase the intracellular concentration of cyclic adenosine monophosphate (cAMP). The most effective agent for enhancing cAMP activity is cholera toxin. This agent causes a 70% increase in the number of AChRs. The increase is not due to an inhibition of degradation, but appears to be related to a direct stimulation of AChR synthesis. The increase in the number of AChRs can be blocked by inhibitors of ribonucleic acid synthesis as well as inhibitors of protein synthesis. The cAMP itself, as well as phosphodiesterase inhibitors and β-adrenergic agonists such as isoproterenol also enhance AChR synthesis (22). This latter observation is of special interest because circulating catecholamines could well influence muscle cAMP levels through β-adrenergic receptor stimulation and thereby lead to stimulation of AChR synthesis. Such enhancement might partially offset the effects of circulating anti-AChR antibodies. Other hormones that influence muscle cAMP metabolism as well as general muscle metabolism could similarly modulate the effects of anti-AChR antibody.

Circumstantial evidence for hormonal or other modulating factors is provided by the clinical syndrome of neonatal MG. The incidence of circulating antibodies among myasthenic mothers should not differ from that among other MG populations (85%). Yet the incidence of neonatal MG is surprisingly low (15%) (23). Many infant offspring of myasthenic mothers have now been studied, and it is clear that anti-AChR antibodies may be present in the infant without any evidence of clinical disease. Conversely, a mother whose MG is in clinical remission but who has high anti-AChR antibody titers may give birth to an infant with classic neonatal MG (24). Thus, host factors clearly play a role in determining the degree of dysfunction when circulating anti-AChR antibodies are present (25).

Part of the explanation for the imprecise correlation of the clinical state with the titers of anti-AChR antibody may be related to the heterogeneity of antibodies present, and the range of antigenic determinants on the AChR. As demonstrated with monoclonal antibody studies described by Dr. Lindstrom (see chapter 17) as well as those from several other laboratories, including those of Dr. Richmond and Dr. Arnason, antibodies against some antigenic determinants can passively transfer EAMG, whereas antibodies against other determinants may well be positive in a radioimmunoassay and not produce disease. Thus, until our radioimmunoassays use the specific AChR antigens, the antibodies to which would correlate well with the clinical state and transfer disease, we should expect present correlations between antibody titer and clinical disease to be somewhat imprecise.

Another possible modulating factor in patients with MG may be related to the degree of cholinergic stimulation and the level of anticholinesterase medication being taken. It is well known that chronic use of anticholinesterase drugs produces a decrease in the number of AChRs in animals (26), and carbamylcholine produces a decrease in the number of AChRs in myotube culture (27). We have studied the effects of both carbamylcholine and myasthenic IgG on AChRs. The effects of both agents are additive. The carbamylcholine effect can be blocked by D-tubocurarine, but the myasthenic antibody effects cannot be blocked by this compound. Carbamylcholine appears to exert its effects by binding at the ACh binding site, whereas AChR antibodies from patients with MG appear to bind at different sites on the receptor. Obviously, each site is associated with a specific diminution in the number of AChRs and the effects are additive. In all of these experiments, long-term effects of carbamylcholine rather than short-term effects of desensitization were being monitored (28).

Thus, the very drugs used to treat MG when administered in high doses for long periods may further disturb neuromuscular junctions already altered by the presence of anti-AChR antibodies. These studies also explain the beneficial clinical effects of "drug holidays" in which patients appear to recover their responsiveness to anticholinesterase medication after being withdrawn for a period of time.

The deleterious chronic effects of carbamylcholine in vitro raise the additional question of whether differences in cholinergic stimulation of various muscles (such as eye muscles) may help explain the differential vulnerability of muscle groups in patients with MG. With this hypothesis, we would assume that the size of the motor unit and extent of cholinergic activity might modulate the loss of AChR produced by antibodies.

An alternative explanation of the extreme sensitivity of eye muscles in MG relates to the possibility of polymorphism in AChRs. The AChRs in eye muscles may be more antigenic or possess more clinically susceptible antigenic groupings, and therefore give rise to enhanced vulnerability of the eye muscles of patients with MG. Alternatively, differences in structure of neuromuscular junctions or extraocular muscle metabolism may help to explain their enhanced vulnerability.

Despite this significant progress, many questions remain to be answered. It is not at all clear what initiates the disease process in the production of anti-AChR antibodies. As pointed out by Dr. Lisak, an alteration in T cells, especially suppressor populations, may contribute. However, it is also possible that alterations in anti-idiotype antibodies may be critical. Thus, anti-idiotype antibodies may not only serve as a meaningful approach to therapy, as described by Dr. Fuchs, but they may also shed light on the etiology of MG. Whether the initiating factor is a virus or some other agent, we still must explain the prominent genetic factors expressed in HL-A studies (29) and the exact way that the thymus is involved. Because AChRs have been described on lymphocytes, it is entirely possible that the diminution in receptors at neuromuscular junctions is not the fundamental point of attack and that the disease MG is really an epiphenomenon. The major problem may well be a disturbance of immune regulation in which lymphocytes are the intended target of circulating anti-AChR antibodies, and the neuromuscular junction is just an innocent bystander.

The next several years should provide as many insights into basic immunologic processes as the last 4 years have provided insight into AChR metabolism. Hopefully, this progress will shed further light not only on the etiology of MG, but also on its therapy and ultimate prevention.

REFERENCES

1. Castleman B: The pathology of the thymus gland in myasthenia gravis. Ann NY Acad Sci 135:496–503, 1966

2. Osserman KE, Genkins G: Studies in myasthenia gravis: review of twenty years experience in over 2,000 cases. Mt Sinai J Med 38:497–537, 1971

3. Patrick J, Lindstrom JM: Autoimmune response to acetylcholine receptor. Science 180:871–872, 1973

4. Lindstrom J, Lennon VA, Seybold ME, et al: EAMG and MG: biochemical and immunochemical aspects. Ann NY Acad Sci 274:254–274, 1976

5. Engel AG, Tsujihota M, Lindstrom J, et al: The motor endplate in MG and EAMG: a quantitative ultrastructural study. Ann NY Acad Sci 274:60–79, 1976

6. Appel SH, Almon RR, Levy N: Acetylcholine receptor antibodies in MG. N Engl J Med 291:1271–1275, 1975

7. Lindstrom JM, Seybold ME, Lennon VA, et al: Antibody to acetylcholine receptor in myasthenia

gravis: prevalence, clinical correlates, and diagnostic value. Neurology (Minneap) 26:1054–1059, 1976

8. Tokya KV, Drachman PB, Pestronk A, et al: Myasthenia gravis: passive transfer from man to mouse. Science 190:397–399, 1975

9. Engel AG, Lambert EA, Howard FM: Immune complexes (IgG and C_3) at the motor endplate in myasthenia gravis. Mayo Clin Proc 52:267–280, 1977

10. Engel AG, Santa T: Histometric analysis of the ultrastructure of the neuromuscular junction in myasthenia gravis and in the myasthenic syndrome. Ann NY Acad Sci 183:35–58, 1971

11. Fambrough DM, Drachman DB, Satyamurti S. Neuromuscular junction in myasthenia gravis: decreased acetylcholine receptors. Science 182:293–295, 1973

12. Elias SB, Appel SH: Acetylcholine receptors in myasthenia gravis: increased affinity for α-bungarotoxin. Ann Neurol 4:250–252, 1978

13. Albuquerque EX, Rash JE, Mayer RF, et al. An electrophysiological and morphological study on the neuromuscular junction in patients with myasthenia gravis. Exp Neurol 51:536–563, 1976

14. Kao I, Drachman DB. Myasthenic immunoglobulin accelerates acetylcholine receptor degradation. Science 1976:527–529, 1977

15. Appel SH, Anwyl R, McAdams MW, et al: Accelerated degradation of cultured rat myotube acetylcholine receptors with myasthenia gravis sera and globulins. Proc Natl Acad Sci USA 74:2130–2134, 1977

16. Anwyl R, Appel SH, Narahashi T: Myasthenia gravis serum reduces acetylcholine sensitivity in cultured rat myotubes. Nature 267:262–263, 1977

17. Stanley EF, Drachman DB: Effect of myasthenia gravis immunoglobulin on acetylcholine receptors of intact mammalian neuromuscular junctions. Science 200:1285–1287, 1978

18. Appel SH, Elias SB, Chauvin P: The role of acetylcholine receptor antibodies in myasthenia gravis. Fed Proc 38:2381–2385, 1979

19. Almon RR, Andrew GG, Appel SH: Serum globulin in myasthenia gravis: inhibition of α-bungarotoxin binding to acetylcholine receptors. Science 186:55–57, 1974

20. Albuquerque EX, Mayer RF, Appel SH, et al: Effects of normal and myasthenia gravis serum factors on innervated and chronically denervated mammalian muscles. Ann NY Acad Sci 274:475–492, 1976

21. Cull-Candy SG, Miledi R, Troutman B: Acetylcholine induced channels and transmitter release at human endplates. Nature 271:74–75, 1977

22. Blosser JC, Appel SH: The regulation of acetylcholine receptor metabolism by cyclic AMP. J Biol Chem 255:1235–1239, 1980

23. Namka T, Brown SB, Grob P: Neonatal myasthenia gravis: report of two cases and review of the literature. Pediatrics 45:488–504, 1970

24. Elias SB, Butler I, Appel SH: Neonatal myasthenia gravis in the infant of a myasthenic mother in remission. Ann Neurol 6:72–75, 1979

25. Elias SB, Appel SH: Current concepts of pathogenesis and treatment of myasthenia gravis. Med Clin North Am 63:745–757, 1979

26. Chang CC, Chen TF, Chuang S-T: Influence of chronic neostigmine treatment on the number of acetylcholine receptors and the release of acetylcholine from the rat diaphragm. J Physiol (Lond) 230:613–618, 1973

27. Noble ND, Brown TN, Peacock JH: Regulation of acetylcholine receptor levels by a cholinergic agonist in mouse muscle cell cultures. Proc Natl Acad Sci USA 75:3488–3492, 1978

28. Ashizawa T, Elias SB, Appel SH: The interaction of myasthenic immunoglobulins and cholinergic agonists on acetylcholine receptors of rat myotubes (abstract). Neurology (NY) 30:388, 1980

29. Feltkamp TEW, Crandenberg-Loonerr PM, Nyinhuis CE, et al: Myasthenia gravis, auto-antibodies, and HL-A antigens. Br Med J 1:131–133, 1974

21
Plasma Exchange and Immunosuppressive Drug Treatment in Myasthenia Gravis

John Newsom-Davis, MD, FRCP

Angela Vincent, MB, MSc

The observation we first reported in 1976 (1) that plasma exchange could induce a short-term remission of myasthenia gravis (MG) appeared to be of interest for three reasons. First, it provided further evidence that a humoral factor was implicated in the pathogenesis of the disease. Second, its ability to control MG symptoms in the short term suggested that it might have clinical application. Third, it offered a possible means of enhancing the effectiveness of immunosuppressive drug treatment by rendering antibody-synthesizing cells more vulnerable to this therapy. Now, some 4 years later, one can say that the evidence that a humoral factor, namely anti-acetylcholine receptor (AChR) antibody, is implicated in MG is reasonably secure (2, 3). Our own group (4–6) and others (7) have documented the inverse relationship between anti-AChR antibody level and clinical state in the period after exchange, consistent with involvement of this antibody in the loss of AChRs that underlies the physiologic defect in MG (8, 9). As to the value of the short-term clinical improvement produced by plasma exchange, many groups have reported similar findings, and the treatment has become widely used in both Europe and North America, although the criteria for its use are perhaps not yet fully agreed. On the final issue, namely whether plasma exchange enhances the effectiveness of immunosuppressive drug treatment, uncertainty exists. This is an important question, because if such synergy were demonstrated, a case could be made for using plasma exchange even in those with mild disease.

This paper describes our experience in treating MG patients with plasma exchange during the past 4 years. We have reported previously that no long-term cumulative benefits attributable to plasma exchange per se were evident when a group of patients receiving immunosuppressive drug treatment were compared to a second group who received repeated plasma exchange in

275

addition (10). We examined this question further by comparing the time course of the increase in anti-AChR antibody concentration after plasma exchange (anti-AChR "recovery") in a control group with that in a group of patients receiving additional immunosuppressive drug treatment.

Thirty-three patients with MG have now been treated with plasma exchange. Seven patients had generalized disease of moderate severity (Osserman Grade IIB), 14 patients had acute severe disease (Grade III), and 12 patients had chronic severe disease (Grade IV). The patients were 17 to 87 years of age, and the duration of the illness ranged from 2 months to 22 years. All but 2 patients had had a thymectomy, and among those for whom pathologic studies were available, 13 showed changes of hyperplasia and 16 had a thymoma. The proportion of patients in each clinical grade with thymoma was approximately the same. Serum anti-AChR antibody concentration was measured using the immunoprecipitation assay as previously described (5) and was, with one exception, increased in all patients.

Our usual regimen for plasma exchange is to undertake a course lasting 3 to 8 days. On each occasion the amount of plasma removed usually corresponds to the plasma volume calculated as 5% body weight. The replacement fluids we use have been described elsewhere (6). In the cases treated in the early part of this study, circulatory access was usually achieved via a Scribner shunt, a constructed arteriovenous fistula, or direct venepuncture. For the last year and a half, however, we have in most cases used femoral vein catheterization for each course of exchange, alternating sides when repeated courses are given. Morbidity has been low (6). However, in one patient, femoral vein thrombosis developed approximately 3 weeks after the vein had been catheterized for a 24-hour period, and this led to fatal complications. We cannot exclude the possibility that the previous catheterization contributed to this.

At the time of assessment of the outcome in these patients, all except one were receiving alternate-day prednisone or azathioprine (2.5 mg/kg of body weight) alone, or a combination of both. One patient was receiving no immunosuppressive drug treatment. Remission was observed in 10 patients (30%), and 14 patients (42%) improved sufficiently that plasma exchange was no longer required. Six patients (18%) were still dependent on plasma exchange and continued to receive regular courses of exchange, usually at 4- to 6-week intervals, for 1.3 to 3.6 years. Two patients were not helped by plasma exchange and immunosuppressive drug treatment; one of them subsequently died of respiratory failure at another institution. The other death was cited previously. The proportion of patients whose disease remitted was greatest among those with acute severe disease (43%), intermediate among those with moderately severe generalized disease (29%), and least in those with chronic severe disease (17%). The patient with no detectable anti-AChR antibody showed a clear response to exchange, suggesting the presence of a humoral factor not detected by the assay.

These data do not provide any evidence that plasma exchange per se had a beneficial influence in the outcome, although most cases showed clear evidence of short-term improvement after each exchange that typically lasted for 3 to 4 weeks.

In an earlier study, we were unable to show that coincident immunosuppressive drug treatment influenced the recovery time of anti-AChR antibody after plasma exchange, as judged by the half-time for antibody recovery (11). This work has now been enlarged and, in collaboration with Dr. Chris Hawkey, cases from the Radcliffe Infirmary, Oxford have been included (12). All values for anti-AChR antibody level were normalized by expressing them as percentages of the preexchange values. We measured the initial decrease in anti-AChR antibody level, the half-time for antibody recovery (the time to reach 50% of the initial decrease), and the recovery by day 28. Twenty patients (10 men and 10 women) were studied. All but 3 patients received alternate-day steroids during the period of the study. The additional immunosuppressive drugs used were azathioprine (2.5 mg/kg), cyclophosphamide (2.5 mg/kg), or cytosine arabinoside (ARA-C, 1 to 5 mg given intravenously for 3 to 4 days immediately after a course of plasma exchange).

In unpaired studies, we first compared the time course of antibody recovery after plasma exchange in a group (n = 12) under control conditions (no additional immunosuppressive drug treatment) with a group (n = 27) receiving additional immunosuppressive drugs. No significant difference in the time course of anti-AChR antibody recovery was observed between them, and this was also true when patients treated with azathioprine and cyclophosphamide were considered separately. In another paired study of 8 patients, the effect of plasma exchange in the presence of azathioprine (2.5 mg/kg) was compared to that of plasma exchange in the same patient when no azathioprine was given. No significant difference was observed in anti-AChR recovery. The same result was found in paired studies of 5 patients receiving ARA-C.

It has been suggested that long courses of exchange may confer additional benefits in MG (13), but we were unable to show any significant difference between the course of antibody recovery after long courses of exchange (more than 14 L) and that after short exchanges (less than 12 L) in unpaired studies. This has since been confirmed by paired studies in 5 patients. A greater initial mean decrease in anti-AChR concentration (80%) was produced by the longer course of exchange than by the shorter course (65%), but the mean values at day 28, expressed as percentages of the initial (preexchange) values, were very similar (89% and 92%, respectively).

These data thus provide no evidence that additional immunosuppressive drug treatment as used here enhances the effectiveness of plasma exchange. Our earlier studies similarly failed to show that repeated plasma exchange leads to long-term cumulative benefits in MG attributable to the plasma exchange itself (10). We therefore suggest that the place of plasma exchange in the management of MG should be based on its ability to produce a short-term remission of symptoms.

Given the relatively high cost of treatment and the fact that it is not wholly without risk to the patient, treatment should be restricted to those with severe disease. We have found it useful in preparing such patients for thymectomy or for controlling symptoms while immunosuppressive drug treatment becomes effective. Repeated courses of exchange at 5- to 6-week intervals have been undertaken for relatively long periods (more than 2 years in 2 patients) and have enabled patients to live independently at home who would otherwise require hospitalization and, possibly, assisted ventilation. At the initiation of immunosuppressive drug treatment, coincident plasma exchange can, by passively reducing anti-AChR antibody concentration, bring forward the time when symptoms are well controlled. But the absence of convincing evidence that plasma exchange has any additional "active" role when given in conjunction with immunosuppressive drug treatment makes it inappropriate, in our view, to consider this treatment in patients whose disability is relatively slight. Until further evidence is produced to the contrary, it is justifiable to accept that the effects of plasma exchange in MG are achieved passively by its ability to decrease serum anti-AChR antibody concentration.

ACKNOWLEDGMENTS

We are grateful to Ms. O Harrington, SRN, and Ms. E Goodger, SRN, for their assistance with most of the exchanges, and to Dr. L Loh, Dr. AJ Pinching, Dr. CD Ward, and Dr. SG Wilson for their help. This work was supported by the Medical Research Council.

REFERENCES

1. Pinching AJ, Peters DK, Newsom-Davis J. Remission of myasthenia gravis following plasma exchange. Lancet 2:1373–1376, 1976

2. Toyka KV, Drachman DB, Griffin DE, et al: Myasthenia gravis: study of humoral immune mechanism by passive transfer to mice. N Engl J Med 296:125–131, 1977

3. Engel AG, Lambert EH, Howard FM. Immune complexes (IgG and C3) at the motor end-plate in myasthenia gravis: ultrastructural and light microscopic localization and electrophysiologic correlations. Mayo Clin Proc 52:267–280, 1977

4. Vincent A, Pinching AJ, Newsom-Davis JM. Circulating anti-acetylcholine receptor antibody in myasthenia gravis treated by plasma exchange (abstract). Neurology (Minneap) 27:364, 1977

5. Newsom-Davis JM, Pinching AJ, Vincent A, Wilson SG. Function of circulating antibody to acetylcholine receptor in myasthenia gravis investigated by plasma exchange. Neurology (Minneap) 28:266–272, 1978

6. Newsom-Davis JM. Plasma exchange in myasthenia gravis. Plasma Ther 1:17–31, 1979

7. Dau PC, Lindstrom JM, Cassel JK, et al: Plasmapheresis and immunosuppressive drug therapy in myasthenia gravis. N Engl J Med 297:1134–1140, 1977

8. Fambrough DM, Drachman DB, Satyamurti S. Neuromuscular junction in myasthenia gravis: decreased acetylcholine receptors. Science 182:293–295, 1973

9. Ito Y, Miledi R, Vincent A, Newsom-Davis JM. Acetylcholine receptors and end-plate electrophysiology in myasthenia gravis. Brain 101:345–368, 1978

10. Newsom-Davis JM, Vincent A, Wilson SG, Ward CD. Long-term effects of repeated plasma exchange in myasthenia gravis. Lancet 1:464–468, 1979

11. Newsom-Davis JM, Ward CD, Wilson SG, et al: Plasmapheresis: short and long-term benefits. In *Plasmapheresis and the Immunobiology of Myasthenia Gravis*. Edited by Dau PC. Houghton Mifflin Professional Publishers, Boston, 1979, pp 199–208

12. Newsom-Davis JM, Hawkey C, Vincent A. Plasma exchange in the treatment of myasthenia gravis. In *Proceedings of an International Symposium on Plasma Exchange Therapy*. Edited by Reuther P. Georg Thieme, Stuttgart (in press)

13. Behan PO, Shakir RA, Simpson JA, et al: Plasma exchange combined with immunosuppressive therapy in myasthenia gravis. Lancet 2:438–440, 1979

22
Plasmapheresis in Myasthenia Gravis

Peter C. Dau, MD

Plasmapheresis is proving to be a valuable new therapy for patients with myasthenia gravis (MG) who have not responded adequately to other methods of treatment. The use of plasmapheresis (1, 2) in the treatment of MG derives its conceptual foundation from a number of diverse observations indicating the presence of pathogenic autoantibody in MG and the possibility of its therapeutic removal with plasmapheresis. An IgG autoantibody against the acetylcholine receptor (AChR) of the specificity appropriate to produce the characteristic blockade of neuromuscular transmission in MG is present in 87% of patients with MG but not in patients with other neuromuscular or autoimmune diseases or in normal controls (3). Immunoglobulin G and C3 are localized to the motor endplate in MG (4). Clinical improvement has been found in MG after thoracic duct drainage, but the disease rapidly reversed on reinfusion of the cell-free lymph of an IgG fraction derived therefrom (5).

The amount of ACh released by nerve terminals at the motor endplates in MG is at least as large as normal (6), but endplate potentials are smaller (7) because of decreased ACh sensitivity of the postsynaptic membrane (8). The AChR content of intercostal muscle in MG is 36% of normal, and the ACh sensitivity is directly proportional to the amount of AChR remaining (9). The loss of AChR is presumably caused by interaction with anti-AChR antibody; an average of 51% of the AChR that remains has antibody bound (9). Although the absolute titer of circulating anti-AChR antibody in MG only correlates roughly with disease severity (3), relative changes in titer of antibody to AChR do correlate well with changes in patients' clinical status (2). It seems reasonable to conclude that the interaction of anti-AChR antibody with AChR at the motor endplate is the major cause of myasthenic weakness (10).

There are two fundamentally different clinical uses of plasmapheresis therapy in MG at the present time. The first is a short-term intensive intervention directed at stabilizing a myasthenic patient whose condition is acutely deteriorating, or improving the condition of a poor-risk patient before thymectomy. Rapid clinical improvement is produced that is transient and independent of any concomitant immunosuppressive drug therapy. The second use of plasmapheresis is as an additional primary therapeutic measure directed toward producing stable clinical remission by permanently reducing the patient's ability to synthesize anti-AChR antibody. Improvement develops gradually, is long term, and is dependent on the concomitant administration of immunosuppressive drugs during both the phase of plasmapheresis and follow-up without plasmapheresis. It is the latter use of plasmapheresis that will be discussed here.

LONG-TERM THERAPY

In my plasmapheresis unit, 50 patients with MG have now completed a series of plasmapheresis as a primary therapeutic modality with the goal of producing long-term clinical improvement. The results in the first 35 patients are presented in Table 1. Except for 5 early patients treated more rapidly because Scribner arteriovenous shunts were in place (11), all patients received an initial series of approximately weekly plasmaphereses that were then terminated, or they were shifted to less frequent maintenance plasmapheresis as circumstances dictated. The end point of the initial series was determined clinically based on three parameters: (a) complete or nearly complete remission; (b) lack of further clinical improvement despite significant residual impairment (especially in chronic MG); and (c) absence of a tendency to develop recurrent symptoms in the few days before the next plasmapheresis. Sometimes toward the end of the initial series of treatments the interval was gradually prolonged to verify this last point. The volume of each exchange was 5% to 6% of body weight (usually 3 to 5 L), and patients received 9.9 g of immune serum globulin by intramuscular injection after each exchange.

In the 35 patients with MG, either the response to conventional therapy (anticholinesterase drugs, corticosteroids, or thymectomy) had been inadequate, or conventional therapy had been deemed contraindicated or inappropriate for reasons such as preexisting diabetes mellitus or hypertension in the case of corticosteroids, advanced patient age, or long-standing MG in the case of thymectomy. Twenty-seven patients had undergone thymectomy (13 for thymomas), and 29 had been treated with corticosteroids. All had generalized disease of at least moderate severity: the Modified Osserman Classification was IIB in 13, III in 7, and IV in 15. Thirteen patients were entirely or partially respirator dependent at the onset of plasmapheresis.

Azathioprine (2.5 to 3.0 mg/kg of body weight/day) was begun on the day of the first plasmapheresis. The dose of corticosteroid used was quite variable and

Table 1. Clinical Results in 35 Myasthenia Gravis Patients Treated with Plasmapheresis

No. of Patients	Condition
24	Stable improvement
4	Relapse, withdrawal of immunosuppression
2	Maintenance plasmapheresis
5	Poor response, inadequate immunosuppression

in many patients was limited by the patient's previous experience with untoward side effects. At the onset of plasmapheresis, the patients were usually already taking the maximal dose of corticosteroids that they had been able to tolerate. In such cases, the preexisting corticosteroid therapy was simply continued; in others, an attempt was made to increase it to 60 to 80 mg of prednisone daily during the initial plasmapheresis, and to taper it to an alternate-day basis (25 to 100 mg) once substantial clinical improvement set in. Thus, during plasmapheresis corticosteroids were unchanged in 19, increased in 7, decreased in 5, and started in 4 patients. Four patients were treated with azathioprine without prednisone; 1 was started on azathioprine without prednisone and later switched to cyclophosphamide because of a poor initial response; 3 patients receiving azathioprine and prednisone were switched to cyclophosphamide and prednisone in an attempt to improve their response; 1 was treated with cyclophosphamide alone; and 1 received pulsed cyclophosphamide and vincristine together with prednisone.

Twenty-four patients eventually attained stable improvement, including 10 patients from the respirator group. All patients became independent of the respirator during their initial series of exchanges. Of patients with stable improvement, 5 became asymptomatic without anticholinesterase medication, 13 had minimal residual symptoms easily controlled by anticholinesterase medication, and 6 had modest to moderate residual weakness. Two of the latter were very chronic cases (duration of 17 and 20 years, respectively) of moderate severity and 2 were patients who had required maintenance plasmapheresis for more than 2 years before becoming stable. The average follow-up in the stable group was 18 months; the shortest follow-up, 9 months. Leaving out the 2 previous maintenance therapy patients who received 41 and 45 exchanges, respectively, the mean number of treatments was 10. Two elderly patients in the stable group died at home from cardiac arrest 6 and 7 months, respectively, after finishing their series of plasmaphereses, and 1 patient died of metastatic thymoma 2.5 months after finishing plasmapheresis. No patient developed any complications during a plasmapheresis that were not readily reversible with prompt medical management (12). Cholinergic reactions were frequent when anticholinesterase medications were administered during plasmapheresis, and they may be attributable in part to the clinical improvement (2) and decrease in plasma cholinesterase (13) that occur during plasmapheresis. The major undesirable side effect from plasmapheresis therapy to date has been enhanced susceptibility to infection. Four patients developed gram-negative pneumonia, and 2 of these, both of whom received more than 20 plasmaphereses in conjunction with prednisone and cyclophosphamide therapy, developed evidence of cytomegalovirus infection with severe involvement. A third patient developed a mildly symptomatic cytomegalovirus infection. Details of the cytomegalovirus infections are described later.

EFFECT ON ANTI-AChR ANTIBODY TITERS

Serial anti-AChR antibody titers were measured from all 14 stable patients who had continued to take both azathioprine and prednisone during follow-up and from whom serum samples were available (Fig. 1). The mean decrease in anti-AChR antibody titer registered at the end of plasmapheresis at 11 weeks in this group was 71%, and follow-up titers 5 and 9 months after the onset of plasmapheresis remained virtually unchanged. The mean change in prednisone dosage at the end of the observation period (compared to the preplasmapheresis dosage) was a reduction of 44 to 34 mg/day. These data strongly suggest that the substantial clinical improvement seen in our patients during the phase of plasmapheresis was due to the rapid decrease in anti-AChR antibody titers produced by the combined action of plasmapheresis and immunosuppressive drug therapy. A single plasmapheresis carried out without immunosuppression does not produce sustained clinical improvement or reduction in anti-AChR antibody titer, and the effect of azathioprine on anti-AChR antibody titers and MG symptoms is smaller and more gradual (14, 15).

The long-lasting effect of plasmapheresis combined with prednisone and azathioprine therapy on anti-AChR antibody titers and serum IgG levels in 2 individual patients (cases 5 and 7 from reference 11) attaining stable improvement after 8 and 15 plasmaphereses, respectively, is illustrated in Figures 2 and 3. The first patient, a 56-year old woman, had a 3-year history of moderately severe, generalized MG refractory to thymectomy for thymoma and prednisone therapy (60 mg on alternate days). She has now been asymptomatic for 40 months, and the prednisone dosage has been reduced to 25 mg on alternate days; azathioprine, from 200 mg daily to 150 mg daily. The second patient, a 26-year old woman, had a 16-month history of severe, generalized MG requiring artificial respiration and tube feeding despite thymectomy for thymoma and prednisone therapy (80 mg daily). Currently, 28 months after finishing a series of 15 plasmaphereses, she is asymptomatic without anticholinesterase medication, despite reduction of the dosage of prednisone to 20 mg on alternate days.

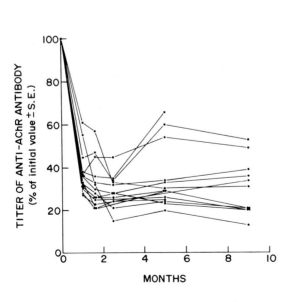

Fig. 1. Serial determinations of titer of antibody to acetylcholine receptor (anti-AChR) in patients with myasthenia gravis (MG) during and after a series of plasmaphereses combined with immunosuppressive drug therapy. Titer of antibody to AChR, expressed as a percentage of the initial value, is plotted as a function of time in 14 patients with MG who attained stable improvement by means of plasmapheresis in combination with prednisone and azathioprine. (Reprinted with permission from Dau PC, Lindstrom JM, Denys EH: Plasmapheresis in neurologic diseases. In *Therapeutic Plasma and Cytapheresis.* Edited by Taswell HF, Pineda AA. U.S. Government Printing Office, Washington DC, in press.)

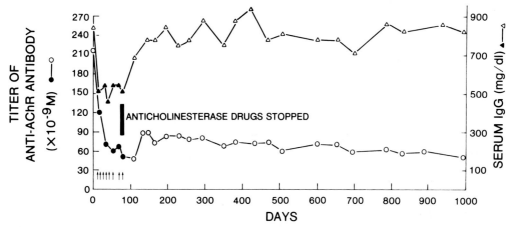

Fig. 2. Serial determinations of titer of antibody to acetylcholine receptor (anti-AChR) and serum IgG in a patient with myasthenia gravis during and after a series of plasmaphereses with immunosuppressive drug therapy. The antibody was measured at the beginning of each plasmapheresis (closed circles) or during follow-up without plasmapheresis (open circles). Serum IgG was measured at the beginning of each plasmapheresis (closed triangles) or without plasmapheresis (open triangles). Plasmapheresis are indicated by arrows. (Reprinted with permission from Dau PC: Plasmapheresis therapy in myasthenia gravis. Muscle Nerve 3:468–482, 1980.)

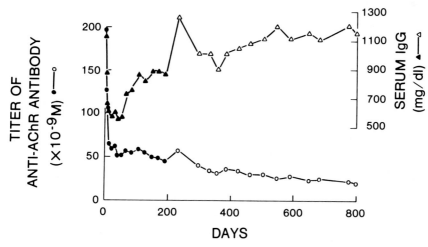

Fig. 3. Serial determinations of titer of antibody to acetylcholine receptor (anti-AChR) and serum IgG in a patient with myasthenia gravis during and after a series of plasmapheresis combined with immunosuppressive drug therapy. The antibody was measured at the beginning of each plasmapheresis (closed circles) or during follow-up without plasmapheresis (open circles). Serum IgG was measured at the beginning of each plasmapheresis (closed triangles) or during follow-up without plasmapheresis (open triangles). (Reprinted with permission from Dau PC: Plasmapheresis therapy in myasthenia gravis. Muscle Nerve 3:468–482, 1980.)

283

MECHANISM OF ACTION

As seen in Figures 2 and 3, three typical phenomena were found in studying anti-AChR antibody titers in patients achieving stable clinical improvement after plasmapheresis and immunosuppressive drug therapy: (*a*) There was rapid initial decrease in anti-AChR antibody titer (to approximately 30% of the original titer). Subsequent plasmaphereses produced little further overall reduction in titer, i.e., reaccumulation (synthesis minus catabolism) of circulating anti-AChR antibody equalled the rate at which it was being removed by plasmapheresis. (*b*) There was a dissociation between the greatly decreased anti-AChR antibody titers and the relatively less depressed total IgG levels. This effect was probably produced at least in part by the replacement of normal immunoglobulin during the phase of plasmapheresis by means of gamma globulin injections. (*c*) After cessation of the series of plasmaphereses, there was little if any increase in anti-AChR antibody titers, although the total IgG levels returned to pretreatment values (16). The ultimate selective depression of anti-AChR antibody titers compared to the total IgG antibody population indicates that the clones of lymphoid cells responsible for the production of the autoantibody might have been selectively depleted by the action of immunosuppressive drugs during the phase of plasmapheresis. After plasmapheresis, the autoreactive lymphoid clones might have been held in check by the continued action of the immunosuppressive drugs, or by partially reestablished suppressor cell control. Concanavalin A–inducible suppressor lymphocyte activity has been reported to be deficient in MG (17). In no case has anti-AChR antibody been completely eliminated from the patient's circulation.

A key early event in the generation of an immune response is clonal expansion through the proliferation of lymphocytes with specificity for the inciting antigen (18). In guinea pigs, specific clonal expansion has also been shown to occur when the feedback inhibition of antibody synthesis is reduced by a decrease in the concentration of a given antibody in the circulation (19). These facts suggest that human autoantibody-producing cells might also be stimulated to enter the mitotic cycle by removing the autoantibody with plasmapheresis. Lymphoid cells producing normal antibodies would be protected from stimulation by administering normal immunoglobulins immediately after each plasmapheresis. If plasmapheresis in humans does stimulate a partially synchronized burst of cell division in autoantibody-producing cells, a more rational approach to drug therapy would be to give pulses of antimitotic chemotherapy after each plasmapheresis, rather than chemotherapy on a continuous basis. Autoantibody-producing clones would find themselves in phases of the cell cycle, for example, the S-phase, which are more sensitive to the cytocidal action of phase- or cycle-specific chemotherapeutic agents such as cyclophosphamide (20), and intermitotic normal lymphoid tissue would be relatively spared. In animals, pulsed chemotherapy has been highly effective in inhibiting the increase in specific antibody titer after exchange transfusion or plasmapheresis (21, 22).

MAINTENANCE PLASMAPHERESIS

Five patients, who had achieved substantial improvement in their MG symptoms during plasmapheresis, showed recurrence of a monotonous constellation of weakness after each plasmapheresis. They would reach a zenith of improvement during the first week after treatment, have a phase of stability lasting for 3 to 10 days, and then begin to experience gradually increasing weakness. Their improvement could be "maintained" with repeated plasmaphereses carried out at 10- to 30-day intervals. Four of these patients received a mean of 53 treatments during a mean of 27 months; 2 of them have now become stable and stopped plasmapheresis for 13 and 7 months, respectively. The fifth patient experienced complete relapse when maintenance plasmaphereses were interrupted after 28 treatments because of the development of allergy to allogeneic g γ-globulin, and immunosuppressive therapy was withdrawn due to side effects. In these 5 patients the severity of the underlying disease process did not allow adequate containment of anti-AChR antibody synthesis by the immunosuppressive drugs after the initial series of plasmaphereses. A net reaccumulation of circulating anti-AChR antibody eventually increased above the level required for the symptomatic recurrence of MG. The patients' improvement has been maintained by periodically reducing the anti-AChR antibody titer with plasmapheresis, so that it did not increase above a mean value of 28% of the original titer. After the initial series of plasmaphereses, the anti-AChR antibody titer as measured just before each plasmapheresis showed no further net decline, i.e., anti-AChR antibody synthesis was equal to catabolism plus the amount of anti-AChR antibody removed by the maintenance plasmaphereses (11).

Figure 4 shows the course of a 51-year-old woman (Case 3 from reference 2) who showed stable improvement for 13 months after stopping maintenance plasmapheresis. She received 41 plasmaphereses during a period of 25 months.

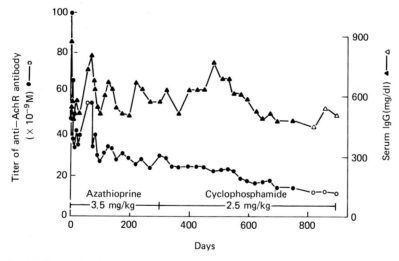

Fig. 4. Serial determinations of titer of antibody to acetylcholine receptor (anti-AChR) and serum IgG in a patient with myasthenia gravis during and after maintenance plasmapheresis. The antibody was measured at the beginning of each plasmapheresis (closed circles) or without plasmapheresis (open circles). The IgG was measured at the beginning of each plasmapheresis (closed triangles) or during follow-up without plasmapheresis (open triangles). (Reprinted with permission from Dau PC: Plasmapheresis therapy in myasthenia gravis. Muscle Nerve 3:468–482, 1980.)

She had had a 7-year history of MG, which became severe 2.5 years before institution of plasmapheresis, necessitating continuous tube feedings and 24 months of artificial respiration. During her initial series of plasmaphereses she became ambulatory, was able to eat again, and was independent of artificial ventilation. Little progress was made in ameliorating her pronounced tendency toward recurrent symptoms, coming on 10 to 14 days after each plasmapheresis, until cyclophosphamide (2.5 mg/kg/day was substituted for azathioprine at the time of her twenty-third treatment. Stable improvement was finally attained when the titer of anti-AChR antibody was decreased to 15% of the original value after approximately 700 days of therapy. During her series of plasmaphereses it was possible to reduce her dose of prednisone from 100 mg to 40 mg on alternate days. Unfortunately, 2 months after her last plasmapheresis, she developed fever and unilateral choreoretinitis. Her complement-fixing titer of antibody to cytomegalovirus was 1:128, and cytomegalovirus was isolated from her urine. The 2 remaining maintenance plasmapheresis patients have now also been switched from azathioprine to cyclophosphamide, with an improved clinical response to plasmapheresis.

IMPORTANCE OF IMMUNOSUPPRESSION

The importance of adequate immunosuppression administered during plasmapheresis is underscored by examining our group of patients whose disease relapsed when their initial series of plasmaphereses was stopped. Four patients were treated using azathioprine alone without concomitant prednisone therapy. They were the only patients in this study treated this way, and all showed only modest improvement with plasmapheresis that was poorly sustained after their series of treatment. However, one of them did later attain stable improvement 3 months after plasmapheresis, probably as a result of thymectomy carried out 2 months before plasmapheresis. Three of them received 8 exchanges and at the time of their seventh exchange their reductions in titer were only 11, 25, and 41%, respectively (Fig. 5), compared to a mean 68% reduction in titer at the time of the seventh exchange in 14 patients receiving both prednisone and azathioprine with their plasmaphereses (Fig. 1). At follow-up 110 to 120 days after the initiation of plasmapheresis, the 3 patients, all of whom continued to take azathioprine alone without prednisone, no longer showed any reduction of anti-AChR antibody titer compared to their pretreatment value, whereas the patients treated with both prednisone and azathioprine maintained their reduced anti-AChR antibody titers during the follow-up period after plasmapheresis. The fourth patient treated with azathioprine alone had a 46% reduction in anti-AChR antibody titer by the time of her tenth plasmapheresis; follow-up titers were not available. Treatment with plasmapheresis and cyclophosphamide alone may be better than treatment with plasmapheresis and azathioprine alone: we observed stable improvement with only minimal residual symptoms in a 73-year-old male diabetic who initially underwent plasmapheresis with azathioprine drug therapy by replacing it with cyclophosphamide (2 mg/kg day) for the seventh through thirteenth exchanges and during follow-up (now 4 months).

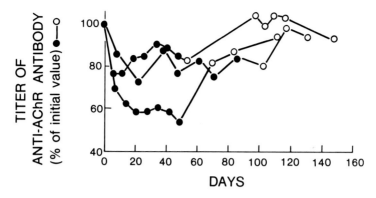

Fig. 5. Serial determinations of titer of antibody to acetylcholine receptor (anti-AChR) in 3 patients with myasthenia gravis who were receiving plasmapheresis combined with azathioprine but without prednisone. The antibody was measured at the beginning of each plasmapheresis (closed circles) or during follow-up without plasmapheresis (open circles). (Reprinted with permission from Dau PC: Plasmapheresis therapy in myasthenia gravis. Muscle Nerve 3:468–482, 1980.)

A clinical course similar to that of the patients treated with azathioprine and plasmapheresis, i.e., modest, poorly sustained improvement, was noted in a fifth patient who received 11 plasmaphereses together with azathioprine and only 15 mg daily of prednisone. Her anti-AChR antibody titers are not shown because anti-AChR antibody was never detectable in her circulation. She definitely had MG, showing a decremental compound action potential response on supramaximal stimulation of the motor nerve of 47% of the deltoid and 19% of the hypothenor muscles. These decremental responses improved after her series of treatments, decreasing to 28% and 11%, respectively; the vital capacity increased from 2.4 to 3.1 L and the arm extended time increased from 20 to 60 seconds. Positive clinical responses to plasmapheresis in patients without detectable anti-AChR antibodies have also been noted by Sanders and coworkers (23) and Newsom-Davis (24). This paradox could be explained by either a level of anti-AChR antibody below the threshold of detection in the circulation that is rapidly taken up by its target organ, or by the presence of another pathogenic antibody that is reactive with a different molecular constituent of the neuromuscular junction, which would not be detected in the assay for anti-AChR antibody. The first hypothesis is favored by the results of analysis of an external intercostal muscle biopsy specimen in our patient, which showed that 12.7% of the AChR was bound to IgG (mean ± SEM, 2.33 ± 1.6%) (9).

The sixth and seventh patients whose disease relapsed partially after their series of plasmaphereses also showed only modest improvement during treatment. Both had increased weakness due to the institution of prednisone therapy; in 1 case it was discontinued during the series of exchanges (11), and in the other, shortly thereafter. After attaining a complete remission during his initial series of plasmaphereses, relapse was provoked by rapid tapering of prednisone in an eighth patient. This 76-year-old man died of respiratory failure complicated by pulmonary embolism and bronchopneumonia despite reinstitution of plasmapheresis together with cyclophosphamide. At autopsy, bilateral *Pseudomonas* pneumonia and evidence of cytomegalovirus infection in the lungs and kidneys were found. A ninth patient developed a bacterial infection of one knee during plasmapheresis and azathioprine had to be withdrawn. A tenth patient experienced severe relapse with respiratory failure and severe bulbar and extremity weakness when prednisone, azathioprine, and cyclophosphamide had to be successively withdrawn because of side effects. She again became independent of the respirator during a series of 8 plasmaphereses carried out in conjunction with chlorambucil therapy (0.1 mg/kg day).

These results underscore the difficulty in adequately treating moderate to severe MG with plasmapheresis unless a full complement of immunosuppressive drugs can also be used. Newsom-Davis (24) also noted relatively poor results in myasthenic patients treated with plasmapheresis and either azathioprine or prednisone alone. Sanders and associates (23) and Keesey (25) have had a relative lack of success in doing plasmapheresis in conjunction with corticosteroids alone. Once control of the myasthenic disease process has been achieved by the combined action of plasmapheresis and immunosuppressive drugs, it must be maintained by the continuous administration of immunosuppressive drugs during the follow-up period. To reduce the incidence of side effects, if the disease has remained well controlled, immunosuppressive medications may gradually be tapered to the minimal dose necessary to prevent recurrent symptoms.

CONCLUSION

From experience with 35 moderately to severely weak myasthenic patients treated with plasmapheresis, it is concluded that plasmapheresis combined with immunosuppressive drug therapy can be a powerful primary therapeutic modality, producing sustained clinical improvement in most patients. The magnitude and duration of the response to plasmapheresis probably depends on 3 factors: (*a*) the intensity of the underlying disease process as reflected in the rate of replacement of anti-AChR antibody removed by plasmapheresis; (*b*) the use of immunosuppressive drugs during plasmapheresis to bring the propensity to synthesize anti-AChR antibody under control; (*c*) the use of an extended series of plasmaphereses, adjusted to the clinical response of each individual patient, to allow adequate time for a synergistic action between immunosuppressive drug therapy and plasmapheresis. Although cytotoxic immunosuppressive drugs such as azathioprine and cyclophosphamide may be used with benefit in MG, they are more rapidly effective and powerful when combined with plasmapheresis. When clinical circumstances warrant the use of cytotoxic immunosuppressive agents in MG, consideration should be given to their use in conjunction with plasmapheresis, to produce a maximal benefit to the patient for a given amount of risk of harmful side effects from cytotoxic chemotherapy.

REFERENCES

1. Pinching AJ, Peters DK, Newsom-Davis J: Remission of myasthenia gravis following plasma exchange. Lancet 2:1373–1376, 1976

2. Dau PC, Lindstrom JM, Cassel CK, et al: Plasmapheresis and immunosuppressive drug therapy in myasthenia gravis. N Engl J Med 297:1134–1140, 1977

3. Lindstrom JM, Seybold MD, Lennon VA, et al: Antibody to acetylcholine receptor in myasthenia gravis. Neurology (Minneap) 26:1054–1059, 1976

4. Engel AG, Lambert EH, Howard FM Jr: Immune complexes (IgG and C3) at the motor end-plate in myasthenia gravis: ultrastructural and light microscopic localization and electrophysiologic correlations. Mayo Clin Proc 52:267–280, 1977

5. Matell G, Bergstrom K, Franksson C, et al: Effects of some immunosuppressive procedures on myasthenia gravis. Ann NY Acad Sci 274:659–676, 1976

6. Ito Y, Miledi R, Molenaar PC, et al: Acetylcholine in human muscle. Proc R Soc Lond [B] 192:475–480, 1976

7. Cull-Candy S, Miledo R, Trautmann A: End plate currents and acetylcholine noise at normal and myasthenic end plates. J Physiol (Lond) 287:247–265, 1979

8. Albuquerque EX, Rosh JE, Mayer RF, Satterfield JR: An electrophysiological and morphological study of the neuromuscular junction in patients with myasthenia gravis. Exp Neurol 51:536–563, 1976

9. Lindstrom JM, Lambert EH: Content of acetylcholine receptor and antibodies bound to receptor in myasthenia gravis, experimental autoimmune myasthenia gravis and Eaton-Lambert syndrome. Neurology (NY) 28:130–138, 1978

10. Lindstrom JM, Dau PC: Biology of myasthenia gravis. Annu Rev Pharmacol Toxicol, 20:337–362, 1980

11. Dau PC, Lindstrom JM, Cassel CK, Clark EC: Plasmapheresis in myasthenia gravis and polymyositis. In *Plasmapheresis and the Immunobiology of Myasthenia Gravis*. Edited by Dau PC. Houghton Mifflin Professional Publishers, Boston, 1979, p 229–247

12. Menke AM, Dau PC: Technical notes on plasmapheresis. In *Plasmapheresis and the Immunobiology of Myasthenia Gravis*. Edited by Dau PC. Houghton Mifflin Professional Publishers, Boston, 1979, p 351–358

13. Paterson JL, Walsh ES, Hall GM: Progressive depletion of plasma cholinesterase during daily plasma exchange. Br Med J 2:580, 1979

14. Lefvert AK, Bergstrom K, Matell G, et al: Determination of acetylcholine receptor antibody in myasthenia gravis. J Neurol Neurosurg Psychiatry 41:394–403, 1978

15. Reuther P, Fulpias BW, Mertens HG, Hertel G: Anti-acetylcholine receptor antibody under long-term azathioprine treatment in myasthenia gravis. In *Plasmapheresis and the Immunobiology of Myasthenia Gravis*. Edited by Dau PC. Houghton Mifflin Professional Publishers, Boston, 1979, p 329

16. Dau PC, Lindstrom JM, Denys EH: Plasmapheresis in neurologic diseases. In *Therapeutic Plasma and Cytapheresis*. Edited by Taswell HF, Pineda AA. U.S. Government Printing Office, Washington DC, (in press)

17. Mischak RP, Dau PC, Gonzales RL, Spitler LE: In vitro testing of suppressor cell activity in myasthenia gravis. In *Plasmapheresis and the Immunobiology of Myasthenia Gravis*. Edited by Dau PC. Houghton Mifflin Professional Publishers, Boston, 1979, p 72

18. Dutton RW, Mischell RI: Cellular events in the immune response: the in vitro response of normal spleen cells to erythrocyte antigens. Cold Spring Harbor Symp Quant Biol 32:407, 1967

19. Sturgill BC, Worzniak MJ: Stimulation of proliferation of 19S antibody-forming cells in the spleens of immunized guinea pigs after exchange transfusion. Nature 228:1304, 1970

20. Winkelstein A: Effects of cytotoxic immunosuppressants on tuberculin-sensitive lymphocytes in guinea pigs. J Clin Invest 56:1587, 1975

21. Bystryn J-C, Schenkein I, Uhr JW: A model for the regulation of antibody synthesis by serum antibody. In *Progress in Immunology*, vol 1. Edited by Amos G. Academic Press, New York, 1971, p 628

22. Terman DS, Garcia-Rinaldi B, Dannerman D, et al: Specific suppression of antibody rebound after extracorporeal immunoadsorption. I. Comparison of single vs combination chemotherapeutic agents. Clin Exp Immunol 34:32–41, 1978

23. Sanders DB, Howard FM, Johns TR, Campa JF: High-dose daily prednisone in the treatment

of myasthenia gravis. In *Plasmapheresis and the Immunobiology of Myasthenia Gravis*. Edited by Dau PC. Houghton Mifflin Professional Publishers, Boston, 1979, p 289–306

24. Newsom-Davis J: Plasma exchange in myasthenia gravis. Plasma Ther 1:17–32, 1979

25. Keesey J: Indications for thymectomy in myasthenia gravis. In *Plasmapheresis and the Immunobiology of Myasthenia Gravis*. Edited by Dau PC. Houghton Mifflin Professional Publishers, Boston, 1979, p 124–136

23
Plasmapheresis Experience in Myasthenia Gravis at the Mount Sinai Medical Center

Peter Kornfeld, MD

Edward P. Ambinder, MD

Adam Bender, MD

Angelos E. Papatestas, MD

Gabriel Genkins, MD

The Myasthenia Gravis Clinic of the Mount Sinai Medical Center has followed 2,200 cases of myasthenia gravis (MG) during the past 30 years. In our institution, management of MG consists, when possible, of early transcervical thymectomy and anticholinesterase drugs, with other forms of therapy reserved for life-threatening symptoms or therapeutic failures, i.e., for patients in whom the preferred approaches produce no good clinical response. Only a small remainder of these severely ill patients with refractory disease exists. Despite the constantly increasing number of myasthenic patients seen, the percentage of refractory cases continues to decrease.

We have limited the use of plasmapheresis to our myasthenic patients whose disease was very severe and generalized, and were refractory to anticholinesterase drugs, thymectomy, and steroids. Randomized studies in 16 such patients confirmed the efficacy of plasmapheresis in this group of patients. None of the 7 control patients improved during observation, whereas all 9 treated patients responded with marked improvement. When the control group was subsequently treated, 3 of 7 responded, for an overall response rate of 75% in this group of 16 patients (5 with thymoma and 11 without thymoma).

All responders showed clinical improvement by the time 6,000 to 8,000 ml of serum had been exchanged. The average volume of plasma exchanged was

2,000 ml. Nonresponders were termed "treatment failures" if no clinical improvement was noted after exchange of 15,000 ml. In responders, relapses after cessation of plasmapheresis occurred within 2 to 6 weeks. Hence, we chose empirically a schedule of exchanges totalling 12,000 to 15,000 ml during a 2-week period, followed by weekly ambulatory 2,000-ml exchanges. Azathioprine (2.5mg/kg) was then added to the previous therapeutic regimen in 6 consenting patients in the hope that this added immunosuppression would allow us to prolong the interval between plasmaphereses. To date, we have not been able to stretch this interval beyond 4 weeks. Although our series is too small to reach definite conclusions, all of the azathioprine-treated patients require plasmapheresis only every 3 to 4 weeks, whereas those not receiving azathioprine have been unable to go more than 2 weeks without plasmapheresis.

Most responders showed a decrease in the serum titer of antibody to the acetylcholine receptor (anti-AChR), but there was no linear correlation between clinical response and absolute antibody titer or the percentage decrease in the antibody titer. As a matter of fact, several patients manifested increasing antibody titers without associated clinical deterioration. Similarly, 2 of the nonresponders had significant decreases in titer. We have shown previously that patients with thymomas or with thymuses with many germinal centers generally have higher serum anti-AChR antibody titers. It was this group that showed the greatest clinical improvement associated with marked decrease in anti-AChR antibody titer. The 4 nonresponders had long-standing MG (5, 7, 11, and 30 years, respectively); 2 had thymomas, and none of the thymuses had shown lymphoid hyperplasia.

Twenty-four per cent of patients manifested toxic side effects, mainly allergic reactions, hypovolemia, or vagovagal responses. No deaths were connected with plasmapheresis. The allergic reactions could be obviated by substituting plasminate and serum albumin for fresh-frozen plasma. Plasma was used in small quantities only during the initial intense phase of plasmapheresis, and no clotting abnormalities were encountered. No significant electrolyte disturbances were observed. Because all patients on chronic plasmapheresis manifest at least a mild degree of normochromic, normocytic anemia, all of our patients receive oral iron supplements.

We do not know how long to keep up the plasmapheresis program in an individual patient and proceed according to the patient's clinical course. Psychological factors play an important role in MG, as in many other chronic diseases, and dependence on plasmapheresis must be prevented. Sham plasmapheresis should be considered in some patients, but obviously presents ethical problems. Our conclusions and recommendations are as follows:

1. Use plasmapheresis only in patients with severe, disabling, generalized MG in whom anticholinesterase drugs, thymectomy, and steroids have failed.

2. Duration of disease, sex, and age should not be selection criteria, although it would seem that patients with shorter duration of MG probably have brighter prospects for improvement with this as well as with all forms of therapy.

3. In view of the lack of direct correlation between clinical state and absolute serum anti-AChR antibody titers and reports of successful plasmapheresis

in patients without increased titers, an increase in anti-AChR antibody titer should not be a criterion for selection.

4. When to stop plasmapheresis or restart plasmapheresis will probably depend on the individual patient's clinical course. Although serum anti-AChR antibody levels may be used as an admittedly imperfect guide, we believe that each patient must serve as his or her own control. We suspect that individual antibody production varies as much as individual anticholinesterase requirements. In our experience, exchange of 2,000 ml of plasma on alternate days during the initial course is effective regardless of body surface area and is associated with the fewest side effects.

5. We have just suggested a prospective randomized plasmapheresis study in postthymectomy myasthenic patients whose thymuses contained many germinal centers or thymomas. These patients generally manifest a long delay between surgery and appearance of clinical improvement and form the nucleus of our refractory patients. We plan to give these patients one course of plasmapheresis (15,000 ml) within 1 month of thymectomy and to observe their behavior during the first postoperative year.

6. We would like to see a study correlating HL-A and Gm typing with plasmapheresis response. This may help to predict which MG patients would be the best candidates for this type of therapy. Anti-AChR antibody is only one immunologic marker and is not necessarily the only or crucial test.

7. Finally, we would like to see a cooperative study using uniform criteria and techniques to delineate group response within a limited number of sharply defined parameters. Parallel plasmapheresis studies with additional immunosuppressants would also appear to be desirable.

24
Plasmapheresis in Myasthenia Gravis: Three Years' Experience

Robert P. Lisak, MD

Several weeks after the report by Pinching and colleagues (1) of the successful use of plasmapheresis in patients with myasthenia gravis (MG), we treated our first patient, a woman with severe, generalized MG. She had periods of rapid deterioration and had failed to show a consistent response to steroids; she had shown no improvement after thymectomy. This patient responded dramatically to plasmapheresis, and thereafter we went on to treat 40 patients on one or more occasions.

These patients were not treated according to any single set protocol (2) and represent patients being treated by 9 neurologists at 3 hospitals. The vast majority of patients have been treated at the Hospital of the University of Pennsylvania in collaboration with Dr. Harold Wurzel and his staff.

Until recently, all adult patients underwent plasmapheresis consisting of 5-L exchange during 2 to 5 days. We have used both discontinuous and continuous flow machines. Recently, we have tried exchanges of 9 to 12 L (vide infra), but data for these patients are not included in the group analysis reported here. With two exceptions, replacement fluid has contained only albumin and saline. Access has been via venipuncture with occasional use of a femoral catheter.

The patients have undergone exchanges 1 to 6 times for various indications; in several patients the indications were different at different times. In some instances there was more than one reason for a particular course of plasmapheresis. All patients had unequivocal MG; the duration of disease varied from 3 months to 20 years. All patients had unequivocal generalized MG. Thirty were women and 10 were men. Sixty courses were performed in thymectomized patients; 20 in patients who had not undergone thymectomy. Forty-four courses were in patients who had already been receiving corticosteroids (15 to 60 mg of prednisone per day or an equivalent alternate-day schedule) for a few days to several years.

Clinical response was seen as early as 2 days after the start of a course of plasmapheresis and as late as 6 days after the last exchange. Some patients responded on some occasions but not on other occasions. The indication for treatment seemed more predictive of outcome of a course of therapy than the individual patient, although this was not invariable.

We performed plasmapheresis for 16 episodes of crisis, with crisis defined as rapid deterioration necessitating respiratory and/or bulbar care. In 15 of 16 patients (94%) there was dramatic improvement; in 1 of 16 (6%), improvement was mild. Some patients had been in crisis at other hospitals for several weeks to as long as 3 months. In 3 instances, the patients underwent repeat plasmapheresis 7 to 10 days after the first treatment, although their condition had not deteriorated, in attempts (generally successful) to obtain further improvement.

We used plasmapheresis 28 times in patients undergoing rapid deterioration (over several weeks) but not requiring ventilatory assistance or oral-nasal-trachael suctioning. Marked improvement was seen in 24 patients (86%), mild to moderate improvement in 2 patients (7%), and no improvement in the remaining 2 subjects (7%).

Slow deterioration during 2 to 6 months was the indication for plasmapheresis on 23 occasions. Marked improvement was noted in 3 instances (12%), mild improvement in 6 (26%), and no improvement in 14 (61%).

On 13 occasions we used plasmapheresis for patients whose condition was stable, but at an unsatisfactory level. Mild improvement was seen in 3 instances (23%) and no improvement was seen in 10 (77%).

We used plasmapheresis during the week before thymectomy on 2 occasions. Each time the patient was rapidly deteriorating; 1 patient was already receiving corticosteroids and the other was not. Marked improvement was noted in both patients after plasmapheresis. One patient also required plasmapheresis therapy in the immediate postoperative period; rapid improvement resulted, although high-dose corticosteroids were given simultaneously.

The duration of the effect has been as short as 3 to 4 weeks or as long as 1 year or more. As yet, we are not sure if the clinical pattern differs, in terms of duration of effect, according to whether the patients (a) were already receiving steroids before plasmapheresis; (b) were given corticosteroids and/or cytotoxic agents (cyclophosphamide or azathioprine) after plasmapheresis; or (c) received only symptomatic agents such as acetylcholinesterase inhibitors. My current practice is to follow a patient not already on corticosteroids after successful plasmapheresis and institute steroids and/or cytotoxic agents only if frequent plasmapheresis is required. We have 7 patients who have not required steroids or cytotoxic agents.

We recently used 9- to 12-L exchanges during 5- to 7-day periods in 5 subjects (1 with slowly progressive disease, 3 with rapidly progressive disease, and 1 with stable mild disease who was already receiving steroids). It is too soon to say whether exchanges of the larger volumes will make any long-term difference.

We are now carefully reviewing our anti-acetylcholine receptor (anti-AChR) antibody data, because we have seen several exceptions to the reports in the literature of a relationship between postplasmapheresis anti-AChR antibody levels and clinical improvement. Some patients with normal levels of anti-AChR antibody, as measured by radioimmunoassay, have improved. In several patients, a return of the antibody level to its pretreatment increased level was not accompanied by clinical deterioration. A decrease in antibody level is not necessarily accompanied by clinical improvement, even over a short period of time. Long-term improvement after plasmapheresis may be related in part to removal of anti-lymphocyte antibodies or other immunoregulatory materials.

The side effects that we have seen with both the 5-L and the 9- to 12-L course have been minimal. One patient had a decrease in hemoglobulin concentration of 2 g/L, but had had borderline anemia before beginning therapy. Several patients experienced transient lightheadedness, and 2 had perioral paresthesias. In 1 of these patients the serum calcium level was 7.4 mg/dl. We have observed no infections, cardiac arrhythmias, emboli, or deterioration related to presumed changes in blood levels of anticholinesterase medications.

REFERENCES

1. Pinching AJ, Peters DK, Newsom-Davis J: Remission of myasthenia gravis following plasma exchange. Lancet 2:1373–1376, 1976
2. Lisak RP, Abramsky O, Schotland DL: Plasmapheresis in the treatment of myasthenia gravis: preliminary study in 21 patients. In *Plasmapheresis and the Immunobiology of Myasthenia Gravis.* Edited by Dau PC. Houghton Mifflin Professional Publishers, Boston, 1979, pp 209–215

25
Plasma Exchange in the Treatment of Myasthenia Gravis

Donald B. Sanders, MD

James F. Howard, Jr., MD

T. R. Johns, MD

During the past 3 years we have performed plasma exchange in 24 patients with myasthenia gravis (MG) at the University of Virginia Medical Center and the North Carolina Memorial Hospital of the University of North Carolina. In all cases, discontinuous exchange of 2.0 to 3.0 L of plasma was performed 3 times per week until maximal improvement was achieved. Anticoagulation during exchange was achieved with acid-citrate-dextrose solution. Replacement solutions usually consisted of normal saline for the first half of the exchange and 5% human albumin solutions for the second half of each exchange. Potassium chloride was added to each liter of replacement fluid. In all but 2 patients, vascular access was via percutaneous puncture of the forearm antecubital vein. Two patients required placement of a GORE-TEX graft for vascular access.

INDICATIONS

Only patients with severe or progressive generalized weakness were considered as candidates for plasma exchange. All patients but 1 had been treated with an adequate course of prednisone (23 patients) or azathioprine (1 patient), and had failed to achieve sustained satisfactory improvement before plasma exchange. The median duration of prednisone or azathioprine therapy before initial plasma exchange was 6 months (range, 0.3 to 150 months). One patient had improved after receiving azathioprine alone for 23 months, but underwent plasma exchange to achieve maximal improvement before cholecystectomy. Another patient required assisted respiration after rapid progression of myasthenic weakness; she received high daily doses of prednisone for only 10 days before plasma exchange, which was performed to improve her respiratory function. Prednisone and/or azathioprine were continued during plasma exchange in all patients but 1.

PATIENTS

There were 7 men 24 to 56 years of age (mean, 36.7 years) and 17 women 15 to 78 years of age (mean, 40.4 years). They had had MG for 0.5 to 18 years (mean, 6.3 years) before plasma exchange.

RESULTS

These 24 patients underwent 47 courses of plasma exchange; and significant improvement occurred during all courses in 23 patients; 1 patient failed to improve during each of 2 courses of exchange. Clinical improvement was defined as increased strength on functional or manual muscle testing while the patient was receiving the same or lower doses of cholinesterase inhibitors than before beginning plasma exchange. Onset of clinical improvement occurred as early as during or within 48 hours after the first exchange in 13 patients during each of 23 courses. All patients who improved did so before the fourth exchange (Fig. 1).

Maximal improvement was seen as early as during or after the first exchange (in 2 patients, both of whom had had at least 2 previous courses of exchange) or as late as after 14 exchanges (Fig. 2). On the average, maximal improvement occurred after a mean ±SD of 5.8 ± 2.6 exchanges. Fifteen patients achieved a state of marked improvement during each of 24 courses of exchange, i.e., they were functionally normal and had only minimal clinically insignificant weakness on manual muscle testing. Nine patients had less but definite improvement after each of 21 courses of exchange. One patient failed to respond to plasma exchange during each of 2 courses of exchange.

The maximal response lasted an average of 2.0 months after exchange (Fig. 3). In 4 patients, the maximal improvement was still being maintained 0.5 to 1 month after completion of the last course of plasma exchange. Maximal improvement lasted less than 1 month after 29 courses of exchange in 11 patients.

Significant improvement over the preexchange state was maintained for or is continuing 7.2 ± 8.2 months after exchange in 23 patients (Fig. 4); 11 of these patients required subsequent courses of exchange. In 18 patients, improvement is continuing an average of 9.9 ± 9.8 months after the last course of exchange.

Thymectomy was performed on 13 patients while they were improved after plasma exchange; 11 are still maintaining exchange-induced improvement 12.7 ± 10.7 months after their last exchange. Six patients had had at least 2 courses of plasma exchange before thymectomy was performed. In all but 1 of these patients, improvement was maintained for a longer period when thymectomy followed plasma exchange than after their previous courses of exchange. In 6

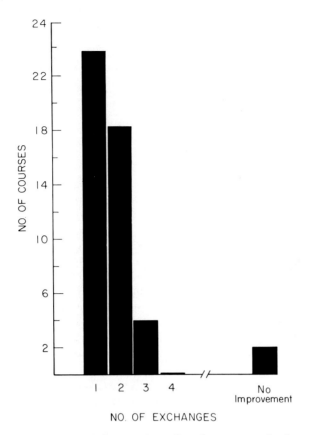

Fig. 1. Frequency histogram of the number of exchanges required to produce initial improvement in 47 courses of plasma exchange. Mean = 1.5 exchanges.

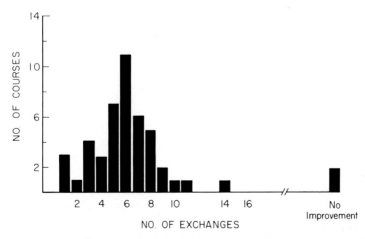

Fig. 2. Number of exchanges required to produce maximal improvement in 47 courses of plasma exchange. Mean = 5.8 exchanges

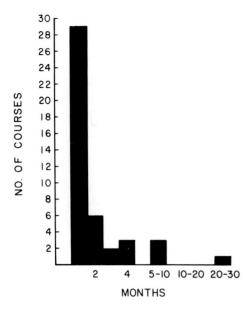

Fig. 3. Duration of maximal improvement after 44 courses of plasma exchange in 23 patients (including 4 patients still maintaining improvement 0.5 to 1 month after last exchange). Mean = 2.0.

patients thymectomy was performed after their first course of plasma exchange. Only 1 of these required subsequent exchange therapy.

Nine patients had progressive improvement after completion of plasma exchange. Six of these patients underwent thymectomy during the postexchange period, and 3 began azathioprine therapy immediately before or shortly after their last course of exchange.

Only 2 patients required more than 3 courses of exchange and are already committed to chronic intermittent plasma exchange to maintain their existence outside the hospital.

ANTI-AChR ANTIBODY TITERS

Assay of precipitating antibodies against human muscle acetylcholine receptor (AChR) was performed on serum specimens from 11 patients before exchange

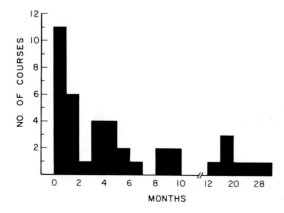

Fig. 4. Duration of improvement after 44 courses of plasma exchange in 23 patients (including 18 patients whose improvement is continuing 9.9 ± 9.8 months after their last exchange). Mean = 7.2 months.

and was abnormal in 8. In all patients with increased levels of anti-AChR antibody who improved clinically during exchange, plasma exchange produced a prompt and significant decrease in the antibody titer. There were no correlations among the initial anti-AChR antibody titer, the percentage reduction in titer after exchange, and the maximal clinical response to exchange. The 1 patient whose condition failed to improve during exchange had no decrease in anti-AChR antibody level after his initial course of exchange, during which he received no immunosuppression. During a second course of exchange, he received azathioprine and had a 52% decrease in anti-AChR antibody titer, but had no significant improvement despite exchange of 31 L of plasma during a period of 26 days. All 3 patients without detectable anti-AChR antibody before exchange had significant improvement after plasma exchange.

COMPLICATIONS AND SIDE EFFECTS

None of our patients had any serious or prolonged side effects of plasma exchange. Several had hypotension or bradycardia during the procedure, and 1 had syncope. These symptoms were usually reversed or avoided by the administration of calcium gluconate during or before exchange, and by administration of 500 to 1,000 ml of normal saline immediately before beginning the exchange procedure. Most patients experienced mild circumoral paresthesias that improved when the rate of reinfusion was reduced.

SUMMARY AND CONCLUSIONS

We used plasma exchange primarily in patients with acquired MG who had severe or progressive generalized weakness and who failed to sustain a satisfactory response to other forms of therapy. These patients represented less than 20% of the patients we treated with high-dose daily prednisone (1). Almost all of the patients with MG whom we treated with plasma exchange had a clinically valuable improvement. In most cases this improvement was only temporary unless thymectomy was performed or immunosuppression therapy was changed after exchange.

Patients who had failed to respond well to previous treatment with both prednisone and thymectomy had the poorest responses to plasma exchange. On the basis of our experience, we cannot say whether thymectomy, with or without previous prednisone therapy, is more likely to be followed by sustained improvement when preceded by plasma exchange.

The main advantage of plasma exchange therapy is that it produces a rapid and predictable improvement in most patients with MG. Even if temporary, this improvement is of considerable benefit to patients undergoing surgery, especially thymectomy performed by the sternal-splitting approach. This surgical procedure has been uneventful in all patients, who usually require no postoperative intensive care and can leave the hospital within 7 to 10 days.

Our experience indicates that patients who undergo thymectomy after plasma exchange also have a more prolonged response to exchange than do others.

This could be a result of patient selection, however, because patients who improved after thymectomy without exchange would not subsequently undergo plasma exchange.

As a result of our experience with plasma exchange, we currently use the following approach to treat patients with acquired MG:

1. The diagnosis is made on the basis of the history, physical examination, and response to cholinesterase inhibitors.
2. Underlying disease is excluded or defined and treated.
3. Cholinesterase inhibitors are given to determine the adequacy of this form of therapy and, in some cases, to confirm the diagnosis.
4. In patients who do not achieve satisfactory function on cholinesterase inhibitors alone, high-dose daily prednisone is recommended. This form of therapy produceds normal function in almost 90% of patients (1).
5. If prednisone is not effective or is contraindicated, azathioprine may be added or used alone.
6. In patients with severe or progressive weakness who do not respond to immunosuppression within 3 to 4 weeks, plasma exchange is considered. We would also consider plasma exchange in any situation in which a rapid though temporary improvement in strength could be of benefit to the patient, e.g., a surgical emergency or respiratory failure potentially requiring tracheostomy.
7. Thymectomy via a sternum-splitting approach is recommended in most patients less than 60 years of age after improvement is maximal. If a thymoma is suspected, surgery is recommended regardless of age.

Because we have found no correlation between anti-AChR antibody level and response to plasma exchange, we do not consider the presence or level of this antibody in determining the indications for exchange.

The main disadvantages of plasma exchange are the logistics and expense of the procedure. In each case, these must be weighed against the immediate and potential long-term benefit to the patient.

REFERENCE

1. Sanders DB, Howard JF, Johns TR, Campa JF: High-dose daily prednisone in the treatment of myasthenia gravis. In *Plasmapheresis and the Immunobiology of Myasthenia Gravis*. Edited by Dau PC. Houghton Mifflin Professional Publishers, Boston, 1979, pp 289–306

26
Panel Discussion: Plasmapheresis

Moderator: Stanley H. Appel, MD

Panelists: John Newsom-Davis, MD, FRCP

Peter C. Dau, MD

Peter Kornfeld, MD

Robert P. Lisak, MD

Donald B. Sanders, MD

Dr. Stanley Appel: We have all now heard something about the extensive differences in the clinical application of plasmapheresis. The first question I would like to address to the panel is this: Has any controlled study been done? Have any of you carried out any study comparing plasmapheresis and immunosuppression? This morning Dr. Newsom-Davis mentioned that plasmapheresis plus immunosuppression may not produce any different effects from immunosuppression alone. Dr. Lisak mentioned that plasmapheresis itself seems to be an immunosuppressant. The major question is, has anyone compared these therapies? Dr. Dau, have you undertaken anything of this sort? Dr. Newsom-Davis?

Dr. Peter Dau: Not in the fashion you would like, I am sure.

Dr. Stanley Appel: I mean well-controlled scientific studies.

Dr. Peter Dau: Well, controlled, yes. Some patients who were doing relatively well on corticosteroids and did not seem to be severely ill enough for plasmapheresis did receive azathioprine in the same dosage as our plasmapheresis patients. We followed serial anti-acetylcholine receptor (AChR) antibody titers in these patients and did, in general, see a gradual decline in titer. But as I mentioned in my talk, the decline in titer was much slower and much smaller than that observed in patients receiving the same drug therapy together with plasmapheresis.

305

Dr. John Newsom-Davis: It would be quite interesting to compare plasma exchange alone versus immunosuppressive drug treatment alone, but there are some theoretical problems. One might expect that plasma exchange alone would lead to antibody rebound, and we have certainly seen this after exchange in 1 or 2 patients who were not adequately immunosuppressed. This makes one very reluctant to embark on a controlled trial of this kind in which patients are randomized between the 2 groups. However, we have used patients as their own controls, first undertaking plasma exchange alone and then going on to look at what happens with coincident suppression. No striking difference was noted between the two.

Dr. Stanley Appel: Dr. Lisak, you implied that you have done a similar study without immunosuppressants. Have you seen the problem of rebound? Do these patients do as well as the patients who are treated only with immunosuppressants?

Dr. Robert Lisak: We have treated patients with just plasmapheresis. We have patients who have not undergone thymectomy during the interval of the treatment and some patients treated with plasmapheresis with prednisone with or without other agents. I hope I said that prednisone is an immunosuppressive drug. When clinicians treat a patient with prednisone they cannot claim that the patient is not immunosuppressed. Where I come from, 60 to 100 mg of prednisone per day is immunisuppressive. We have patients (predominantly those of Dr. Norman Schatz and Dr. Gareth Parry) who are treated predominantly with immunosuppression, without any plasmapheresis. But again, the assignment to treatments is not random, and we do not have the resources to set up a random study.

Plasmapheresis might be somewhat generally immunosuppressive because it removes other immunoregulatory substances, including such antibodies as anti-lymphocyte antibodies. It is possible that in 1 patient we might have allowed the immunoregulatory system to recover by removing antibodies in addition to anti-AChR antibody. We have seen antibody rebound in which the patient gets weaker, but we have also seen antibody rebound in which the patient does *not* get weaker. We do not use the antibody level as a guide to whether or not to repeat plasmapheresis. We have seen antibody rebound in patients who have been on prednisone and Imuran; sometimes they do not rebound any faster without therapy. I think you just have to treat the individual patient unless a cooperative study is set up with very rigorous criteria.

Dr. Stanley Appel: There is no question that we have to make a plea, hopefully to the Muscular Dystrophy Association, to develop just such protocols and to set up just such a study in a very well-controlled fashion. Dr. Kornfeld, did you want to add something?

Dr. Peter Kornfeld: I think Dr. Rickert has reported extensively on work with azathioprine in MG. His clinical results with this form of immunosuppression are just as good as those reported with plasmapheresis today, but I am not certain whether his was a controlled study.

Dr. Stanley Appel: One issue that came up in Dr. Sanders' presentation was the use of plasmapheresis before thymectomy. Does everyone on the panel agree that plasmapheresis has a role before thymectomy, prednisone, and anticholinesterase drugs, or is this just one clinic's special approach?

Dr. Peter Kornfeld: We have done more than 500 thymectomies in the past 25 years. Since plasmapheresis came into vogue, we have not had to resort to plasmapheresis in a single instance to prepare a patient for thymectomy. We have strictly limited the use of plasmapheresis to the very desperately ill patients who failed to respond to any other therapeutic modality. Dr. Sanders' report that preoperative plasmapheresis potentiates the clinical effects of thymectomy is fascinating and deserves further investigation.

Dr. Robert Lisak: We have used plasmapheresis on 2 occasions in the immediate prethymectomy period as opposed to 1 or 2 months beforehand. The patients improved dramatically, and they were both patients whose condition had deteriorated rapidly. They both went smoothly through thymectomy. One of them, a woman with thymoma, required plasmapheresis and steroids after surgery. The other patient, who was already on prednisone, did not require anything more after thymectomy and has done very well. So we find it useful both before and after thymectomy. We have not had to do it that often because, like Dr. Kornfeld's group, most physicians in our group advocate early thymectomy. Therefore, we have not had very many really desperately ill patients go to surgery.

Dr. Peter Kornfeld: What exactly did the plasmapheresis do to the patient? What did it allow you to do that you could not have done before? What was it that the plasmapheresis really did to "prepare" the patient for surgery? I am not sure I understand that.

Dr. Robert Lisak: Both were patients who were on maximal anticholinesterase therapy and had suboptimal vital capacity. We had operated on patients like that in the past before plasmapheresis and sometimes they had an extremely rocky postoperative course. We do not do it routinely before thymectomy. We would usually use prednisone several months before in a patient who we think needs steroids before thymectomy, although we do not routinely treat with steroids either. However, unstable prethymectomy patients who have received all of these agents will also receive plasmapheresis to obtain temporary improvement. We use it for symptomatic improvement in patients who are not doing so well on whatever else they are on.

Dr. Donald Sanders: Let me just make a point about the 13 patients we treated with plasma exchange followed by thymectomy. All achieved a state of marked improvement with exchange that they carried through the surgical procedure, which was uneventful in all cases. Eleven of those patients are still maintaining their plasma exchange-induced improvement. I do not think we would see such a response in these patients with thymectomy without plasma exchange. The average period of follow-up now is 10 months.

Dr. Peter Kornfeld: Were these thymoma patients?

Dr. Donald Sanders: Only 1 of these patients had a thymoma.

Dr. Stanley Appel: One of the implications of the use of plasmapheresis was presented by Dr. Newsom-Davis, namely that in addition to being an effective tool, it might also shed light on our notions about the role of circulating antibodies. There are, from various clinics, a small but definable number of patients who have very low titers of circulating anti-AChR antibodies by our routine assays and in fact may well benefit from plasmapheresis. The question that I would like to address to the panel is, how does plasmapheresis benefit those patients?

Dr. John Newsom-Davis: We have had 1 such patient who had no detectable anti-AChR antibody but responded well to plasma exchange. One explanation is that the solubilized human receptor used in the immunoprecipitation assay lacks the critical antigenic determinants. That is the simplest explanation, but obviously there are others.

Dr. Stanley Appel: Any other comments? Dr. Lisak?

Dr. Robert Lisak: Our first patient had no anti-AChR antibody titer as determined by Drs. Brenner and Abramsky. I think that Dr. Newsom-Davis' explanation is probably correct; we know there is not a perfect correlation between antibody titer and clinical disease in patients. The difference may be one of antibody immunoglobulin class or subclass, or of antigenic specificity, or a combination of these. I think Dr. Sanders might want to comment. He has some data about the correlation with passive transfer to animals as opposed to anti-AChR titers and clinical improvement which suggest that Dr. Newsom-Davis' comment is correct.

Dr. Donald Sanders: In our lab Dr. James Howard has demonstrated that serum from 1 of our 3 patients with no anti-AChR antibody, who improved with exchange, was capable of transferring a defect of neuromuscular transmission to immunologically tolerant rats and that the serum-borne factor was reduced by plasma exchange. I think this fits in well with Dr. Newsom-Davis' explanation.

Dr. Peter Kornfeld: Dr. Newsom-Davis, did you imply that solubilization of receptor in the assay procedure caused alteration or denaturation of the active determinants for those patients in whom no antibody could be detected? Dr. Sanders' comment suggests that these antibodies could be detected in vivo, where the active determinants are presumably still intact. Or are we dealing with yet another antigen-antibody reaction?

Dr. Stanley Appel: The problem is not one of denaturating an antigenic group. One need not implicate denaturation at all. The antibody might be directed to a different antigen that might induce disease. What is being measured in the radioimmunoassay is not the specific antigen that might be responsible for the disease process when the antibody is present.

I would now like to raise an issue mentioned by Dr. Sanders that should not be at the top of the list at a scientific conference, but must be included here: cost. Plasmapheresis is an expensive procedure, in terms of the psychological and emotional consequences, the potential side effects, and the physical cost to the patient. In addition, financial cost is quite considerable. Dr. Dau, what does it cost to do a plasmapheresis at your institution, and who pays for it?

Dr. Peter Dau: The current is about $800; generally, third-party carriers pay for it.

Dr. Stanley Appel: Is it $800 per exchange?

Dr. Peter Dau: That is correct.

Dr. Stanley Appel: What is the total cost for an average series of exchanges to a patient who will presumably benefit from this treatment?

Dr. Peter Dau: It would be $8,000.

Dr. Stanley Appel: Dr. Kornfeld?

Dr. Peter Kornfeld: Our average cost has been $700 to $725, including the cost of replacement fluids. A large part of this cost has been picked up by the Muscular Dystrophy Association as well as by third-party carriers. We figure that the cost of a patient who receives chronic plasmapheresis is $15,000 to $20,000 per year.

Dr. Robert Lisak: The cost at our institution, using albumin and saline, is about $1,300 per 2-L exchange. The price can be reduced by about one-third if fresh frozen plasma is used, because it is less expensive. However, we have chosen not to use it because of the possible side effects, so the cost is about $1,300 for 2 L.

Dr. Stanley Appel: And for the whole patient exchange?

Dr. Robert Lisak: We consider 5 L to be one course. We can do the procedure on an outpatient basis, so in some instances the inpatient cost can be saved. For inpatients you have to add the price of the room, which I believe in most institutions is about $260 or more for a semiprivate room. The procedure is expensive. Alternatively, you could figure out what the cost is for 3 months in the intensive care unit for a patient in crisis as opposed to plasmapheresis. If we can select patients who would be helped by plasmapheresis, the investment would be worthwhile. It is the $5,000 to $8,000 per 2-week run in a person who is not likely to benefit that is unjustified.

Dr. Stanley Appel: I think that is an important point. I do not want just to illustrate one side here or suggest that there are costs without any benefits or indicate that if we did not spend the $8,000, we would incur no expense. In fact, the alternatives such as time in the intensive care unit imply considerable costs.

Dr. Donald Sanders: We do all of our exchanges in the hospital and that certainly affects the cost (on the average, $10,000 to $20,000 per patient course). I should add that we have found it necessary to embark on a course of chronic repeated exchanges in only 2 patients to date. All the rest of them either have remained sufficiently improved to lead an independent existence, or the time from their last exchange is too short to say.

Dr. John Newsom-Davis: The cost is indeed an important matter. One of the reasons for using the procedure principally in those who are very severely disabled is the savings achieved if they can leave the intensive care unit and live independently at home. It is much more difficult to justify plasma exchange in economic terms in those who are less severely affected.

Dr. Stanley Appel: I think this might be an appropriate time to ask for questions from the audience. We welcome any comments you would like to make or any questions you would like to address to any of the panelists.

Dr. Ivan Diamond: I would like to comment on the fact that the absolute level of anti-AChR antibody does not appear to correlate directly with the severity of disease. This antibody can be measured, because we have developed specific probes to recognize the AChR. Therefore, we can use it as an antigen to recognize the antibody. We know that the AChR is only one component of the postsynaptic membrane and that this structure contains many other proteins in addition to the receptor protein. Some of these proteins must play a role in mediating or modulating the response of the receptor in the postsynaptic membrane. There is a great change in the postsynaptic membrane during the course of MG, so that many structural or functional proteins are affected in this disorder. If we were able to identify other proteins in the postsynaptic membrane, we would be able to develop new assays to search for specific antibodies directed against postsynaptic proteins associated with the AChR. Some of these antibodies might be responsible for severe myasthenic symptoms in patients who do not have very high titers of antireceptor antibody but who respond to immune suppression and plasmapheresis. Indeed, changes in proteins associated with the AChR might play an important role in the pathogenesis of the disease.

Dr. Stanley Appel: I would like briefly to discuss this point. Whereas looking at membrane proteins other than the AChR may provide an additional way of approaching the changes, it may not be necessary to do so. As pointed out by Dr. Lindstrom, there is such a vast array of antigenic determinants on the AChR that our radioimmunoassay, using control receptor as the antigen, may not give us as much information as would a radioimmunoassay using a specific antigenic determinant. Future monoclonal antibody studies that correlate levels of antibody with the passive transfer of disease to animals might give us a better idea of which antigenic groupings are the most appropriate to use for such clinical tests. I believe it is more reasonable for us to rule out all ways in which the AChR could be involved before implicating the involvement of other membrane proteins in the postsynaptic changes. For the moment, there is still much that we need to learn about antigenic groups on the AChR.

Dr. Sara Fuchs: One specificity that we definitely do not look at in the radioimmunoassay of human patients is the antibodies to the cholinergic binding site, because the radioimmunoassay is based on the bungarotoxin labeling of the receptor. If this particular specificity is of importance, we are definitely not looking at it.

Dr. Stanley Appel: Well, many groups do look at that. We have looked at that; Dr. Drachman talked about looking at it. Clearly, a very high percentage of so-called blocking antibodies are present, but I would agree that these are not uniformly tested in most radioimmunoassays.

Dr. Paul Schultz: The panelists have told us of some impressive cases of patients who have been able to come off ventilators after plasmapheresis, but most of these cases seem to represent medication failures. What has not been mentioned is the possibility of compliance failures; patients may appear to be taking their medication when, in fact, they are not.

Dr. Peter Dau: Most of these patients are so desperate and so sick and this is such a severe illness that in my experience they are very faithful about taking their medication. Any deviation from the schedule is a very upsetting experience for them.

Dr. Peter Kornfeld: I echo Dr. Dau's findings completely.

Dr. Donald Sanders: Steroid side effects usually demonstrate the patient's compliance to prednisone and the question of compliance does not arise with thymectomy.

Dr. Angela Vincent: I just have one point to make on the assay for anti–cholinergic binding site antibodies of the human AChR. It is quite simple to assay for this antibody because the human AChR has more than one bungarotoxin binding site; if you saturate only half the binding sites in your receptor preparation, you can measure the binding of antibodies to the unlabeled bungarotoxin binding site. By using less bungarotoxin in the whole assay system you get low backgrounds; your total number of available bungarotoxin binding sites is increased because you have only saturated half the sites and you can detect antibodies that bind to the bungarotoxin site by precipitation of the labeled toxin on the other side of the receptor.

Dr. Stanton Elias: The fact that this panel discussion has to take place is itself very disappointing to me. We can no longer make single reports of therapeutic trials and do so only to our colleagues. These reports are now immediately picked up by the national press and by national television. There is a large audience waiting for physicians to provide miracle cures for any number of diseases, and they create a giant demand for therapies that have not been proved effective. I wonder whether the fact that treatments are being published as possibilities without controlled studies represents a critical commentary about the adequacy of our own journals. The controlled study should come first, followed by publication of the results. We should not create an aura of expectation and false hopes by reporting a single therapeutic trial, especially in a disease such as MG, for which standard therapies are very effective.

Dr. Stanley Appel: Would any one like to comment? Obviously this position has considerable support.

Dr. Peter Dau: I would just mention that it is very difficult to organize randomized prospective studies. One must begin somewhere, and I think that the primary consideration must be an attempt to relieve human suffering. I agree that if the preliminary data are inconclusive, and merely suggest that a given therapeutic intervention is effective, then prospective randomized studies are in order.

Dr. Peter Kornfeld: I agree fully with Dr. Dau's order of priorities.

Dr. Robert Lisak: I also agree with Dr. Dau's comments. Among the so-called type A, type B, and type C studies, most investigators would agree that type C studies are now needed in MG. But the history of the way plasmapheresis developed, as Dr. Dau just said, requires that it be done, at least at first, in an uncontrolled manner. In my opinion there are some other neurologic diseases in which doing anything but a controlled study is ludicrous, but I would not put MG in that category.

Dr. John Newsom-Davis: I certainly think it is justifiable to report apparently effective treatment in a small uncontrolled group. It is surely up to the physician to respond responsibly if approached by the media.

Dr. Peter Kark: I would like to raise a different ethical issue. In view of the panel's discrepant results, I wonder whether, in any future large-scale and stratified study, it might not be ethically important to include as controls either minimal volume exchange or reinfusing the patient's own plasma?

Dr. Stanley Appel: Any comments from any of the panelists?

Dr. Peter Kornfeld: Besides doing sham plasmapheresis, such studies should also include reinfusing the patient's own plasma, infusion of plasmanate, serum albumin, and so on.

Dr. Robert Lisak: I think we do need the controlled studies, but I do not think that reinfusion of plasma must be part of the control protocol.

Dr. W. King Engel: I would just like to emphasize the uncertainty regarding azathioprine. We hear that some members of the panel favor it and some do not use it. In addition, the dose is important, because Dr. Kornfeld mentioned 2.5 mg/kg whereas we use 3 mg/kg. In some patients, even that is not enough. Ideally, one should titrate the dose of azathioprine against some indicator such as leukopenia. In any therapeutic trial the actual dose of azathioprine will be as important as uniformity.

Dr. Audrey Penn: I would like to ask the panel to address the question I think they started with: Do you really feel that, regardless of how we do it, plasmapheresis improves the patient? In our studies with Drs. Rowland and Clark of 17 patients, we examined a variety of protocols differing in number of exchanges, timing, and amount of plasma removed. We have had an experience similar to that of several panelists, but the anti-AChR antibody titers tend to come down gradually over a couple of weeks to about 50% of baseline and then rebound after about 10 days. We do not plan exchanges in terms of the anti-AChR antibody titers, but rather in terms of clinical response. The patients report a clinical response subjectively. That is one of the problems requiring controls. With a whirring machine at the bedside, patients can report a response and then be devastated again the next day. I am particularly concerned about patients who get nothing but anticholinesterase drugs. We have had 3 such patients; they had severe disease and their condition remained unstable. We had to get them ready for thymectomy, which required tracheostomy. We then initiated immunosuppressive agents in the intensive care unit postoperatively. Dr. Newsom-Davis said he would just as soon use immunosuppression alone, if I understood him correctly. Do we know that this procedure is worth the expense and effort? If it is, how can we maximize its effects using the minimal number of treatments?

Dr. John Newsom-Davis: It would be interesting to know whether there is general acceptance of the proposition that a reasonable proportion of patients undergoing an adequate course of exchange do actually improve. That seems to be the view of most of the panelists. Perhaps this should be the first point on which to agree before considering other ways in which the treatment might be helpful.

Dr. Richard Edwards: As we hear of the possible alternative treatments, I would like to emphasize that it is not a question of whether or not to plasmapherese. There may be a way in which conventional treatment can be optimized as a result of very careful observations of muscle function. In any possible trial of plasmapheresis such careful measurements of muscle function are, I think, absolutely essential. I have a patient who was in a wheelchair for several years. As a result of very careful measurements of muscle function, force measurement, and responses to electrical stimulation, it was possible to optimize the treatment so that she is now leading a completely independent life. Dr. Newsom-Davis knows this patient and I bring this point to your attention simply because we have the means now to quantify human muscle function very precisely and I would urge you to bear these function measurements in mind in any trial of therapy in the future.

Dr. David Yaffe: I have a question as an outsider; maybe it will be too naive. To prevent complications of infusion of foreign plasma, is it not possible to develop an immune-adsorbent system in which the patient's own plasma is transferred, cleaned up, and returned to the patient?

Dr. Peter Kornfeld: Our present methodology is rather crude; hopefully, future hemabsorption techniques will be more sophisticated.

Dr. Robert Lisak: There is a report of doing something like that in lupus, Dr. Yaffe. An attempt was made to remove immune complexes and anti-DNA antibodies. The use of such specific immunoabsorption came up at a MDA meeting a few months ago. All panel members were there. There were three problems. First, the specific antigen would have to be relatively pure. As far as I know, the antigen that is purified is from torpedo fish or eel and there is very little antibody in myasthenic serum, at least by current assays of binding to AChR from those sources. Second, once the patient's serum is going through the column, the antigen must be put on the column carefully; otherwise, you might activate the patient's complement system and start an in vitro antigen-antibody reaction on the column. Theoretically it could be dangerous to infuse activated complement back into the patient. Third, the construction of the column is problematic. Dr. Newsom-Davis has some comments concerning this.

Dr. John Newsom-Davis: Large amounts of receptor would be needed to clear the serum of someone with an average level of anti-AChR antibody. Clearly, one would need a technique in which the antibody could be eluted from the column. A potentially better solution might be the hollow fiber plasma separation technique, with which it may be possible through a cascade system to remove selectively the immunoglobulin fraction.

Dr. Alan Pestronk: One of the reasons we are reluctant to use cytotoxic immunosuppressive drugs such as azathioprine is the possibility that they may increase the incidence of neoplasia. Is there any evidence that that actually occurs in patients with MG as opposed to renal transplant patients?

Dr. Peter Dau: To my knowledge, there is not. In the large study by McEwon and Felty, 4,000 patients were treated with azathioprine for autoimmune diseases and there was not an increased incidence of any form of cancer. The increased incidence of lymphoma has been seen exclusively in patients subjected to chronic antigenic stimulation through allografts.

Dr. Peter Kornfeld: In our experience, the incidence of neoplasia is much higher in myasthenic than nonmyasthenic patients. Papatestas has reported that for a young myasthenic woman the chance of developing carcinoma of the breast is 5 times higher than that for an age-matched nonmyasthenic woman. It has been shown that if such a patient undergoes thymectomy, her chances of subsequently developing carcinoma of the breast are the same as that of the general population. The incidence of lymphomas, lymphatic leukemia, and various other carcinomas is also greater in MG. When you deal with a select population such as patients with MG, who are more prone to other autoimmune disturbances and neoplasia, other studies are not applicable.

Dr. Robert Lisak: In addition to the allograft stimulation discussed by Dr. Dau, the drug dosages used in myasthenic patients are still fairly low compared to what some of the transplant patients receive. Moreover, renal transplant patients are more immunosuppressed. Uremia itself is immunosuppressive. Renal transplant patients also receive antilymphocyte globulin at some centers. With regard to other side effects, we have had more trouble with hepatotoxicity than decreasing the white blood cell count. I would also point out that chronic use of cyclophosphamide carries a risk of sterility, especially in young women and young men.

Dr. Robert Miller: I wish to elaborate on what Dr. Richard Edwards said with regard to the anti-AChR antibody measurement. Everyone agrees that the absolute titer is poorly correlated with the clinical severity. In a dynamic sense, the clinical course correlates fairly well with the change in antibody level, although even that is not absolute. As Dr. Dau indicated, many patients with no antibody respond to plasmapheresis dramatically in a manner similar to the response of patients who have detectable antibody titers. This means that reports showing simply the change in antibody as an indicator of clinical change are not complete enough. We have analyzed vital capacity and arm outstretch time and have observed dramatic changes within as little as 36 to 48 hours after the first exchange. Therefore, I would make a plea for these kinds of objective measures, as Dr. Edwards has already done.

Dr. Jose Ochoa: There seems to be a limited role for plasma exchange in selected cases of Guillain-Barré syndrome, at least in atypical cases or very severe cases that run a progressive course. A few cases are reported in the literature. We reported 1 patient who unquestionably responded to plasma exchange, although the response was transient. Only when azathioprine was added was the improvement sustained. Theoretically, the interesting point is that, in addition to the stable organic demyelinating disorder, a humoral factor appears to contribute to a reversible nerve block in chronic Guillain-Barré syndrome. Have any members of the panel had any similar experience?

Dr. Robert Lisak: We have not treated any patients with acute Guillain-Barré syndrome; if they get better, I would not know how to interpret it. Dr. William Bank, Dr. Arthur Asbury, Dr. Mark Brown, Dr. Richard Lewis, and I have treated 5 patients with chronic demyelinating neuropathy with plasmapheresis before steroids. I think 2 patients improved and 3 did not, and the 2 that did improve did not do so spectacularly. The evidence of circulating antibody in chronic neuropathy or acute Guillain-Barré syndrome is fragmentary. I think Guillain-Barré syndrome must be studied in a controlled manner from the very first. There was a report several years ago in *Lancet* about using azothiaprine in acute Guillain-Barré syndrome; 5 out of 6 patients got better. The major question was, why didn't the other patient?

Dr. Stanley Appel: I would like to make one closing comment. I would plea for a controlled study of the value of plasmapheresis in MG. This morning a range of clinical approaches has been discussed. Obviously, all of us have our own biases with respect to the usefulness of various therapeutic approaches in MG. It is quite clear that there really are no scientific data concerning the validity of one approach compared to another, when to start plasmapheresis, and when not to use it. The cost is expensive from every point of view: psychologically, physically, and financially. I hope that by the next International Muscular Dystrophy Association Conference or even sooner, we will have controlled data that not only will validate plasmapheresis as a procedure, but will also help us understand the basis for its usefulness. If such data are important in MG, for which we have suggestive indications of its usefulness under appropriate circumstances, then controlled studies are even more imperative in other diseases, for which there are even far fewer indications and far less scientific data that plasmapheresis may have any value. Thank you all for your participation and your interest.

Part IV

MEMBRANES AND MUSCULAR DYSTROPHY

Section A
Physical and Physiological Aspects

27
Biophysical Probes of Surface Membranes: Application to Disease

Franklyn G. Prendergast, PhD

There is increasing evidence that the plasma membrane may be the locus of abnormalities that cause disease. A growing body of information suggests, e.g., that several of the dystrophic muscle diseases are due to defects in the plasma membrane of muscle cells. However, a more recent hypothesis is that the defects are not only expressed in plasma membranes of muscle, but also affect the plasma membrane structure and/or function of other cell types, i.e., are "generalized membrane defects." The manifestation of the disorder as a disease of muscle would indicate that from a functional standpoint this is the most susceptible of all the tissues.

We are primarily concerned in this paper with a discussion of how these defects may be investigated. Our focus is on investigation of the plasma membrane at the molecular level and, in particular, we address the use of spectroscopic techniques for such studies.

Of the spectroscopic approaches now available, those most suited for study of natural membranes are the magnetic resonance techniques, nuclear magnetic resonance (NMR) and electron spin resonance (ESR), and fluorescence spectroscopy. The last two mentioned rely on the introduction into the membrane of a molecule that serves as a "reporter" group or "probe" of the biologic membrane, although the intrinsic fluorescence of membrane proteins may also be used. The expectation is that perturbation of the probe's environment will result in an alteration in the ESR or fluorescence signal, which in turn may be interpreted in terms of changes in the structure and/or dynamics of the membrane. By design, probes may be made that selectively label either the lipid milieu or the proteins, and in either case be noncovalently or covalently attached to lipid and/or protein moieties of the membrane.

The purpose of this essay is to review the principles on which the use of fluorescence and ESR probes is based, to examine the nature of the data obtained in well-defined model membrane systems, and finally to consider the data that have been obtained in studies of membranes from normal persons

321

and patients with disease. Barchi (1) has provided a similar review on the subject. We conclude that, although extrinsic probes can be used to great effect, the data must be interpreted with considerable caution.

THE NATURE OF FLUORESCENCE EMISSION

We do not intend to provide here a detailed description of the fundamental principles of fluorescence and ESR spectroscopy. However, application of the fluorescence or ESR technique to the study of biologic systems cannot be properly understood without some discussion of the nature of the spectroscopic signals and their analysis.

The absorption of light by a molecule results in the promotion of an electron to a higher energy level (Fig. 1). This transition is rapid (approximately 10^{-15} seconds) relative to the rate expected for nuclear oscillations, and the molecule as a whole may be said to be promoted from an unexcited (ground) state to an excited state.

The nature of overlap of the potential energy surfaces of the ground and excited states is such that the electron is taken to a high vibrational energy level in the excited state (Fig. 1). Return of this electron to the ground state occurs from the lowest vibrational level of the excited state and requires that the excess vibrational energy be dissipated. This excess vibrational energy is lost by exchange with solvent molecules (thermal relaxation) or by partition among the various degrees of freedom in the polyatomic molecule. The result of these relaxation processes is that the molecule attains a zero vibrational level of the excited state (Fig. 1), which it may relax to the ground state by a variety of routes. Direct relaxation to the ground state (denoted in the figure as a process with rate constant k_f) results in emission of a photon, and the phenomenon is called fluorescence. The other mechanisms for dissipation of energy compete with the process leading to fluorescence. Most notably, the reorientation of solvent (or environmental) dipoles in response to the altered electronic structure of the excited molecule leads to further lowering of the excited state energy. Because energy is dissipated throughout the electronic relaxation processes, the emission spectrum of the fluorophore is shifted toward lower energy (i.e., toward the red) relative to the absorption spectrum (Stokes' shift). Competing processes such as solvent reorientation cause a further loss of energy and therefore a further shift in the spectrum toward the red. All of these factors inevitably also affect the rate of the fluorescent emissive process. We may define a useful parameter, the fluorescence lifetime (τ_f) such that

$$\tau_f = \frac{1}{(k_f + k_{nr})} \tag{1}$$

where k_f is the rate of decay by fluorescence, and k_{nr} is the rate constant for the nonradiative decay of Si_1^* (Fig. 1) and is, in fact, the sum of the rate constants for internal conversion processes and intersystem crossing. We may note that any molecule in the environment, whether it be solvent or another dissolved solute, theoretically could influence the rate of fluorescence emission through interaction with the ground or excited state fluorophore. When the fluorescence

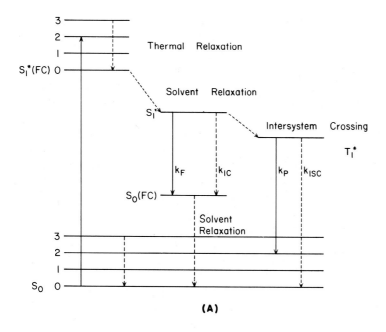

(A)

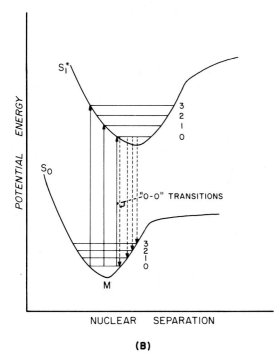

(B)

Fig. 1. Diagrammatic representation of the electronic and vibrational energy levels and transitions between them **(A)** and the potential energy profiles for the ground and excited state of a hypothetical fluorophore **(B)**. Absorption and emission are depicted by solid lines; processes resulting in heat loss are shown by broken lines. Franck-Condon states not in equilibrium with solvent are shown by (FC).

emission is diminished by such interaction, the process is termed fluorescence quenching.

If there is an interaction only in the excited state, the process necessarily occurs during the fluorescence lifetime and adds another term to k_{nr} in equation 1. Because τ_f is inversely proportional to k_f and k_{nr}, and k_f is invariant, then an increase in k_{nr} results in a shortening of τ_f. When τ_f is altered by collision with an extrinsic molecule (solute or solvent), the process is termed dynamic or collisional quenching. It will be intuitively apparent that one may use specific quenching agents to alter deliberately the fluorescence intensity and/or lifetime.

An important aspect of the absorption process is its directionality: absorption occurs along a specific direction relative to the molecular coordinates of the fluorophore. Fluorescence emission is similarly associated with a particular molecular direction. Under ideal circumstances the absorption of light and fluorescence emission occur along the same axis and in the same plane of the molecule. In reality, this ideal seldom holds true (at least with respect to the orientation of their molecular coordinates).

It should now be apparent that the fluorescent signal contains a wealth of information. Obviously, the environment of the probe profoundly influences the nature of the fluorescent signal; in turn, the fluorescence of the probe reflects, albeit indirectly, the dynamic properties of the environment. Several parameters related to that signal may be measured: fluorescence intensity and spectra, fluorescence lifetimes, and the variation in any or all of these that may be induced by fluorescence quenching. However, one of the most commonly measured parameters, fluorescence anisotrophy, relates to directionality of fluorescence signal, i.e., the degree of polarization of the emitted light.

Let us consider molecules of a fluorophore (cylindrically symmetric) dissolved in a rigid but transparent glass and therefore randomly distributed. We may assume that the absorption of light occurs along the long axis of the molecule and that emission is colinear with absorption. If the fluorophores are now excited by vertically polarized light, the molecules with their absorption moments aligned with the electric vector of the exciting light will be preferentially excited. Because the molecules are rigidly fixed and fluorescence emission is along the same axis as absorption, the light emitted is perfectly polarized. If, however, the molecule is free to rotate during its fluorescence lifetime, then the emitted light will have a significant horizontal component and will be partially depolarized relative to the exciting light. The extent to which the signal is depolarized is clearly dependent on the fluorescence lifetime and on the rate of rotation of the probe.

The example used here is obviously idealized. In reality, the absorption and emission processes are almost never colinear, meaning that the absorption and emission transition moments are displaced relative to each other, say by an angle, θ. This means that fluorescence emission occurs at an angle relative to the axis of absorption and the signal is therefore partially depolarized even though the symmetry axis of the probe may be rigidly fixed in a glass (e.g., propylene glycol at $-70°$ C). The polarization term (p) and the anisotrophy term (r) are defined by the following relations:

$$p = \frac{I_\parallel - I_\perp}{I_\parallel + I_\perp} \tag{2}$$

$$r = \frac{I_\parallel - I_\perp}{I_\parallel + 2I_\perp} \tag{3}$$

where $I_\parallel$ and $I_\perp$ refer to the measured intensities of the parallel and perpendicular components of emitted light, respectively. The anisotrophy term (r) is somewhat more useful in that it is related to the total fluorescence intensity (defined by $I_{\parallel} + 2I_{\perp}$) and because anisotrophy values are additive (2). The anisotrophy of a probe rendered immobile in a glass is termed the limiting (or zero time) anisotrophy (r_0) and has a theoretical maximum of 0.4; the corresponding polarization term (p_0) has a theoretical maximum of 0.5. As pointed out earlier, this theoretical maximum is attained only for the ideal case in which the probe does not rotate and has colinear absorption and emission dipoles. However, some fluorophores, notably 1,6-diphenyl hexa-1,3,5-triene (DPH) and derivatives, and the parinaric acids exhibit very high r_0 values (0.392 and 0.386, respectively) (3). The parameter r_0 is essential for any calculation that involves estimation of motion of fluorescent probes, because the fluorescence anisotrophy term may be used in conjunction with the Perrin-Weber and Stokes-Einstein equations to calculate a microviscosity parameter, at least for the probe embedded in an isotropic solvent (4, 5).

From these discussions it should be apparent that the extent of polarization of DPH fluorescence could provide a useful measure of the dynamics of the probe in its particular volume element irrespective of the system in which it is found. It must be remembered that the probe itself helps to create a microenvironment unique to itself and at best only indirectly reflects the behavior of the molecules that comprise that microenvironment. However, if the perturbation induced by the probe is minimal, then it should truly act as a "reporter" of the behavior of the whole system in which the fluorophore is a guest.

ELECTRON SPIN RESONANCE

In this review we are mainly interested in the use of fluorescence probes for the study of biologic membranes. For that reason, and because several excellent reviews are available on ESR, we will provide only a brief outline of the theory and principles of use of the technique (6–9).

The motion of an electron is associated with a magnetic moment (the dipole moment) which will be aligned with the lines of force when the molecule is placed in a magnetic field. By application of microwave radiation while a strong magnetic field is being maintained, the electron may be induced to reverse the orientation of its dipole moment from being parallel to being antiparallel (or vice versa) to the lines of force of the magnetic field ("spin flipping"). The wavelength of the electromagnetic (microwave) radiation that induces this spin flip is termed the resonance frequency. At equilibrium most electrons in a system will be oriented with parallel spins and will effectively absorb radiant energy.

Electronic transitions of the type described here are energetically most probable where there is a single electron in an orbit, i.e., with free radicals in which there is an unpaired electron that will readily undergo such resonance-induced transitions (hence, *electron spin resonance*). The ESR principle is illustrated in Figure 2. An electron, however, is also under the influence of the electric and magnetic effects of the atomic nucleus, and because the nuclear magnetic moment is quantized, there will be a number of discrete resonance absorption peaks for an unpaired electron that reflect the number of permissible states of the nuclear magnetic moment. There are, for example, three permis-

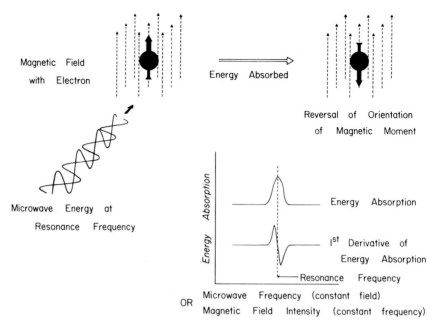

Fig. 2. The spinning electron is characterized by a dipole moment that will lie aligned with the magnetic lines of force of a strong magnetic field. On absorption of microwave electron magnetic energy (which occurs only at a definite resonance frequency), the electron acquires sufficient energy that its dipole moment is flipped to lie antiparallel to the magnetic field. When a varying frequency of electromagnetic radiation is directed at a free electron in a constant magnetic field, a peak of energy absorption occurs (lower right panel) at the resonance frequence at which this "spin-flip" occurs. For ease of analysis, the absorption data are usually presented as the first derivative of the absorption spectrum. (Adapted from figure 3 of Barchi RL: Physical probes of biological membranes in studies of the muscular dystrophies. Muscle Nerve 3:82–97, 1980.)

sible states for the nitrogen nucleus, which means that the ESR spectrum of the commonly used nitroxide radicals shows three peaks; ESR spectra are usually presented as the first derivatives of the absorption spectra.

These electron nucleus interactions are termed "hyperfine interactions" and the individual peaks are related by the hyperfine splitting values. The hyperfine splitting, in turn, is sensitive to the electronic state of neighboring atomic nuclei and hence may, for example, be used to detect changes in polarity (which influences the electronic distribution in molecules). It will be apparent that the nuclear hyperfine splitting will also be sensitive to the position and orientation of the unpaired electron relative to other atoms in the molecule.

These molecular positional effects may be averaged if the probe molecule containing the unpaired electron tumbles at a rate that is fast (rotational correlation time of 10^{-9} second) relative to the time required for an electronic transition. Immobilization of the probe in random orientation relative to the applied magnetic field results in a spectrum that is merely the sum of all possible spectra, each exhibiting a unique positional effect. The result is a broadened, more diffuse spectrum. These are two extremes of motion, and it

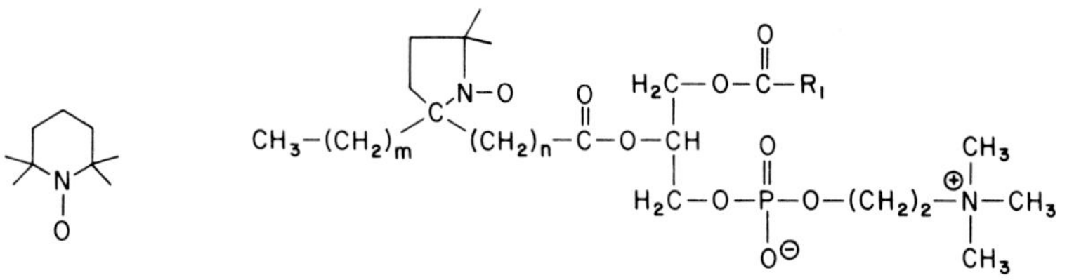

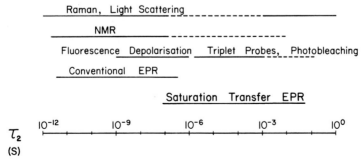

Fig. 3. Typical nitroxide electron spin resonance probes: 1, TEMPO; 2, a typical nitroxide phospholipid.

will be apparent that analysis of line shape will provide information on the motion of the probe. More detailed discussions of these features of ESR spectral analysis are available (10–12).

Many types of molecules (and atoms) contain unpaired electrons. The most commonly used probes for biologic studies on membranes are the nitroxides; typical examples are shown in Figure 3. The spectrum of the free probe in solution differs from that of the probe bound to a fatty acid or a protein, because the environment and motions are altered. An additional effect is noted where the probe's motions are restricted, i.e., are ordered, whence a parameter termed the "order parameter" (S) may be introduced. In a perfectly ordered system, the motion of the probe is highly restricted and $S = 1$, whereas if the probe is tumbling freely in an isotropic manner, $S = 0$.

LIMITATIONS IN THE ANALYSIS OF MOTION

There are clear limitations on the use of both fluorescence and ESR techniques for quantitative resolution of rates of motion. These are schematically illustrated in Figure 4. For example, fluorescence studies are limited by the fluorescence lifetime: events much faster or slower than the fluorescence lifetime are invisible to this technique. Additional limitations are imposed by an inadequate theoretical framework for analyzing fluorescence or ESR data on anisotropic rotations, especially in situations where the motions of the probes are hindered.

Raman, Light Scattering

NMR

Fluorescence Depolarisation   Triplet Probes, Photobleaching

Conventional   EPR

Saturation Transfer EPR

10^{-12} 10^{-9} 10^{-6} 10^{-3} 10^{0}

τ_2
(S)

Fig. 4. Time frames in which different spectroscopic methods are capable of resolving molecular events. NMR, nuclear magnetic resonance.

Both theoretical and practical techniques, however, are constantly being developed. For example, a new saturation transfer ESR technique allows study of motion on the millisecond time scale (Fig. 4), and an optical method that features measurement of time-resolved phosphorescence anisotropy affords similar analytic capabilities. Discussion of both of these is beyond the scope of this review.

STUDYING MEMBRANE STRUCTURE

When dried phospholipid interacts with water, the lipid takes on a variety of physical forms (13, 14). At high water content, phospholipids form bilayer structures that may be multilamellar liposomes or unilamellar vesicles, depending on the method used in the preparation. The lipid bilayers so formed are models of the lipid component of plasma membranes. However, all natural membranes are markedly heterogeneous with respect to types of phospholipid present, to the amount of cholesterol and other nonphosphate lipid moieties, and to the nature and amount of protein bound. The membrane is also spatially heterogeneous, in that the outer and inner monolayers of the bilayer are often of markedly different compositions, which is not surprising given the vectorial nature of many membrane enzyme and transport systems. The model of Singer and Nicholson provides the best overall description of plasma membrane structure according to the information available at present (Fig. 5).

Many studies, however, have been performed on artificial lipid bilayers to facilitate interpretation of data from natural membranes. Lipid bilayers composed of a single phospholipid that has saturated fatty acyl chains (in ester linkage) at the α- and β-carbons of the glycerol moiety exhibit thermotropic phase transitions: they are in a gel-like state at low temperatures, but with an increase in temperature cooperatively attain a second state in which the system may be described as "liquid crystalline," as in the melting of butter (Fig. 6) (15). The transition occurs over a small temperature range (approximately 2 to 4° C

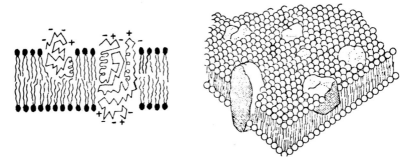

Fig. 5. Schematic representation of the Singer-Nicholson fluid mosaic model of biologic membranes. On the left side of the figure, the proteins are shown as they might interact with the hydrophilic and hydrophobic components of the lipid bilayer. On the right, proteins are shown as inclusions in a "sea" of lipid.

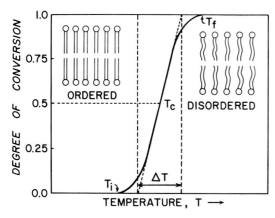

Fig. 6. Idealized representation of the phase transition as it might be detected by the change in a biophysical parameter such as the fluorescence anisotropy. At a degree of conversion of 1, the system is in a new phase. T_i is the initial temperature; T_f, the final temperature; T_c, the midpoint (transition) temperature; $\triangle T$, width, in °C or °K, of the phase transition.

in a highly cooperative manner. The temperature at the midpoint of this transition may be regarded as the phase-transition temperature (Tc).

The term "fluidity" is widely used to describe the relative freedom of motion of the phospholipids in a bilayer. Above Tc the lateral diffusive motions of phospholipids are markedly enhanced, from which we may infer that the bilayer is considerably more fluid at temperatures greater than Tc than at temperatures less than Tc. But it is equally important to realize that the transition may also be regarded as an order-disorder change, meaning that the intrinsic packing of the fatty acyl chains, so highly ordered at temperatures less than Tc, is disrupted at temperatures greater than Tc. The value of Tc depends on length (in methylene units) and degree of unsaturation of the fatty acyl chains, on head group structure of the phospholipid, and on the presence of other types of lipid, notably cholesterol. In general, as the degree of unsaturation increases, the extent of disorder at any given temperature also increases.

As pointed out before, natural membranes are perhaps best characterized by their heterogeneity. Lipids from a natural membrane do not usually show a unique phase transition, and the dynamics of the system are such that the membranes almost invariably appear to be "fluid" by the criteria usually used to define that term. There are certainly a number of factors that could, in a local region of a biomembrane, result in a greater or lesser degree of order; such "domain" effects might be important in the isothermal regulation of membrane function.

Proteins that are intrinsic to the membrane, i.e., interact with hydrophilic and hydrophobic domains of the lipid bilayer, necessarily influence the packing and, hence, order of the lipids. In some instances specific lipids associate with a protein; in such situations that protein may constantly be surrounded by a particular "boundary" lipid. In other situations, the boundary layer of lipid is determined by stochastic processes, and the lifetime of any particular lipid in that boundary layer will be largely (but not completely) determined by the bulk diffusion rate of the lipid molecule in the bilayer. However, there are mutual interactions in such a lipid-protein system; alterations in the physical state of the lipid can markedly influence the structure and dynamics of the protein bound in the lipid. One may readily envisage lipid-promoted protein conformational adaptions, but the nature and mechanisms of such adaptations are yet to be described.

RATIONALE FOR USING SURFACE FLUORESCENCE AND ESR PROBES IN STUDY OF BIOMEMBRANE STRUCTURE

In the search for a generalized membrane defect in the plasma membrane of cells from patients with disease, most of the emphasis has been on the study of membrane fluidity. The notion has been, and is, that a generalized membrane defect might be manifest as a change in the physical dynamics of the plasma membrane, which in turn might be reflected as a decrease or increase in the apparent freedom of motion of phospholipids and membrane proteins. Both ESR and fluorescence probes have been used in such studies. As we stated earlier, the fundamental principles on which the use of ESR and fluorescence probes is predicated are in essence the same. The rationale for use of fluorescence probes in the study of membrane "fluidity" is discussed below.

As stated earlier, when the axis of the emission dipole is displaced by rotation during the fluorescence lifetime of a flourophore, the effect of the displacement on the fluorescent signal may be measured as a change in the polarization of the emitted light relative to the exciting light. The basic equation for calculating the degree of polarization (anisotropy) was given in equation 3. The anisotropy parameter so determined may be used with the Perrin-Weber equation (equation 4) to calculate the apparent rotational rate of the probe, and the rotational rate of the probe may then be inserted into the Stokes-Einstein equation to calculate an apparent microviscosity parameter, η. The equation is

$$\frac{r_o}{r} = 1 + \frac{3\tau}{\rho} = 1 + C(r)\frac{T\tau}{\eta} \tag{4}$$

where ρ is the rotational correlation time, τ is the fluorescence lifetime, T is the temperature in degrees Kelvin, and $C(r)$ is a parameter related to the molecular shape and the position of the transition dipole relative to the principal diffusion axes of the molecule. For a sphere, $C(r) = k/V$, where k is Boltzmann's constant and V is the effective molar volume of the sphere; for all other molecular shapes $C(r)$ is inconstant. The microviscosity parameter is denoted η. The other symbols have their usual meaning.

The relationships are deceptively simple and at first glance it appears that the microviscosity parameters so derived should reasonably reflect the overall viscosity properties of the solvent in which the probe is dissolved. To some extent this is true, but there are distinct limitations in the application of the Stokes-Einstein equation. To apply this equation realistically to the analysis of fluorophore motion, the fluorophore or other objects rotating in the solvent must be rotating isotropically, the solvent should be isotropic, and the rotating molecule should be significantly larger (in molecular dimensions) than the molecules of solvent. If the rotating molecule is much smaller than the solvent molecules, an anomalously low viscosity parameter will be deduced.

One should also realize that the parameter being measured in a fluorescence or spin-labeled experiment is usually the rotational correlation time, which gives only a measure of rotational diffusion rate and says little of the translational motion of the probe or the viscosity of the system that opposes translational motion of a solute. Nonetheless, the use of steady-state polarization to determine the rotational rate of fluorescence probes in isotropic solvents and in artificial and biologic membranes has continued apace.

Early experiments had shown that when DPH was dissolved in a saturated lipid, e.g., dimyristoylphosphatidylcholine, the apparent phase behavior of this lipid, could readily and accurately be detected and measured as it was heated. Figure 7 illustrates the pattern of change in anisotropy of DPH dissolved in a number of phospholipids that exhibit a phase change. Until recently, these anisotropy changes have been interpreted in terms of a change in the rotational rate of the probe: the rotational rate increases dramatically at the phase transition temperature of the lipid bilayer. From this change in rotational rate and through application of the Stokes-Einstein equation, an apparent microviscosity change was calculated (16–19). The apparent microviscosity of the lipid was considerably less when it was in the fluid state than when it was in the gel state. For this reason, the lipid bilayer is said to be "fluid" above the phase-transition temperature Tc.

Phospholipids such as dioleoylphosphatidylcholine, or a mixed acid phospholipid such as 1-palmitoyl-2-oleoylphosphatidylcholine, do not exhibit phase transitions in the temperature range 2 to 50°. In these lipids the anisotropics of DPH are less than they would be in a lipid below the phase transition. Consequently we may view such lipids to be essentially "fluid" in the physiological temperature range.

It is important to note that these conclusions regarding lipid dynamics are based on data gathered under steady-state conditions. But the rate of decay of anisotropy may also be determined by following the time dependence of $I_\parallel$ and $I_\perp$ after an extremely short excitation pulse. Alternatively, because the anisotropy

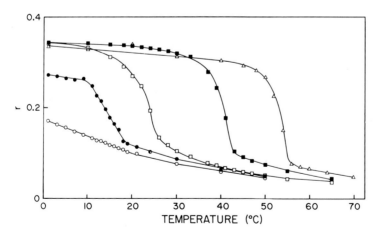

Fig. 7. Variation in steady-state anisotrophy (r_{ss}) of diphenylhexatriene (DPH) with temperature. The DPH was embedded in dioleoylphosphatidylcholine (○), dielaidoylphosphatidylcholine (●), dimyristoylphosphatidylcholine (□) dipalmitoylphosphatidylcholine (■), and distearoylphosphatidylcholine (△). The graph shows typical (experimental) phase-transition profiles.

is dependent on τ, variation in τ through use of quenching agents (e.g., oxygen) changes r; measurements of r (τ) can, in principle, also provide time-resolved fluorescence anisotropy data.

Time-resolved and lifetime-resolved measurements of anisotropy of DPH in lipid bilayers have altered our concepts of the motion of the fluorescent probes in such structures (20–26). Time-resolved measurements have shown that the anisotropy of DPH embedded in lipid bilayers did not decrease to zero at times that were long compared to the fluorescence lifetime (as would be predicted from the Perrin-Weber equation), but decreased instead to some distinctly nonzero, limiting value (Fig. 8). From these data it is apparent that, when embedded in the gel phase of a phospholipid (i.e., below Tc), DPH does not rotate freely. It cannot tumble end-over-end in the manner expected for motion of that probe in an isotropic liquid, but rotates within a restricted volume in the bilayer.

Intuitively, one can imagine that a cylindrical molecule such as DPH, oriented with its long axis normal to the plane of the membrane, would be constrained by the fatty acyl chains of the phospholipids that run approximately parallel to the long axis of the DPH molecule (27). The constraint would be most severe in the gel state. However, melting of the phospholipid chains at Tc would increase the probability for motion of DPH and therefore for displacement of the emission dipole of that molecule during its fluorescence lifetime. As a consequence, the anisotropy parameter r would decrease at Tc.

If the value of r at times that were long compared to the value of τ_f obtained time-resolved anisotropy measurements (26) measured the extent to which the probe motion was constrained then, logically, at Tc the absolute value of the limiting anisotropy would also decrease. A variety of experiments (20–23) have clearly demonstrated that this is so; namely, that at Tc the limiting anisotropy value (denoted r_∞) for the hindered motion of DPH changes rather markedly in a manner akin to that observed for the (usually measured) steady-state anisotropy parameter (r_{ss}).

These time-resolved data have been corroborated by the findings of Lakowicz and Prendergast (24) and Lakowicz and colleagues (25, 26), who used a technique known as differential polarized phase fluorometry and oxygen quenching (to achieve lifetime-resolved anisotropies) to measure the molecular motions of DPH in lipid bilayers. Their data allowed calculation of r_∞, and the values obtained agreed precisely with those obtained by time-resolved methods.

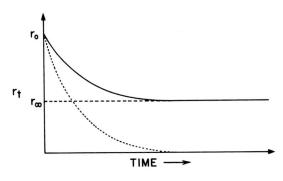

Fig. 8. Theoretical time-decay curves for anisotropy of diphenyl-hexatriene in lipid bilayers (solid line) and in isotropic solvents (broken line). The r_t on the ordinate refers to anisotropy at time t; r_o, the anisotropy when no motion of the probe occurs during the fluorescence lifetime; r_∞, the limiting anisotropy value that results from hindrance of the motion of the probe.

They also showed that above Tc, or if DPH was dissolved in an intrinsically "fluid" lipid such as dioleoylphosphatidylcholine, r_∞ values were small. Subsequently, a number of workers have shown that r_∞ is, in fact, a measure of the order parameter, which is a term familiar to users of ESR and NMR techniques. The precise relationship is given as

$$\frac{r}{r_o} = S^2 \tag{5}$$

where S is the order parameter. Although the values differ, *patterns* of change in r_∞ and steady-state anisotropy (r_{ss}) are identical.

At temperatures much greater than the phase transition temperature of a particular lipid, or in lipid bilayers composed of a phospholipid such as dioleoylphosphatidylcholine (which has unsaturated fatty acyl chains), r_∞ approaches zero more rapidly than does r_{ss}, indicating that r_{ss} measures more than lipid order. Recent theoretical work of Lipari and Szabo (28), Jähnig (29), Heyn (30), and Engel and Prendergast (31) has quite clearly demonstrated that r_∞ reflects the average static angular distribution of the probe and does not yield any information regarding the rate of motion of the probe. Prendergast and Engel (32) have recently provided a detailed account of the nature and significance of r_∞ values in fluorescence probe studies of bilayer.

The similarity in profiles (and of actual values) of r_{ss} and r_∞ shows the large dependence of r_{ss} on orientational factors rather than rate of motion. Clearly, this finding profoundly influences the use of r_{ss} to calculate "microviscosity" parameters in bilayers. The data given in Figures 9 and 10 further illustrate the problems inherent in the use of r_{ss} to measure microviscosity when the probe's motion is hindered. The data show that the rotational rate calculated from measurements of r_{ss} alone differ rather markedly from those calculated by a model that takes into account the fact that the probe's motion is hindered.

The value of the fluorescence anisotropy of DPH in membranes, however, depends not only on the degree of saturation of the fatty acyl chains that comprise the membrane, but also on the presence in the lipid of other components. For example, cholesterol markedly affects the anisotropy of the probe, as does the presence of proteins. These inclusions in an otherwise homogeneous membrane create structural heterogeneity; because a probe such as DPH is likely to partition into all regions relatively equally, the anisotropy signal measured reflects the variety of probe populations that result. In other words, at all temperatures, irrespective of the intrinsic Tc of the bilayer, r_{ss} and r_∞ will inevitably reflect the effects of protein and/or other inclusions such as cholesterol or other phospholipids.

The extent to which inclusions affect the signal is determined by the molar ratio of the host lipid to the inclusions. Whereas the actual (quantitative) ratio of the two components may be predetermined in any given experiment, the *effective* ratio is more difficult to determine. For example, the effect of proteins embedded in lipid bilayers is not limited to lipids immediately in the vicinity of the protein, but extends some ill-defined distance into the lipid bilayer. This means that the packing behavior of the lipid is altered for some poorly defined distance away from the protein; furthermore, lipid molecules influenced by the protein do not have the same (bulk) properties as the host lipid.

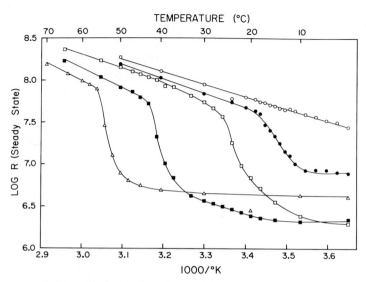

Fig. 9. Rotational rates (R) of diphenylhexatriene (plotted as log R) as a function of temperature for the probe embedded in lipid bilayers composed of dioleoylphosphatidylcholine (○), dielaidoylphosphatidylcholine (●), dimyristoylphosphatidylcholine (□), dipalmitoylphosphatidylcholine (■), and distearoylphosphatidylcholine (△) and calculated from steady-state anisotropy (r_{ss}) data. Note the marked increase in rotational rate (predicted from r_{ss} data) at the phase-transition temperature.

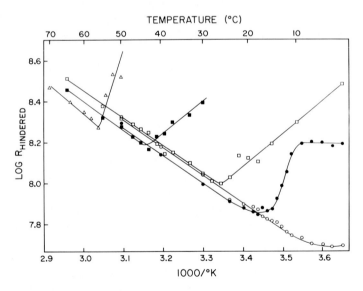

Fig. 10. Plots of the rotational rate of diphenylhexatriene in the same lipids described in Figure 9, but calculated from differential polarized phase lifetimes. The absolute values for the rates differ markedly from those given in Figure 9, and the profiles are also completely different. Symbols: dioleoylphosphatidylcholine (○), dielaidoylphosphatidylcholine (●); dimystearoylphosphatidylcholine (□); dipalmitoylphosphatidylcholine (■); distearoylphosphatidylcholine (△).

334

The experiments required to quantify the effects of various lipid: protein ratios on the motion of the fluorescent probe have not been done. In natural membranes, which are markedly heterogeneous with respect to both lipid content and protein content, the anisotropy signals from an embedded probe, irrespective of whether they are steady-state, time-resolved, or lifetime-resolved, must reflect an extremely heterogeneous environment. Because anisotropy signals are additive, the chance of observing a change in fluorescence anisotropy for a probe dissolved in a natural membrane is directly proportional to the volume of the perturbed domain relative to the total volume, provided that DPH partitions with equal probability into all domains. For this reason, it would be difficult to predict whether one could or should expect to find a difference between normal and abnormal membranes unless one could predict that the abnormality was derived from some generalized defect in lipid production and/ or destruction that affects relatively large domains or even the entire membrane.

Lipids isolated from natural membranes seldom exhibit a phase transition in a physiological temperature range. This results largely from the heterogeneity of lipid types, the presence of cholesterol, and the structure of natural phospholipids. The last mentioned are usually mixed acid phospholipids with a saturated fatty acyl group in the R_1 position and an unsaturated fatty acyl group in the R_2 position; these groups render the membrane fluid at essentially all temperatures, or at least considerably more fluid than would the corresponding saturated phospholipid (Fig. 11). Both the absolute amount of inclusions in a lipid bilayer and the spatial distribution of these components in the bilayer affect the apparent motion of a fluorescent or spin-labeled probe. For example, proteins may be distributed throughout the bilayer, be limited to one monolayer, be distributed in some crude lattice over the surface, or be clumped in one

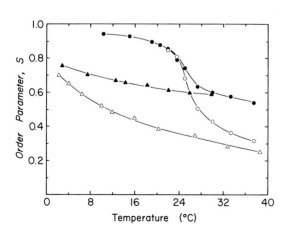

Fig. 11. Plots of the order parameter (see text) of diphenyl-hexatriene (DPH, open symbols) and 1[4-trimethylaminophenyl]-6-phenyl-hexa-1,3,5-triene (TMA-DPH, closed symbols) embedded in dimyristoylphosphatidylcholine (DMPC, circles) and 1-palmitoyl-2-oleoylphosphatidylcholine (POPC, triangles). The TMA-DPH is located at the lipid-water interface and cannot rotate as freely as DPH at temperatures greater than the midpoint (phase-transition) temperature (T_c). The POPC showed no discernible phase transition at any of the temperatures studied here, but the apparent "fluidity" of the bilayers of POPC and DMPC are substantially the same at temperatures greater than T_c for the saturated lipid (DMPC).

region of the membrane. Each pattern will affect the signal from a fluorescent probe in a different way. It is not difficult, for example, to perceive how a cytoskeletal system, which is attached to the entire surface of the inner monolayer of the membrane, could profoundly alter the dynamics of a probe embedded in the bilayer.

The distribution of a fluorescence probe in intact cells poses another problem. A molecule such as DPH, which is only minimally soluble in water, readily partitions into the lipid bilayer, presumably into the hydrocarbon region formed by the tails of the fatty acyl groups of the phospholipid. Diphenylhexatriene, however, is sufficiently soluble in the lipid milieu that it will readily transfer from the plasma membrane to intracellular membranes and therefore be distributed fairly readily throughout all cellular compartments, including intracellular lipid droplets. Any signal measured from such a population of fluorophores reflects the sum of anisotropies from several environments and cannot be ascribed solely to DPH dissolved in the plasma membrane. Because the last-mentioned location is the focus of our interest in the study of disease processes in muscle, interpreting data from studies using DPH as a probe of plasma membrane structure and dynamics is problematic.

This particular difficulty with the use of DPH can be mitigated if isolated plasma membranes are used, but then one must contend with problems inherent in the preparation of plasma membranes. The isolated plasma membrane has properties rather different from those of the intact cellular membrane. In ESR experiments, the problem of probe location is no less severe, but may be ameliorated through the use of probes with a charged moiety attached, e.g., the doxyl- or nitroxyl-labeled fatty acids. A similar tack can be used with fluorescence probes.

Fluorescence Data

Several studies have recently been reported in which fluorescence and ESR probes have been used to study the structure and dynamics of membranes from cells of normal persons and from patients with disease, mostly muscular dystrophy. Both fluorescence and ESR experiments were performed in essentially the same way: cells were incubated with an appropriate probe; the spectroscopic signal from the probe, presumably ensconced in the plasma membrane, was detected, measured, and analyzed. There have been relatively few studies in which fluorescence probes have been used to investigate membranes of cells exhibiting dystrophic disease.

Chalikian and Barchi (33), working on the premise that fluorescence techniques were inherently more sensitive than those of ESR, investigated the properties of red blood cell (RBC) membranes from patients with myotonic dystrophy. They hoped to find differences between the cells of these patients and those of normal subjects that were at least qualitatively similar to differences previously described by Butterfield and coworkers (38–42), who had used ESR probes (see later). Chalikian and Barchi (33) used 4 probes, DPH, anilinonaphthalene sulfonate (ANS), D-equilinen, and α-parinaric acid, to investigate the dynamics of RBC membranes from patients with myotonic dystrophy. Their rationale was that the probes should partition into different regions of the lipid bilayer component of the membrane and therefore allow study of any area of the membrane that might show a difference in structure and/or dynamics. D-equilenin was chosen, e.g., because it grossly resembles the cholesterol molecule and might be expected to partition in a manner similar to that of cholesterol. The authors examined the fluorescence spectral and polarization properties of these probes as a function of temperature and found that there were no significant differences between the RBC membranes of normal persons and patients with disease.

Initial studies by Shaw (unpublished observations) were also performed with DPH as probe to investigate fibroblast cell membranes. Cells from normal subjects and from patients with muscular dystrophy were grown in tissue culture for an equal number of passages; cell membranes were then isolated from the tissue cultures. Shaw measured steady-state anisotropy and differential polarized phase lifetimes to determine the nature of molecular motion of DPH in these cell membranes. The data showed quite convincingly that there were essentially no differences between the two populations of cell membranes. As Shaw has pointed out, however, if the membranes were "abused" during the membrane preparation, (e.g., if they were exposed to agents such as ethylenediamine tetra-acetic acid or ethyleneglycol tetra-acetic acid during the preparative process), then fairly significant differences could be observed between the two populations.

It is not at all clear why harsh preparative methods should differentially affect the normal and diseased cell membranes or whether this indicates a fundamental difference in the plasma membrane architecture. We have used the same techniques as Shaw, but studied the motion of fluorescence probes in the membranes of myotubes grown in tissue culture. The cells were examined as they grew on coverslips. Data gathered on steady-state anisotropies and differential phase lifetimes showed no differences between normal and diseased cells when DPH was used as a probe (Table 1). Experiments were then conducted with all-*trans* β-parinaric acid; again, no differences were observed.

Although Huntington's disease (HD) is not a disease of muscle per se, it is worthwhile commenting on fluorescence studies that have been done on fibroblasts, lymphocytes, and RBCs from patients with this hereditary neurologic disease. These data have been reported by Pettegrew and coworkers (34, 35). The authors used predominantly ANS as a probe and measured spectra, fluorescence intensities, and anisotropies of ANS bound to the plasma membrane. The authors reported that cells grown to the fourth passage showed a 30-fold increase in ANS fluorescence intensity when bound to the plasma membrane of diseased cells. In addition, they reported a very significant blue shift in the spectrum, which they interpreted as being due to partitioning of the ANS into "more hydrophobic" domains in cells from patients with HD. Lakowicz and Sheppard (36) recently repeated the experiments of Pettegrew and colleagues, but could not corroborate the original findings. Lakowicz and Sheppard, however, extended their studies to use of DPH and a new probe, laurdan, which exhibits dramatic spectral shifts in response to changes in the polarity of the environment of the probe. They chose laurdan because of its remarkable sensitivity to the environment, in the hope that if the probes were at all able to partition into different regions of the membrane, this should show up more readily in the spectral behavior of laurdan than in the fluorescence spectra of ANS. However, in no instance did Lakowicz and Sheppard observe any

Table 1. Representative Fluorescence Depolarization of Diphenylhexatriene in Membranes and Cells from Patients with Duchenne Muscular Dystrophy (DMD) and Normal Control Subjects

Subjects	Parameter	Temperature, °C 16	30
Patients with DMD	r_∞	0.207(S)	0.156(S)
		0.218	0.166
Normal controls	r_∞	0.231(S)	0.180(S)
	r_∞	0.212	0.160
Patients with DMD	r_{ss}	0.225(S)	0.173(S)
		0.236	0.179
Normal controls	r_{ss}	0.240	0.175

Data are unpublished observations of Shaw and Prendergast. Values from Shaw are for myoblast membranes and are shown by (S). The other data are from Prendergast, from experiments done on intact myoblasts. For the latter, the value at 16°C was interpolated. At comparable temperatures the anisotropy values for diphenylhexatriene (DPH) in vesicles of egg lecithin showed r_∞ values of 0.044 and 0.017, respectively. No significant differences between patients with DMD and normal subjects were noticed in the fluorescence lifetime or the logarithm of the rotational rates of DPH.

Abbreviations: r_∞, the limiting anisotropy value for the hindered motion of diphenylhexatriene; r_{ss}, steady-state anisotropy value.

differences between normal and diseased cells, irrespective of whether fluorescence spectra intensity or anisotropies were used to investigate the behavior of the probes.

The overwhelming conclusion from these preliminary studies is that, in contrast to the data from ESR, the fluorescence techniques have so far failed to show any significant differences between normal cell membranes and the membranes of cells from patients with dystrophy or HD. As we shall see shortly, ESR data have shown rather marked differences. It is not at all simple to rationalize the disparities in the data obtained by the two techniques; if anything, fluorescence should be far more sensitive than ESR and the perturbation of the fluorescence signal should in no way be less easily observed than the perturbation of the ESR signal.

ESR Data

Electron spin resonance probes were the first to be used in the investigation of the membrane properties of cells derived from patients with muscle disease. Most of the work has been done by Butterfield and coworkers (37–41). Most of the published data have been concerned with myotonic dystrophy and Duchenne muscular dystrophy, and in some instances, cells from animals made dystropic with diazacholesterol were examined. Butterfield and associates showed that there was a minor but significant difference in the behavior of a spin-labeled probe in the lipid milieu of cells from patients with myotonic dystrophy compared to normal subjects. Red blood cells were used for these experiments.

Gaffney and coworkers (42) have recently studied the "fluidity" of intact RBC

membranes from patients with myotonic dystrophy. They used 5-nitroxylstear-
ate as a probe for ESR experiments. In a carefully performed series of
experiments, these workers were not able to verify the findings of Butterfield
and coworkers. Similarly, Swift et al. (43) examined the membranes of cells
derived from goats with myotonic dystrophy and were unable to find any
significant differences between normal and dystrophic animals. The data for
myotonic dystrophy, then, are equivocal, and it seems likely that the earlier
reports of a generalized defect in this disease may not be accurate.

The results are less equivocal for cells derived from patients with Duchenne
muscular dystrophy. Data obtained with both conventional ESR and a new
technique, saturation transfer ESR, have shown differences between normal
and diseased cell membranes. The initial studies were done by Butterfield and
associates (39, 41) with conventional ESR and showed that there was a significant
increase in "fluidity" in the cells of patients with muscular dystrophy.

Sato and associates (44) also showed marked differences in the apparent
motional freedom of a nitroxide moiety located close to the methyl terminus of
a stearic acid moiety when this probe was embedded in RBCs from normal
subjects and those with Duchenne muscular dystrophy. Recently, Wilkerson et
al. (45) used saturation transfer ESR to examine the motional behavior of 5-
nitroxylstearate (5-NS) dissolved in the membranes of RBCs from patients with
Duchenne muscular dystrophy as compared to those of normal persons.
Saturation transfer ESR can detect motion that occurs on a much slower time
scale than would be detected by either fluorescence or conventional ESR. The
molecules of 5-NS appeared to cluster in the membranes of the RBCs from
patients with Duchenne muscular dystrophy in such a manner that the spin
signal was broadened (due to spin-spin interaction) and that the rate of
migration of the 5-NS (indicated by decreased broadening) was apparently
considerably slower in these membranes than normal membranes (Fig. 12). The
differences were significant, but the apparent molecular basis for this phenomenon is not clear.

It could be that the fatty acid probes tend to partition into a unique
environment in the membrane created by an appropriate defect and that either
lateral diffusion or transmembrane transport of the fatty acid thereafter is
retarded in the cells of the patients with muscular dystrophy. In any event,
these data provide the most clear evidence to date for the existence of a defect
in RBCs of patients with any kind of dystrophy. Most significantly, they suggest
that there may be a generalized membrane abnormality. One must presume
that the next stage will be to examine the membranes of other cell types and
ultimately, the muscle membrane itself, to see whether similar phenomena may
be observed.

Again, it is useful to point out that ESR experiments have also shown an
apparent generalized membrane defect in the cells of patients with HD.
Butterfield and coworkers (46) used probes attached to sulfhydryl groups of
proteins to examine the cells of patients with HD and showed marked differences
in the apparent order parameter calculated for these probes. When probes of
the lipid region were used, the cells of normal and diseased patients appeared
the same.

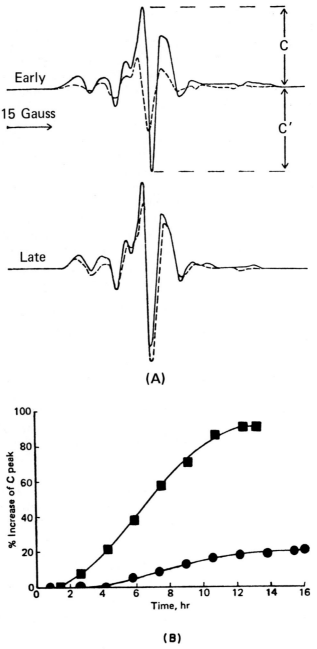

Fig. 12. **(A)** Tracings at early and late time points of representative saturation transfer EPR (ST-EPR) spectra for erythrocytes from a patient with Duchenne muscular dystrophy (broken line) and a control subject (solid line). **(B)** Relative change in the ST-EPR C peaks (see A) as a function of time after labeling; (●), control subject; (■), patient with Duchenne muscular dystrophy. (Reprinted with permission from Wilkerson LS, Perkins RC Jr, Roelofs R, et al: Erythrocyte membrane abnormalities in Duchenne muscular dystrophy monitored by saturation transfer electron paramagnetic resonance spectroscopy. Proc Natl Acad Sci USA 75:838–841, 1978.)

340

SEARCH FOR A GENERALIZED MEMBRANE DEFECT

The evidence presented above is sufficiently equivocal to suggest that we reexamine our rationale for asserting that there should be or is a generalized membrane defect in (some) hereditary diseases. The notion is attractive and certainly logical, in that the phenotypic expression of a genetically based membrane disorder may very well be reflected in abnormalities of the structure and/or function of a multiplicity of cell types. On the other hand, we might anticipate that the mutation responsible for hereditary diseases such as muscular dystrophy results from a point mutation, which in turn is likely to influence only one or at most a very few gene products.

We may continue this line of reasoning to infer that a single protein or at least a single component of a multiprotein system is likely to be influenced. If this protein were an enzyme, especially one involved in lipid metabolism, then we might anticipate that either an increase or a decrease in enzyme activity could induce moderate to severe abnormalities in the lipid bilayer component of the plasma membrane and thereby cause marked changes in membrane structure and/or function. However, analyses of the lipid milieu of the plasma membrane of cells from patients with dystrophy have yielded no evidence that the lipid architecture is significantly altered, at least in composition or spectroscopic data (see above). In any event, the membrane is sufficiently "plastic" to be able to tolerate fairly substantial alterations in its basic lipid makeup without severe perturbation of function.

Admittedly, the damage might be especially severe in highly localized regions (or microdomains) that contribute only a small portion of the total lipid content of the membrane and hence may not be detected by conventional techniques for lipid analysis. The latter argument is not readily refuted and will be a difficult problem to resolve. We take the tack, however, that a point mutation in a gene which codes for a single membrane-bound protein, possibly an enzyme or a transport system, is likely. It is then relatively easy to envisage a gene product that is relatively or absolutely specific for skeletal muscle and that the structural abnormality in this protein system is the molecular basis for the dysfunction of that organ. This situation is not difficult to imagine, because we know that there are tissue-specific systems, e.g., isozymes of creatine kinase or lactic dehydrogenase, and it is now clear that skeletal and cardiac troponin T are distinctly different molecular species.

Obviously, if the defect is in some key protein, then the system finally "runs down" as a consequence of the malfunctioning of that particular protein and leads eventually to cell destruction and cell death. If we adhere to the notions that a generalized membrane defect may occur and that a single genetic mutation is responsible for the disease, then we might productively focus our attention on a protein system that could influence overall membrane structure and/or dynamics. For example, an abnormality of the cytoskeletal system could certainly manifest itself as a perturbation in the organization and/or dynamics of membrane-bound proteins or lipids and could do so in a variety of tissues.

No data have yet been adduced from either electron microscopic examination or biochemical studies. Nevertheless, the idea remains an attractive one, if only because there are a number of ways to determine whether some aspect of cytoskeletal control is awry. It is also possible that excessive phopholipid production or destruction (e.g., by an abnormal phospholipase A_2) may result in destruction of the integrity of the lipid milieu and become manifest as a defect that is generalized with respect to both an entire cell surface and to cell types.

FUTURE APPROACHES USING SURFACE PROBES

The criticisms that we have leveled at the data gathered so far are in no way related to the possible usefulness of biophysical techniques in the study of disease processes. Clearly, the sensitivity of conventional ESR, saturation transfer ESR, and fluorescence make them attractive techniques for investigating cells of normal persons and patients with disease. It seems appropriate, however, to suggest some further diversification in the use of these techniques and considerably more caution in the interpretation of the data.

With both ESR and fluorescence, the specificity of the probes must be increased; for example, it may be possible to label the plasma membrane of cells with a fluorescent or spin-labeled probe that should only very slowly, if at all, be transported across the plasma membrane into the intracellular milieu and hence into other membranes. This might be readily achieved through the use of a charged fluorescent species, although some charged species, such as ANS, do sometimes traverse the plasma membrane. Alternatively, it might be possible to use a fluorescently or spin-labeled phospholipid that can be inserted into the plasma membrane through the action of a phospholipid-exchange protein.

A useful fluorescent probe that we do not think crosses the membrane to any significant extent is shown in Figure 13. This trimethylamino analogue of DPH has recently been fully characterized by Prendergast and colleagues (47) and shows great promise for investigating the plasma membrane, in that it appears

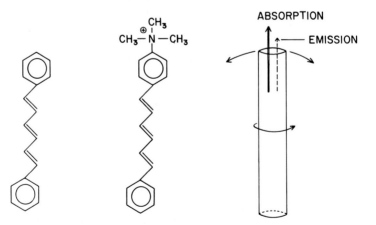

Fig. 13. Chemical structures of diphenylhexatriene (*left*) and 1[4-trimethylaminophenyl]-6-phenyl-hexa-1,3,5-triene (*middle*). Schematic drawing (*right*) shows the (approximate) directions of the absorption and emission dipoles.

to partition only into the outer leaflet of the plasma membrane when applied to intact cells. This particular molecule shares all the spectral advantages of DPH, including a high extinction coefficient and high quantum yield, a reasonably long fluorescence lifetime in membranes (approximately 7 nsec), and virtual colinearity of the absorption and emission dipoles.

Greater emphasis must be placed on the study of membrane proteins by ESR and fluorescence spectroscopic techniques. Labeling of a specific protein is difficult, but the class of proteins that contain sulfhydryl groups can be isolated because the sulfhydryl group forms a locus for labeling with thiol-specific agents. The full brunt of spectroscopic techniques may then be brought to bear to examine the structure and dynamics of these membrane proteins and how they respond to perturbation in membrane structure. For fluorescence spectroscopy this requires the measurement of as many fluorescence parameters as possible, including fluorescence lifetimes, differential polarized lifetimes, fluorescence anisotropy, fluorescence intensity and spectra, and where possible, the use of lifetime-resolved anisotropy measurements.

Clearly, one need not study motion alone; as much or more information might be available from differences in spectral profiles of probes bound in membranes from normal and diseased cells. Conventional or saturation transfer ESR experiments should be done. Whether fluorescence or ESR techniques are used, it is clear that interpretations of membrane structure and dynamics ought not be made on the basis of a single type of spectroscopic investigation. Moreover, it is essential that spectroscopic data be validated by structural data gathered with more "conventional" biochemical techniques and by studies designed to investigate functional abnormalities in the diseased cell.

ACKNOWLEDGMENTS

I wish to thank Ms. Evonne Webster for helping with the preparation of this manuscript and Mr. Peter J Callahan for preparing the figures. This work was supported in part by the Muscular Dystrophy Association and the Mayo Foundation. This work was done during the tenure of an Established Investigatorship of the American Heart Association. The author is a Searle Foundation Scholar. Thanks are also due to Dr. K Prendergast and Dr. J Blinks for continuing support.

REFERENCES

1. Barchi RL: Physical probes of biological membranes in studies of the muscular dystrophies. Muscle Nerve 3:82–97, 1980
2. Weber G: Rotational brownian motion and polarization of the fluorescence of solutions. Adv Protein Chem 8:415–459, 1953
3. Prendergast FG: Patterns of "motion" of α and β parinaric acids and their methyl esters in lipid bilayers as determined by differential polarized phase fluorometry. Biochemistry Submitted for publication
4. Shinitzky M, Dianoux AC, Gitler C, Weber G: Microviscosity and order in the hydrocarbon region of micelles and membranes determined with fluorescent probes. I. Synthetic micelles. Biochemistry 10:2106–2113, 1971

5. Shinitzky M, Inbar M: Microviscosity parameters and protein mobility in biological membranes. Biochim Biophys Acta 433:133–149, 1976

6. Gaffney BJ, McFarland B: The molecular basis of fluidity in membranes. Chem Phys Lipids 8:303–313, 1972

7. Gaffney BJ, Chen S-C: Spin label studies of membranes. Methods Membr Biol 8:291–358, 1977

8. Mehlhorn RJ, Keith AD: Spin labeling of biological membranes. In *Membrane Molecular Biology.* Edited by Fox CF, Keith AD. Sinauer Press, Stamford, CT, 1972

9. Berliner LJ (ed): *Spin Labeling: Theory and Applications.* Academic Press, New York, 1976

10. Levine YK: Physical studies of membrane structure. Prog Biophys Mol Biol 24:1–74, 1972

11. Ohnishi SI: A spin-label study of biological membranes with special emphasis on calcium-induced lateral phase separation. Adv Biophys (Tokyo) 8:35–81, 1975

12. Schreier S, Polnaszek C, Smith ICP: Spin labels in membranes: problems in practice. Biochim Biophys Acta 515:375–436, 1978

13. Chapman D, Williams RM, Ladbrooke BD: Physical studies of phospholipids. VI. Thermotropic and lyotropic mesomorphism of some 1,2-diacyl-phosphatidylcholines (lecithins). Chem Phys Lipids 1:445–475, 1967

14. Luzzatti V, Tardieu A: Lipid phases: structure and structural transitions. Annu Rev Phys Chem 25:79–94, 1979

15. Fontell K: Liquid crystalline behaviour in lipid water systems. Prog Chem Fats Other Lipids 16:145–162, 1978

16. Shinitzky M, Barenholz Y: Fluidity parameters of lipid regions determined by fluorescence polarization. Biochim Biophys Acta 515:367–394, 1978

17. Lentz BR, Barenholz Y, Thompson TE: Fluorescence depolarization studies of phase transitions and fluidity in phospholipid bilayers. I. Single component phosphatidylcholine liposomes. Biochemistry 15:4521–4528, 1976

18. Lentz BR, Barenholz Y, Thompson TE: Fluorescence depolarization studies of phase transitions and fluidity in phospholipid bilayers. II. Two-component phosphatidylcholine liposomes. Biochemistry 15:4529–4537, 1976

19. Shinitzky M, Barenholz Y: Dynamics of the hydrocarbon layer in liposomes of lecithin and sphingomyelin containing dicetylphosphate. J Biol Chem 249:2652–2657, 1974

20. Kinosita K, Kawato S, Ikegami A: A theory of fluorescence depolarization decay in membranes. Biophys J 20:289–305, 1977

21. Kawato S, Kinosita K, Ikegami A: Effect of cholesterol on the molecular motion in the hydrocarbon region of lecithin bilayers studied by nanosecond fluorescence techniques. Biochemistry 17:5026–5031, 1978

22. Chen LA, Dale RE, Roth S, et al: Nanosecond time-dependent fluorescence depolarization of diphenylhexatriene in dimyristoyl-lecithin vesicles and the determination of "microviscosity." J Biol Chem 252:2163–2169, 1977

23. Dale RE, Chen LA, Brand L: Rotational relaxation of the "microviscosity" probe diphenylhexatriene in paraffin oil and egg lecithin vesicles. J Biol Chem 252:7500–7510, 1977

24. Lakowicz JR, Prendergast FG: Quantitation of hindered rotations of diphenylhexatriene in lipid bilayers by differential polarized phase fluorometry. Science 200:1399–1401, 1978

25. Lakowicz JR, Prendergast FG, Hogen D: Differential polarized phase fluorometric investigations of diphenylhexatriene in lipid bilayers: quantitation of hindered depolarizing rotations. Biochemistry 18:508–519, 1979

26. Lakowicz JR, Prendergast FG, Hogen D: Fluorescence anisotropy measurements under oxygen quenching conditions as a method to quantify the depolarizing rotations of fluorophores: application to diphenylhexatriene in isotropic solvents and in lipid bilayers. Biochemistry 18:520–527, 1979

27. Andrich MP, Vanderkooi JM: Temperature dependence of 1,6-diphenyl 1,3,5-hexatriene fluorescence in phospholipid artificial membranes. Biochemistry 15:1257–1262, 1976

28. Lipari E, Szabo A: Effect of librational motion on fluorescence depolarization and nuclear magnetic resonance relaxation in macromolecules and membranes. Biophys J 30:489–506, 1980

29. Jähnig F: Structural order of lipids and proteins in membranes: evaluation of fluorescence anisotropy data. Proc Natl Acad Sci USA 76:6361–6365, 1979

30. Heyn MP: Determination of lipid order parameters and rotational correlation times from fluorescence depolarization experiments. FEBS Lett 108:359–364, 1979

31. Engel LW, Prendergast FG: Theoretical analysis of fluorescence parameters for the evaluation of molecular motion. Biochemistry Submitted for publication

32. Prendergast FG, Engel LW: Values for and significance of order parameters and "cone angles" of fluorophore rotation in lipid bilayers. Biochemistry Submitted for publication

33. Chalikian DM, Barchi RL: Fluorescent probe analysis of erythrocyte membrane physical properties in myotonic muscular dystrophy. Neurology (NY) 30:277–285, 1980

34. Pettegrew JW, Nichols JS, Stewart RM: Fluorescence spectroscopy on Huntington's fibroblasts. J Neurochem 33:905–911, 1979

35. Pettegrew JW, Nichols JS, Steward RM: Studies of the fluorescence of fibroblasts from Huntington's disease: evidence of a membrane abnormality. N Engl J Med 300:678, 1979

36. Lakowicz JR, Sheppard JR: Fluorescence spectroscopic studies of Huntington's fibroblast membranes. Submitted for publication

37. Butterfield DA, Roses AD, Cooper ML et al: A comparative electron spin resonance study of the erythrocyte membrane in myotonic muscular dystrophy. Biochemistry 13:5078–5082, 1974

38. Butterfield DA, Chesnut DB, Roses AD, et al: Electron spin resonance studies of erythrocytes from patients with myotonic muscular dystrophy. Proc Natl Acad Sci USA 71:909–913, 1974

39. Butterfield DA, Chesnut DB, Appel SH, et al: Spin label study of erythrocyte membrane fluidity in myotonic and Duchenne muscular dystrophy and congenital myotonia. Nature 264:159–161, 1976

40. Butterfield DA, Roses AD, Appel SH, et al: Electron spin resonance studies of membrane proteins in erythrocytes in myotonic muscular dystrophy. Arch Biochem Biophys 177:226–234, 1976

41. Butterfield DA: Electron spin resonance investigations of membrane proteins in erythrocytes in muscle diseases. Biochim Biophys Acta 470:1–7, 1977

42. Gaffney BJ, Drachman DB, Lin DC, et al: Spin label studies of erythrocytes in myotonic dystrophy: no increase in membrane fluidity. Neurology (NY) 30:272–276, 1980

43. Swift LL, Atkinson JB, Perkins RC Jr, et al: Electron paramagnetic resonance and saturation transfer electron paramagnetic resonance studies on erythrocytes from goats with and without hereditable myotonia. J Membr Biol 52:165–172, 1980

44. Sato B, Nishikida K, Samuels L, et al: ESR studies of erythrocytes from patients with Duchenne muscular dystrophy. J Clin Invest 61:251–259, 1978

45. Wilkerson LS, Perkins RC Jr, Roelofs R, et al: Erythrocyte membrane abnormalities in Duchenne muscular dystrophy monitored by saturation transfer electron paramagnetic resonance spectroscopy. Proc Natl Acad Sci USA 75:838–841, 1978

46. Butterfield DA, Purdy MJ, Markesbery WR: Electron spin resonance, hematological, and deformability studies of erythrocytes from patients with Huntington's disease. Biochim Biophys Acta 551:452–458, 1979

47. Prendergast FG, Callahan PJ, Haugland RP: 1-(4'-trimethylaminophenyl)-6-phenyl-hexa-1,3,5-triene (TMA-DPH): synthesis, fluorescence properties, and use as a probe of lipid bilayers. Biochemistry Submitted for publication

DISCUSSION

Dr. Donald Wood: Would you comment on the problems of using these kinds of probes in a system such as muscle, which has a variety of types of membranes, such as surface membranes, tubular membranes, and sarcoplasmic reticulum membranes? What kinds of approaches might be useful in identifying the location of the probe and interpreting data from these probes in such a multimembrane system?

Dr. Franklyn Prendergast: That is a superb question and identifies perhaps the most formidable problem in the use of fluorescence or spin-label probes for the study of any cellular system. The fundamental difficulty is how to localize the probe to a particular environment, and if possible, to localize the probe to lipid domains, i.e., to keep it away from protein so that the signal makes some sense. A probe such as diphenylhexatriene (DPH) is fairly promiscuous: it will partition anywhere. Consequently, as a function of time, the probe partitions and repartitions until it is everywhere in the cell. One obvious way to achieve specific labeling is to put a charge on the probe molecule. The trimethyl ammonium diphenylhexatriene (TMA-DPH) derivative was chosen for just that reason; it will partition uniquely into the outer leaflet of the bilayer and only very slowly enter the cell. It also maintains the excellent spectroscopic properties of DPH while getting away from the promiscuity of DPH. This is very, very important. Even parinaric acid, being a fatty acid, is subject to transport across the bilayer and consequently to metabolism and redistribution as a function of time. The same thing might occur to some of the spin-label probes. Another strategy is to use protein-sensitive probes, both those that will be transported across a membrane and get to both sides of the bilayer, and those that will localize just to the outside. Dr. Butterfield has been doing some of that work and can describe it in detail. I think this is a very intelligent approach.

Dr. Alan Horwitz: Two points ought to be reemphasized for this nonspecialist audience. The first is the concept of microviscosity that is rampant in the current literature. One is actually dealing with an anisotropic probe situated in an anisotropic environment. The probe is the same size as are the solvent molecules, and there are probably many local environments unevenly visited by the probe. In this system the concept of "microviscosity" or "apparent micro-viscosity" is misleading, a point you have made very well. The second point concerns the complexity of the fluid state. Reports claiming a change in fluidity between two membranes usually do not make their meaning clear. Does it mean there is different acyl chain ordering? Does it mean there are different lateral diffusion rates? Does it mean there are different phase equilibria? Is the probe visiting different environments? It is important to keep this complexity in mind when reading papers using membrane probes. You made these points very well, and your discussion should help us interpret this literature meaningfully.

Dr. Franklyn Prendergast: Your point is critically important. You can get an apparent change in fluidity simply by moving the proteins around, with no change in the lipid system at all. It is critically important to realize this, because the calculated values of microviscosity can have little significance simply because the Stokes-Einstein equation has been inappropriately applied in a system where there is such severe anisotropy. One final comment: natural membranes are inherently fluid. The reason is that the fatty-acyl group in the 2 position of most phospholipids is unsaturated, and that single change makes all the difference to the fluid parameters of the membrane. What you see in a natural membrane or in lipid extracted from a natural membrane, apart from the effects of cholesterol, is a progressive decrease in all of the so-called fluid parameters, e.g., as temperature is varied; but at all temperatures the membrane appears disordered and, hence, "fluid." This is important, because membrane-bound enzymes may show apparent phase transitions in terms of function while the lipid exhibits no phase transition whatever.

Dr. Daniel Drachman: I appreciate your comment on the difficulties of determining microviscosity, but let me ask perhaps the most difficult question to answer. Can you enlarge on the one sentence in which you dealt with the published or unpublished studies of "fluidity" in red blood cell membranes from a variety of diseases? Can you just give us a brief critique of that?

Dr. Franklyn Prendergast: That is a loaded question! I think Dr. Larry Dalton has done that for me very efficiently in his use of saturation transfer electron paramagnetic resonance (EPR), and I think Dr. Butterfield would agree with Dalton's implicit conclusion. That implicit conclusion is that what has been seen in EPR studies of Duchenne red blood cell membranes may not be at all related to membrane fluidity; rather, it may represent a time-dependent redistribution of probe molecules in the system that resembles changes in freedom of motion of the probe. If so, it is a simple case of misinterpreting the data. The point is, however, that there were differences between normal and diseased cell membranes (if the data can be validated). As I said before, there are so many things that can produce apparent changes in fluidity that the problem with the published data may not be related to the quality of the data but rather to their interpretation.

28

Lateral Distribution of Ionic Channels in the Cell Membrane of Skeletal Muscle

W. Almers, PhD

R. Fink, PhD

N. Shepherd, PhD

Electric excitability depends in large measure on the operation of ionic channels, a class of molecules (polypeptides or proteins) capable of forming small holes through which the appropriate ions may pass across cell membranes. Here, we will discuss their distribution over the cell membrane. In general, this distribution is uneven, despite the view that the matrix wherein ionic channels reside, the lipid bilayer, is fluid at physiologic temperatures. In the postsynaptic membrane of a neuromuscular junction, for example, acetylcholine (ACh)-sensitive (cholinergic) channels are locked closely together in an almost crystalline array and show no measurable lateral mobility. However, uneven distribution is found also with extrasynaptic ionic channels, either transiently during development and after denervation, or as a permanent feature of adult tissue. This review will focus on extrasynaptic channels.

Table 1 lists the major ionic channels that have been found in the cell membrane of skeletal muscle by electrophysiologic techniques. Most of these are also found in other excitable cells. The list may not be exhaustive. Adrian and colleagues (1) postulated the existence of an additional K^+-channel with slow time and voltage dependence, and Palade and Almers (2) have described a permeability mechanism for monovalent cations that is blocked by external Ca^{2+} but not by tetrodotoxin (TTX). These channels are not considered here since they have not been described in detail and their physiologic roles are unclear.

Table 1. Ionic Channels in Muscle Membrane

Type	Function	Antagonists or Blockers
Cholinergic channel	Synaptic transmission	Curare, α-bungarotoxin
Na^+ channel	Action potential	Tetrodotoxin
Delayed K^+ channel	Action potential	Tetraethylammonium
Cl^- channel	Resting potential	Anthracine-9-COOH
Inward rectifier K^+ channel	Resting potential	Ba^{2+}, Cs^+, Rb^+
Ca^{2+} channel	Unknown	D-600, nifedipine

DISTRIBUTION ALONG A MUSCLE FIBER

The distribution of extrasynaptic channels over the sarcolemma is generally assumed to be uniform, but this view may reflect mainly a lack of experimental information. In the few instances in which the matter has been tested, the data suggest otherwise.

Extrajunctional Chemosensitive Channels

In frog skeletal muscle acetylcholine (ACh), activated channels occur not only at the neuromuscular junction but also at the ends of fibers. Figure 1 shows data of Katz and Miledi (3) and concerns these "extrajunctional" cholinergic channels. Plotted on the abscissa is the distance from the tendon end; the ordinate gives the change in membrane potential produced by localized iontophoretic application of a fixed quantity of ACh. The experiment shows that the density of cholinergic channels declines steeply with distance from the tendon, dropping e-fold within approximately 70 μ. Similar results are obtained in locust muscle where excitatory channels open in response to interaction of glutamate with D-receptor (4). As with cholinergic channels in vertebrate muscle, extrajunctional glutaminergic channels in locus muscle are concentrated near the tendon ends. Judging by the response to local application of glutamate, the density of extrajunctional channels declines e-fold within 30 μm from the tendon.

After denervation of vertebrate muscle, extrajunctional cholinergic channels appear over the entire sarcolemma. In mice, some of these new extrajunctional ACh receptors are crowded together in patches so that their local density

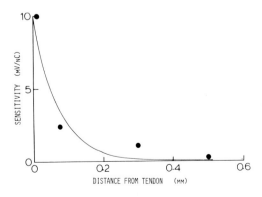

Fig. 1. Gradient of sensitivity to acetylcholine (ACh) at the muscle-tendon junction. Data are from Katz & Miledi (3) and are replotted on different coordinates. The solid line represents an exponential function declining e-fold in 70 μm. Sensitivity is given as millivolts (mV) per nanocoulomb (nC).

approaches that believed to exist in the innervated endplate region (5). Patches are 1 to 30 μm in diameter, and are found least frequently near the tendons and in the region occupied by the former endplate. In tissue-cultured rat myotubes, receptors within a patch show a lateral mobility of less than 10^{-12} cm^2/sec (6).

Sodium Channels

Slow muscle fibers of the frog ordinarily have no TTX-sensitive Na$^+$ channels, but they acquire them after denervation (7). An interesting recent paper by Schalow and Schmidt (8) reported that 9 to 14 days after denervation of slow fibers, Na$^+$ channels were found in discrete membrane areas, mostly in the middle of the fiber and close to the denervated, degenerating endplate. This discrete localization appeared to be largely transient, because the Na$^+$ channels ultimately spread virtually over the entire fiber. However, even 4 weeks after denervation, action potentials near the tendon ends tended to be smaller than those in the middle of the fiber, suggesting that some irregularities in distribution persist over long times, perhaps indefinitely. In Schalow and Schmidt's experiments, Na$^+$ channels could not readily be activated locally, and the localization of Na$^+$ channels in their work is limited in resolution to about a millimeter by the electric "cable properties" of a muscle fiber.

It is not clear whether frog twitch fibers have relatively fewer Na$^+$ channels near the tendon end. Comparison of sodium current (I_{Na}) measurements from 250-μm sections at the end (9) with others from sections at least 1 mm distant from the end (10) suggests that this might be so.

After denervation, mammalian muscle fibers show an intermittent spontaneous activity called "fibrillation." Fibrillation appears to be due to discrete patches of membrane extending less than 100 to 200 μm along a fiber and capable of spontaneous depolarizations called "fibrillatory origin potentials" (11). Fibrillatory origin potentials are TTX-sensitive, and their frequency and amplitude depend on membrane potential and previous history of electric activity, with active periods lasting 10 to 20 hours followed by inactive periods lasting 24 to 36 hours (12). Membrane patches capable of giving fibrillatory origin potentials were found most frequently near the former endplate, and next most frequently near the tendons. Patches of this kind appear to be stable, remaining stationary for 4 to 11 hours.

DISTRIBUTION BETWEEN SARCOLEMMA AND TRANSVERSE TUBULAR SYSTEM

The cell membrane of a muscle fiber is much more extensive than it appears, for example, under a dissection microscope. This is due to the presence of the transverse tubular system (TTS), and also because the sarcolemma itself is folded and contains numerous caveoli (small vesicles open to the extracellular space). The contribution of folds and caveoli to total cell membrane area is best referred to the surface of a smooth circular cylinder with the same radius as that of the muscle fiber. In a frog twitch muscle (sartorius) at physiologic

Table 2. Membrane Areas of Sarcolemma and Transverse Tubular System

Area	Values Given	Values Used
Total sarcolemma,[a] cm^2/cm^2 of smooth cylinder surface	$1.61^b - 1.81^c$	1.7
Sarcolemma proper	$1.06^b - 1.08^c$	1.07
Caveoli	$0.55^b - 0.73^c$	0.63
Transverse tubular system, cm^2/ml fiber volume	$2,200^b$ $2,800^d$	2,200

[a] A circular fiber cross section was assumed, so the values given could be higher inasmuch as this assumption is incorrect. Sarcolemma proper excludes caveoli.
[b] Reference 44.
[c] Reference 45.
[d] Reference 46.

sarcomere length (2.4 μ), this contribution is such that for every cm^2 of cylinder surface there are 1.7 cm^2 of sarcolemmal membrane (Table 2). Even larger is the contribution of the TTS, a network of narrow, tubelike invaginations of the sarcolemma. The tubules contained in 1 ml of fiber volume have enough membrane to cover 2,200 cm^2 (frog sartorius, Table 2). Since the number of tubules per unit fiber volume is constant, the tubule membrane area per unit cylinder surface grows linearly with fiber diameter, being given by 1,100 a/cm, where a is the fiber radius in cm. Total cell membrane area is the sum of sarcolemmal and tubular areas, and it exceeds the surface of our reference cylinder by the factor A_0,

$$A_0 = 1.7 + 1100 \text{ a/cm} \tag{1}$$

The ratio of tubular to sarcolemmal area is (647 a/cm) if caveoli are included and (1,028 a/cm) if they are not.

In rabbit skeletal muscle, the chemical composition of both sarcolemmal (13) and TTS membranes (14), has been investigated and can be compared. Lipid composition in the two membrane fractions is similar or identical, as if lipids are in diffusional equilibrium, but the TTS has two to three times less protein per mg of lipid than does the sarcolemma. Consistent with this suggestion of protein concentration gradients between sarcolemma and TTS, electrophysiologic analysis has shown that ionic channels are unevenly distributed, some being concentrated mostly in the sarcolemma, others in the membranes of the TTS. Most of our information on this point comes from two general approaches.

The first (and conceptually simplest) method is to disrupt the continuity between TTS and sarcolemma by sudden withdrawal of external glycerol from glycerol-loaded fibers. The mechanism of this effect is not well understood, and the degree of disruption can be highly variable. However, after successful glycerol treatment, most of the formerly continuous network of tubules is fragmented, and the lumen of the fragments is no longer accessible to extracellular markers (15). The membrane capacity falls to 2 to 4 $\mu F/cm^2$ of cylinder surface from the usual 6 to 8 $\mu F/cm^2$, indicating that all or at least a substantial amount of tubular membrane is no longer electrically a part of the cell membrane (16, 17). In fibers so treated, it is hoped that the sarcolemma can be studied in isolation, and whatever electrical property is missing is attributed to the tubular membrane.

The second method makes use of the fact that diffusional exchange between external fluid and the TTS lumen is relatively slow. Ion movements through ionic channels in the tubular membrane will, therefore, cause depletion or accumulation of the permeant ion, and electrical effects thought to be consequences of such concentration changes can be analyzed. With a given ionic channel, for instance, the fraction of electric conductance subject to accumulation and depletion effects can then be attributed to the transverse tubules.

Calcium Channels

Excitable membranes generally contain Ca^{2+} channels, which are closed at the resting potential and open in response to cell membrane depolarization. Skeletal muscle is no exception (2, 18, 47), and Figure 2 shows Ca^{2+} current (I_{Ca}) across the voltage-clamped muscle cell membrane. The Ca^{2+} channels are first opened with a strong depolarization to $+70$ mV. At $+70$ mV, total current is outward because I_{Ca} is small due to the small inward driving force for Ca^{2+}. On partial repolarization to -10 mV, however, there is a large transient inward current

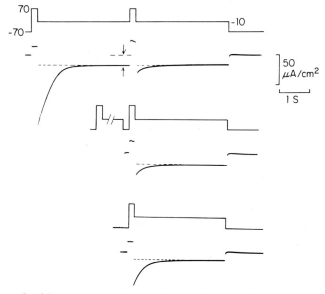

Fig. 2. Decline of calcium current (I_{Ca}) under maintained depolarization and recovery from this effect. The figure shows three pairs of traces. In each pair, the upper trace shows membrane potential; the lower trace, membrane current versus time. *Upper left*: A brief positive prepulse is given to open calcium channels; during this time there is a small outward current. The fiber is then repolarized to -10 mV, and a large inward transient I_{Ca} results. *Right*: The sequence of potential changes is repeated after intervals of 0 second (top), 0.2 second (middle), and 2 seconds (bottom); the longer the interval, the larger the second transient. Except for the top trace, current and voltage during the first sequence in each pair have been omitted. Vaseline-gap voltage clamp technique. (From unpublished data of Almers W, Fink R, Palade PT.)

(carried by Ca^{2+}) that declines to a steady value. Apparently, the decline is due not to a voltage-dependent closing of Ca^{2+} channels, but rather, to Ca^{2+} depletion from the lumen of the transverse tubules (48). The evidence is as follows. (a) The current decreases fastest at intermediate potentials, where currents are largest, and becomes slow under strong depolarization. Membrane potential–dependent processes generally show the opposite behavior, being fastest at extreme potentials. Under these and a large variety of other experimental perturbations, the rate of decline apparently depends on the current itself and only indirectly on potential. (b) At constant external Ca^{2+} activity, decline is slowed in proportion to the Ca^{2+}-buffering strength of the external solution. (c) The charge carried by the transient portion of inward current in Figure 2 (upper left) closely equals that on the Ca^{2+} ions expected to be dissolved in the tubule lumen.

If the decrease of I_{Ca} in Figure 2 is due to Ca^{2+} depletion from the tubules, some or all of the Ca^{2+} channels must reside there. At least 80% of the channels must be in the TTS because the current declines to 20% of its initial value. At least some of the remaining 20% must also be tubular, because Ca^{2+} depletion in the TTS is unlikely to be complete. Driven by radial concentration gradients, Ca^{2+} is expected to diffuse continually into the TTS from the outside, and diffusional entry of Ca^{2+} must, in the steady state, equal the tubular current. This diffusional entry is related to the initial rate at which I_{Ca} recovers while current is interrupted. Figure 2 shows current transients recorded at various intervals after a depleting pulse.

Inasmuch as the time integral of the transient current represents the amount of Ca^{2+} removed from the TTS, the corresponding time integral during a second pulse should be a measure of the Ca^{2+} gained during recovery. Figure 3 plots charge under the second transient against recovery interval. The data can be fitted by a diffusion equation (solid line), and the dashed line is an exponential chosen to be tangential to the recovery curve near the origin. Its slope there represents a current almost identical to the final current in Figure 2 (arrows, upper left). To explain the observed rate of recovery in Figure 3, one must, therefore, attribute almost the entire steady current in Figure 2 (left) to the TTS. It follows that the vast majority of Ca^{2+} channels reside in the TTS, and that the density of Ca^{2+} channels in the TTS probably exceeds that in the sarcolemma. Presence of Ca^{2+} channels in the TTS is also suggested by the finding that glycerol treatment causes a loss of I_{Ca} along with a roughly proportional loss in membrane capacity (19). The physiologic role of Ca^{2+} channels in the TTS is not clear.

Delayed Potassium Channels

A single action potential is accompanied by release of K^+ into the bathing fluid amounting to approximately 15 pmol/cm^2 of cylinder surface (26) and predominantly occurring through delayed K^+ channels. In skeletal muscle, trains of action potentials are followed by after-depolarizations lasting a few hundred milliseconds. The early literature attributed this effect to K^+ accumulation in the TTS (27), and Kirsch and colleagues (28) have recently obtained strong evidence for this view. Comparing the amplitude of after-depolarizations with

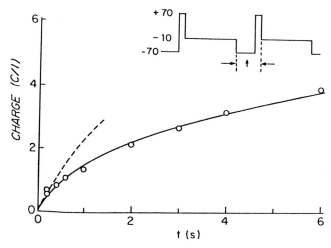

Fig. 3. Analysis of transient currents (current trace minus dashed line in Figure 2). *Ordinate.* Charge carried by the second current transient (righthand traces in Figure 2) in coulombs per liter (C/l) fiber volume. *Abscissa.* Recovery interval as defined in the inset solid curve: theoretical prediction for diffusion into a cylinder of a substance applied outside at time $(t) = 0$; the curve gives the amount of substance taken up by the cylinder and was drawn with an apparent diffusivity of $\kappa = 10^{-6}$ cm^2/sec for Ca^{2+}. Same experiment as Figure 2.

potential changes caused by step changes of external K$^+$ concentration, they calculated the tubular K$^+$ concentration at the end of a train of action potentials, and hence the amount of K$^+$ deposited in the TTS during activity. This amount was half the total K$^+$ released (26), and the authors concluded that some, perhaps half, of the delayed K$^+$ channels must reside in the tubules.

Inward Rectifier Potassium Channels

This ionic channel provides the K$^+$ permeability of the resting muscle membrane, and has long been suspected to be present in the transverse tubules (20). In the absence of permeant anions, the electric conductance of the resting membrane is thought to be due entirely to this channel. Because this conductance diminishes 2- to 4-fold after glycerol treatment, it has been concluded that 50% to 75% of inward rectifier sites reside in the transverse tubules (21). An analysis of K$^+$ depletion in muscle tubules as described above for Ca^{2+} channels leads to a similar conclusion (22).

The most recent and most ingenious analysis is that of Schneider and Chandler (23), who investigated the relationship between inward rectifier conductance and effective membrane capacity (C_{eff}). If C_{eff} is defined as electric charge supplied to the cell membrane divided by the sarcolemmal potential displacement, it is easy to see that C_{eff} should depend on the efficiency of potential spread into the TTS. When the tubule membrane conductance is low, sarcolemmal potential displacement will be experienced completely and uniformly by the tubule membranes, and C_{eff} should equal C_m, i.e., the product of total cell membrane area (sarcolemma plus tubules) times specific capacity.

When the TTS membrane conductance is high, on the other hand, tubules will act as leaky cables, a sarcolemmal potential step will suffer attenuation in the TTS, and the charge stored on the tubular membrane (and hence C_{eff}) will be less. Using C_{eff} to measure the efficiency of potential spread into the TTS, Schneider and Chandler (23) could calculate the conductance of the tubular membrane by cable theory. They could show that inward rectifier conductance is distributed between sarcolemma and TTS in the same proportion as the total membrane capacity C_m. Because specific membrane capacities in tubules and sarcolemma are probably the same, it follows that inward rectifier sites are distributed evenly over sarcolemma and tubular membranes.

Chloride Channels

The distribution of Cl^- channels is not known with precision. Early experiments on glycerol-treated fibers (21) gave the impression that Cl^- conductance resides entirely in the sarcolemma. Later experiments (24) showed that the resting membrane conductance per unit cylinder surface grows with fiber diameter. Because the same is true of the tubule membrane area, and because most of muscle membrane's resting conductance is attributed to the Cl^- channel, the finding suggests that at least some Cl^- channels reside in the tubules. A similar correlation of resting membrane conductance with fiber diameter is seen when the inward rectifier is blocked by replacing external K^+ with Rb^+, and all conductance is due to Cl^- (Almers W: unpublished observations). Experiments on rat muscle fibers show a loss of Cl^- conductance after glycerol treatment as if more than 60% (25) of the Cl^- conductance resided in the tubules. On the whole, available evidence suggests the presence of at least some Cl^- channels in the tubules, but it is difficult to be precise.

Table 3 summarizes present data on the distribution of ionic channels between sarcolemma and TTS membranes (column 1). Using the average diameter of fibers used in these experiments (last column), the ratio of tubular to sarcolemmal membrane areas (including caveoli) was calculated as discussed in connection with equation 1. Given the fraction of channels in the TTS together with the fractional membrane area of the TTS, one can calculate the average density of channels there relative to that in the sarcolemma.

Sodium Channels: A Graded Density Profile in the TTS?

Estimates of the Na^+ channel density in the TTS have been derived from experiments on glycerol-treated fibers (29) and from electrical measurements (10, 30). The first approach uses TTX, a substance that specifically blocks Na^+ channels by binding to them in a one-to-one fashion. Uptake of the toxin can be measured by radio- or bioassay, and analyzed to give the number of binding sites and the dissociation constant for the toxin-receptor complex (31, 32).

In normal frog sartorius muscle the amount of toxin bound at saturation corresponds to 300 to 400 binding sites per μm^2 of smooth cylinder surface, but after the TTS is disconnected by glycerol treatment, toxin binding is diminished to approximately 45%. No such effect is seen in crayfish nerve, which has no TTS. Toxin binding by glycerol-treated muscle is restored to

Table 3. Ionic Channels in Frog Twitch Muscle: Distribution over Transverse Tubular System and Sarcolemma

Channel	Fraction in TTS (%)	Average Density TTS/Sarcolemma[a]	Average Fiber Diameter (μm)
Extrajunctional cholinergic	Unknown	—	—
Na^+	12[c]	0.02–0.03	127–139[b]
	55[d]	0.43–0.69	55
Delayed K^+	50[e]	0.4	~90
Inward rectifier K^+	78[f]	~1	~80
	75[g]	~1	80–120
Cl^- (rat)	>60[h]	~1	~60
$Ca^{2+(48)}$	92–100	>3	97

[a] Densities were calculated as discussed in connection with equation 1.

[b] Fiber diameter was corrected to apply approximately to physiologic sarcomere length (2.4 μm) by assuming fiber shortening to occur at constant volume.

[c] Reference 10.

[d] Reference 29.

[e] Reference 28.

[f] Reference 30.

[g] Reference 23.

[h] Reference 25.

normal if the tissue is homogenized (and the disconnected tubules are "opened up") before exposure to the toxin. Therefore, the diminished binding by glycerol-treated, but otherwise intact, muscle results because half of the binding sites become inaccessible, as they would if they resided in the TTS. These experiments therefore indicate that at least 55% of the Na^+ channels are located in the TTS.

The fibers used in these experiments had an average diameter of 55 μm, and therefore 1.78 or 2.83 times more tubular than sarcolemmal area, depending on whether or not caveoli are included (see Table 1 and discussion connected with equation 1). Therefore, the average density of Na^+ channels in the TTS relative to the sarcolemma is 0.43 if Na^+ channels are excluded from caveoli, and 0.69 if they reside at equal density in caveoli and sarcolemma proper. These figures could be higher because the glycerol treatment might not have disconnected all transverse tubuli.

Calculations show (10, 30) that if tubular Na^+ channels were evenly distributed, they should have conspicuous electric effects. This is because the tubule lumen acts as a resistance in series with the tubular membranes that is largest for centrally located tubuli and less for more peripheral ones. Because of this series resistance, a change in sarcolemmal potential will reach the central portion of the TTS after a delay of a few milliseconds, so Na^+ channels there will be affected later than sarcolemmal or peripheral ones. Also, tubular Na^+ channels are expected to "escape" potential control by a voltage clamp and thus produce currents of different kinetics. Effects of this kind should be particularly conspicuous in fibers of large diameter, where tubular membranes are relatively more extensive and much of the TTS is located at greater electrical distance from the surface.

Under voltage clamp, small effects of the predicted kind are observed in large fibers, but they are smaller than expected if the density of Na$^+$ channels in the TTS is uniform and as large as the toxin-binding data would suggest (29). Assuming uniform distribution in the TTS, Hille and Campbell (10) estimate from their electrical measurements that the tubular density of Na$^+$ channels is approximately 0.013 times that in a smooth sarcolemma without caveoli. If Na$^+$ channels invade the caveoli, Hille and Campbell's estimate would become 0.013 × 1.7 = 0.022. Thus, the relative density estimated from electrical measurements is approximately 30 times smaller than is suggested by the effect of glycerol treatment on TTX binding.

The conflict between these two measurements can probably be explained if the tubular Na$^+$ channels are mostly concentrated in the peripheral portions of the TTS. Figure 4 shows a possible profile, with the density of Na$^+$ channels in the TTS relative to that on the sarcolemma plotted as a function of radial coordinate. The curves are given by

$$\text{Relative density } = \frac{I_0(r/\lambda_T)}{I_0(a/\lambda_T)} \qquad (2)$$

where r is the distance from the center; a is the fiber radius; $I_0(x)$ is the modified Bessel function of order zero and argument x; and λ_T is a constant whose possible significance is stated below. Such a relationship would be predicted if Na$^+$ channels were inserted only into the sarcolemma and had to invade the tubular membranes by lateral diffusion. With a finite lifetime, not all Na$^+$ channels will survive long enough to reach the center, so the channel density there will be less than in the sarcolemma or in peripheral portions of the TTS. Indeed, λ_T in this model gives an average radial distance a channel may expect to cover on its lifelong journey into the TTS. This distance depends on the product of lateral diffusion coefficient, D, and average lifetime, τ_{Na}, of sodium

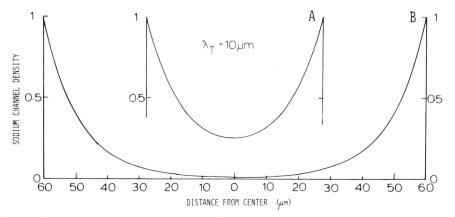

Fig. 4. Hypothetical profiles for the number of sodium channels per unit membrane area in the transverse tubular system. Profiles apply to two fibers of circular cross section with diameters of 55 μm (curve A) and 120 μm (curve B). Curves were drawn according to equation 4 with λ_T as indicated.

channels:

$$\lambda_T = \sqrt{0.33\tau_{Na}D} \tag{3}$$

where the "network factor" 0.33 takes account of the fact that diffusion paths along transverse tubules are tortuous (33). Equations [2] and [3] can be obtained by a treatment similar to that given for Ca^{2+}-diffusion in transverse tubules (48).

In Figure 4, fiber radii have been chosen to approximate those in the experiments of Jaimovitch and colleagues (29) (55 μm, curve A) or Hille and Campbell (10) (120 μm, curve B), and the curves were drawn with $\lambda_T = 10$ μm. For curve A, this gives an average density of 0.6, i.e., 0.6 times that of the sarcolemma, as in Jaimovitch and assocites (29). The density is 0.25 in the center and approaches 1.0 on the periphery; 80% of all tubular Na^+ channels are within 10 μm of the sarcolemma. In curve B, the central density is 0.015, the average density is 0.3, and 80% of all channels are located within 15 μm of the sarcolemma.

We can now suggest why tubular Na^+ currents fail to stand out prominently in voltage-clamp recordings even though their density is expected to be large. If Na^+ channels are distributed as in Figure 4, there would be little resistance in series with most of them and they would behave electrically like sarcolemmal channels. On the other hand, because glycerol treatment affects tubuli regardless of radial position, all of them could become inaccessible to TTX after the treatment.

Uniform-distribution and peripheral-location models for tubular Na^+ channels also make different predictions for the effect of fiber diameter. Under uniform distribution, the number of tubular Na^+ channels per unit cylinder surface should increase with diameter, just as a membrane capacity does. The average distance (and electric resistance) between tubular channels and sarcolemma should also increase. As a consequence, fiber diameter should have a strong effect on the shape of the muscle action potential, particularly the early after-depolarization, which is believed to be due to the activity of tubular Na^+ channels. Such an effect is not found experimentally (30). Under the peripheral-location hypothesis, on the other hand, neither the number of tubular Na^+ channels per unit cylinder surface nor their average distance from the sarcolemma is expected to vary strongly over the range of diameters observed (50 to 120 μm). This might explain why the shape of the action potential does not depend strongly on fiber diameter.

DISTRIBUTION AND LATERAL MOBILITY

It is not clear how the uneven distribution of ionic channels comes about, but it is of interest that for some ionic channels, the observed gradients in density are probably not too steep to be consistent with measured lateral mobilities. One such example is the extrajunctional cholinergic channels concentrated at the tendon end of frog twitch fibers. Suppose, for the sake of argument, that new channels are inserted only at the extreme tendon end, and that channels, once inserted, are free to diffuse down the fiber. If their average lifetime, τ, is finite, then so is the average distance they can diffuse along the sarcolemma before they die off. For one-dimensional diffusion and first-order kinetics for death of cholinergic channels, this distance is

$$\lambda S = \sqrt{\tau D_{\text{ch}}} \qquad (4)$$

where D_{ch} is the lateral diffusion coefficient for cholinergic receptors. Channel density as a function of distance can be shown to be given by

$$\text{Density} = A \exp(-x/\lambda S) \qquad (5)$$

where $x = 0$ at the tendon end and A is a constant proportional to the rate at which receptors are inserted. The average lifetime, τ, for extrajunctional receptors is of the order of 10^5 seconds: for rat diaphragm in vivo, $\tau = 24$ hours (34); for rat and chick myotubes, $\tau = 32$ to 35 hours (35). The lateral diffusion coefficient in rat myotubes is of the order of 10^{-10} cm^2/sec (36). These values suggest that $\lambda_S \simeq 33$ μm, similar to (but less than) the value of 70 μm suggested by the data of Katz and Miledi (3) (Fig. 1).

Evidently, both the survival time and the diffusion coefficient of cholinergic receptors are sufficiently low to prevent lateral diffusion from establishing uniform receptor density. Thus, the observed longitudinal gradients of receptor density do not conflict with lateral mobility.

With Na$^+$ channels, survival time and lateral mobility are unknown, but if they are the same as with cholinergic channels, the characteristic distance λ_T for radial spread in a model as in Figure 4 and equations 2 and 3 would be approximately 18 μm. This is of the same order of magnitude as suggested in Figure 4 on the basis of TTX binding data (29).

LATERAL MOBILITY OF SODIUM CHANNELS

In an attempt to measure lateral mobility of Na$^+$ channels in the sarcolemma, we took advantage of a finding (37, 38) that Na$^+$ channels can be destroyed irreversibly by irradiation with ultraviolet (UV) light. In frog myelinated nerve, the action spectrum for this effect shows a maximum at 280 nm, as if UV light attacked an aromatic amino acid in a protein.

Figure 5A shows approximately to scale a piece cut from a single fiber (stippled). Threads of stopcock grease or vaseline 150 to 200 μm thick are laid across the fiber to isolate electrically a narrow (60-μm) section in the middle. This section is bathed in Ringer solution while the cut ends on either side are soaking in isotonic CsF. Recording transmembrane potential through the one cut end and injecting electric current through the other, the central section can be voltage-clamped as described by Hille and Campbell (10). The experimental records in Figure 5 (bottom) show current flowing through Na$^+$ channels versus time; they were recorded during step depolarizations from -90 mV to approximately 10 mV. The large trace was recorded before, the smaller one after an approximately 10-second exposure of the central compartment to UV light (280 nm). The time course of current is unchanged, but its amplitude is diminished approximately 10-fold.

The entire shaded area in Figure 5 (left) was irradiated by the UV beam, but

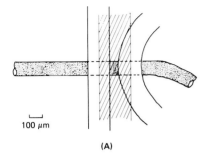

(A)

100 µm

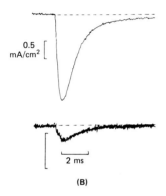

0.5 mA/cm²

2 ms

(B)

Fig. 5. (A) Schematic drawing of fiber (stippled) with grease seals in place. A quartz coverslip was placed over the seals to exclude a grease film that might otherwise have formed at the air-water interface of the central compartment. A beam of ultraviolet light could be generated to irradiate the shaded area. The beam was focused in the center of the fiber. **(B)** Sodium current during a depolarizing step from -90 mV to 0 mV first before, then after, 10-second irradiation with 280-nm light. In the lower trace, five sweeps were graphically superimposed.

measurements showed that the grease strongly absorbed UV light (a 170-µm layer attenuated the beam more than 100-fold). Consequently, we expect that the UV light reaches effectively only a 60-µm ring of membrane around the muscle fiber. If lateral diffusion of Na$^+$ channels proceeds rapidly, one may expect them to move into this ring of membrane from the protected membrane underneath the grease seals, leading to a slow recovery of Na$^+$ current from the central compartment. Figure 6 tests this point, plotting peak Na$^+$ current during successive depolarizations against time. Sodium current remained constant for 20 minutes, then declined 10-fold during irradiation, but showed no significant recovery thereafter.

To analyze the experiment quantitatively, let us assume that the grease seals cast a sharp shadow on the fiber, allowing Na$^+$ channels to be destroyed only in a ring of sarcolemma of the same width, b, as the central compartment. Current is collected from a wider area of width $(b + 2d)$, however, because the strings of grease are rounded and hide beneath them narrow strips of membrane of width d, one on each side, that are in electric continuity with the central pool but receive no UV light. When lateral diffusion occurs after irradiation, it will first occur between the protected and the irradiated zone, leading to no gain in Na$^+$ channels in the membrane area from which we collect current. New channels will be gained only after the protected zone has been partially depleted, and a gradient in density has been established between it and the membrane in direct contact with the grease seals. Therefore, recovery of Na$^+$ current is

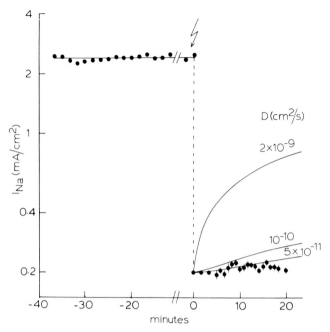

Fig. 6. Peak amplitude of sodium currents (I_{Na}) during repeated step depolarizations as in Figure 5B. Irradiation with 280-nm light at the arrow. Theoretical curves show predicted recovery of I_{Na} if Na^+ channels can move into the irradiated patch by lateral diffusion in the sarcolemma and with diffusion coefficients (D) as indicated. No allowance was made for sarcolemmal folding, for the presence of caveoli, or for the possibility of diffusional exchange between transverse tubules and sarcolemma.

expected to occur after a delay. Starting from equation 4 in Carslaw and Jaeger (39), one can show that the average density of channels contained in the membrane from which we collect current, v, is given by the following equation:

$$v = \frac{V}{b + 2d}\left\{ d\, \text{erfc}(-d/T) + (b + d)\, \text{erfc}\left(\frac{b + d}{T}\right) \right.$$
$$\left. - \frac{T}{\sqrt{\pi}}\left[\exp\left(\frac{-(b + d)^2}{T^2}\right) - \exp\frac{-d^2}{T^2} \right] \right\} \quad (6)$$

where erfc(x) is the error function complement of argument x,

$$T = 2\sqrt{Dt} \quad (7)$$

and V is the density before irradiation; v and V are assumed to be proportional to the total current collected.

Equation 6 contains only measurable quantities except for d and D, the lateral diffusion coefficient. An upper limit for d can be obtained by attributing the entire Na^+ current remaining after irradiation to the protected zone underneath the grease seals. For the experiment in Figure 6, this suggests that $d = 2.7\ \mu m$, so $v/V = 0.1$ when $t = 0$. D is adjusted empirically, and the curves in Figure 6 are plots of equation 6 with values for D as indicated. A value of $D = 4 \times 10^{-9}$ cm^2/sec was measured for rhodopsin in frog and toad rod outer segments (40), which clearly is too high to fit our data. However, $D = 10^{-10}$ cm²/sec, the value measured for cholinergic channels in rat myotubes, may be consistent with them. The experiment suggests that lateral diffusion of Na⁺ channels in the sarcolemma along an adult frog twitch fiber is as slow as, or slower than, diffusion of cholinergic channels along rat myotubes.

CONCLUSION

Among the ionic channels found in skeletal muscle, most are unevenly distributed over the cell membrane. In some cases, such distribution probably has physiologic significance. It is not difficult to imagine, for instance, that the distribution of Na⁺ channels between sarcolemma and TTS may be carefully optimized. With too few functional Na⁺ channels in the TTS, radial spread of an action potential there is strongly decremental, so that the electric signal in central portions of the TTS is too small for reliable control of contractile activation (41, 42). With too many Na⁺ channels, on the other hand, one expects that the inevitably delayed activity in the TTS may become strong enough to reexcite the meanwhile repolarized sarcolemma. The fiber would give multiple action potentials in response to a single nerve impulse, a generally undesirable result. Similarly, having too many delayed K⁺ channels in the TTS could result in excessive K⁺ accumulation during nerve impulses (33), giving rise to large after-depolarizations (28). These in turn may result in repetitive discharges similar to those observed in goats with congenital myotonia (43). Keeping the density of K⁺ channels in the TTS low may thus be physiologically significant. In other cases, however, the benefits of uneven distribution are unclear. It is hard to see, for instance, why Ca²⁺ channels should be concentrated in the TTS or cholinergic channels near the tendon end.

It is still unknown how a cell decides which ionic channels go where. Here we explored the hypothesis that discrete location results from discrete insertion into the membrane, but this possibility is only one among many. Nevertheless, our analysis suggests that for ACh receptors and Na⁺ channels, the observed lateral concentration gradients are not inconsistent with a fluid lipid bilayer matrix. On the basis of (admittedly incomplete) data on lifetime and mobility, it would appear that channels remain discretely localized simply because they do not survive long enough to diffuse very far.

ACKNOWLEDGMENT

We thank Ms. Lea Miller for her expert secretarial help and Dr. Bertil Hille and Dr. Peter Detwiler for reading the manuscript. This work was supported by U.S. Public Health Service grant no. AM-17803.

REFERENCES

1. Adrian RH, Chandler WK, Hodgkin AL: Slow changes in potassium permeability in skeletal muscle. J Physiol (Lond) 208:645–668, 1970

2. Palade PT, Almers W: Slow Na^+ and Ca^{++} currents across the membrane of frog skeletal muscle fibres. Biophys J 21(abstr):168a, 1978

3. Katz B, Miledi R: Further observations on the distribution of acetylcholine-reactive sites in skeletal muscle. J Physiol (Lond) 170:379–388, 1964

4. Cull-Candy SG: Glutamate sensitivity and distribution of receptors along normal and denervated locust muscle fibres. J Physiol (Lond) 276:165–181, 1978

5. Ko PK, Anderson MJ, Cohen MW: Denervated skeletal muscle fibers develop discrete patches of high acetylcholine receptor density. Science 196:540–542, 1977

6. Axelrod D, Ravdin P, Koppel DE, et al: Lateral motion of fluorescently labeled acetylcholine receptors in membranes of developing muscle fibers. Proc Natl Acad Sci USA 73:4594–4598, 1976

7. Miledi R, Stefani E, Steinbach AB: Introduction of the action potential mechanism in slow muscle fibers of the frog. J Physiol (Lond) 217:737–754, 1971

8. Schalow G, Schmidt H: Local development of action potentials in slow muscle fibres after complete or partial denervation. J Physiol (Lond) 203:445–457, 1979

9. Adrian RH, Chandler WK, Hodgkin AL: Voltage clamp experiments in striated muscle fibres. J Physiol (Lond) 208:607–644, 1970

10. Hille B, Campbell DT: An improved vaseline gap voltage clamp for skeletal muscle fibers. J Gen Physiol 67:399–416, 1976

11. Purves D, Sakmann B: Membrane properties underlying spontaneous activity of denervated muscle fibres. J Physiol (Lond) 239:125–153, 1974

12. Purves D, Sakmann B: The effect of contractile activity on fibrillation and extrajunctional acetylcholine-sensitivity in rat muscle maintained in organ culture. J Physiol (Lond) 237:157–182, 1974

13. Mahrla Z, Zachar J: Lipid composition of isolated external and internal skeletal muscle membranes. Comp Biochem Physiol 47B:493–502, 1974

14. Lau YH, Caswell AH, Brunschwig J-P, et al: Lipid analysis and freeze-fracture studies on isolated transverse tubules and sarcoplasmic reticulum subfractions of skeletal muscle. J Biol Chem 254:540–546, 1979

15. Franzini-Armstrong C, Venosa RA, Horowicz P: Morphology and accessibility of the transverse tubular system in frog sartorius muscle after glycerol treatment. J Membr Biol 14:197–212, 1973

16. Gage PW, Eisenberg RS: Capacitance of the surface and transverse tubular membrane of frog sartorius muscle fibers. J Gen Physiol 53:265–278, 1969

17. Chandler WK, Rakowski RF, Schneider MF: Effects of glycerol treatment and maintained depolarization on charge movement in skeletal muscle. J Physiol (Lond) 254:285–316, 1976

18. Sanchez JA, Stefani E: Inward calcium current in twitch muscle fibres of the frog. J Physiol (Lond) 283:197–209, 1978

19. Nicole-Siri L, Sanchez JA, Stefani E: Effect of glycerol treatment on the calcium current of frog skeletal muscle. J Physiol (Lond) 305:87–96, 1980

20. Hodgkin AL, Horowicz P: The effect of sudden changes in ionic concentrations of the membrane potential of single muscle fibres. J Physiol (Lond) 153:370–385, 1960

21. Eisenberg RS, Gage PW: Ionic conductances of the surface and transverse tubular membranes of frog sartorius fibers. J Gen Physiol 53:279–297, 1969

22. Almers W: The decline of potassium permeability during extreme hyperpolarization in frog skeletal muscle. J Physiol (Lond) 225:57–83, 1972

23. Schneider MF, Chandler WK: Effects of membrane potential on the capacitance of skeletal muscle fibers. J Gen Physiol 67:125–164, 1976

24. Hodgkin AL, Nakajima S: The effects of diameter on the electrical constants of frog skeletal muscle fibres. J Physiol (Lond) 221:105–120, 1972

25. Palade PT, Barchi RL: Characteristics of the chloride conductance in muscle fibers of the rat diaphragm. J Gen Physiol 69:325–342, 1977

26. Hodgkin AL, Horowicz P: Movements of Na^+ and K^+ in single muscle fibres. J Physiol (Lond) 145:405–432, 1959

27. Freygang WH, Goldstein DA, Hellman DC: The after-potential that follows trains of impulses in frog muscle fibers. J Gen Physiol 47:929–952, 1964

28. Kirsch GE, Nichols RA, Nakajima S: Delayed rectification in the transverse tubules. J Gen Physiol 70:1–21, 1978

29. Jaimovitch E, Venosa RA, Shrager P, et al: Density and distribution of tetrodotoxin receptors in normal and detubulated frog sartorius muscle. J Gen Physiol 67:399–416, 1976

30. Adrian RH, Peachey LD: Reconstruction of the action potential of frog sartorius muscle. J Physiol (Lond) 235:103–131, 1973

31. Almers W, Levinson SR: Tetrodotoxin binding to normal and depolarized frog muscle and the conductance of a single sodium channel. J Physiol (Lond) 247:483–509, 1975

32. Ritchie JM, Rogart RB: The binding of saxitoxin and tetrodotoxin to excitable tissue. Rev Physiol Biochem Pharmacol 79:1–50, 1978

33. Almers W: Potassium concentration changes in the transverse tubules of vertebrate skeletal muscle. Fed Proc 39:1527–1532, 1980

34. Berg DK, Hall ZW: Loss of α-bungarotoxin from junctional and extrajunctional acetylcholine receptors in rat diaphraghm muscle in vivo and in organ culture. J Physiol (Lond) 252:771–789, 1975

35. Devreotes PN, Fambrough DM: Acetylcholine receptor turnover in membranes of developing muscle fibers. J Cell Biol 65:335–358, 1975

36. Axelrod D, Ravdin PM, Podleski T: Control of acetylcholine receptor mobility and distribution in cultured muscle membranes: a fluorescence study. Biochim Biophys Acta 511:23–28, 1978

37. Fox JM: Selective blocking of the nodal sodium channels by ultraviolet radiation. I. Phenomenology of the radiation effect. Pfluegers Arch 351:287–301, 1974

38. Oxford GS, Pooler JP: Ultraviolet photoalteration of ion channels in voltage-clamped lobster giant axons. J Membr Biol 20:13–30, 1975

39. Carslaw HS, Jaeger JE: *Conduction of Heat in Solids*, 2nd ed. Clarendon Press, Oxford, 1959, p 54

40. Poo M, Cone RA: Lateral diffusion of rhodopsin in the photoreceptor membrane. Nature 247:438–441, 1974

41. Costantin LL: The role of sodium current in the radial spread of contraction in frog muscle fibers. J Gen Physiol 55:703–715, 1970

42. Bastian J, Nakajima S: Action potential in the transverse tubules and its role in the activation of skeletal muscle. J Gen Physiol 63:257–278, 1974

43. Adrian RH, Bryant SH: On the repetitive discharge in myotonic muscle fibers. J Physiol (Lond) 240:505–515, 1974

44. Mobley BA, Eisenberg BR: Sizes of components in frog skeletal muscle by methods of sterology. J Gen Physiol 66:31–46, 1975

45. Dulhunty AF, Franzini-Armstrong C: The relative contributions of the folds and caveolae to the surface membrane of frog skeletal muscle fibres at different sarcomere lengths. J Physiol (Lond) 250:513–539, 1975

46. Peachey LD: The sarcoplasmic reticulum and transverse tubules of the frog's sartorius. J Cell Biol 25:209–231, 1965

47. Almers W, Palade PT: Slow calcium and potassium currents across frog muscle membrane: Measurements with a vaseline-gap technique. J Physiol (Lond) 312: in press, 1981

48. Almers W, Fink R, Palade PT: Calcium depletion in frog muscle tubules: The decline of calcium current under maintained depolarization. J Physiol (Lond) 312: in press, 1981

DISCUSSION

Dr. Andrew Engel: Decreased density of Na^+ channels in the transverse (T) tubules in the center of the fiber is a very provocative hypothesis, but it would be nice to confirm it cytochemically; ^{3}H-labeled tetrodotoxin (TTX) and autoradiography come to mind.

Dr. Wolfard Almers: We have tried that and did not get enough binding. You have to average about 10,000 serial sections to do that, which seemed prohibitive. It would be better, maybe, to use an iodinated scorpion toxin, which has a higher activity. That would certainly be worth doing.

Dr. Robert Rakowski: I am not sure that you entirely resolved the discrepancy between measurements of Na^+ channel density based on glycerol shock technique and the measurement based on a model calculation of Na^+ current. Is it not true, e.g., that the glycerol shock technique, when used routinely, does not produce 100% detubulation? One would expect to find a very high apparent surface density because many of the tubules are not disconnected from the surface.

Dr. Wolfhard Almers: I would disagree. I think the measurement sets the lower limit on the density in the tubule, because as you say, not all tubules are disconnected.

Dr. Edson Albuquerque: Did you find TTX-insensitive sites dispersed along the T-tubular system in a way similar to that observed on the presynaptic membrane? Could these TTX-insensitive sites explain some of the discrepancy seen between the very inner portions of the T-tubular system and the area at the interface with the sarcolemmal membrane?

Dr. Wolfhard Almers: Electrically, all Na^+ currents and innervated adult frog twitch fibers are TTX sensitive. When you apply TTX, the current all goes away, so it is believed that there are no TTX-insensitive Na^+ channels in these fibers. There are some in denervated rat muscle fibers, but not in frog twitch fibers.

29
Biochemical Characterization of the Sarcolemmal Sodium Channel

Robert L. Barchi, MD, PhD

The signal for initiation of skeletal muscle contraction spreads outward from the neuromuscular junction as a regenerative action potential along the muscle surface and into the transverse tubular system to reach the sites of excitation-contraction coupling. This action potential is the result of transient local changes in membrane conductance first to sodium ions (Na^+) and subsequently to potassium ions (K^+) (1). These conductance changes are produced by separate ion-specific channels through the membrane that change their characteristics as a reproducible function of transmembrane potential and time (2). To understand fully the mechanisms that produce the action potential, it is ultimately necessary to identify and isolate the intrinsic membrane proteins that form these unique voltage-dependent channels.

Isolation of the voltage-dependent Na^+ channel from excitable membranes has proved difficult for several reasons. First, the channel is usually identified by virtue of the ionic currents it controls; measurement of such currents requires an intact membrane and an ion concentration gradient. Once the integrity of the membrane is destroyed during the process of isolation, this functional means of identification is lost. A second major difficulty that has arisen during the course of purification efforts involves the potential instability of this channel complex once it is removed from its native membrane environment.

A solution to the first of these problems is provided by the availability of several classes of naturally occurring neurotoxins that bind with high specificity to the Na^+ channel complex. Saxitoxin (STX) and tetrodotoxin (TTX) are small polar toxins that bind to the channel and block the movement of ions through it without modifying the conformational changes associated with the gating process (3). The current hypothesis is that these toxins actually insert themselves partially into the outer opening of the channel itself, and thus they provide a valuable indicator for the presence of this structure. Equilibrium dissociation constants for the binding of these two toxins to the Na^+ channel are in the low nanomolar range for most tissues studied, and at these concentrations toxin binding is quite specific. Unfortunately, this binding is rapidly reversible, so that equilibrium binding determinations must be used if either STX or TTX binding is to be used as a marker for the Na^+ channel during purification.

Both STX and TTX can now be prepared in radiolabeled form (4, 5). Titration of STX is considerably easier and yields a product with high specific activity and biologic purity. Saxitoxin binding to isolated sarcolemma can be quantified by rapid filtration on micropore glass filters as long as care is taken to wash membrane fragments sufficiently rapidly that back-exchange of bound toxin is avoided (6). In many cases complete binding curves sufficient for Scatchard or double-reciprocal analysis can be constructed with less than 1 mg of purified membrane protein.

The binding of ^3H-STX to rat muscle sarcolemma has properties that are dependent on ionic strength, pH, temperature, and the cation composition of the incubation medium (7). In normal Ringer's solution at pH 7.5 and 0° C, the equilibrium dissociation constant (K_d) for STX binding is 1.4×10^{-9} M. Toxin binding to the voltage-dependent channel in sarcolemma is competitively inhibited by monovalent cations in the sequence $Tl^+ > Li^+ > Na^+ > K^+ > Rb^+ > Cs^+$.

Calcium and magnesium also inhibit binding in an apparently competitive fashion. The K_d exhibits a positive Q_{10} of 1.3, moving toward higher STX values with increasing temperature. The rate constant for the dissociation (k^{-1}) and association (k^{+1}) processes are quite temperature dependent in rat sarcolemma, with Q_{10} values of 2.6 and 1.9, respectively. The toxin binding site contains a titratable residue that, when protonated, blocks the binding of STX. In sarcolemma this residue has an apparent pK of 6.0.

SOLUBILIZING THE CHANNEL

As identified by STX-binding ability, 50% to 75% of the membrane voltage-dependent Na^+ channels can be solubilized from purified sarcolemma using non-ionic detergents of medium chain length such as Triton X-100, NP-40, or Lubrol PX (8). Effective solubilization can also be obtained with sodium cholate, although the channels are less stable in this detergent than in those previously mentioned. This solubilized channel STX-binding component (SBC) may represent all or only a portion of the original Na^+ channel complex. For various reasons (see later), we believe that this component is, in fact, a major portion of the channel if not the entire channel; this bias is indicated by the interchangable usage of "SBC" and "solubilized channel" in the remainder of this discussion. The reader is cautioned, however, to keep the limitations of this assumption in mind.

Because effective solubilization of the Na^+ channel precludes use of the usual filtration assays, a different approach is required to determine specific STX binding to the solubilized channel protein. Binding is quantified using a modification of the microcolumn technique of Lefkowitz and associates (9) with

2.5-ml columns of Sephadex G-25. Gel filtration is carried out rapidly (<30 seconds) by centrifugation of these minicolumns overlayered with the samples to be assayed for toxin binding. Unbound STX partitions into the gel matrix as a sample moves through the column and is retained; bound toxin is spun through with the column-excluded volume. This approach allows for rapid separation of bound and free toxin and quantification of specifically bound toxin in the solubilized system.

The equilibrium dissociation binding constant for STX to the solubilized SBC is the same as that obtained in intact sarcolemma (8). This binding constant is temperature dependent, with a Q_{10} of approximately 1.4 within the temperature range 0 to 15° C. Rate constants for dissociation of the toxin-channel complex measured at temperatures between 0 and 10° C also correspond to those measured in intact sarcolemma. Competitive inhibition of STX binding by monovalent cations is seen after solubilization with the same sequence of cation binding as was observed in intact membranes. This sequence is not dependent on the phospholipid used to form mixed detergent-lipid micelles [phosphatidylcholine (PC), phosphatidylethanolansine (PE), Asolectin] and therefore does not appear to reflect a secondary effect on surface charge.

Stability of SBC

Stability of the solubilized Na^+ channel depends critically on temperature and on the presence of phospholipid in its environment. An optimal ratio of phospholipid molecules to detergent molecules must be maintained during solubilization and subsequent manipulation of the channel, or STX binding is lost. During initial solubilization, phospholipid is provided by endogenous lipid in the sarcolemma; subsequently, exogenous phospholipid must be provided for running buffers and other diluents (8, 10). Adjustment of the membrane protein concentration relative to detergent concentration during solubilization to maintain detergent:phospholipid molar ratios in the range of 5:1 to 7:1 provides the best stability for the solubilized channel. In our laboratory, we routinely use a final detergent concentration of 1% NP-40, a final sarcolemma concentration of 1.5 mg/ml 0.5 mM calcium, and 20 mM HEPES (pH 7.4) for initial solubilization. Under these conditions, approximately 60% of the total sarcolemmal STX binding sites are obtained in solution after centrifugation for 1 hour at 100,000 ×g.

Further manipulation of the solubilized channel SBC requires continued maintenance of an optimal phospholipid:detergent environment. If the solubilized SBC is diluted with buffer containing detergent alone, phospholipid molecules will be exchanged from the initial mixed detergent-phospholipid micelles into the pure detergent micelles. Under these circumstances, rapid loss of specific STX binding capacity is observed. Our typical buffers contain contain 0.1% NP-40 with phospholipid added for a detergent:lipid molar ratio of 5:1. Phosphatidylcholine, phosphatidylethanolamine, or mixed soybean phosphatides are effective in preserving channel stability, whereas phosphatidyl serine or cholesterol alone is not.

In the presence of an optimal detergent:phospholipid ratio the solubilized Na^+ channel SBC has a half-life at 0° C in excess of 48 hours. Increasing temperature markedly reduces stability. Typical rate constants for decay of specific binding activity at 15° C averaged 0.027 min^{-1} and increased to 0.14 min^{-1} at 25° C.

Column Chromatography

The solubilized Na$^+$ channel SBC from sarcolemma carries a significant negative charge at neutral pH. The solubilized SBC is retained by diethylamino-ethyl Sephadex and can be eluted with an ionic strength gradient generated with choline chloride. Unfortunately, in this system a significant percentage of total membrane protein is also retained by the column and elutes in a similar ionic strength range as the solubilized SBC. Relatively little effective purification is obtained, and this column is not really useful as a step in an overall purification protocol.

Based on these results, however, several column matrices exhibiting weaker ion-exchange properties were investigated. The most effective of these was a column synthesized with a guanidinium group attached to a 19-atom spacer arm having relatively hydrophilic characteristics and immobilized to sepharose beads (Fig. 1). The solubilized SBC is quantitatively retained by this column, but binding characteristics of the functional group are sufficiently weak that more than 95% of the total sarcolemmal membrane protein passes through the column without being adsorbed, and significant enrichment of the SBC is obtained (8).

The concentration of STX binding sites in crude muscle homogenates ranges between 0.1 and 0.3 pmol of STX bound per mg of protein. Purification of sarcolemma yields 20- to 40-fold improvement in specific activity, with toxin binding values of 5 to 9 pmol/mg in purified membranes being typical. When solubilized sarcolemma is applied to the guanidinium column, the material not retained by the column has STX binding capacities of less than 0.5 pmol/mg of protein if column binding capacity is not exceeded. Subsequent elution of the guanidinium column with a 100 to 800 mM gradient of choline chloride displaces a symmetric peak of STX binding material having a maximal specific activity of 80 to 140 pmol/mg of protein, roughly 10- to 20-fold higher than the initial sarcolemma and 500- to 1,000-fold higher than crude homogenate.

Because the voltage-dependent Na$^+$ channel is by definition an intrinsic membrane protein, it seemed reasonable to assume that it would contain sugar residues on its externally exposed terminal. Based on this possibility, the binding of the SBC to immobilized lectins was investigated. A total of 12 lectins were studied having specificities for a variety of sugar residues (Table 1). Significant binding of the solubilized channel was noted to four of these.

Eighty per cent or more of the solubilized SBC could be retained by concanavalin A immobilized to sepharose beads. However, it proved difficult to dissociate this bound SBC with reasonable concentrations of mannose or α-methyl-D-mannoside, possibly because of multisite attachment of the lectin to the channel. This binding strongly suggests the presence of mannose or glucose residues in the glycosylated portion of the Na$^+$ channel.

Solubilized SBC was also quantitatively retained by a column containing immobilized wheat germ agglutinin (WGA) (Fig. 2). This column has highest

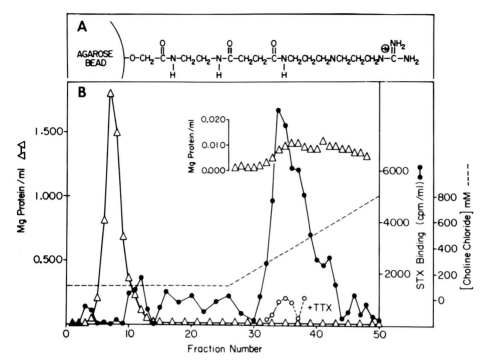

Fig. 1. (A) A weak anion-exchange column was synthesized by immobilizing a guanidinium functional group to agarose beads by a 19-atom flexible hydrophilic spacer. (B) Ion-exchange chromatography of solubilized sarcolemma on a 2.6×8 cm column of agarose beads containing the functional group in A. The column was equilibrated in 0.1% NP-40/phosphatidylcholine, 100 mM choline chloride, 50 mM KH_2PO_4 (pH 7.4). Sarcolemma was solubilized (2 mg of protein per ml) with 1% NP-40, and a total of 20 mg were applied at a flow of 4 ml/min. The column was eluted at 3 ml/min with a 100 to 800 mM choline chloride gradient in the column running buffer; 8-ml fractions were collected. Symbols: $\triangle$, protein; $\bullet$, total ^{3}H-STX binding; $\bigcirc$, nonspecific ^{3}H-STX binding.

specificity for N-acetylglucosamine residues with lower affinity for sialic acid. The SBC bound to this immobilized lectin was not displaced by increasing ionic strength (0 to 800 mM choline chloride) but was specifically displaced by a relatively low concentration of N-acetylglucosamine (20 mM).

Treatment of intact sarcolemma with the enzyme neuraminidase, producing progressive cleavage of terminal N-acetylneuraminic acid residues from exposed glycoproteins, results in correspondingly less binding of subsequently solubilized SBC to the WGA column. Conversely, treatment of intact sarcolemma with terminal glucosidase, an enzyme that cleaves terminal N-acetylglucoside residues, has no effect on binding of the solubilized SBC to this column. Thus, it appears that binding to the WGA column may be mediated by terminal sialic acid residues rather than by terminal or internal N-acetylglucosamine residues.

More than 95% of the membrane protein from crude solubilized sarcolemma passes through a column of immobilized WGA without being bound, whereas the solubilized SBC can be quantitatively retained if the capacity of the gel is not exceeded. Subsequent elution of the column with a gradient of N-acetyl-

Table 1. Binding of Solubilized Saxitoxin Binding Component (SBC) to Immobilized Lectins

Lectin	Specificity	% SBC Bound	Lectin Density (mg lectin/ml gel)	Apparent Binding Capacity (pmol/ml gel)
Concanavalin A	D-Glucose, D-mannose 8-methyl derivatives	85–90	10	4.0
Wheat germ agglutinin	(N-acetylglucosamine)n N-acetylneuraminic acid	100	5	2.0
Lens culinaris (lentil)	D-Mannose, D-glucose, methyl derivatives	30	2	0.20–0.85
Ricinus communis (Type 1) (castor bean)	Lactose, β-methyl-D-galactose	25	4	0.85
Ulex europeus	α-L-(−)-Fucose	8	4	0.16
Helix pomatia	N-acetyl galactosamine	Variable	1	Variable
Glycine max (soybean)	N-acetyl galactosamine	0	4	0
Dalichos biflorus (Anti-A or horse gram)	N-acetyl galactosamine	0	2	0
Abrus precatorius (Jequirity bean)	D-galactose	0	1	0
Arachis hypogaea (peanut)	D-galactose	0	5	0
Bandeiraea simplificolia I	D-galactose	0	4	0

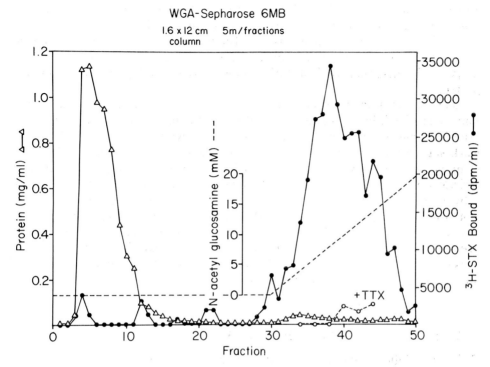

Fig. 2. Affinity chromatography of solubilized sarcolemma on a column containing wheat germ agglutinin immobilized to Sepharose 6B beads. The column (1×3 cm) was equilibrated in 0.1% NP-40/phosphatidylcholine, 400 mM choline chloride, and 50 mM KH_2PO_4 (pH 7.4). Sarcolemma was solubilized (2 mg of protein per ml) with 1% NP-40, and 30 mg were applied to the column in running buffer at a flow of 1 ml/min. The column was eluted with a 0 to 20 mM gradient of N-acetylglucosamine at the same flow; 5-ml fractions were collected. Symbols: $\triangle$, total protein; $\bullet$, total ^{3}H-STX binding.

glucosamine (0 to 20 mM) results in nearly quantitative recovery of the bound SBC. This column in itself allows 15- to 20-fold enrichment of the sarcolemmal SBC.

Purifying SBC

A scheme for purification of the SBC of the mammalian Na^+ channel from sarcolemma was devised using the two column procedures discussed above (8). The initial step in purification involves isolation of sarcolemma from rat muscle; this isolation step provides a significant increase in specific activity of Na^+ channels and is a prerequisite for successful purification. Purified sarcolemma is solubilized under optimal conditions in Triton X-100 or NP-40 and is chromatographed on an ion-exchange column containing the immobilized guanidinium groups described above. The peak eluted from this column with a choline chloride gradient is applied directly to a second column containing immobilized wheat germ lectin without prior concentration or dialysis. After sufficient washing, the lectin column is eluted with a shallow gradient of N-

acetylglucosamine (0 to 20 mM), and the peak of specific STX binding is collected and concentrated by Amincon pressure filtration. Quantification for a typical purification scheme is given in Table 2. Overall purification of 6,000-fold or more from crude homogenate can be obtained. Peak specific activities range in the neighborhood of 1,500 pmol of STX binding/mg of membrane protein.

Final channel purity can be roughly estimated based on independent determinations of minimal channel molecular weight (mus). One such estimate is available from electron inactivation studies of Levinson and Ellory (11); this work suggests a minimum MW of 230,000 daltons for the SBC of the Na^+ channel. Assuming MW of 250,000 daltons, theoretical peak STX binding activity would be 4,000 pmol/mg of purified protein. Because STX binding activity decays with time during purification, some nonbinding channel protein would be expected to copurify with the identifiable SBC. In light of observed sedimentation behavior, the MW of the channel is also likely to be somewhat greater than the minimal estimate referred to previously. Based on these considerations, we believe that the SBC obtained with this protocol is probably 50% pure and may well exceed that value.

SIZE OF SOLUBILIZED NA$^+$ CHANNEL SBC

Estimates of the apparent size of the solubilized channel can be obtained by chromatography on gel filtration columns such as Sepharose 6B. When sarcolemma is solubilized and run directly on such a column, a significant amount of membrane protein and of the specific STX binding material is eluted in the void volume of the column. A single major included peak of STX binding is also observed (12). The average retention value for this peak ranges between 0.22 and 0.28 and is slightly dependent on which non-ionic detergent is used for solubilization. Purified sarcolemmal SBC run on this column in Lubrol-Px also elutes in the same range with a retention coefficient (K_{av}) of 0.26. When compared to the elution behavior of known protein standards, this K_{av} would correspond to that expected for a globular protein having a Stokes radius of approximately 95 Å and MW of 500,000 to 600,000 daltons (Fig. 3A). When solubilized in Triton X-100 or NP-40, the apparent stokes radius is slightly smaller, averaging about 86 Å. The detergent-solubilized SBC will certainly run at an anomalously large apparent size, however, because of the mixed phospholipid-detergent micelle in which it resides. In addition, any asymmetry of the molecule will contribute to its apparent size, because gel filtration will depend to a large extent on the longest axial dimension of the molecule.

An independent estimate of molecular size can be obtained by observing the sedimentation behavior of the solubilized or purified SBC in the ultracentrifuge (12). Solubilized SBC from sarcolemma was analyzed using the Ames centrifugation technique (13), and its behavior was compared to that of a number of proteins of known $S_{20,w}$ (12). After centrifugation for 16 hours and fractionation, these gradients demonstrated a single sharp peak of specific STX binding activity. This peak consistently migrated at a point suggesting an $S_{20,w}$ between 9.1 and 9.9 (Fig. 3B). For a soluble globular protein, this would correspond to

Table 2. Purification of Saxitoxin Binding Component

Fraction	Protein		Total Binding Sites		Specific Activity	Purification Fold	
	mg	%	pmol	%	(pmol/mg)		
Muscle homogenate	—	—	—	—	0.25	1	
Isolated sarcolemmal fraction (total)	125.0	100	767.0	100	6.1	24	1
Solubilized sarcolemma (total)	94.8	76.0	516.0	67.3	5.4	21	0.89
Guanidinium column (pooled peak)	2.93	2.4	259.0	34.7	89	356	14.6
Wheat germ agglutinin–Sepharose column							
Pooled peak	0.150	0.09	118.0	17.4	1,079	4,316	177
Peak tube	0.0149		22.5		1,510	6,040	248

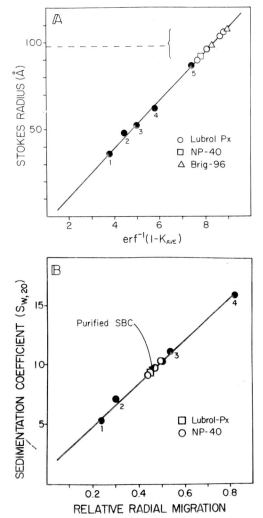

Fig. 3. **(A)** A summary of chromatographic behavior of the sodium channel saxitoxin binding component (SBC) on Sepharose 6-B columns after solubilization in various non-ionic detergents. In each case the corresponding detergent was present at a 0.1% concentration in the column running buffer. Data are expressed after the method of Ackers (14) to allow comparison with the results of Agnew and colleagues (10) with the sodium channel from eel electroplax. Standards are: 1, lactoperoxidase; 2, aldolase; 3, catalase; 4, ferritin; 5, thyroglobulin. **(B)** Summary of sedimentation behavior data for the solubilized SBC from sarcolemma and for the SBC after purification as outlined in text. (Purified SBC, X). Standards are: 1, lactoperoxidase; 2, lactate dehydrogenase; 3, catalase; 4, β-galactosidase.

an apparent Stokes radius of approximately 60 Å and MW of 250,000 to 350,000 daltons. The purified SBC sediments had an apparent $S_{20,w}$ of 9.6 (8). Thus, both the behavior on gel filtration columns and the apparent $S_{20,w}$ of the Na^+ channel SBC is unchanged by purification. The presence of detergent associated with the solubilized SBC will tend to increase its partial specific volume somewhat above the typical value of 0.73 for soluble proteins. This may produce lower $S_{20,w}$ values for the solubilized material in detergent solution than would be attributed to the protein itself. Molecular asymmetry, however, would be expected to contribute less to behavior in this system than with gel filtration.

It appears that the true MW of the solubilized Na^+ channel SBC is in the vicinity of 300,000. Actual determination of this value, however, requires sedimentation studies of purified material in $D_2O = H_2O$ mixtures that effectively neutralize the contribution of detergent to the sedimentation behavior.

Preliminary experiments suggest a partial specific volume of 0.83 for the sodium channel-detergent micelle. Calculations based on this and other data indicate a MW of 314,000 for the sodium channel protein.

SDS Gel Electrophoresis Pattern

Sodium dodecyl sulfate gel electrophoresis of purified sarcolemmal membranes reveals a reproducible pattern containing 50 to 75 identifiable bands of varying intensity. Peak fractions containing the Na^+ channel SBC from the initial guanidinium column show SDS gel electrophoresis patterns considerably different from those of the native sarcolemma; these, however, still contain many proteins ranging in MW from less than 20,000 to more than 200,000. Peak fractions from the final WGA column having STX binding specific activities in excess of 1,000 pmol/mg of protein contain in the best preparations; only 4 significant bands correspond to proteins of approximate MW 55,000, 47,000, 40,000, 37,000 (8). Several other very faint but variable bands are occasionally observed. It is premature to assume that these polypeptides are subunits of the Na^+ channel itself. One or more may represent contaminating copurified protein. Proteolytic clipping of the channel protein may occur during purification, resulting in the production of several smaller fragments from one initially larger fragment. Considerable additional work must be done before definitive statements can be made concerning subunit composition and MW in the purified material.

FUTURE DIRECTIONS

A primary goal at this time is the definitive analysis of MW, geometry and subunit composition, and stochiometry of the purified channel complex. The next major step to be attempted will be the reconstitution of functional purified Na^+ channels into phospholipid vesicles and eventually into black lipid bilayers in a manner that allows study of their current gating properties. In related studies, the development of monoclonal antibodies to the purified channel could provide new tools for the purification itself; more importantly, they will open new avenues for accurate localization of Na^+ channels in situ at the light and electron microscopic level in a variety of tissues.

REFERENCES

1. Hodgkin AL, Huxley AF: A quantitative description of membrane current and its application to conduction and excitation in peripheral nerve. J Physiol (Lond) 117:500–544, 1952

2. Armstrong C: Ionic pores, gates and gating currents. Rev Biophys 7:179–210, 1975

3. Ritchie JM, Rogart RB: The binding of saxitoxin and tetrodotoxin to excitable tissues. Rev Physiol Biochem Pharmacol 79:1–51, 1977

4. Hafemann DR: Binding of radioactive tetrodotoxin to nerve membrane preparations. Biochim Biophys Acta 266:548–556, 1972

5. Ritchie JM, Rogart RB, Strichartz GR: A new method for labelling saxitoxin and its binding to nonmyelinated fibers of the rabbit vagus, lobster walking leg and garfish olfactory nerves. J Physiol (Lond) 261:477–494, 1976

6. Weigele JB, Barchi RL. Analysis of saxitoxin binding in isolated rat synaptosomes using a rapid filtration assay. FEBS Lett 91:310–314, 1978

7. Barchi RL, Weigele JB: Characteristics of saxitoxin binding to the sodium channel in sarcolemma isolated from rat skeletal muscle. J Physiol (Lond) 295:383–397, 1979

8. Barchi RL, Cohen SA, Murphy LE. Purification of the excitable membrane sodium channel STX binding component from sarcolemma. Proc Natl Acad Sci USA 77:1306–1310, 1980

9. Lefkowitz RJ, Harber E, O'Hara D: Identification of the cardiac beta-adrenergic receptor protein: solubilization and purification by affinity chromatography. Proc Natl Acad Sci USA 69:2828–2832, 1972

10. Agnew WS, Levinson SR, Brabson JS, Raftery MA: Purification of the tetrodotoxin-binding component associated with the voltage-sensitive sodium channel from *Electrophorus electricus* electroplax. Proc Natl Acad Sci USA 75:2606–2610, 1978

11. Levinson SR, Ellory JC: Molecular size of the tetrodotoxin binding site estimated by irradiation-inactivation. Nature [New Biol] 245:122–123, 1973

12. Barchi RL, Murphy LE: Size characteristics of the solubilized sodium channel STX binding site from mammalian sarcolemma. Biochim Biophys Acta 597:391–398, 1980

13. Martin RG, Ames BN: A method for determining the sedimentation behavior of enzymes: application to protein mixtures. J Biol Chem 236:1372–1379, 1961

14. Ackers GK: A new calibration procedure for gel filtration columns. J Biol Chem 242:3237–3238, 1967

DISCUSSION

Dr. Edson Albuquerque: When you isolated your tetrodotoxin (TTX)-bound Na$^+$ channel, did you measure binding of Na$^+$ channel agonists like batrachotoxin or scorpion toxin to see whether the putative channel has recognition sites for these toxins? How many lipid molecules do you need to assure the stability of the putative TTX channel? Some information for you is that we may have an irreversible binding toxin for the Na$^+$ channel.

Dr. Robert Barchi: I would love to have some of your polypeptide toxin! Returning to the first point, I would also like to have the opportunity to study batrachotoxin binding; if we can get some batrachotoxin from you, that would be the experiment to do. As far as scorpion toxins are concerned, the binding of those polypeptide toxins is, as you know, voltage dependent. Once you take the channel out of the membrane, you destroy the voltage gradient. These toxins simply do not bind under these conditions, so you can not do that experiment. The batrachotoxin binding study would be the one to do. I'd love to have some tritiated batrachotoxin to do that experiment.

Dr. Edson Albuquerque: We found that toxin binds to the putative channel, but it seems that only a fraction of the Na$^+$ channel is attached with some affinity to benzo-batrachotoxin. This affinity of benzo-batrachotoxin for the TTX putative channel is apparently increased when lipid is added to the mixture to assure stability of the TTX channel unit.

Dr. Robert Barchi: Let me just answer your other questions. Dr. Catterall has looked at the photoaffinity labeling of Na$^+$ channels with iodinated polypeptide toxin in the intact membrane and then taken the membrane apart. He finds binding to something that looks about the same overall size as our solubilized saxitoxin binding component does. We had some differences in terms of the final SDS gels, but I do not think we have any differences in terms of the apparent size of the molecule on sepharose chromotography or sedimentation assay. That suggests that they behave very similarly, but as you know, those two toxins bind to totally different parts of the molecule. They are not competitive with each other, which I consider to be at least suggestive evidence that we do not have just a small piece of the channel. As far as the amount of lipid required for stability of the solubilized channel, you need about one phospholipid molecule (phosphatidylcholine or phosphatidylethanolamine, not phosphatidylserine) per five detergent molecules in the mixed micelle to get a stabilized channel. If you do not have at least that ratio, stability is lost. I do not know whether the channel dissociates or what, but the saxitoxin binding disappears and as far as we are concerned, the molecule becomes transparent.

Dr. Clifford Andrew: Have you stained any of your polyacrylamide gels with periodic acid–Schiff stain to identify which of the three polypeptides of the isolated Na$^+$ channel are glycoproteins?

Dr. Robert Barchi: We are still in the very preliminary stages of that. What we are working with now is iodinated lectins (iodinated concanavalin A and iodinated wheat germ agglutinin). I think that at least two of the bands I showed you are glycoproteins, but I would rather not stick my neck too far out on that.

Dr. John Bird: Have you tried coupling any of the toxins with the 50,000- to 60,000-dalton proteins that you isolated?

Dr. Robert Barchi: Do you mean, have we tried binding the toxin to the proteins after we isolate them?

Dr. John Bird: Right.

Dr. Robert Barchi: Well, when we purified the channel in its final form, we do toxin binding assays to determine its specific activity, so before we denature with SDS, toxin clearly binds and we are talking about 1,500 pmol of binding per mg of protein. After the purified channel is denatured with SDS, we have not tried to do specific binding, but I would be surprised if you could see anything at that point. Current thinking is that the binding site for the saxotoxin is really in the channel and is probably formed by the tertiary and quaternary structure of that protein. When you destroy this tertiary and quaternary structure by SDS and reduction of disulfide bonds, you would probably lose the binding site. The other problem is that when you do these SDS gels, the amount of protein that you actually have on the gels is very low and the amount that you can recover to do subsequent binding studies might be too low for adequate resolution. Another approach would be to try to crosslink the toxins into the protein before you take it apart. That has not worked. A third approach is to try to do site-specific labeling or site-protective labeling in conjunction with toxins. I think that will work, and we are in the process of attempting such experiments.

30
Physical Basis of Myotonia

S. H. Bryant, PhD

The excitability of skeletal muscle membranes is so profoundly altered in the condition known as myotonia that the fibers tend to fire in response to normally subthreshold stimuli and respond with trains of repetitive action potentials and an afterdischarge following cessation of stimulation. Myotonia is seen most frequently in the human muscle diseases *myotonia dystrophica* and *myotonia congenita*. In myotonia congenita the myotonia is the principal sign of the disease, whereas in the more common form, myotonia dystrophica, there is muscle weakness, muscle wasting, and several other somatic manifestations. Myotonia occurs in other rare human diseases such as *paramyotonia congenita* and hyperkalemic periodic paralysis, and it may be seen as a consequence of administration of drugs such as clofibrate, diazacholesterol, and certain carboxylic acids.

The clinical signs of myotonia are an abnormal electromyographic pattern consisting of repetitive trains of action potentials known as "dive-bomber" activity, a prolonged contraction of muscle fibers in response to direct mechanical percussion, and an aftercontraction following voluntary efforts that can interfere with normal movement. In most cases of myotonia the stiffness and delayed relaxation are greater after a period of muscle inactivity and the myotonia lessens with repeated muscle activations, a phenomenon known as "warm up" (1–3). The abnormal contractions in myotonia are undoubtedly due in part to the repetitive action potentials, but abnormal excitation-contraction coupling may play a role. For example, in paramyotonia the abnormal contractions can occur in cooled muscle when repetitive firing is inhibited (4). In addition, many of the carboxylic acids that induce myotonia can cause twitch potentiation and delayed relaxation of contraction independent of their ability to cause abnormal repetitive firing (5, and Valle JR, Bryant SH: unpublished observations).

Myotonia has been reported to occur naturally in muscle disease in only a few animal species (6–8). The best known and most thoroughly studied has been the nondystrophic hereditary myotonia of goats (2, 5, 9). Caprine myotonia resembles human myotonia congenita in most aspects, including a low resting membrane chloride conductance, which is the major factor accounting for the myotonic excitability (2, 9, 10).

The physical model for myotonic behavior derived from earlier electrophysiologic studies and tested by computer simulations has had as its basis the assumption of g_{Na} and g_K kinetics measured in frog muscle (11–16). These Na^+ kinetic parameters lead to a slight overlapping of the activation, m, and the inactivation, h, variables in their steady state. This results in small steady-state depolarizing Na^+ currents near the threshold for excitation that contribute to instability and production of repetitive action potentials. The presence of a large Cl^- leak conductance g_{Cl} having an equilibrium potential near the stable resting potential leads to normal excitability, because it shunts these Na^+ currents, reducing their effectiveness for reexciting the fiber. Absence of g_{Cl} leads to a myotonic excitability characterized by low threshold and repetitive firing. The myotonic afterdischarge that follows a train of stimulated impulses is brought about by the late after-depolarization due to accumulation of K^+ in the transverse tubules (13, 17). The late after-depolarization is too small (~ 0.1 mV/impulse) to be of physiologic importance in normal fibers. In the myotonic fiber, where g_{Cl} is lacking, the late after-depolarization amounts to approximately 1 mV/impulse and decays over a period of seconds. Thus, a late after-depolarization can occur in the myotonic fiber after a short voluntary stimulation that is sufficient to give a prolonged afterdischarge of action potentials with development of an after-contraction (13).

The remainder of this paper will describe our recent experiments, which attempt to provide insight into two of the basic questions regarding the physical basis of myotonia. The first question concerns the nature of the chloride conductance channels and the mechanism by which the conductance is decreased in myotonia. The second consideration involves the kinetics of the voltage-dependent Na^+ and K^+ conductance channels in normal and myotonic goat skeletal muscle membranes. All of the simulations of the myotonic response published to date have had to assume Na^+ and K^+ kinetics derived from frog or squid data (14–16). Only recently have data from voltage-clamped mammalian fibers been available, and these were from rat fibers (18–20). The use of frog or rat data would not be so serious a consideration in myotonia simulations were it not for the fact that the simulations are very sensitive to small changes in the kinetic parameters. In fact, whether or not a simulation becomes realistically myotonic when g_{Cl} is decreased can depend on these small changes in kinetics (16).

CHLORIDE CHANNEL IN MYOTONIA

With the finding that there is a low g_{Cl} in some naturally occurring and in some drug-induced myotonias, and that this low Cl^- conductance is necessary for myotonic excitability, it is natural to ask about the condition of the Cl^- channel in these two situations (2, 12, 21–23). That is, are the channels blocked by an occluding substance, or is the selectivity for Cl^- ions altered? In the case of the hereditary myotonias with low g_{Cl} are the channels simply decreased in number? In mammalian skeletal muscle the Cl^- channel density appears to be about the same for surface and transverse tubular membranes (24, 25). Thus, the major portion of g_{Cl} (60% to 90%) in mammalian skeletal muscle fibers is tubular.

For myotonia induced by anthracene-9-carboxylic acid, there is evidence that this agent blocks g_{Cl} by altering the natural ionic preference of the channels. In control membranes the sequence of anionic permeabilities or conductances is $Cl^- > Br^- > I^-$, whereas the effect of anthracene-9-carboxylic acid is to produce complete reversal of the sequence ($I^- > Br^- > Cl^-$) or partial reversal (e.g., $I^- > Cl^- > Br^-$), depending on the concentration (23). Because the absolute permeability of the channel to I^- is low, g_{Cl} would be very low at moderate concentrations of anthracene-9-carboxylic acid (50% inhibition at 1.1 $\times$ 10^{-5} M) (23). It has been proposed that the myotonia inducer acts in the membrane in the vicinity of the ion selectivity filter to change the channel preference (22, 23). This conclusion is different from that drawn by Bryant and Morales-Aguilera (12), whose studies suggested that the agent simply occluded the Cl^- channel.

We have recently repeated the types of measurement made by Palade and Barchi (23) on normal and myotonic goat external intercostal fibers using essentially the same methodology (26). Relative permeabilities were monitored by observing the direction and magnitude of the potential change that occurred when a foreign anion was quickly substituted for Cl^- in a fast-flow low-volume chamber. Relative conductances were determined by cable analysis estimates of the membrane conductances averaged over many fibers in physiologic solutions containing Cl^-, I^-, Br^-, or methylsulfate as the principal anion. A summary of the qualitative effects on both permeability and conductance is given in Table I. It should be noted that the permeability and conductance sequences of the myotonic fibers are essentially normal. Furthermore, as in normal fibers, there occurs complete or partial reversal of the sequences in the presence of anthracene-9-carboxylic acid.

We have concluded from these preliminary studies that there are fewer Cl^- channels in myotonic fibers. That is, g_{Cl} is not low in myotonic fibers because of the presence of a naturally occurring myotonia inducer resembling the carboxylic acids. The reason for the decreased number of channels is not apparent. Possibly the channels are synthesized at an abnormally low rate, or perhaps there is interference with incorporation of the channels into the

Table 1. Anion Conductance and Permeability Sequences in Myotonic and Normal Goat Muscle Fiber Membranes

		Control	*A9C + TTX*
Myotonic Goat			
	g_{an}	$Cl^- > Br^- \geq I^- > MeSO_4^-$	$MeSO_4^- > Br^- \geq I^- > Cl^-$
	P_{an}	$Cl^- > Br^- > I^- > MeSO_4^-$	$I^- > MeSO_4^- > Cl^- > Br^-$
Normal Goat			
	g_{an}	$Cl^- > Br^- > I^- > MeSO_4^-$	$Br^- > I^- > Cl^-$
	P_{an}	$Cl^- > Br^- > I^- \geq MeSO_4^-$	$I^- > Cl^- > MeSO_4^- > Br^-$

Abbreviations: A9C, anthracene-9-carboxylic acid; TTX, tetrodotoxin; g_{an}, conductance of the anions indicated; P_{an}, permeability of the membrane to the anions indicated.

membrane because of membrane lipid alteration. Earlier studies also suggested the possibility that the motor nerve may play a role, because in mammalian skeletal muscle fiber innervation controls the membrane g_{Cl} (27–30); probably, both impulses and trophic factors are involved.

SODIUM CHANNEL IN MYOTONIA

There were no remarkable differences in the rate of rise of the action potential or in the overshoot in myotonic fibers compared with normal fibers (2). We recently reported that resting P_{Na} was also normal in myotonic fibers (31). The latter measurements are too insensitive to detect the subtle changes in g_{Na} that could affect myotonic excitability. Experiments were therefore performed with TE DeCoursey to examine the Na^+ currents in myotonic and normal goat skeletal muscle fibers with the Hille-Campbell voltage-clamp method (32). The original procedure was used with 0.1 M CsF in all of the pools except the test pool, which contained normal physiologic solution. Under these conditions K^+ currents are effectively abolished; after the digitized current records were corrected for capacity and leak current with a computer, the remaining current was a relatively pure Na^+ current that could be fitted very well by least-squares methods to the conventional Hodgkin and Huxley m^3h model (33). Cut fibers from external intercostal and gastrocnemius fibers were studied at 12° C. Preliminary accounts of these results have appeared (34, 35).

It was found that the instantaneous and peak current-voltage curves as well as the Na^+ activation parameters were normal in the myotonic fibers. The voltage for half-maximal Na^+ activation (m_∞^3) occurred at approximately -45 mV, with $\bar{\alpha}_m$ equal to 0.06 msec^{-1} and $\bar{\beta}_m$ equal to 0.2 msec^{-1}. $\bar{\alpha}_m$ and $\bar{\beta}_m$ are the forward and backward rate constant parameters, respectively, as defined in Adrian et al. (36). On the other hand, Na^+ inactivation was slower in the myotonic fibers, the effect being greater in gastrocnemius fibers compared with external intercostal fibers. When the rate constants of inactivation h were determined by least-squares fits to the data, the slower inactivation of the myotonic fibers was shown to be largely accounted for by a reduction of $\bar{\beta}_h$. $\bar{\beta}_h$ is the backward rate constant parameter for inactivation, as defined by Adrian et al. (36). This finding indicates that inactivation gates close more slowly in the myotonic fiber.

Steady-state inactivation, h_∞, was determined with the variable prepulse method and fitted to the following Boltzmann-type relation, after the analysis of Adrian and colleagues (36):

$$h_\infty = 1/(1 + \exp[(V - V_h)/k_h])$$

The half-maximal potential, V_h, was similar in myotonic and normal fibers and was equal to that calculated by fitting to kinetic data. V was the membrane potential, and k_h a slope factor. In myotonic fibers the slope of the h_∞ curve was less steep (mean ± SEM $k_h = 14 \pm 0.7$ mV in 8 myotonic fibers, compared with 12 ± 0.6 mV in 9 normal fibers; $P < 0.05$). A slow (seconds) inactivation process was also observed in both normal and myotonic fibers.

POTASSIUM CHANNEL IN MYOTONIA

In an early study we reported that resting K^+ conductance was increased approximately 2-fold in myotonic goat fibers (12). Because this conductance increased with a more negative resting potential, it probably represented an increase in the number of inward rectifying channels. This increased resting g_k would, of course, tend to compensate for some of the loss of g_{Cl} in these fibers and lessen the tendency toward myotonia. In more recent work with a more highly inbred strain of myotonic goats (possibly a recessive type) this increased resting g_k has not always been seen (Bryant SH: unpublished observations).

In collaboration with JR Valle we have investigated the outward rectifying channels in the myotonic fibers using the voltage clamp (37). Both the 3-electrode end-of-fiber voltage clamp and the cut fiber 3 vaseline-gap voltage clamp were used after significant modification of these original techniques (32, 36). In the case of the 3-electrode method, to place the electrodes accurately at the tendon end of the goat intercostal fibers, it was first necessary to perform a careful microdissection to remove fat cells and connective tissue, which accumulate in this region. This procedure is tedious and requires 2 to 4 hours before setting the electrodes. A less tiring method and now our standard approach is to use the Hille-Campbell technique, which requires only the stripping of short 4- to 6-mm lengths of fiber from the biopsy specimen (32). To record K^+ currents it was necessary to use special solutions for dissection and in the fiber end pools, because the original CsF method effectively blocks all K^+ currents. The solutions that we used in the K^+ current studies were based on those developed at UCLA by J Vergara (personal communication) for this purpose. The principal ingredients are: ethylene glycol bis(β-amino-ethyl ether)N,N,N',N'-tetra-acetic acid, glutamate, adenosine triphosphate, Tris maleate buffer, $MgCl_2$, and KCl. Tetrodotoxin (1×10^{-6} M) was added to block Na^+ currents after installation of the fiber in the clamp and initial testing for adequate clamping.

The average peak K^+ currents at 0.0 mV are 2-fold greater in myotonic fibers (0.9 mA/cm^2) than control fibers (1.8 mA/cm^2). However, the threshold voltage ($\simeq$53 mV) is the same for both types of fiber. These results suggest that myotonic fibers have a 2-fold higher density of outward rectifying K^+ channels. The results of analysis of the kinetics of K^+ activation are incomplete at this time, but the steady-state potassium activation n_∞ curves of the myotonic fibers have a small shift toward hyperpolarization, and preliminary observations suggest minor shifts in kinetic parameters.

Potassium inactivation as a result of long depolarizing pulses appears to be different from normal in myotonic fibers. An initial delay shown in this figure has frequently been seen to precede the usual exponential time course of the K^+ current decay. None of the normal fibers showed this phenomenon.

IONIC CONDUCTANCE ABNORMALITIES IN MYOTONIA

At my presentation at the previous conference in this series, I concluded that although the mathematical simulations of low chloride conductance were impressive, the investigators had to assume kinetics and limiting conductances for Na^+ and K^+ (9). The preliminary results discussed in this paper represent the first attempts to measure the Na^+ and K^+ currents directly in a naturally occurring myotonia.

We have not yet used a sophisticated model such as the one published by Adrian and Marshall (16) to explore the effects of the cation kinetic differences we have reported here, but we have substituted our new values into a simple nonpropagating membrane action potential model with the following qualitative results. The alterations in the Na^+ kinetics we observed, i.e., lower threshold to long pulses and increased tendency to fire repetitively, tend to increase the degree of myotonia. The differences in the slopes of the inactivation (h_∞) curves would increase the overlap at the bases of the h_∞ and $m_\infty{}^3$ curves. This greater overlap is important, because it results in the myotonic fiber having a larger steady-state depolarizing Na^+ current in the threshold region as well as a decreased rate of inactivation. Both of these effects would be expected to increase the myotonia. The slow inactivation process observed for Na^+ could play a role in the termination of trains of action potentials in myotonic fibers.

It was not intuitively obvious that the effect of an increase in outward rectification, $\bar{g}_K$, should increase the myotonia by increasing the maximal frequency of impulses in a myotonic train of action potentials. We have since tested the effects of 4-aminopyridine (10^{-6} to 10^{-5} M) on the ability of rat fibers treated with anthracene-9-carboxylic acid to fire repetitively (Bryant SH: unpublished observations). When outward rectification is blocked with the 4-aminopyridine, the membrane responds to long depolarizing pulses with fewer repetitive impulses in the train and a smaller late after-depolarization (unpublished observations). Without outward rectification, the membrane tends to depolarize to inactivation levels (≈ 40 mV), which inhibits further repetitive firing because the large increase in potassium conductance with each action potential is necessary to reset the membrane potential below threshold between repetitive impulses. With lower g_K, there should be lessened tubular K^+ accumulation, a necessary condition for production of the myotonic afterdischarge (13, 17).

The cation conductance abnormalities we have observed in myotonic goat fibers are in a direction of "promoting" myotonia but are insufficient in and of themselves to induce myotonia in the presence of a normal chloride conductance. Thus, the decrease in g_{Cl} remains the principal underlying factor for allowing myotonia to occur in the goat model, but for quantitative and realistic modeling of the myotonia, the cation abnormalities described must also be considered.

The fact that we can now report some abnormality in every ionic channel studied (K^+ inward and outward rectifying channels, Na^+ channels, and Cl^- channels) leads us to speculate that there may be some abnormality in the structure of the membrane that is basic to all of these channel alterations. It seems unlikely that a single autosomal genic defect in caprine myotonia would produce alterations in each of several protein channels. Some reports have suggested that there are membrane chemical abnormalities in myotonic goat membranes, but these findings cannot be related directly to the problem of altered excitability (38–40).

ACKNOWLEDGMENTS

This work was supported by a grant from the Muscular Dystrophy Association and by U.S. Public Health Service Grant NS-03178 from the National Institutes of Health.

REFERENCES

1. McComas AJ: *Neuromuscular Function and Disorders*, ed 1. Butterworths, London, 1977, pp 123–132

2. Bryant SH: The electrophysiology of myotonia, with a review of congenital myotonia of goats. In *New Developments in Electromyography and Clinical Neurophysiology*, vol 1. Edited by Desmedt JE. S Karger, Basel, 1973, pp 420–450

3. Walton JN: *Disorders of Voluntary Muscle*. Little, Brown and Co., Boston, 1974, pp 561–613

4. Ricker K, Hertel G, Langescheid K, et al: Myotonia not aggravated by cooling: force and relaxation of the adductor pollicis in normal subjects and in myotonia as compared to paramyotonia. J Neurol 216:9–20, 1977

5. Bryant SH: Myotonia in the goat. Ann NY Acad Sci 317:314–325, 1979

6. Brown GL, Harvey AM: Congenital myotonia in the goat. Brain 62:341–363, 1939

7. Entrikin RK, Bryant SH: Suppression of myotonia in dystrophic chicken muscle by phenytoin. Am J Physiol 237:C131–C136, 1979

8. Steinberg G, Botelho S: Myotonia in a horse. Science 137:979–980, 1962

9. Bryant SH: The physiological basis of myotonia. In *Pathogenesis of Human Muscular Dystrophies*. Edited by Rowland LP. Excerpta Medica, Amsterdam, 1977, pp 715–728

10. Lipicky RJ, Bryant SH, Salmon JH: Cable parameters, sodium, potassium, chloride, and water content, and potassium efflux in isolated intercostal muscle of normal volunteers and patients with myotonia congenita. J Clin Invest 50:2091–2103, 1971

11. Bryant SH: Cable properties of external intercostal muscle fibres from myotonic and nonmyotonic goats. J Physiol (Lond) 204:539–550, 1969

12. Bryant SH, Morales-Aguilera A: Chloride conductance in normal and myotonic muscle fibers and the action of monocarboxylic aromatic acids. J Physiol (Lond) 219:367–383, 1971

13. Adrian RH, Bryant SH: On the repetitive discharge in myotonic muscle fibers. J Physiol (Lond) 240:505–515, 1974

14. Bretag AH: Mathematical modelling of the myotonic action potential. In *New Developments in Electromyography and Clinical Neurophysiology*, vol 1. Edited by Desmedt JE. S Karger, Basel, 1973, pp 464–482

15. Barchi RL: Myotonia: an evaluation of the chloride hypothesis. Arch Neurol 32:175–180, 1975

16. Adrian RH, Marshall MW: Action potentials reconstructed in normal and myotonic muscle fibers. J Physiol (Lond) 258:125–143, 1976

17. Almers W: Potassium concentration changes in the transverse tubules of vertebrate skeletal muscle. Fed Proc 39:1527–1532, 1980

18. Adrian RH, Marshall MW: Sodium currents in mammalian muscle. J Physiol (Lond) 268:223–250, 1977

19. Duval A, Leoty C: Ionic currents in fast skeletal muscle. J Physiol (Lond) 278:403–423, 1978

20. Pappone P: Voltage clamp experiments in normal and denervated mammalian skeletal muscle fibres. J Physiol (Lond) 306:377–410, 1980

21. Barchi RL: Muscle membrane chloride conductance and the myotonic syndromes. In *Contemporary Clinical Neurophysiology* (EEG Suppl. No. 34). Edited by Cobb WA, Van Duijn H. Elsevier, Amsterdam, 1978, pp 559–570

22. Furman RE, Barchi RL: The pathophysiology of myotonia produced by aromatic carboxylic acids. Ann Neurol 4:357–365, 1978

23. Palade PT, Barchi RL: On the inhibition of muscle membrane chloride conductance by aromatic carboxylic acids. J Gen Physiol 69:879–896, 1977

24. Palade PT, Barchi RL: Characteristics of the chloride conductance in muscle fibers of the rat diaphragm. J Gen Physiol 69:325–342, 1977

25. Dulhunty AF: Distribution of potassium and chloride permeability over the surface and t-tubule membranes of mammalian skeletal muscle. J Membr Biol 45:293–310, 1979

26. Bryant SH, Owenburg K: Characteristics of the chloride channel in skeletal muscle from myotonic and normal goats. Fed Proc 39:579, 1980

27. Bryant SH, Camerino D: Chloride conductance of denervated gastrocnemius fibers from normal goats. J Neurobiol 7:229–240, 1976

28. Camerino D, Bryant SH: Effects of denervation and colchicine treatment on the chloride conductance of rat skeletal muscle fibers. J Neurobiol 7:221–228, 1976

29. Lorkovic H, Tomanek RJ: Potassium and chloride conductances in normal and denervated rat muscles. Am J Physiol 232:C109–C114, 1977

30. DeCoursey TE, Younkin SG, Bryant SH: Neural control of chloride conductance in rat extensor digitorum longus muscle. Exp Neurol 61:705–709, 1978

31. DeCoursey TE, Bryant SH, Owenburg KM: Dependence of membrane potential on extracellular ionic concentrations in myotonic goats and rats. Am J Physiol (in press)

32. Hille B, Campbell DT: An improved vaseline gap voltage clamp for skeletal muscle fibers. J Gen Physiol 67:265–293, 1976

33. Hodgkin AL, Huxley AF: A quantitative description of membrane current and its application to conduction and excitation in nerve. J Physiol (Lond) 117:500–544, 1952

34. DeCoursey TE, Bryant SH: Sodium currents in normal and myotonic mammalian skeletal muscle fibers. Biophys J 25:69a, 1979

35. Bryant SH, DeCoursey TE: Sodium currents in cut skeletal muscle fibres from normal and myotonic goats. J Physiol 307:31p–32p, 1980

36. Adrian RH, Chandler WK, Hodgkin AL: Voltage clamp experiments in striated muscle fibres. J Physiol (Lond) 208:607–644, 1970

37. Valle R, Bryant SH: Potassium conductance in myotonic and normal mammalian skeletal muscle fibers. Fed Proc 39:2073, 1980

38. Winer N, Klachko DM, Baer RD, et al: Studies on the pathogenesis of myotonia. Clin Res 13:326, 1965a

39. Swift LL, Atkinson JB, LeQuire VS: The composition and calcium transport activity of the sarcoplasmic reticulum from goats with and without heritable myotonia. Lab Invest 40:384–390, 1979

40. Swift LL, Atkinson JB, Perkins RC, et al: Electron paramagnetic resonance and saturation transfer electron paramagnetic resonance studies on erythrocytes from goats with and without heritable myotonia. J Membr Biol 52:165–172, 1980

DISCUSSION

Dr. Donald Wood: The question I have relates to the fact that these are inherited disorders that presumably arise from a single gene defect leading to a single protein defect. Do you now think, given the apparent multiplicity of the conductance abnormalities you see in K^+ and Cl^-, that there is a specific defect in these channels, or that there is some generalized membrane disorder, e.g., of the surface membrane, that is independent of the channels but affects these channels?

Dr. Shirley Bryant: I am gland you asked that, because I did not have time to present my last few slides. Taking a cue from Drs. Barchi and Palade, who showed that in model myotonias the drugs that block Cl^- channels altered their permeability and conductance sequences, we have recently used this approach with the myotonic goat and normal goat fibers. The few channels that remained in the myotonic goat fibers had normal permeability and the same conduction sequences, so the channel did not appear to be greatly altered. Possibly, there are simply fewer channels. However, in other experiments it was not clear whether these channels were actually absent, because they could be recovered. For instance, after dehydration of myotonic goats, we might be able to recover some Cl^- channels. We do not know where they come from. The multiplicity of membrane channel defects does make it appear that there are some problems with the membrane per se. Maybe, as you suggest, there are normal channels sitting in, and modified by, an abnormal membrane.

Section B
Biochemical Aspects

31
Acetylcholine Receptor Phosphorylation in the Postsynaptic Membrane

Ivan Diamond, MD, PhD

Adrienne S. Gordon, PhD

C. Geoffrey Davis, BA

Gilbert Magilen, PhD

Dale Milfay, MS

Acetylcholine (ACh) released at the neuromuscular junction (NMJ) reacts with the acetylcholine receptor (AChR) to produce changes in the properties of the receptor and the postsynaptic membrane. However, the molecular mechanisms that regulate receptor functions such as the opening and closing of specific ion pores or desensitization of the receptor response are not understood. We have discovered that the membrane-bound AChR is reversibly phosphorylated by endogenous protein kinase (1, 2) and phosphatase (3) activities in AChR-enriched membranes. Phosphorylation in AChR-enriched membranes appears to be inhibited by cholinergic ligands and stimulated by potassium (1), agents known to react specifically with the AChR (4–6). Our data suggest that changes in the level of AChR phosphorylation may be related to changes in the physiologic properties of the AChR in the postsynaptic membrane.

The phosphate donor for the phosphorylation of the AChR is ATP (7). Both ACh and ATP are stored in synaptic vesicles and released into the synaptic cleft at the NMJ (8, 9). Because phosphorylation of specific proteins is a key cellular regulatory mechanism, ATP released at the NMJ could play a role in regulating or mediating the function of the AChR and the postsynaptic membrane. In this report we characterize some of the properties of the membrane kinase and

393

phosphatase that control reversible phosphorylation and dephosphorylation in postsynaptic membranes.

AChR-ENRICHED MEMBRANES

When the electric organ of *Torpedo californica* was homogenized and the resulting membranes were purified by ultracentrifugation, several membrane fractions (A, B, C, D, and E) were recovered (7). We determined which fraction was enriched in AChR by using *Naja naja siamensis* toxin, a specific nicotinic cholinergic antagonist. The distribution of toxin binding in the various fractions was also compared to other membrane markers. Fraction D had nearly a 15-fold increase in receptor activity and fraction C was enriched 5-fold. In contrast to the distribution of AChR, acetylcholinesterase (AChE) was enriched in fraction A and Na, K-ATPase activity was enriched in fractions B and E. Thus, fraction D, the fraction most enriched in AChR, contained the lowest levels of Na, K-ATPase and AChE activity (7). This suggested that fraction D was enriched in membranes of postsynaptic origin.

If phosphorylation regulates receptor function in the postsynaptic membrane, then receptor-enriched membranes should contain endogenous protein kinase activity. When all of the fractions were examined for endogenous membrane protein phosphorylation by incubating the membranes with γ-^{32}P-ATP in the presence of Mg^{2+}, fraction D exhibited maximal phosphorylation (Fig. 1). Several of the phosphorylated polypeptides had molecular weights corresponding to subunits of the purified AChR. Significant phosphorylation of the same polypeptides was also demonstrated in fraction C, but was markedly reduced in fraction B and virtually absent from fraction A. Thus, fraction D, a specialized membrane preparation enriched in AChR, also showed maximal endogenous membrane protein phosphorylation.

PHOSPHORYLATION OF THE AChR

In the experiments described above, we found phosphorylation of several major polypeptides with molecular weights the same as those of subunits of the AChR. In addition, phosphorylation of these polypeptides appeared to be regulated by K^+ and cholinergic ligands (1). These results suggested that the membrane-bound AChR itself might be a substrate for the endogenous protein kinase. To investigate this possibility directly, we used antibodies prepared against the purified AChR to prove that several of the phosphorylated polypeptides are components of the AChR (2). The technique we used was two-dimensional immunoelectrophoresis as described by Converse and Papermaster (10). Acetylcholine receptor-enriched membranes were incubated with γ-^{32}P-ATP and Mg^{2+} and the reaction was terminated by the addition of sodium dodecyl sulfate (SDS). The solubilized membranes were then electrophoresed in duplicate in SDS polyacrylamide gels (Fig. 2). The gels were cut into longitudinal strips along the sample wells; one gel was stained for protein, and another was

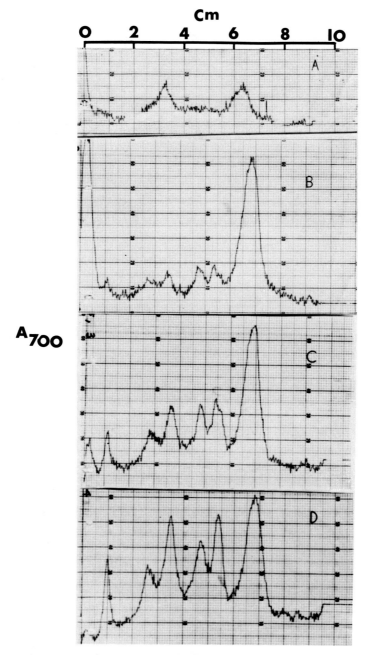

Fig. 1. Endogenous phosphorylation of membrane fractions A through D. Densitometric scan at 700 nm of autoradiographs of dried sodium dodecyl sulfate (SDS) polyacrylamide gels. Membranes were incubated for 0.5 minutes at 0° C with γ-^{32}P-labeled adenosine triphosphate and Mg^{2+}. The reaction was stopped by the addition of SDS, and the phosphorylated polypeptides were separated by SDS polyacrylamide gel electrophoresis (8).

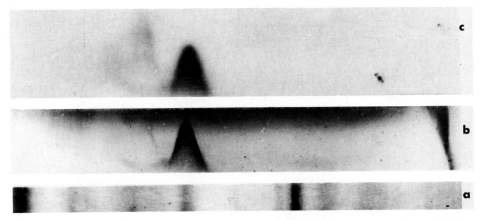

Fig. 2. Two-dimensional immunoelectrophoresis of acetylcholine receptor (AChR)-enriched membranes phosphorylated in situ (2). (**a**) Coomassie blue–stained sodium dodecyl sulfate (SDS) gel. (**b**) Coomassie blue–stained agarose gel after immunoelectrophoresis of the SDS strip into agarose-containing goat anti-AChR. (**c**) Autoradiography of gel shown in b.

subjected to immunoelectrophoresis at right angles into two layers of agarose. The first layer contained 1.5% Lubrol PX to remove excess SDS and the second contained goat anti-AChR antiserum.

Polypeptides derived from the AChR that were present in optimal concentrations formed immunoprecipitates with the anti-AChR antiserum and were recognized as "rockets." Figure 2b shows a major Coomassie blue–stained rocket corresponding to the 65,000-dalton polypeptide of the AChR. Control gels run against preimmune serum showed no rockets. Autoradiography of the dried gel (Fig. 2c) demonstrated that the same polypeptide precipitated by anti-AChR antiserum contained ^{32}P. This experiment provided unambiguous evidence that the 65,000-dalton component of the AChR was phosphorylated in situ by an endogenous membrane protein kinase present in AChR-enriched membranes. This is the first component of a membrane receptor protein to be identified as a substrate for an endogenous membrane protein kinase. Unlike most other phosphorylated membrane proteins studied, the phosphorylated substrate in our studies is a subunit of a postsynaptic membrane protein whose function is known and which has been biochemically characterized. Therefore, we anticipate that it will soon be possible to begin to correlate phosphorylation of the membrane-bound AChR with the function of the receptor in the postsynaptic membrane.

We have also investigated some of the factors that regulate protein kinase activity in the postsynaptic membrane (7). Figure 3 shows that ATP is the specific phosphate donor for phosphorylation of the membrane-bound AChR. With guanosine triphosphate as the phosphate donor, only the 100,000-dalton band was phosphorylated; no receptor phosphorylation was seen. We also used histone and casein to study phosphorylation of exogenous substrates by the membrane-bound protein kinase present in AChR-enriched membranes. Histone and casein could be phosphorylated by the membrane-bound protein kinase present in AChR-enriched membranes, and the amount of ^{32}P-PO$_4$ incorporated into either soluble protein was proportional to the amount of membrane protein added. We have previously shown that endogenous phosphorylation in these membranes is independent of cyclic adenosine monophosphate (cAMP) (1), and cAMP did not stimulate phosphorylation of casein or histone (7). These results suggested that the protein kinase that phosphorylates the AChR in the postsynaptic membrane is not a cAMP-dependent enzyme.

THE DEPHOSPHORYLATION REACTION

If phosphorylation of the membrane-bound AChR is an important regulatory event at the synapse, then dephosphorylation of the AChR must also occur in situ. Therefore, the AChR-enriched membranes should have endogenous membrane phosphoprotein phosphatase activity that can dephosphorylate the AChR. We first studied phosphoprotein phosphatase activity using casein labeled with ^{32}P-PO$_4$ as exogenous substrate (3). Release of ^{32}P from phosphorylated casein occurred after incubation with AChR-enriched membranes. Boiled membrane control preparations or phosphorylated casein without membranes did not show release of radioactivity during this same time interval. The effect of activators and inhibitors on protein phosphatase activity in AChR-enriched membranes was investigated extensively. The data indicated that this membrane protein phosphatase was similar to other cAMP-independent protein phosphatases (3).

If phosphatase activity is important in regulating the level of AChR phosphorylation, then the membrane-bound enzyme should dephosphorylate the membrane-bound receptor. We used two different assay systems to study this question. In the first, we measured time-dependent release of ^{32}P-PO$_4$ from

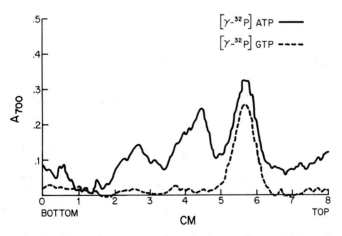

Fig. 3. Comparison of equal concentrations and specific activities of γ-^{32}P-labeled adenosine triphosphate and γ-^{32}P-labeled guanosine triphosphate as phosphate donors for the phosphorylation of the acetylcholine receptor (7).

Table 1. Dephosphorylation of the Membrane Bound Acetylcholine Receptors[a]

Condition	Exp A (pmol ^{32}P-PO_4 released)	Exp B (^{32}P-PO_4 in 65,000-dalton subunit of AChR) A_{700}
Control time zero	0.57 ± 0.03	4.5
NaCl (0.1 M)	0.74 ± 0.02	2.8
NaF (0.1 M)	0.50 ± 0.03	4.2

[a] Membranes were initially phosphorylated as described by Gordon and colleagues (1). The phosphorylated membranes were then incubated for 10 minutes at 37°C in either 200 mM NaCl or NaF. Exp A: Reaction was stopped by addition of trichloroacetic acid, and ^{32}P-PO_4 released was measured by extraction into isobutanol and liquid scintillation counting of the organic layer. Exp B: Reaction was stopped by addition of sodium dodecyl sulfate (SDS) and mercaptoethanol to final concentrations of 3.7% and 4%, respectively. The samples were then subjected to SDS gel electrophoresis and autoradiography as described previously (1).

AChR-enriched membranes that had been phosphorylated in the presence of γ-^{32}P-ATP and Mg^{2+}. Table 1 shows that ^{32}P-labeled inorganic phosphate was released from the phosphorylated membranes during incubation at 4° C. This reaction was also inhibited by fluoride ion. Thus, the enzyme does dephosphorylate endogenous membrane protein.

In the second assay, we measured changes in the level of phosphorylation of the membrane-bound AChR directly after incubation at 4° C for 10 minutes. Subsequent SDS gel electrophoresis of the phosphorylated membranes showed that a major subunit of the AChR had been dephosphorylated, because there was less covalently bound ^{32}P-PO_4 (Table 1). As before, endogenous dephosphorylation of the AChR was also inhibited by 0.1 M NaF. Therefore, the AChR-enriched membranes contain both endogenous protein kinase and phosphatase activities that regulate the level of phosphorylation of the AChR in situ.

POSTSYNAPTIC ATP-BINDING PROTEINS

The purified AChR of *T. californica* has 4 subunits, but only the 40,000-dalton polypeptide binds ACh. The function of the other polypeptides is unknown. We reasoned that one of the other AChR subunits might have protein kinase or phosphatase activity. Therefore, we set out to determine whether subunits of the AChR or membrane polypeptides associated with the AChR were the enzymatic subunits of the protein kinase and phosphoprotein phosphatase. Because our data showed that both the kinase and the phosphatase had ATP-binding sites, we used arylazido-β-alanyl ATP as a photoaffinity ligand to identify these sites (11). These experiments were done in collaboration with Dr. Ferdinand Hucho and Dr. Richard Guillory. Arylazido-β-alanyl ATP was synthesized as described by Jeng and Guillory (12) using either unlabeled ATP or α-^{32}P-ATP. The AChR-enriched membranes were incubated with the photoaffinity label and then irradiated so that the label remained covalently bound to the polypeptide containing the ATP binding sites. The polypeptides were then separated by SDS polyacrylamide gel electrophoresis and the dried gels were autoradiographed to determine which polypeptides reacted with the ATP analogue. Figure 4 shows that the AChR-enriched membranes used in this study contained approximately 8 major polypeptides, including 4 subunits of the AChR (α, β, γ, δ). After photoirradiation, the ATP photoaffinity analogue, arylazido-β-alanyl α-^{32}P-ATP, reacted with only 3 polypeptides and none of these were components of the AChR. In the absence of irradiation, there was no incorporated radioactivity (data not shown). Thus, comparison of the Coomasie blue–stained gel (Fig. 4B) with the autoradiograph (Fig. 4A) of the gel showed that the affinity ligand–labeled bands migrate with molecular weights of 45,000, 55,000 and 100,000 daltons.

The specificity of binding of the photoaffinity label for ATP binding sites was also investigated (11). Unlabeled ATP at increasing concentrations correspondingly inhibited the reaction of the labeled photoaffinity compound with the membranes. On the other hand, arylazido-β-alanine, i.e, the photolabel without the ATP moiety, did not cause a significant decrease in reactivity of the radioactive affinity label. These results strongly suggest that the analogue was acting as a photoaffinity probe of adenine nucleotide binding sites in AChR-enriched membranes.

The 100,000-dalton band probably is the Na, K-ATPase that has the same molecular weight (13). This band is not a component of the AChR but is present in variable amounts in receptor-enriched membrane preparations and does have an ATP binding site. The 45,000- and 55,000-dalton labeled bands are probably related to the protein kinase and protein phosphatase activities present in the receptor-enriched membranes. Because ATP is a substrate for the protein kinase reaction, this enzyme must have an ATP binding site. The phosphatase is inhibited by ATP, so it probably also has a specific recognition site for the nucleotide.

If the photoaffinity ATP analogue reacts with protein kinase in the membrane, it would be expected to inhibit protein kinase activity. When this was investigated directly, the photoaffinity label had a striking inhibitory effect on AChR phosphorylation in receptor-enriched membranes (11). The membrane-bound AChR was phosphorylated in situ with γ-^{32}P-ATP as described in Figure 1. Increasing concentrations of unlabeled photoaffinity ligand progressively in-

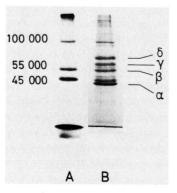

Fig. 4. Photoaffinity labeling of acetylcholine receptor–enriched membranes with arylazido-β-alanyl adenosine triphosphate (ATP) (11). Protein (1 mg/ml) was suspended in 15 mM Tris-HCl (pH 7.5) containing 10 mM ouabain and 0.225 mM arylazido-β-alanyl α-P^{32}-ATP. Irradiation was performed 4 times for 15 seconds each at room temperature. The samples were chilled in ice after each 15-second irradiation. Sodium dodecyl sulfate (SDS) electrophoresis was carried out in 7.5% acrylamide gels: autoradiograph (A) and Coomasie blue–stained SDS polyacrylamide gel (B).

hibited receptor phosphorylation. Because we know that the ATP analogue does not bind to the AChR (Fig. 4), the ATP photoaffinity label must have been reacting with the membrane kinase to inhibit phosphorylation of the membrane-bound AChR.

We have determined that ATP inhibits phosphatase activity in the same membrane preparation. However, because of methodologic limitations we have not been able to study the interaction of the ATP photoaffinity label with this endogenous membrane phosphoprotein phosphatase. Therefore, we cannot assign a specific function to the 45,000- and 55,000-dalton bands labeled by the ATP photoaffinity probe. We can conclude, however, that at least one of these bands appears to be the kinase and that neither is a component of the purified AChR. We are now in the process of purifying the 45,000- and 55,000-dalton bands so that we can generate specific antibodies against these polypeptides. We anticipate that the antibodies will allow us to determine the function of each of these polypeptides. Once we establish that such antibodies inhibit specific enzyme activities, we will be able to identify the kinase and phosphatase and use the antibodies to manipulate the level of phosphorylation of the AChR in situ.

EXOGENOUS PHOSPHORYLATION IN MAMMALIAN MUSCLE CELLS IN CULTURE

The role of ATP released at the NMJ has not received a great deal of attention by contemporary investigators (8, 9). There is physiologic evidence that exogenous ATP increases the sensitivity of muscle to ACh and causes a significant reduction in the muscle resting membrane potential (14, 15). It is possible that ATP released at the NMJ produces these physiologic effects because it is used by a surface membrane protein kinase to phosphorylate key postsynaptic and/ or sarcolemmal proteins. Roses and collaborators (16) suggest that changes in membrane protein phosphorylation might play a role in myotonic and Duchenne muscular dystrophy. These findings, taken together with our studies on AChR phosphorylation, prompted us to study the effect of exogenous ATP on mammalian muscle cells in culture as a potential model system for investigating the pathogenesis of muscular dystrophy.

We first examined membrane protein phosphorylation in tissue culture using the rat myogenic cell line, L-8. Myoblasts differentiate into fused myotubes enriched in AChR. We found that ATP added to the outside of L-8 myotubes supports phosphorylation of several sarcolemmal membrane proteins (Fig. 5). Phosphorylation is detected at 1 minute and increases for at least 10 minutes. Control experiments with ^{32}P-PO$_4$ show that inorganic phosphate does not support phosphorylation of most of these polypeptides. Because ATP does not readily cross biologic membranes, our data suggest that exogenously added ATP is used as a phosphate donor by an external membrane protein kinase to phosphorylate sarcolemmal membrane proteins. In the *Torpedo* electric organ we have been able to prove that the receptor undergoes reversible phosphorylation in the postsynaptic membrane. Therefore, we attempted to determine whether the AChR in muscle cell cultures is phosphorylated using anti-AChR

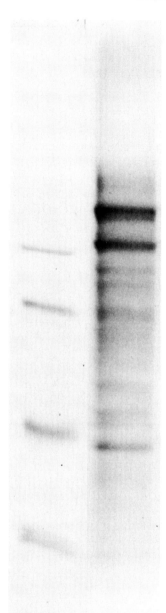

Fig. 5. Phosphorylation of differentiated muscle cell surface proteins. *Left*: 92,000- 69,000- 45,000- and 30,000- dalton ^{14}C-labeled standard marker proteins. *Right*: Autoradiograph of a sodium dodecyl sulfate (SDS) polyacrylamide gel of phosphorylated L-8 muscle cells. Differentiated L-8 myotubes (150 µg of protein) were washed 3 times with buffer (140 mM NaCl, 5.4 mM KCl, 5 mM MgCl$_2$, 1.8 mM CaCl$_2$, 1 mg/ml glucose, and 15-mM HEPES buffer, pH 7.4) and reacted with buffer containing 5 µM γ-^{32}P-labeled adenosine triphosphate for 2 minutes at 37° C. The reaction was stopped by removal of the reaction medium, solubilization of the cells in SDS, and boiling for 1 minute. The autoradiograph of the dried gel was exposed for 5 days.

antibodies. Because of the small number of AChRs in these cells our results were not definitive, but it appeared that the receptor was not phosphorylated to any great extent.

A direct effect of exogenously added ATP on muscle membrane protein phosphorylation suggests a critical role in regulating membrane function. The ATP released into the synaptic cleft at the neuromuscular junction may play a major role in development, differentiation, or stabilization of the AChR at the neuromuscular junction. It may also modulate or mediate the effect of ACh on other postsynaptic muscle membrane proteins. Defects in membrane protein phosphorylation may be related to the pathogenesis of membrane abnormalities in several neuromuscular disorders. We believe that this model system in cell culture will provide a new and fruitful avenue for investigating the role of sarcolemmal protein phosphorylation in neuromuscular disorders.

ACKNOWLEDGMENTS

The labeling experiments with arylazido-β-alanyl ATP were done in collaboration with Dr. Ferdinand Hucho, Universitat Konstanz, and Dr. Richard Guillory, University of Hawaii. This work was supported by grants from the National Institutes of Health, NATO, the National Science Foundation, the Muscular Dystrophy Association of America, and the Los Angeles and California Chapters of the Myasthenia Gravis Foundation.

REFERENCES

1. Gordon AS, Davis CG, Diamond I: Phosphorylation of membrane proteins at a cholinergic synapse. Proc Natl Acad Sci USA 74:263–267, 1977

2. Gordon AS, Davis CG, Milfay D, et al: Phosphorylation of the acetylcholine receptor by an endogenous membrane protein kinase in receptor-enriched membranes of *Torpedo californica*. Nature 267:539–540, 1977

3. Gordon AS, Milfay D, Davis CG, et al: Protein phosphatase activity in acetylcholine receptor-enriched membranes. Biochem Biophys Res Commun 87:876–883, 1979

4. Grunhagen H-H, Changeux J-P: Studies on the electrogenic action of acetylcholine with *Torpedo marmorata* electric organ. J Mol Biol 106:497–516, 1976

5. Weber M, David-Pfeuty T, Changeux J-P: Regulation of binding properties of the nicotinic receptor protein by cholinergic ligands in membrane fragments from *Torpedo marmorata* Proc Natl Acad Sci USA 72:3443–3447, 1975

6. Gibson RE, Juni S, O'Brien RD: Monovalent ion effects on acetylcholine receptor from *Torpedo californica*. Arch Biochem Biophys 179:183–188, 1977

7. Gordon AS, Davis CG, Milfay D, et al: Membrane-bound protein kinase activity in acetylcholine receptor-enriched membranes. Biochem Biophys Acta 600:421–431, 1980

8. Silinsky EM. On the association between transmitter secretion and release of adenine nucleotides from mammalian motor nerve terminals. J Physiol (Lond) 247:145–162, 1975

9. Ribeiro JA: ATP: related nucleotides and adenosine on neurotransmission. Life Sci 22:1373–1380, 1978

10. Converse CA, Papermaster D: Membrane protein analysis by two-dimensional immunoelectrophoresis. Science 189:469–472, 1975

11. Gordon AS, Guillory R, Diamond I, et al: ATP-binding proteins in acetylcholine receptor-enriched membranes. FEBS Lett 108:37–39, 1979

12. Jeng ST, Guillory RT: The use of aryl azido ATP analogs as photoaffinity labels for myosin ATPase. J Supramolec Struct 3:448–468, 1975

13. Jean DH, Albers RW, Koval GJ. Sodium-potassium-activated adenosine triphosphatase of *Electrophorus* electric organ. J Biol Chem 250:1035–1040, 1975

14. Saji Y, Escalona de Motta G, del Castillo J: Depolarization and potentiation of responses to acetylcholine elicited by ATP on frog muscle. Life Sci 16:945–954, 1975

15. Ewald DA: Potentiation of post-junctional cholinergic sensitivity of rat diaphragm muscle by high-energy-phosphate adenine nucleotides. J Membr Biol 29:47–65, 1976

16. Roses AD, Herbstreith MH, Appel SH: Membrane protein kinase alteration in Duchenne muscular dystrophy. Nature 254:350–351, 1975

DISCUSSION

Dr. Michael Bárány: I should like to mention that one can measure phosphatase activity through ^{32}P-phosphate incorporation as follows: if you know how much phosphate is bound to the receptor, as can be measured easily by sensitive techniques, and if you know the specific activity of the ^{32}P-ATP, then you can measure how much of the total phosphate is ^{32}P-phosphate. From this you can calculate the rate of phosphatase activity, because a protein that can be specifically labeled with ^{32}P-ATP must contain nonradioactive bound phosphate in its natural environment. That is, the nonradioactive phosphate must be split by the phosphatase to protein and phosphate, and this protein is then the substrate for the ^{32}P-ATP transfer by the protein kinase. Therefore, the ^{32}P incorporation into a protein labeled physiologically is the sum of two reactions, the first reaction via the protein phosphatase and the second reaction via the protein kinase.

Dr. Ivan Diamond: Yes, we are aware of this approach. However, several problems complicate the matter in our system. We do not know how much phosphate is originally present on the receptor. Also, there is a great deal of endogenous phosphatase activity in our preparation. This makes it difficult to use the approach you suggest.

Dr. Vanda Lennon: Was the ^{32}P-labeled protein precipitable by antibodies to AChR in the tissue culture studies?

Dr. Ivan Diamond: We have used antibody raised against the mammalian receptor to precipitate 95% of the receptor protein in this preparation, but we did not find ^{32}P in the immune precipitate. The problem with these experiments, however, is that the concentration of receptors is much lower than that in the electric organ and the sensitivity of our assay may not be great enough to detect small amounts of receptor phosphorylation. Therefore, we cannot rule out receptor phosphorylation. However, we are very much interested in the other sarcolemmal polypeptides phosphorylated by the external addition of ATP to the L-8 myotubes.

Dr. Alfred Stracher: How did you rule out the possibility that what you considered to be a phosphatase reaction might actually be a proteolytic event?

Dr. Ivan Diamond: We looked very carefully for evidence of proteolysis. There was no change in the SDS gel pattern after the incubation. We also showed that this was specific phosphate by extraction in molybdate, so we knew we were dealing with a phosphatase rather than another enzyme system.

Dr. Douglas Fambrough: This is more a plea than a question. There are many cases in which the nucleotide sugars or ATP are provided exogenously to look at metabolic events that one would guess were going on inside the cells. It has been kind of a mystery that our common sense tells us that ATP is not going to go across lipid bilayers well and yet one can observe phosphorylation of phosphatidyl inositides, for example. It looks as though, when you give ATP, somehow the γ-^{32}P-phosphate is winding up on internal structures. The same kind of thing is true for the glyceryl transferases and sugars. I have always been interested in what people think about this. I would appreciate all comments over the week plus yours right now.

Dr. Ivan Diamond: We were very worried about that. The argument is that we may be looking at internal phosphorylation. Perhaps ATP is degraded and free phosphate goes into the cell and then is incorporated into ATP pools to phosphorylate proteins inside the cell. Although only 2% of the ATP was hydrolyzed in 1 minute, we still did several controls to check this possibility. When we added ^{32}P-labeled inorganic phosphate, it took about 10 minutes instead of 1 minute to see any labeled bands. The phosphate had to enter intracellular pools and be synthesized into ATP. Also, the bands that were phosphorylated by phosphate were totally different from those phosphorylated by ATP. Moreover, we iodinated the cell surface by lactoperoxidase, which does not enter cells. Most of the phosphorylated bands were found to be iodinated by the lactoperoxidase. This suggests that the proteins phosphorylated by externally added ATP were available on the surface of the cell.

It is also possible, but not likely, that ATP is transported into the cell. We see phosphorylation very quickly. We also see it with minute amounts of STP in micromolar concentrations. The small amount of ATP that would enter the cell would be diluted by millimolar concentrations of ATP in the cell, and the specific activity would become so low that you might not detect anything. We think the fact that this occurs quickly, that it occurs on proteins that are on the surface of the cell, and that inorganic phosphate gives a different band pattern suggests that we are studying exogenous protein phosphorylation. This may have physiologic significance. Dr. Buchtal, who is here, has published papers showing quite clearly that ATP has an effect on the surface of the muscle cell: it lowers the threshold for depolarization. There are known effects of ATP on the surface of cells, and yet this has been virtually unexplored in muscle. I do not think we can ignore the fact that ATP is localized to synaptic vesicles, is released into the synaptic cleft, and is found to support phosphorylation of key postsynaptic proteins. Protein phosphorylation has been found to regulate many other systems and probably plays an important role on the surface of muscle as well.

Dr. Stanley Appel: In line with the question that Dr. Lennon asked about what other membrane components are being phosphorylated, one of your slides showed that with NaCl more phosphate was lost than could be accounted for by the receptor. I did not see how much phosphate was lost from the receptor, but presumably the amount of phosphate on the receptor is only one tiny fraction and the phosphate may activate the release of a much larger amount. What is that percentage and what other proteins are we talking about?

Dr. Ivan Diamond: That slide did not have the information you are mentioning. The amount of phosphate in the receptor was in arbitrary units based on densitometric scans. The amount of phosphate released from the receptor was not tiny. The gels showed that only the receptor changed its level of phosphorylation during the incubation, so we think most of the phosphate released was derived from the receptor.

32
Duchenne Erythrocyte Calcium Transport

David Pleasure, MD

Joan Mollman, MD

The calcium (Ca) content of non-necrotic muscle fibers from patients with Duchenne muscular dystrophy is increased (1, 2), but the sarcoplasmic concentration of calcium ions (Ca^{2+}) has not been measured in such muscle fibers. If it, too, were elevated, the resultant activation of proteinases and phospholipases and interference with mitochondrial function might help to explain the muscle fiber necrosis (3–10).

Muscle fiber Ca^{2+} concentration is modulated by cytosolic Ca buffers, by intracellular compartmentalization in sarcoplasmic reticulum and mitochondria, and by the balance between sarcolemmal Ca^{2+} permeability (and Na^+-Ca^{2+} exchange) and sarcolemmal outward Ca^{2+} transport (11–20). This complex regulatory system makes biochemical studies of Ca in muscle technically demanding.

The mature red blood cell (RBC), which lacks mitochondria and microsomes, is a more favorable cell for studies of plasma membrane Ca transport than is the skeletal muscle fiber. Erythrocytes can be readily and repeatedly sampled, and secondary pathologic changes that complicate interpretation of biochemical data dealing with Duchenne skeletal muscle are not present. Four recent studies indicate that the kinetic properties of the Duchenne RBC plasma membrane Ca^{2+} transport system differ from those of normal control RBCs (21–24).

NORMAL RBC CALCIUM TRANSPORT SYSTEM

In the RBC, the cytosolic Ca^{2+} concentration is maintained at less than 1 μm by a plasma membrane-associated Ca pump (25). The two best characterized components of this pump are a Ca^{2+}-stimulated, Mg^{2+}-dependent adenosine triphosphatase (Ca,Mg-ATPase), oriented in the plasma membrane so that Ca^{2+} and nucleotide binding sites face inward, and calmodulin, a cytosolic protein that (in the presence of Ca) binds to the Ca,Mg-ATPase and stimulates its activity (26–36).

Erythrocyte calmodulin, an acidic protein of molecular weight 17,000 daltons, is very similar in amino acid composition and peptide pattern to the calmodulin of brain, and probably also to the calmodulins of skeletal muscle and other tissues (32). Calmodulin has 4 high-affinity binding sites for Ca; Ca binding causes a marked conformational change in calmodulin (32, 37). Formation of the calmodulin-Ca^{2+}-Ca,Mg-ATPase complex causes a several-fold increase in the V_{max} of the Ca,Mg-ATPase for ATP hydrolysis and of the Ca pump for Ca translocation (27–29, 31, 32, 35, 36).

The RBC Ca,Mg-ATPase has been extracted from plasma membrane with non-ionic detergent and partially purified by affinity chromatography. The purified enzyme retains the capacity to bind calmodulin (30, 31, 33, 34). Incubation of the solubilized enzyme with γ-^{32}P-labeled ATP results in self-phosphorylation (34).

Kinetic properties of the human RBC Ca,Mg-ATPase have been studied extensively. Variations in experimental design, however, have led to disagreement about kinetic mechanism and to considerable scatter in reported kinetic constants. Factors that seem responsible for these discrepancies include the following:

1. Method of plasma membrane isolation. Seemingly trivial variations such as choice of lysing buffer, presence or absence of a Ca chelator in the washes, and duration and conditions of storage of the membranes before use have profound effects on the affinity of the Ca,Mg-ATPase for Ca^{2+} and $MgATP^{2-}$ (38–40). This may be due to changes in amount of calmodulin remaining bound to the membrane fraction after processing as well as to alterations in the organization of the membrane surrounding the enzyme.

2. Composition of the assay medium. Concentrations of Ca^{2+}, Mg^{2+}, $MgATP^{2-}$, and monovalent cations are important in governing Ca,Mg-ATPase activity (41, 42). There has been no uniformity in choice of assay conditions, and few investigators have established optimal concentrations of all relevant ionic species. To obtain valid kinetic data, it is of particular importance that an adequate Ca^{2+} buffer be included in the medium and that the dissociation constant of the buffer-Ca complex be corrected for pH and ionic strength effects (43). Optimally, actual Ca^{2+} concentrations should be measured (42, 44–46).

Experimental design becomes more stringent when Ca^{2+} transport is to be studied. Detection of vectoral Ca^{2+} movements requires that plasma membrane be sealed. The normal geometry of the RBC, with Ca^{2+}, nucleotide, and calmodulin binding sites facing inward, makes precise control and measurement of concentrations of these species difficult. The best approach to this problem is to invert and then reseal plasma membrane, forming inside-out vesicles (47). In this way, levels of Ca^{2+}, $MgATP^{2-}$ and other species of interest can be regulated, and Ca^{2+} transport can be measured by assaying intravesicular Ca content (27–29, 35, 42, 48).

The most detailed study of Ca transport by normal human RBC plasma membrane was carried out using the inside-out resealed vesicle technique and depending on ATP to buffer Ca^{2+}. The transport system has a single affinity for Ca^{2+}, with K_m of 3.4 μm. Concentrations of Ca^{2+} above 100 μm caused substrate inhibition. Optimal pH was 6.9 to 7.3. Half-maximal Ca^{2+} transport was observed with a $MgATP^{2-}$ concentration of 1.0 mM. The nucleotide data suggested a complex kinetic mechanism (42). Calcium transport by RBC inside-out plasma membrane vesicles is stimulated by addition of calmodulin to the medium (27–29, 35).

DUCHENNE RBC CALCIUM TRANSPORT

In 1977, Hodson and Pleasure (21) reported studies of the Ca,Mg-ATPase of RBC plasma membrane fragments prepared from 11 children with Duchenne dystrophy and 11 age-matched male control subjects. Membranes were prepared by hypotonic lysis, and assays were run on the day the blood was drawn. Membranes from each Duchenne patient were studied simultaneously with those from his control subject. Assays were performed in a buffer solution containing 2.7 mM $MgATP^{2-}$ and 0.5 mM Ca^{2+}. Specific activity of the Duchenne Ca,Mg-ATPase was 21% above that of the pair-matched control subjects ($P < 0.01$).

Further studies of the Duchenne RBC Ca,Mg-ATPase, reported in the same paper, were with variable concentrations of $MgATP^{2-}$, maintaining Ca^{2+} at 0.5 mM. Nonlinear double-reciprocal plots of Ca,Mg-ATPase activity versus $MgATP^{2-}$ suggested negative cooperativity or some more complex mechanism. The apparent K'_{MgATP} of the Duchenne enzyme was 0.36 mM; that of the control enzyme, 0.83 mM ($P < 0.01$). The implication of this result is that the greater activity of the Duchenne Ca,Mg-ATPase, when measured at 2.7 mM $MgATP^{2-}$, is a result of saturation of the nucleotide site of the Duchenne enzyme, but not the lower-affinity site of the normal control enzyme (21).

Several flaws in experimental design of this study should be pointed out. No control patients with neuromuscular or other diseases were studied; thus, the specificity of the Duchenne kinetic alteration was not established. The assays were performed with 0.5 mM Ca^{2+}, a concentration well into the substrate inhibitory range. The level of calmodulin remaining in the membrane fragments was not determined, nor was the effect of exogenous calmodulin on the Duchenne and control membranes.

Two 1979 studies confirmed the increased activity of the Duchenne RBC plasma membrane Ca,Mg-ATPase. Ruitenbeek (22) prepared RBC membranes from Duchenne patients, normal control subjects, and children with myotonic dystrophy. The membranes, obtained by hyptonic lysis, were washed with 0.6 mM ethylenediamine tetra-acetic acid (EDTA), frozen, and stored for as long as 18 months. Assays used 0.18 or 0.97 mM $MgATP^{2-}$ and 0.6 mM Ca^{2+}. Specific activity of the Duchenne Ca,Mg-ATPase was approximately 80% above that of the normal Ca,Mg-ATPase; that of membranes from myotonic patients was increased to a similar extent. Exogenous calmodulin stimulated the control and Duchenne enzymes by a similar percentage.

The experimental design of the Ruitenbeek study (22) was not ideal. The membranes were subjected to an EDTA wash, which is known to affect the kinetics of the Ca,Mg-ATPase (38) and were then stored for long periods. As in the paper by Hodson and Pleasure (21), the Ca^{2+} concentration was in the inhibitory range (42).

Luthra and coworkers (23) measured Ca,Mg-ATPase activity of both saponin-lysed RBCs and freeze-thawed RBC plasma membranes from 24 patients with Duchenne dystrophy, 25 with myotonic dystrophy, and control subjects of similar ages. Assays were done on the day blood samples were drawn. Concentrations of Ca^{2+} and $MgATP^{2-}$ cannot be calculated from the data provided. Because they observed substantial stimulation of the RBC Ca,Mg-ATPase without addition of Ca to the medium, however, it appears likely that their assay medium was contaminated by Ca^{2+} from an indeterminate source. Activity of the Duchenne RBC Ca,Mg-ATPase was increased to an extent similar to that reported by Hodson and Pleasure (21). In contrast with Ruitenbeek's study (22), Luthra and colleagues (23) found the specific activity of the Ca,Mg-ATPase of RBCs from patients with myotonic dystrophy to be less than that of normal control RBCs. Addition of RBC cytosol, as a source of calmodulin, stimulated the control, Duchenne, and myotonic dystrophy Ca,Mg-ATPases by similar percentages.

Most recently, Mollman and associates (24) measured Ca^{2+} transport by inside-out resealed RBC vesicles from 8 patients with Duchenne dystrophy and 8 age-matched normal male control subjects. Duchenne-control pairs were run simultaneously. The medium contained 2.7 mM $MgATP^{2-}$ and 0.25 to 25 μm Ca^{2+}. Both the K_m for Ca^{2+} and the V_{max} for Ca transport by the Duchenne vesicles were greater than normal. Studies of disease controls, of the affinities of the Duchenne and control vesicle calcium transport systems for $MgATP^{2-}$, and the effects of exogenous calmodulin on Ca transport by the Duchenne and control vesicles are now in progress.

SUMMARY

Three studies of the RBC Ca,Mg-ATPase from patients with Duchenne muscular dystrophy have shown that its activity is greater than the RBC Ca,Mg-ATPase from age-matched normal control subjects. There is a correspondingly greater than normal rate of Ca transport by Duchenne RBC plasma membrane vesicles. The molecular basis for this alteration, its disease specificity, and its biologic significance remain to be established.

REFERENCES

1. Mokri B, Engel AG: Duchenne dystrophy: electron microscopic findings pointing to a basic or early abnormality in the plasma membrane of the muscle fiber. Neurology (Minneap) 25:1111–1120, 1975

2. Maunder-Sewry CA, Dubowitz V: Myonuclear calcium in carriers of Duchenne muscular dystrophy: an x-ray microanalysis study. J Neurol Sci 42:337–347, 1979

3. Wrogemann K, Pena SDJ: Mitochondrial calcium overload: a general mechanism for cell-necrosis in muscle diseases. Lancet 1:672–673, 1976

4. Kar NC, Pearson CM: A calcium-activated neutral protease in normal and dystrophic human muscle. Clin Chim Acta 73:293–297, 1976

5. Anderson DR, Davis JL, Carraway KL: Calcium-promoted changes of the human erythrocyte membrane: involvement of spectrin, transglutaminase and a membrane-bound protease. J Biol Chem 252:6617–6623, 1977

6. Chien KR, Abrams J, Serroni A, et al: Accelerated phospholipid degradation and associated membrane dysfunction in irreversible, ischemic liver cell injury. J Biol Chem 253:4809–4817, 1978

7. Publicover SJ, Duncan CJ, Smith JL: The use of A23187 to demonstrate the role of intracellular calcium in causing ultrastructural damage in mammalian muscle. J Neuropathol Exp Neurol 37:544–557, 1978

8. Wrogemann K, Hayward WAK, Blanchaer MC: Biochemical aspects of muscle necrosis in hamster dystrophy. Ann NY Acad Sci 317:30–45, 1979

9. Kameyama T, Etlinger JD: Calcium-dependent regulation of protein synthesis and degradation in muscle. Nature 279:344–346, 1979

10. Azanza JL, Raymond J, Robin JM, et al: Purification and some physicochemical and enzymic properties of a calcium ion-activated neutral proteinase from rabbit skeletal muscle. Biochem J 183:339–347, 1979

11. St. Louis PJ, Sulakhe PV: Adenosine triphosphate-dependent calcium binding and accumulation by guinea pig cardiac sarcolemma. Can J Biochem 54:946–956, 1976

12. Barchi RL, Bonilla E, Wong M: Isolation and characterization of muscle membranes using surface-specific labels. Proc Natl Acad Sci USA 74:34–38, 1977

13. Langer GA: Events at the cardiac sarcolemma: localization and movement of contractile-dependent calcium. Fed Proc 35:1274–1278, 1976

14. Endo M: Calcium release from the sarcoplasmic reticulum. Physiol Rev 57:71–108, 1977

15. Blaustein MP: Sodium-calcium exchange and the regulation of cell calcium in muscle fibers. Physiologist 19:525–540, 1976

16. Tada M, Yamamoto Y, Tonomura Y: Molecular mechanism of active calcium transport by sarcoplasmic reticulum. Physiol Rev 58:1–79, 1978

17. Pleasure D, Wyszynski B, Sumner A, et al: Skeletal muscle calcium metabolism and contractile force in vitamin D-deficient chicks. J Clin Invest 64:1157–1167, 1979

18. Pitts BJR: Stoichiometry of sodium-calcium exchange in cardiac sarcolemma vesicles: coupling to the sodium pump. J Biol Chem 254:6232–6235, 1979

19. Racker E: Fluxes of Ca^{2+} and concepts. Fed Proc 39:2422–2426, 1980

20. Fiskum G, Lehninger AL: The mechanisms and regulation of mitochondrial Ca^{2+} transport. Fed Proc 39:2432–2436, 1980

21. Hodson A, Pleasure D: Erythrocyte cation-activated adenosine triphosphatases in Duchenne muscular dystrophy. J Neurol Sci 32:361–369, 1977

22. Ruitenbeek W: Membrane-bound enzymes of erythrocytes in human muscular dystrophy. J Neurol Sci 41:71–80, 1979

23. Luthra MG, Stern LZ, Kim HD: $(Ca^{++} + Mg^{++})$-ATPase of red cells in Duchenne and myotonic dystrophy: effect of soluble cytoplasmic activator. Neurology (NY) 29:835–841, 1979

24. Mollman JE, Cardenas JC, Pleasure DE: Alteration of calcium transport in Duchenne erythrocytes. Neurology (in press)

25. Schatzmann HJ, Burgin H: Calcium in human red blood cells. Ann NY Acad Sci 307:125–147, 1978

26. Luthra MG, Au KS, Hanahan DJ: Purification of an activator of human erythrocyte membrane $(Ca^{2+} + Mg^{2+})$-ATPase. Biochem Biophys Res Commun 77:678–687, 1977

27. Macintyre JD, Green JW: Stimulation of calcium transport in inside-out vesicles of human erythrocyte membranes by a soluble cytoplasmic activator. Biochim Biophys Acta 510:373–377, 1978

28. Hinds TR, Larsen FL, Vincenzi FF: Plasma membrane Ca^{2+} transport: stimulation by soluble proteins. Biochem Biophys Res Commun 81:455–461, 1978

29. Larsen FL, Vincenzi FF: Calcium transport across the plasma membrane: stimulation by calmodulin. Science 204:306–309, 1979

30. Haaker H, Racker E: Purification and reconstitution of the Ca^{2+}-ATPase from plasma membranes of pig erythrocytes. J Biol Chem 254:6598–6602, 1979

31. Lynch TJ, Cheung WY: Human erythrocyte Ca^{2+}-Mg^{2+}-ATPase: mechanism of stimulation by Ca^{2+}. Arch Biochem Biophys 194:165–170, 1979

32. Jarrett HW, Kyte J: Human erythrocyte calmodulin: further chemical characterization and the site of its interaction with the membrane. J Biol Chem 254:8237–8244, 1979

33. Niggli V, Ronner P, Carafoli E, et al: Effects of calmodulin on the $(Ca^{2+} + Mg^{2+})$ATPase partially purified from erythrocyte membranes. Arch Biochem Biophys 198:124–130, 1979

34. Niggli V, Penniston JT, Carafoli E: Purification of the $(Ca^{2+}$-$Mg^{2+})$-ATPase from human erythrocyte membranes using a calmodulin affinity column. J Biol Chem 254:9955–9958, 1979

35. Vincenzi FF, Larsen FL: The plasma membrane calcium pump: regulation by a soluble Ca^{2+} binding protein. Fed Proc 39:2427–2431, 1980

36. Muallem S, Karlish SJD: Regulatory interaction between calmodulin and ATP on the red cell Ca^{2+} pump. Biochim Biophys Acta 597:631–636, 1980

37. Dedman JR, Potter JD, Jackson RL, et al: Physicochemical properties of rat testis Ca^{2+}-dependent regulator protein of cyclic nucleotide phosphodiesterase: relationship of Ca^{2+}-binding, conformational changes, and phosphodiesterase activity. J Biol Chem 252:8415–8422, 1977

38. Wolf HU: Effects of ethylenediamine tetra-acetate and deoxycholate on kinetic constants of the calcium ion-dependent adenosine triphosphatase of human erythrocyte membranes. Biochem J 130:311–314, 1972

39. Farrance ML, Vincenzi FF: Enhancement of $(Ca^{2+} + Mg^{2+})$-ATPase activity of human erythrocyte membranes by hemolysis in isosmotic imidazole buffer. I. General properties of variously prepared membranes and the mechanism of the isosmotic imidazole effect. Biochim Biophys Acta 471:49–58, 1977

40. Katz S, Roufogalis BD, Landman AD, et al: Properties of $(Mg^{2+} + Ca^{2+})$-ATPase of erythrocyte membranes prepared by different procedures: influence of Mg^{2+}, Ca^{2+}, ATP, and protein activator. J Supramolec Struct 10:215–225, 1979

41. Scharff O: Stimulating effects of monovalent cations on activator-dissociated and activator-associated states of Ca^{2+}-ATPase in human erythrocytes. Biochim Biophys Acta 512:309–317, 1978

42. Mollman J, Pleasure DE: Calcium transport in human inside-out erythrocyte vesicles. J Biol Chem 255:569–574, 1980

43. O'Sullivan WJ, Smithers GW: Stability constants for biologically important metal-ligand complexes. In *Methods in Enzymology*, vol 63, part A. Edited by Purich DL. 1979, pp 294–336

44. Kendrick NC, Ratzlaff RW, Blaustein MP: Arsenazo III as an indicator for ionized calcium in physiological salt solutions: its use for determination of the CaATP dissociation constant. Anal Biochem 83:433–450, 1977

45. Scarpa A, Brinley FJ, Tiffert T, et al: Metallochromic indicators of ionized calcium. Ann NY Acad Sci 307:86–111, 1978

46. Yingst DR, Hoffman JF: Changes of intracellular Ca^{++} as measured by arsenazo III in relation to the K permeability of human erythrocyte ghosts. Biophys J 23:463–471, 1978

47. Kant JA, Steck TL: Cation-impermeable inside-out and right-side-out vesicles from human erythrocyte membranes. Nature [New Biol] 240:26–28, 1972

48. Sarkadi B, Macintyre JD, Gardos G: Kinetics of active calcium transport in inside-out red cell membrane vesicles. FEBS Lett 89:78–82, 1978

DISCUSSION

Dr. Wilfried Mommaerts: The use of these inside-out vesicles was very ingenious, but one does not quite know what may happen while making them. Would you consider using the Gardos technique as a control?

Dr. David Pleasure: The Gardos technique involves loading the cells with Ca^{2+} in the presence of ionophore, then getting rid of the ionophore by washing with albumin solutions so that one can watch the Ca^{2+} being pumped out. It is a good technique. The problem is that one cannot control the $MgATP^{2-}$ or Ca^{2+} levels inside the cell in the way that one would like for steady-state kinetic measurements. One can get some idea of what is going on and, hopefully, find an abnormality, but one is dealing with shifting levels of all the various substrates and it becomes a madhouse trying to figure out kinetic constants.

Dr. Alfred Stracher: I have two comments. First, I was surprised to hear that calmodulin is a constituent of RBCs. Second, you imply that calmodulin may actually be a membrane-bound protein. Would you comment on that?

Dr. David Pleasure: The second part first: if I said that, I bite my tongue. Calmodulin is a cytosolic protein present in a concentration greater than 1 μm inside the RBC. By peptide mapping and amino acid composition, it appears to be identical with brain calmodulin. Calmodulin is bound to the plasma membrane only in the presence of Ca^{2+} but then forms a ternary complex with Ca,Mg-ATPase or with other Ca^{2+}-dependent enzymes. In the RBC, calmodulin is present in great excess over the Ca,Mg-ATPase. In the normal physiologic state, all of the Ca,Mg-ATPases are probably saturated with calmodulin. Whereas the calmodulin level is well above 1 μM in the RBC, it has been estimated that there are only about 5,000 Ca,Mg-ATPases per RBC.

Dr. Anthony Means: Unfortunately, there is considerable misconception about the location of calmodulin in cells. When one prepares an extract of cells, clearly, a lot of protein is present in the supernatant fluid. But if you evaluate by immunocytochemistry or indirect immunofluorescence microscopy, the localization of this protein in any tissue, including RBCs is 90% or more with membranes. The second point is that the association of Ca^{2+} with this protein produces a conformational change that exposes an extremely lipophilic surface. This explains the activity of the phenothiazines mentioned earlier in the week and most probably explains why, in the presence of Ca^{2+}, you have so much of the protein associated with a plasma membrane like that of the RBC. The final point is that even if you extract RBC membranes or any other plasma membrane with 10 mM ethyleneglycol tetra-acetate, a significant percentage of calmodulin determined by radioimmunoassay is still associated with the membrane. So I would caution that it is a little premature to assume either a cytosolic location of calmodulin in the RBC or whether changes in calmodulin localization play a role in any disease state.

Dr. David Pleasure: Those points are well taken. One is concerned that the calmodulin Ca^{2+} might be so sticky that it is binding nonspecifically to the membrane, but the recent studies indicating that calmodulin Ca^{2+} combines with the reasonably well-purified Ca,Mg-ATPase suggests that there is a specificity to it, in any event.

Dr. Michael Merickel: It is nice to find what appears to be consistent differences between normal and dystrophic RBCs. However, we would really like to understand what is going on in muscle. Could you comment on this increased Ca,Mg-ATPase activity in terms of muscle? Would you expect it to change Ca^{2+}

gradients, buffering capacity, and maybe some of the electrical excitability parameters of muscle?

Dr. David Pleasure: You are really asking two questions. The first question is, can we be sure, because there have been four studies in a row that show an abnormality in Ca,Mg-ATPase, that it is really so? I do not think we can be completely sure if we look back into the history of RBCs in Duchenne dystrophy. The first several studies on ouabain binding also tended to confirm each other. You have to keep an open mind until these studies have really been carried out in great detail without the flaws that I mentioned. It is premature to try to decide, even in the RBC, what the increased K_m and increased V_{max} of the Ca,Mg-ATPase and Ca^{2+} transport system means. Under almost any conceivable circumstance that one can plot out, it looks like the Duchenne RBC ought to be able to pump more Ca^{2+} than the normal RBC; therefore, one could not explain the accumulation of Ca^{2+} in the Duchenne RBC by this factor alone. At the very least, this indicates that there is something wrong with the membrane in Duchenne dystrophy, which I think most of us are now coming to believe. I do not know what it means as far as the mechanism by which Ca^{2+} gets into Duchenne muscle and chews it up.

33

Increased ^{32}P-Phosphorylation of Spectrin Peptides in Duchenne Muscular Dystrophy

A. D. Roses, MD

M. E. Mabry, MD

M. H. Herbstreith, BS

P. V. Shile, BA

C. V. Balakrishnan, PhD

Biophysical and biochemical observations involving the red blood cell (RBC) from patients with Duchenne muscular dystrophy (DMD) and myotonic muscular dystrophy (MyD) have supported the concept that the RBC membrane may be altered in these diseases (1–5). An alteration in the ^{32}P-phosphorylation of the RBC membrane protein spectrin Band 2 in DMD was reported by our laboratory in 1975 (6). Subsequent conflicting reports appeared in the literature (7–9), each of which contained important methodologic differences (10–12). In this communication, we report that the increased ^{32}P-phosphorylation of Band 2 can be demonstrated in peptide fractions prepared by either tryptic or cyanogen bromide (CnBr) cleavage of purified spectrin. No unique ^{32}P-labeled DMD peptides have been identified.

METHODS

Methods for endogenous protein kinase assays and spectrin isolation have been reported previously (13). Additional detailed methods of tryptic and CnBr cleavage of purified spectrin are contained in communications describing each set of experiments (14, 24–25).

413

RESULTS

Figure 1 illustrates background information, defines the nomenclature of the system, and presents a summary of previously reported Band 2 ^{32}P-phosphorylation data. These data were obtained by cutting the Coomassie blue–stained band 2 protein from duplicate or triplicate gels, solubilizing, and quantifying the radioactivity by scintillation spectroscopy.

Purified spectrin (Bands 1 and 2) was prepared as previously described after endogenous protein kinase incubations (13). The purified spectrin was then

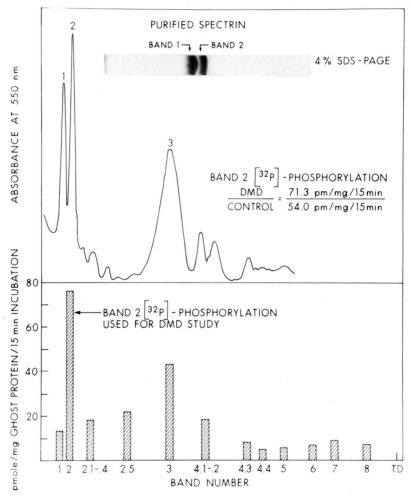

Fig. 1. *Upper panel*: Densitometry recording of a Coomassie blue–stained 6% sodium dodecyl sulfate (SDS)-polyacrylamide gel of solubilized erythrocyte ghost membrane. There are no differences between the patterns for patients with Duchenne muscular dystrophy (DMD) and control subjects. *Lower panel*: A typical pattern for ^{32}P labeling of each of the indicated gel bands. Note that Band 2 labeling is approximately twice that of Band 3 (see *Discussion*). The insert illustrates a Coomassie blue–stained 4% SDS-polyacrylamide gel of purified spectrin Bands 1 and 2 (13). The top inserted data have been previously reported (24).

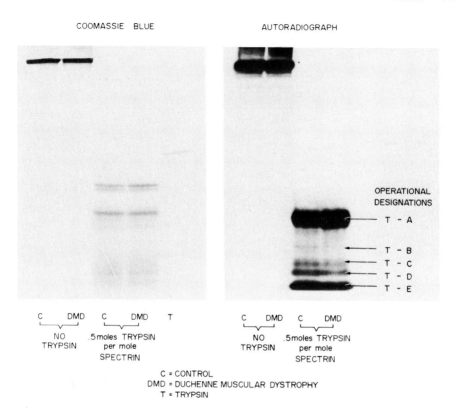

COOMASSIE BLUE   AUTORADIOGRAPH

OPERATIONAL
DESIGNATIONS

T - A

T - B
T - C
T - D
T - E

C   DMD   C   DMD   T   C   DMD   C   DMD

NO   .5moles TRYPSIN   NO   .5moles TRYPSIN
TRYPSIN   per mole   TRYPSIN   per mole
           SPECTRIN   SPECTRIN

C = CONTROL
DMD = DUCHENNE MUSCULAR DYSTROPHY
T = TRYPSIN

Fig. 2. ^{32}P-phosphorylated tryptic peptides of purified spectrin. Coomassie blue-staining pattern and autoradiograph of 5%/15% stacking slab gel electrophoresis of tryptic peptides of purified spectrin. No consistent qualitative differences were demonstrated (no unique peptides), but the ^{32}P-phosphorylation of Band T-A was greater in patients with Duchenne muscular dystrophy than in control subjects (Table 1). *Left channels*: Purified spectrin. *Right channels*: Tryptic peptides.

subjected to cleavage by trypsin or CnBr. Figure 2 demonstrates the Coomassie blue staining pattern and an autoradiograph of stacking slab acrylamide gels (5%/15%) of tryptic peptides. No qualitative differences between DMD and control preparations could be demonstrated, i.e., there were no unique DMD ^{32}P-labeled peptides. The major broad band (T-A) contains several peptides, but this peptide fraction was more highly ^{32}P-phosphorylated in DMD spectrin preparations (Table 1).

To analyze ^{32}P-peptide specificity in DMD, we use CnBr cleavage techniques rather than trypsin or clostripain. The latter two enzymes produce many small peptides, but CnBr, which cleaves polypeptides at methionine residues, produces approximately 30 peptides per spectrin band. Because the purified spectrin preparations contain both Bands 1 and 2, we could expect at least 60 peptides (if peptides from Band 1 and 2 were completely different). Because we were interested in defining the ^{32}P-labeled peptides of interest, CnBr cleavage produces a smaller number of larger-sized ^{32}P-peptides for analysis.

Figure 3 illustrates a Coomassie blue–stained sodium dodecyl sulfate-poly-acrylamide stacking gel of the CnBr cleavage peptides from spectrin. There

Table 1. Comparison of ^{32}P-phosphorylation of Spectrin and Tryptic Peptide A (T-A)

	Spectrin DMD/Control	Peptide T-A DMD/Control
Mean	1.18	1.17
SEM	0.05	0.05
No. of pairs	11	10

Statistical analysis of data from 11 consecutive, prospective paired experiments by two-tailed paired t test of log ^{32}P incorporation, expressed as pmol of ^{32}P incorporated/mg of spectrin or T-A. The 95% confidence interval for spectrin: 8% to 28% increase in ^{32}P incorporation ($0.001 < P < 0.005$). The 95% confidence interval for T-A: 7% to 28% increase in ^{32}P incorporation ($0.001 < P < 0.005$).

were no differences in the stained peptide patterns between patients with DMD and control subjects. The three adjacent autoradiographs are all from the same sample developed for 24, 48, and 96 hours, respectively. If only A1 were illustrated, it would appear that more than 90% of the ^{32}P-radioactivity migrated with Band CN-A. In fact, however, autoradiography cannot be used to quantify incorporated radioactivity unless the radioactivity calculated from densitometry absorption is linearly related to the number of counts. Figure 3 illustrates the inherent quantitative error in this method. Therefore, all ^{32}P incorporation calculated in our experiments was quantified by cutting and solubilizing duplicate gels and counting the radioactivity by scintillation spectroscopy. Approximately 60% of the total radioactivity applied to the gel migrated in Band CN-A (26).

Table 2 presents the quantitative data from 13 consecutive prospective paired experiments. The band labeled CN-A contained at least three distinct ^{32}P-phosphorylated polypeptide chains of very similar apparent molecular weights (21,500 to 23,000 daltons). This band was the only gel fraction in which significant differences between DMD and control ^{32}P-labeled peptides could be demonstrated. The data are presented as pmol of ^{32}P incorporated per µg of protein.

Densitometry measurements of the Coomassie blue–stained gels demonstrated that less than 2% of both DMD and control peptide protein migrated

Table 2. ^{32}P-Phosphorylation of Spectrin CnBr Band (CN-A)

DMD	10.7 ± 2.0
Control	8.9 ± 1.6

Data are given presented as mean ± SEM pmol of ^{32}P incorporated/mg of total peptide protein. In 13 consecutive, prospective paired experiments, p < 0.03.

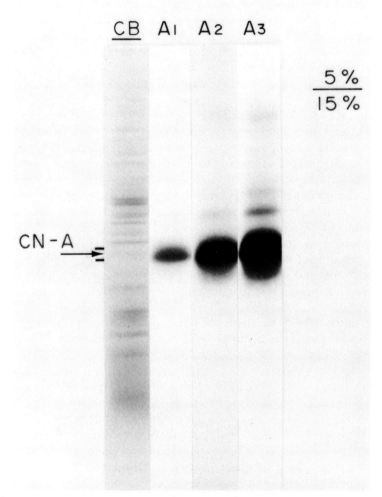

Fig. 3. Cyanogen bromide cleavage of purified spectrin. Coomassie blue-staining pattern and autoradiographs of 5%/15% stacking slab gel electrophoresis of CnBr peptides of purified spectrin. The major ^{32}P-labeled Band CN-A comigrates with at least three faintly stained Coomassie blue peptides of apparent molecular weight 21,500 to 23,000 daltons. No qualitative differences (no unique peptides) were demonstrated, but the ^{32}P-phosphorylation of Band CN-A was greater in patients with Duchenne muscular dystrophy than in control subjects (Table 2). CB, Coomassie blue–stained peptides; A_1, 24-hour autoradiograph of CB gel; A_2, 48-hour autoradiograph of CB gel; A_3, 96-hour autoradiograph of CB gel.

at the CN-A band (26). Thus, this band represented less than 2% of the total spectrin protein but contained approximately 60% of the ^{32}P-phosphorylation.

SUMMARY

We have presented data that extend previous reports of increased ^{32}P-phosphorylation of DMD RBC spectrin Band 2 by endogenous protein kinase. We have confirmed these data by demonstrating increased ^{32}P-phosphorylation in a peptide fraction of isolated spectrin. The increased ^{32}P-phosphorylation takes place at a peptide that represents less than 2% of the total peptide protein, which implies that a particular site on the molecule is involved. Whether this represents a site where a mutation is represented or whether there is a difference in the in vivo starting state of phosphorylation remains to be investigated.

The implications for the relationship of these data to the pathogenesis of DMD in skeletal muscle is entirely speculative. We plan to investigate the possible linkage by using immunologic probes prepared against abnormally ^{32}P-phosphorylated peptides to investigate human muscle. At this time, however, we have no data and therefore prefer not to advance broad speculations concerning the relationship of spectrin to skeletal muscle.

Of critical importance to this conference, however, is the validity of our original data. In a recent review, Rowland (15) listed three reports that apparently failed to confirm our data (7–9). Responses to each have been published, but a brief description would be of value to this audience (10–12). Iyer and colleagues (7) used a method of RBC ghost preparation that produced resealing during incubation. In addition, they did not differentiate lipid and protein phosphorylation, an important consideration in view of the long incubation times used. The methods were so dramatically different that any comparison of data is virtually impossible.

The methodology used by Fisher and coworkers (8) was also different from ours. Although they stated that "endogenous protein kinase was assayed according to Roses, et al" (13), in fact, quite different methods were used. The effects of differences in technique can be readily appreciated by examining the data presented by Fisher and associates. Studies of RBC ghost membrane endogenous protein kinase in multiple laboratories have repeatedly demonstrated greater (2- to 3-fold) ^{32}P-phosphorylation of Band 2 compared to Band 3, expressed as pmol/mg of ghost protein/unit time (10, 16–21). Fisher and associates reported virtually identical levels of ^{32}P-phosphorylation for Bands 2 and 3 in both control subjects and patients; the Band 2 levels were well below values expected for 5-minute incubations. Because Fisher and colleagues used extremely hypotonic incubation buffers, one possible explanation for their unusual data may be the extraction of Band 2 into the buffer, separating it from the membrane and making it unavailable for ^{32}P-phosphorylation by the endogenous protein kinase. A number of other systematic errors could also explain the differences between their published (control and DMD) data and those of other groups.

The third report, by Falk and associates (9), is actually a corroboration of our data. The scant data presented demonstrated an increase of approximately 18% in the ^{32}P-phosphorylation of DMD Band 2. Their point was that this test could not be used for individual carrier detection. They are absolutely correct, although they misinterpreted our discussion (12). This point was clearly made in our original communication and by the accompanying editorial (22, 23).

We therefore believe that when sound, sensitive techniques have been applied, increased ^{32}P-phosphorylation of DMD RBC Band 2 has been demonstrated. Our peptide experiments presented in this communication support the original data. Possible interpretations of increased ^{32}P-phosphorylation of DMD RBC Band 2 depend on additional experiments. Speculations concerning the relationship of these data to the clinically significant disease in muscle are premature.

ACKNOWLEDGMENTS

We thank the patients, controls subjects, and staff of the Duke Neuromuscular Research Clinic. We thank Ms. Mickey Harris for secretarial assistance. These experiments were supported in part by grant NS 13455 from the National Institute of Neurological and Communicative Disorders and Stroke and by a Clinical Research Grant from the Muscular Dystrophy Association. Dr. ME Mabry was a student in the Neurosciences Study Program of Duke University School of Medicine during the period of these experiments. Mr. PV Shile was a Special Premedical Fellow of the Duke Neurobiology Program.

REFERENCES

1. Roses AD, Hartwig GB, Mabry M, et al: Red blood cell and fibroblast membranes in Duchenne and Myotonic muscular dystrophy. Muscle Nerve, 3:36–54, 1980

2. Tsung P, Palek J. Red cell membrane protein phosphorylation in hemolytic anemias and muscular dystrophy. Muscle Nerve 3:55–69, 1980

3. Plishker GA, Appel SH: Red blood cell alterations in muscular dystrophy: the role of lipids. Muscle Nerve 3:70–81, 1980

4. Barchi RL: Physical probes of biological membranes in studies of the muscular dystrophies. Muscle Nerve 3:82–97, 1980

5. Schotland DL, Bonilla E, Wakayama, Y: Applicaton of the freeze fracture technique to the study of human neuromuscular disease. Muscle Nerve 3:21–27 1980

6. Roses AD, Herbstreith MH, Appel SH: Membrane protein kinase alteration in Duchenne muscular dystrophy. Nature 254:350–351, 1975

7. Iyer SL, Hoenig PA, Sherblom AP, Howland, JL: Membrane function affected by genetic muscular dystrophy. Biochem Med 18:384–391, 1977

8. Fisher S, Tortolero M, Piau JP, Delaunay J, Shapira G: Protein kinase and adenylate cyclase of erythrocyte membrane from patients with Duchenne muscular dystrophy. Clin Chim Acta 88:437–440, 1978

9. Falk RS, Campion D, Futhrie D: Phosphorylation of red cell membrane proteins in Duchenne muscular dystrophy. N Engl J Med 300:258, 1979

10. Vickers JD, Rathbone MP, Roses AD: Alterations of erythrocyte ghost protein phosphorylation in Duchenne and myotonic muscular dystrophy. Biochem Med 20:434–439, 1978

11. Roses AD: Erythrocyte membrane autophosphorylation in Duchenne muscular dystrophy: effect of two methods of erythrocyte ghost preparation on results. Clin Chim Acta 95:69–73, 1979

12. Roses AD: More on phosphorylation of red-cell membranes in muscular dystrophy. N Engl J Med 300:114, 1979

13. Roses AD, Herbstreith MH, Metcalf BS, Appel SH: Increased phosphorylated components of erythrocyte membrane spectrin band II with reference to Duchenne muscular dystrophy. J Neurol Sci 30:167–178, 1976

14. Roses AD, Herbstreith M, Shile P: The isolation of abnormally [^{32}P]-phosphorylated cyanogen bromide cleavage products of erythrocyte membrane spectrin in Duchenne muscular dystrophy. Neurology (NY) 30:423, 1980

15. Rowland LP: Biochemistry of muscle membranes in Duchenne muscular dystrophy. Muscle Nerve 3:3–20, 1980

16. Guthrow C, Rasmussen H: Phosphorylation of an endogenous membrane protein by an endogenous membrane-associated cyclic adenosine, 5'-monophosphate dependent protein kinase in human erythrocyte ghosts. J Biol Chem 247:8145–8153, 1972

17. Roses AD, Appel SH: Erythrocyte protein phosphorylation. J Biol Chem 248:1408–1411, 1973

18. Rubin CS, Erlichman J, Rosen OM: Cyclic adenosine 3',5'-monophosphate dependent protein kinase of human erythrocyte membranes. J Biol Chem 247:6135–6139, 1972

19. Rubin CS, Rosen OM: Protein phosphorylation. Annu Rev Biochem 44:831–888, 1975

20. Avruch J, Fairbanks G: Phosphorylation of endogenous substrates by erythrocyte membrane protein kinase. I. A monovalent cation-stimulated reaction. Biochemistry 13:5507–5514, 1974

21. Marchesi VT, Futhmayr H, Tomita JM: The red cell membrane. Annu Rev Biochem 45:667–697, 1976

22. Roses AD, Roses MJ, Miller SE: Carrier detection in Duchenne muscular dystrophy. N Engl J Med 294:193, 1976

23. Shohet SB, Layzer RB: The "muscle" of the red cell. N Engl J Med 294:222–227, 1976

24. Roses AD, Appel SH: Erythrocyte spectrin peak II phosphorylation in Duchenne muscular dystrophy. J Neurol Sci 29:185–193, 1976

25. Mabry ME, Roses AD: Increased [32P]-phosphorylation of tryptic peptides of erythrocyte spectrin in Duchenne muscular dystrophy. Muscle and Nerve (in press)

26. Roses AD, Shile PE, Herbstreith MH, Balakrishnan CV: Indentification of abnormally [32P]-phosphorylated cyanogen bromide cleavage product of erythrocyte membrane spectrin in Duchenne muscle dystrophy. Neurology (in press)

DISCUSSION

Dr. Robert Barchi: In the final figure describing the phosphorylation of the CnBr fragment from spectrin Band 2, you showed about a 20% increase in phosphorylation, but before that, you showed about a 20% increase in phosphorylation of total membrane protein.

Dr. Allen Roses: Total Band 2 protein; the initial numbers were for Band 2, and there was approximately a 20% increase. We also saw approximately the same increase in our isolated peptide bands CN-A.

Dr. Robert Barchi: Is that essentially the only CnBr fragment of Band 2 that is phosphorylated?

Dr. Allen Roses: No, it is not the only one that is phosphorylated, but it is the only CnBr peptide that shows the difference in phosphorylation. The phosphorylation values for the other CnBr peptides are the same in control subjects and patients with Duchenne muscular dystrophy (DMD).

Dr. Robert Barchi: The problem I have is with the numbers. If that fragment is only one of many fragments that is phosphorylated, and if phosphorylation of that one is increased by 20%, why isn't the increase less than 20% when you look at the total phosphorylation of Band 2?

Dr. Allen Roses: One would suspect that you would be taking away some of the phosphorylated background of Band 2 that would be equal, so you would expect the proportion to be slightly greater, not slightly less. Our statistical methods with multiple experiments just do not allow us to see that difference. The CN-A does represent about 60% of the total Band 2 protein phosphorylation; we would not be able to see a statistically significant difference between this and, let us say, one-third more. There is too much variation between experiments.

Dr. Barry Wilson: Some years ago, serum effects were shown for ATP. Is there any effect on the phosphorylation of normal RBCs when you incubate them in serum from dystrophic patients?

Dr. Allen Roses: The phosphorylation of whole membrane or the CnBr fragments?

Dr. Barry Wilson: The whole membrane.

Dr. Allen Roses: When you add serum, you add phosphatases, and what you get is uninterpretable because of the phosphoprotein phosphatase available in the serum. We did not do those experiments very carefully because we would not know how to interpret them once they were done. We have done some switching experiments, but they were uninterpretable.

Dr. Paul Horowicz: First, is there any alteration in the morphology or fragility of these RBCs, and second, is there any change in the binding of spectrin to Band 3, or whatever people now believe it binds to, on phosphorylation or dephosphorylation?

Dr. Allen Roses: Some differences in morphology have been reported. We reported that when fresh cells are taken right out of a butterfly and fixed, there is a difference in the morphologic reaction to specific fixatives. If you look at wet preparations of RBCs from patients with DMD and control subjects, there are no morphologic differences at all. They all look normal. With respect to osmotic fragility, some papers now say that there are some differences. I do not know. We were never able to find a difference. With regard to the other problem, we have been looking with Dr. Vann Bennett, who described a spectrin binding protein, to see whether there are differences in DMD. With respect to whether there is any abnormality in the association of spectrin with the RBC membrane, we did find differences under certain conditions of extraction. Dr. YaNagano, working in my laboratory, has data to demonstrate differences in the extractability of spectrin. Our interpretation is that in DMD there may be a slight change in charge, which may have some effect on the extractability. I might relate this to the Ca-ATPase data, in that this difference in extraction may play a role. The preparation of inside-out ghosts involves the extraction of spectrin in each of the experiments reported by Dr. Pleasure.

Dr. Douglas Fambrough: At the last meeting, you reported that carriers and patients with DMD were equal and different from normal subjects in this phosphorylation property. How is that holding up?

Dr. Allen Roses: We are doing a blind study of carriers at the present time. I cannot tell you what the data will say, but we are certainly running this experiment over a series of carriers. We plan to run 7 definite carriers, 7 probable carriers, and 14 possible carriers (the same group reported in 1976).

Dr. Michael Bárány: It would be very helpful to know the phosphate content of spectrin of normal and dystrophic RBCs. If the spectrin from dystrophic cells contains less bound phosphate than that of normal cells, the rate of the kinase reaction would be faster for dystrophic than normal cells.

Dr. Allen Roses: We tried to dephosphorylate the isolated spectrin by treating it with phosphoprotein phosphatase and then rephosphorylating the material with purified protein kinase. We tended to get equal amounts of ^{32}P-phosphate into spectrin. One of the big problems with rephosphorylating spectrin is that you cannot reconstitute the endogenous system. The amount of phosphate that we could get back on was but 2% of what we were able to do if we phosphorylated the spectrin in situ in the membrane. We found essentially no difference in that 2%. We do not know about the other 98% of phosphorylatable sites that we could not rephosphorylate in our attempts at reconstitution.

34
Adenylate Cyclase in Human Genetic Myopathies

Joseph H. Willner, MD

Cesare Cerri, MD

Donald S. Wood, PhD

In the past decade many researchers interested in human genetic myopathies, particularly muscular dystrophies, have turned from studies of contractile proteins or intermediary metabolism to studies of surface membranes. In this discussion we will focus on a single membrane-bound enzyme, adenylate cyclase, which has been studied in several genetic myopathies.

Ideally, biochemical studies would be done on sarcolemma isolated from pathologic muscle: lipid composition would be analyzed; kinetics of membrane-bound enzymes would be determined; number and affinity of receptors would be characterized. Practically, these studies have been difficult to accomplish because biopsy sizes are limited and yields of membranes are generally low, sarcolemma not contaminated with other membranes has not been isolated, and isolation of membranes may result in changes in activity of the enzyme to be studied.

Two attempted solutions, neither free of problems nor replacing the eventual need for study of sarcolemma, have emerged. One has been to assume that expression of the genetic defect is not limited to muscle and to analyze erythrocyte (1) or lymphocyte (2) membranes. The other has been to study lipid composition of sarcolemma or activity of sarcolemma-bound enzymes in homogenates of muscle, without isolating membranes.

Only one component of sarcolemma, adenylate cyclase, has been extensively studied in homogenates from human myopathies. Behind many of these studies was a belief that alterations in enzyme activity could reflect changes in sarcolemmal chemistry (4), and that problems of measuring a sarcolemmal enzyme in crude homogenates were surmountable. For adenylate cyclase, the problems included uncertain localization in muscle cells, because activities in sarcoplasmic reticulum (5) and transverse tubules (6) relative to sarcolemma (7) are unknown;

uncertain localization in muscle tissue, because relative contributions from nonmuscle cells are unknown and may vary in disease; possibly different properties in red and white muscle fibers (8, 9); and instability of enzyme activity during homogenization and assay (see later). Given these limitations, studies of homogenate adenylate cyclase are, inevitably, an imprecise probe of sarcolemmal biochemistry. However, they are a probe offering several unique advantages: unlike spin resonance probes, adenylate cyclase is normally present in membranes and cannot cause artifactual perturbations; the enzyme can be monitored without isolation of membranes; soluble factors that may influence membrane or enzyme behavior are not discarded.

The significance of studies of adenylate cyclase in human myopathies will be considered in the light of the regulation and function of the enzyme in normal skeletal muscle, and the methodologic problems of studying activity in homogenates and isolated membranes.

ADENYLATE CYCLASE IN SKELETAL MUSCLE

Adenylate cyclase synthesizes cyclic adenosine monophosphate (cAMP) from Mg-adenosine triphosphate (MgATP) (10, 11), providing a mechanism for extracellular control of cellular protein phosphorylation. Specific plasmalemmal receptors permit regulation of adenylate cyclase by monoamines and peptides. Only a single receptor that regulates adenylate cyclase has been recognized in skeletal sarcolemma, a β_2 receptor (12, 13) that permits activation of adenylate cyclase by epinephrine.

Only a fraction of phosphoproteins are substrates for a cAMP-dependent protein kinase, and in still fewer proteins is phosphorylation of known physiologic significance. The number of muscle proteins for which phosphorylation by cAMP-dependent protein kinase has known physiologic significance is even more limited (Table 1), although several contractile proteins (18–20), sarcolemmal proteins (21), and enzymes, such as phosphofructokinase (22), have been identified as substrates of this enzyme.

Table 1. Muscle Proteins Regulated by cAMP Catalyzed Phosphorylation

Substrate Protein	Effect of Phosphorylation by cAPK[a]
Phosphorylase kinase (β-subunit)[b]	Activation
Phosphorylase kinase (α-subunit)[b]	May contribute to activation
Glycogen synthetase (several sites)[b]	Inhibition
Protein phosphatase inhibitor[c]	Activation
Histone[d]	Derepression of protein synthesis
Phospholamban[e]	Stimulation of Ca^{2+} transport in sarcoplasmic reticulum

[a] cAPK = cyclic adenosine monophosphate–dependent protein kinase.
[b] Reference 14.
[c] Reference 15.
[d] Reference 16.
[e] Reference 17.

Because of the limitations of sarcolemmal preparations, mechanisms identified in other tissues for regulation of adenylate cyclase have been little examined in muscle. In isolated membrane preparations (13) or in homogenates (see later), guanosine triphosphate (GTP) or its GTPase-resistant analogue, guanosine imididodiphosphate (GppNHp), stimulates basal activity or enhances the response to catecholamines. The probable mechanism, demonstrated with other cells, is a requirement for GTP in coupling of β receptors to catalytic subunits of adenylate cyclase (23, 24).

Adenosine in fat cell membranes binds to receptors capable of activating or inhibiting adenylate cyclase (25). In homogenates of human muscle we found maximal inhibition of enzyme activity by adenosine at a concentration of 1.25 mM, which is unlikely to be of physiologic importance.

Regulation of adenylate cyclase by divalent cations, however, is likely to be physiologically important for muscle. The magnesium ion (MG^{2+}) may have a specific binding site in the catalytic subunit (26); enzyme activation by Mg^{2+} measured with human muscle homogenates was consistent with this behavior (see later). Stimulation of adenylate cyclase by Mg^{2+} occurs at physiologic concentrations of this cation, but whether intracellular Mg^{2+} fluctuates significantly in healthy or diseased muscle is not known.

With preparations of either enriched sarcolemma (7) or crude homogenate (27) submicromolar concentrations of Ca^{2+} inhibit enzyme activity, implying that adenylate cyclase could be inhibited during muscle contraction. In a membrane-enriched preparation of pancreatic islet cells, Ca^{2+} also inhibited adenylate cyclase, but addition of exogenous calmodulin resulted in activation of adenylate cyclase by Ca^{2+} (28). Because it is not known whether activation of adenylate cyclase by a Ca^{2+}-calmodulin complex is a general property of the enzyme or is peculiar to pancreas and brain (29), it is appropriate that regulation of the muscle enzyme by Ca^{2+} be reevaluated with a physiologic preparation of muscle or with sarcolemma supplemented with calmodulin.

These brief comments but superficially indicate the complex regulation of adenylate cyclase, which is better reviewed in several recent publications (30, 31). They serve, however, to introduce our recent study of adenylate cyclase in normal human muscle, which was begun not only because regulation of adenylate cyclase is better understood in 1980 than 1972, but also because discrepancies in past measurements of enzyme activity in normal human muscle have made it difficult to evaluate reports of altered enzyme activity in human myopathies.

ADENYLATE CYCLASE IN NORMAL HUMAN MUSCLE

Past studies of adenylate cyclase in normal human muscle (32–37) found basal activities ranging from 2.9 to 20 pmol/mg of noncollagen protein (NCP)/min, and catecholamine-activated activity ranged from 1.08 to 256 pmol/mg/min. No two groups used the same method of homogenization of muscle or conditions for enzyme assay; we decided to determine whether these variables could account for the variation in reported activities.

Stability During Homogenization

For these studies we homogenized muscle in sucrose (27%, wt/vol), 0.4 mM ethyleneglycol tetra-acetate (EGTA), 10 mM Tris (pH 7.5). In this buffer, enzyme activity was stable at 4° C for more than 1 hour. To evaluate methods of tissue disruption, we varied duration or intensity of homogenization to maximize enzyme activity. Homogenization in an all-glass homogenizer consistently gave lower activity than optimal homogenization with a Teflon-glass homogenizer with identical clearance or with a Polytron homogenizer. These latter two methods resulted in identical values. Activity was dramatically reduced with pulverization of frozen muscle before homogenization, sonication of homogenate, or prolonged homogenization with any of the methods described.

The type of homogenization differed in previous studies, and could account for some of the variation in results. This variation was not due to thermal denaturation during homogenization, because all homogenates were kept at 4° C. It is possible that membrane particle size with a multicomponent membrane-bound enzyme or vesicle conformation may influence activity: disruption of membranes may cause disruption of enzyme or impair access of substrate to catalytic site.

Stability of Homogenate Enzyme

Several different buffers were used in previous studies (32–38). We found that inclusion of a divalent cation chelator was obligatory to prevent loss of basal enzyme activity, which occurred rapidly at 4° C between the time of homogenization and assay (Fig. 1). Either ethylenediamine tetra-acetate or EGTA stabilized activity; in subsequent studies we used EGTA to avoid the need to correct for chelation of Mg^{2+}. This protective action of the chelators remains unexplained. Addition of Ca^{2+} in excess to chelator capacity inhibited, but did not destabilize, enzyme activity; Mn^{2+} was without effect.

Catecholamine-activation also deteriorated at 4° C. Addition of 100 μM GTP variably, or 10 μM GppNHp dependably, stabilized responses to catecholamines (Fig. 1). Guanyl nucleotides had the same effect if they were added immediately after homogenization or just before assay; they probably replaced GTP lost from the catalytic site, either by diffusion or GTPase activity.

Either 0.15 M KCl or 27% sucrose (38) in the homogenizing medium yielded stable enzyme activities, but activity was 25% higher with KCl.

Components of Assay

Temperature and pH

At 37° C activity was 4 times higher than at 30° C. Maximal basal and isoproterenol-stimulated activities occurred at pH 7.6 and 7.8, respectively.

Phosphodiesterase Inhibition

Theophylline gave highest apparent enzyme activity at a concentration of 20 mM, but activity then was 28% lower than in assays in which 1 mM cAMP was used to prevent ^{32}P-cAMP from hydrolysis. Higher concentrations of cAMP

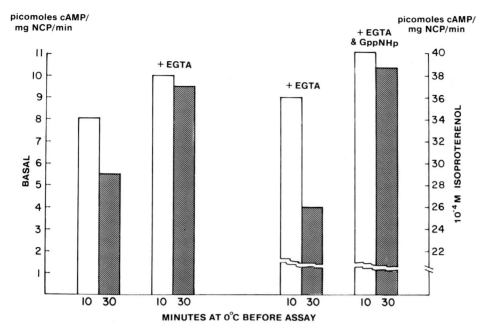

Fig. 1. Lability of homogenate adenylate cyclase. Addition of 400 μM ethyleneglycol tetra-acetate (EGTA) to homogenates prevents lability of adenylate cyclase, which occurs rapidly in homogenates, despite storage in ice. Response of adenylate cyclase to isoproterenol is independantly labile at this temperature, apparently because of loss of guanyl nucleotide necessary for coupling of the β receptor to catalytic subunits of the enzyme. cAMP, cyclic adenosine monophosphate; GppNHp, guanosine imididodiphosphate; NCP, noncollagen protein.

caused lower apparent enzyme activities. Theophylline may be a suboptimal choice as a phosphodiesterase inhibitor in adenylate cyclase assays, because it stimulates adenosine receptors that inhibit adenylate cyclase activity (25).

Regenerating System for ATP
To maintain constant substrate concentrations despite ATPase activity, a regenerating system for ATP is commonly used. Phosphoenol pyruvate-pyruvate kinase and creatine phosphate-creatine kinase were indistinguishable in this assay, although differences had been observed with other tissues (39).

ATP and Divalent Cations
Activity was not detected in the absence of Mg^{2+}. With 0.5 mM $MgCl_2$ and 1 mM ATP, activity was present, but was not stimulated by isoproterenol. At 1 mM $MgCl_2$, basal activity increased and stimulation by isoproterenol became evident. At 4 mM $MgCl_2$, isoproterenol-stimulated activity was maximal; at higher concentrations of $MgCl_2$, isoproterenol-stimulated activity declined progressively, although basal activity continued to increase at concentrations of $MgCl_2$ above 10 mM. No differences were found between $MgSO_4$ and $MgCl_2$. When either the $MgATP/Mg^{2+}$ ratio or the total Mg concentration was constant, the concentration of Mg^{2+} did not effect the K_m for MgATP. The K_m in the

presence of GppNHp was identical to the K_m under basal conditions (0.28 mM MgATP).

When Ca^{2+} was added to the assay mixture or to the homogenate in amounts exceeding the chelating capacity of EGTA (free Ca^{2+} concentration of 10 or 100 μM), activity was inhibited by 20% or 60%, respectively. The effect was the same whether Ca^{2+} was added to the assay mixture or to the homogenate.

Because the affinity of Mg^{2+} for ATP increases with pH in the range of 7.0 to 8.6 (40), an increase of pH within this range increases the concentration of MgATP. If the concentration of MgATP was kept constant by correcting for the effect of pH on the affinity constant, basal activity did not increase with increasing pH. Dependence of enzyme activity on pH was therefore partially due to variations in concentrations of MgATP, Mg^{2+}, and ATP^{-4}.

The influence of Mg on adenylate cyclase activity is bimodal: the substrate is probably MgATP rather than free ATP (11), but with constant concentration of MgATP, V_{max} increased with Mg^{2+}. A possible explanation would be an inhibition of the enzyme by free ATP (41, 42) because increasing Mg^{2+} when MgATP is held constant decreases the concentration of free ATP. A more satisfactory explanation is to assume an allosteric regulatory site for Mg^{2+} (11, 26, 42), which would explain increased V_{max} when free Mg^{2+} increased and, if this site is on the catalytic unit, different effects of Mg^{2+} on basal and isoproterenol-stimulated activity but identical effects on basal and guanylnucleotide-stimulated activities.

Adenosine

At a concentration of 1.25 mM, adenosine inhibited adenylate cyclase activity by 50%. Adenosine deaminase could reverse inhibition by exogenous adenosine but did not affect activity in the absence of added adenosine, indicating that endogenous adenosine was not interfering with assay of adenylate cyclase.

Reproducibility

To determine values for normal adult human muscle under optimal conditions, we measured enzyme activity in 14 muscles, 5 obtained under general anesthesia and 9 with local anesthesia. We homogenized muscles to a concentration of 3% to 5% (wt/vol) in 10 mM Tris, 0.15 M KCl, 0.4 mM EGTA (pH 7.6) with a Potter-Elvehjem homogenizer and Teflon pestle. In a final volume of 100 μl, activity was measured at 37° C (pH 7.6) with 1.0 mM ATP (30 to 50 cpm of ^{32}P/pmol), 2.0 mM $MgCl_2$, 20 mM creatine phosphate, 100 U/ml creatine kinase, 35 mM Tris, 1.25 U/ml adenosine deaminase, and 1.0 mM cAMP. The cAMP was separated from ATP by column chromatography (43). Type of anesthesia had no significant effect on activity. The mean ± SD basal activity was 10.88 ± 3.61 (range, 6.00 to 16.2); isoproterenol-stimulated activity assayed in the presence of 10^{-4} M Gpp(NH)p, 41.6 ± 23.3 (range, 16.8 to 101), for an increase over basal activity of 4.0 ± 1.9fold.

Reproducibility of this method was assessed by 5 assays on 2 different days of a piece of human vastus lateralis muscle (kept frozen in liquid nitrogen). Two pieces were homogenized using maximal speed for 5 seconds on the Polytron and three, with the Teflon glass homogenizer for 30 seconds. Values of triplicate determinations of the same homogenate varied less than 5% of the mean. The standard deviation of values around a mean of 8.20 was 1.19 pmol/mg protein/min.

Conclusions

We have reviewed in detail our studies of adenylate cyclase in muscle homogenates to clarify the variables that must be considered in studies of this enzyme. The absence of uniform conditions in different laboratories has undoubtedly resulted in variation in results.

It should be emphasized that we do not claim a "correct" method, if by "correct" is meant an in vitro assay that reproduces in vivo conditions. Content of cAMP and activity of cAMP-dependent protein kinase are low in unstimulated muscle (44). Adenylate cyclase under unstimulated conditions is, in other words, a relatively quiescent enzyme. We found that in muscle homogenates, as in other tissues, basal activity is highly dependent on free Mg^{2+} concentration. The Mg^{2+} concentration we used in the above studies was selected, not because it resulted in a "correct" activity, but because it provided a basal activity that was readily measured and permitted good stimulation by catecholamines.

ADENYLATE CYCLASE IN ISOLATED MEMBRANES

Whether homogenates or isolated membranes should be used to study muscle adenylate cyclase will not be easily resolved. The enzyme in muscle may be regulated by intracellular GTP, ADP-ribose (46), and calmodulin, all of which are lost to an unknown extent in different membrane preparations. Determination of kinetic properties in isolated membranes provides meaningful information about the enzyme in those membranes, but, as is true for any purified enzyme, extrapolation back to how the intact enzyme works may be an act of faith.

Potential loss of intracellular regulators of enzyme activity is only one problem in studying isolated membranes. Two others are membrane purity and enzyme lability. Density gradients are virtually unavoidable in membrane isolation, and one problem is to assure that the experimental variable (disease, denervation, drug administration) has no effect on the buoyant density of membranes in the gradient. Another problem is to know the origin of the enzyme to be studied. Reiss and Katz (47) reported that adenylate cyclase in cardiac sarcoplasmic reticulum differs from the sarcolemmal enzyme. If this is true in skeletal muscle, undetected contamination of sarcolemma with other membranes may create inaccurate conclusions about function of adenylate cyclase in sarcolemma.

The method of Severson and co-workers (7), which is commonly used at least to initiate isolation of sarcolemma for subsequent study of adenylate cyclase, does not use a metal chelator, which we found essential to prevent lability of the enzyme. Table 2 lists reported values in membrane fractions. It is difficult to compare different reports because the techniques of both assay and isolation varied. Differences between starting tissues probably matters less, because neither Severson (7), using isolated membranes nor we, comparing homogenates of rat, rabbit, and human muscle, found differences as large as those reported for different membrane preparations. Nearly all of these studies used LiBr to

Table 2. Adenylate Cyclase in Muscle Surface Membrane

Reference	Preparation	Method Reference	Adenylate Cyclase Activity (pmol/mg/min)		
			Basal	Catechol-Stimulated	NaF
Severson et al. (7)	Rabbit leg SL	(7)			810.4 (8 mM NaF)
Mawatari et al. (27)	Human SL	(7)	40.7	89.8 (100 μM E)	817.1 (8 mM NaF)
Rodan et al. (48)	Chick pectoralis SL	(7)	4.02		
Festoff et al. (8)	Rat EDL SL	(51)	10.3	12.1[a]	112[a]
	Rat soleus SL	(51)	16.8	31.8	143
Novom and Lewinstein (49)	Rabbit gastrocnemius SL	(7)	230	600 (1 μM E)	
Caswell et al. (6)	Rabbit sacrospinalis, heavy microsomes = T tubules	(6)	13	39 (10 μM I)	111 (5 mM NaF)
Smith et al. (50)	Rat SL	(52)	51	160 (0.1 μM I)	1,750 (20 mM NaF)
Reddy et al. (37)	Human SR	(5)	41.3	72 (10 μM I)	933 (10 mM NaF)
	Human SL (PL)	(5)	30.7	105 (10 μM I)	1,120 (10 mM NaF)
	Further purified SL (PL$_1$)	(5)	45.3	160 (10 μM I)	3,240 (10 mM NaF)
Narayanan et al. (26)	Rabbit SL	(7)	38		164 (5 mM NaF)
Reddy et al. (9)	Rabbit EDL SL	(5)	166	273 (10 μM I)	3,368 (5 mM NaF)
	Rabbit soleus SL	(5)	149	528 (10 μM I)	3,343 (5 mM NaF)
Wei et al. (41)	Guinea pig leg SL	(7)	120	220 (10 μM I)	

Abbreviations: SL, sarcolemma; E, epinephrine; EDL, extensor digitorum longus; I, isoproterenol; PL, plasmalemma.

[a] Concentration not stated.

extract myofilament protein; other methods for preparing sarcolemma for study of adenylate cyclase have generally yielded inferior results. Some authors reported "enriched" membrane preparations with activity not much different from the mean of 10.9 we found in whole homogenate, probably because of enzyme lability during membrane isolation. Conversely, claims of membrane enrichment in membrane preparations based on increased specific activity of adenylate cyclase may be compromised by lability being greater in homogenates stored at 4° C than in membranes during isolation, and activity in homogenates being determined only after isolation of membranes.

ADENYLATE CYCLASE IN HUMAN MYOPATHIES

The concentration of adenylate cyclase in surface membranes has made it a logical enzyme to study in myopathies believed to be membrane disorders. Because of uncontrolled variables in membrane isolation, we believe that homogenates are now the most reasonable preparation for initial studies of muscle disease. Most studies of human myopathies have used homogenates, but all past studies were of an enzyme that was probably labile during homogenization and was certainly labile in the interval between homogenization and assay.

Duchenne Dystrophy

Six laboratories have reported studies of adenylate cyclase in homogenates of Duchenne muscle (Table 3). Each used a different method of assay, and no two laboratories achieved similar results. Because Duchenne muscle contains both degenerating and regenerating muscle cells as well as fat and connective tissue, all of which possess adenylate cyclase activity, some investigators have questioned the meaning of these observations. The discrepancies in reported values from different laboratories have also done little to inspire confidence that this enzyme is abnormal in Duchenne muscle.

Some of these concerns about studies of Duchenne muscle were partially answered by study of muscle cells in culture, erythrocyte membranes, and carrier muscle. In cultured Duchenne muscle cells in the myotube stage of dvelopment, Mawatari and associates (53) found abnormal enzyme activity: stimulation by epinephrine was reduced, isoproterenol inhibited activity, and basal activity was increased. Because the enzyme was normal in cells from other diseases, was not due to contaminating cells or muscle at different stages of development, and was expressed at an early stage of cellular development, which preceded morphologic signs of cellular degeneration, it is difficult to dismiss this observation. It remains the only observation that abnormal sarcolemmal chemistry or morphology is expressed in Duchenne muscle at this stage of development; given the potential importance of the observation and the relative ease of isolating sarcolemma from cultured cells, it is curious that no effort has been made either to replicate or to extend this study. Three laboratories (54–56) found in erythrocyte ghosts patterns of abnormality of adenylate cyclase similar to those in cultured muscle, bolstering the significance

Table 3. Adenylate Cyclase in Muscle Homogenates

| | | | | Addition | |
| | | | | Catecholamine[a] | NaF |
Reference	Subjects	No.	None	$(10^{-4}$ M)	$(10^{-2}$ M)
Mawatari et al. (27)	Normal	(7)	2.9	16.1	52.3
	Duchenne	(6)	2.6	4.3	20.5
Susheela et al. (33)	Normal	(3)	—	1.08	0.85
	Duchenne	(5)	—	0.31	0.25
Canal et al. (32)	Normal	(16)	5.4	—	42.8
	Duchenne	(4)	2.3	—	26.9
Takahashi et al. (36)	Normal	(1)	20.0	29.0	53.8
	Duchenne	(2)	15.5	18.3	48.4
			21.0	28.6	31.8
Willner et al. (35)	Normal	(8)	10.4	33.6	58.5
	Duchenne	(8)	5.2	6.6	21.5
Khokhlov and Malakhovsky (34)	Normal	(7)	4.1	256.0	1,000.0
	Duchenne	(6)	3.0	26.0	196.0

To obtain the data shown, published values were reduced to common denominator and expressed as pmol/mg of protein/min. Individual results are given for the data of Takahashi and associates (3); all other data are means. Mawatari et al. (27), Canal et al. (32), and Willner et al. (35) used noncollagen protein as reference; Susheela et al (33) and Takahashi et al (36) used total protein. Khokhlov and Malakhovsky used noncollagen protein as the reference, but used a membrane fraction rather than whole homogenates.

[a] Mawatari et al (27), Takahashi et al (36), and Khoklov and Malakhovsky (34) used epinephrine; Susheela et al (33) and Willner et al (35) used isoproterenol.

of the observation made with myotubes. A laboratory that did not confirm (57) used EGTA in the buffer for preparation of red cells, which, as shown by Roses (58) for studies of protein kinase in erythrocytes, may remarkably alter results.

Using a then standard method of homogenization, we studied muscle of genetically possible Duchenne carriers who had abnormal serum enzymes (35). Tissues were histologically free of "dystrophic" changes. The study was controlled for duration of time between homogenization and assay, and for duration of homogenization. Stimulation of adenylate cyclase by isoproterenol was significantly less in carrier muscle than control muscle, but basal activity was normal. However, an all-glass homogenizer was used and a calcium chelator was not included in the homogenate; this study must be repeated to provide data comparable to our more recent observations.

Another concern arises from our study of enzyme lability. It was possible that lower basal activity in one earlier study of Duchenne muscle could have been due to increased enzyme lability. In fact this is not the case. We found that basal activity of Duchenne muscle homogenates prepared in the presence of EGTA with a Potter-Elvejhem and Teflon pestle was lower than control activity $(3.24 \pm 1.6$, compared to 10.9 ± 3.6 pmol/mg of noncollagen protein/min). It is still possible that this measurement lacks meaning, if, as recently reiterated by Samaha and associates (59) noncollagen protein is an inappropriate reference base for Duchenne muscle. However, the response of the enzyme to catecholamines is a measurement independent of reference base; we have confirmed that it is, indeed, reduced (activation in Duchenne homogenates, 1.7-fold; in control homogenates, 4.0-fold).

No studies have related this enzyme abnormality to the pathogenesis of Duchenne dystrophy. It may be a biochemical correlate to the structural abnormalities in sarcolemma. Its usefulness as a tool for probing biochemical changes in sarcolemma and its relation to other abnormalities in Duchenne muscle remain to be determined.

Myotonic Dystrophy

Mawatari and associates (27) reported that epinephrine-stimulated adenylate cyclase in homogenates of muscle from patients with myotonic dystrophy was less than control (p < .02), whereas basal activity was normal (27); this difference was not considered meaningful, in comparison to the difference between Duchenne and control muscle (p < .001). Reddy and colleagues (60) isolated sarcolemma from biopsy specimens, controlling for possible artifactual redistribution of sarcolemma from myotonic dystrophy muscle into other subcellular fractions. They reported that basal activity in sarcolemma from 5 patients was 30% to 60% reduced, compared to sarcolemma from control muscle. However, they did not assess recovery of enzyme activity, and it would be important to know that the same yield of activity was achieved from diseased and control muscle. Otherwise, a disease-related difference in lability of the enzyme could account for differences observed in basal activity by Reddy and coworkers (60) with sarcolemma, but not by Mawatari and colleagues (27) with homogenate.

Thyrotoxic Periodic Paralysis

There have been 2 studies of a total of 3 patients with thyrotoxic periodic paralysis. Tagaki and coworkers (61) reported that enzyme activity in a sarcoplasmic reticulum fraction decreased more than 40% during paralysis induced by glucose and insulin. Activity before paralysis did not differ from the control value (n = 2). Because the number of bands of sarcoplasmic reticulum protein on SDS-acrylamide gels also changed during paralysis and other measured enzyme activities also declined, the reference base for adenylate cyclase rather than the enzyme activity might have changed. Koehler and associates (62) studied homogenates of muscle from 2 patients between attacks. They reported 35% and 85% reductions of activity.

Malignant Hyperthermia

Persons who are susceptible to attacks of malignant hyperthermia have an underlying myopathy (63). When inheritance can be established, an autosomal dominant pattern usually emerges (64). Some susceptible individuals have an electrophysiologically or morphologically distinct myopathy, such as central core disease (65). Most, including those we studied, have muscle that lacks definition by these tests and is usually classified instead according to physiologic tests, such as the response of isolated muscle strips to caffeine (66). Attacks of malignant hyperthermia usually occur in response to anesthetic agents, but have been reported to occur after emotional or physical stress (67). Between attacks, this myopathy commonly is without signs or symptoms; musculoskeletal abnormalities, strabismus, increased body temperature without infection, muscular hypertrophy, and cramps may be nonspecific signs or symptoms (68).

Our studies of cAMP metabolism in muscle of persons who are susceptible to malignant hyperthermia stemmed from our observation with chemically skinned fibers (see chapter 42) that abnormal function of sarcoplasmic reticulum was the cause of the hypersensitive response of isolated muscle strips to caffeine. Increased rate of Ca^{2+} accumulation, which had been demonstrated in one study of isolated sarcoplasmic reticulum (69), was one of several possible explanations for this response. A physiologic mechanism for stimulating Ca^{2+} transport by sarcoplasmic reticulum of rabbit (70) and human slow-twitch muscle (Wood DS, Willner JH, Salviati G: unpublished observations) is mediated by cAMP. Halothane (directly) (Willner JH, Vuillemoz Y: unpublished data) and stress (indirectly, by catecholamine release) could stimulate skeltal muscle adenylate cyclase. Pyrophosphate, a product of the hydrolysis of ATP by adenylate cyclase, was reported increased in serum of persons who are susceptible to malignant hyperthermia (71). These observations provided a possible mechanism for the abnormality of sarcoplasmic reticulum and a suggestion that this mechanism could be involved in pathogeneis of the syndrome.

Our initial studies (45) are reproduced in Table 4. Basal and catecholamine-activated activities were increased in muscle homogenates, due to an increased V_{max} with no change K_m. Interpretation of kinetic studies with a crude enzyme may be limited; but for reasons stated above, studies with isolated membranes may not be superior. For these studies we prepared muscle without EGTA, but duration of homogenization and interval between homogenization and assay were controlled. Activity was measured with 5 mM total Mg and 1 mM total ATP. The cAMP content of muscle was also increased (Table 4). Because cAMP activates a protein kinase which, in turn, activates phosphorylase kinase, we measured the relative proportions of phosphorylase b and a. The increased phosphorylase activity we found (72) was not phosphorylase b stimulated by AMP, because the AMP content was normal, and was probably not due to

Table 4. Biochemical Studies in Malignant Hyperthermia

Measurement	Control	n^a	MH	n^a	P value
cAMP content (pmol/mg NCP)	2.94 ± 0.80	8	9.95 ± 3.23	5	< .05
Adenylate cyclase activity (pmol/ mg NCP/min)					
Basal	5.54 ± 1.77	8	16.7 ± 5.67	5	< .005
10^{-4} Iso	9.26 ± 4.25	8	41.1 ± 10.1	5	< .001
cAMP phosphodiesterase activity (nmol/mg/10 min)	3.63 ± 1.84	8	2.88 ± 1.39	5	< .05
Phosphorylase a/Total (%)	2.63 ± 2.02	34	45.6 ± 26.2	8	< .0005

Abbreviations: cAMP, cyclic adenosine monophosphate; NCP, noncollagen protein; Iso, isoproterenol; n, number of patient muscles assayed.

[a] Data are mean ± SD.

activation of phosphorylase kinase by Ca^{2+}, since two laboratories have reported normal Ca content in muscle from patients susceptible to attacks of malignant hyperthermia (73, 74).

We have now begun to measure activity with the more reliable conditions we described above. We have not yet generated enough data, but preliminary experiments indicate that, due to a shift in the K_a for Mg^{2+} in muscle of persons susceptible to malignant hyperthermia, increased adenylate cyclase activity is only evident at low Mg^{2+} concentrations in the assay.

In skinned fibers from human skeletal muscle, only a fraction of fibers are responsive to removal of endogenously produced cAMP by addition of exogenous cAMP phosphodiesterase, or to addition of exogenous cAMP. In muscle from one survivor of malignant hyperthermia, skinned fibers with sarcoplasmic reticulum Ca^{2+} uptake responsive to cAMP had more rapid Ca^{2+} uptake than similarly responsive fibers in control muscle (see chapter 46 this volume).

CONCLUSION

In the past decade there have been a number of efforts to study adenylate cyclase in muscle from patients with myopathies generally considered to be membrane disorders. As the properties and regulation of this enzyme in normal human muscle continue to be clarified, the significance and interpretation of abnormal activity in human myopathies should emerge more clearly. Even with the limitations of many past studies, they have provided strong evidence that some human genetic myopathies may be expressed in sarcolemma.

ACKNOWLEDGMENTS

We would like to express our appreciation to Dr. Lewis P. Rowland for his insights, criticism, and support. This work was supported by grants from the Muscular Dystrophy Association. JH Willner is the recipient of a Teacher-Investigator Development Award from the National Institute of Neurological and Communicative Disorders and Stroke. C Cerri is the recipient of a postdoctoral fellowship from the Muscular Dystrophy Association.

REFERENCES

1. Roses AD: Erythrocytes in dystrophies. In *Pathogenesis of Human Muscular Dystrophies.* Edited by Rowland LP. Excerpta Medica, Amsterdam, 1977, pp 648–655

2. Pickard NA, Gruener HD, Verrey HL: Systemic membrane defect in the proximal muscular dystrophies. N Engl J Med 299:841–846, 1978

3. Kunze D, Olthoff D: Der lipidgenalt menschlicher skelettmuskulatur bei primaren und sekundaren myopathien. Clin Chim Acta 29:455–462, 1970

4. Rowland LP: Pathogenesis of muscular dystrophies. Arch Neurol 33:315–321, 1976

5. Schutze W, Winterberger V, Krause EG, et al: Localization of adenylate cyclase in muscle tissues at the fine structure level. Ergebn Exp Med 28:215–216, 1978

6. Caswell AH, Baker SP, Boyd H, et al: β-adrenergic receptor and adenylate cyclase in transverse tubule of skeletal muscle. J Biol Chem 253:30–54, 1978

7. Severson DI, Drummond GI, Sulakhe PV: Adenylate cyclase in skeletal muscle: kinetic properties and hormonal stimulation. J Biol Chem 247:2949–2958, 1972

8. Festoff BW, Oliver KL, Reddy NB: In vitro studies of skeletal muscle membranes: adenylate cyclase of fast and slow twitch muscle and effects of denervation. J Membr Biol 31:331–343, 1977

9. Reddy NB, Oliver KL, Engel WK: Differences in catecholamine-sensitive adenylate cyclase and β-adrenergic receptor binding between fast and slow twitch skeletal muscle membranes. Lif Sci 24:1765–1772, 1979

10. Sutherland EW, Rall TW, Menon T: Adenyl cyclase. I. Distribution, preparation, and properties. J Biol Chem 237:1220–1238, 1962

11. Neer EJ: Interaction of soluble brain adenylate cyclase with manganese. J Biol Chem 254:2089–2096, 1979

12. Reddy NB, Oliver KL, Festoff BW, et al: Adenylate cyclase system of human skeletal muscle: characteristics of catecholamine stimulation and nucleotide regulation. Biochim Biophys Acta 540:348–401, 1978

13. Nambi P, Drummond GI: Catecholamine and guanine nucleotide activation of skeletal muscle adenylate cyclase. Biochim Biophys Acta 583:287–294, 1979

14. Soderling TR: Regulatory function of protein multisite phosphorylation. Mol Cell Endocrinol 16:157–179, 1979

15. Nimmo GA, Cohen P: The regulation of glycogen metabolism: phosphorylation of inhibitor-1 from rabbit skeletal muscle and its interaction with protein phosphatase III and II. Eur J Biochem 87:353–365, 1978

16. Langan TA: Cyclic AMP and histone phosphorylation. Ann NY Acad Sci 185:166–180, 1971

17. Tada M, Ohmori F, Kimoshita N, et al: Cyclic AMP regulation of active calcium transport across membranes of sarcoplasmic reticulum: role of the 20,000 dalton protein phospholamban. In *Advances in Cyclic Nucleotide Research*, vol 9. Edited by George CWJ, Ignarro LJ. Raven Press, New York, 1977, pp 35–370

18. Noir ASG, Wilkinson JM, Perry SV: The phosphorylation sites of troponin I from white skeletal muscle of the rabbit. FEBS Lett 42:253–256, 1974

19. Silver PJ, DiSalvo J: Adenosine 3′:5′ monophosphate-mediated inhibition of myosin light chain phosphorylation in bovine aortic actomyosin. J Biol Chem 254:9951–9954, 1979

20. Bárány M, Bárány K: Phosphorylation of the myofibrillar proteins. Ann Rev Physiol 42:275–292, 1980

21. Walsh DA, Clippinger MS, Sivarmakrishnan S, et al: Cyclic adenosine monophosphate dependent and independent phosphorylation of sarcolemma membrane proteins in perfused rat heart. Biochemistry 18:871–877, 1979

22. Requelme PT, Hosey MM, Marcus F, et al: Phosphorylation of muscle phosphofructokinase by the catalytic subunit of cyclic AMP-dependent protein kinase. Biochem Biophys Res Commun 85:1480–1487, 1978

23. Levitzky A: The mode of coupling of adenylate cyclase to hormone receptor and its modulation by GTP. Biochem Pharmacol 27:2083–2088, 1978

24. Abramowitz J, Iyengar T: Guanylnucleotide regulation of hormonally responsive adenylyl cyclase. Mol Cell Endocrinol 16:129–146, 1979

25. Londos C, Cooper DMF, Schlegel W, et al: Adenosine analogs inhibit adipocyte adenyl cyclase by a GTP-dependent process: basis for actions of adenosine and methylxanthines on cyclic AMP production and lipolysis. Proc Natl Acad Sci USA 75:5362–5364, 1978

26. Narayanan N, Wei J. Sulakhe PV: Differences in the cation sensitivity of adenylate cyclase for heart and skeletal muscle: modification by guanyl nucleotides and isoproterenol. Arch Biochem Biophys 197:18–29, 1979

27. Mawatari S, Takagi A, Rowland LP: Adenyl cyclase in normal and pathologic human muscle. Arch Neurol 30:96–102, 1974

28. Valverde I, Vanderweers A, Ansaeyuld R, et al: Calmodulin activation of adenylate cyclase in pancreatic islets. Science 206:225–227, 1979

29. Brostrom MA, Brostrom CO, Breckenride BM, et al: Calcium-dependent regulation of brain adenylate cyclase. Adv Cyclic Nucleotide Res 9:85–100, 1978

30. Abramowitz J, Iyengar R, Birnbaumer L: Guanyl nucleotide regulation of hormonally-responsive adenylyl cyclases. Mol Cell Endocrinol 16:129–146, 1979

31. Ross EM, Haga T, Howlett AC, et al: Hormone-sensitive adenylate cyclase: resolution and reconstitution of some components necessary for regulation of the enzyme. In *Advances in Cyclic Nucleotide Research*, vol 9. Edited by George WJ, Ignarro LJ. Raven Press, New York, 1978, pp 53–68

32. Canal N, Frattola L, Smirne S: The metabolism of cyclic 3'-5' adenosine monophosphate (cAMP) in diseased muscle. J Neurol 208:259–265, 1975

33. Susheela AK, Kaul RD, Sachdeva K, et al: Adenyl cyclase activity in Duchenne dystrophic muscle. J Neurol Sci 24:361–363, 1975

34. Khokhlov AP, Malakhovsky VK: Characteristics of cyclic 3'-5' AMP turnover in patients with progressive muscular atrophy. Vopr Med Khim 24:754–758, 1978

35. Willner JH, Cerri CG, Somer H, et al: Adenyl cyclase: abnormal in Duchenne carrier muscle (abstract). IVth Int Cong Neurmusc Dis, Abs 478:Montreal, 1978

36. Takahashi K, Takao H, Takai T: Adenylate cyclase in Duchenne and Fukuyama type of dystrophy. Kobe J Med Sci 24:193–198, 1978

37. Reddy NB, Oliver KL, Festoff BW, et al: Adenylate cyclase system of human skeletal muscle: subcellular distribution and general properties. Biochim Biophys Acta 540:371–388, 1978

38. Iyengar R, Swartz TL, Birnbaumer L: Coupling of glucagon receptor to adenylate cyclase: requirement of a receptor-related guanyl nucleotide binding site for coupling. J Biol Chem 254:1119–1123, 1979

39. Garbers DL, Johnson RA: Metal and metal-ATP interactions with brain and cardiac adenylate cyclase. J Biol Chem 250:8449–8456, 1975

40. Bartfai T: Preparation of metal-chelate complexes and the design of steady-state kinetic experiments involving metal nucleotide complex. In Adv Cyclic Nucleotide Res 10:219–242, 1979

41. Wei JW, Narayanan N, Sulakhe VP: Adenylate cyclase of guinea pig skeletal muscle sarcolemma: comparison of the properties of the enzyme with Mg and Mn as divalent cation cofactors. Int J Biochem 10:109–116, 1979

42. Stolc V: Control of adenylate cyclase by divalent cations and agonists. Biochim Biophys Acta 569:267–276, 1979

43. White AA, Karr DB: Improved two step method for assay of adenylate and guanylate cyclase. Anal Biochem 85:451–460, 1977

44. Keely SL: Prostaglandin E_1 activation of heart cAMP-dependent protein kinase: apparent dissociation of protein kinase activation from increases in phosphorylase activity and contractile force. Mol Pharmocol 15:235–245, 1978

45. Willner JH, Cerri CG, Wood DS: Malignant hyperthermia: abnormal cyclic AMP metabolism in skeletal muscle. Neurology (NY) 29:57, 1979

46. Brady RO, Fishman PH: Biotransducers of membrane-mediated information. In Adv Enzymol 35:303–323, 1979

47. Reiss DS, Katz AM: Hormone sensitivity of adenylate cyclase activity in cardiac sarcolemma and sarcoplasmic reticulum preparations. J Mol Cel Cardiol 11:1095–1107, 1979

48. Rodan SB, Hentz RL, Sha'afi RI, et al: The activity of membrane bound enzymes in muscular dystrophic chick. Nature 252:589–591, 1979

49. Novom S, Lewinstein C: Adenylate cyclase and guanylate cyclase of normal and denervated skeletal muscle. Neurology (Minneap) 27:869–874, 1977

50. Smith PB, Grefrath SP, Appel SH: β-Adrenergic receptor-adenylate cyclase of denervated sarcolemma membrane. Exp Neurol 59:361–371, 1978

51. Festoff BW, Engel WK: In vitro analysis of the general properties and junctional receptor characteristics of skeletal muscle membranes: isolation, purification and partial characterization of sarcolemma fragments. Proc Natl Acad Sci USA 71:2435–2439, 1974

52. Andrew CC, Alman RR, Appel SH: Phosphatidylinositol turnover in muscle membranes following denervation. J Neurochem 23:1077–1080, 1974

53. Mawatari S, Miranda A, Rowland LP: Adenyl cyclase abnormality in Duchenne muscular dystrophy: muscle cells in culture. Neurology (Minneap) 67:1016–1021, 1976

54. Mawatari S, Schonberg M, Olarte M, et al: Biochemical abnormalities of erythrocyte membrane in Duchenne dystrophy-ATPase and adenyl cyclase. Arch Neurol 33:489–493, 1976

55. Wacholtz MC, Doible SG, Jackowsky S, et al: Adenylate cyclase and ATPase activities in red cell membranes of patients and genetic carriers of Duchenne muscular dystrophy. Clin Chim Acta 96:255–259, 1979

56. Lane RJM, Maskrey P, Nicholson GA: An evaluation of some carrier detection techniques in Duchenne muscular dystrophy (abstract) 488, 4th Int. Congress on Neuromuscular Diseases, Montreal, 1978

57. Fischer S, Tortolero M, Piau JP, et al: Protein kinase and adenylate cyclase of erythrocyte membrane proteins from patients with Duchenne muscular dystrophy. Clin Chim Acta 88:437–440, 1978

58. Roses AD: Erythrocyte membrane autophosphorylation in Duchenne muscular dystrophy: effect of two methods of erythrocyte ghost preparations on results. Clin Chim Acta 95:69–73, 1979

59. Samaha FJ, Davis B, Nagy BF: Adenosine triphosphate and creatine phosphate levels in Duchenne dystrophic muscle. Neurology (NY) 30:423, 1980

60. Reddy NM, Oliver KL, Engel WK: Alterations in the sarcolemmal adenylate cyclase activity (AC-a) in myotonia. Neurology (Minneap) 27:378, 1977

61. Takagi A, Schotland DL, DiMauro S, et al: Thyrotoxic periodic paralysis:function of sarcoplasmic reticulum and muscle glycogen. Neurology (Minneap) 23:1008–1016, 1973

62. Koehler JP, Triner L, Vuillemoz Y: Adenyl cyclase, phosphodiesterase cyclic AMP system in thyrotoxic periodic paralysis, thyrotoxic myopathy and sporadic hypokalemic periodic paralysis. Neurology (Minneap) 23:408, 1973

63. Isaacs H, Barlow MB: Malignant hyperpyrexia during anaesthesia: possible association with subclinical myopathy. Br Med J 1:275–277, 1970

64. King JO, Denborough MA, Zapf PW: Inheritance of malignant hyperpyrexia. Lancet 1:365–370, 1972

65. Denborough MA, Dennett X, Anderson RMcD: Central core disease and malignant hyperpyrexia. Br Med J 1:272–273, 1973

66. Kalow W, Britt BA, Richter A: The caffeine test of isolated human muscle in relation to malignant hyperthermia. Can Anaesth Soc J 24:678–694, 1977

67. Wingard DW: Malignant hyperthermia: a human stress syndrome? Lancet 1:1450–1451, 1974

68. Jardon OM, Wingard DW, Barak AJ: Malignant hyperthermia: a potentially fatal syndrome in orthopaedic patients. J Bone Joint Surg 61:1064–1070, 1979

69. Dhalla NS, Sulakhe PV, Clinch NF, et al: Influence of fluothane on calcium accumulation by the heavy microsomal fraction of human skeletal muscle: comparison with a patient with malignant hyperpyrexia. Biochem Med 6:333–343, 1972

70. Kirchberger M, Tada M: Effects of adenosine 3′-5′-monophosphate dependent protein kinase on sarcoplasmic reticulum isolated fom cardiac and slow and fast contracting skeletal muscles. J Biol Chem 251:725–734, 1976

71. Wormr DE, Armstrong DA, Solomons CC: Serum levels of inorganic pyrophosphate as a laboratory aid in assessing malignant hyperthermia risk. In *Second International Symposium on Malignant Hyperthermia.* Edited by Aldrete AA, Britt BA. Grune & Stratton, New York, 1978, pp 261–268

72. Willner JH, Wood DS, Cerri C, et al: Increased myophosphorylase a in malignant hyperthermia. N Engl J Med 303:138–140, 1980

73. Britt BA, Endrenyi L, Barclay RL, et al: Total calcium content of skeletal muscle isolated from humans and pigs susceptible to malignant hyperthermia. Br J Anaesth 47:647–653, 1975

74. Bennett D, Cain PA, Ellis FR, et al: Calcium and magnesium contents of malignant hyperpyrexia-susceptible muscle. Br J Anaesth 49:979–981, 1977

DISCUSSION

Dr. N. Bojji Reddy: I would like to make a small correction to your statement that Ca^{2+} activates adenylate cyclase in most tissues. To date, Ca^{2+} is known to stimulate only in a few tissues such as brain, so one expects not to see Ca^{2+} activation of adenylate cyclase in muscle. Adenylate cyclase is actually activated in sarcolemma in the presence of ethyleneglycol tetra-acetate (EGTA), which suggests that membrane-bound Ca^{2+} and perhaps calmodulin have an adverse effect on adenylate cyclase. Regarding your studies on adenylate cyclase stability in homogenates, did you use any proteolytic inhibitors such as phenylmethysulfonyl fluoride (PMSF) that could give us an idea of whether proteolytic activity has anything to do with your stability? At what temperature did you look at the stability of the enzyme?

Dr. Joseph Willner: Remarkably, instability appeard on ice at 4° C. The addition of proteolytic inhibitors had no effect on the instability of the enzyme either in our system or, as shown by Drummond, in cardiac sarcolemma. Now to the first question: the issue of calmodulin regulation of adenylate cyclase in muscle really requires reevaluation. You may have seen a recent paper in *Science* by Balverde and coworkers regarding pancreatic islet cells. They showed that, in the absence of calmodulin, neither homogenates nor membranes were stimulated by Ca^{2+}. The adenylate cyclase was inhibited by Ca^{2+}. When calmodulin was added back, the result was a Ca^{2+}-stimulated enzyme. This sort of experiment has not been done in muscle, probably because sarcolemma has not been adequately looked at yet. The whole question must be readdressed. I do not have the references here, but I do not think it is true that the only Ca^{2+}-activated adenylate cyclase has been in brain.

Dr. N. Bojji Reddy: To follow up another question on malignant hyperthermia, did you look at the cAMP-phosphodiesterase activity in your preparations? I have evidence in skeletal muscle of malignant hyperthermic pigs that there is an increase in cAMP phosphodiesterase and that it can be inhibited by dantrolene sodium, which is used in the management of human malignant hyperthermia. Have you done some of these studies in your human biopsy specimens?

Dr. Joseph Willner: Only in a very cursory way. We originally looked at phosphodiesterase in a whole homogenate, looking only at the low-affinity form of phosphodiesterase; we found a slight but unimpressive increase. We also tried separating out cytoplasmic from membrane-bound phosphodiesterase, and the difference still was not very impressive; it was not the sort of difference we got looking at adenylate cyclase.

Dr. Stanley Appel: Have you begun to dissect out which of the many different steps could have given rise to the decreased basal cyclase and the decreased activation of cyclase? Admittedly, it is a horrendous task, but as you point out, someone has to do it and you already have very good beginning data that confirm the original observation. Where do you think the difficulty in the activation lies? Why is the basal level so decreased?

Dr. Joseph Willner: I do not know about the basal level. As I mentioned before, the reference is noncollagen protein, but because all these other tissues are there, you do not know whether you are really looking at muscle protein. I prefer to look at the actual activation of the enzyme, and the next step is to go from homogenates to isolated membranes, perhaps using carrier muscle that does not have all the contaminating cells in it. We have some preliminary evidence that activation of the enzyme in carrier muscle was abnormal. Using sarcolemma from carrier muscle, we can begin to answer the question you were asking. I think that is the way it has to go. Looking at homogenates is limited, but is a useful initial step.

Dr. Alfred Stracher: I think you should not rule out the possibility of proteolysis as one of the effects by adding just a single inhibitor. Adding just one inhibitor; e.g., PMSF, may not be sufficient to inhibit some of the variety of proteases that may exist. Another comment: in some of our experiments in blood platelets even 1 mM EGTA has not been sufficient to inhibit proteolysis. It has been necessary to use as much as 10 mM EGTA to prevent proteolysis in platelet proteins.

Dr. Joseph Willner: I do not know the mechanism of the instability of the enzyme in homogenates. It might be proteolysis, and you are right in saying that the addition of one inhibitor does not prove a case. Using higher concentrations of EGTA we found the same stability of the enzyme. We found that 1 mM EDTA or 0.4 mM EGTA was adequate to do it.

Dr. Klaus Wrogemann: A question regarding conversion of phosphorylase b to a in malignant hyperthermia. Could it be that these patients, when they come in for the biopsy, are simply under greater stress in the wake of the hazardous condition they carry, and that this could explain the increased conversion from b to a?

Dr. Joseph Willner: Do you mean they are under greater stress than you or I would be during a biopsy?

Dr. Klaus Wrogemann: Yes, because they know whenever they go into the hospital they are in greater danger of something happening to them. Even though they do not undergo general anesthesia, they might be more scared.

Dr. Joseph Willner: I think that is possible, but it would not explain the abnormality of adenylate cyclase. It may be that the enzyme is activated, causing an increased amount of phosphorylase in the muscle, or it may be a secondary phenomenon occurring during the biopsy. We found the same increase in phosphorylase a in Dr. Britt's patients, whose biospies were carried out under general anesthesia, which reduces the likelihood that this increased phosphorylase a was entirely stress induced.

35
Protein Phosphorylation in Neurons

Paul Greengard, PhD

Pietro De Camilli, MD

Studies carried out during the past 10 years have provided a great deal of evidence that protein phosphorylation is of paramount importance in biologic regulation (1). These studies indicate that protein phosphorylation is a final common pathway mediating certain of the actions of large numbers of regulatory agents and other biologically active substances (Fig. 1). In the case of the nervous system in particular, protein kinases have been found that are activated specifically by each of the three known types of intracellular second messenger, cyclic adenosine monophosphate (cAMP), cyclic guanosine monophosphate (cGMP), and calcium (Ca). We believe that these three types of protein kinase mediate many of the actions of neurotransmitters that are expressed through second-messenger systems. These various protein kinases have been purified and characterized, and we are now engaged in a study of their endogenous substrates.

Endogenous substrates have been found for each of these three classes of protein kinases in nervous tissue. To date, a total of a dozen or so neuron-specific endogenous substrates have been detected. We are currently engaged in the purification and characterization of these various substrates and in studies attempting to establish their physiologic roles. Rather than presenting an overview of all of these substrates, we shall summarize here the results of studies of just one of these substrates, as a way of illustrating the type of approach that is currently being used in this area. This substrate protein is a doublet that has been referred to as Protein I (2). It is the most prominent substrate for cAMP-dependent protein kinase in brain tissue. It is also a prominent substrate for Ca-calmodulin-dependent protein kinase(s) in brain tissue. It is present in most, if not all, neurons and it has a unique localization within these neurons: it is localized primarily to the nerve terminal region, where it is associated with neurotransmitter-containing vesicles. It is relevant to the field of muscular dystrophy that the distribution of Protein I includes the cholinergic nerve

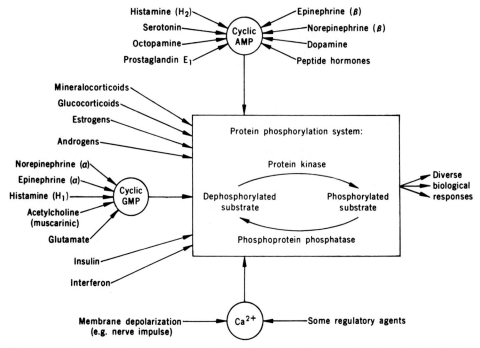

Fig. 1. Schematic diagram of postulated role played by protein phosphorylation in mediating some of the biologic effects of a variety of regulatory agents.

terminals that innervate skeletal muscle. It seems very likely that Protein I is involved in regulating some important aspect of the function of the neurotransmitter-containing vesicles in many types of axon terminals, including those at the neuromuscular junction.

PROTEIN I

In experiments that led to the discovery of Protein I (3, 4), a synaptic membrane fraction was incubated for a few seconds with radioactive γ-^{32}P-adenosine triphosphate (ATP), in the absence or presence of cAMP. The reaction was then terminated by the addition of the detergent sodium dodecyl sulfate (SDS), which also solubilized the membrane proteins. These proteins were then separated from one another by SDS-polyacrylamide gel electrophoresis and were analyzed by protein staining and autoradiography. Figure 2 illustrates an experiment of this type. Of the many protein bands present in this synaptic fraction, the phosphorylation of only a few was markedly affected by the presence of cAMP. Two of these proteins, referred to as Proteins Ia and Ib, have very similar properties, and we collectively call this doublet Protein I. Protein I has been purified to homogenity from bovine brain by Ueda and Greengard (2) and from rat brain by DeGennaro (DeGennaro LJ, Greengard P: unpublished data). Some of the physicochemical properties of Protein I purified from bovine brain are shown in Table 1. Particularly noteworthy are

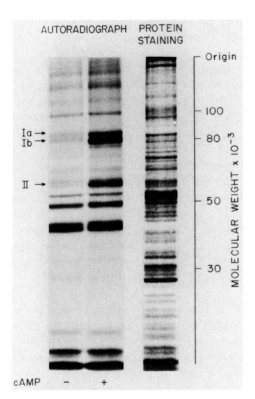

Fig. 2. Effect of cyclic AMP on endogenous protein phosphorylation in a synaptic membrane fraction from rat caudate nucleus. The synaptic membrane fraction was incubated with 7 μM γ-^{32}P-ATP for 15 seconds at 30° C in the absence or presence of 10 μM cyclic AMP. The reaction was terminated by the addition of sodium dodecyl sulfate (SDS), which also solubilized the membrane proteins. An aliquot of the reaction product was then subjected to SDS-polyacrylamide gel electrophoresis to separate the membrane proteins from one another. The separated proteins were located in the gel by standard procedures of protein staining. Autoradiography was then carried out to locate the protein bands into which radioactive phosphate had been incorporated. *Left.* Phosphorylation of endogenous proteins in the absence (−) or presence (+) of cyclic AMP. *Right.* Protein staining. (Modified, with permission, from Sieghart W, Forn J, Greengard P: Ca^{2+} and cyclic AMP regulate phosphorylation of same two membrane-associated proteins specific to nerve tissue. Proc Natl Acad Sci USA 76:2475–2479, 1979.)

the observations that Proteins Ia and Ib maintained a constant molar proportion of 1:2 throughout purification to homogeneity, that both peptides are extremely basic, having isoelectric points greater than 10, and that the peptides have unusual structural features. Thus, a variety of physicochemical studies indicate that each of the peptides contains a globular region that is insensitive to collagenase as well as an elongated proline-rich tail that is rapidly and specifically degraded by highly purified collagenase (2, and DeGennaro LJ, Greengard P: unpublished data).

Table 1. Physicochemical Properties of Bovine Brain Protein I

	Protein IA	*Protein IB*
Molar proportion	1	2
Molecular weight	86,000	80,000
Isoelectric point	10.3	10.2
Stokes radius	59 Å	59 Å
Shape	Highly elongated	Highly elongated
Other structural features	A globular collagenase-insensitive region and an elongated proline-rich collagenase-sensitive tail	

Calcium/Calmodulin-Dependent Protein Kinases

Experiments with Protein I led to the discovery of a new class of enzymes, Ca/calmodulin-dependent protein kinases. It is well established, from work in numerous laboratories, that entry of Ca into the nerve terminal affects several physiologic processes including the biosynthesis (5) and release (6–9) of neurotransmitters. It seemed possible that certain of the effects of Ca at the nerve terminal might be associated with alterations in protein phosphorylation. For this reason, Krueger and associates (10) studied the effect of Ca on protein phosphorylation in synaptosomes, i.e., isolated, viable nerve terminals that contain synaptic vesicles, cytoplasm, and mitochondria.

In these experiments, synaptosomes were preincubated with radioactive inorganic phosphate for 30 minutes to label the intrasynaptosomal ATP pool, and then incubated for 30 seconds in the absence or presence of veratridine, K^+, and Ca^{2+} as indicated in Figure 3. The synaptosomal proteins were then analyzed by SDS-polyacrylamide gel electrophoresis and autoradiography. Veratridine and K^+ were used in these experiments because they depolarize the plasma membrane of synaptosomes, leading to the opening of voltage-sensitive Ca^{2+} channels in the plasma membrane and resulting in an influx of Ca^{2+} (11–13).

As shown in Figure 3, influx of Ca^{2+} into the synaptosomes under these experimental conditions led to an alteration in the state of phosphorylation of several proteins. The most prominent effect of Ca^{2+} influx was on two proteins that had electrophoretic mobilities identical to those of authentic Protein Ia and Protein Ib. Subsequent studies by Werner Sieghart and colleagues (14), using peptide mapping and immunoprecipitation techniques, demonstrated that this pair of proteins, the phosphorylation of which was affected by Ca^{2+} influx, was indeed identical to Proteins Ia and Ib, the substrates that were phosphorylated by cAMP-dependent protein kinase.

When, in the experiment of Figure 3, Ca was omitted from the incubation medium, veratridine and K^+ were without a detectable effect on phosphorylation of synaptosomal proteins, indicating that the effect of these depolarizing agents was achieved through the influx of Ca^{2+}, possibly through altering the state of activity of a Ca dependent protein kinase. More direct evidence for this possibility was obtained by a study of protein phosphorylation in synaptosomal lysates (15, 16). Thus, when a synaptosomal lysate was incubated with radioactive ATP, the addition of Ca^{2+} resulted in stimulation of the phosphorylation of a large number of protein bands, including Proteins Ia and Ib (Fig. 4, lanes 1 and 2). In fact, many more proteins were observed to undergo Ca-dependent phosphorylation in such lysates than in the experiments with intact synaptosomes. The phosphorylation of some of these proteins, including Proteins Ia and Ib, undoubtedly reflects endogenous physiologic processes. However, the phosphorylation of certain other of these proteins might have resulted from the artifactual juxtaposition of protein kinase and substrate proteins that would not ordinarily come into contact within the cell, but did so as a result of the lysis procedure. In control experiments, it was shown that the effect of Ca^{2+} on Protein I phosphorylation was due to stimulation of a protein kinase rather than to inhibition of a protein phosphatase.

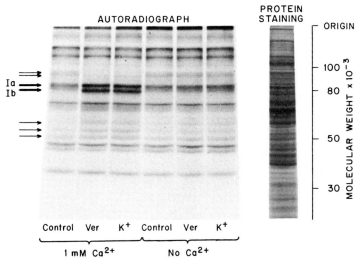

Fig. 3. Effect of veratridine and of high K^+, in the absence and presence of Ca^{2+}, on the phosphorylation of endogenous proteins in crude synaptosomal preparation from rat cerebral cortex. The synaptosome fraction was preincubated with ^{32}P-labeled inorganic phosphate for 30 minutes in the absence of Ca^{2+}. Aliquots of this suspension were then incubated for 30 seconds in the absence (Control) or presence of 100 μM veratridine (Ver) or 60 mM K^+; 1 mM Ca^{2+} was present where indicated. The incubation was terminated by the addition of sodium dodecyl sulfate (SDS), and the samples were subjected to SDS-polyacrylamide gel electrophoresis. The positions of Proteins Ia and Ib are indicated by bold arrows. Light arrows indicate the positions of other protein bands, the phosphorylation of which was inhibited (upper two arrows) or stimulated (lower three arrows) by veratridine or high K^+. (Reprinted with permission from Krueger BK, Forn J, Greengard P: Depolarization-induced phosphorylation of specific proteins, mediated by calcium ion flux in brain synaptosomes. J Biol Chem 252:2764–2773, 1977.)

Having demonstrated Ca-dependent protein kinase activity in the synaptosomal lysate, which contained membranes (synaptic membranes plus synaptic vesicles) and synaptosomal cytoplasm, it became possible to study the enzyme system involved. The effect of subsynaptosomal fractionation of the synaptosomal lysate on Ca-dependent protein phosphorylation was determined. The Ca-dependent phosphorylation observed in lysed synaptosomes was lost on preparation of cytoplasm-free membranes (Fig. 4, lanes 3 and 4). This phenomenon was not due to inactivation of the Ca-dependent protein kinase during experimental manipulations, because it could be regained by addition of an amount of boiled (Fig. 4, lanes 5 and 6) or unboiled synaptosomal cytoplasm commensurate with the amount of membrane protein present. This sample of boiled cytosol, which conferred Ca-dependent phosphorylation on cytosol-free membranes, did not exhibit any endogenous phosphorylation when incubated in the absence of membranes (Fig. 4, lane 7), nor did it show any protein kinase activity using added histone, protamine, or casein as substrate. Thus, the Ca-dependent phosphorylation in synaptic membranes required a soluble heat-stable factor present in synaptosomal cytosol.

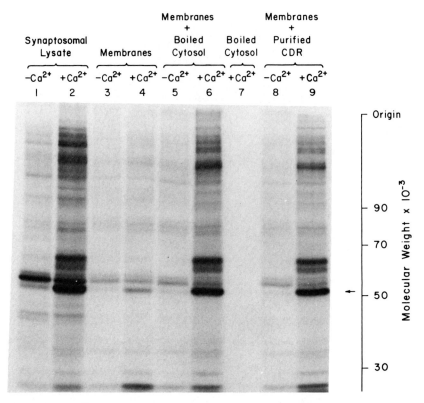

Fig. 4. Effect of Ca^{2+}, synaptosomal cytoplasm, and purified calmodulin on endogenous protein phosphorylation of brain membranes. Incubation was carried out for 10 seconds at 30° C; the reaction was terminated by the addition of sodium dodecyl sulfate (SDS), and an aliquot of the sample was analyzed for protein phosphorylation by SDS-polyacrylamide gel electrophoresis and autoradiography. (Reprinted with permission from Schulman H, Greengard P: Stimulation of brain membrane protein phosphorylation by calcium and an endogenous heat-stable protein. Nature 271:478–479, 1978.)

The biochemical mechanisms underlying the physiologic effects of Ca were not well understood at the time of this work. A common feature of those systems that had been investigated at the molecular level, however, was the involvement of a Ca-binding protein (17). For example, the trigger for contraction of skeletal muscle had been shown to be the interaction of Ca with troponin C (a Ca-binding protein) (18). A similar but distinct Ca-binding protein (calmodulin, or Ca-dependent regulator) had been found to regulate the activity of cyclic nucleotide phosphodiesterase (19, 20) and of a detergent-solubilized preparation of adenylate cyclase (21, 22) from mammalian brain. It therefore seemed possible that a similar function might be served by the factor in the synaptosomal cytosol. Indeed, the heat stability of the stimulating factor in the cytosol suggested a possible relationship to calmodulin. Therefore, calmodulin was purified to homogeneity by the method of Teo and associates (23), based on its ability to activate phosphodiesterase, to test its effect in the Ca-dependent protein phosphorylation system. Addition of this protein to washed synaptosomal membrane fractions restored Ca-dependent protein phosphorylation (Fig. 4, lanes 8 and 9). The pattern of phosphorylation obtained on addition of calmodulin was indistinguishable from that obtained on addition of boiled synaptosomal cytoplasm (compare Fig. 4, and lanes 6 and 9), suggesting that the two factors are functionally equivalent.

Stimulation of endogenous protein phosphorylation in synaptic membrane fractions was dependent on the presence of both Ca and either the cytosol factor or calmodulin. Thus, Ca in the absence of boiled cytosol and boiled cytosol in the absence of Ca were ineffective, whereas addition of both Ca and boiled cytosol restored phosphorylation (Fig. 4, compare lanes 3, 4, 5, and 6). Analogous results were obtained with calmodulin (Fig. 4, compare lanes 3, 4, 8 and 9).

This endogenous kinase activator, like calmodulin, was extremely heat stable, nondialyzable, resistant to DNAase and RNAase, and sensitive to trypsin (15). Moreover, the activator for phosphodiesterase and the activator for Ca-dependent protein kinase copurified from cytosol to homogeneity (16). In addition, the ability of the cytosol to activate the Ca-dependent protein kinase could be quantitatively accounted for by its content of calmodulin. This series of studies indicated that there was a Ca-dependent protein kinase present in the membrane fraction of the synaptosomes that required calmodulin, present in the cytosol, for activity.

Some of the properties of Protein I as a substrate for cAMP-dependent and Ca/calmodulin-dependent protein kinases, based on the studies just summarized, as well as on recent studies of Huttner and associates (24, 25) and Kennedy and Greengard (26), are as follows:

1. Manifests multiple-site phosphorylation, with at least one site in the globular region and at least two sites in the tail region.
2. A principal substrate for (Type II) cyclic AMP-dependent protein kinase, being phosphorylated in globular region.
3. A principal substrate for two calcium/calmodulin-dependent protein kinases, being phosphorylated both in globular and in tail regions.

Almost simultaneously with publication of the results on the existence of Ca/calmodulin-dependent protein kinase activity in brain tissue (15), other research groups published results indicating that myosin light chain kinase (27–29) and phosphorylase kinase (30) were also Ca/calmodulin-dependent enzymes. Because it seemed that this new class of enzyme might be of general importance, the particulate fractions from a large number of tissues were examined for Ca/calmodulin-dependent protein kinase activity (16). Results of that survey indicated that there was a Ca/calmodulin-dependent protein kinase present in the membrane fraction of every tissue examined, and that this enzyme phosphorylated a tissue-specific array of substrate proteins (16). It therefore seems very likely that this class of enzymes, which was found by studying the Ca-dependent phosphorylation of neuronal substrates, is involved in mediating many of the actions of Ca acting as a second messenger in various tissues. However, rather than describing recent developments in research in that area further, we would like at this point to return to a discussion of our studies of protein phosphorylation in the nervous system and of Protein I in particular.

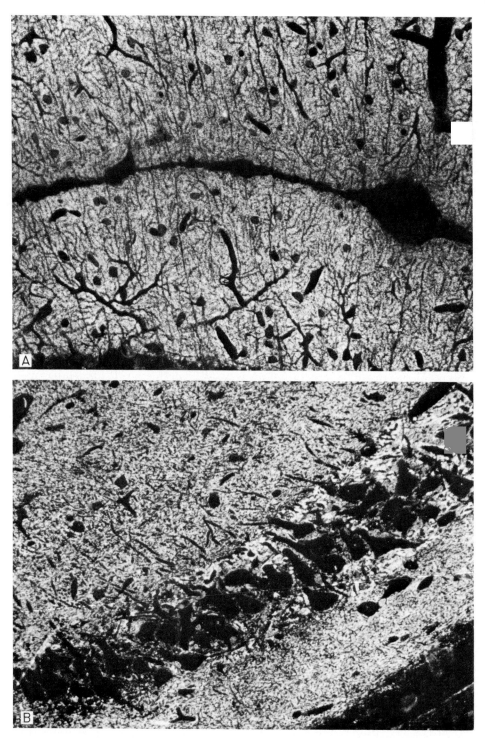

Fig. 5. Immunofluorescent localization of Protein I in rat brain (**A**) Cerebellar cortex
(1-μm plastic section). The molecular layers of two adjacent folia are shown. Bright
immunofluorescence of the neuropil (white in the figure) is seen against the dark
background of nonsynaptic regions. In the latter, one can see Purkinje cell dendrites,
cell bodies of neuronal and glial cells, and blood vessels. (magnification ×420.)

448

Distribution of Protein I

Our knowledge concerning the distribution of Protein I is based largely on earlier immunocytochemical studies using an immunoperoxidase technique (31, 32) and on more recent studies using an immunofluorescence technique (33), (De Camilli P, Greengard P: unpublished data). These morphologic studies indicate that Protein I is present only in the nervous system both central and peripheral. Within the nervous system, it is present only in neurons and is concentrated in the synaptic region. Within the synaptic region, it is associated primarily with synaptic vesicles. Recent immunofluorescence studies indicate that Protein I is present in most, if not all, synapses, including synapses where it was not detected previously (31), such as the neuromuscular junction and the outer plexiform layer of the retina. Such studies also indicate that Protein I appears simultaneously with synapse formation during development. Some of the results obtained by immunofluorescence are illustrated in Figures 5–7.

Recently, Susan E. Goelz and Eric J. Nestler have developed a sensitive and precise radioimmunoassay for Protein I. This procedure has been applied to a study of the amount of Protein I in various subcellular fractions of rat cerebral cortex (Huttner WB, De Camilli P, Greengard P: unpublished data). It was found that Protein I represents approximately 0.4% of the total protein present in the cerebral cortex. Protein I was most highly enriched in synaptic vesicle fractions, in agreement with the results of earlier studies (34). Very little Protein I was present in the cytosol. Interestingly, Protein I represented almost 4% of the total protein of the crude synaptic vesicle fraction. When one considers that this crude synaptic vesicle fraction was contaminated by other subcellular organelles, and that some Protein I might have been lost from the vesicles during their isolation, it seems possible that the true content of Protein I associated with the synaptic vesicles might be even higher. The high concentration of Protein I associated with the vesicle fraction strongly suggests that Protein I is important in some aspect of the functioning of synaptic vesicles.

Physiologic Studies of Protein I

Results of some physiologic studies of Protein I can be summarized as follows:

1. In whole animals, convulsants increase and depressants decrease state of phosphorylation
2. In intact slices of brain, depolarizing agents and cyclic AMP increase state of phosphorylation
3. In specific anatomical regions of central and peripheral nervous system, the relevant neurotransmitters (serotonin, dopamine) increase state of phosphorylation.

In untreated whole animals, Protein I was found to exist partially (approximately 33%) in the phosphorylated form, and partially (approximately 67%) in

---

(**B**) Hippocampus (1-μm plastic section). Cell bodies and major dendrites of pyramidal cells in dark silhouette against the immunoreactive neuropil (white in the figure). Note the absence of immunoreactivity in the axon bundles at the lower right. (magnification ×410.)

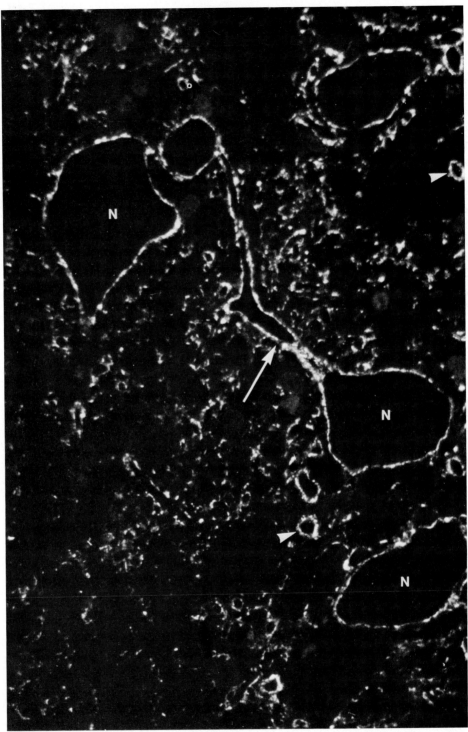

Fig. 6. Immunofluorescent localization of Protein I in axon terminals of the rat brain stem (1-μm plastic section). Dots of immunoreactivity reveal the outlines of several large neurons (N) and their major dendrites. The arrow indicates a dendrite sectioned longitudinally, and the arrowheads indicate two other dendrites sectioned perpendicularly. (magnification ×1100.)

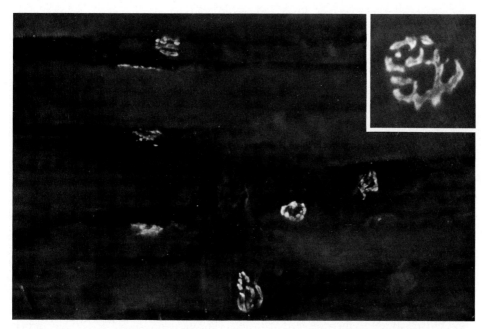

Fig. 7. Immunofluorescent localization of Protein I in rat diaphragm (20-μm thick frozen section). Bright immunoreactivity is present on motor end plates. Striated muscle fibers (running horizontally in the figure) and branches of the phrenic nerve from which the nerve terminals visible in the picture originate can be identified by their pale autofluorescence. Note that the immunoreactivity is confined to the axon terminals. (Magnification ×380.) Inset: higher magnification of a single motor end plate. (Magnification ×910.)

the dephosphorylated form, and these proportions could be altered by in vivo administration of appropriate pharmacologic agents (35).

In unstimulated slices of rat cerebral cortex incubated in vitro for 1 hour, the cAMP-sensitive phosphorylation site on Protein I appeared to be almost entirely in the dephosphorylated form (36). Two depolarizing agents, K^+ and veratridine, both of which cause influx of Ca^{2+} into, and neurotransmitter release from, presynaptic nerve terminals, were tested for their ability to affect the state of phosphorylation of Protein I in slices of rat cerebral cortex. Both depolarizing agents caused large increases in the amount of phosphoProtein I in such slices. The effect of various concentrations of K^+ on phosphoProtein I levels is shown in Figure 8A; a half-maximal increase in Protein I phosphorylation occurred in the presence of 25 to 30 mM K^+. A maximally effective concentration of K^+ caused the phosphorylation of approximately 60% of the total Protein I present in the slices. The increase in phosphorylation of Protein I in the presence of high K^+ was rapid; the effect was more than half-maximal in the shortest time studied (10 seconds), and a maximal effect was observed within 20 seconds of incubation (Fig. 8B). In the continued presence of K^+, dephosphorylation of Protein I then occurred.

The dephosphorylation of Protein I in the continued presence of the depolarizing agent can be interpreted in the following way. It is well established that, under conditions of maintained depolarization, the voltage-sensitive Ca

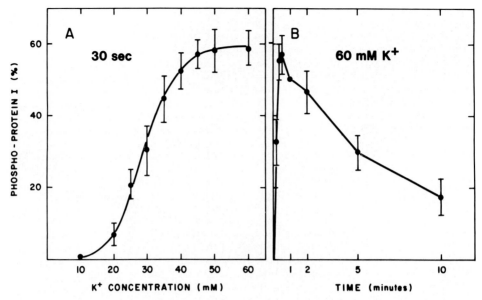

Fig. 8. Formation of phosphoProtein I from dephosphoProtein I in rat cerebral cortex slices incubated (**A**) in the presence of various concentrations of K^+ for 30 sec and (**B**) in the presence of 60 mM K^+ for various times. Data are expressed as 100 X phosphoProtein I/total Protein I. Each point represents the mean ± SEM of determinations on 6 samples incubated, extracted, and assayed separately. (Reprinted with permission from Forn J, Greengard P: Depolarizing agents and cyclic nucleotides regulate the phosphorylation of specific neuronal proteins in rat cerebral cortex slices. Proc Natl Acad Sci USA 75:5195–5199, 1978

channels present in the plasma membrane close (37). Presumably the free intracellular Ca^{2+} is then sequestered, resulting in inactivation of the Ca/calmodulin-dependent protein kinase. As a result, the Protein I phosphatase can now effectively dephosphorylate its substrate protein. Consistent with this interpretation, if the K^+ depolarization is maintained for only 30-second intervals, then the effect of depolarization on Protein I phosphorylation can be repeatedly produced. Thus, by alternating the incubation medium bathing rat cerebral cortical slices through many cycles of high (60 mM) and low (5 mM) K^+ concentration, it is possible repeatedly to bring about the alternate phosphorylation and dephosphorylation of Protein I. Such results indicate that Protein I is not an inert structural protein, but rather that its state of phosphorylation is rapidly attuned to the state of polarization of the neuronal plasma membrane.

Although it was possible to demonstrate that depolarizing agents and cAMP affect the state of phosphorylation of Protein I in slices of whole cerebral cortex (36), it has been much more difficult to demonstrate effects of specific neurotransmitters on the state of phosphorylation of Protein I in nervous tissue. However, recently it has been possible to do so in both the central and peripheral nervous systems, by using well-defined, relatively homogeneous preparations of nervous tissue. Thus, Dolphin and Greengard (38) have demonstrated that serotonin brings about the phosphorylation of Protein I in slices of rat facial motor nucleus. Moreover, Nestler and Greengard (39) have demonstrated that dopamine is capable of increasing the state of phosphorylation of Protein I in bovine superior cervical ganglia. In addition, Ivar Walaas has demonstrated that dopamine stimulates the phosphorylation of Protein I in slices of rat caudate nucleus and substantia nigra (Walaas I, Greengard P: unpublished data). We will briefly describe the results obtained with serotonin on the state of phosphorylation of Protein I in slices of facial motor nucleus.

The facial motor nucleus is a relatively homogeneous portion of the central nervous system that has been studied extensively by McCall and Aghajanian in recent years (40–42). Virtually the only type of neuronal cell body present in the facial motor nucleus is the motor neuron that sends axons to innervate the facial musculature. This region of the brain is virtually devoid of any interneurons, which greatly simplifies the task of analysis. The major type of afferent input (90% to 98% of the afferent nerve fibers) to this motor neuron consists of excitatory fibers, which are believed to utilize an amino acid as the neurotransmitter. A minor input (approximately 2% of the afferent fibers) is composed of serotonergic nerve fibers (42). Because immunohistochemical studies (De Camilli P, Dolphin AC: unpublished data) suggest that terminals containing Protein I are much more abundant than serotonergic terminals in the facial nucleus, it would appear that much of the Protein I in this region of the brain is present in the major excitatory afferent input. Consistent with this interpretation, destruction of the serotonergic fibers by 5,7-dihydroxytryptamine does not significantly decrease the level of Protein I in the facial motor nucleus, determined either by phosphorylation or by radioimmunoassay (Dolphin AC, Goelz SE, Greengard P: unpublished data).

The effect of serotonin on the state of phosphorylation of Protein I was studied in quartered sections of the facial motor nucleus. The formation of phosphoProtein I from dephosphoProtein I in such preparations, as a function of 5-hydroxytryptamine (5-HT) concentration, is shown in Figure 9. The stimulation of phosphorylation caused by 5-HT was potentiated by isobutyl-

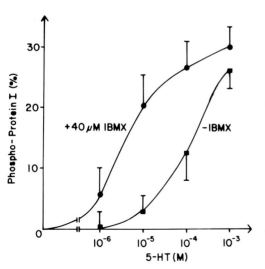

Fig. 9. Formation of phosphoProtein I from dephosphoProtein I in slices of rat facial nucleus incubated in the presence of various concentrations of 5-hydroxytryptamine (5-HT). Experimental slices were incubated in the presence of the indicated concentration of 5-HT, in the presence (●) or absence (■) of 4×10^{-5} M IBMX. Paired control slices were incubated in the absence of 5-HT, in the presence or absence of 4×10^{-5} M IBMX, respectively. (Reprinted with permission from Dolphin AC, Greengard P: Serotonin stimulates the phosphorylation of Protein I, a synapse-specific protein, in the facial motor nucleus of rat brain. Nature, 289:76–79, 1981.)

methylxanthine (IBMX) at a concentration (4×10^{-5} M), which alone caused little alteration in the state of phosphorylation of Protein I. In the presence of this concentration of IBMX, the maximal effect of 10^{-3} M 5-HT was to convert $30.1 \pm 3.7\%$ (n = 9) of Protein I from the dephospho- to the phospho- form; the half-maximally effective concentration (EC_{50}) of 5-HT was 4×10^{-6} M.

That 5-HT affected Protein I phosphorylation by interaction with specific receptors was indicated by the ability of mianserin, an antagonist at central 5-HT receptors (43–45), to block the phosphorylation of Protein I induced by 5-HT. However, mianserin, at the concentration used (10^{-5} M), also caused a slight phosphorylation of Protein I when incubated with slices in the absence of 5-HT. This and other classic serotonin antagonists have been found to be partial agonists of 5-HT-sensitive adenylate cyclase in brain, in that they stimulate adenylate cyclase at concentrations of 10^{-5} M and more (45).

The results obtained with 5-HT in the facial motor nucleus suggest that this neurotransmitter can alter the state of phosphorylation of Protein I in the terminals of the main afferent excitatory pathway (38). This effect of 5-HT may reflect the functional equivalent of an axo-axonic communication between the terminals of the serotonergic fibers and the terminals of the main afferent excitatory pathway. However, the possibility cannot be ruled out that 5-HT can affect the state of phosphorylation of Protein I in the motor neuron somas, even though immunocytochemical evidence suggests that the concentration of Protein I is very low in neuronal cell bodies.

Possible Roles for Protein I

It has been shown, in the studies just summarized, that Protein I is a major phosphoprotein in the nervous system, that it is present in very high concentrations in nerve terminals, where it seems to be associated with synaptic vesicles, that it is phosphorylated by both cAMP-dependent and Ca/calmodulin-dependent protein kinases, and that its state of phosphorylation in intact cells is altered rapidly and extensively by depolarizing agents and by specific neurotransmitters. Therefore, it seems quite possible that Protein I is involved in regulating some function of neurotransmitter vesicles. Some of these functions are listed in Table 2. Certain of these possible roles for Protein I are less attractive than others. For example, because Protein I appears to be present in most nerve terminals, it seems unlikely that it would be involved in regulation of the

Table 2. Some Events Associated with the Function of Synaptic Vesicles That Might Be Regulated by Protein I

Neurotransmitter biosynthesis
Neurotransmitter uptake
Neurotransmitter storage
Vesicle translocation
Vesicle membrane interaction with plasma membrane
Release of neurotransmitter (exocytosis)
Recovery of vesicle membrane from plasma membrane

---

biosynthesis of neurotransmitters, each of which has its own specific biosynthetic pathway.

We are currently attempting to test the hypothesis that Protein I is involved in regulating the release of neurotransmitter from the nerve terminal, either by affecting the translocation of vesicles to the plasma membrane or by affecting the interaction of the vesicle membrane with the plasma membrane. This hypothesis is attractive for several reasons. Both Ca and cAMP have been shown to potentiate the release of neurotransmitters from various neurons under a variety of experimental conditions. For example, a burst of neuronal activity has been shown to increase the amount of neurotransmitter released in response to a single nerve impulse, in several types of neuronal preparations, by a Ca-dependent process known as "posttetanic potentiation" (46). Similarly, cAMP and regulatory agents that act through increasing cAMP levels have been shown to increase the amount of neurotransmitter released in response to a single nerve impulse in several types of neuronal preparation, including nerve terminals at both vertebrate (47) and invertebrate (48) neuromuscular junctions, as well as innervated nerve terminals at axo-axonic synapses (49). Because Ca and cAMP each stimulate the phosphorylation of Protein I, a major protein of synaptic vesicles, it seems possible that the phosphorylation of Protein I might be involved in the molecular processes that underlie these two types of physiologic potentiation of neurotransmitter release.

The experimental data support the idea that Protein I is associated in vivo primarily with synaptic vesicles. In addition, several types of experiment indicate that Protein I is an extrinsic protein, located on the outer or cytoplasmic surface of the vesicle membrane. In support of this interpretation, Protein I can be phosphorylated in intact vesicles by Ca/calmodulin-dependent and cAMP-dependent protein kinases added to the vesicle fraction. Moreover, exposure of intact vesicles to appropriate proteolytic enzymes causes the release of Protein I fragments from the vesicles. Finally, Protein I can be extracted from the vesicles by conditions used to extract extrinsic proteins. Such results raise the possibility that Protein I, located on the cytoplasmic surface of the synaptic vesicle membrane, interacts with an extravesicular component, perhaps a cytoskeletal protein or the plasma membrane itself, and that the rate or extent of this interaction is affected by the state of phosphorylation of Protein I (Huttner WB, De Camilli P, Greengard P: unpublished data). Through such a mechanism, Protein I might conceivably mediate some of the effects of Ca and of cAMP on neurotransmitter release.

CONCLUSION

Large amounts of correlative data indicate a relationship between the state of phosphorylation of a particular protein and the state of activation of a given physiologic process, in neurons as well as in several nonneuronal systems that carry out physiological processes analogous to those occurring nerve cells. In addition, in collaboration with two other groups of workers (50, 51) it has been demonstrated that the injection of highly purified catalytic subunit of cAMP-dependent protein kinase into appropriate neurons and neurosecretory cells

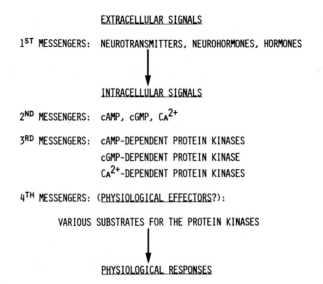

Fig. 10. Signals in the brain.

mimics the physiologic response to synaptic activation of these cells. These latter studies have provided direct evidence for a causal relationship between protein phosphorylation and physiologic response in these cells. These results support the idea that through the detection, purification, and characterization of substrate proteins for cAMP-dependent, cGMP-dependent, and Ca-dependent protein kinases in the nervous system, and the elucidation of the physiologic roles of these substrate proteins, a detailed understanding will be achieved of the molecular mechanisms by which nerve cells respond to various stimuli with specific physiologic responses.

The scheme shown in Figure 10 summarizes our current concepts about what is inside the black box that we call the neuron. The neuron responds to extracellular signals or first messengers with a physiologic response that is mediated through a series of intracellular signals. It may be that some of the protein kinase substrates, i.e., fourth messengers, that we have found, are the immediate effectors that regulate physiologic responses. It may be that other substrate proteins, or fourth messengers, are still one or more steps removed from the final physiologic process, i.e., there may be even more messengers intercalated between the phosphorylated substrate proteins and the final physiologic response. In any case, it now seems possible to determine which neurotransmitters, working through which phosphorylated proteins, produce which physiologic responses, and to learn much about the molecular mechanisms involved.

ACKNOWLEDGMENTS

We are pleased to acknowledge the Muscular Dystrophy Association of America for their generous support of the work described in this article.

REFERENCES

1. Greengard P: Phosphorylated proteins as physiological effectors. Science 199:146–152, 1978

2. Ueda T, Greengard P: Adenosine 3′,5′-monophosphate-regulated phosphoprotein system of neuronal membranes. I. Solubilization, purification and some properties of an endogenous phosphoprotein. J Biol Chem 252:5155–5163, 1977

3. Johnson EM, Ueda T, Maeno H, Greengard P: Adenosine 3′,5′-monophosphate-dependent phosphorylation of a specific protein in synaptic membrane fractions from rat cerebrum. J Biol Chem 247:5650–5652, 1972

4. Ueda T, Maeno H, Greengard P: Regulation of endogenous phosphorylation of specific proteins in synaptic membrane fractions from rat brain by adenosine 3′,5′-monophosphate. J Biol Chem 248:8295–8305, 1973

5. Patrick RL, Barchas JD: Stimulation of synaptosomal dopamine synthesis by veratridine. Nature 250:737–739, 1974

6. Katz B, Miledi R: A study of synaptic transmission in the absence of nerve impulses. J Physiol (Lond) 192:407–436, 1967

7. Douglas WW: Stimulus-secretion coupling: the concept and clues from chromaffin and other cells. Br J Pharmacol 34:451–474, 1968

8. Katz B: *The Release of Neural Transmitter Substances.* Charles C Thomas, Springfield, IL, 1969

9. Baker PF, Hodgkin AL, Ridgway EB: Depolarization and calcium entry in squid giant axons. J Physiol (Lond) 218:709–755, 1971

10. Krueger BK, Forn J, Greengard P: Depolarization-induced phosphorylation of specific proteins, mediated by calcium ion influx, in rat brain synaptosomes. J Biol Chem 252:2764–2773, 1977

11. Ulbrict W: The effect of veratridine on excitable membranes of nerve and muscle. Ergeb Physiol Biol Chem Exp Pharmakol 61:18–71, 1969

12. Blaustein MP, Johnson EM, Jr, Needleman P: Calcium-dependent norepinephrine release from presynaptic nerve endings in vitro. Proc Natl Acad Sci USA 69:2237–2240, 1972

13. Blaustein MP: Effects of potassium, veratridine and scorpion venom on calcium accumulation and transmitter release by nerve terminals in vitro. J Physiol (Lond) 247:617–655, 1975

14. Sieghart W, Forn J, Greengard P: Ca^{2+} and cyclic AMP regulate phosphorylation of same two membrane-associated proteins specific to nerve tissue. Proc Natl Acad Sci USA 76:2475–2479, 1979

15. Schulman H, Greengard P: Stimulation of brain membrane protein phosphorylation by calcium and an endogenous heat-stable protein. Nature 271:478–479, 1978

16. Schulman H, Greengard P: Ca^{2+}-dependent protein phosphorylation system in membranes from various tissues, and its activation by "calcium-dependent regulator." Proc Natl Acad Sci USA 75:5432–5436, 1978

17. Kretsinger RH: Calcium-binding proteins. Annu Rev Biochem 45:239–266, 1976

18. Ebashi S: Regulatory mechanism of muscle contraction with special reference to the Ca-troponin-tropomyosin system. Essays Biochem 10:1–36, 1974

19. Cheung WY: Cyclic 3′,5′-nucleotide phosphodiesterase: demonstration of an activator. Biochem Biophys Res Commun 38:533–538, 1970

20. Kakiuchi S, Yamazaki R: Calcium-dependent phosphodiesterase activity and its activating factor (PAF) from brain: Studies on cyclic 3′,5′-nucleotide phosphodiesterase (III). Biochem Biophys Res Commun 41:1104–1110, 1970

21. Brostrom CO, Huang Y-C, Breckenridge BMcL, Wolff DJ: Identification of a calcium-binding protein as a calcium-dependent regulator of brain adenylate cyclase. Proc Natl Acad Sci USA 72:64–68, 1975

22. Cheung WY, Bradham LS, Lynch TJ, et al: Protein activator of cyclic 3′,5′-nucleotide phosphodiesterase of bovine or rat brain also activates its adenylate cyclase. Biochem Biophys Res Commun 66:1055–1062, 1975

23. Teo TS, Wang TH, Wang JH: Purification and properties of the protein activator of bovine heart cyclic adenosine 3′,5′-monophosphate phosphodiesterase. J Biol Chem 248:588–595, 1973

24. Huttner WB, Greengard P: Multiple phosphorylation sites in protein I and their differential regulation by cyclic AMP and calcium. Proc Natl Acad Sci USA 76:5402–5406, 1979

25. Huttner WB, DeGennaro LJ, Greengard P: Differential phosphorylation of multiple sites in purified protein I by cyclic AMP–dependent and calcium-dependent protein kinases. J Biol Chem in press, 1981

26. Kennedy MB, Greengard P: Two calcium/calmodulin-dependent protein kinases, which are highly concentrated in brain, phosphorylate protein I at distinct sites. Proc Natl Acad Sci USA in press, 1981

27. Dabrowska R, Sherry JMF, Aromatorio DK, Hartshorne DJ: Modulator protein as a component of the myosin light chain kinase from chicken gizzard. Biochemistry 17:253–258, 1978

28. Yagi K, Yazawa M, Kakiuchi W, et al: Identification of an activator protein for myosin light chain kinase as the Ca^{2+}-dependent modulator protein. J Biol Chem 253:1338–1340, 1978

29. Perry SV, Cole HA, Frearson N, et al: Phosphorylation of the myofibrillar proteins. Proc 12th FEBS Meeting, Volume 54, Cyclic Nucleotides and Protein Phosphorylation in Cell Regulation. Edited by Krause EG, et al. Pergamon Press, Oxford and New York, 1979, pp 147–159

30. Cohen P, Burchell A, Foulkes JG, et al: Identification of the Ca^{2+}-dependent modulator protein as the fourth subunit of rabbit skeletal muscle phosphorylase kinase. FEBS Lett 92:287–293, 1978

31. De Camilli P, Ueda T, Bloom FE, et al: Widespread distribution of protein I in the central and peripheral nervous system. Proc Natl Acad Sci USA 76:5977–5981, 1979

32. Bloom FE, Ueda T, Battenberg E, Greengard P: Immunocytochemical localization in synapses of protein I, an endogenous substrate for protein kinases in mammalian brain. Proc Natl Acad Sci USA 76:5982–5986, 1979

33. De Camilli P, Cameron R, Greengard P: Localization of protein I by immunofluorescence in the adult and developing nervous system. J Cell Biol 87:72a, 1980

34. Ueda T, Greengard P, Berzins K, et al: Subcellular distribution in cerebral cortex of two proteins phosphorylated by a cAMP-dependent protein kinase. J Cell Biol 83:308–319, 1979

35. Strombom U, Forn J, Dolphin AC, Greengard P: Regulation of the state of phosphorylation of specific neuronal proteins in mouse brain by *in vivo* administration of anesthetic and convulsant agents. Proc Natl Acad Sci USA 76:4687–4690, 1979

36. Forn J, Greengard P: Depolarizing agents and cyclic nucleotides regulate the phosphorylation of specific neuronal proteins in rat cerebral cortex slices. Proc Natl Acad Sci USA 75:5195–5199, 1978

37. Baker PF: Transport and metabolism of calcium ions in nerve. Prog Biophys Mol Biol 24:177–223, 1972

38. Dolphin AC, Greengard P: Serotonin stimulates the phosphorylation of protein I, a synapse-specific protein, in the facial motor nucleus of rat brain. Nature 289:76–79, 1981

39. Nestler EJ, Greengard P: Dopamine and depolarizing agents regulate the state of phosphorylation of protein I in the mammalian superior cervical sympathetic ganglion. Proc Natl Acad Sci USA 77:7479–7483, 1980

40. McCall RB, Aghajanian GK: Serotonergic facilitation of facial motoneuron excitation. Brain Res 169:11–27, 1979

41. McCall RB, Aghajanian GK: Denervation supersensitivity in the facial nucleus. Neuroscience 4:1501–1510, 1979

42. Aghajanian GK, McCall RB: Serotonergic synaptic input to facial motoneurons: localization by electron-microscopic autoradiography. Neuroscience 5:2155–2162, 1980

43. Vargaftig BB, Coignet JL, de Vos CJ, et al: Mianserin hydrochloride: peripheral and central effects in relation to antagonism against 5-hydroxytryptamine and tryptamine. Eur J Pharmacol 16:336–346, 1971

44. Nelson DL, Herbert A, Bourgoin S, et al: Characteristics of central 5-HT receptors and their adaptive changes following intracerebral 5,7-dihydroxytryptamine administration in the rat. Mol Pharmacol 14:983–995, 1978

45. Enjalbert A, Hamon M, Bourgoin S, Bockaert J: Postsynaptic serotonin-sensitive adenylate

cyclase in the central nervous system. II. Comparison with dopamine- and isoproterenol-sensitive adenylate cyclases in rat brain. Mol Pharmacol 14:11–23, 1978

46. Rosenthal JE: Post-tetanic potentiation at the neuromuscular junction of the frog. J Physiol (Lond) 203:121–133, 1969

47. Miyamoto MD, Breckenridge BMcL: A cyclic adenosine monophosphate link in the catechol-amine enhancement of transmitter release at the neuromuscular junction. J Gen Physiol 63:609–624, 1974

48. Kravitz EA, Battelle B-A, Evans PD, et al: Octopamine neurons in lobsters. Neurosci Symp 1:67–81, 1975

49. Klein M, Kandel ER: Presynaptic modulation of voltage-dependent Ca^{2+} current: mechanism for behavioral sensitization in Aplysia californica. Proc Natl Acad Sci USA 75:3512–3516, 1978

50. Kaczmarek LK, Jennings KR, Strumwasser F, et al: Microinjection of catalytic subunit of cyclic AMP-dependent protein kinase enhances calcium action potentials of bag cell neurons in cell culture. Proc Natl Acad Sci USA 77:7487–7491, 1980

51. Castellucci VF, Kandel ER, Schwartz JH, et al: Intracellular injection of the catalytic subunit of cyclic AMP-dependent protein kinase simulates facilitation of transmitter release underlying behavioral sensitization in Aplysia. Proc Natl Acad Sci USA 77:7492–7496, 1980

DISCUSSION

Dr. Alan Emery: I would like to suggest that the very beautiful technique you have could be applied in an entirely different field. As you know, we can now diagnose prenatally spina bifida and anencephaly by looking at alpha-fetopro-tein levels in amniotic fluid. However, this test is not specific. Occasionally you get positive results for conditions when you would not wish to terminate the pregnancy. One way around this has been to look at the cells in the amniotic fluid and try to differentiate by morphologic criteria spina bifida from other conditions, but these methods but have not been successful. With your cyto-chemical technique, especially because it is specific for the nervous system, I wonder whether you could look for Protein I in amniotic fluid and, specifically, look at it in amniotic fluid cells in neural tube defects?

Dr. Paul Greengard: We certainly think that Protein I is an organ-specific marker, and it certainly could have a lot of applications based on that property. For example, you can examine tissues that are very sparsely innervated by nerve fibers and demonstrate Protein I by a sufficiently sensitive radioimmunoassay procedure. When you do the immunocytochemistry, all of the Protein I may be accounted for in terms of the nerve fibers. We hope to confirm this by denervating tissues and showing that Protein I disappears.

Dr. Gerald Fischbach: Is the change in phosphorylation on the K^+-induced depolarization a change in the specific activity of the phosphorylation, or is the level of Protein I changing?

Dr. Paul Greengard: The short-term physiologic experiments have to do with the state of phosphorylation of Protein I. There is no change in absolute level. We are now carrying out studies with various preparations to see whether we can get changes in the total level of Protein I. These studies include examination of neuronal differentiation, as well as chronic alterations in neuronal activity.

Dr. Gerald Fischbach: One last philosophical question. Transmitter release occurs on the time scale of 0.5 msec after depolarization. Is phosphorylation fast enough to account for that?

Dr. Paul Greengard: One possibility, which I do not favor at this time, is that the wave of depolarization at the nerve terminal, which causes Ca^{2+} to enter, causes the phosphorylation of Protein I and that phosphorylation directly leads to the release of the neurotransmitter. A second possibility is that Protein I phosphorylation is modulatory and not essentially related to neurotransmitter release. A third possibility is that Protein I phosphorylation is actually involved obligatorily in the sequence of events leading to neurotransmitter release, but that it happens earlier on than the impulse-coupled release process. According to this concept, the phosphorylation of the Protein I primes the fusion process, but does not immediately trigger the release process.

Dr. Stanley Appel: Is Protein I ever found in the presynaptic membrane? According to the notion of exocytosis, we might expect to find it there at some time, especially with prolonged activity.

Dr. Paul Greengard: We do occasionally see images compatible with this notion. Dr. Pietro deCamilli and I plan to test the effect of neuronal activity on the cytochemical distribution of Protein I.

Dr. Stephen Thesleff: Do you know whether aminopyridines, which immensely enhance transmitter release, interfere with Protein I directly or by some secondary mechanisms?

Dr. Paul Greengard: We have not examined that yet.

Dr. Daniel Drachman: You answered half of my question already. Have you looked at the Eaton-Lambert syndrome also?

Dr. Paul Greengard: No.

Section C
Morphologic Aspects

36

Myasthenic Antibodies Alter the Arrangement of Acetylcholine Receptors in Cultured Rat Myotubes: Freeze-Fracture Studies

David W. Pumplin, PhD

Daniel B. Drachman, MD

The freeze-fracture technique has yielded new insights into the structure of membranes. Freeze-fracture provides en face views of large contiguous areas of membrane at high resolution, complementing the on-edge views of thin-section electron microscopy. A method for fracturing cells growing in tissue culture (1) has been applied to the study of developing chick or rat myotubes. Using this technique, Cohen and Pumplin (2) found that regions of myotubes having a high concentration of acetylcholine receptors (AChRs), identified by binding of fluorescent-labeled α-bungarotoxin (α-BuTx), coincided with the presence of large (10-nm) angular intramembrane particles. In myotubes grown in tissue culture, a high concentration of the particles was associated with increased sensitivity to iontophoretically applied ACh (3). The particles are also strikingly similar in both appearance and concentration to those seen at the tops of postjunctional folds of neuromuscular junctions of the frog (4) and rat (5), again a location coincident with α-BuTx binding (6). Furthermore, the particles at postjunctional folds have been directly labeled with ferritin-coupled α-BuTx (7). These findings strongly suggested that the 10-nm angular particles are or contain AChRs. The foregoing observations indicated that the distribution of AChRs can be studied over large areas of myotube membrane at, or close to, the level of individual molecules, by means of the freeze-fracture technique.

In this study, we used freeze-fracture methods to study the effects of anti-AChR antibodies from patients with myasthenia gravis (MG) on the distribution of AChRs in cultured rat myotubes. The basic abnormality in MG is a decrease in the number of AChRs at neuromuscular junctions (8) due to an autoimmune reaction directed against the receptors (reviewed in 9). Most patients with MG have circulating antibodies to AChR (10). These antibodies have been shown to play an important role in the pathogenesis of the disease, because the basic features of MG can be passively transferred to animals by injection of the purified IgG from human patients (11). The presence of anti-AChR antibodies is associated with a decrease in the number of available AChRs at neuromuscular junctions and in a simplification of the postjunctional folds (8–12). Several mechanisms have been described by which AChR loss can occur (13). One such mechanism is the acceleration of the rate of degradation of AChRs. When IgG from myasthenic patients is applied to rat myotubes in tissue culture or transferred to intact mice, a 2- to 3-fold increase in the rate of AChR degradation occurs, resulting in a decrease of receptors (14–17). This effect requires cross-linking of AChRs by divalent antibody (IgG or $F(ab)'_2$); monovalent Fab fragments do not accelerate degradation (18).

In this study, we asked two questions: How does cross-linking by myasthenic IgG alter the distribution of AChRs in myotubes? Can alterations in the distribution of AChRs suggest mechanisms for their increased rate of degradation?

METHODS

Cultures were prepared by standard methods (19). Hind limb muscles of 19-day-old rat fetuses were dissociated by mechanical and trypsin treatment, and cultured in Earle's minimal essential medium supplemented with 10% horse serum, penicillin (100 U/ml), streptomycin (100 U/ml), and amphotericin B (2.5 μg/ml). The myotubes were grown in 35-mm plastic Petri dishes on gelatin-coated plastic or glass coverslips. Circles 4 mm in diameter were scored on the glass coverslips before coating with gelatin. Fibroblasts were nearly eliminated by preplating the dissociated cell suspensions, and by treating the cultures with cytosine arabinoside (10^{-5} M) for 48 hours after 2 days in culture. Cultures were maintained at 37° C in an atmosphere of 10% CO_2 in air.

Six days after plating, the cultures were treated with medium containing approximately 1 mg/ml of IgG or Fab fragments from myasthenic patients or control subjects. Cultures were exposed to the antibody preparations for 1 to 8 hours at 37° C in a 10% CO_2 atmosphere. They were subsequently fixed for 1 hour with 5% glutaraldehyde in 0.15 M cacodylate buffer (pH 7.4). Fixed cultures were equilibrated with 33% glycerol in water, and 4-mm circles were broken out of the scored glass coverslips or cut out of the plastic coverslips. The circles were inverted onto a drop of 30% polyvinyl alcohol (Gelvatol 20–30, Monsanto, New York, NY) in 33% glycerol and placed on a Balzers specimen carrier. The resulting sandwich was frozen in liquid Freon-22 subsequently freeze-fractured using the complementary-replica holder in a Balzers 360 M apparatus at −119° C and a vacuum of 10^{-6} mm Hg.

Replicas were cleaned in sodium hypochlorite solution and picked up on slotted Formvar coated grids for examination in the electron microscope.

For fluorescence observations of antibody effects, cultures were exposed to

10^{-7} M tetramethylrhodamine-labeled α-Butx (TMR-α-BuTx) for 1 hour before antibody treatment as described previously. After antibody treatment, cultures were rinsed with the culture medium three times for 10 minutes each, and then fixed for 30 minutes in 2% formaldehyde (freshly prepared from paraformaldehyde) in cacodylate buffer. Fluorescence was viewed and photographed with the standard filters for tetramethylrhodamine. Essentially all of the label was confined to the myotubes.

RESULTS

Light Microscopy

The distribution of AChRs on myotubes, and its alteration by myasthenic IgG, was studied with α-BuTx conjugated with the fluorescent ligand tetramethylrhodamine (TMR-α-BuTx). Fluorescence microscopy using TMR-α-BuTx showed diffuse labeling with a few sharply defined bright spots in untreated control myotubes (Fig. 1a). The bright areas are presumed to be "hot spots," because similar dense accumulations of AChRs have previously been identified by iontophoretic application of ACh (20) and by autoradiography with ^{125}I-α-BuTx (21) in cultured skeletal muscle. Incubation of myotubes for 1 hour with myasthenic IgG resulted in a striking redistribution of the fluorescent TMR-α-BuTx (Fig. 1b). The fluorescence was concentrated in small bright dots and larger patches; the remaining areas of the myotubes appeared somewhat darker than in controls. Treatment with the monovalent antibody fragment Fab prepared from myasthenic patients' IgG had no effect (Fig. 1c). However, cultures first incubated with myasthenic patients' Fab followed by anti-human IgG showed a redistribution of the pattern of fluorescence essentially identical to that produced by myasthenic IgG (Fig. 1d). This shift in the fluorescence pattern closely resembled that seen in myotubes treated with anti-AChR antibodies from animals with experimental autoimmune myasthenia gravis (22, 23).

Electron Microscopy

Both P and E faces of the sarcolemma of rat myotubes contained large (10-nm) angular particles that were assumed to be AChRs for the reasons given previously. These particles were more prevalent in the P face, with a distribution similar to that in chick myotubes (2). Quantitative results were obtained solely from P faces. The particles were found in four configurations: singly; grouped into clusters comprising 2 to 60 particles spaced 120 to 140 Å apart; in aggregates of 10 to 100 clusters spaced approximately 0.5 to 1 μm apart (see Fig. 3.); and as members of hot spots (see Fig. 4). A cluster of 25 to 30 particles corresponds to a dot of fluorescence in the light microscope; aggregates and hot spots appear as larger patches of fluorescence.

The incidence of individual clusters was determined in freeze-fractured material by photographing random areas of myotubes (with no hot spots or aggregates) at a magnification too low to see individual particles. The number

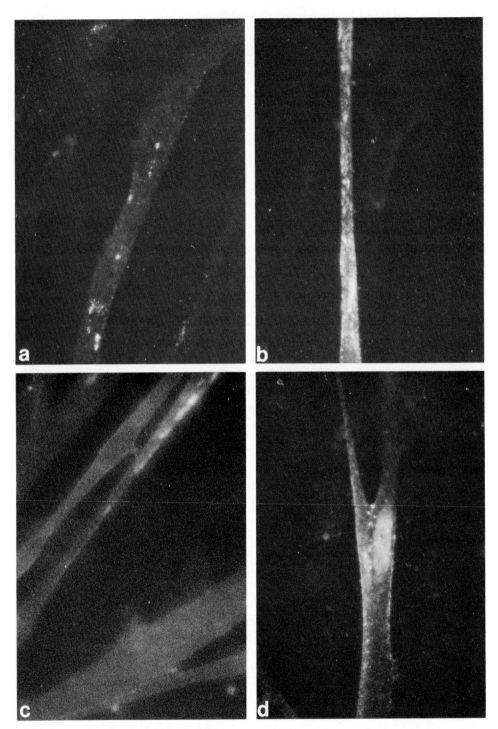

Fig. 1. Fluorescence due to tetramethyl-rhodamine-α-bungarotoxin bound to myotubes. Control myotubes (**a**) showed a diffuse distribution of fluorescence, with only a few bright spots presumably indicating hot spots and/or aggregates. Treatment for 1 hour

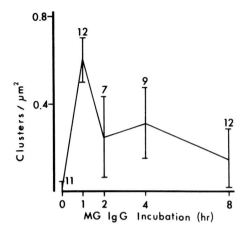

Fig. 2. Time course of the effect of exposure to myasthenic IgG on the incidence of individual clusters of acetylcholine receptor particles in randomly chosen areas of myotubes without hot spots or aggregate enlargements. No more than three areas were counted on any one myotube. Note the marked increase in incidence of clusters at 1 hour, followed by a decrease to near control levels by 2 hours. Bars indicate ±1 SD, and the number of observations is given for each time point.

of clusters was then counted in photographic enlargements. Control myotubes contained a low incidence of clusters (Fig. 2), confirming the impression from fluorescence microscopy that most AChRs are dispersed in the membranes. The incidence of clusters initially increased sharply in myotubes incubated for 1 hour with myasthenic IgG; with longer incubation times, the incidence of clusters decreased rapidly (Fig. 2).

The incidence of aggregates and their total area was determined by exhaustively searching randomly selected myotubes at high power (24,000×) and photographing the entire areas occupied by aggregates. The total area of the myotube examined was determined from micrographs made at low power (2,400×) in which only the outlines of the myotubes could be seen. Aggregates were present at a low incidence in control myotubes; they increased rapidly in myotubes incubated with myasthenic IgG, and subsequently decreased to very low levels after more prolonged incubation (Table 1).

We also investigated another membrane feature, consisting of large depressions approximately 100 nm in diameter, which often contained AChR particles (Fig. 3). These depressions are of particular interest because they are the appropriate size to be "coated pits," or coated vesicles caught by fixation in the act of merging with (pinching off from) the sarcolemma. Coated pits have been described in freeze-etched fibroblasts (24) and have been implicated in the endocytosis of a variety of surface receptors (25, 26).

We determined the incidence of 100-nm depressions within aggregates, in hot spots, and in randomly chosen areas of myotube membrane not containing either feature (Table 2). Depressions were approximately 10 times more

←————————————————————————————

with myasthenic IgG (**b**) produced a greatly increased number of bright spots, corresponding to the increased incidence of clusters and aggregates of acetylcholine receptors. Treatment with Fab fragments of IgG from the same myasthenic patient (**c**) did not alter the control pattern of diffuse fluorescence with a few bright spots. Myotubes treated with Fab followed by antihuman IgG (**d**) again showed an increase in bright dots and patches of fluorescence and a decrease in the diffuse fluorescence, similar to that of myotubes exposed to intact myasthenic IgG. All micrographs were exposed, developed, and printed in as similar a way as possible. (Original magnification ×500.)

Table 1. Time Course of Aggregate Formation in Myotubes Exposed to Myasthenic IgG

Culture Exposed to	% of Total Area Occupied by Aggregate[a]	Total Area Examined (μm^2)[b]	No. of Fibers Examined
Medium alone	3.0	13,800	7
Myasthenic IgG			
1 hour	17	7,500	3
2 hour	16	6,200	2
8 hour	0.1	15,800	6

[a] Aggregates were photographed at high magnification, and the total area occupied was determined from a montage.

[b] The total myotube area examined was determined from a montage made from low-magnification micrographs.

prevalent in aggregates and hot spots than in comparable areas of the remaining membrane.

Hot spots consisted of readily identified large collections of densely concentrated AChR particles (750 to 1,000/μm^2) extending several tens of micrometers along myotubes and having sharp boundaries at which the concentrations of particles fell to the "background" level of 10/μm^2. Within hot spots on control myotubes the particles had a characteristic even distribution (Fig. 4a). The interparticle distance was relatively constant, but particles were not packed tightly. This arrangement of particles was too evenly dispersed to be random (2, 27). When myotubes were treated with myasthenic IgG, AChR particles in hot spots were redistributed into tightly packed clusters separated by areas free of such particles (Fig. 4b). The new particle distribution was too uneven to be random (27). This redistribution began within 2 hours of exposure to myasthenic IgG; no further change in the distribution occurred after 4 hours of exposure. The effect occurred only in the presence of divalent anti-AChR antibodies,

Table 2. Incidence of 100-nm Depressions[a]

	No. of Cultures	Membrane Area Examined (μm^2)	Depressions/μm^2
Within hot spots			
Control myotubes	8	820	0.108
Myasthenic IgG–treated myotubes	10	910	0.129
Within aggregates			
Control	6	210	0.081
Myasthenic IgG–treated	8	480	0.088
Membrane not in hot spot or aggregate	4	2,900	0.011[b]

[a] Micrographs were taken at random intervals along a myotube. Micrographs containing portions of aggregates or hot spots were excluded from this analysis.

[b] Significantly different from other incidence ($P < 0.01$ by Mann-Whitney U test). Other incidences did not differ significantly.

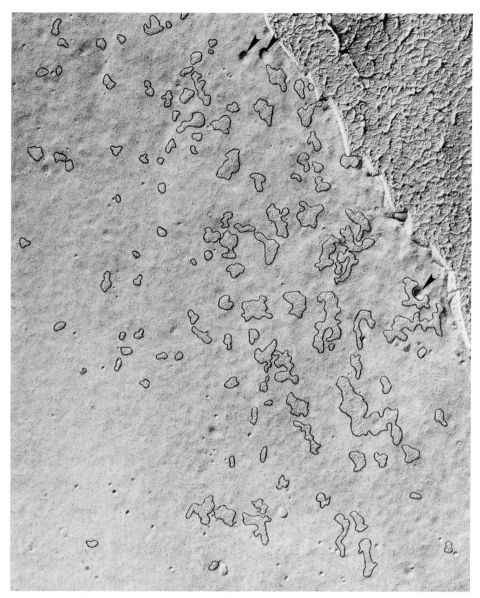

Fig. 3. Aggregate of clusters of acetylcholine receptor particles on a myotube treated for 1 hour with myasthenic IgG. Individual clusters are outlined for clarity. The incidence of clusters decreases sharply at the lower left of the micrograph, indicating the border of the aggregate. Such borders were sufficiently well marked to allow quantification of the membrane area contained in an aggregate. Large depressions (coated pits) were preferentially found in the aggregates (large arrows). (Original magnification ×23,000.)

469

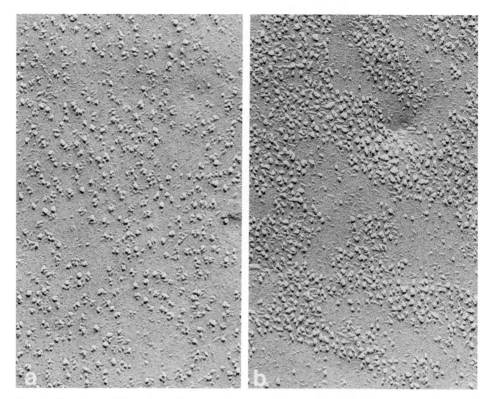

Fig. 4. Portions of hot spots found on cultured myotubes. Illustrated are a control myotube (**a**) and myotubes incubated for 2 hours at 37° C with myasthenic IgG (**b**). The 10-nm angular particles are relatively evenly spaced in control myotubes (**a**), but become increasingly clustered by exposure to the antibody. All hot spots had well-defined borders (a portion is shown at the lower right in **a**) at which the concentration of large particles decreased sharply. Small "background" particles are present in the "spaces" between clusters. (Original magnification ×91,000.)

evidently requiring cross-linking of AChRs. Thus, IgG and F(ab)'$_2$ fragments caused receptor redistribution at hot spots, whereas monovalent Fab fragments did not. However, the latter could in turn be cross-linked by a second "piggy-back" anti-human IgG, and this caused redistribution of particles similar to that due to myasthenic patients' IgG.

DISCUSSION

Treatment of myotubes in culture with myasthenic IgG accelerates the rate of degradation of AChRs (14–17) by a mechanism requiring cross-linking of the receptors (18). The present freeze-fracture observations on myotubes treated with myasthenic IgG suggest a possible mechanism for this acceleration, with redistribution of AChRs into clusters and aggregates, followed by endocytosis, via coated pits as outlined in Fig. 5.

The formation of clusters and aggregates resembles the process of patching of surface antigens that is known to occur on lymphocytes (28, 29). It is reasonable to suppose that the increase in number and size of clusters results directly from cross-linking of AChRs by the myasthenic IgG, because (a) only divalent antibodies induce cluster formation, and (b) the mean distance between particles within a cluster closely approximates the span of an IgG molecule. The mechanism of aggregate formation is less clear. Aggregates consist of particle clusters spaced several hundred nanometers apart, similar to the patches that develop in T-lymphocytes treated with an anti-θ or anti-H$_2$ antibody (29). The distance between individual clusters in an aggregate is far too large to be accounted for by direct interaction between proteins of adjacent clusters, or by antibody bridges between clusters. How then does aggregation take place?

At least two theories have been suggested to explain the similar redistribution of surface receptors in lymphocytes undergoing patching or capping (30). Cross-linking by divalent antibodies has been shown to restrict the random lateral movement of intramembrane antigens (in a fibroblast system) (31). The cross-linked molecules may be passively swept along by lipid currents, accumulating at a point where membrane lipids and/or proteins are internalized and recycled (32). Alternatively, it has been proposed that cytoskeletal elements attach to the clusters and propel them to aggregation sites (33).

Along with the increased incidence of aggregates in muscle cells treated with myasthenic IgG, there was a concomitant increase in the total number of coated pits, because these were found preferentially in aggregates. Such coated pits appear to play an important role in the endocytosis of intramembrane proteins (reviewed in 25). Assuming that the surface lifetime of coated pits is not changed by myasthenic IgG, their incidence may be an index of the rate of endocytosis. Therefore, the observed increase in coated pits supports recent evidence suggesting that endocytosis is the step that determines the rate of AChR loss in both normal and antibody-treated skeletal muscle (34, 35).

Hot spots in normal myotubes contain AChR particles that are evenly spaced in a nonrandom distribution, as described above. The distance between particles is too great to allow for direct AChR-AChR interactions, suggesting that the arrangement of particles is dictated by an underlying cytoskeleton. This is further supported by the observation that the lifetime of a hot spot (several days) (36) is far longer than that of individual AChRs (18 to 22 hours) (37). The fact that myasthenic antibodies are capable of altering the arrangement of AChRs within the hot spots suggests that a high-affinity interaction between AChRs and the antibodies disrupts the AChR-cytoskeleton scaffold. Again,

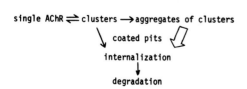

Fig. 5. Proposed scheme for removal and degradation of acetylcholine receptors (AChRs), as described in text. Cross-linking of AChRs by myasthenic IgG favors the formation of clusters, which are in turn gathered to form aggregates. Internalization is more rapid from aggregates (indicated by relative size of arrows) due to the larger number of coated pits.

cross-linking is required for this effect: only divalent antibodies produce rearrangement of the particles; monovalent Fab fragments do not. We were unable to determine whether this rearrangement leads to loss of some AChRs within the hot spots, although the hot spots clearly do not disappear after treatment with myasthenic IgG.

In conclusion, the present studies suggest the following scheme, by which antibody-dependent rearrangement of AChRs can lead to their rapid loss;

1. The normal sarcolemmal membrane contains mainly individual AChRs, in equilibrium with relatively few clusters and aggregates. Rapid lateral motion of AChRs occurs within the sarcolemmal membrane.

2. In the presence of divalent antibody, AChRs are cross-linked to form clusters of as many as 60 particles.

3. Many of the clusters are rearranged to form aggregates.

4. The presence of aggregates induces the formation of increased numbers of coated pits, which serve as vehicles for the endocytosis of the AChRs.

5. The endocytosed (internalized) AChRs are degraded by lysosomal enzymes. Endocytosis, rather than lysosomal degradation, appears to be the step that determines the rate of AChR loss.

6. Within the hot spots, AChRs are also rearranged when exposed to myasthenic IgG, from an evenly spaced ordered pattern to one of clusters with intervening empty spaces. The effect of this rearrangement on AChR loss is not yet certain.

The mechanisms elucidated in the cultured skeletal muscle system may also apply to the accelerated loss of AChRs at intact neuromuscular junctions, and may shed light on the many other cell systems in which a variety of ligands can trigger endocytosis of surface receptors.

ACKNOWLEDGMENTS

We thank RN Adams for his skilled technical assistance, DM Fambrough for a gift of TMR-α-BuTx, TS Reese for use of the electron microscope and darkroom facilities, and C Barlow and MJ Klein for help in preparation of the manuscript. D. Pumplin is supported by grant NS-15513 from the National Institutes of Health. D Drachman is supported by grants 5 PO1 NS 10920 and 5 RO1 HD04817 from the National Institutes of Health.

REFERENCES

1. Pauli BU, Weinstein RS, Soble LW, et al: Freeze fracture of monolayer cultures. J Cell Biol 72:763–769, 1977

2. Cohen SA, Pumplin DW: Clusters of intramembrane particles associated with binding sites for α-bungarotoxin in cultured chick myotubes. J Cell Biol 82:494–516, 1979

3. Yee AG, Fischbach G, Karnovsky M: Clusters of intramembranous particles on cultured myotubes at sites that are highly sensitive to acetylcholine. Proc Natl Acad Sci USA 75:3004–3008, 1978

4. Heuser JT, Reese TS, Landis DMD: Functional change in frog neuromuscular junctions studied with freeze-fracture. J Neurocytol 3:109–131, 1974

5. Rash JE, Ellisman MH: Macromolecular specializations of the neuromuscular junction and the nonjunctional sarcolemma. J Cell Biol 63:567–586, 1974

6. Fertuck HC, Salpeter MM: Quantitation of junctional and extrajunctional acetylcholine receptors by electron microscope autoradiography after ^{125}I-α-Bungarotoxin binding at mouse neuromuscular junctions. J Cell Biol 69:144–158, 1976

7. Rash JE, Hudson CS, Ellisman MH: Ultrastructure of acetylcholine receptors at the mammalian neuromuscular junction. In *Cell Membrane Receptors for Drugs and Hormones.* Edited by Straub RW, Bolis L. Raven Press, New York, 1978

8. Fambrough DM, Drachman DB, Satyamurti S: Neuromuscular junction in myasthenia gravis: decreased acetylcholine receptors. Science 182:293–295, 1973

9. Drachman DB: Myasthenia gravis. N Engl J Med 298:136–142, 186–193, 1978

10. Lindstrom JM, Seybold ME, Lennon VA, et al: Antibody to acetylcholine receptor in myasthenia gravis: prevalence, clinical correlates, and diagnostic value. Neurology (Minneap) 26:1054–1059, 1976

11. Toyka KV, Drachman DB, Griffin DE, et al: Myasthenia gravis: study of humoral immune mechanisms by passive transfer to mice. N Engl J Med 296:125–131, 1977

12. Engel AG, Tsujihata M, Lambert EH, et al: Experimental autoimmune myasthenia gravis: a sequential and quantitative study of the neuromuscular junction ultrastructure and electrophysiologic correlations. J Neuropathol Exp Neurol 35:569–587, 1976

13. Drachman DB, Adams, RN, Stanley EF, et al: Mechanisms of acetylcholine receptor loss in myasthenia gravis. J Neurol Neurosurg Psychiatry 43:601–610, 1980

14. Kao I, Drachman DB: Myasthenic immunoglobulin accelerates acetylcholine receptor degradation. Science 196:527–529, 1977

15. Appel SH, Anwyl R, McAdams MW, et al: Accelerated degradation of acetylcholine receptor from cultured rat myotubes with myasthenia gravis sera and globulins. Proc Natl Acad Sci USA 74:2130–2134, 1977

16. Bevan S, Kullberg RW, Heinemann SF: Human myasthenic sera reduce acetylcholine sensitivity of human muscle cells in tissue culture. Nature 267:263–265, 1977

17. Stanley EF, Drachman DB: Effect of myasthenic immunoglobulin on acetylcholine receptors of intact mammalian neuromuscular junctions. Science 200:1285–1287, 1978

18. Drachman DB, Angus CW, Adams RN, et al: Myasthenic antibodies cross-link acetylcholine receptors to accelerate degradation. N Engl J Med 298:1116–1122, 1978

19. Yaffe D: Rat skeletal muscle cells. In *Tissue Culture: Methods and Applications.* Edited by Kruse Jr P, Patterson MK. Academic Press, New York, 1973, pp 106–113

20. Fischbach GD, Cohen SA: The distribution of acetylcholine sensitivity over uninnervated and innervated muscle fibers grown in cell culture. Dev Biol 21:147–162, 1973

21. Sytkowski AJ, Vogel Z, Nirenberg MW: Development of acetylcholine receptor clusters on cultured muscle cells. Proc Natl Acad Sci USA 70:270–274, 1973

22. Lennon VA: Immunofluorescence analysis of surface acetylcholine receptors on muscle: modulation by auto-antibodies. In *Cholinergic Mechanisms and Psychopharmacology.* Edited by Jenden DJ. Plenum Press, New York, 1978, pp 77–92

23. Prives J, Hoffman L, Tarrab-Hazdai R, et al: Ligand induced changes in stability and distribution of acetylcholine receptors on surface membranes of muscle cells. Life Sci 24:1713–1718, 1979

24. Orci L, Carpenter J-L, Perrelet A, et al: Occurrence of low density liproprotein receptors within large pits on the surface of human fibroblasts as demonstrated by freeze-etching. Exp Cell Res 113:1–13, 1978

25. Goldstein J, Anderson R, Brown M: Coated pits, coated vesicles and receptor mediated endocytosis. Nature 279:679–684, 1974

26. Willingham MC, Maxfield FR, Pastan IH: α_2-macroglobulin binding to the plasma membrane of cultured fibroblasts: diffuse binding followed by clustering in coated regions. J Cell Biol 82:614–625, 1979

27. Dixon WJ, Massey FJ: Introduction to statistical analysis. 2nd ed. McGraw-Hill, New York, 1957

28. Schreiner GF, Unanue ER: Membrane and cytoplasmic changes in B lymphocytes induced by ligand-surface immunoglobulin interaction. Adv Immunol 24:38–165, 1976

29. Karnovsky MJ, Unanue ER: Mapping and migration of lymphocyte surface macromolecules. Fed Proc 32:55–59, 1973

30. Edidin M: Molecular motions and membrane organization and function. In *Membrane Structure and Function*. Edited by Finean JB, Michell RH. Comprehensive Biochemistry, in press

31. Wolf DE, Henkart P, Webb WW: The diffusion, patching, and capping of stearoylated dextrans on 3T3 cell plasma membranes. Biochemistry in press

32. Bretscher MS: Directed lipid flow in cell membranes. Nature 260:21–22, 1976

33. Taylor RB, Duffus WPH, Raff MC, dePetris S: Redistribution and pinocytosis of lymphocyte surface immunoglobulin molecules induced by anti-immunoglobulin antibody. Nature [New Biol] 233:225–229, 1971

34. Libby P, Bursztajn S, Goldberg AJ: Degradation of the acetylcholine receptor in cultured muscle cells: selective inhibitors and the fate of undegraded receptors. Cell 9:481–491, 1980

35. Drachman DB, Pestronk A, Stanley EF, et al: Mechanisms of acetylcholine receptor loss in myasthenia gravis. To be published In *Diseases of the Motor Unit*, Elsevier Press, New York

36. Anderson MJ, Cohen MW: Nerve-induced and spontaneous redistribution of acetylcholine receptors on cultured muscle cells. J Physiol (Lond) 268:757–773, 1977

37. Devreotes PN, Fambrough DM: Acetylcholine receptor turnover in membranes of developing muscle fibers. J Cell Biol 65:335–358, 1975

DISCUSSION

Dr. Vanda Lennon: If I understood your beautiful data in the last slide, it implied that the receptors in the preexisting hot spots were redistributed by antibody. Is that right?

Dr. David Pumplin: Yes.

Dr. Vanda Lennon: This is a little surprising, in view of the photobleaching recovery data of Axelrod, which showed that the receptors labeled by fluorescent bungarotoxin were not mobile over many hours, in contrast to the non–hot spot receptors.

Dr. David Pumplin: It may be just a local shift. The particles do not have to move that far. This would be a shift over, say, a few tens of nanometers rather than a shift over a micrometer or more.

Dr. Vanda Lennon: A second point is that when I looked at the redistribution of receptors induced by anti-receptor antibodies from rat, 24 hours later I could still see hot spots that appeared to be on the membrane.

Dr. David Pumplin: Perhaps I did not make that clear: the aggregates disappear, but the hot spots do not. We find hot spots even after aggregates are gone, and that is after 8 hours of exposure to antibody. I have not looked at longer intervals.

37
Freeze-Fracture Studies in Human Muscular Dystrophy

Eduardo Bonilla, MD

Donald L. Schotland, MD

Yoshihiro Wakayama, MD

A number of biochemical and ultrastructural studies have suggested membrane abnormalities in human muscular dystrophy (1, 2). In Duchenne muscular dystrophy (DMD) there is a marked increase in serum creatinine phosphokinase activity (3) and a reduction in the response of adenyl cyclase to epinephrine (4). Electron microscopic studies have shown focal defects of the muscle cell surface membrane in non-necrotic fibers (5, 6), and cytochemical studies have demonstrated entry of peroxidase and procian yellow through the defects (5, 7). Freeze-fracture studies have demonstrated changes in the distribution and number of intramembranous particles in the muscle plasma membrane (2, 8–10), and lectin cytochemistry has shown focal alterations in concanavalin A binding in a population of dystrophic muscle fibers (11). In DMD a significant decrease in the ability of sarcoplasmic reticulum to accumulate calcium has been demonstrated (12–14). In myotonic dystrophy (MyD) a reduction in muscle cell surface protein kinase (15) and an alteration in the lipid composition of the muscle plasma membrane have been reported (16). In addition, electron microscopic studies have shown focal proliferations of the transverse (T)-tubular system in fibers without other structural abnormalities (17).

Additional evidence of membrane abnormalities in human muscular dystrophy, in particular DMD, has been obtained from studies of red blood cells. These cells demonstrate an abnormal response of adenyl cyclase to epinephrine (18), an increase in the activity of protein kinase (19), and biophysical (20) as well ultrastructural abnormalities of the hydrophobic domain of the membrane (21). Thus, current lines of research in human muscular dystrophy point towards a membrane defect.

The freeze-fracture technique is a powerful tool for studying the ultrastructural organization of biologic membranes. Branton (22) has previously shown that the fracture pathway follows the midline of the membrane through the

475

hydrophobic phospholipid interior. The fracture faces reveal intramembranous particles that are now considered to represent proteins with functional and structural roles in the membrane (23, 24).

We have therefore used the freeze-fracture technique in an attempt to analyze the changes in the internal structure of the muscle plasma membrane in muscle biopsy specimens from patients with three well-characterized forms of human muscular dystrophy.

METHODS

Quadriceps muscle biopsy specimens were obtained from 7 patients with DMD, including 2 preclinical cases; 5 patients with facioscapulohumeral muscular dystrophy (FSH), and 5 patients with MyD. All of the patients in these groups had characteristic clinical, electromyographic, and pathologic features of these diseases.

For control data normal human quadriceps muscle was obtained from 8 male children 4 to 15 years of age who were undergoing orthopedic operations, and 1 normal adult. Histochemical studies of these biopsy specimens were normal.

The specimens were removed at resting length in a U-shaped muscle clamp or attached to a stick and were fixed immediately in 3% glutaraldehyde in 0.1 M phosphate buffer (pH 7.4). Under the dissecting microscope, fascicles were carefully removed, cut into small blocks, and gradually infiltrated in glycerol up to a concentration of 30%. Freezing was carried out in the liquid phase of Freon 22, cooled with liquid nitrogen. Fracture was performed at $-110°$ C in a Balzer BAF-301 freeze-fracture apparatus at a vacuum of 6×10^{-7} mm Hg and immediately replicated with platinum and carbon using electron beam guns. The thickness of the replicas was regulated with a quartz crystal thin film monitor. The tissue was digested in a commercial bleaching solution (Clorox). The detached replicas were washed twice in distilled water and finally picked up on uncoated 300-mesh grids (25). In some instances the control and disease specimens were fractured simultaneously. The material was examined and micrographed in a Zeiss EM-10 electron microscope operated at 60 kV.

Replicas meeting the following criteria were analyzed: (a) presence of smooth extracellular space; (b) presence of different populations of intramembranous particles; and (c) very fine background texture (26).

Double-blind particle, orthogonal array, and caveolae counts/μm^2 were carried out on areas of the protoplasmic (P) face and extracellular (E) face of the plasma membranes on prints at 160,000× and 50,000× magnification. Particles were marked as counted to avoid scoring the same particle more than once. Only particles that cast clearly defined shadows were counted. These were usually 60 to 120 Å in diameter. Each print was counted two or three times (on triplicate micrographs by different persons), and the average number of particles was used. Orthogonal arrays in the P face were identified as aggregates of four or more 60- to 70-Å particles and in the E face as aggregates of four or more 60- to 70-Å pits. Plasma membranes from a minimum of 10 fibers (5 P faces and 5 E faces) were studied in each biopsy specimen. The randomness of the sample was ensured by photographing any area of the fracture that was recognized as muscle plasma membrane. The muscle plasma membrane was recognized by the following criteria: (*a*) presence of orthogonal arrays; (*b*) continuity with the internal cytoplasm of the muscle fiber; or (*c*) presence of the sarcomere outline in the fracture face.

RESULTS

Both the P and E faces of the normal muscle plasma membrane contain openings that correspond to caveolae. At higher magnifications the P face characteristically shows large particles 100 to 120 Å in diameter, a population of individual smaller particles, and orthogonal arrays composed of aggregates of 60- to 70-Å particles. All particles appear distributed in a uniform fashion (Fig. 1A) with a group mean ± SEM density of 1,564 ± 66 particles/μm^2, excluding subunits of orthogonal arrays. The group mean ± SEM density including subunits of orthogonal arrays was 2020 ± 88 particles/μm^2. The E-face particles were less numerous (Fig. 1B), with a group mean ± SEM density of 778 ± 37 particles/μm^2; corresponding pits of the orthogonal arrays were present. The median density of orthogonal arrays was 13.2 aggregates/μm^2 with a mid-range of 6 to 22 aggregates/μm^2 (25 to 75% of the counts). The group mean density of caveolae was 18.6 ± 2.5 caveolae/μm^2.

In contrast to the findings in the normal control specimens, the plasma membrane from DMD muscle showed a significant diminution in the number of intramembranous particles. This finding was noted in both P and E faces (Fig. 2). The group mean particle density in the P face was 1060 ± 44 particles/μm^2 ($P < 0.001$) excluding subunits of orthogonal arrays. The group mean density including subunits of orthogonal arrays was 1066 ± 44 particles/μm^2 ($P < 0.001$). The group mean particle density in the DMD E face was 583 ± 39 particles/μm^2 ($P < 0.002$). The median density of orthogonal arrays was 0 arrays/μm^2 with a midrange of 0 to 0.5 arrays/μm^2 ($P < 0.0001$ for pairwise comparison by Dunn's method). The group mean density of caveolae in DMD was 27.2 ± 3.1 caveolae/μm^2 ($P < 0.002$).

In FSH the group mean density of intramembranous particles in the P face, excluding subunits and orthogonal arrays, was 1,413 ± 143 particles/μm^2 ($P > 0.1$) and did not differ significantly from the control density. In contrast, the group mean density including subunits of orthogonal arrays was 1561 ± 185 particles/μm^2 ($P < 0.001$) and was diminished. The density of intramembranous particles in the FSH E face was 657 ± 53 particles/μm^2 ($P > 0.1$) and was not decreased. The median density of FSH orthogonal arrays was 4 arrays/μm^2 with a midrange of 0 to 11 arrays/μm^2 ($P < 0.001$ for pairwise comparison by Dunn's method) (Fig. 3). The group mean density of caveolae in FSH was 18.9 ± 2.3 caveolae/μm^2 ($P > 0.1$).

No significant differences were noted in the intramembranous particle and orthogonal array densities in MyD plasma membranes (Fig. 4). The group mean particle density in the MyD P face, excluding subunits of orthogonal arrays, was 1,635 ± 110 particles/μm^2 ($P > 0.1$). The group mean density including subunits of orthogonal arrays, was 2100 ± 134 particles/μm^2 ($P > 0.1$). The group mean density in MyD E faces was 755 ± 57 particles/μm^2 ($P > 0.1$). The

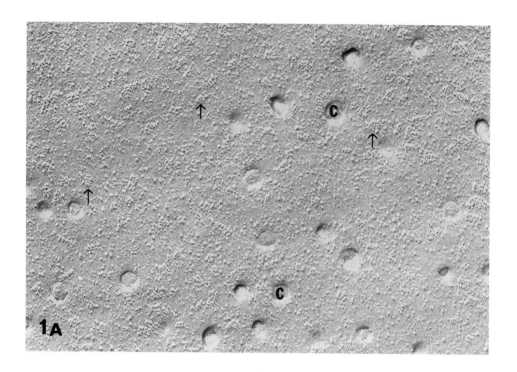

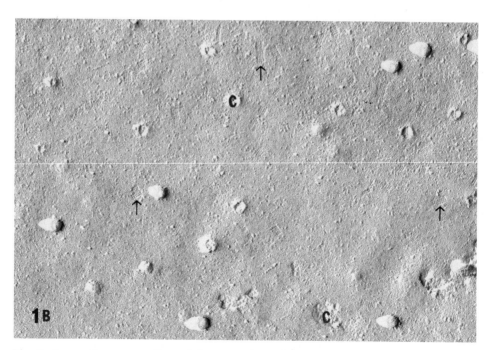

Fig. 1. Freeze-fracture replicas of the normal muscle plasma membrane. **(A)** The P face shows orthogonal arrays (arrows), caveolae (C), and other intramembranous particles. **(B)** The E face shows pits of orthogonal arrays (arrows), fewer intramembranous particles, and caveolae (C). (Original magnification A and B, ×80,000.)

478

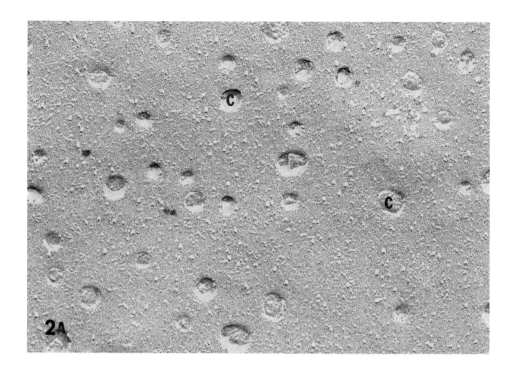

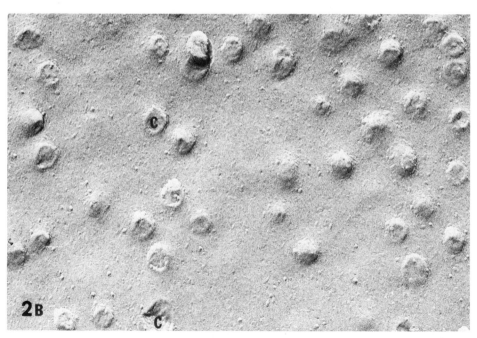

Fig. 2. Freeze-fracture replicas of muscle plasma membrane for a biopsy specimen from a patient with Duchenne muscular dystrophy. (**A**) The P face shows a diminution of intramembranous particles and an increase in caveolae (C). (**B**) The E face shows also a diminution of intramembranous particles and an apparent increase in caveolae (C). (Original magnification A and B, ×80,000.)

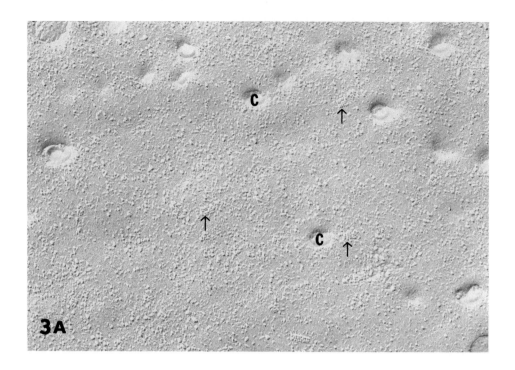

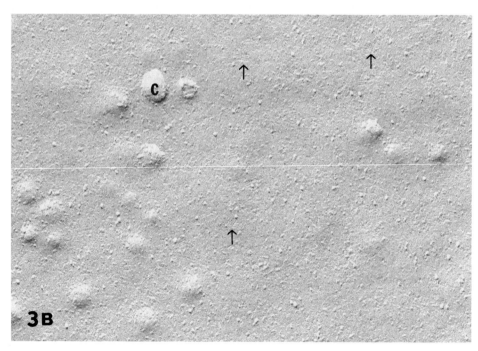

Fig. 3. Freeze-fracture replicas of muscle plasma membrane for a biopsy specimen from a patient with facioscapulohumeral muscular dystrophy. **(A)** The P face. **(B)** The E face. Both faces show a diminution of orthogonal arrays and their pits (arrows). The caveolae (C) appear normal. (Original magnification ×80,000.)

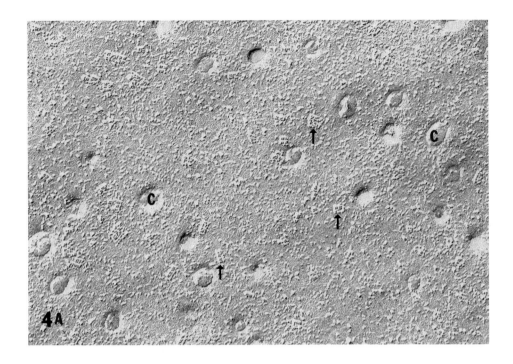

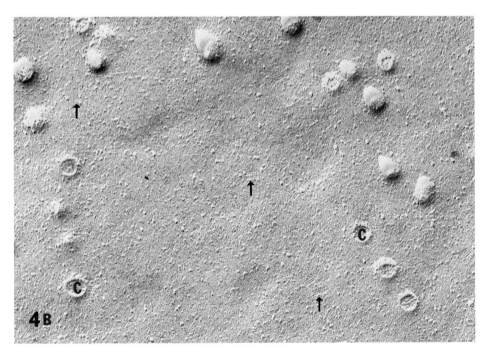

Fig. 4. Freeze-fracture replicas of muscle plasma membrane for a biopsy specimen from a patient with myotonic dystrophy. **(A)** The P face. **(B)** The E face. Both faces appear similar to those of the control plasma membrane. Orthogonal arrays (arrows) and their pits (arrows), and (C) are indicated. (Original magnification ×80,000.)

median density of orthogonal arrays was 15.5 arrays/μm^2 with a midrange of 8 to 24 arrays/μm^2 ($P > 0.1$ for pairwise comparison by Dunn's method). The group mean density of caveolae in MyD was 18.6 ± 3.9 caveolae/μm^2 ($P > 0.1$).

DISCUSSION

In previous freeze-fracture studies of human muscular dystrophy, changes in the number and distribution of intramembranous particles of the muscle plasma membrane have been reported. Schotland and colleagues (8) studied the quadriceps muscle in 8 cases of DMD and in 5 normal control subjects and reported a significant depletion in the number of intramembranous particles in DMD plasma membrane. In another group of patients, a depletion of orthogonal arrays was also observed (27). Ketelsen (9) studied 1 case of human muscular dystrophy and reported an increase in the number of intramembranous particles in the muscle surface membrane. Yoshioka and Okuda (10) studied 1 case of DMD and also reported an increase in the number of particles in the muscle plasma membrane.

In the present study we analyzed the ultrastructure of the muscle plasma membrane in 7 new cases of DMD, 5 cases of FSH, 5 cases of MyD, and 9 new control subjects.

The findings indicate that there is a significant diminution in the number of particles and orthogonal arrays and an increase in the number of caveolae in the surface membrane of a population of muscle fibers from patients with DMD. It should be noted that the intramembranous particle density, excluding subunits of orthogonal arrays, was not decreased in 5 patients with FSH.

It is of interest that no significant differences were found in this study between patients with MyD and control subjects with respect to number of intramembranous particles, orthogonal array density, on caveolar density. These results do not preclude an abnormality at other levels of membrane organization in this disease.

The depletion of orthogonal arrays noted in plasma membrane from patients with DMD and with FSH is particularly interesting. In human muscle plasma membrane the orthogonal arrays are consistently associated with the inner membrane leaflet or P face, and complementary pits appear on corresponding E faces. Whether the orthogonal arrays seen in freeze replicas of human muscle plasma membrane are associated with specializations on the outer surface of the membrane or with structures in the underlying cytoplasm could not be determined. Because of the consistent association of the orthogonal arrays with the P fracture face, however, it seems likely that they represent proteins located at the inner surface of the plasma membrane. The function and the biochemical identity of these conspicuous specializations of the muscle plasma membrane remain to be established.

Orthogonal arrays of 60- to 70-Å particles were first observed in hepatocytes and were found subsequently in plasma membrane of intestinal epithelial cells, skeletal muscle cells, glial cells, and cardiac muscle cells (29–33). It has also been noted that orthogonal arrays are not observed in the neuromuscular junction in rat skeletal muscle but are present in other areas (31). However, Heuser and coworkers (34) have found orthogonal arrays at the neuromuscular junction; because they are also present in the plasma membrane of other cells that do not propagate action potentials, such as the hepatocyte, their possible role in the conduction of the action potential remains to be established.

Ellisman and associates (35) reported that orthogonal arrays were more numerous in the plasma membrane of rat fast twitch muscle fibers than in the plasma membrane of slow twitch fibers. In this study we noted a median density of 13.2 orthogonal arrays/μm^2, with a midrange of 6 to 22 arrays/μm^2 in normal human muscle. Clearly defined peaks corresponding to fiber types, as reported by Schmalbruch (36) were not noted, but plasma membranes with low and high densities of orthogonal arrays as reported by Shafiq and coworkers (37) were observed. Frozen sections stained with adenosine triphosphatase at pH 9.4 in the control preparations revealed 45.4% type I fibers and 54.6% type II fibers.

The results of this investigation show that loss of orthogonal arrays is not specific for DMD, because a significant decrease in orthogonal array density was also observed in FSH. Further support for the nonspecificity of this finding was obtained from our preliminary studies of 2 cases of myositis in which orthogonal array density was also decreased. These data may indicate that the muscle plasma membrane reverts to an immature form during the course of these diseases, because orthogonal arrays appear shortly after birth in developing rat muscle (28).

It is worth noting that we found a significant increase in caveolar density in DMD. The significance of this finding is not clear, because little is known about the function of the caveolae in skeletal muscle. The possibility that they are involved in uptake and transport of proteins is not generally accepted (38). On the other hand, recent studies have shown that a proportion of caveolae in vertebrate muscle correspond to T-tubular system openings (39, 40). It is also interesting that in dystrophic chickens an increase in caveolar density associated with extensive proliferation of T-tubular system networks have been reported (41–43). Whether the increase in the caveolar density noted in DMD is also associated with proliferation of the T-tubular system is unknown. Further work on this issue is being carried out.

In conclusion, DMD appears to be the only disease so far in which there is a decrease in intramembranous particles and orthogonal array density and an increase in caveolar density in a population of fibers in quadriceps muscle. The significance of these findings remains to be established.

ACKNOWLEDGMENTS

This work was supported by a Research Center Grant from the Muscular Dystrophy Association of America and by grants NS-08075, NS-14471, and 5 M01RR00040 from the U.S. Public Health Service. The authors thank Peggy VanMeter for skillful technical assistance and Sylvia Dunn for typing the manuscript.

REFERENCES

1. Rowland LP: Pathogenesis of muscular dystrophies. Arch Neurol 33:315–321, 1976

2. Schotland DL, Bonilla E, Wakayama Y: Application of the freeze-fracture technique to the study of human neuromuscular disease. Muscle Nerve 3:21–27, 1980

3. Dreyfus JC, Schapira F: Biochemical study of muscle in progressive muscular dystrophy. J Clin Invest 33:794–797, 1954

4. Mawatari S, Takagi A, Rowland LP: Adenyl cyclase in normal and pathologic human muscle. Arch Neurol 30:96–102, 1974

5. Mokri B, Engel AG: Duchenne dystrophy: electron microscopic findings pointing to a basic or early abnormality in the plasma membrane of the muscle fiber. Neurology (Minneap) 25:111–120, 1975

6. Schmalbruch H: Segmental fiber breakdown and defects of the plasmalemma in diseased human muscle. Acta Neuropathol (Berl) 33:129–141, 1975

7. Bradley WG, Fulthorpe JJ: Studies of sarcolemmal integrity in myopathic muscle. Neurology (NY) 28:670–677, 1978

8. Schotland DL, Bonilla E, VanMeter M: Duchenne dystrophy: alteration in plasma membrane structure. Science 196:1005–1007, 1977

9. Ketelsen UP: The plasma membrane of human skeletal muscle cells in the pathological state. In *Recent Advances in Myology*. Edited by Bradley WG, Gardner-Medwin D, Walton JN. Excerpta Medica, Amsterdam, 1975, pp 446–454

10. Yoshioka M, Okuda R: Human skeletal muscle fibers in normal and pathological states: freeze etch replica observations. J Electron Microsc (Tokyo) 26:103–110, 1977

11. Bonilla E, Schotland DL, Wakayama Y: Duchenne dystrophy: focal alterations in the distribution of concanavalin A binding sites at the muscle cell surface. Ann Neurol 4:177–123, 1978

12. Samaha F, Gergely J: Biochemical abnormalities of the sarcoplasmic reticulum in muscular dystrophy. N Engl J Med 280:184–188, 1969

13. Peter JB, Worsfold M: Muscular dystrophy and other myopathies: sarcotubular vesicles in early disease. Biochem Med 2:364–371, 1969

14. Takagi A, Schotland DL, Rowland LP: Sarcoplasmic reticulum in Duchenne dystrophy. Arch Neurol 28:380–384, 1973

15. Roses AD, Appel S: Muscle membrane protein kinase in myotonic muscular dystrophy. Nature 250:245–247, 1974

16. Peter JB, Fiehn W, Nagatomo T, et al: Studies of sarcolemma from normal and diseased skeletal muscle. In *Exploratory Concepts in Muscular Dystrophy*. Edited by Milhorat AT. Excerpta Medica, Amsterdam, 1974, pp 479–490

17. Schotland DL: An electron microscopic investigation of myotonic dystrophy. J Neuropathol Exp Neurol 29:241–252, 1970

18. Mawatari S, Schonberg M, Olarte M: Biochemical abnormalities of erythrocyte membrane in Duchenne dystrophy. Arch Neurol 30:96–102, 1974

19. Roses AD, Herbstreith MH, Appel S: Membrane protein kinase alteration in Duchenne muscular dystrophy. Nature 254:350–351, 1975

20. Sato B, Nishikida K, Samuels LT, et al: Electron spin resonance studies of erythrocytes from patients with Duchenne muscular dystrophy. J Clin Invest 61:251–259, 1978

21. Wakayama Y, Hodson A, Pleasure D, et al: Alteration in erythrocyte membrane structure in Duchenne muscular dystrophy. Ann Neurol 4:253–256, 1978

22. Branton D: Fracture faces of frozen membranes. Proc Natl Acad Sci USA 55:1048–1056, 1966

23. Marchesi VT, Tillack TW, Jackson RL, et al: Chemical characterization and surface orientation of the major glycoprotein of the human erythrocyte membrane. Proc Natl Acad Sci USA 69:1445–1449, 1972

24. MacLennan DH, Seeman P, Iles GH, et al: Membrane formation by the adenosine triphosphatase of sarcoplasmic reticulum. J Biol Chem 246:2702–2710, 1971

25. Franzini-Armstrong C: Freeze fracture of skeletal muscle from the tarantula spider. J Cell Biol 61:501–513, 1974

26. Staehelin LA: Analysis and critical evolution of the information contained in freeze-etch micrographs. In *Freeze-Etching Techniques and Applications.* Edited by Benedetti EM, Farvard P. Société Française de Microscopie Electronique, Paris, 1973, pp 107–134

27. Schotland DL, Bonilla E, Wakayama Y: Pathogenesis of muscle cell damage in the dystrophies: morphologic aspects including freeze fracture studies. In *Current Topics in Nerve and Muscle Research.* Edited by Aguayo AJ, Karpati G. Excerpta Medica, Amsterdam, 1979, pp 29–38

28. Hudson SC, Rash JE, Albuquerque EX: A thin section and freeze fracture study of mammalian neuromuscular junction development. J Cell Biol 75:116a, 1977

29. Kreutsiger GO: Freeze etching of intracellular junctions of mouse liver. Proc Elec Microsc Soc Am 26:234–235, 1968

30. Staehelin LA: Three types of gap junctions interconnecting intestinal epithelial cells visualized by freeze etching. Proc Natl Acad Sci USA 69:1318–1321, 1972

31. Rash JE, Ellisman MH: Studies of excitable membranes. I. Macromolecular specializations of the neuromuscular junction and the non-junctional sarcolemma. J Cell Biol 63:567–586, 1974

32. Landis MD, Reese TS: Arrays of particles in freeze fractured astrocytic membranes. J Cell Biol 60:316–320, 1974

33. McNutt NS: Ultrastructure of the myocardial sarcolemma. Circ Res 37:1–13, 1975

34. Heuser JE, Reese TS, Landis MD: Functional changes in frog neuromuscular junctions studied with freeze fracture. J Neurocytol 3:108–131, 1974

35. Ellisman MH, Rash JE, Staehelin LA, et al: Studies of excitable membranes. II. A comparison of specializations of neuromuscular junctions and non-junctional sarcolemma of mammalian fast and slow twitch fibers. J Cell Biol 68:752–774, 1976

36. Schmalbruch H: "Square arrays" in the sarcolemma of human skeletal muscle fibers. Nature 281:145–146, 1979

37. Shafiq SA, Leung B, Schutta HS: A freeze-fracture study of fiber types in normal human muscle. J Neurol Sci 42:129–138, 1979

38. Dulhunty AF, Franzini-Armstrong C: The relative contributions of the folds and caveolae to the surface membrane of frog skeletal muscle fibers at different sarcomere lengths. J Physiol (Lond) 250:513–539, 1975

39. Franzini-Armstrong C, Landmesser L, Pilar G: Size and shape of transverse tubule openings in frog twitch muscle fibers. J Cell Biol 64:493–497, 1975

40. Rayns DG, Simpson FO, Bertaud WS: Surface features of striated muscle. II. Guinea pig skeletal muscle. J Cell Sci 3:475–482, 1968

41. Costello BR, Shafiq SA: Freeze fracture study of muscle plasmalemma in normal and dystrophic chickens. Muscle Nerve 2:191–201, 1979

42. Malouf NN, Sommer JR: Chicken dystrophy: the geometry of the transverse tubules. Am J Pathol 84:299–316, 1976

43. Beringer T: Stereologic analysis of normal and dystrophic avian myofibers. Exp Neurol 61:380–394, 1978

DISCUSSION

Dr. Jerry Shay: Have you ever looked at any obligate carriers of Duchenne muscular dystrophy (DMD) for orthogonal arrays or intermembranous particles?

Dr. Eduardo Bonilla: No, not so far.

Dr. Carl Pearson: Would you tell us about the age of these 5 patients with

DMD? Were they all very young, or were some older? Is there any correlation in this regard with some of your findings?

Dr. Eduardo Bonilla: As a matter of fact, we have studied 2 preclinical cases, one 6 months old and the other 1 year old. The oldest patient was 8 years old. The findings were similar in all cases.

Dr. Alan Emery: Someone has asked whether you looked at carriers; this is terribly important. If you are looking for a carrier detection test that will be useful in an X-linked disease, you should be able to demonstrate cellular mosaicism. This would be possible in RBCs, because if there is a significant reduction in the number of membrane particles only in DMD, then there might be two populations of particle counts in carriers. I do not know of any other parameter currently being studied for which it might be possible to demonstrate cellular mosaicism in carriers of this disease.

Dr. Eduardo Bonilla: I agree with you. We have those studies in mind.

Dr. Anthony Martonosi: You hinted briefly at the differences in intramembranous particle density and in the density of orthogonal arrays between red and white muscle fibers. You also mentioned that the particle densities did not indicate two distinct fiber types in DMD. What did you find in your histochemical studies of fiber types? Your observations would appear to be consistent with a predominance of red slow fibers with a diminished intramembranous particle density and the absence of orthogonal arrays in DMD.

Dr. Eduardo Bonilla: Portions of our control biopsy specimens were studied histochemically. Using ATPase at pH 9.4, 45% of the fibers were type I and 54% were type II. In the DMD specimens 42% of the fibers were type I and 57% were type II. Obviously, I cannot completely rule out the possibility that we might be fracturing only type I fibers in DMD.

Dr. Anthony Martonosi: In principle, it should be possible to initiate experiments in which well-defined fiber types would be studied morphologically using some independent enzymologic criteria for identifying the fibers that are selected for electron microscopy.

Dr. Eduardo Bonilla: I agree.

Dr. Daniel Drachman: Dr. Schotland or Dr. Bonilla, have you ever transplanted Duchenne dystrophic muscle into nude mice? If so, have you seen any abnormality that you could attribute to Duchenne muscular dystrophy (DMD) at an early stage of development that would be relevant to the culture situation?

Dr. Donald Schotland: We have not transplanted DMD muscle into nude mice as yet.

Dr. Michael Brooke: One of the excellent aspects of this study is that it compares two very similar populations of cells. One problem in the investigation of DMD muscle is the control. As Dr. Martonosi mentioned in his paper, the fiber type composition in DMD is completely different from that of most controls that can be used. The number of 2C fibers is large, and Type 1 fibers predominate. The only control you could use for DMD, then, would be a neonate with the undifferentiated type 2C fiber. One of the tremendous advantages of your studies is the comparison of homogeneous groups. The next step is to compare the newborn with DMD with a newborn control in which the fiber type may be roughly similar. To compare a 6-year-old patient with DMD with a 6-year-old control subject almost begs the question, because the fiber types are so completely different.

38
Freeze-Fracture Electron Microscopic Study of Cultured Muscle Cells in Duchenne Dystrophy

Mitsuhiro Osame, MD

Andrew G. Engel, MD

Charles J. Rebouche, PhD

Robert E. Scott, MD

Various morphologic abnormalities of the muscle fiber plasma membrane have been reported in Duchenne muscular dystrophy (DMD). These include holes in the plasma membrane in non-necrotic muscle fibers (1–3), focal decreases in concanavalin A binding sites overlying the plasma membrane (4), a decrease in the numerical density of intramembranous particles (IMPs) and orthogonal particle arrays, and an increase in the density of caveoli in the freeze-fractured plasma membrane (5, and chapter 37, this volume). A depletion of IMPs has also been noted in the erythrocyte plasma membrane in DMD (6). The present study was designed to determine whether IMPs are depleted in the plasma membrane of the cultured muscle cell in DMD. Such a depletion occurring early in ontogenesis would support the concept that a genetically determined abnormality resides in the muscle fiber plasma membrane, and would suggest that depletion of IMPs represented a very early and probably important structural alteration in the pathogenesis of the disease.

CLINICAL DATA

Specimens of lateral vastus muscle were obtained from 6 boys, 2 to 9 years of age, with DMD. The diagnosis was based on the clinical features, the increased

489

serum level of creatine phosphokinase, and the electromyographic and histologic findings. Control muscle specimens were obtained from limbs of 4 men and 2 women, 8 to 41 years of age. None of these subjects had objective evidence of muscle disease on the basis of manual muscle testing, serum enzyme levels, electromyography, and histologic studies of muscle.

METHODS

Muscle Cultures

Muscle cultures were established by the explant technique, as described by Witkowski and coworkers (7). Cultures were grown on 25-mm round polystyrene coverslips in medium 199 supplemented with 10% heat-inactivated horse serum, 2.5% chick embryo extract, 15 mM HEPES buffer, penicillin (100 U/ml), streptomycin (100 μg/ml), and Fungizone (1.25 μg/ml).

Approximately 2 to 3 weeks after explanation, confluent or nearly confluent layers of cells were obtained. These were fixed with 1% glutaraldehyde in 0.1 M phosphate buffer (pH 7.2) for 15 minutes at room temperature and then rinsed with several changes of 0.1 M cacodylate buffer (pH 7.3). Subsequently, the specimens were equilibrated with 15% buffered glycerol for 30 minutes. After this, selected areas (see later) of the coverslips were excised and processed for freeze fracture by the technique of Pauli and colleagues (8).

Freeze-Fracture Procedures

Specimens were fractured in a Balzer's 300 instrument at stage temperatures ranging from -114 to $-116°$ C and at pressures ranging from 10^{-7} to 2×10^{-7} mbar. The conditions chosen were just above the "ice line" (9), i.e., the line obtained by plotting the vapor pressures of ice against the temperature according to the equation cited by Washburn (9), so that they slightly favored sublimation, instead of condensation, of water vapor. Immediately after fracture, the specimen was shadowed at a 40° angle with a deposit of platinum-carbon 2 nm thick and then backed with a deposit of carbon 20 nm thick, emitted from electron-beam guns. Thickness of the deposited films was regulated by a quartz crystal thin-film monitor. A permanent record of the thickness and rate of deposition of the films was obtained by a millivolt recorder connected to the voltage output terminals of the quartz crystal control unit. The replicas were retrieved and cleansed by conventional methods, mounted on 200-mesh copper grids and examined in a Philips model 300 electron microscope.

Precise Phase Microscopic to Freeze Fracture Electron Microscopic Correlation

Because explants of human muscle in culture yield mononuclear cells, which can be either myoblasts or fibroblasts, and because the numeric density of IMPs as well as other structural features of the plasma membrane could be different

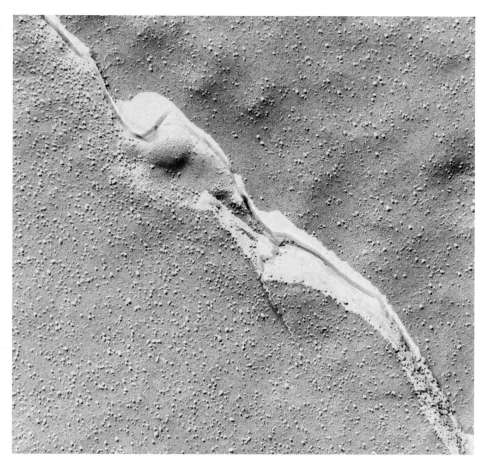

Fig. 1. (*P*) fracture faces of plasma membranes of two separate but adjacent cells. The *P* face at lower left, derived from a myotube, displays more intramembranous particles than the *P* face at upper right, which was derived from a mononuclear cell. The method for determining the cell of origin of the replicated membrane leaflet is explained in the text and is illustrated in Figures 2 and 3. (Original magnification ×73,000.)

for each cell type (Fig. 1), it was essential to know the cell of origin of each replicated membrane leaflet observed in the electron microscope. For this reason, we devised a method for precise correlation of freeze-fracture electron microscopic with phase microscopic images. Corners of selected areas, approximately 1.7 × 1.7 mm in size, were demarcated on the plastic coverslips with pinholes during the period of buffer rinse. Phase micrographs of these areas were taken at an original magnification of 90×, and enlargements of the phase micrographs were assembled into a montage (Fig. 2, left panel). After glycerination of the specimen, the demarcated areas were excised with iris scissors, care being taken to include the pinhole landmarks. Subsequently, electron micrographs were made of the entire retrieved replica at an original magnification of 270× in the "scanning mode," without an objective lens aperture but

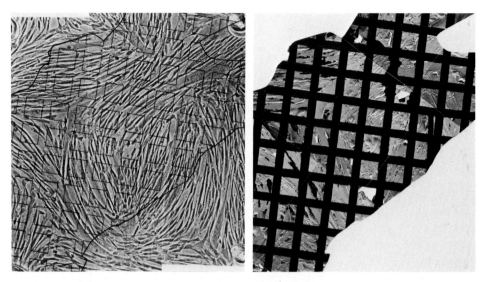

Fig. 2. *Left.* Montage of phase micrographs of cultured muscle cells growing on plastic coverslip. Four corners of photographed field are demarcated by pinholes. *Right.* Montage of low-magnification electron micrographs made of entire retrieved replica. Image of pinhole landmark appears in left upper corner. Contours of larger cells in phase micrograph can be readily matched with corresponding regions in replica. Outlines of entire replica and its supporting grid are superimposed on phase montage.

with a 200-μm diffraction lens aperture. The enlarged electron micrographs were also assembled into a montage (Fig. 2, right panel) so that the final magnifications of the two montages were identical. Using at least two pinhole landmarks or, if the entire replica was not retrieved, outlines of at least two easily identifiable cells in different regions of the replica, the two montages were aligned and matched. After this, a transparent image of the contour of the entire replica and of the copper supporting grid was superimposed on the phase montage (Fig. 2, left panel). At this point, every area and cell in the phase montage could be matched to the corresponding membrane leaflet seen in the electron microscope, and every membrane leaflet seen in the electron microscope could be assigned to its cell of origin (Figs. 2 and 3). Further selected regions of individual cells and cell-cell contacts could be identified and then studied at a higher magnification.

Sampling Procedures

Only replicas that showed satisfactory complementarity, as evidenced by pits in the external (*E*) membrane faces, were retained for analysis. To avoid bias in selecting membranes in the electron microscope, cells and cell regions to be studied were predetermined in the phase montages. The selected regions on a given cell were always nearest the central part of the cell. Predetermined areas were photographed at an electron optical magnification of approximately

40,000× without further selection. Only one micrograph was obtained from each cell for IMP counts. Three to five mononuclear cells and three to five myotubes were sampled in each replica. With few exceptions, sampling was continued in each case until 10 to 20 separate myotube protoplasmic (P) faces, myotube E faces, mononuclear cell P faces, and mononuclear cell E faces had been photographed. Particle counts were done at a final magnification of 100,000× on coded pictures by observers who had not seen the prints previously. A transparent sheet marked by a 10×10-cm grid made of 1×1-cm squares was placed on the central part of each picture. All identifiable IMPs were counted in each square in which the membrane surface was adequately shadowed and was not interrupted by caveoli, exposed sarcoplasm, or dirt.

Particle sizes were analyzed in P faces on myotubes from 1 control subject and 1 patient with DMD. For this part of the study, control and DMD myotubes were simultaneously fractured and replicated. The P faces of 10 randomly selected myotubes were analyzed in each case. Each myotube was represented by a single micrograph. Dimensions of IMPs were measured in electron micrographs enlarged 200,000× (Fig. 4) viewed through a 7× measuring magnifier scaled at 0.1-mm intervals (final magnification, 1,400,000×). A transparent 10×5-cm sheet divided into 1-cm squares was placed over the center of each micrograph. The width of IMPs (widest diameter perpendicular to the direction of shadowing) was measured in individual squares, beginning at the upper left square and then proceeding row by row, until 100 particles were measured in each micrograph. Thus, diameters of 1,000 IMPs were measured in each case. Large (12- to 17-nm) particles aggregated in characteristic clusters and representing putative acetylcholine receptors (10, 11) were excluded from this analysis.

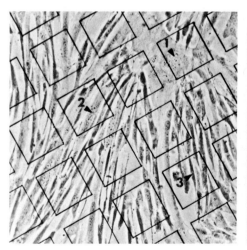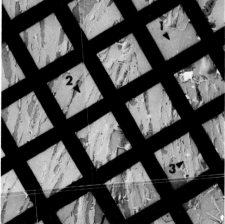

Fig. 3. Correlation of phase microscopic montage (*left*) with electron microscopic montage (*right*). As an example, myotubes (arrows 1 and 2) and mononuclear cell (arrow 3) seen on the left can be definitively matched to corresponding membrane leaflet seen on the right. (Original magnification both figures ×270.)

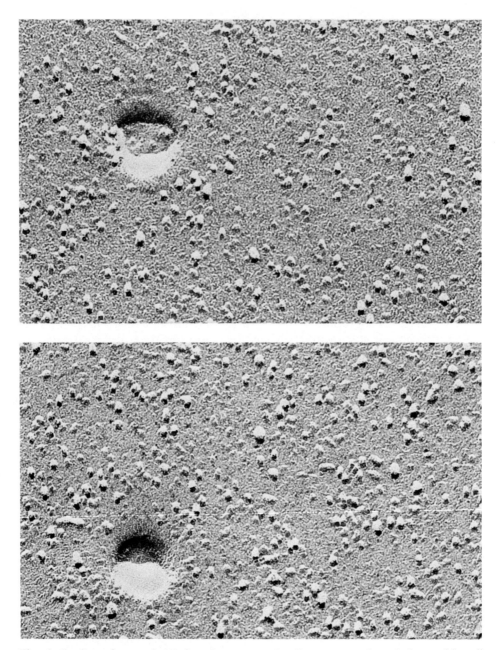

Fig. 4. Region of myotube *P* face from control cell (*upper panel*) and dystrophic cell (*lower panel*). (Original magnification ×200,000.)

RESULTS

No qualitative differences were noted by simple inspection between corresponding leaflets of control and DMD cells of the same type (Fig. 4). The numerical density of IMPs was determined in *P* faces of 202 myotubes and 220 mononuclear cells and in E faces of 133 myotubes and 146 mononuclear cells. No significant differences were found between P faces of control and DMD myotubes, or between P faces of control and DMD mononuclear cells; and the same conclusions were reached for E faces of myotubes and mononuclear cells from control and dystrophic subjects (Table 1, Fig. 5). However, for both control and dystrophic cells, the mean P-face particle density was higher for myotubes than for mononuclear cells. The difference between mononuclear cells and myotubes was significant for the control cells ($P < 0.02$), but failed to reach significance for the dystrophic cells ($P = 0.053$).

The frequency distribution of IMPs according to their size, determined in P faces of simultaneously fractured myotubes of 1 patient and 1 control subject, were virtually identical. At least 5 classes of particles were resolved according to size in both DMD and control membranes (Fig. 6).

Additional observations were as follows: P faces of DMD myotubes contained a mean $\pm$ SEM of 0.92 ± 0.20 caveoli/μm^2. The corresponding value for control myotubes was 0.98 ± 0.14 caveoli/μm^2. These values were not significantly different. Cell-cell contacts between mononuclear cells and between mononuclear cells and myotubes displayed tight junctions, gap junctions (Fig. 7), and "nude spots," the latter presumably indicative of recent or incipient membrane fusion (12). No qualitative difference could be observed in these

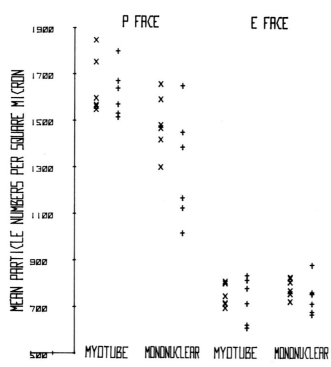

Fig. 5. Mean counts of intramembranous particles (IMPs) for control (+) and dystrophic (×) subjects. The distribution of particle counts is similar in corresponding leaflets of control and dystrophic cells of the same type. For both control and dystrophic cells, P-face particle counts show a higher distribution in myotubes than in mononuclear cells.

Table 1. Density of Intramembranous Particles (no./μm^2)

Source	P Fracture Face				E Fracture Face			
	Myotube Mean ± SD	n^a	Mononuclear Cell Mean ± SD	n	Myotube Mean ± SD	n	Mononuclear Cell Mean ± SD	n
Duchenne								
1	1,847 ± 225	24	1,657 ± 244	15	800 ± 137	10	804 ± 136	10
2	1,562 ± 143	26	1,418 ± 211	15	808 ± 150	14	825 ± 137	12
3	1,568 ± 141	15	1,592 ± 201	12	694 ± 125	12	754 ± 133	12
4	1,752 ± 118	14	1,467 ± 248	31	715 ± 121	7	720 ± 128	17
5	1,597 ± 194	14	1,481 ± 224	12	745 ± 74	10	821 ± 116	13
6	1,548 ± 126	18	1,300 ± 112	13	712 ± 92	9	767 ± 104	11
Group Mean ± SD	1,646 ± 124		1,486 ± 127		746 ± 48		782 ± 42	
Control								
1	1,571 ± 153	14	1,124 ± 266	19	713 ± 108	9	664 ± 95	11
2	1,799 ± 91	17	1,650 ± 230	25	620 ± 181	10	710 ± 115	12
3	1,531 ± 160	14	1,016 ± 165	20	607 ± 65	10	675 ± 78	12
4	1,639 ± 122	13	1,385 ± 182	15	813 ± 153	13	877 ± 121	11
5	1,671 ± 235	20	1,449 ± 282	16	778 ± 132	11	752 ± 83	10
6	1,515 ± 181	13	1,167 ± 266	27	833 ± 121	18	759 ± 134	15
Group Mean ± SD	1,621 ± 106		1,299 ± 237		738 ± 84		740 ± 78	

[a] Number of fracture faces analyzed.

496

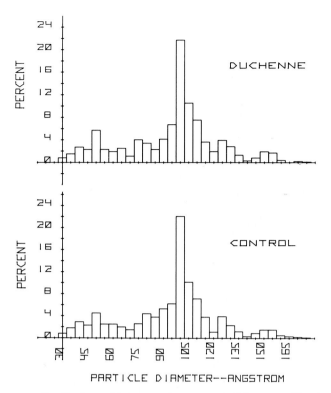

Fig. 6. Frequency distribution of intramembranous particles according to size in *P* faces of myotubes from a patient with Duchenne muscular dystrophy and a control subject. The two distributions are virtually identical. Putative acetylcholine receptor particles occurring in clusters were excluded from this analysis.

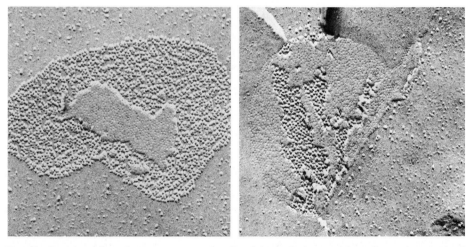

Fig. 7. Gap junctions between control cells (*left*) and dystrophic cells (*right*). In both panels cleavage plane steps from *P* face of one cell to *E* face of adjacent cell with corresponding change from convex particles to concave pits in the gap junctions. (Original magnification: left panel, ×71,000; right panel, ×69,000.)

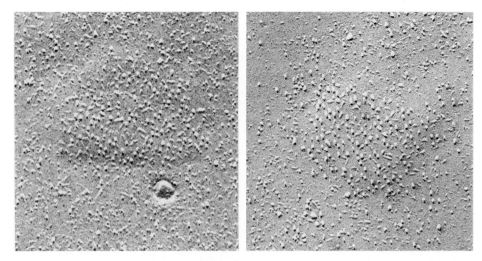

Fig. 8. Clusters of putative acetylcholine receptor particles on control (*left*) and dystrophic (*right*) myotube *P* faces. (Original magnification ×71,600.)

features in control and DMD cells. Clusters of 12- to 17-nm particles, typical of acetylcholine receptors in cultured cells (10, 11), were found on plasma membranes of control and DMD myotubes and were similar in size and abundance in both groups (Fig. 8). Orthogonal particle arrays, present on plasma membrane leaflets of mature muscle fibers in vivo, were not found in either control of DMD myotubes or mononuclear cells in vitro.

DISCUSSION

This study shows no structural abnormality in the freeze-fractured plasma membrane of the cultured muscle cell in DMD. Therefore, the abnormalities observed in mature muscle fibers in this disease must arise at a later stage of differentiation, or are secondary to other events that do not take place in cultured cells.

Had we observed a depletion of IMPs in our study, we would have concluded that an early, or possibly basic, abnormality was expressed in the plasma membrane of the cultured muscle cell. On the other hand, the fact that we obtained negative data does not detract from the possible significance of previous observations made on mature muscle fibers. Further classes of IMPs may exist that are not expressed in plasma membrane of the aneurally cultured muscle cell but occur only in the mature and/or innervated muscle fiber. For example, orthogonal particle arrays were not observed in the cultured cells. Such arrays are present in mature muscle fibers in vivo, and are significantly reduced in number in DMD. Further studies will be required to determine whether the depletion of IMPs in mature muscle fibers in DMD is a cause or a consequence of the muscle fiber injury, and what role this depletion plays in muscle cell death in the disease.

ACKNOWLEDGMENT

This work was supported in part by a Research Center Grant from the Muscular Dystrophy Association and by Research Grant NS 6277 from the National Institutes of Health. We thank Ms. Linda Bremner for preparation of this manuscript.

REFERENCES

1. Mokri B, Engel AG: Duchenne dystrophy: electron microscopic findings pointing to a basic or early abnormality in the plasma membrane of the muscle fiber. Neurology (Minneap) 25:1111–1120, 1975

2. Schmalbruch H: Segmental breakdown and defects of the plasmalemma in diseased human muscle. Acta Neuropathol (Berl) 33:129–141, 1975

3. Carpenter S, Karpati G: Duchenne muscular dystrophy: plasma membrane loss initiates muscle cell necrosis unless it is repaired. Brain 102:147–161, 1979

4. Bonilla E, Schotland DL, Wakayama Y: Duchenne dystrophy: focal alterations in the distribution of concanavalin A binding sites at the muscle cell surface. Ann Neurol 4:117–123, 1978

5. Schotland DL, Bonilla E, Wakayama Y: Application of the freeze-fracture technique to the study of human neuromuscular disease. Muscle Nerve 3:21–27, 1980

6. Wakayama Y, Hodson A, Pleasure D, et al: Alteration in erythrocyte membrane structure in Duchenne muscular dystrophy. Ann Neurol 4:253–256, 1978

7. Witkowski JA, Durbridge M, Dubowitz V: Growth of human muscle in tissue culture: an improved technique. In Vitro 12:98–106, 1976

8. Pauli BU, Weinstein RS, Soble LW, Alroy J: Freeze-fracture of monolayer cultures. J Cell Biol 72:763–769, 1977

9. Washburn EW: The vapor pressures of ice and water up to 100°C. In *International Critical Tables of Numerical Data*, vol 3, Physics, Chemistry and Technology. Edited by Washburn EW. McGraw Hill, New York, 1928, p 210

10. Peng HB, Nakajima Y: Membrane particle aggregates in innervated and noninnervated cultures of *Xenopus* embryonic muscle cells. Proc Natl Acad Sci USA 75:500–504, 1978

11. Yee AG, Fischbach GD, Karnovsky MJ: Clusters of intramembranous particles on cultured myotubes at sites that are highly sensitive to acetylcholine. Proc Natl Acad Sci USA 75:3004–3008, 1978

12. Kalderon N, Gilula NB: Membrane events involved in myoblast fusion. J Cell Biol 81:411–425, 1979

DISCUSSION

Dr. Eduardo Bonilla: Did you see any orthogonal arrays in the control preparations?

Dr. Mitsuhiro Osame: We saw no orthogonal arrays in our membranes.

Dr. Jerry Shay: What were your culture conditions?

Dr. Mitsuhiro Osame: Dr. Rebouche will answer that.

Dr. Charles Rebouche: They were cultured in normal horse serum.

Dr. Jerry Shay: Have you ever tried culturing them in the patient's serum?

Dr. Charles Rebouche: No, we have not.

Dr. Alan Horwitz: If I understand you correctly, there is no significant change in either the number of particles per cell or their size. Have you done a radial distribution analysis to see whether there is a difference in the distribution? This could be done either by measuring nearest neighbor radii and averaging, or by using grids of different sizes and looking at the magnitude of fluctuations about the mean density per square on the grid.

Dr. Mitsuhiro Osame: We found no difference of this kind.

Dr. Alan Horwitz: Is there any quantitative evidence indicating a distributional change?

Dr. Mitsuhiro Osame: You mean hot spots?

Dr. Alan Horwitz: I mean any sort of distributional inhomogeneity. The total number of particles per cell might be the same, but there might be a little patch here, a cluster there, a hexagonal array over there, and so on.

Dr. Mitsuhiro Osame: So far as we observed, there was no difference between them in distribution.

Dr. Alan Horwitz: But you have not quantified that?

Dr. Andrew Engel: If you would like us to quantify something, you have to explain what you are thinking of quantifying.

Dr. Alan Horwitz: Well, for example, one way to analyze these distributions quantitatively would be to put grids of varying size on top of your freeze-fracture picture and then count the number of particles within each section of the grid. This would give you a mean and the magnitude of 2 fluctuations about the mean, which could be compared from cell to cell or to random statistics.

Dr. Andrew Engel: This type of analysis is a way of looking for clustering of particles, as was done by Weiss, e.g., on bladder epithelial cells. We have looked for evidence of this kind and did not find it.

Dr. Donald Wood: Your work, along with that of others, begs the question of when an abnormality that might be considered primary would be expressed in the muscle and how it comes about that the surface membranes do appear to develop abnormalities.

Dr. Mitsuhiro Osame: If the observed changes in membrane particles in biopsy specimens represented altered gene product, then cultured cells could be expected to show this. The lack of abnormality in cultured cells suggests that changes in membrane particles in mature muscle fibers are secondary or reactive.

Dr. Joan Mollman: At the recent Academy of Neurology Meetings one paper reported that some enzymes defect present early in culture disappeared later in culture. I would offer as an alternative to your lack of difference in particle densities that the abnormality was actually present very early and disappeared. Have you looked at very early cultures?

Dr. Andrew Engel: The population of cultured cells is heterogeneous. Some cells are still in the myoblast stage, and we did compare myoblasts to myotubes. Just how old a particular myotube or myoblast is, we cannot say.

39
Freeze-Fracture Studies of Experimentally Damaged Skeletal Muscle Fibers

H. Schmalbruch, MD

In Duchenne muscular dystrophy segmental necrosis of muscle fibers is initiated by local defects of the plasma membrane (1, 2). The lipid composition and the physical properties of cell membranes of muscle fibers and also of nonmuscle cells was reported to be abnormal in affected persons and in carriers of Duchenne dystrophy (3). Freeze fractures of the plasma membranes of muscle fibers and erythrocytes of patients with Duchenne muscular dystrophy revealed a decrease in the number of intramembranous particles (4–6 and chapter 37 of this volume). Similar changes were found in dystrophic mice and chicken (7–9). These findings seem to support the hypothesis that the basic defect in Duchenne dystrophy is an abnormality of the cell membranes that does not affect muscle fibers alone.

The interpretation of the results of freeze-fracture (and biochemical) studies is hampered by the fact that dystrophic muscles are histologically nonhomogeneous. "Intact" fibers undergo segmental necrosis, which is followed by activation of satellite cells and regeneration. Hence, a dystrophic muscle consists of "intact" fibers, necrotizing fibers, and a variable number of regenerating fibers at different degrees of maturity. At present, no safe criteria exist to distinguish these fibers in freeze fractures. Moreover, little is known about the effect of improper treatment of tissue samples on the freeze-fracture image. The state of mitochondria, a common criterion for judging the preservation of a given fiber in electron micrographs of thin sections, cannot be evaluated in freeze fractures.

In this paper, sarcolemmal changes caused by delayed fixation, by exocytosis of autophagic vacuoles, and by regeneration are described. Changes due to delayed fixation, i.e., hypoxia, are probably related to commencing necrosis.

503

MORPHOLOGIC METHODS

Rat soleus and extensor digitorum longus muscles were used. In some experiments, biopsy samples from human vastus muscles were also used. Whenever possible, the muscles were fixed by vascular perfusion with 2.5% glutaraldehyde in 0.1 M phosphate buffer. To rinse the vascular bed and to prevent contracture, perfusion was started with Ringer solution containing heparin and procaine (for details, see reference 10). Muscles to be fixed by immersion were stretched in adjustable holders to 130% equilibrium length. Specimens fixed for 15 minutes to 24 hours (usually, 20 hours) were immersed in 30% glycerol for 30 minutes, frozen in nitrogen slush, and at $-100°$ C fractured and replicated in a Balzers BAE 120 unit with a double fracture device (11). Samples from all muscles were postfixed in osmium tetroxide, embedded in Epon, and studied in semithin and thin sections for light and electron microscopy.

RESULTS

Delayed Fixation

Rat soleus muscles were fixed by perfusion, or by immersion after the muscle had been stored for as long as 60 minutes in Ringer's solution at 7 to $37°$ C. In some rats the muscles were excised 30 or 60 minutes after death and then fixed by immersion.

Freeze fractures of the sarcolemma of fibers fixed by vascular perfusion showed randomly distributed intramembranous particles. The incidence of particles attached to the P face was 1,500 to $2,000/\mu m^2$, as counted on prints magnified $\times 2,000,000$. Pits of the membrane ("caveolae") represented openings of T tubules and of pinocytotic vesicles. Their incidence was 10 to $20/\mu m^2$, in different parts of the same fiber. In muscles left in situ for 30 minutes or incubated for 30 minutes in Ringer's solution without oxygenation, the P face of the plasma membrane of numerous muscle fibers showed band-like particle-free areas (Fig. 1) (12). These particle-free areas were more prominent when the muscles were incubated for 60 minutes, and when the temperature of the Ringer's solution was $37°$ C instead of 7 or $20°$ C.

In specimens kept for 60 minutes at $37°$ C, the sarcolemma of each fiber appeared abnormal. After 30 minutes of incubation, the density of intramembranous particles was unchanged. After 60 minutes it was normal in most fibers, but in some the number was reduced (600 to $1,000/\mu m^2$ of P face). In these fibers, particle-free areas were confluent and did not appear band-like. This indicates that band-like particle-free areas were initially due to clustering rather than loss of particles; eventually, the number of particles decreased. Areas with pronounced clustering tended to show fewer caveolae than did regions with random distribution of particles. Plasma membranes of adjacent endothelial cells never showed clustering of particles or other abnormalities.

Thin sections of specimens that showed pronounced clustering in freeze fracture revealed relatively discrete changes. Some mitochondria were slightly swollen; the sarcoplasmic reticulum appeared normal.

In several biopsy specimens of normal human muscle that had been fixed

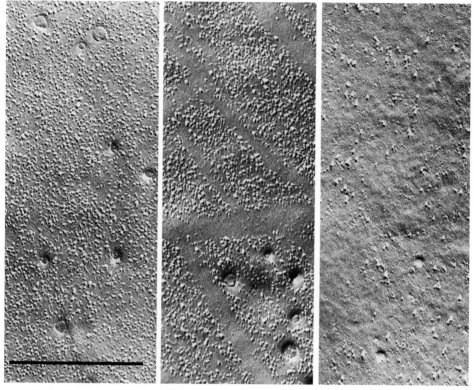

Fig. 1.   Rat soleus muscle. P faces of the sarcolemma of fibers fixed by vascular perfusion of the living animal (left) and by immersion after 60-minute incubation without oxygen (middle and right). Note band-like particle-free areas (middle) and loss of intramembraneous particles (right). Caveolae of the plasma membrane are scarce after delayed fixation (bar, 0.5 μm).

without delay at room temperature, band-like particle-free areas were encountered. These were never seen in biopsy specimens fixed at 5° C. In human muscles, particle-free areas became abundant when the muscle was stored for 30 to 60 minutes before fixation.

Exocytosis of Autophagic Vacuoles

Chloroquine and chlorphentermine (a sympathomimetic previously used as an anorectic) cause generalized lipidosis and a necrotizing myopathy initiated by the formation of myeloid bodies and autophagic vacuoles; the content of these vacuoles is expelled from the muscle fiber by exocytosis (13, 14).

Autophagocytosis and exocytosis were studied by freeze fracture in the soleus and extensor digitorum longus muscles of rats treated with chlorphentermine or chloroquine (10, 15). To avoid coexistence of necrotic and regenerating fibers, the animals received sublethal doses (50 to 100 mg/kg/day) of one of the drugs for only 5 to 10 days. Semithin cross sections passing through the entire muscle were cut, and muscles containing many necrotic fibers were excluded.

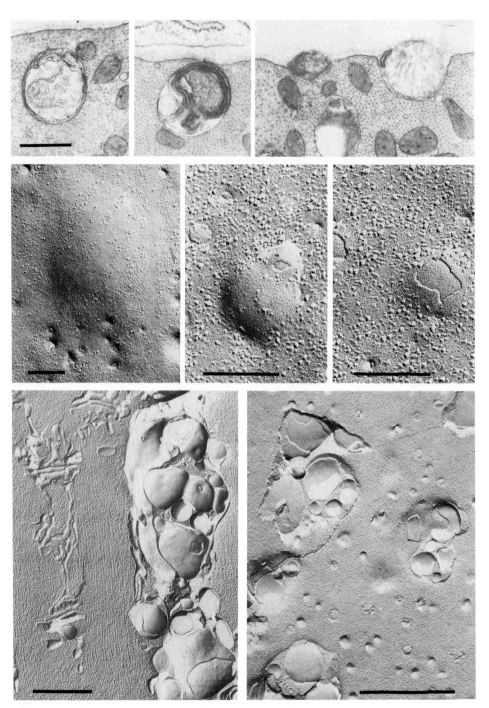

Fig. 2. *Top*: Soleus muscle of a rat treated with chloroquine for 8 days (total, 530 mg/kg). Small autophagic vacuoles together with sarcolemma are shown. Each vacuole contains remnants of a mitochondrion and a myelin figure. The 3 micrographs represent different stages of exocytosis (bar, 0.5 μm). *Middle*: Soleus muscle of rat treated with chloroquine for 6 days (total, 500 mg/kg). The P face of the sarcolemma shows bulges

506

Electron micrographs of thin sections showed numerous autophagic vacuoles containing myeloid bodies and, frequently, single mitochondria (Fig. 2). The diameter of the vacuoles ranged from less than 0.5 to several μm. In the soleus muscle, all fibers were affected. In the extensor digitorum longus muscle, changes were seen exclusively in fibers rich in mitochondria.

In freeze fracture, autophagic vacuoles showed one or several globules with a common surrounding membrane. The fracture face of the limiting membrane carried intramembranous particles; the surface of the globules was smooth. The globules were usually multilayered, i.e., consisted of concentric protein-free bilayers of polar lipids. Exocytosis as seen in thin sections (Fig. 2) implies that the limiting membrane of the vacuole fuses with the sarcolemma and that an orificium is formed through which the content of the vacuole is expelled into the extracellular space.

In freeze fractures of the P face, the sarcolemma sites of commencing exocytosis were marked by bulges. Often, the fracture face left the sarcolemma and exposed the underlying vacuole with its lipid content. The membrane bulge was cleared of intramembranous particles. After fusion and formation of an orificium the limiting membrane of the vacuole formed a pouch of the sarcolemma, which often contained remnants of smooth lipid layers. Numerous globules consisting of concentric smooth membranes were found in the interstitium.

Regeneration

Muscle fiber necrosis is followed by regeneration, provided myogenic cells, i.e., satellite cells, have survived. The principle of regeneration is the same as that in fetal myogenesis: satellite cells, i.e., myoblasts, divide and fuse to myotubes, which mature to myofibers. Myoblasts within the gap between viable fragments of a necrotic fiber may fuse with these fragments and may, under favorable conditions, restore the continuity of the fiber. Myonuclei do not proliferate and do not participate in regeneration.

I have studied regeneration in rat soleus muscles that had been injured by local injection of Ringer's solution at 70° C. This caused widespread fiber necrosis, but left satellite cells and the vascular supply largely intact. Phagocytosis and myoblast proliferation were most prominent during the first 2 days. At the fourth day, clusters of myotubes and myoblasts were found within the persisting basal lamina tubes of necrotic fibers (Fig. 3). Numerous cells contained myofilaments, and cross striations were visible in semithin sections by light microscopy. The new muscle cells had not yet formed basal laminae, and adjacent cells were often separated by 20-nm clefts only. During subsequent days adjacent myotubes

<hr />

and clearing of particles in sites of commencing exocytosis (bars, 0.2 μm). *Bottom*: Extensor digitorum longus muscle of rat treated with chlorphentermine for 4 days (total, 300 mg/kg). Autophagic vacuoles between myofibrils (left). The vacuoles consist of several globules formed by smooth lipid layers, and a limiting membrane with particles. Note t tubules and sarcoplasmic reticulum. The P face of the sarcolemma (right) shows autophagic vacuoles in different stages of exocytosis. One intracellular vacuole is exposed because the overlying membrane is broken away; 3 vacuoles are already extracellular and form pouches of the sarcolemma (bars, 1 μm).

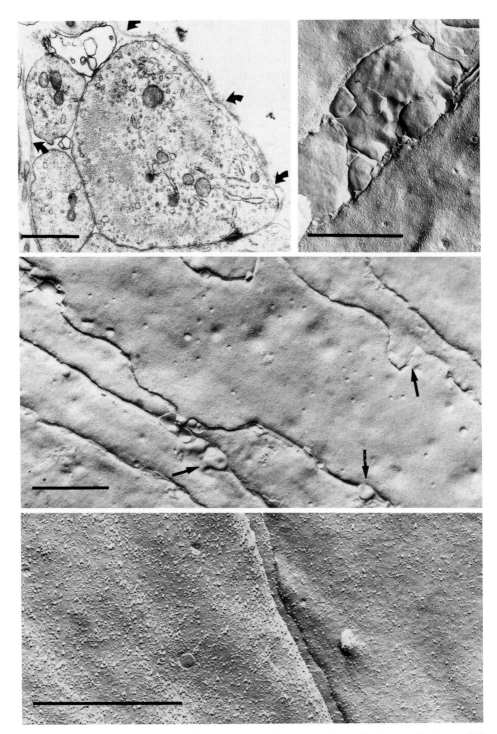

Fig. 3. Soleus muscle of rat, fixed 4 days after local injection of Ringer solution at 70° C (bars, 1 μm). *Top*: (Left) Closely attached myotubes and myoblasts within the persisting basal lamina (arrows) of a necrotic fiber. (Right) Note extracellular myelin figures, which appear smooth in the freeze fracture. *Middle*: P faces of myoblasts and myotubes forming a strand of myogenic cells. Note short lateral projections and single smooth vesicles between adjacent cells (arrows). *Bottom*: P faces of 2 adjacent myotubes or young myofibers to demonstrate the different density of intramembranous particles.

508

detached and formed basal laminae or fused laterally. In many cases, lateral fusion was incomplete and the outcome was a branched or "split" muscle fiber (16).

Muscles fixed by vascular perfusion 4 days after the lesion were studied in freeze fractures. At this time many myogenic cells in different stages of development were present, and most phagocytes that might confuse the freeze-fracture image had disappeared. It was easiest to relate the freeze-fracture image to the histologic picture when the muscles were fractured longitudinally.

Several criteria identified nonmuscle cells. Endothelial cells were flat; the plasma membrane showed numerous circular openings of pinocytotic vacuoles; and intramembranous particles appeared more distinct than did particles on fracture faces of muscle fibers. Occasionally, tight junctions were found between endothelial cells. Phagocytes were characterized by microvilli, and because of their uneven surface, the fracture face usually passed through the cytoplasm. The cytoplasm contained autophagic vacuoles enclosing concentric particle-free membranes; the nuclei were more or less lobulated. Erythrocytes were rare and only present in places so severely injured that no regeneration had taken place. They were easily identified by their smooth surface and the high density of intramembranous particles.

Most of the remaining cells were probably myoblasts or myotubes. Two different patterns were observed. Some cells were polygonal, not oriented, and always associated with cells of the same type. The cell surface showed few blunt projections, and the projections of adjacent cells interdigitated. Nuclei were loss lobulated than those of phagocytes; phagocytotic vacuoles were rare and, when present, small. The cytoplasm contained vesicles and tubules of a membranous reticulum. The plasma membranes revealed relatively few intramembranous particles, and pinocytotic vesicles were scarce. The membranes were connected by gap junctions that were found preferentially between the blunt projections. These cells were probably prefusion myoblasts.

In other places, cells formed parallel strands (Fig. 2). Some of these cells were long and stretched through the entire replica; others were spindle shaped and were 20 to 100 μm long. These cells had few lateral projections; gap junctions were lacking. The long cells had many intramembranous particles and caveolae, and resembled mature muscle cells. In membranes of the spindle-shaped cells, intramembrane particles tended to be more scarce and caveolae were absent in large areas. The incidence of particles attached to the P face varied from 600 to 1,300/μm². These strands correspond to clusters of myotubes and myoblasts, and hence were more mature myogenic cells than were the polygonal cells connected by gap junctions. It is reasonable to assume that the long cells were the most mature cells within a strand.

The extracellular space often contained large membranes that were smooth and showed neither caveolae nor intramembranous particles. Most of these large membranes formed multilayered cisternae or globules. The diameters ranged from 0.1 to more than 10 μm. Smooth extracellular membranes were most prominent in muscles studied 2 days after the lesion and probably represented lipid bilayers formed by remnants of cell membranes of necrotic cells. In sections, they appeared as extracellular myelin figures; their shape was less regular than that seen in freeze fractures, probably because of the strong solvents used during embedding.

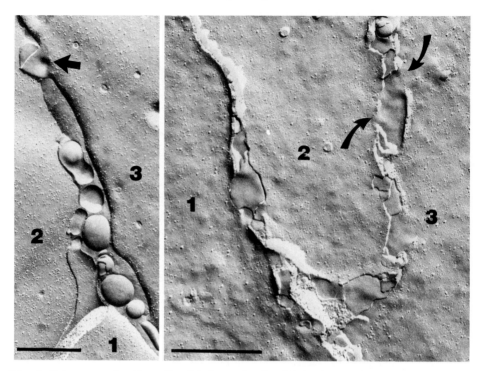

Fig. 4. Soleus muscle of rat, fixed 4 days after local injection of Ringer solution at 70° C (bars, 0.5 μm). (Left) P faces and (Right) E faces of adjacent myogenic cells (1, 2, 3) and smooth lipid vesicles between these cells. In the left micrograph, one vesicle is continuous with a cell membrane (arrow); in the right micrograph, a particle-free membrane forms a bridge between adjacent cells (arrows).

Between the cells of a strand, chains of smooth lipid vesicles ranging from 0.05 to 1 μm in diameter were present. Some of these vesicles were multilayered, but many seemed to be single layered. Frequently, they were continuous with the cell membranes of adjacent cells; occasionally, they formed bridges between 2 cells (Fig. 4).

DISCUSSION

The findings described in this report illustrate the variability of the array and incidence of intramembranous particles of the sarcolemma.

Delayed fixation of normal rat and human muscle causes clustering of intramembranous particles of the sarcolemma and the formation of band-like particle-free areas. After 60 minutes of hypoxia the number of particles decreases and caveolae disappear. Particle-free areas are produced in unfixed lymphocytes by glycerol (17), in Tetrahymena by low temperature (18), and in chicken erythrocytes by incubation with Sendai virus at 4° C but not at 37° C (19).

Because clustering in muscle fibers was more pronounced at 37° C than at 7° C, and because typical band-like particle-free areas were present in specimens frozen without glycerination, these findings were not due to glycerol or low temperature. Moreover, other factors that either increase the fluidity of the membrane lipids or disorganize their array cause clustering of proteins (20). Whether clustering after delayed fixation was directly due to hypoxia, or to acidosis or lack of adenosine triphosphate, is unknown.

In rat muscles, clustering is obvious after 30 minutes of hypoxia; this is consistent with the fact that mammalian muscle kept in vitro without oxygenation is irreversibly damaged after 30 minutes. The formation of band-like particle-free areas by clustering is probably an early sign of necrosis. It is noteworthy that large particle-free areas of the sarcolemma were found in muscle fibers of a patient with necrotizing myopathy. This patient was suspected to have had an abortive attack of malignant hyperthermia (21).

Clustering of particles occurring in biopsy samples of normal human muscle has a practical aspect as well. It indicates that the time necessary to fix all fibers within a biopsy sample is sufficient to produce morphologic changes of the sarcolemma, at least at room temperature. It is therefore advisable to fix biopsy samples to be studied by freeze fracture at low temperature.

The initial change of the plasma membrane in sites of exocytosis of autophagic vacuoles is the formation of a patch of lipid bilayer devoid of intramembranous particles. This facilitates fusion with the limiting membrane of the vacuole. Membrane fusion preceded by clearing of intramembranous particles was reported for a variety of cellular events and was investigated extensively in secretory cells during exocytosis of specific granules (22–24). Nevertheless, a recent study of exocytosis in sea urchin eggs "quick frozen" without fixation and glycerination suggests that the particle-free patches of the membrane are artifacts caused by glycerol (25). Even if this is true for cells of homoiothermal animals as well, the fact that glycerol produces such patches indicates that the molecular structure of the membrane is locally perturbed. Fusion of adjacent membranes requires that the bilayer structure is changed and that hydrophobic groups of the lipid molecules become exposed (26). Whether this implies removal of the proteins remains obscure (27).

Freeze fractures of regenerating muscles show that the incidence of intra-membranous particles of the P face and the incidence of caveolae increases with maturity of the myogenic cells and muscle fibers. This is consistent with the morphologic features of cultured myoblasts and myotubes (28–30). The P face of cultured prefusion myoblasts shows 400 particles/μm^2 compared to 900/μm^2 in myoblasts that are able to fuse (31). Satellite cells of normal rat muscle have fewer membrane particles and caveolae than do the adjacent muscle fibers (10). In fibroblasts of the chicken cornea, the incidence of P face particles increases during development, from 600 to 1300/μm^2 (32).

In injured muscles, extracellular membranes devoid of particles were observed to form vesicles; these were lipid bilayers probably derived from the debris of membranes. In sections they appeared as myelin figures, both inside and outside the basal lamina tubes of the necrotic fibers. Between myotubes and myoblasts chains of single-layered and multilayered lipid vesicles were present. Frequently, these vesicles were continuous with the cell membranes; occasionally, they formed bridges between adjacent cells. One might speculate that these extracellular lipid vesicles are involved in cell fusion and act as intermediaries.

In vitro, artificially generated single-layered and multilayered lipid vesicles (liposomes) fuse with cell membranes and stimulate fusion of mononucleated mammalian cells (33–37). This speculation differs from the mechanism for fusion of cultured myoblasts proposed by Kalderon and Gilula (29), who believe that myoblasts produce intracellular lipid vesicles that become incorporated into the cell membrane as particle-free patches. Particle-free patches of the plasma membrane are then assumed to fuse with similar patches of membranes of adjacent cells.

ACKNOWLEDGMENTS

I wish to thank Mrs. Marianne Bjærg for skilled technical help. This work was supported by grants from the Danish Medical Research Council.

REFERENCES

1. Mokri B, Engel AG: Duchenne dystrophy: electron microscopic findings pointing to a basic or early abnormality in the plasma membrane of the muscle fiber. Neurology (Minneap) 25:1111–1120, 1975

2. Schmalbruch H: Segmental fiber breakdown and defects of the plasmalemma in diseased human muscles. Acta Neuropathol (Berl) 33:129–141, 1975

3. Rowland LP: Pathogenesis of muscular dystrophies. Arch Neurol 33:315–321, 1976

4. Schotland DL, Bonilla E, Van Meter M: Duchenne dystrophy: alteration in muscle plasma membrane structure. Science 196:1005–1007, 1977

5. Schotland DL, Bonilla E, Wakayama Y: Application of the freeze-fracture technique to the study of human neuromuscular disease. Muscle Nerve 3:21–27, 1980

6. Wakayama Y, Hodson A, Bonilla E, et al: Freeze-fracture studies of erythrocyte plasma membrane in human neuromuscular diseases. Neurology (NY) 29:670–675, 1979

7. Shafiq SA, Leung SA, Schutta HS: Reduced density of intramembrane particles of erythrocytes of dystrophic chickens. J Neurol Sci 30:299–302, 1976

8. Atkinson BG, Shivers RR, Nixon B, et al: The erythrocyte plasma membrane in murine muscular dystrophy: a scanning electron microscopic and freeze fracture study. Can J Zool 57:983–986, 1979

9. Shivers RR, Atkinson BG: Freeze-fracture analysis of intramembrane particles of erythrocytes from normal, dystrophic, and carrier mice. Am J Pathol 94:97–102, 1979

10. Schmalbruch H: The early changes in experimental myopathy induced by chloroquine and chlorphentermine. J Neuropathol Exp Neurol 39:65–81, 1980

11. Schmalbruch H: Satellite cells of rat muscles as studied by freeze-fracturing. Anat Rec 191:371–376, 1978

12. Schmalbruch H: Delayed fixation alters the pattern of intramembrane particles in mammalian muscle fibers. J Ultrastruct Res 70:15–20, 1980

13. MacDonald RD, Engel AG: Experimental chloroquine myopathy. J Neuropathol Exp Neurol 29:479–499, 1970

14. Drenckhahn D, Lüllmann-Rauch R: Experimental myopathy induced by amphiphilic cationic compounds including several psychotrophic drugs. Neuroscience 4:549–562, 1979

15. Schmalbruch H: Early changes in chlorphentermine myopathy of rat studied by freeze fracturing. Muscle Nerve 1:421–422, 1978

16. Schmalbruch H: The morphology of regeneration of skeletal muscles in the rat. Tissue Cell 8:673–692, 1976

17. McIntyre JA, Gilula NB, Karnovsky MJ: Cryoprotectant-induced redistribution of intramembranous particles in mouse lymphocytes. J Cell Biol 60:192–203, 1974

18. Kitajima Y, Thompson Jr. GA: Tetrahymena strives to maintain the fluidity interrelationships of all its membranes constant: electron microscope evidence. J Cell Biol 72:744–755, 1977

19. Volsky DJ, Loyter A: Role of Ca^{++} in virus-induced membrane fusion: Ca^{++} accumulation and ultrastructural changes induced by Sendai virus in chicken erythrocytes. J Cell Biol 78:465–479, 1978

20. Ahkong QF, Fisher D, Tampiou W, et al: Mechanisms of cell fusion. Nature 253:194–195, 1975

21. Schmalbruch H: A freeze-fracture study of the plasma membrane of muscle fibers of a patient with chronic creatine kinase elevation suspected for malignant hyperthermia. J Neuropathol Exp Neurol 38:407–418, 1979

22. Lagunoff D: Membrane fusion during mast cell secretion. J Cell Biol 57:232–250, 1973

23. Lawson D, Raff MC, Gomperts B, et al: Molecular events during membrane fusion: a study of exocytosis in rat peritoneal mast cells. J Cell Biol 72:242–259, 1977

24. Orci L, Perrelet A, Friend DS: Freeze-fracture of membrane fusions during exocytosis in pancreatic B-cells. J Cell Biol 75:23–30, 1977

25. Chandler DE, Heuser J: Membrane fusion during secretion: cortical granule exocytosis in sea urchin eggs as studied by quick-freezing and freeze-fracture. J Cell Biol 83:91–108, 1979

26. Cullis PR, De Kruijff B: Lipid polymorphism and the functional roles of lipids in biological membranes. Biochim Biophys Acta 559:399–420, 1979

27. Tilney LG, Clain JG, Tilney MS: Membrane events in the acrosomal reaction of limulus sperm: membrane fusion, filament-membrane particle attachment, and the source and formation of new membrane surface. J Cell Biol 81:229–253, 1979

28. Kalderon N, Epstein ML, Gilula NB: Cell-to-cell communication and myogenesis. J Cell Biol 75:788–806, 1977

29. Kalderon N, Gilula NB: Membrane events involved in myoblast fusion. J Cell Biol 81: 411–425, 1979

30. Cohen SA, Pumplin DW: Clusters of intramembrane particles associated with binding sites for α-bungarotoxin in cultured chick myotubes. J Cell Biol 82:494–516, 1979

31. Dahl G, Schudt C, Gratzl M: Fusion of isolated myoblast plasma membranes: an approach to the mechanism. Biochim Biophys Acta 514:105–116, 1978

32. Hasty DL, Hay ED: Freeze-fracture studies of the developing cell surface. I. The plasmalemma of the corneal fibroblast. J Cell Biol 72:667–686, 1977

33. Martin F, MacDonald R: Liposomes can mimic virus membranes. Nature 252:161–163, 1974

34. Pagano RE, Huang L, Wey C: Interaction of phospholipid vesicles with cultured mammalian cells. Nature 252:166–167, 1974

35. Papahadjopoulos D, Mayhew E, Poste G, et al: Incorporation of lipid vesicles by mammalian cells provides a potential method for modifying cell behaviour. Nature 252:163–165, 1974

36. Poste G, Papahadjopoulos D: Lipid vesicles as carriers for introducing materials into cultured cells: influence of vesicle lipid composition on mechanism(s) of vesicle incorporation into cells. Proc Natl Acad Sci USA 73:1603–1607, 1976

37. Tyrrell DA, Heath TD, Colley CM, et al: New aspects of liposomes. Biochim Biophys Acta 457:259–302, 1976

DISCUSSION

Dr. Eduardo Bonilla: Did you study regeneration in a mixed muscle or in a fast muscle?

Dr. Henning Schmalbruch: There were a number of experimental models. Chloroquine lesions were studied in the soleus and also in the extensor digitorum longus muscles. Regeneration was investigated in the solens muscle only.

Dr. Allen Roses: I am somewhat bothered by a paper that appeared in February or March 1980 in *Nature* in which a Euopean group freeze-fractured lipid multilamellar structures and produced a P face and an E face that had bumps or particles in the absence of protein. With regard to the question of whether there are some differences in a particular disease or not, is it possible in diseased muscle, e.g., Duchenne muscle, in which there is a lot of lipid, that the freezing step might introduce a consistent freezing artifact resulting in a difference in the number of bump or particle counts?

Dr. Henning Schmalbruch: Are you referring to a paper from a Dutch group showing that if phase transformation of lipids takes place one might get a 60-Å particle attached to one face and not to the other?

Dr. Andrew Engel: I think the paper mentioned by Dr. Roses shows intramembranous lipid particles attributed to inverted micelles due to phase transformation, as Dr. Schmalbruch said.

Dr. Allen Roses: Could freezing different tissues from muscle biopsy specimens with different lipid compositions, perhaps reflected in their membranes, lead to a systematic artifact that would account for the differences seen in biopsy tissue versus tissue culture, without having to resort to developmental or other speculative arguments?

Dr. Henning Schmalbruch: I do not think so. Inverted micelles in membranes are smaller. Another question is whether all of these particles are proteins, as we all believe. I do not think that loss of particles has anything to do with freezing.

Dr. Arthur Asbury: Dr. Schmalbruch, do you think that the abnormalities seen by Dr. Bonilla and Dr. Schotland in biopsy specimens from patients with Duchenne muscular dystrophy (DMD) could be explained on the basis of damaged or regenerating fibers?

Dr. Henning Schmalbruch: I think it is possible, but I do not know. What is strange is the absence of square arrays in DMD muscles. In fetal human muscle you do not find square arrays. This suggests that many fibers in DMD muscle are immature. I did not study biopsy specimens from DMD muscles as systematically as Dr. Bonilla did.

Dr. Arthur Asbury: One issue was the number of caveolae; it was increased in DMD biopsy specimens and seemed to be decreased in damaged or regenerating muscles. Is that correct?

Dr. Henning Schmalbruch: There is great variation even within the same normal fiber. You might find 5 caveolae/μm^2 in one part of the fiber and 20 caveolae/μm^2 in another part. It is true that in necrotic fibers and in regenerating fibers caveolae are rare or even absent from large areas. If Dr. Bonilla finds a higher number, that must mean something.

Dr. Donald Fischman: As you are aware, Kalderon and Gilula described similar lipid, particle-free vesicles in developing muscles of chick cultures, and there has been some controversy about the significance of those observations based on the quick-freeze experiments of Heuser and Reese. In view of the possible lability and artifactual nature of these structures, how is it going to be possible to pursue some of the pathologic material, to say nothing of the regeneration and cell culture investigations, without doing quick-freeze experiments?

Dr. Henning Schmalbruch: I agree that the idea that extracellular lipid vesicles are involved in myoblast and myotube fusion sounds unlikely, although I do not think it is more unlikely than the hypothesis proposed by Kalderon and Gilula in 1979. It claims that particle-free patches of the plasma membranes, which represent sites of fusion, arise from fusion with intracellular lipid vesicles. The extracellular smooth vesicles I have shown are present in unglycerinated specimens as well. I cannot tell whether they are continuous with plasma membranes. It is unknown whether the particle-free patches in myoblast membranes are due to glycerol, as in sea urchin eggs. The fluidity of membranes depends, among other things, on temperature and lipid composition; both are different in sea urchin eggs and myoblasts.

40
Micropuncture Lesions of Skeletal Muscle Cells: A New Experimental Model for the Study of Muscle Cell Damage, Repair, and Regeneration

George Karpati, MD

Stirling Carpenter, MD

Despite a large amount of careful descriptive microscopic work in skeletal muscle diseases, much remains to be discovered about the temporal sequence and causal relationships of the reactions of muscle cells to injury. We have devised an experimental model that is suitable for studying the effects of injury to skeletal muscle cells. In this type of injury (micropuncture), damage to the plasma membrane is a definite factor and probably the most important factor in triggering the changes that follow. The effects of plasma membrane damage are of particular interest at present, because of observations suggesting that plasma membrane breakdown initiates necrosis in Duchenne muscular dystrophy (1–4).

METHODS

In adult rats anesthetized with intraperitoneal sodium pentobarbital (Nembutal), the gastrocnemius muscle was surgically exposed. The fine fascia over the muscle was removed. Micropuncture needles were made of a fine tungsten

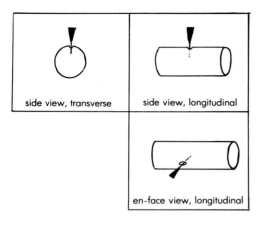

side view, transverse

side view, longitudinal

en-face view, longitudinal

Fig. 1. Schematic view of micropuncture in 3 main axes.

wire approximately 2 mm long, with one end of the wire embedded in a plastic stem 2 cm long. The tip of the wire was 8 to 10 μm in diameter. The plastic stem was held by a hand-operated micromanipulator, so that it could be moved in three planes. Within an area of 10 × 5 mm under microscopic control (25 × magnification), multiple punctures were made in the muscle cells, either in a random distribution or in 1 to 6 parallel rows running 2 mm apart at right angles to the long axis of the muscle.

During each puncture, 1 to 2 mm of the tip of the wire were driven into the muscle. In some animals, instead of the tungsten wire, a microelectrode pipette with a 5-μm tip was used. Each time a muscle was pierced, a brief twitching was observed. This could be eliminated by first placing a few drops of 2% lidocaine on the surface of the exposed muscle. Occasionally, a minute bleeding point developed during the micropuncture, probably from piercing a capillary. When this occurred, the site was abandoned and a new one was selected.

Specimens were removed at the following intervals after micropuncture: less than 10 minutes (containing the immediate lesions), 30 minutes, and 2, 6, 8, 10, 24, and 48 hours. Specimens to be embedded in epoxy resin were fixed in situ with Karnovsky's fixative for 10 minutes, removed, divided into a thin slab, and fixed for an additional hour. Semithin sections were stained with paraphenyl-enediamine and viewed with phase optics. Blocks were taken with different orientation with regard to the micropuncture paths so that the lesions could be examined in different views (Fig. 1).

Other micropunctured specimens were prepared for cryostat sections and stained with hematoxylin and eosin, glyoxal-*bis*-hydroxyanil (GBHA) technique for calcium (5), for the activity of reduced nicotinamide adenine dinucleotide (NADH)–tetrazolium reductase, and of acid phosphatase. In some experiments, within a few minutes after completion of the micropunctures, a solution of 150 mg of horseradish peroxidase (Sigma type II) was injected in 1 ml of saline solution through a plastic tube placed in the abdominal aorta. Thirty minutes later, the muscle sample was removed. The cryostat sections were then reacted for peroxidatic activity by the method of Graham and Karnovsky (6). Some blocks for epoxy resin embedding were exposed to lanthanum nitrate tracer in the fixative solution.

In some animals, starting before and continuing during the micropuncture procedure, a saturated (15%) solution of ethylenediamine tetra-acetic acid (EDTA) was infused through the abdominal aorta, and concomitantly a slow drip of the same solution was applied to the surface of the surgically exposed muscle. These specimens were fixed in a calcium-free fixative, removed within 15 minutes after micropuncture, and processed for cryostat sections or epoxy resin embedding.

Some animals were injected intraperitoneally with leupeptin (375 mg/kg of body weight) or pepstatin (1,500 mg/kg of body weight) 6 hours before and 1 and 10 hours after micropuncture. These samples were removed for epoxy resin embedding 12 hours after micropuncture.

RESULTS

Immediately after Puncture

In specimens fixed within 10 minutes after completion of the micropuncture procedure the punctures were relatively easy to find and identify. In longitudinal epoxy semithin sections, each micropuncture tract near the surface of a muscle fiber was bordered by a collar of intense myofibrillar hypercontraction (Fig. 2). Where the puncture tract passed deeper in the fiber, this hypercontraction was lacking. The hypercontraction appeared to have two different effects in various specimens. Sometimes, it enlarged the superficial part of the puncture path into a funnel-shaped cavity approximately 10 × 5 μm (Fig. 3). In other cases,

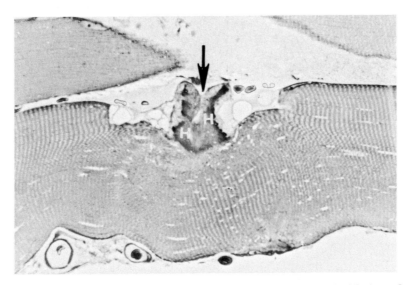

Fig. 2. Semithin epoxy section showing longitudinal view of a typical lesion of muscle fiber (side view) immediately after micropuncture. The superficial part of the puncture tract (arrow) is bordered by dark zones of intense myofibrillar hypercontraction (H). Symmetrically adjacent to these areas are large superficial cavities. Deep in the muscle fiber there are numerous lucent spaces; the deeper part of the puncture path is not shown. (Paraphenylenediamine stain; phase optics; original magnification ×800.)

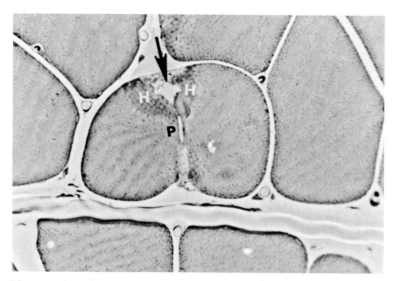

Fig. 3. Epoxy section showing cross-sectional view of a muscle fiber lesion immediately after micropuncture. Areas of hypercontraction (H) surround a cavity (arrow) near the surface of the fiber; the deeper portion of the puncture tract (P) is not bordered by hypercontraction. (Paraphenylenediamine stain, phase optics; original magnification ×800.)

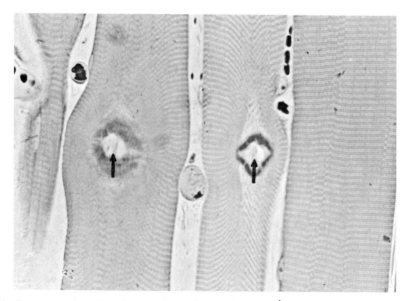

Fig. 4. Epoxy section showing en face view of two lesions immediately after micropuncture (arrows). The collars of hypercontraction surrounding them near the surface of the fiber are dark. (Paraphenylenediamine stain, phase optics; original magnification ×800.)

the puncture path was only slightly enlarged, but symmetric, more or less triangular, cavities were produced next to the surface on either side of the hypercontraction zone along the long axis of the fiber (Fig. 2). Dilated spaces extended for a variable distance around the area of the micropuncture. The larger of these were clearly elongated in the long axis of the muscle fiber. Views of the puncture path en face near the surface and in the depths of muscle fibers confirmed the impression gained from longitudinal or transverse sections cut parallel to the plane of puncture (Fig. 4).

Cryostat sections confirmed the features seen in epoxy sections. The GBHA method for calcium showed the lesions particularly well. Precipitated calcium was deposited in the regions of myofibrillar hypercontraction and possibly in some of the adjacent cytoplasm as well (Fig. 5). Activation of lysosomes was not seen at this time. The NADH–tetrazolium reductase reaction revealed prominent activity in the zones just lateral to the myofibrillar hypercontraction (Fig. 6),

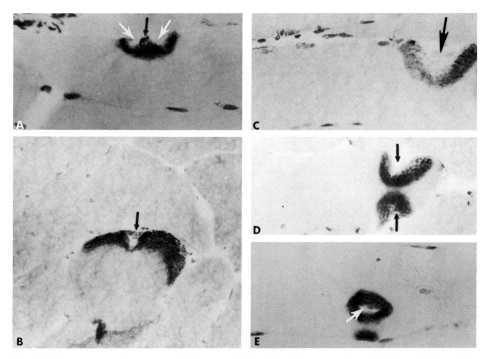

Fig. 5. Cryostat sections reacted for precipitated calcium produce bright-red granular staining (all views of the lesions were obtained immediately after micropuncture; original magnification ×800). **(A)** Side view of a lesion in a longitudinally sectioned fiber; black arrow points to the puncture path, which is obscured; white arrows indicate tear cavities. Calcium deposition is extensive. **(B)** In a transversely cut muscle fiber, calcium deposition extends for a considerable distance circumferentially from the puncture cavity (arrow). **(C)** Longitudinally sectioned muscle fiber shows a large puncture cavity (arrow); the calcium deposition roughly corresponds to the zone of myofibrillar hypercontraction. **(D)** Oblique view of a transfixed fiber showing that both entry and exit puncture cavities (arrows) are surrounded by calcium deposits, but they are not present in the center of fiber. **(E)** En face view of longitudinal section; the enlarged puncture tract (arrow) is surrounded by a collar of calcium deposits.

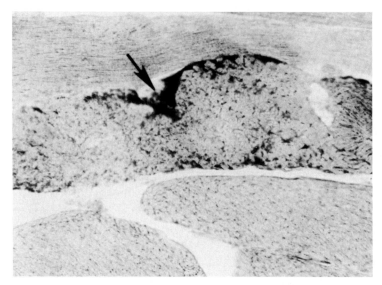

Fig. 6. Two hours after micropuncture, heavy diformazan deposition is present around an enlarged puncture path (arrow). Coarse, irregularly distributed reaction products replaced the normal intermyofibrillar pattern in a muscle fiber segment adjacent to the puncture. (Staining for reduced nicotinamide adenine dinucleotide–tetrazolium reductase; (original magnification ×350).

where electron microscopy showed damaged mitochondria and loops of proliferated membranes.

In specimens exposed to horseradish peroxidase, segments of muscle fibers showed a diffuse staining for several hundred micrometers to either side of the micropuncture lesion (Fig. 7). This implies entry of the tracer at the site of

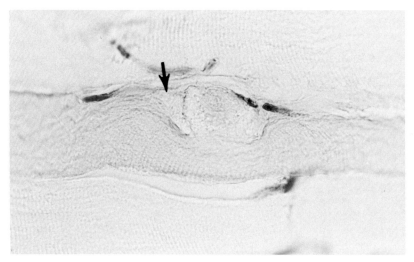

Fig. 7. A segment of muscle fiber adjacent to a micropuncture lesion (arrow) displays peroxidative activity after intraarterial loading with horseradish peroxidase. (Graham-Karnovsky stain; (original magnification ×350).

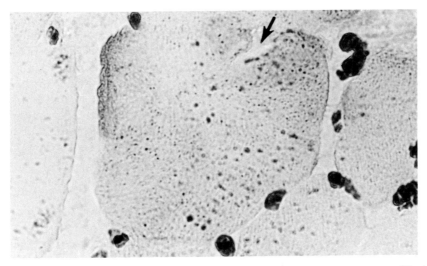

Fig. 8. Horseradish peroxidase injected intraarterially during micropuncture filled the lumen of multiple small, dilated spaces. A portion of the puncture tract is marked by the arrow. The strongly reacting sites surrounding muscle fibers correspond to capillaries. (Graham-Karnovsky stain; original magnification ×800).

membrane breakage where the puncture was performed and diffusion into the aqueous cytoplasm.

Vacuolar spaces, as noted previously, were present in the fiber around the punctured area. When these were small, the tracer appeared to fill their lumen (Fig. 8), but when they were quite large, the tracer seemed only to outline their walls (Fig. 9).

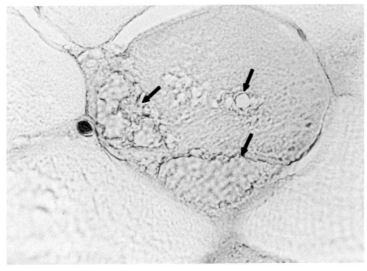

Fig. 9. Horseradish peroxidase injected intraarterially during micropuncture outlined the walls of large, dilated spaces (arrows). (Graham-Karnovsky stain; original magnification ×800).

Electron microscopy of the lesions immediately after puncture suggested that there was considerable indentation of the surface membrane, including basal lamina, along the puncture tract (Fig. 10). In the tear cavities produced symmetrically just lateral to the zone of hypercontraction, much lanthanum tracer was seen along with very numerous membranous profiles. On the deep surface of the tear cavities, there was an irregular membrane that was continuous with the plasmalemma of the neighboring segment of the muscle (Fig. 11). Various dilated electron-lucent spaces were found. Some of these, close to the puncture path and just beyond the zone of hypercontraction, were clearly dilated, injured mitochondria (Fig. 11). Extending some distance away from the micropuncture path are other large dilated spaces whose nature is not immediately obvious (Fig. 12). At first view, these spaces could be interpreted as either transverse (T)-tubular dilatations, dilated sarcoplasmic reticulum, or fluid in the intermyofibrillar aqueous cytoplasm. Studies of cryostat sections stained with horseradish peroxidase suggested that many of the spaces at least communicated with the T tubules (Figs. 8, 9). Electron microscopy revealed some dilatation of T tubules in punctured fibers. Further study of these dilated spaces is needed.

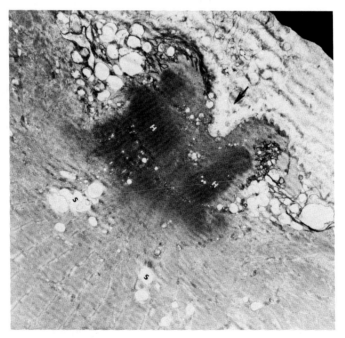

Fig. 10. Electron micrograph of a longitudinal section of a muscle fiber immediately after micropuncture. This section goes through part of the collar of hypercontraction (H) that surrounds the superficial part of the puncture path. Lateral to the masses of hypercontracted myofibrils are numerous vacuolar spaces, many of which are probably injured mitochondria. The specimen was loaded with lanthanum during fixation, and dark staining of the lanthanum can be seen among the numerous membranous profiles superficial and lateral to the hypercontracted areas. In the deeper portion of the fiber, there are membrane-bound dilated spaces (S). (Original magnification ×8,000.)

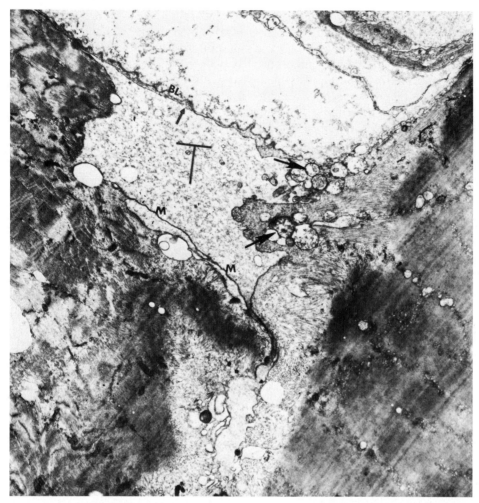

Fig. 11. Electron micrograph showing one of the "tear cavities" (large T) found next to the area of hypercontraction in the long axis of the muscle fiber. The puncture path was beyond the right-hand border of the picture. Dilated damaged mitochondria (large arrows) are present medial to the cavity. The basal lamina (BL) is continuous over the cavity, but the plasma membrane is interrupted (small arrow). A membrane seems to line the deeper portions of the cavity (M). (Original magnification ×20,000.)

Evolution of Micropuncture Lesions

Six hours after micropuncture, relatively extensive segments of necrosis were seen, even in muscle fibers that could only have had one puncture. The necrotic segment (from which Z-discs were missing) and the surviving stump were not yet demarcated from each other by any membrane (Fig. 13). Dilated spaces, some of which appeared definitely to communicate with T tubules, were seen in the stumps. In one fiber at 6 hours, the beginning of demarcation of the necrotic segment from the viable stump by membrane lined clefts appeared to be underway (Fig. 14).

Ten hours after micropuncture, almost all of the necrotic segments were clearly demarcated from the surviving stumps by a single membrane (Figs. 15, 16). Vacuolar spaces were now mostly absent from the stumps. Macrophages appeared in the necrotic segments approximately 10 hours after micropuncture.

In specimens from animals perfused with the calcium chelator EDTA, immediate lesions have not so far been identified in epoxy sections. In some transverse cryostat sections, thin puncture tracts have been seen in a few muscle fibers, but adjacent myofibrillar hypercontractions or tear cavities appear to be absent (Fig. 17). Because animals do not survive for long after EDTA infusion,

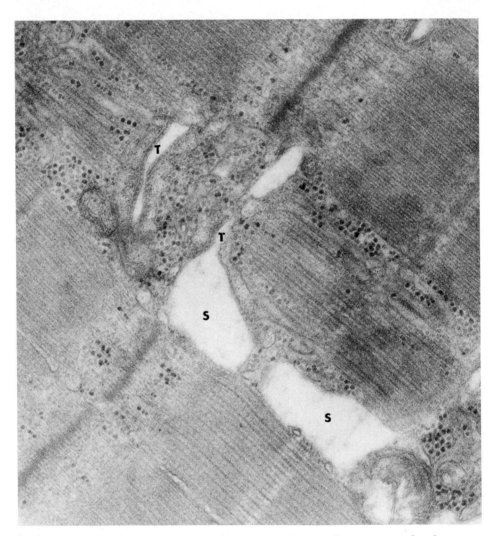

Fig. 12. Electron micrograph of a specimen taken 2 hours after puncture showing some of the numerous dilated spaces (S) that were present in non-necrotic portions of punctured fibers. They appear here to arise from or at least connect with transverse tubules (T). (Original magnification ×50,000.)

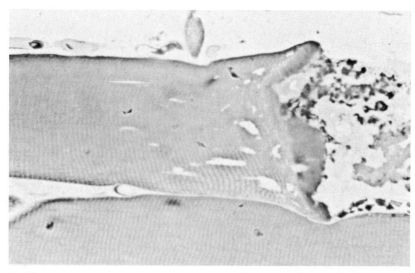

Fig. 13. Epoxy section of a specimen taken 6 hours after puncture, showing the transition from a necrotic segment (right) to the non-necrotic stump. The necrosis does not appear to be demarcated by a membrane. Dilated spaces are present in the stump. (Paraphenylenediamine stain, phase optics; original magnification ×800.)

observation of the effects of initial calcium chelation on the later development of lesions will not be possible.

The administration of the protease inhibitors leupeptin and pepstatin neither prevented the development of extensive segmental necrosis after micropuncture nor appeared to influence it in any way.

Lesions produced by 5-μm glass micropipettes appeared identical to those produced by 10-μm tungsten wires. Micropunctures in young rats (20 days of age) showed no lesser incidence of necrosis.

DISCUSSION

While the microscopic abnormalities produced in a muscle cell by micropuncture are quite varied, we believe that the most important feature is the damage to the plasma membrane. We have evidence from tracers of abnormal communication between the extracellular space and the interior of the muscle cell. This communication would allow the entry of calcium-rich extracellular fluid into the muscle cell, resulting in the massive deposition of calcium (presumably as phosphate salts) seen in the vicinity of the micropuncture, probably mainly on myofibrils. The myofibrillar hypercontraction is probably triggered by the high calcium concentration, because it was not seen in the deeper portions of the path where the increase in calcium concentration would be less. The myofibrillar hypercontraction itself probably has an additional injurious effect, resulting either in enlargement of the puncture path or in the production of new tears up and down the long axis of the muscle fiber. These tears may give

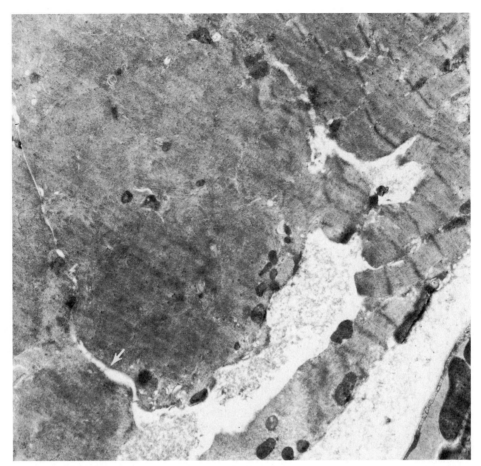

Fig. 14. Electron micrograph of a longitudinal section of a muscle fiber 6 hours after puncture. There is partial demarcation of the non-necrotic portion of the fiber at the top right of the picture from the necrotic portion by a membrane that appears to begin as an elongated cistern (white arrow). (Original magnification ×10,000.)

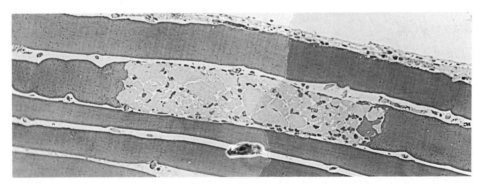

Fig. 15. Epoxy section from a specimen removed 18 hours after puncture. The pale necrotic segment is well demarcated from the surviving stumps of the muscle fiber on either end. Numerous macrophages have entered the necrotic segment. (Paraphenylenediamine stain, phase optics; original magnification ×400.)

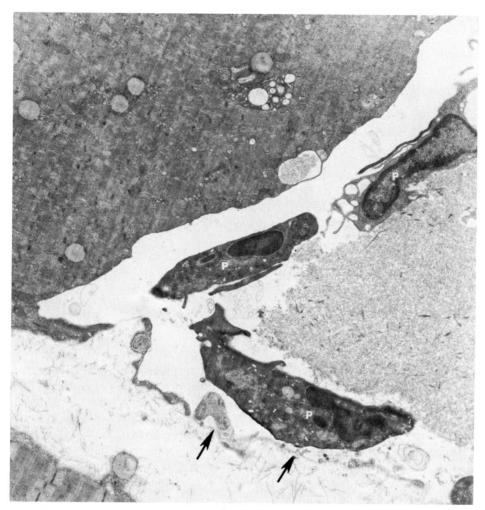

Fig. 16. Electron micrograph taken through the membrane demarcating the necrotic segment (right) from the surviving stump of the fiber seen in Figure 18, 18 hours after puncture. Three mononuclear phagocytes (P) are present adjacent to the necrotic debris. The basal lamina persists (arrows) over the necrotic segment. (Original magnification ×6,250.)

further access of the calcium-rich extracellular fluid to the interior of the fiber. The very swollen mitochondria seen in the immediate vicinity of the puncture could well have been damaged by the calcium, which they would be unable to exclude. Abundant irregular loops of membrane, present next to the myofibrillary tears, appeared to represent some new formation of membranes. They were associated with lanthanum deposition so that they were probably derived from T-tubular membranes. We do not know the mechanism that triggered this membranous proliferation.

The experiments of others have suggested that an influx of calcium mediates cell death caused by various membrane poisons (7). The effects of calcium chelation on the lesion immediately after puncture are still under study.

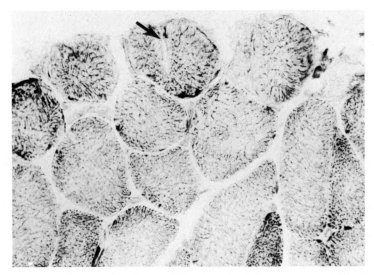

Fig. 17. Only a fine puncture tract (arrow) marks the site of a micropuncture done after and during perfusion with the calcium chelator ethylenediamine tetra-acetic acid. (Reduced nicotinamide adenine dinucleotide–tetrazolium reductase; original magnification ×350.)

The presence of dilated spaces in the muscle fibers around the puncture area is of great interest. In Duchenne muscular dystrophy, fibers that have lost their surface membrane but do not yet show any other necrotic changes routinely show dilatation of some membrane-bound spaces (4). In a number of other conditions in which necrosis of muscle fibers is common, "vacuoles" may be seen as an apparent nonspecific reaction. The dilatation of membrane-bound spaces around the micropuncture may be explained by a phenomenon known as "calcium-induced potassium release." This has been described in several cell types, including skeletal muscles, (8, and chapter 70, this volume), but its molecular mechanism is unknown. In muscle, an influx of calcium would drive potassium out through the plasma membrane and into the T tubules (9). The excess potassium does not diffuse out of the T-tubular system readily, so that an increased concentration of this ion might draw water with it to enlarge T tubules. Some of the dilated spaces 2 hours after puncture did appear to connect with T tubules.

Almost all micropuncture lesions appeared to result in segmental necrosis. Thus far, we have not found evidence that the fiber can avert necrosis by repairing the plasmalemmal damages associated with the immediate lesion. It is of particular interest that the administration of the inhibitors of the calcium-activated endogenous proteases, which have been implicated in the mediation of muscle damage (10–12), did not arrest necrosis. The distance over which necrosis spread from the actual site of micropuncture was surprising. The necrosis appeared to stop spreading only when it was successfully limited by a new membrane produced by the stump. This process of demarcation appeared to start between 6 and 10 hours after the injury.

The micropuncture model should also be useful for examining regeneration after segmental necrosis. We have noted the survival of satellite cells in necrotic segments, but as long as 12 hours after puncture, there appears to be no activation of regenerative myoblasts.

ACKNOWLEDGMENTS

We thank Mr. Steven Prescott and Miss Barbara Nuttal for their technical assistance. Mr. Eddy Puodziynas prepared the micropuncture needles. This study was supported by the Medical Research Council of Canada, the Muscular Dystrophy Association of Canada, and the Killam Memorial Fund of the Montreal Neurological Institute.

REFERENCES

1. Mokri B, Engel AG: Duchenne dystrophy: electron microscopic findings pointing to a basic or early abnormality in the plasma membrane of the muscle fiber. Neurology (Minneap) 25:1111–1120, 1975

2. Schmalbruch H: Segmental fiber breakdown and defects of the plasmalemma in diseased human muscles. Acta Neuropathol (Berlin) 33:129–141, 1975

3. Schotland DL, Bonilla E, Wakayama Y: Application of the freeze-fracture technique to the study of neuromuscular disease. Muscle Nerve 3:21–27, 1980

4. Carpenter S, Karpati G: Duchenne dystrophy: plasma membrane loss initiates muscle cell necrosis unless it is repaired. Brain 102:147–161, 1979

5. Kashiwa HK: Calcium in cells of fresh bone stained with glyoxal-bis-(2-hydroxyanil). Stain Technol 41:49–55, 1966

6. Graham RC, Karnovsky MJ: The early stages of absorption of injected horseradish peroxidase in the proximal tubules of mouse kidney: ultrastructural cytochemistry by a new technique. J Histochem Cytochem 14:291–302, 1966

7. Schanne F, Kane AB, Young EE, et al: Calcium dependence of toxic cell death: a final common pathway. Science 206:700–702, 1979

8. Fink R, Lütgau HCH: The effect of metabolic poisons upon the membrane resistance of striated muscle fibers. J Physiol (Lond) 234:29P–30P, 1973

9. Almers W: Potassium concentration changes in the transverse tubules of vertebrate skeletal muscle. Fed Proc 39:1527–1532, 1980

10. McGowan EB, Shafiq SA, Stracher A: Delayed degeneration of dystrophic and normal muscle cell cultures treated with pepstatin, leupeptin and antipain. Exp Neurol 50:649–657, 1976

11. Goldberg AL, DeMartino GN, Libby P: Influence of thyroid hormones and protease inhibitors on protein degradation in skeletal muscle. In Current Topics in Nerve and Muscle Research. Edited by Aguayo AJ, Karpati G. Excerpta Medica, Amsterdam-New York, 1979, pp 53–60

12. Kar NC, Pearson CM: Muscular dystrophy and activation of proteinases. Muscle Nerve 1:308–313, 1978

DISCUSSION

Dr. Henning Schmalbruch: Dr. Karpati, I like this model very much. Did you continue your study? Did you see regeneration? I am sure these gaps will be closed by strands of myoblasts dividing within the gaps. One connection or two or three strands of cells is what is called "fiber splitting." In your paper in *Brain* about these defects, you state that the defects have no relation to segmental contracture.

Dr. George Karpati: Let me respond to the first question. This model lends itself very nicely to the study of regenerative processes; no doubt we shall do this, but we have not yet reached that stage. We have seen surviving satellite cells in the necrotic segments, so there is no doubt that regeneration will ensue. Time does not allow me to go into the controversy about "delta lesions" in Duchenne muscular dystrophy (DMD) that you referred to. I think there are differences between the micropuncture lesions and the "delta lesions" that have been described in DMD. For example, it is quite uncertain whether the delta lesions arise in vivo or after removal of muscle. The most similar feature between the experimental lesions and necrosis in DMD is the dilated spaces.

Dr. Richard Almon: There are many elements in your micrographs that look very similar to the effects of the Ca^{2+}-activated protease that disarrays the T-tubular system. Have you looked for that enzyme in those areas of damage?

Dr. George Karpati: No, we have not measured this enzyme. However, we have used a modification of our experimental design in which we treated animals with inhibitors of the Ca^{2+}-activated protease, both before and after micropuncture. We gave the maximal tolerable doses of leupeptin and pepstatin intraperitoneally and then scrutinized the specimens for the prevalence and time course of necrosis. There was no recognizable difference from untreated animals. I am not prepared to say that Ca^{2+}-activated proteases may not have some role in contributing to necrosis in this model or other models, but by enzyme inhibition, we could not avert necrosis or modify it in any way that we could recognize.

Dr. Andrew Engel: Did I understand you correctly that these are quite different from what you see in DMD?

Dr. George Karpati: Some of the components of the immediate micropuncture lesions share certain features with muscle cell lesions in DMD. The most important one is the dilated spaces. In early DMD, necrotic fibers are almost always present, as they are here. Of course, segmental necrosis is a feature of both the micropuncture model and DMD.

Dr. Andrew Engel: I am trying to clarify whether or not you are suggesting that this is a model for studying DMD.

Dr. George Karpati: This is a model to study certain mechanisms that take place in muscle cells in DMD. I do not think that I can justify a claim that this is necessarily a precise replica of the DMD lesion.

Dr. Richard Edwards: What is the effect of micropuncture on the contractile properties of the fiber? Does contraction have a particularly bad effect on the development of the morphologic changes? Because muscle is not a passive tissue, we must logically consider whether any pathologic change is ameliorated or exacerbated by the physiologic activity of the cell.

Dr. George Karpati: The intense myofibrillar contraction indicates that we are dealing with live myofibrils, and the hypercontraction evoked secondary deleterious effects. We have modified this model by depolarizing the membranes before micropuncture with systemic ouabain or succinyl choline. We have not analyzed the specimens yet. The results may be interesting.

Dr. Alfred Stracher: Two quick questions. What was the medium in which you punctured the muscle? Where do you suppose the Ca^{2+} is coming from that you see deposited around that puncture?

Dr. George Karpati: The puncture was done in the natural surroundings of the muscle. No external medium was introduced. The tissue was wet, not dry. The Ca^{2+} comes from the extracellular space; plenty of it is found there.

41
Universal Involvement of Complement in Muscle Fiber Necrosis

Andrew G. Engel, MD

Gregory Biesecker, PhD

Muscle fiber necrosis is a stereotyped response in vivo to a variety of pathogenic stimuli. It can be defined as an irreversible injury to all organelles of the entire fiber, a segment of the fiber, or a circumscribed region of the fiber that is subsequently either absorbed or removed by macrophages

Although muscle fiber necrosis occurs commonly in many neuromuscular disorders, the factors that initiate it and the subsequent sequence of events that ultimately lead to necrosis are not well understood. In one disorder, Duchenne muscular dystrophy (DMD), defects in the plasma membrane occur in non-necrotic muscle fibers (1–3). Such defects allow ingress of extracellular fluid (1, 4), which may initiate a sequence of events that leads to fiber necrosis. It has not been established that similar small defects in the plasma membrane represent the initial morphologic change in fiber necrosis in all myopathies. On the other hand, necrotic fibers in any disorder are denuded of their plasma membrane, which suggests that destruction of large segments of the plasma membrane represents a final common pathway in diverse disorders.

In various muscle diseases focal increases in calcium exist in circumscribed regions of non-necrotic fibers (5) and there is abnormal deposition of calcium in all necrotic fibers (5, 6). Excess intracellular calcium may play an important role in propagating the events that lead to fiber necrosis by inhibiting the normal respiratory activities of mitochondria (7, 8), by activation of a calcium-dependent neutral protease (9, 10), by depolymerizing microtubules (11), and by overwhelming the calcium uptake capability of the sarcoplasmic reticulum (12, 13).

In this study we direct attention to another mechanism involved in muscle fiber destruction. We demonstrate that complement activation invariably occurs and that complement always participates in muscle fiber necrosis.

535

METHODS

Sixty-six muscle biopsy specimens that contained necrotic fibers were studied. The following cases were represented: DMD, 13; other dystrophies, 15; inflammatory myopathies, 31; idiopathic myoglobinuria, 4; myophosphorylase deficiency, 1; other myopathies, 2. Serial cryostat sections were cut from each specimen. One or more sections in each series were stained trichromatically, and the remainder were used for immunocytochemical studies. The following were localized: the neoantigenic determinants of C5b-9 membrane attack complex (MAC), C9, C3, C4, C1q, and IgG.

Human MAC was isolated from rabbit erythrocytes lysed by human serum (14). Antibodies to MAC were raised in rabbits. The antibodies were rendered specific for the neoantigenic determinants presented by the quaternary structure of MAC by adsorption with fresh human plasma covalently linked to Sepharose 4B. The specificity of the adsorbed antibody for the neoantigenic determinants of MAC and its lack of reactivity toward circulating complement components were determined by Ouchterlony analysis and radioimmunoassay (15).

MAC neoantigen(s) were localized by the indirect immunoperoxidase method with the specific antibody as the primary immunoreagent and with peroxidase-labeled goat anti-rabbit IgG as the secondary immunoreagent. Controls consisted of treatment of the primary immunoreagent with MAC; substitution of preimmune rabbit serum for the primary immunoreagent; omission of either primary or secondary immunoreagent; and omission of H_2O_2 from the diaminobenzidine medium.

C9 and C3 were localized by the direct immunoperoxidase method with antibodies raised in rabbits (16, 17).

C1q and C4 were localized by the indirect immunoperoxidase method with rabbit anti-human C1q (Bio-Rad Laboratories) and rabbit anti-human C4 (Behring Diagnostics) as the primary immunoreagents, and with peroxidase-labeled goat anti-rabbit IgG as the secondary immunoreagent. Controls consisted of substitution of preimmune rabbit serum for the primary immunoreagent; omission of either primary or secondary immunoreagent; and omission of H_2O_2 from the diaminobenzidine medium.

IgG was localized with peroxidase-labeled staphylococcal protein A, as previously described (17).

RESULTS

The Necrotic Fiber

In trichromatically stained fresh-frozen sections, the necrotic fiber is defined by the following criteria: (a) green to green-blue color (normal color, deep blue); (b) absent, attenuated, or clumped intermyofibrillar membranous network; (c) the necrotic fiber may or may not be invaded by macrophages; and (d) a necrotic fiber remnant and regenerating elements can occur immediately adjacent to each other within confines of an area previously occupied by a non-necrotic fiber (Fig. 1).

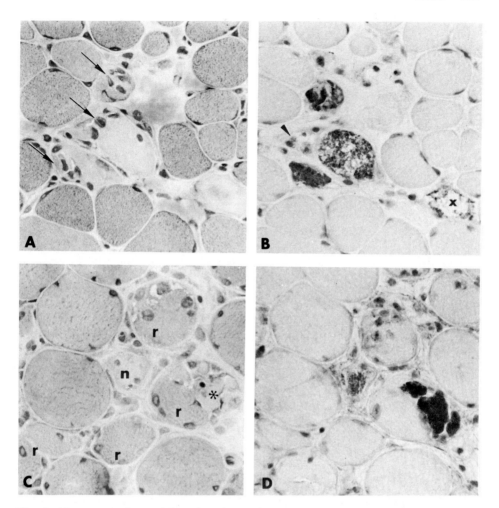

Fig. 1. Nonconsecutive serial sections in Duchenne muscular dystrophy (A and B) and dermatomyositis (C and D) stained trichromatically (A and C) and reacted for (MAC) (B and D). In A, 4 necrotic fibers are present, 3 of which are invaded by macrophages (arrows). In B, the necrotic fibers react strongly for MAC. Macrophages (arrowhead) react faintly for MAC. Empty space (x) represents artifact due to dropping out of part of fiber during the preparation of the slide. In C, there are 4 regenerating fibers (r) with prominent nuclei and nucleoli, a necrotic fiber (n). A necrotic fiber remnant (asterisk) is adjacent to regenerating elements within confines of an area previously occupied by a non-necrotic fiber. In D, necrotic material reacts for MAC. (Original magnification A–D, ×380.)

Localization of MAC Neoantigen(s)

MAC was found in all necrotic fibers and in none of the non-necrotic fibers in all biopsy specimens (Figs. 1B, 1D, 2G, 3B, 3D, 4B, 4D, and 5B). The portions of the necrotic fibers not replaced by macrophages reacted vividly (Fig. 1B). Regenerating elements, identified by their prominent nuclei and pink-blue cytoplasm, did not react for MAC even when immediately adjacent to necrotic

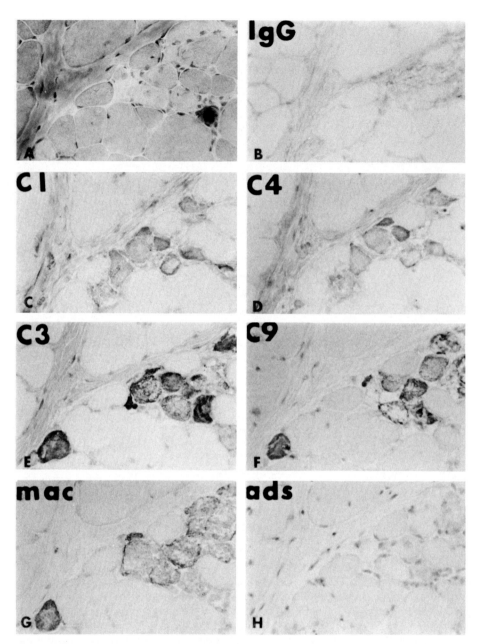

Fig. 2. Serial sections in Duchenne muscular dystrophy stained trichromatically (A) and reacted for IgG (B), C1q (C), C4 (D), C3 (E), C9 (F), MAC (G), and for MAC after adsorption of the primary immunoreagent with MAC (H). The sections are not arranged in the same sequence in which they were cut. A cluster of necrotic fibers is present at the upper right, and a single necrotic fiber is imaged at the lower left in all sections except C and D, where the field does not include this fiber. Necrotic fibers react strongly for C9 and MAC. Adsorption of anti-MAC with MAC abolishes the cytochemical localization of MAC. Abundant C3 is detected in the necrotic fibers. The reaction for C1q and C4 exceeds the background in only a few of the necrotic fibers. None of the necrotic fibers show reaction for IgG greater than the background staining. (Original magnification all sections, ×240.)

538

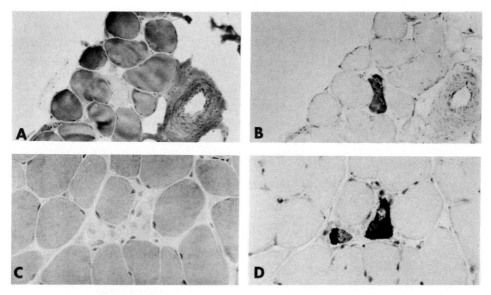

Fig. 3. Sections in Becker's dystrophy (A and B) and limb girdle dystrophy (C and D) stained trichromatically (A and C) and reacted for (MAC) (B and D). Note intense reaction for MAC confined to necrotic fibers. (Original magnifications: A and B, × 100; C and D, × 240.)

fiber remnants (Fig. 1D). Macrophages invading necrotic fibers reacted faintly (Fig. 1B), vividly, or not at all. Background staining was essentially absent. Treatment of the primary immunoreagent with MAC abolished the cytochemical reaction (Fig. 2H).

Localization of C9

The terminal component of the lytic complement pathway is C9, and each MAC contains six C9 molecules. However, C9 is also present in small amounts in the interstitial fluid, which can permeate the necrotic fiber. Therefore, the localization of C9 on a target surface is substantive only if the intensity of the reaction clearly exceeds the background staining. In our study, C9 was localized to all necrotic fibers in all specimens with negligible background staining. The reaction was as strong as that for MAC (Fig. 2F), or only slightly weaker.

Localization of C3

In all specimens C3 was localized to all necrotic fibers, with slight background staining. In 57 of 66 specimens the intensity of the reaction in the fibers was considerably stronger than the background staining (Figs. 2E, 4F). However, in 1 of 13 cases of DMD, 4 of 12 cases of limb girdle dystrophy, 3 of 31 cases of inflammatory myopathy, and in the case of myophosphorylase deficiency the reaction in necrotic fibers was only slightly more intense than background staining.

Localization of C1q and C4

Demonstration of these components in necrotic fibers at a level significantly exceeding background staining would indicate activation of the classical pathway. However, C1q could become dissociated from the activating substance and the concentration of C4 remaining on the target surface might be too low for detection. Therefore lack of substantive localization of these complement components does not preclude involvement of the classical pathway in fiber necrosis.

In most necrotic fibers the intensity of the reaction for either C1q or C4 did not exceed background staining. However, in occasional biopsy specimens in each disease group there were some necrotic fibers in which the intensity of the reaction was greater than background staining (Figs. 2B, 2C).

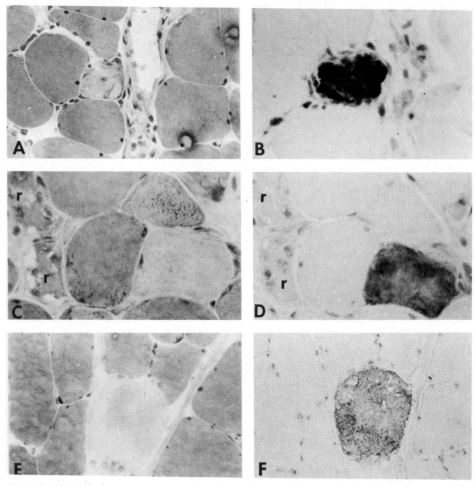

Fig. 4. Sections in dermatomyositis (A and B), polymyositis (C and D), and scleroderma (E and F) stained trichromatically (A, C, and E), and reacted for (MAC) (B and D) and for C3 (F). Reaction for MAC and C3 occured in necrotic but no other fibers. Note regenerating fibers (r) in C and D. Background staining is negligible. (Original magnifications: A, ×250; B, C, D, ×400; E, F, ×250.)

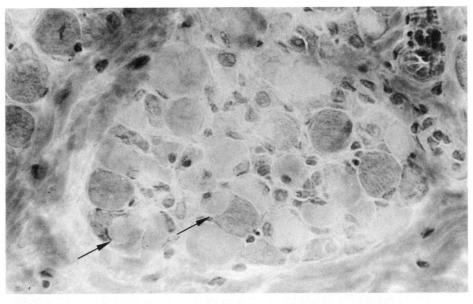

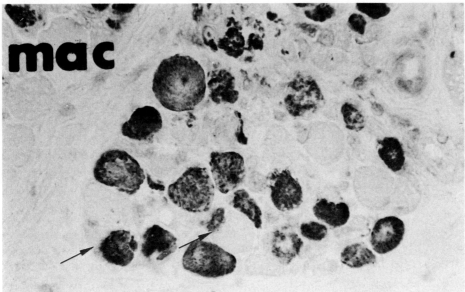

Fig. 5. Recent attack of myoglobinura, shown in serial sections. Upper panel is stained with trichrome; lower panel is reacted for (MAC). All necrotic fibers contain abundant MAC. Contours of several fibers contain necrotic material and regenerating elements (arrows). (Original magnification ×800.)

Localization of IgG

Substantive localization of IgG in a necrotic fiber would be consistent with the notion that the classical pathway is activated when IgG, attached to antigenic sites, binds C1q (18). However, because IgG is abundant in the interstitial fluid, the localization must distinctly exceed background staining to have any significance. In 56 of 66 biopsy specimens there were no significant IgG deposits in necrotic fibers (Fig. 2B). However, in 10 specimens (1 of 13 cases of Duchenne dystrophy, 1 of 12 cases of limb-girdle dystrophy, 3 of 4 cases of myoglobinuria, and 5 of 31 cases of inflammatory myopathy) the reaction for IgG in at least some necrotic fibers clearly exceeded the intensity of the background stain.

DISCUSSION

Complement activation can occur through either the classical pathway (via C1q, C1s, C1r, C2, and C3) or the alternative pathway (interaction of C3 with factors B, D, and properdin (18, 19). Either pathway leads to the formation of a C5 convertase: C4b2a3b for the classical pathway and C3bBbC3bP for the alternative pathway (C4b, C2a, C3b, and Bb representing cleavage products of C4, C2, C3, and factor B, respectively). Both C5 convertases generate C5a and C5b, and C5b initiates self-assembly of the C5b-9 membrane attack complex (MAC); MAC, a highly stable, cyclindrically shaped, phospholipid-binding molecule, induces focal and irreversible membrane lesions (14, 20, 21). Complement activation products have additional effects. Thus, C5a is chemotactic for macrophages, enhancing their migration to sites where C5 is split (22); Bb immobilizes and spreads macrophages that reach the target surface (22); and target-bound C3b enhances phagocytosis by interacting with specific macrophage receptors (opsonization) (23).

Previous immunofluorescence studies showed no consistent or specific association between muscle fiber necrosis and deposition of complement. However, C3 was observed in degenerating (24, 25) as well as normal (25, 26) fibers, and the reaction was often accompanied by staining for IgG or IgM (24, 26). These findings were believed to be of little importance (24), or to be related to nonspecific binding of plasma proteins to damaged muscle cells (25).

Our findings clearly establish that complement is universally involved in muscle fiber necrosis. The localization of MAC neoantigen(s) in all necrotic fibers has five important implications for events occurring during fiber necrosis:

1. There is ingress of complement components into the fiber.
2. The lytic pathway becomes activated.
3. MAC is assembled.
4. MAC binds to target surfaces within the fiber.
5. Complement reaction products (C5a, C3b, and perhaps Bb) are formed, which recruit macrophages and stimulate phagocytosis of the necrotic fiber.

Furthermore, the cytochemical localization of MAC cannot be due to nonspecific adsorption of complement precursors because these are not recognized by the antibody used to detect MAC neoantigen(s).

The main questions now pertain to how and why complement is activated in the course of fiber necrosis. The localization of C3 in necrotic fibers implicates either the classical or the alternative pathway, whereas the variable localization of C1q and C4 neither proves nor disproves involvement of the classical pathway. The classical pathway might be activated by C1q binding to immune complexes. For example, antistriational (27), antimyoglobin (28), and antinuclear (29) autoantibodies, which are known to circulate in certain disorders, could recognize specific antigens in damaged fibers and thus trigger the classical pathway. This could have occurred in a small proportion of our cases in which there was strong IgG localization in necrotic fibers. However, a number of antibody-independent mechanisms of complement activation could operate in all cases.

C1q, which initiates the classical pathway, binds to intermediate (10-nm) cytoskeletal filaments in cultured human fibroblasts rendered permeable to serum by detergents (30); C1q also binds to C-reactive protein attached to choline phosphatides (31). Human heart mitochondria incubated with human serum activate both complement pathways (32). Cultured human kidney cells injured by heat (56° C for 1 hour) activate the alternative pathway (33). Proteases can cleave C3 and factor B and may thus initiate the alternative pathway (34). Proteolytic degradation of C3 or C5 may either initiate the alternative pathway or lead to the assembly of MAC directly (35, 36). Finally, stripping of sialic acid residues from sheep erythrocytes activates the alternative pathway (37, 38). The last finding is particularly intriguing because it suggests that altered biologic membranes may "self-destruct" by triggering the alternate pathway.

Although further studies will be required to define the manner in which complement is activated in the course of muscle fiber necrosis, one can infer that exposure of complement proteins to intracellular organelles (mitochondria, intermediate filaments), altered biologic membranes, or proteolysis could cause activation. Regardless of which machanism(s) activate it, it is now clear that complement participates in fiber necrosis by lysis of membranous organelles and by promoting efficient removal of critically injured fibers by macrophages. Finally, cell necrosis in general may involve the participation of complement.

ACKNOWLEDGMENTS

We thank Ms. LouAnn Gross for expert technical assistance and Ms. Linda Bremner for preparation of this manuscript.

REFERENCES

1. Mokri B, Engel AG: Duchenne dystrophy: electron microscopic findings pointing to a basic or early abnormality in the plasma membrane of the muscle fiber. Neurology (Minneap) 25:1111–1120, 1975
2. Schmalbruch H: Segmental fiber breakdown and defects of the plasmalemma in diseased human muscles. Acta Neuropathol (Berl) 33:129–141, 1975

3. Carpenter S, Karpati G: Duchenne muscular dystrophy: plasma membrane loss initiates muscle cell necrosis unless it is repaired. Brain 102:147–161, 1979

4. Bradley WG, Fulthorpe JJ: Studies of sarcolemmal integrity in myopathic muscle. Neurology (Minneap) 28:670–677, 1978

5. Bodensteiner JB, Engel AG: Intracellular calcium accumulation in Duchenne dystrophy and other myopathies: a study of 567,000 muscle fibers in 114 biopsies. Neurology (Minneap) 28:439–446, 1978

6. Oberc MA, Engel WK: Ultrastructural localization of calcium in normal and abnormal skeletal muscle. Lab Invest 36:566–577, 1977

7. Wrogemann K, Blanchaer MC, Jacobson BE: Calcium-associated magnesium-responsive defect of oxidative phosphorylation by skeletal muscle mitochondria of B10 14.6 dystrophic hamsters. Life Sci 9:1167–1173, 1979

8. Wrogemann K, Hayward WAK, Blanchaer MC: Biochemical aspects of muscle necrosis in hamster dystrophy. Ann NY Acad Sci 317:30–43, 1979

9. Busch WA, Stromer MH, Goll DE, Suzuki A: Ca^{2+}-specific removal of Z lines from rabbit skeletal muscle. J Cell Biol 52:367–381, 1972

10. Azanza JL, Raymond J, Robin JM, et al: Purification and some physicochemical and enzymatic properties of a calcium ion-activated neutral proteinase from rabbit skeletal muscle. Biochem J 183:339–347, 1979

11. Schliwa M: The role of divalent cations in the regulation of microtubule assembly: in vivo studies on microtubules of the helizoan axopodium using the ionophore A23187. J Cell Biol 70:527–540, 1976

12. Endo M: Calcium release from sarcoplasmic reticulum. Physiol Rev 57:71–108, 1977

13. Carafoli E, Patriarca P, Rossi CS: Comparative study of the role of mitochondria and the sarcoplasmic reticulum in the uptake and release of Ca^{++} by the rat diaphragm. J Cell Physiol 74:17–30, 1969

14. Biesecker G, Podack ER, Halverson CA, Muller-Eberhard HJ: C5b-9 dimer: isolation from complement lysed cells and ultrastructural identification with complement-dependent membrane lesions. J Exp Med 149:448–458, 1979

15. Biesecker G, Curd JG, Müller-Eberhard HJ: Neoantigens of the dimeric (C5b-9) membrane attack complex and SC5b-9 complex of complement: Quantitative analysis by radioimmunoassay. J Immunol 124:1514, 1980

16. Sahashi K, Engel AG, Lambert EH, et al: Ultrastructural localization of the terminal and lytic ninth complement component (C9) at the motor endplate in myasthenia gravis. J Neuropathol Exp Neurol 39:160–172, 1980

17. Engel AG, Lambert EH, Howard FM: Immune complexes (IgG and C3) at the motor end-plate in myasthenia gravis. Ultrastructural and light microscopic localization and electrophysiologic correlations. Mayo Clin Proc 52:267–280, 1977

18. Müller-Eberhard HJ: Complement. Annu Rev Biochem 44:697–724, 1975

19. Müller-Eberhard HJ, Schreiber RD: Molecular biology and chemistry of the alternative pathway of complement. Adv Immunol 29:1–53, 1980

20. Bhakdi S, Tranum-Jensen J: Molecular nature of complement lesions. Proc Natl Acad Sci USA 75:5655–5659, 1978

21. Podack ER, Biesecker G, Müller-Eberhard HJ: Membrane attack complex of complement: generation of high-affinity phospholipid binding by fusion of five hydrophilic plasma proteins. Proc Natl Acad Sci USA, 76:897–901, 1979

22. Bianco C, Götze O, Cohn ZA: Regulation of macrophage migration by products of the complement system. Proc Natl Acad Sci USA 76:888–891, 1979

23. Gigli I, Nelson RA Jr: Complement dependent immune phagocytosis. I. Requirements for C'1, C'4, C'2, C'3. Exp Cell Res 51:45–67, 1968

24. Whitaker JN, Engel WK: Vascular deposits of immunoglobulin and complement in idiopathic inflammatory myopathy. N Engl J Med 286:333–338, 1972

25. Heffner RR, Barron SA, Jenis EH, et al: Skeletal muscle in polymyositis. Arch Pathol Lab Med 103:310–313, 1979

26. Oxenhandler R, Adelstein EH, Hart MN: Immunopathology of skeletal muscle: the value of direct immunofluorescence in the diagnosis of connective tissue disease. Hum Pathol 8:321–328, 1977

27. Peers J, McDonald RI, Dawkins RL: The reactivity of antistriational antibodies associated with thymoma and myasthenia gravis. Clin Exp Immunol 27:66–73, 1977

28. Nishikai M, Homma M: Circulating autoantibody against human myoblobin in polymyositis. JAMA 237:1842–1844, 1977

29. Notman DD, Kurata N, Tan EM: Profiles of antinuclear antibodies in systemic rheumatic diseases. Ann Intern Med 83:464–469, 1975

30. Linder E, Lehto VP, Stenma S: Activation of complement by cytoskeletal intermediate filaments. Nature 278:176–178, 1979

31. Kaplan MH, Volanakis JE: Interaction of C-reactive protein complexes with the complement system. I. Consumption of human complement associated with the reaction of C-reactive protein with pneumococcal C-polysaccharide and with the choline phosphatides, lecithin and sphyngomyelin. J Immunol 112:2135–2147, 1974

32. Giclas PC, Pinckard RN, Olson MS: In vitro activation of complement by isolated human heart subcellular membranes. J Immunol 122:146–151, 1979

33. Baker PJ, Osofsky SG: Activation of human complement by heat-killed, human kidney cells grown in cell culture. J Immunol 124:81–86, 1980

34. Taylor FB, Ward PA: Generation of chemotactic activity in rabbit serum by plasminogen-streptokinase mixtures. J Exp Med 126:149–158, 1967

35. Bokisch VA, Müller-Eberhard HJ, Cochrane CG: Isolation of fragment (C3a) of the third component of human complement containing anaphylatoxin and chemotactic activity and description of an anaphylatoxin inactivator of human serum. J Exp Med 129:1109, 1969

36. Budzko DB, Bokisch VA, Müller-Eberhard HJ: A fragment of the third component of human complement and anaphylatoxin activity. Biochemistry 10:1166–1172, 1971

37. Pangburn MK, Müller-Eberhard HJ: Complement C3 convertase: cell surface restriction of βIH control and generation of restriction on neuraminidase-treated cells. Proc Natl Acad Sci USA 75:2416–2420, 1978

38. Fearon DT: Regulation by membrane sialic acid of βIH-dependent decay dissociation of amplification C3 convertase of the alternative complement pathway. Proc Natl Acad Sci USA 75:1971–1975, 1978

DISCUSSION

Dr. Sergio Pena: You did not see complement in any fiber that was not abnormal by light microscopy?

Dr. Andrew Engel: We did not see the membrane attack complex in fibers that we had judged normal by light microscopy.

Dr. Sergio Pena: Would that mean that complement is probably not an initiator but rather a propagator of necrosis?

Dr. Andrew Engel: That is certainly correct.

Dr. Henning Schmalbruch: Dr. Engel, you stated in one of your slides that the complement must have access to the necrotic fiber and you showed that complement had access in different diseases. In a paper (Schmalbruch, Acta

Neuropathol 1975) published simultaneously with yours (Mokri and Engel, Neurology 1975), I reported finding membrane defects in DMD and in other disorders as well.

Dr. Andrew Engel: All I showed you in this presentation was that necrosis of muscle fibers, from whatever cause, involves activation of complement.

Dr. Stanley Appel: Could you tell us which mechanism you think is the most likely in this system? Are all of them relevant, or is one (namely, the activation of proteases), more important than the other?

Dr. Andrew Engel: It is clear that complement activation is involved in muscle fiber necrosis due to whatever cause. This nicely explains why macrophages invade fibers, which has not been analyzed thus far, and how membranous components are lysed. We should recognize, however, that this is only one mechanism involved in fiber necrosis. Proteases and complement probably act in concert.

Dr. George Karpati: You have shown membrane attack complex in macrophages that were phagocytosing. Was membrane attack complex present in macrophages that were in the interstitial space and not actively engaged in phagocytosis?

Dr. Andrew Engel: I did not see anything, but perhaps I should reexamine our material to answer your question.

Dr. King Engel: I noticed in most of your pictures of DMD that there were several necrotic fibers grouped together. Do you have any explanation as to why that is?

Dr. Andrew Engel: Grouped necrotic fibers are nice to show on photographs of serial sections. There were also isolated nectoric fibers in DMD.

Part V

MUSCLE AND CALCIUM

42

The Role of the Plasma Membrane in the Control of Cellular Calcium Metabolism

David B. P. Goodman, MD, PhD

David M. Waisman, PhD

Jeffrey Gimble, PhD

Howard Rasmussen, MD, PhD

The critical role for calcium (Ca) as a coupling factor in cell activation was first appreciated in physiologic studies of muscle (1) and nerve (2). Since these initial findings in excitable tissues, the ubiquitous role of Ca^{2+} as a second messenger in the activation of a variety of differentiated cells has become evident (3). For Ca^{2+} to function in its unique role as an intracellular regulator, the concentration of this ion in the cytosol must not only be tightly controlled, but also be capable of undergoing rapid change. To achieve this, multiple cellular mechanisms have evolved including specific membrane ion channels, carriers, and pumps. This discussion will focus on the role of the plasma membrane in regulating intracellular Ca metabolism.

Several aspects of overall cellular Ca metabolism should be appreciated before the specific role of the plasma membrane is discussed (4). First, Ca is distributed asymmetrically within the various subcellular compartments. Second, most of the intracellular Ca exists in mitochondria and microsomes as a nonionic, rapidly exchangeable phosphate salt; and finally, the asymmetric distribution of Ca is maintained by a complex set of factors including cellular energy change, the Na distribution across the plasma membrane, and extracellular pH and phosphate concentration.

The Ca^{2+} in the cytosol is the critical pool that subserves the cellular messenger function. In the resting non-activated cell, the concentration of cytosolic Ca^{2+} is 10^{-8} to 10^{-7} M (3). Because there is approximately a 10^4- to 10^5-fold concentration gradient for Ca^{2+} across the plasma membrane, this cellular membrane, as well as the endoplasmic reticulum and the mitochondria

549

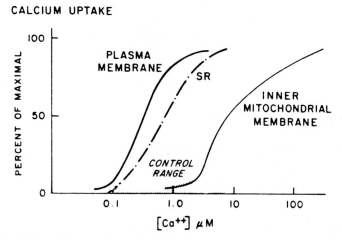

Fig. 1. The activity of the various subcellular membrane calcium pumps as a function of Ca^{2+} concentration. As the cell is activated, intracellular Ca^{2+} concentration increases and the activity of the specific membrane pumps increases to control Ca^{2+} concentration within a narrow range.

possess Ca^{2+} pumps directionally oriented to reduce cytosolic Ca^{2+} (Fig. 1). It is the combined activities of these Ca^{2+} pumps and the entry of Ca^{2+} back into the cytosol that determines the level of cytosolic Ca^{2+}.

CALCIUM ENTRY

There are at least three channels or pathways by which Ca^{2+} enters the cytosol across the plasma membrane. There is a membrane potential–independent, relatively specific Ca^{2+} channel that is altered when certain hormones interact with their receptors (5). This nondepolarizing hormone receptor interaction results in entry of Ca^{2+} into mammalian and fly salivary gland, hepatocytes, and mast cells. In many cells, particularly those activated by acetylcholine, hormone-receptor interaction results in a depolarization of the plasma membrane. This depolarization of the plasma membrane leads to an increase in the permeability of a potential-dependent, relatively specific Ca^{2+} channel and a consequent increase in cytosolic Ca^{2+}. This pathway, observed in nerve, cardiac and smooth muscle, pancreatic islets, and chromaffin granules, is blocked by certain heavy metals and by verapamil. Finally, Ca^{2+} may enter across the plasma membrane after membrane depolarization via the Na^{2+} channel. This is the "early calcium channel" in nerve that is blocked by blocking the Na^+ channel with tetrodotoxin (6).

CALCIUM EFFLUX

There are two active, energy-dependent mechanisms for extruding Ca^{2+} out of the cytosol across the plasma membrane: a Ca^{2+}/Na^+ or Ca^{2+}/H^+ antiporter, and a specific Ca, Mg-ATPase. A Na^+/Ca^{2+} exchange has been demonstrated in excitable tissues (7) as well as in erythrocytes (8). Until recently the study of this process has been based on isotope efflux data in nerve (9) and muscle (10, 11) preparations and studies of mechanical responses in muscle (12). However, the preparation of isolated membrane vesicles derived from cardiac sarcolemma has allowed definition of the properties of the Ca^{2+}/Na^+ antiporter (13). Cardiac membrane vesicles take up Ca^{2+} when loaded initially with Na^+. Dissipation of the Na^+ gradient by passive diffusion or by incubation with a monovalent cation ionophore decreases Ca^{2+} uptake. Additionally, increasing the external Na^+ blocks Ca^{2+} uptake into the vesicles and accelerates Ca^{2+} efflux from the vesicles. These observations provide strong evidence for the operation of a Na^+/Ca^{2+} antiporter in the sarcolemmal membrane. The Ca^{2+} accumulates within the vesicles only when it can exchange for Na^+ and vice versa.

A direct competition between Na^+ and Ca^{2+} for the antiporter probably accounts for observations that Na^+ blocks Na^+-dependent Ca^{2+} uptake. In intact tissue, the driving force for this Ca^{2+}-Na^+ exchange is provided by the Na^+ gradient generated by the Na, K-ATPase. More detailed studies using membrane vesicles will allow precise definition of the stoichiometry, kinetics, and electrogenicity of this Ca^{2+}/Na^+ exchange. It should also be noted that this Ca^{2+}/Na^+ antiporter system in bovine heart has recently been solubilized, partially purified, and reconstituted back into artificial liposomes (14).

The possible importance of Ca^{2+}/Na^+ exchange in regulating cellular Ca metabolism can be studied by altering the Na^+ gradient or by using cardiac glycosides such as ouabain that block the Na, K-ATPase and thus reduce the Na^+ gradient across the membrane. Thus, ouabain enhances insulin and neurohypophyseal hormone secretion as well as cardiac and smooth muscle contraction (3, 7), but has no effect on the Ca-mediated increase in renal gluconeogenesis (4) and actually inhibits phytohemagglutin-induced lymphocytic transformation (15).

There is an additional effect of Ca on the plasma membrane that should be noted. An increase in cytosolic Ca^{2+} concentration leads to an increase in the permeability of the plasma membrane to K^+ (16, 17). A decrease in the K^+ gradient across the membrane would activate the Na, K-ATPase and lead to a decrease in intracellular Na^+ and thus to an increase in Ca^{2+} efflux via the Ca^{2+}/Na^+ antiporter. This could be viewed as a negative feedback loop controlling the increase in Ca^{2+}.

Plasma membrane vesicles isolated from the eukaryotic microorganism *Neurospora* also carry out ATP-dependent Ca^{2+} uptake (18). The fact that this Ca^{2+} accumulation is inhibited by the proton conductor carbonylcyanide *m*-chlorophenylhydrazone and that the ATPase is a proton pump provides strong evidence for Ca^{2+} transport being driven by the proton motive force generated by the proton-translocating ATPase via a Ca^{2+}/H^+ antiporter. Additional evidence for the role of the Ca^{2+}/H^+ antiporter comes from experiments employing nigericin. This monovalent cation ionophore allows an electrochemical exchange of K^+ and protons (19). Thus, in the presence of nigericin and external K^+, any proton gradient across the membrane vesicles generated by the proton-translocating ATPase should be dissipated. If Ca^{2+} accumulation is driven by a Ca^{2+}/H^+ antiporter, then nigericin and K^+ should inhibit Ca^{2+} uptake. Because ATP-dependent Ca^{2+} accumulation is inhibited by nigericin and K^+ together, but is unaffected by K^+ or nigericin separately, it appears that a proton gradient is a major driving force for Ca^{2+} accumulation via a Ca^{2+}/H^+ antiporter (20). Until recently, most evidence suggested that eukaryotic cells use a Ca^{2+}/Na^+ antiporter and that prokaryotic cells employ Ca^{2+}/H^+ antiporters. However, the recent reports of a Ca^{2+}/Na^+ antiporter (21) and an ATP-linked Ca^{2+} pump (22) in prokaryotes and the eukaryotic Ca^{2+}/H^+ antiporter described above make such generalizations less clear.

Membrane vesicles have also been used to study the enzymatic and transport properties of the Ca^{2+}-ATPase Ca^{2+} pump (23). The most extensively studied plasma membrane Ca^{2+} pump is the Ca^{2+}-ATPase in the human erythrocyte (24). Study of this system has been greatly facilitated by the recent development of rapid techniques for reproducibly isolating inside-out membrane vesicles (25). This system is of particular interest because the Ca receptor protein calmodulin activates the Ca^{2+}-ATPase and Ca^{2+} transport in this system (24).

Schatzman (26) and Schatzman and Vincenzi (27) first suggested that the Ca^{2+}-activated ATPase in the erythrocyte was the biochemical expression of the Ca^{2+} pump. This activity was shown to be regulated by a soluble protein (28) that underwent a Ca-dependent association with the membrane (29, 30). It was subsequently demonstrated that this Ca-binding protein was calmodulin and that it mediated a Ca-dependent activation of the Ca^{2+}-ATPase (31). Recently, our laboratory has been investigating the regulation of the human erythrocyte Ca^{2+} pump by calmodulin.

Inside-out resealed vesicles (IOV) from human erythrocytes are prepared by a modification of the procedure originally described by Steck and Kant (25). A time course for IOV Ca^{2+} uptake is shown in Figure 2. In the absence of added calmodulin, Ca^{2+} is accumulated at approximately 3.8 nmol/min/unit of acetylcholinesterase (AChE). Addition of calmodulin results in a 3-fold increase in the rate of Ca^{2+} accumulation. These values agree favorably with other reports in IOV (32, 33), resealed ghosts (33–35), and intact erythrocytes (36, 37), suggesting that the Ca^{2+} pump is perturbed minimally during IOV preparation. In addition, more than 95% of the accumulated Ca is quickly released when the vesicles are treated with the Ca ionophore A23187, and in the absence of added ATP, no significant Ca accumulation occurs. The intravesicular volume in this IOV preparation is 5 μl/unit of AChE. Consequently, after a 30-minute incubation the Ca concentration inside the IOV is 60 mM, representing a 400-fold concentration gradient across the membrane.

The activation of the erythrocyte Ca^{2+} pump by increasing concentrations of calmodulin is presented in Figure 3. The concentration of calmodulin necessary to stimulate the Ca^{2+} pump half maximally is 60 ng/ml. Addition of bovine brain modulator binding protein, a protein that specifically binds calmodulin (38), completely inhibits the activation of the Ca^{2+} pump by calmodulin. However, modulator binding protein did not alter Ca^{2+} pump activity in the absence of exogenous calmodulin. This result suggests that Ca^{2+} transport in the absence of added exogenous calmodulin is not due to residual calmodulin in the IOV preparation.

The dependence of Ca^{2+} accumulation on the Ca^{2+} concentration in the

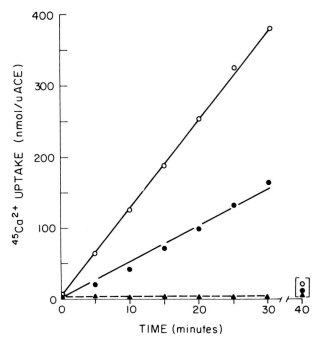

Fig. 2. The time course of calcium uptake into inside-out human erythrocyte vesicles. Vesicles were incubated in the presence (○) or absence (●) of calmodulin (1.45 μg/ml). When ATP was deleted from the incubation medium (▲), no uptake was observed. Addition of 1 μM A23187 (a calcium ionophore) after 30 minutes of incubation resulted in the rapid release of the previously accumulated calcium during the next 10 minutes. (Reproduced with permission from Waisman DM, Gimble JM, Goodman DBP, et al: Studies of the Ca^{2+} Transport Mechanism of Human Erythrocyte Inside-Out Plasma Membrane Vesicles. I. Regulation of the Ca^{2+} pump by calmodulin. J Biol Chem 256:409–414, 1981.

medium was determined using a calcium-ethyleneglycol tetra-acetate (EGTA) buffer system (Fig. 4). Under these conditions, the apparent K_m (Ca) was 0.62 Ca^{2+}/EGTA in the presence of calmodulin and 0.44 in the absence of calmodulin. These Ca/EGTA ratios correspond to 0.8 and 0.4 μM free Ca^{2+}, respectively (39). Calmodulin enhances V_{max} approximately 5-fold. Because the resting free Ca^{2+} concentration in the erythrocyte is believed to be less than 1 μM (40), a physiologic function for this Ca^{2+} pump is apparent.

The ratio of Ca^{2+} transported to ATP hydrolyzed has been reported to vary from 2/1 (36, 41) to 1/1 (32, 34, 35, 42). The Mg^{2+}-ATPase activity determined under conditions identical to those used for Ca uptake is 2.75 nmol hydrolyzed/min/unit of AChE. The Ca^{2+},Mg^{2+}/ATPase activity is 11.3 and 2.4 nmol of inorganic phosphate/min/unit of AChE, respectively, in the presence and absence of calmodulin. Thus, either with or without added calmodulin, a stoichiometry of 0.9 Ca^{2+} transported per ATP hydrolyzed can be calculated. These results suggest that calmodulin is not altering the efficiency of the Ca^{2+} pump.

When the Ca^{2+} concentration was altered using a Ca-EGTA buffer system,

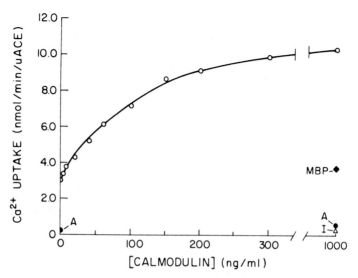

Fig. 3. The effect of increasing concentrations of calmodulin on calcium uptake into inside-out human erythrocyte vesicles. Inclusion of modulator binding protein (MBP) reduced Ca^{2+} uptake to a level seen in the absence of added calmodulin. The effects of deletion of adenosine triphosphate (A) and addition of the calcium ionophore A23187 (I) are also shown. (Reproduced with permission from Waisman DM, Gimble JM, Goodman DBP, et al: Studies of the Ca^{2+} Transport Mechanism of Human Erythrocyte Inside-Out Plasma Membrane Vesicles. I. Regulation of the Ca^{2+} Pump by Calmodulin J. Biol. Chem. 256:409–414, 1981.)

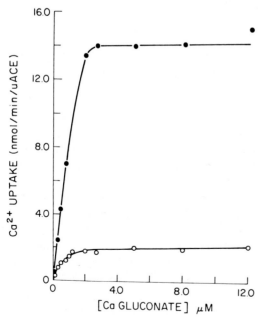

Fig. 4. The effect of increasing calcium concentration on Ca^{2+} uptake into inside-out human erythrocyte vesicles. Vesicles were incubated in a Ca-ethyleneglycol tetra-acetate buffer system in the presence (•) or absence (○) of 1.45 µg/ml calmodulin. The incubation was carried out for 25 minutes.

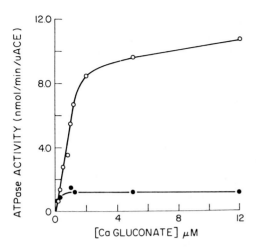

Fig. 5. The effect of increasing calcium concentration on Ca, Mg-ATPase activity in inside-out human erythrocyte vesicles. Vesicles were incubated in a Ca-ethyleneglycol tetra-acetate buffer system in the presence (○) or absence (●) of 1.45 μg/ml calmodulin. The incubation was carried out for 25 minutes. (Reproduced with permission from Waisman DM, Gimble JM, Goodman DBP, et al: Studies of the Ca²⁺ Transport Mechanism of Human Erythrocyte Inside-Out Plasma Membrane Vesicles. I. Regulation of the Ca²⁺ Pump by Calmodulin J. Biol. Chem. 256:409–414, 1981.)

apparent K_m (Ca) values of 0.62 Ca/EGTA and 0.40 were determined for the ATPase in the presence and absence of calmodulin, respectively (Fig. 5). These Ca/EGTA ratios correspond to 0.8 and 0.4 μM free Ca^{2+} respectively (39). This similarity in apparent K_m (Ca) for the Ca^{2+} pump and Ca^{2+}-ATPase is additional evidence that the Ca^{2+}-ATPase represents the Ca^{2+} pump.

In addition to providing further evidence that the properties of the Ca^{2+}-ATPase and those of transmembrane Ca^{2+} movement are similar, our present results provide further support for the concept that calmodulin mediates Ca^{2+}-dependent activation of the erythrocyte plasma membrane Ca^{2+} pump. Both the present results and those of other investigators (24) show that in a Ca-EGTA buffer system, when the pump is activated by calmodulin, both the V_{max} and the K_m of the process for Ca^{2+} increase. The observation that the K_m of the pump increases after calmodulin treatment is of particular interest.

On cell activation, there is good evidence that cytosolic Ca^{2+} concentration increases sharply initially and then decays to a new steady-state level only slightly greater than that seen in the resting cell (3). One can hypothesize that because the K_m (Ca) is increased by calmodulin, this Ca^{2+} receptor protein controls the rate of Ca^{2+} efflux out of the cell across the plasma membrane to balance a sustained increase in the rate of influx, such that a new higher steady state of Ca^{2+} concentration is maintained while protecting the cell against the continuous entry of Ca^{2+}. The association of calmodulin with the membrane pump alters its properties such that two results are achieved: (*a*) an increased rate of Ca^{2+} entry across the plasma membrane is balanced by an increase in the rate of Ca^{2+} removed from the cell by the plasma membrane Ca^{2+} pump; (*b*) during this increased cycling of Ca^{2+} the steady-state level of Ca^{2+} is maintained at a higher level than in the non-activated cell.

In previous studies it was not clear whether the basal rates of Ca^{2+} transport and the Ca^{2+}-ATPase were due to residual membrane-bound calmodulin, and whether in the complete absence of calmodulin the rate of Ca^{2+} transport would be nil. The present results using modulator binding protein indicate that addition of this calmodulin-inhibiting protein completely inhibits the effect of added calmodulin but has no effect on the rate of basal transport or ATPase activity. These results imply that calmodulin does not regulate the basal activity of the pump. Similar results have been reported by Larsen and coworkers (42).

The mediation of the Ca^{2+}-linked regulation of the erythrocyte Ca^{2+} pump by Ca^{2+} suggests that calmodulin may function as a cytosolic Ca^{2+} sensor. Recently, Kuo and coworkers (43) have demonstrated the regulation of the synaptic plasma membrane Ca^{2+} pump by calmodulin. Hormonal regulation of the synaptic membrane Ca^{2+} pump has not been reported. However, the observation that the adipocyte plasma membrane Ca^{2+} pump is inhibited by insulin (44) and that chronic exposure of the rat erythrocyte to catecholamines results in calmodulin translocation from the cytosol to the plasma membrane (Clayberger CA, Goodman DBP, Rasmussen H: unpublished data) suggests that calmodulin may play a critical role in hormonal regulation of plasma membrane Ca^{2+} transport.

This review has attempted to summarize the current understanding of the role of the plasma membrane in the control of cellular Ca metabolism. Most information has been derived from relatively indirect experimental systems using intact tissue. The recent development of techniques for isolating plasma membrane vesicles from both excitable and nonexcitable tissues and studying the transport and enzymatic properties of these membranes should allow precise definition of the role of this membrane in cellular Ca metabolism.

ACKNOWLEDGMENTS

This work was supported by Grants AM 19813 and AM 27184 from the United States Public Health Service. Dr. Goodman is an Established Investigator of the American Heart Association. Dr. Waisman is a Postdoctoral Fellow of the Muscular Dystrophy Association of Canada.

REFERENCES

1. Fatt P, Ginsborg BL: The ionic requirements for the production of action potentials in crustacean muscle fibres. J Physiol (Lond) 142:516–543, 1958
2. del Castillo J, Katz B: Biophysical aspects of neuro-muscular transmission. Prog Biophys 6:121–170, 1956
3. Rasmussen H, Goodman DBP: Relationships between calcium and cyclic nucleotides in cell activation. Physiol Rev 57:421–509, 1977
4. Rasmussen H, Goodman DBP, Friedmann N, et al: Ions and the control of metabolic processes. In Handbook of Physiology, Sec 7, Endocrinology, vol VII. Edited by Aurbach GD. American Physiological Society, Washington DC, 1976 pp 225–264
5. Borle A: Calcium metabolism at the cellular level. Fed Proc 32:1944–1950, 1973
6. Baker PF: The regulation of intracellular calcium in giant axons of Loligo and Myxicola. Ann NY Acad Sci 307:250–268, 1978
7. Blaustein MP: The interrelationship between sodium and calcium fluxes across cell membranes. Rev Physiol Biochem Pharmacol 70:33–82, 1974
8. Parker JC: Sodium and calcium movements in dog red blood cells. J Gen Physiol 71:1–17, 1978
9. Baker PF: Regulation of intracellular Ca and Mg in squid axons. Fed Proc 35:2589–2595, 1976

10. Jundt H, Porzig H, Reuter H, et al: The effect of substances releasing intracellular calcium ions on sodium-dependent calcium efflux from guinea-pig auricles. J Physiol (Lond) 246:229–253, 1975

11. Wendt IR, Langer GA: The sodium calcium relationship in mammalian myocardium: effect of sodium deficient perfusion on calcium fluxes. J Mol Cell Cardiol 9:551–564, 1977

12. Luttgan HC, Niedergerke R: The antagonism between Ca and Na ions in the frog's heart. J Physiol (Lond) 143:486–505, 1958

13. Reeves HP, Sutko JF: Sodium-calcium ion exchange in cardiac membrane vesicles. Proc Natl Acad Sci USA 76:590–594, 1979

14. Miyamoto H, Racker E: Solubilization and partial purification of the Ca^{2+}/Na^+ antiporter from the plasma membrane of bovine heart. J Biol Chem 255:2656–2658, 1980

15. Quastel MR, Kaplan JG: Lymphocyte stimulation: the effect of ouabain on nucleic acid and protein synthesis. Exp Cell Res 62:407–420, 1970

16. Romero PJ, Whittam R: The control by internal calcium of membrane permeability to sodium and potassium. J Physiol (Lond) 214:481–507, 1971

17. Sarkadi B, Szasz I, Gardos G: The use of ionophores for rapid loading of human red cells with radioactive cations for cation-pump studies. J Membr Biol 26:357–370, 1976

18. Stroobant P, Dame JB, Scarborough GA: The *Neurospora* plasma membrane Ca^{2+} pump. Fed Proc 39:2437–2441, 1980

19. Pressman BC: Biological applications of ionophores. Annu Rev Biochem 45:501–530, 1976

20. Stroobant P, Scarborough GA: Active transport of calcium in *Neurospora* plasma membrane vesicles. Proc Natl Acad Sci USA 76:3102–3106, 1979

21. Belliveau JW, Lanyi JK: Calcium transport in *Halobacterium halobium* envelope vesicles. Arch Biochem Biophys 186:98–105, 1978

22. Kobayashi H, VanBrunt J, Harold FM: ATP-linked calcium transport in cells and membrane vesicles of *Streptococcus faecalis*. J Biol Chem 253:2085–2092, 1978

23. Morcos NC, Jacobson AL: Interaction of sodium with sarcolemmal calcium system. Can J Biochem 56:1–6, 1978

24. Vincenzi FF, Larsen FL: The plasma membrane calcium pump: regulation by a soluble Ca^{2+} binding protein. Fed Proc 39:2427–2431, 1980

25. Steck TL, Kant JA: Preparation of impermeable ghosts and inside out vesicles from human erythrocyte membranes. In *Methods in Enzymology*, vol 31. Edited by Fleischer S, Parker L. Academic Press, New York, 1974, pp 172–180

26. Schatzmann HJ: ATP-dependent Ca^{++} extrusion from human red cells. Experientia 22:364–365, 1966

27. Schatzmann HJ, Vincenzi FF: Calcium movements across the membrane of human red cells. J Physiol (Lond) 201:369–395, 1969

28. Bond GH, Clough DL: A soluble protein activator of (Mg^{2+} and Ca^{2+})-dependent ATPase in human red cell membranes. Biochim Biophys Acta 323:592–599, 1973

29. Farrance ML, Vincenzi FF: Enhancement of (Ca^{2+}-Mg^{2+})-ATPase activity of human erythrocyte membranes by hemolysis in isosmotic imidazole buffer. I. General properties of variously prepared membranes and the mechanism of the isosmotic imidazole effect. Biochim Biophys Acta 471:49–58, 1977

30. Farrance ML, Vincenzi FF: Enhancement of (Ca^{2+}-$Mg:s2^+$)-ATPase activity of human erythrocyte membranes by hemolysis in isosmotic imidazole buffer. II. Dependence on calcium and a cytoplasm activator. Biochim Biophys Acta 471:59–66, 1977

31. Jarrett HW, Penniston JT: Purification of the Ca^{2+}-stimulated ATPase activator from human erythrocytes. J Biol Chem 253:4676–4682, 1978

32. Larsen FL, Vincenzi FF: Calcium transport across the plasma membrane: stimulation by calmodulin. Science 204:306–309, 1979

33. Sarkadi B, Schubert A, Gardos G: Effects of calcium-EGTA buffers on active calcium transport in inside-out red cell membrane vesicles. Experientia 35:1045–1047, 1979

34. Larsen FL, Hinds TR, Vincenzi FF: On the red blood cell Ca^{2+} pump: an estimate of stoichiometry. J Membr Biol 41:361–376, 1978

35. Schatzmann HJ: Dependence on calcium concentration and stoichiometry of the calcium pump in human red cells. J Physiol (Lond) 235:551–569, 1973

36. Sarkadi B, Szasz I, Gerloczy A, et al: Transport parameters and stoichiometry of active calcium ion extrusion in intact human red cells. Biochim Biophys Acta 461:93–107, 1977

37. Ferreira HG, Lew VL: Use of ionophore A23187 to measure cytoplasmic Ca^{2+} buffering and activation of the Ca^{2+} pump by internal Ca^{2+}. Nature 259:47–49, 1976

38. Watterson DM, Garrelson WS, Keller PM, et al: Structural similarities between the Ca^{2+}-dependent regulatory proteins of 3'5'-cyclic nucleotide/phosphodiesterase and actinomyosin ATPase. J Biol Chem 251:4501–4513, 1976

39. Owens JD: The determination of the stability constant for calcium-EGTA. Biochim Biophys Acta 451:321–325, 1976

40. Schatzmann HJ: Active calcium transport and Ca^{2+} activated ATPase in human red cells. Curr Top Membr Transport 6:125–168, 1975

41. Quist EE, Ronfogalis BD: Determination of the stoichiometry of the calcium pump in human erythrocytes using lanthanum as a selective inhibitor. FEBS Lett 50:135–139, 1975

42. Larsen FL, Raess BU, Hinds TR, et al: Modulator binding protein antagonizes activation of $(Ca^{2+}\text{-}Mg^{2+})$ ATPase and Ca^{2+} transport of red blood cell membranes. J Supramolec Struct 9:269–274, 1978

43. Kuo CH, Ichida S, Matsuda T, et al: Regulation of ATP-dependent Ca-uptake of synaptic plasma membranes by Ca-dependent modulator protein. Life Sci 25:235–240, 1979

44. Pershadsingh HA, McDonald JM: Direct addition of insulin inhibits a high affinity Ca^{2+} ATPase in isolated adipocyte plasma membranes. Nature 281:495–497, 1979

DISCUSSION

Dr. Donald Wood: For the cell, there are two problems. One is to release calcium into the myofilament space to activate the contractile apparatus when tension is initiated, and the other, of course, is to remove that calcium during relaxation. Different membranes may be involved to different extents in both processes. Would you comment on the role of calcium transport by the plasma membrane in relaxation of either cardiac or skeletal muscle?

Dr. David Goodman: The point that you make is a critical one, that of defining the role of a specific membrane in a specific cell type. The importance of a particular subcellular membrane is going to be determined by the amount of that membrane present, by the specific activity of the pump in that membrane and the affinity of that pump for calcium, and by the metabolic state in which the specific subcellular membrane finds itself. Consequently, you cannot say absolutely that a specific cell membrane is or is not involved in a process or that any one membrane is more important than another under all circumstances. Clearly, when a cell is loaded with calcium because of previous anoxia, then the mitochondrial membrane pump may be more important than the plasma membrane in reducing the concentration of cytosolic calcium.

Dr. John Gergely: You mention the mitochondria. I thought that Somlyo found no accumulation in mitochondria using the electromicroprobe. Do you agree with this?

Dr. David Goodman: Well, I do not agree or disagree and I will let Dr. Martonosi answer that question when he gives his talk. With regard to the microprobe itself, analysis of data obtained with the microprobe suggests that the level of sensitivity of that technique may not be sufficient to detect changes within a physiologic range of concentrations. It is necessary to detect a change in the concentration of cytoplasmic ionized calcium between 10^{-8} and 10^{-6} M; you may not be able to see that by microprobe. Also, you are talking about free ionized calcium, and much of the calcium that is in the cytoplasm may actually be bound. You cannot differentiate free from bound calcium with the microprobe.

43
Optical Studies of Excitation-Contraction Coupling in Muscle

F. Bezanilla, PhD

J. L. Vergara, PhD

Several membrane systems are involved in the chain of events linking excitation with contraction, and changes in the voltage across these membranes play an important role. We have attempted to study changes in membrane potential using potentiometric dyes introduced by Cohen and associates (1).

One way to classify potentiometric dyes is by their ability to penetrate the plasma membrane. The permeant dyes can stain internal membranes and give signals when the membrane potential changes (2).

The present discussion will include only two impermeant dyes, WW781 (3) and WW375 (1). These two dyes are expected to stain the surface membrane and the tubular membranes of skeletal muscle fibers, and we have used them to study the electrical characteristics of the transverse tubular system (T-system) of single skeletal twitch muscle fibers of the frog. Some of the results presented here have been reported recently (4).

Segments of single fibers dissected from semitendinosus muscle of *Rana catesbeiana* were voltage clamped with the triple-gap technique described by Hille and Campbell (5), using a fiber optic bundle to illuminate the muscle fiber. Details of the technique have been described by Vergara and colleagues (2).

When fibers were stained with WW781, we found a large change in fluorescence associated with the action potential, with a similar but delayed time course consistent with the notion that most of the signal was coming from the tubular membrane.

Under voltage clamp, during hyperpolarizing pulses, the optical signal had a nearly exponential time course when a step of voltage was imposed at the surface membrane. Its time course followed very closely the slow component of the capacitative current across the muscle membrane, indicating that the signal was coming from the T-system. The same result was observed for small depolarizing pulses, but when the depolarization elicited sodium currents, new components were observed in the optical signal that had the time course of the small delayed inward current attributed to sodium conductance in the tubular system. For larger depolarizing pulses, the optical signal showed a much faster rate of rise, which could be explained as a fast depolarization of the tubular membrane produced by the tubular sodium currents. At the "off" of a depolarizing pulse, the optical signal was slower than the "off" of a hyperpolarizing pulse; this can be explained by a turn-off of the sodium conductance (sodium "tails") of the tubules, which keeps the membrane depolarized for a longer time.

These results were obtained in full-sodium Ringer's solution or in a modified Ringer's solution with half the sodium ions replaced by tetramethylammonium ion (TMA), indicating that the extra component of the optical signal for depolarizing pulses is not the result of failure of membrane potential control *along* the muscle fiber. Full replacement of sodium by TMA or addition of tetrodotoxin abolished sodium currents and eliminated the extra component of the optical signal; the steady-state values of the fluorescence signal were linearly related to the imposed voltage.

We compared our experimental fluorescence signals measured with WW781 in the absence of sodium and potassium conductances with predictions of a distributed tubular model of the muscle fiber based on the radial model developed by Adrian and associates (6). When the membrane parameters were adjusted to fit the time course of the fluorescence signal to the integral of the tubular potential, an excellent fit was obtained for the time course of the slow capacitative current.

Fibers stained with WW375 gave a different type of optical signal. For both hyperpolarizing and depolarizing pulses, the rise and fall times of the absorption signal were much faster than the signal obtained with WW781. The time course of the optical signal followed the time course of the voltage clamp pulse within the response time of the photodetector electronics. This result seems to indicate that WW375 stained the surface membrane and did not stain the tubular membranes significantly within the staining periods used in our experiments.

When sodium currents were present, the absorption signal from fibers stained with WW375 showed no indication of an extra component, even when a secondary inward current was recorded during the depolarizing voltage clamp pulse. This result provides further support for the notion that the surface membrane potential was well controlled all along the fiber in the pool where membrane potential is measured and controlled and membrane current is measured, i.e., pool A of Hille and Campbell (5).

The studies with impermeant dyes have provided direct recordings of the changes in membrane potential of the T-system; the fit of the data with the radial model of the tubular system has given values for the T-system parameters in the absence of sodium conductance. The optical recording of the tubular potential in the presence of sodium currents has provided strong evidence for a regenerative sodium conductance in the T-system membrane and has shown that the tubular potential escapes from surface potential control during voltage clamp. The optical records obtained with fibers stained with WW781 have shown that the physiologic function of the T-system sodium conductance is to accelerate the tubular depolarization during the propagation of the surface action potential for a more effective coupling through the triad. Further fitting of the optical data to the electrical model of the T-system including the sodium conductance, should allow us to determine the density of the sodium channels on the tubular membrane walls.

ACKNOWLEDGMENTS

This work was supported by U.S. Public Health Service grant AM25201 and grant C781030 from the Muscular Dystrophy Association. We thank Dr. A Waggoner for providing us with the dyes WW781 and WW375.

REFERENCES

1. Cohen LB, Salzberg BM, Dávila HV, et al: Changes in axon fluorescence during activity: molecular probes of membrane potential. J Membr Biol 19:1–36, 1974

2. Vergara J, Bezanilla F, Salzberg B: Nile Blue fluorescence signals from cut single muscle fibers under voltage or current clamps conditions. J Gen Physiol 72:775–800, 1978

3. Cohen LB, Kamino K, Lesher S, et al: Possible improvements in optical methods for monitoring membrane potential. Biol Bull 153:419, 1977

4. Vergara J, Bezanilla F. Optical studies of E-C coupling with potentiometric dyes. In: *Regulation of Muscle Contraction: Excitation-Contraction Coupling*. Edited by Grinnell AD, Brazier MAB. Academic Press, New York, 1980

5. Hille B, Campbell DT: An improved vaseline gap technique clamp for skeletal muscle fibers. J Gen Physiol 67:265–293, 1976

6. Adrian RH, Chandler WK, Hodgkin AL: The kinetics of mechanical activation in frog muscle. J Physiol (Lond) 204:207–230, 1969

44

Regulation of Cytoplasmic Calcium Concentration by Sarcoplasmic Reticulum

Anthony N. Martonosi, MD

The free cytoplasmic Ca^{2+} concentration in resting skeletal muscle, nerve, and other cells, is several orders of magnitude lower than the Ca^{2+} concentration in the extracellular fluid. This Ca^{2+} gradient is maintained by the coordinated action of a complex system of adenosine triphosphate (ATP)-energized Ca^{2+} pumps, Na^+-Ca^{2+} and H^+-Ca^{2+} exchange systems, Ca^{2+} channels, and Ca^{2+}-binding components located in the surface membranes, sarcoplasmic reticulum, mitochondria, myofibrils, and cytosol (1, 2). The maintenance of cytoplasmic Ca^{2+} concentration requires a delicate balance between the cellular concentration, Ca^{2+} affinity, and transport or binding activity of each of these components (Fig. 1).

The contractile activity of skeletal and cardiac muscle is defined by the cytoplasmic free Ca^{2+} concentration (3–5). In resting muscle, much of the intracellular Ca^{2+} is sequestered within the sarcoplasmic reticulum and perhaps in other intracellular organelles.

During contraction the depolarization of the surface membrane and transverse (T) tubules triggers the release of Ca^{2+} from intracellular storage sites, the cytoplasmic Ca^{2+} concentration increases, and Ca^{2+} binding to troponin initiates the complex set of reactions that leads to actin-myosin interaction and shortening (6).

Relaxation is caused by the reabsorption of Ca^{2+} into the sarcoplasmic reticulum through an ATP-dependent Ca^{2+} pump, which is capable of decreasing the cytoplasmic Ca^{2+} concentration to 10^{-7} to 10^{-8} M and generating a Ca^{2+} activity gradient of 1,000-fold or more across the sarcoplasmic reticulum membrane (7–9).

The contribution of mitochondria to the regulation of cytoplasmic Ca^{2+} concentration is likely to vary in different types of muscles (1, 10). In normal

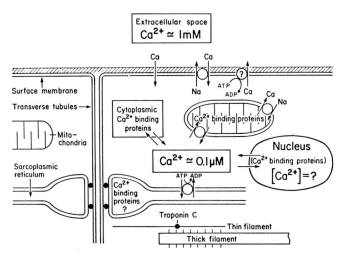

Fig. 1. Systems participating in the regulation of cytoplasmic Ca^{2+} concentration in skeletal muscle.

fast-twitch skeletal muscle the sarcoplasmic reticulum is so abundant that its Ca^{2+} transport activity largely accounts for the physiologic fluctuations in cytoplasmic Ca^{2+} concentration, and the contribution of mitochondria to the Ca^{2+} regulation may be minor (1, 11). On the other hand, in slow-twitch skeletal, cardiac, and embryonic muscles, the Ca^{2+} transport activity of sarcoplasmic reticulum is limited and Ca^{2+} transport by mitochondria could have physiologic significance (1, 11).

The Ca^{2+} transport activity of sarcoplasmic reticulum vesicles isolated from muscles of patients with Duchenne muscular dystrophy is reduced in comparison with control muscles of healthy persons (12–17). Similar differences were observed in genetically dystrophic mice and chicken muscles (18–38). The diminished Ca^{2+} transport activity of dystrophic muscle microsomes is usually viewed as part of a generalized membrane defect (39), suggested to be an early and perhaps primary phenomenon in the pathogenesis of the disease.

In view of the large differences in the abundance and Ca^{2+} transport activity of sarcoplasmic reticulum in *normal* muscles of different contraction-relaxation velocities (40–46), and in the endoplasmic reticulum of other tissues, the question must be raised as to whether the decreased Ca^{2+} transport activity of sarcoplasmic reticulum in dystrophic muscle represents the pathologic property of diseased muscle cells or arises from an increase in the relative amount of slow muscle fibers and adipose and connective tissue cells in the diseased muscle.

The purpose of this report is to evaluate data from the literature pertinent to this question, and to point out further avenues of investigation that may help to solve the problem.

THE STRUCTURE OF SARCOPLASMIC RETICULUM

The sarcoplasmic reticulum of skeletal muscle contains three morphologically (47) and functionally distinct regions (Fig. 2):

1. The junctional sarcoplasmic reticulum, which forms the specialized triad junctions with the T-tubules, where the excitatory stimulus is transmitted to the sarcoplasmic reticulum causing Ca^{2+} release.

2. The cisternae, which have an electron-dense content in their interior that may represent storage sites for accumulated Ca^{2+}.

3. The longitudinal elements of the sarcoplasmic reticulum, which are narrow tubules that connect the cisternae through the center of the sarcomere and across the Z-line.

The Ca^{2+}-transport ATPase is evenly distributed through the cisternae and longitudinal tubules, whereas the junctional sarcoplasmic reticulum contains specialized elements and probably does not participate in Ca^{2+} transport.

Fragmented sarcoplasmic reticulum preparations obtained by differential centrifugation contain microsomes derived from all three regions of sarcoplasmic reticulum, together with T tubules and surface membrane elements. These microsome preparations were used for most studies reported so far on dystrophic muscle. The crude microsomal preparations can be resolved into fractions containing T tubules, terminal cisternae (heavy microsome), and longitudinal tubules (light microsome) by sucrose gradient centrifugation (48). The various fractions differ in Ca^{2+} transport activity and protein composition, and their detailed analysis has only begun. The Ca^{2+}-transport ATPase (Ca-ATPase) is more or less uniformly distributed among the various fractions, including the putative T tubules (48–52).

The Ca-ATPase molecules are asymmetrically distributed in the membrane. Electron microscopic studies by freeze fracture (53), negative staining (54, 55), and tannic acid fixation (56) indicate that a major portion of the ATPase polypeptide is exposed on the cytoplasmic side of the bilayer. A similar disposition of the Ca-ATPase is suggested by the electron density profiles of pelleted microsomal material analyzed by x-ray diffraction (57).

Negative staining of fragmented sarcoplasmic reticulum vesicles using potassium phosphotungstate reveals 40-Å particles on the cytoplasmic surface of the

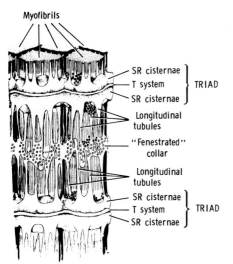

Fig. 2. The structure of sarcoplasmic reticulum. SR, sarcoplasmic reticulum; T system, transverse tubular system.

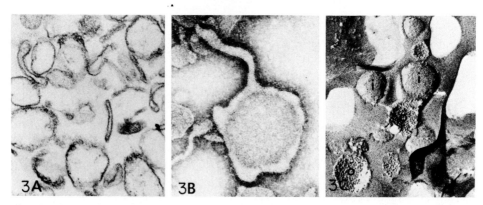

Fig. 3. Electron micrographs of fragmented sarcoplasmic reticulum. **(A)** Thin section. **(B)** Negative staining with potassium phosphotungstate. **(C)** Freeze-fracture (I, inside or luminal; O, outside or cytoplasmic fracture face). × A 71,000, B 140,000, C 71,000

membrane (Fig. 3), each of which probably represents a portion of the ATPase polypeptide that projects from the membrane into the water phase (54, 55). The density of 40-Å surface particles is close to 16,000/μm^2 of surface area in microsomes isolated from adult fast-twitch skeletal muscle (58). The 40-Å surface particles are not visible in negatively stained microsomes isolated from 10- to 12-day-old chicken embryos, which contain little Ca-ATPase (59).

By freeze-etch electron microscopy, 85-Å intramembranous particles are seen in the sarcoplasmic reticulum of whole muscle (47, 60), in isolated sarcoplasmic reticulum vesicles (53, 58, 61), and in reconstituted vesicles containing only the purified Ca-ATPase (56, 58). It is reasonably well established that these particles represent the Ca-ATPase complex. The 85-Å particles are more frequent in the cytoplasmic than in the luminal leaflet of the bilayer (Fig. 3), in agreement with the proposition that much of the mass of the Ca-ATPase polypeptide is on the cytoplasmic side of the membrane. The density of the 85-Å intramembranous particles is approximately 4,000/μm^2 of surface area, i.e., approximately one-fourth the density of the 40-Å surface particles seen by negative staining (58, 61). Because both sets of particles are related to the Ca-ATPase, it was suggested that the 85-Å intramembranous particles are clusters of several (probably four) ATPase molecules. Interactions between ATPase molecules were also observed in detergent-solubilized sarcoplasmic reticulum material by ultracentrifugation (62) and in reconstituted ATPase vesicles by fluorescence energy transfer measurements (63). The formation of ATPase oligomers may account for the half of the sites' reactivity (64) and the cooperative kinetic behavior of ATPase activity and Ca^{2+} transport derived from steady-state and transient state kinetic studies (65).

The density of 85-Å intramembranous particles is only 200 to 400/μm^2 of membrane surface area in the skeletal muscles of 10- to 14-day-old chicken embryos (60), where the Ca-ATPase and Ca^{2+} transport activities are barely detectable (66). The density of 85-Å particles increases 10- to 20-fold during development into mature muscle, parallel with the increase in the Ca-ATPase content of the sarcoplasmic reticulum (66, 67).

Sarcoplasmic reticulum of the red slow-twitch skeletal muscle is characterized by low Ca-ATPase content and poor Ca^{2+} transport activity (40–44); this is reflected in a significantly lower density of intramembranous 85-Å particles compared with fast-twitch white skeletal muscle (45, 46).

Therefore, the large changes in the concentration of Ca-ATPase and in the density of 85-Å freeze-etch particles are regular features of the sarcoplasmic reticulum in developing muscles, and major differences in Ca-ATPase content characterize muscles of different phenotypes.

THE FUNCTION OF SARCOPLASMIC RETICULUM

The transport of Ca^{2+} by sarcoplasmic reticulum is coupled to the hydrolysis of ATP through a Mg^{2+}, Ca^{2+}-activated ATPase that is the major intrinsic protein component of sarcoplasmic reticulum membranes. For each mole of ATP hydrolyzed, two Ca^{2+} atoms are transferred across the membrane (8). Steady-state and rapid kinetic studies established the minimal reaction sequence for Ca^{2+} translocation shown in Figure 4 (68).

Random interaction of the enzyme with Ca^{2+} and Mg-ATP on the cytoplasmic side (Step 1) leads to the formation of the E $<^{2Ca}_{ATP}$ complex with apparent dissociation constants of about 0.1 and 1.0 μM for Ca^{2+} and ATP, respectively (7). The binding of Ca^{2+} and ATP induces a conformational change in the enzyme that is detectable by changes in tryptophan fluorescence (69) and SH group reactivity (70) and by the altered mobility of protein-bound spin labels (71).

The rapid cleavage of ATP is coupled with the phosphorylation of an aspartyl residue (72) at the active site (Step 2). The process is reversible, resulting in ATP-ADP exchange (8).

The phosphorylation of the enzyme is followed by the translocation of Ca across the membrane, a decrease in the affinity of Ca^{2+} binding sites (Step 3) (73), and the release of Ca^{2+} on the inside (luminal) membrane surface (Step 4).

The cycle is completed by the isomerization of the phosphoenzyme (Steps 5 and 6) and the eventual cleavage of phosphoprotein with the release of inorganic phosphate on the cytoplasmic surface (74). The rate-limiting step of the overall process is one of the steps following Ca^{2+} translocation, and appears to be related to the hydrolysis of phosphoprotein (75).

The Ca^{2+} pump is capable of lowering the cytoplasmic Ca^{2+} concentration to or below 10^{-8} M and establish an electrochemical Ca^{2+} gradient of 1,000-

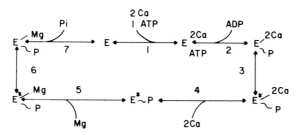

Fig. 4. Reaction sequence for calcium translocation in the sarcoplasmic reticulum.

fold or greater across the membrane (8). The process is reversible, and the release of each two Ca^{2+} atoms from the sarcoplasmic reticulum permits the synthesis of 1 mol of ATP from ADP and inorganic phosphate (9, 76). During reversal of Ca^{2+} transport, the enzyme is phosphorylated by inorganic ortho-phosphate, yielding a phosphoenzyme intermediate that shares many of the properties of the phosphoenzyme formed with ATP (9).

The Ca-ATPase is an intrinsic membrane protein that requires phospholipids for activity. Depletion of membrane phospholipids by treatment with phospho-lipase C and A, or by extraction with detergents, reversibly inhibits the ATPase activity and Ca^{2+} transport (77). Inhibition of Ca^{2+} transport activity was also observed after exchange of membrane phospholipids with dipalmitoyl or dimyristoylphosphatidylcholine when tested below the temperature of gel-liquid transition (78, 79). These observations establish a plausible relationship between the fluidity of the lipid-phase of the membrane and the mobility of the enzyme required for Ca translocation and the hydrolysis of phosphoprotein intermediate (79).

Interactions between lipoprotein complexes are common in biologic mem-branes and presumably contribute to the wide range of cooperative phenomena expressed in excitability, receptor functions, transport processes, and enzyme activity. The following evidence suggests that cooperative interactions are also important in the case of the Ca-ATPase. The steady-state concentration of phosphoenzyme intermediate under optimal conditions for ATPase activity and Ca^{2+} transport is close to 0.5 mol/mol of enzyme, suggesting "half of the sites" reactivity. Cooperativity is also evident in the dependence of ATPase activity on ATP concentration (80, 81). Electron microscope (58), ultracentrifuge (62), gel exclusion chromatography (82), and fluorescence energy transfer data (63) suggest that the Ca-ATPase molecules interact with each other in the membrane to form oligomers (presumably tetramers) that are in equilibrium with mono-mers and dimers. The protein-protein interactions reflected in the kinetic and hydrodynamic properties of the Ca-ATPase are influenced by the composition of the lipid phase (62) and are expected to depend critically on the concentration of Ca-ATPase in the membrane (83).

In addition to the Ca-ATPase, sarcoplasmic reticulum membranes contain at least two calcium binding proteins, glycoproteins, and several proteolipids (52). The role of these components in the process of Ca^{2+} translocation is not clearly understood.

This brief survey of the principal characteristics of the Ca^{2+} transport system of sarcoplasmic reticulum emphasizes the close relationship between Ca^{2+} transport, ATPase activity, the concentration of ATPase enzyme in the mem-brane, and the composition of membrane lipids. Changes in all these aspects may alter the rate of Ca^{2+} transport and may contribute to the properties of dystrophic sarcoplasmic reticulum.

SARCOPLASMIC RETICULUM IN MUSCULAR DYSTROPHY

Among the earliest morphologic manifestations of various forms of muscular dystrophy are the "vacuolation" and "dilation" of sarcoplasmic reticulum and

T tubules (84–87) and changes in the ultrastructure of the surface membrane in muscle cells (88–93) and in erythrocytes (94). Ultrastructural differences were also reported between microsome fractions isolated from normal and dystrophic chicken and mouse muscles (24, 29, 31, 33–35).

The interpretation of the morphologic changes is complicated by the variable time course of the disease, sampling problems related to fiber type composition, and the possibility of secondary changes either in vivo or after biopsy. Isolated membrane fractions are notoriously heterogeneous, with possible contributions from surface membranes, T tubules, and mitochondrial outer membranes, in addition to sarcoplasmic reticulum. The massive infiltration of dystrophic muscle by connective and adipose tissue makes quantitative evaluation of biochemical data uncertain.

For these reasons, the ultrastructural, biochemical, and physiologic data are difficult to correlate. Some of the changes attributed to dystrophy may in fact be normal properties of muscle fibers which are spared by the dystrophic process and represent an increasing proportion of the muscle mass as the disease progresses; others could be due to contaminating connective tissue cells.

The Duchenne type human dystrophy and the genetic dystrophies of chicken and mice will be discussed separately.

Chicken Dystrophy

Although earlier observations indicated an increased rate of Ca^{2+} uptake and elevated Ca storage capacity in pectoralis muscles of 4- to 6-week-old dystrophic chicken (24, 25), recent studies suggest a significant decrease in the rate of Ca^{2+}-dependent ATP hydrolysis (26, 36), the initial velocity (36) and steady-state level (33, 34, 36) of Ca^{2+} uptake, and the maximal steady-state concentration of phosphoenzyme intermediate (26, 36) in dystrophic microsomes (Table 1). The average density of 85-Å intramembranous freeze-etch particles, assumed to represent the Ca-ATPase, decreases in proportion to the decrease in Ca^{2+} transport activity (33).

A unique morphologic feature of chicken muscular dystrophy is the proliferation of T tubules and junctional membranes (31, 35, 87), which are characterized by low intramembranous particle density and low Ca^{2+} transport activity (35). The tubular networks become visible in mature fibers after the myogenesis is completed (38). The proliferation of T tubules is probably related to the increased density and less regular disposition of caveolae on the surface membranes of dystrophic chicken muscle (91).

The Ca, Mg-dependent ATPases isolated from normal and dystrophic chicken microsomes are identical in molecular weight, proteolytic peptide pattern, enzyme activity, and Ca^{2+} and Mg^{2+} dependence (28, 37). The calsequestrins isolated from the two sources bind identical amounts of Ca (37). Therefore, the two principal sarcoplasmic reticulum proteins appear to be normal in dystrophic chicken muscle.

It was suggested that the low Ca^{2+} transport capacity and 85-Å particle density of dystrophic chicken microsomes are due to the admixture of relatively large amounts of junctional sarcoplasmic reticulum and T-tubule elements (31, 34, 35). This interpretation is supported by the high cholesterol and sphingo-

Table 1. Functional and Morphologic Characteristics of Sarcoplasmic Reticulum in Normal and Dystrophic Muscles

| | Yield of Microsomes (mg protein/g muscle) | ATPase Activity (µmol substrate/mg/min) | | | Ca Transport | | | $E \sim p$[a] (nmol/mg protein) | 85-Å Particles (no./µm²) | Reference |
| | | Total | Ca-Insensitive | Ca-Sensitive | Initial Rates (µmol/mg/min) | Total Uptake (µmol Ca/mg protein) | | | | |
						Without Oxalate	With Oxalate			
Chicken										
Normal	0.29	2.53	2.19	0.49	0.28			3.26	—	Hanna and Baskin (26)
Dystrophic	0.44	1.35	1.30	0.08	0.94			1.45	—	
Normal	—	7.2	3.0	4.2	3.12	0.043		3.13	1320	Verjovski-Almeida, Inesi 1979 (36), Scales Sabbadini 1979 (35)
Dystrophic	—	7.2	4.8	2.4	1.45	0.029		1.95	990	
Normal	0.57	3.04	1.31	1.73	1.45	0.125		—	3700	Scales et al. (34)
Dystrophic	0.83	3.15	0.98	2.16	2.35	0.065		—	2500	
Normal	0.326	3.0	—	—	—	0.072		—	5150	Sabbadini et al. (33)
Dystrophic	0.153	3.0	—	—	—	0.02	—	—	3700	
Mouse										
Normal	1.6	0.68	0.41	0.27	0.30	0.06	2.86			Sreter et al. (19)
Dystrophic	2.7	1.25	0.98	0.27	0.10	0.03	0.89			
Normal	2.17	0.88	0.39	0.49		0.062	2.05			Martonosi (20)
Dystrophic	1.94	0.75	0.56	0.19		0.037	0.81			
Normal	0.96	2.7	—	—		0.062	4.0	2.8	3100	Mrak and Baskin (29)
Dystrophic	0.97	2.8	—	—		0.046	1.4– 1.8	1.51	3100	Mrak and Baskin (30)
Human										
Normal	—	0.84	—	—	0.38		2.04			Samaha and Gergely (13)
Duchenne Dystrophy	—	0.38	—	—	0.19		0.68			
Myotonic Dystrophy	—	0.69	—	—	0.53		2.12			
Normal	—		0.10	—	0.5		4.3			Takagi et al. (15)
Duchenne Dystrophy	—		0.07	—	0.05– 0.4		1.1			

[a] Steady-state concentration of phosphoprotein ($E \sim P$).

myelin and low dipalmitoylphosphatidylcholine content of dystrophic microsomes (22).

The striking overproduction of T tubules in dystrophic chicken muscle is phenomenologically similar to the development of labyrinthine tubular networks in denervated rat skeletal muscle (95) or in cultured chicken muscle (67, 96). After denervation of rat gastrocnemius muscle, there is a transient increase in the Ca^{2+} transport activity of isolated microsomes, followed by a decrease; 42 days after denervation the concentration of phosphoprotein, which indicates the Ca-ATPase content, decreased from 2 nmol/mg of protein to 0.3 nmol/mg of protein (42).

These observations indicate some similarity between denervated (11) and dystrophic muscles with respect to T tubule and sarcoplasmic reticulum involvement, suggesting that "functional denervation" may contribute to the pathogenesis of the disease.

It is a common observation that type II (white) muscle fibers are preferentially affected in muscular dystrophy (97–100). During normal development of chicken muscle the oxidative-glycolytic αR type fibers are replaced by glycolytic αW type fibers. Ashmore and Doerr (100) suggested that the degenerative changes are expressed only in the αW fiber population. The large proportion of αR fibers in dystrophic chicken muscle (87) may arise from selective destruction of αW fibers or slow conversion of αR into αW fibers. The net result is the persistence of embryonic histochemical and biochemical characteristics in dystrophic chicken muscle even in adult animals.

The Ca^{2+} transport activity and Ca-ATPase content of red (40–44) and embryonic muscle microsomes (59, 66, 67) is low (Table 2). This is also reflected in the smaller number of intramembranous 85-Å particles in red (45, 46) as compared with white muscles and in embryonic (59, 60) as compared with adult muscles.

The predominance of oxidative-glycolytic, embryonic fiber types in dystrophic muscle may contribute to the low Ca-ATPase content and the reduced number of intramembranous 85-Å particles in the isolated microsomes. If this interpretation is correct, the biochemical observations on dystrophic chicken muscle merely reflect the normal characteristics of the predominant red fiber type, which is resistant to the dystrophic process. As the consequences of denervation are also less pronounced in red than white muscle fibers (11), these considerations are also consistent with the possible role of functional denervation in the pathogenesis of chicken dystrophy.

Mouse Dystrophy

Dystrophic mouse microsomes are characterized (Table 1) by a decreased rate of Ca^{2+} transport and Ca^{2+} uptake capacity (17, 19, 20, 30), a decrease in the maximal steady-state concentration of phosphoenzyme intermediate (30), and a decrease in Ca-sensitive ATPase activity (18–20, 30). The yield of microsomes from dystrophic muscle increases together with an increase in Ca-insensitive ATPase activity (18–20).

Ultrastructurally, swelling of the sarcoplasmic reticulum represents one of the early signs of the disease (29, 101, 102). The swollen regions of the

Table 2. Calcium Transport and Calcium-Activated ATPase Activity

Type of Muscle	Reference	Ca Uptake[a] (μmol Ca/mg protein)	Ca-Activated ATPase Activity (μmol Pi/mg protein/min)	Phosphorylated Intermediate (nmol Pi/mg protein)
Chicken				
Embryonic (14 days) pectoralis muscle	66	0.21	0.04	0.22
Adult superficial pectoralis (white muscle)	66	2.40	0.70	2.20
Adult anterior latissimus dorsi (red muscle)	—	0.30	0.52	0.45
Rabbit				
Adult adductor magnus, vastus lateralis (white muscle)	40	3.95	1.01	6.07
Adult soleus, semitendinosus, crureus, intertransversarius (red muscle)	40	0.20	0.54	0.84

[a] Calcium uptake was measured in the presence of 5 mM oxalate. For other details, see references.

sarcoplasmic reticulum are apparently deficient in intramembranous freeze-etch particles (29), but no abnormalities of the T tubules were detected in freeze-fracture replicas (29).

The prolonged relaxation time and slow fatigue of dystrophic mouse muscles is consistent with the sparing and accumulation of slow fiber types (97, 103). The increased yield and reduced Ca^{2+} transport activity of dystrophic mouse microsomes are consistent with the characteristics of sarcoplasmic reticulum vesicles isolated from predominantly red muscles (40–46).

Duchenne Dystrophy

The first study of the Ca^{2+} transport of sarcoplasmic reticulum in diseased human muscle was carried out by Sugita and colleagues (12), who observed a decrease in Ca^{2+} transport and an increase in Ca^{2+}, Mg^{2+}-ATPase activity in Duchenne dystrophy and in myositis. The Na^+, K^+-ATPase activity was unaffected. The possibility was raised that the T tubules could be the site of the leakage into the blood of cytoplasmic enzymes such as ATP:creatine phosphotransferase.

In a more extensive series of studies, Samaha and Gergely (13) found a decrease in the initial rate of Ca^{2+} transport, total Ca^{2+} uptake, and ATPase activity in Duchenne dystrophic microsomes isolated either from the gastrocnemius or from the vastus lateralis muscles of 8 patients (Table 1). The initial rate of Ca^{2+} uptake was increased in 4 cases of myotonic dystrophy, with no change in total Ca^{2+} capacity and a slight decrease in ATPase activity compared with control microsomes of 15 normal persons.

Similar observations were made by Peter and Worsfold (14), who also noted that the Ca^{2+} transport activity of sarcoplasmic reticulum and the oxidative phosphorylation by mitochondria are normal in myotonic dystrophy (104).

A more detailed characterization of muscle microsomes from Duchenne dystrophic patients was reported by Takagi and associates (15). The Ca^{2+} uptake capacity of Duchenne dystrophic microsomes was drastically reduced both in the presence and in the absence of Ca-precipitating anions, with relatively slight change in the Mg^{2+}-activated ATPase (Table 1). Decreased Ca^{2+} uptake was also observed in microsomes isolated from Becker dystrophy (2 cases), limb girdle dystrophy (2 cases), polymyositis (2 cases), and 1 of 2 cases of facioscapulohumeral dystrophy. Normal Ca^{2+} uptake was observed in amyotrophic lateral sclerosis (2 cases) and in one case of chronic polyneuropathy.

The total lipid content of microsomes was slightly increased in Duchenne dystrophy with a decrease in phosphatidylcholine and an increase in sphingomyelin content. In view of the massive infiltration of dystrophic muscle by adipose and connective tissue, the phospholipid composition of microsomes isolated from connective tissue was also analyzed. It was estimated that a mixture representing equal parts of normal muscle microsomes and microsomes from connective tissue would give approximately the same phospholipid composition as was found in sarcoplasmic reticulum of dystrophic muscle. Because the Ca^{2+} transport activity of adipose and connective tissue microsomes is rather weak, this degree of contamination would also explain the deficient Ca^{2+} transport activity of Duchenne dystrophic microsomes.

These studies clearly demonstrate the need for better methods for obtaining purified sarcoplasmic reticulum membranes from dystrophic muscle and for analyzing their heterogeneity.

Because the purity of the microsome preparations from diseased muscle is ill-defined, the slight changes in protein composition observed by sodium dodecyl sulfate-polyacrylamide gel electrophoresis are of doubtful significance (15, 16).

The prolonged relaxation times of muscles affected by Duchenne dystrophy (105, 106) suggests a predominance of type I fibers, which is observed histochemically in 90% of the patients with Duchenne muscular dystrophy (107). In view of the poor Ca^{2+} transport activity of microsomes isolated from normal red skeletal muscles, meaningful evaluation of Ca^{2+} transport data on dystrophic membranes would require some knowledge of the fiber type composition of the starting material used for the isolation of microsomes.

THE SURFACE MEMBRANES IN DUCHENNE DYSTROPHY

Changes in the ultrastructure of surface membrane may contribute to the leakage of cytoplasmic enzymes into the blood and could promote the dystrophic process through increased Ca^{2+} influx into the muscle cells. No definitive information is available on either of these problems. Two morphologic findings must be mentioned.

Perhaps the most striking ultrastructural change in surface membranes of dystrophic chicken muscle is the increased number and irregular arrangement of the caveolae (91), which may be related to the proliferation of T-tubule network (31, 87).

Conflicting findings were reported regarding the density of intramembranous freeze-etch particles on muscle cell surface membranes in Duchenne dystrophy. Schotland and colleagues (89, 90) found a decrease in particle density for both faces of sarcolemma in the quadriceps muscle of 14 patients with Duchenne dystrophy whereas Yoshioka and Okuda (92) observed a substantial increase in the particle density in 1 case; Ketelson (93) also reported an increase in 1 case of human muscular dystrophy. Sampling of different fiber types may account for this discrepancy. The density of surface membrane particles increases during embryonic development (60). The number of these particles differs in red and white muscles, and the orthogonal arrays of surface particles that are characteristic of white muscle surface membrane are absent from red and dystrophic muscles (90).

No information is available concerning the identity of intramembranous particles with known components of the surface membrane. Their size heterogeneity suggests contributions by several proteins.

The Ca^{2+} pumps and Na^{+}-Ca^{2+} exchange systems in the surface membrane of muscle cells must play an important role in the maintenance of total cell Ca within normal limits. It is tempting to speculate that a decrease in the concentration of an ATP-dependent Ca pump in the surface membrane may accompany the deficient Ca^{2+} transport of sarcoplasmic reticulum. Because of the difficulties in isolating pure surface membranes from skeletal muscle, reliable biochemical data on the enzymatic activity and composition of normal and dystrophic surface membranes are scarce.

CONCLUSIONS

During the past decade a massive amount of basic information about the structure, composition, and transport activity of sarcoplasmic reticulum in different muscles has been accumulated, providing a solid foundation for future definitive studies on the involvement of these membranes in muscular dystrophy.

The survey of currently available information indicates gross deficiency of Ca^{2+} transport in sarcoplasmic reticulum preparations isolated from dystrophic human, chicken, and mouse muscle. It is evident, however, that these changes cannot be regarded with certainty as primary manifestations of a genetic defect in the sarcoplasmic reticulum. In fact, there are good reasons to assume that the deficient Ca^{2+} transport may arise from a combination of factors that are not primary features of the disease. Among these are:

1. A change in the fiber type composition of dystrophic muscle. The muscles used in these studies contain a mixture of white and red fibers, with widely different Ca^{2+} transport activities. A preferential destruction of white muscle

fibers in dystrophic muscles could account for the diminished Ca^{2+} transport activity, without invoking a genetic defect directly affecting sarcoplasmic reticulum.

2. Immature muscle fibers. The presence of a greater proportion of young, regenerating muscle fibers in dystrophic tissue with relatively low Ca^{2+}-transport ATPase content would lower the Ca^{2+} transport activity of dystrophic microsomes compared with normal muscles of the same age.

3. Contamination by adipose and connective tissue. Dystrophic muscles contain large amounts of adipose and connective tissue; microsomes isolated from them are likely to contain significant membrane contamination of nonmuscle origin. This may explain not only the diminished Ca^{2+} transport, but also the differences in phospholipid and cholesterol composition between normal and dystrophic microsomes.

4. Contamination by non–sarcoplasmic reticulum membranes. Sarcoplasmic reticulum membranes isolated from red and dystrophic muscles are likely to contain greater contamination by other membrane elements (mitochondrial outer membranes, surface membranes, T tubules) than are white muscle microsomes. This is suggested by the fact that the yield of microsomes from red and dystrophic muscles is usually greater than that from their white and normal counterparts, but no definitive identification of the contaminating membranes has been achieved.

5. Lysosomes. The picture is further complicated by the increased lysosome content of dystrophic muscles with the possibility of degradative changes in the isolated membranes by proteolytic or phospholipase enzymes, with inhibition of Ca^{2+} transport activity.

Solution of these problems will require development of new techniques for the analysis of biochemical changes in single fibers of well-defined fiber type. Existing methods must be refined for the separation and characterization of distinct membrane elements from small samples of biopsy material.

Further effort is necessary in the purification and characterization of surface membranes from normal and dystrophic muscle fibers.

The biochemical studies on isolated membrane fractions should be systematically correlated with ultrastructural and histochemical analysis of intact muscles to obtain information about fiber type composition, variability of morphologic features between muscle fibers of the same sample, and the extent of degenerative changes.

Application of powerful new electrophysiologic techniques to living single fibers of dystrophic muscle may help to define the changes in T tubules and junctional sarcoplasmic reticulum which feature prominently in certain types of dystrophy. Methods have become available for measurement of changes in cytoplasmic free Ca^{2+} concentration in normal and dystrophic living muscle fibers.

The influence of innervation on the relative amounts of various types of membranes such as T tubules and junctional sarcoplasmic reticulum, within the muscle cell should be better defined.

A good start has been made, but a coordinated multidisciplinary effort is required to evaluate the significance of the available information on sarcoplasmic reticulum in muscular dystrophy and to expand it into a critical assessment of the role of membranes in the pathogenesis of the disease.

ACKNOWLEDGMENTS

This work was supported by research grants from the National Institutes of Health (AM 26545) and the National Science Foundation (PCM 7919502) and by a research grant in aid from the Muscular Dystrophy Association.

REFERENCES

1. Carafoli E, Crompton M: The regulation of intracellular Calcium. Curr Top Membr Transport 10:151–216, 1978
2. Requena J, Mullins LJ: Calcium movements in nerve fibres. Q Rev Biophys 12:371–460, 1979
3. Ebashi S: Excitation-contraction coupling. Annu Rev Physiol 38:293–313, 1976
4. Fozzard HA: Heart excitation-contraction coupling. Annu Rev Physiol 30:201–220, 1977
5. Weber A: Energized Ca transport and relaxing factors. Curr Top Bioenergetics 1:203–254, 1966
6. Lymn RW: Kinetic analysis of myosin and actomyosin ATPase. Annu Rev Biophys Bioeng 8:145–163, 1979
7. Yamamoto T, Takisawa H, Tonomura Y: Reaction mechanism for ATP hydrolysis and synthesis in sarcoplasmic reticulum. Curr Top Bioenerg 9:179–236, 1979
8. Hasselbach W: The sarcoplasmic calcium pump. A model of energy transductions in biological membranes Top Curr Chem 78:1–56, 1979
9. deMeis L, Vianna AL: Energy interconversion by the Ca^{2+} dependent ATPase of the sarcoplasmic reticulum. Annu Rev Biochem 48:275–292, 1979
10. Fiskum G, Lehninger AL: The mechanism and regulation of mitochondrial Ca^{2+} transport. Fed Proc 39:2432–2436, 1980
11. Martonosi A: Biochemical and clinical aspects of sarcoplasmic reticulum function. Curr Top Membr Transport 3:83–197, 1972
12. Sugita H, Okimoto K, Ebashi S, Okinaka S: Biochemical alterations in progressive muscular dystrophy with special relevance to the sarcoplasmic reticulum. In *Exploratory Concepts in Muscular Dystrophy and Related Disorders.* Edited by Milhorat AT. Excerpta Medica, Amsterdam, New York, 1967, pp 321–326
13. Samaha F, Gergely J: Biochemical abnormalities of the sarcoplasmic reticulum in muscular dystrophy. N Engl J Med 280:184–188, 1969
14. Peter JB, Worsfold M: Muscular dystrophy and other myopathies: sarcotubular vesicles in early disease. Biochem Med 2:364–371, 1969
15. Takagi A, Schotland DL, Rowland LP: Sarcoplasmic reticulum in Duchenne muscular dystrophy. Arch Neurol 28:380–384, 1973
16. Samaha FJ, Congedo CZ: Two biochemical types of Duchenne dystrophy: sarcoplasmic reticulum membrane proteins. Ann Neurol 1:125–130, 1977
17. Wood DS, Sorenson M, Eastwood AB, et al: Duchenne dystrophy: Abnormal generation of tension and Ca^{2+} regulation in single skinned fibers. Neurology (Minneap) 28:447–457, 1978
18. Sreter FA, Martonosi A, Gergely J: Sarcoplasmic reticulum in dystrophic mouse and chicken. Fed Proc 23:530, 1964
19. Sreter FA, Ikemoto N, Gergely J: Studies on the fragmented sarcoplasmic reticulum of normal and dystrophic mouse muscle. In *Exploratory Concepts in Muscular Dystrophy and Related Disorders.* Edited by Milhorat AT. Excerpta Medica, Amsterdam, New York, 1967, pp 289–298

20. Martonosi A: Sarcoplasmic reticulum. VI. Microsomal Ca^{2+} transport in genetic muscular dystrophy of mice. Proc Soc Exp Biol Med 127:824–828, 1968

21. Hsu QS, Kaldor G: Studies on the sarcoplasmic reticulum of normal and dystrophic animals. Proc Soc Exp Biol Med 131:1398–1402, 1969

22. Hsu QS, Kaldor G. Studies on the lipid composition of the fragmented sarcoplasmic reticulum of normal and dystrophic chicken. Proc Soc Exp Biol Med 138:733–737, 1971

23. Kaldor G, Hsu QS: Studies on the fragmented sarcoplasmic reticulum and "natural" tropomyosin of normal and dystrophic chickens. Proc Soc Exp Biol Med 149:362–366, 1975

24. Baskin RJ: Ultrastructure and Ca transport in dystrophic chicken muscle microsomes. Lab Invest 23:581–589, 1970

25. Sylvester R, Baskin RJ: Kinetics of calcium uptake in normal and dystrophic sarcoplasmic reticulum. Biochem Med 8:213–227, 1973

26. Hanna SD, Baskin RJ: Calcium transport and phosphoenzyme formation in sarcoplasmic reticulum isolated from normal and dystrophic chickens. Biochem Med 17:300–309, 1977

27. Crowe LM, Baskin RJ: Stereological analysis of developing sarcotubular membranes. J Ultrastruct Res 58:10–21, 1977

28. Hanna SD, Baskin RJ: Comparison of the $Ca^{2+} + Mg^{2+}$ ATPase proteins from normal and dystrophic chicken sarcoplasmic reticulum. Biochim Biophys Acta 540:144–150, 1978

29. Mrak RE, Baskin RJ: Ultrastructure of dystrophic mouse sarcoplasmic reticulum. Biochem Med 19:277–293, 1978

30. Mrak RE, Baskin RJ: Calcium transport and phosphoenzyme formation in dystrophic mouse sarcoplasmic reticulum. Biochem Med 19:47–70, 1978

31. Malouf NN, Sommer JR: Chicken dystrophy. The geometry of the transverse tubules. Am J Pathol 84:299–316, 1976

32. Ettienne EM, Singer RH: Ca^{2+} binding, ATP-dependent Ca^{2+} transport and total tissue Ca^{2+} in embryonic and adult avian dystrophic pectoralis. J Membr Biol 44:195–210, 1978

33. Sabbadini R, Scales D, Inesi G: Ca^{2+} transport and assembly of protein particles in sarcoplasmic membranes isolated from normal and dystrophic muscle. FEBS Lett 54:8–12, 1975

34. Scales D, Sabbadini R, Inesi G: The involvement of sarcoplasmic membranes in genetic muscular dystrophy. Biochim Biophys Acta 465:535–549, 1977

35. Scales DJ, Sabbadini RA: Microsomal T system: a stereological analysis of purified microsomes derived from normal and dystrophic skeletal muscle. J Cell Biol 83:33–46, 1979

36. Verjovski-Almeida S, Inesi G. Rapid kinetics of calcium ion transport and ATPase activity in the sarcoplasmic reticulum of dystrophic muscle. Biochim Biophys Acta 558:119–125, 1979

37. Yap JL, MacLennan DH: Characterization of the adenosine-triphosphatase and calsequestrin isolated from sarcoplasmic reticulum of normal and dystrophic chickens. Can J Biochem 54:670–673, 1976

38. Allen ER, Murphy BJ: Sarcotubular development in dystrophic skeletal muscle cells. Cell Tissue Res 194:125–130, 1978

39. Rowland LP: Biochemistry of muscle membranes in Duchenne muscular dystrophy. Muscle Nerve 3:3–20, 1980

40. Sreter FA: Temperature, pH and seasonal dependence of Ca uptake and ATPase activity of white and red muscle microsomes. Arch Biochem Biophys 134:25–33, 1969

41. Sreter FA, Luff AR, Gergely J: Effect of cross reinnervation on physiological parameters and on properties of myosin and sarcoplasmic reticulum of fast and slow muscles of the rabbit. J Gen Physiol 66:811–821, 1975

42. Sreter FA: Effect of denervation on fragmented sarcoplasmic reticulum of white and red muscle. Exp Neurol 29:52–64, 1970

43. Heilmann C, Pette D: Molecular transformations in sarcoplasmic reticulum of fast twitch muscle by electrostimulation. Eur J Biochem 93:437–446, 1979

44. Wang T, Grassi AO, Schwartz A: Kinetic properties of calcium adenosine triphosphatase of sarcoplasmic reticulum isolated from cat skeletal muscles. J Biol Chem 254:10675–10678, 1979

45. Beringer T: A freeze fracture study of sarcoplasmic reticulum from fast and slow muscle of the mouse. Anat Rec 184:647–663, 1976

46. Bray DF, Rayns DG: A comparative freeze-etch study of the sarcoplasmic reticulum of avian fast and slow muscle fibers. J Ultrastruct Res 57:251–259, 1976

47. Franzini-Armstrong C: Structure of sarcoplasmic reticulum. Fed Proc 39:2403–2409, 1980

48. Lau YH, Caswell AH, Brunschwig JP: Isolation of transverse tubules by fractionation of triad junctions of skeletal muscle. J Biol Chem 252:5565–5574, 1977

49. Lau YH, Caswell AH, Brunschwig JP, et al: Lipid analysis and freeze fracture studies on isolated transverse tubules and sarcoplasmic reticulum subfractions of skeletal muscle. J Biol Chem 254:540–546, 1979

50. Caswell AH, Lau YH, Garcia M, Brunschwig JP: Recognition and junction formation by isolated transverse tubules and terminal cisternae of skeletal muscle. J Biol Chem 254:202–208, 1979

51. Lau YH, Caswell AH, Garcia M, Letellier L: Ouabain binding and coupled sodium, potassium and chloride transport in isolated transverse tubules of skeletal muscle. J Gen Physiol 74:335–349, 1979

52. Michalak M, Campbell KP, MacLennan DH: Localization of the high affinity calcium binding protein and an intrinsic glycoprotein in sarcoplasmic reticulum membranes. J Biol Chem 255:1317–1326, 1980

53. Deamer DW, Baskin RJ: Ultrastructure of sarcoplasmic reticulum preparations. J Cell Biol 42:296–307, 1969

54. Ikemoto N, Sreter FA, Nakamura A, Gergely J: Tryptic digestion and localization of calcium uptake and ATPase activity in fragments of sarcoplasmic reticulum. J Ultrastruct Res 23:216–232, 1968

55. Martonosi A: Sarcoplasmic reticulum. V. The structure of sarcoplasmic reticulum membranes. Biochim Biophys Acta 150:694–704, 1968

56. Wang CT, Saito A, Fleischer S: Correlation of ultrastructure of reconstituted sarcoplasmic reticulum membrane vesicles with variation in phospholipid to protein ratio. J Biol Chem 254:9209–9219, 1979

57. Herbette L, Marquardt J, Scarpa A, Blasie JK: A direct analysis of lameller x-ray diffraction from hydrated oriented multilayers of fully functional sarcoplasmic reticulum. Biophys J 20:245–272, 1977

58. Jilka RL, Martonosi AN, Tillack TW: Effect of the purified $(Mg^{2+} + Ca^{2+})$ activated ATPase of sarcoplasmic reticulum upon the passive Ca permeability and ultrastructure of phospholipid vesicles. J Biol Chem 250:7511–7524, 1975

59. Martonosi A: Membrane transport during development in animals. Biochim Biophys Acta 415:311–333, 1975

60. Tillack TW, Boland R, Martonosi A: The ultrastructure of developing sarcoplasmic reticulum. J Biol Chem 249:624–633, 1974

61. Scales D, Inesi G: Assembly of ATPase protein in sarcoplasmic reticulum membranes. Biophys J 16:735–751, 1976

62. Moller JV, Lind KE, Anderson JP: Enzyme kinetics and substrate stabilization of detergent-solubilized and membraneous $(Ca^{2+} + Mg^{2+})$-activated ATPase from sarcoplasmic reticulum. J Biol Chem 255:1912–1920, 1980

63. Vanderkooi JM, Ierokomos A, Nakamura H, Martonosi A: Fluorescence energy transfer between Ca^{2+} transport ATPase molecules in artificial membranes. Biochemistry 16:1262–1267, 1977

64. Martonosi A: The mechanism of Ca transport in sarcoplasmic reticulum. In *Calcium Transport in Contraction and Secretion.* Edited by Carafoli E, Clementi F, Drabikowski W, Margreth A. North-Holland Publishing Co, Amsterdam 1975, pp 313–327

65. Inesi G, Kurzmack M, Coan C, Lewis DE: Cooperative calcium binding and ATPase activation in sarcoplasmic reticulum vesicles. J Biol Chem 255:3025–3031, 1980

66. Boland R, Martonosi A, Tillack TW: Developmental changes in the composition and function of sarcoplasmic reticulum. J Biol Chem 249;612–623, 1974

67. Martonosi A, Roufa D, Boland R, et al: Development of sarcoplasmic reticulum in cultured chicken muscle. J Biol Chem 252:318–332, 1977

68. Froehlich JP, Taylor EW: Transient state kinetic effects of calcium ion on sarcoplasmic reticulum adenosine triphosphatase. J Biol Chem 251:2307–2315, 1976

69. Dupont Y, Leigh JB: Transient kinetics of sarcoplasmic reticulum Ca^{2+} + Mg^{2+} ATPase studied by fluorescence. Nature 273:396–398, 1978

70. Ikemoto N, Morgan JF, Yamada S: Ca^{2+}-controlled conformational states of the Ca^{2+} transport enzyme of sarcoplasmic reticulum. J Biol Chem 253:8027–8033, 1978

71. Coan C, Verjovski-Almeida S, Inesi G: Ca regulation of conformational states in the transport cycle of spin-labeled sarcoplasmic reticulum ATPase. J Biol Chem 254:2968–2974, 1979

72. Degani C, Boyer PD: A borohydride reduction method for characterization of the acyl phosphate linkage in proteins and its application to sarcoplasmic reticulum adenosine triphosphatase. J Biol Chem 248:8222–8226, 1973

73. Ikemoto N: Behavior of the Ca^{2+} transport sites linked with the phosphorylation reaction of ATPase purified from the sarcoplasmic reticulum. J Biol Chem 251:7275–7277, 1976

74. Knowles AF, Racker E: Properties of a reconstituted calcium pump. J Biol Chem 250:3538–3544, 1975

75. Martonosi A, Lagwinska E, Oliver M: Elementary processes in the hydrolysis of ATP by sarcoplasmic reticulum membranes. Ann NY Acad Sci 227:549–567, 1974

76. Hasselbach W: The reversibility of the sarcoplasmic calcium pump. Biochim Biophys Acta 515:23–53, 1978

77. Martonosi A, Donley JR, Pucell AG, Halpin RA: Sarcoplasmic reticulum. XI. The mode of involvement of phospholipids in the hydrolysis of ATP by sarcoplasmic reticulum membranes. Arch Biochem Biophys 144:529–540, 1971

78. Nakamura H, Jilka RL, Boland R, Martonosi A: Mechanism of ATP hydrolysis by sarcoplasmic reticulum and the role of phospholipids. J Biol Chem 251:5414–5423, 1976

79. Hidalgo C, Thomas DD, Ikemoto N: Effect of the lipid environment on protein motion and enzymatic activity of sarcoplasmic reticulum Ca-ATPase. J Biol Chem 253:6879–6887, 1978

80. Dupont Y: Kinetics and regulation of sarcoplasmic reticulum ATPase. Eur J Biochem 72:185–190, 1977

81. Boyer PD, Ariki M: ^{18}O-probes of phosphoenzyme formation and cooperativity with sarcoplasmic reticulum ATPase. Fed Proc 39:2410–2414, 1980

82. Lemaire M, Møller JV, Tanford C: Retention of enzyme activity by detergent-solubilized sarcoplasmic Ca^{2+}-ATPase. Biochemistry 15:2336–2342, 1976

83. Martonosi A: Protein-protein interactions in sarcoplasmic reticulum: functional significance. In *Membrane Proteins*. Edited by Nicholls P, Møller JV, Jørgensen PL, Moody AJ. Pergamon Press, New York, 1978, pp 135–148

84. VanBreemen VL: Ultrastructure of human muscle. II. Observations on dystrophic striated muscle fibers. Am J Pathol 37:333–342, 1960

85. Pearce GW: Tissue culture and electron microscopy in muscle disease. In *Disorders of Voluntary Muscle*. Edited by Walton JN. Little Brown, Boston, 1964, pp 220–254

86. Milhorat AT, Shafiq SA, Goldstone L: Changes in muscle structure in dystrophic patients, carriers and normal siblings seen by electron microscopy; correlation with levels of serum creatine-phosphokinase (CPK). Ann NY Acad Sci 138:246–292, 1966

87. Beringer T: Stereologic analysis of normal and dystrophic avian αW myofibers. Exp Neurol 61:380–394, 1978

88. Mokri B, Engel AG: Duchenne dystrophy: electron microscopic findings pointing to a basic or early abnormality in the plasma membrane of the muscle fiber. Neurology (Minneap) 25:1111–1120, 1975

89. Schotland DL, Bonilla E, Van Meter M: Duchenne dystrophy: alteration in muscle membrane structure. Science 196:1005–1007, 1977

90. Schotland DL, Bonilla E, Wakayama Y: Application of the freeze fracture technique to the study of human neuromuscular disease. Muscle Nerve 3:21–27, 1980

91. Costello BR, Shafiq SA: Freeze-fracture study of muscle plasmalemma in normal and dystrophic chickens. Muscle Nerve 2:191–201, 1979

92. Yoshioka M, Okuda R. Human skeletal muscle fibers in normal and pathological states: freeze-etch replica observations. J Electron Microscopy (Tokyo) 26:103–110, 1977

93. Ketelsen U-P: Ultrastructure of dystrophic skeletal muscle. Isr J Med Sci 13:107–120, 1977

94. Shafiq SA. Leung B, Schulta HS: Reduced density of intramembrane particles in erythrocytes of dystrophic chickens. J Neurol Sci 30:299–302, 1976

95. Pellegrino C, Franzini C: An electron microscope study of denervation atrophy in red and white skeletal muscle fibers. J Cell Biol 17:327–349, 1963

96. Ishikawa H: Formation of elaborate networks of T-system tubules in cultured skeletal muscle with special reference to the T-system formation. J Cell Biol 38:51–66, 1968

97. Brust M: Relative resistance to dystrophy of slow skeletal muscle of the mouse. Am J Physiol 210:445–451, 1966

98. Cosmos E, Butler J: Differentiation of fiber types in muscle of normal and dystrophic chicken. In *Exploratory Concepts of Muscular Dystrophy and Related Disorders* Edited by Milhorat AT. Excerpta Medica, Amsterdam, New York, 1967, pp 197–204

99. Shafiq SA, Askanas V, Milhorat AT: Fiber types nd preclinical changes in chicken muscular dystrophy. Arch Neurol 25:560–571, 1971

100. Ashmore CR, Doerr L: Postnatal development of fiber types in normal and dystrophic skeletal muscle of the chick. Exp Neurol 30:431–446, 1971

101. Banker BQ: A phase and electron microscopic study of dystrophic muscle. II. The pathological changes in the newborn Bar Harbor 129 dystrophic mouse. J Neuropathol Exp Neurol 27:183–209, 1968

102. Platzer AC, Powell JA: Fine structure of prenatal and early postnatal dystrophic mouse muscle. J Neurol Sci 24:109–126, 1975

103. Sandow A, Brust M: Contractility of dystrophic mouse muscle. Am J Physiol 194:557–563, 1958

104. Peter JB, Worsfold M: Oxidative phosphorylation and calcium transport by sarcotubular vesicles in myotonic dystrophy. Biochem Med 2:457–460, 1969

105. McComas AJ, Sica REP, Currie S: An electrophysiological study of Duchenne dystrophy. J Neurol Neurosurg Psychiatry 34:461–468, 1971

106. Roe RD, Yamaji K, Sandow A: Contractile responses of dystrophic muscles of mouse and man. In *Exploratory Concepts in Muscular Dystrophy and Related Disorders*. Edited by Milhorat AT. Excerpta Medica, Amsterdam, New York, 1967, pp 299–304

107. Dubowitz V, Brooke MH: In *Muscle Biopsy: A Modern Approach*. WB Saunders, Philadelphia, 1973, p 168

DISCUSSION

Dr. Frank Sreter: I wonder whether changes in the fiber distribution might also play a role in the decreased calcium uptake of the sarcoplasmic reticulum from dystrophic muscle. We recently found that even among the fast fibers, calcium uptake ability of type 2A fibers had only about 35% or 40% of the calcium uptake ability of 2B fibers.

Dr. Anthony Martonosi: In addition to the single fiber typing, of course, age differences may also contribute. If there is significant regeneration in a dystrophic muscle, as there is usually, the younger fibers would contain much less calcium transport activity in the sarcoplasmic reticulum.

Dr. Frederick Samaha: I would like to emphasize the need to do single-fiber studies, because the differences among the various fiber types in human muscle with regard to sarcoplasmic reticulum transport have not been demonstrated and the matter is confused. For example, when studying myosin light chains in human skeletal muscle, you think you are dealing with a mixture of all of these fiber types; yet all I can isolate are two light chains (and it is not a mixture of fast and slow light chains). We need to demonstrate what the various fiber types do in terms of calcium transport and then translate this fiber by fiber to dystrophic muscle.

Dr. Anthony Martonosi: The differences in calcium transport activity will probably result from contributions by fiber type, age, adipose and connective tissue, and contaminating membrane elements; some effort should be made to coordinate all of these contributions in the final evaluation of the differences.

Dr. Frederick Samaha: I agree.

Dr. Alan McComas: Do you think that the difference you showed in calcium-transporting activity between fast- and slow-twitch muscle is entirely responsible for the very much greater post-activation potentiation of the twitch in fast-twitch muscle? Apropos of that, Dr. Belanger and I have shown that this difference in post-activation potentiation between fast- and slow-twitch muscle is very obvious in human muscle as well as in animal muscle.

Dr. Anthony Martonosi: I do not know.

Dr. Frank Jolesz: This is not a question, but a comment. With regard to Dr. Samaha's results with human single fibers, we checked approximately 100 human single fibers and found that fast single fibers contain 3 light chains; slow single fibers, 2 light chains. So there is no difference between human and rabbit single fibers with respect to the number of light chains (LC). Even the mobility of the LC_1 is the same in slow- and fast-twitch human single fibers. The only difference is the mobility of LC_2 fast and LC_2 slow and the presence of LC_3 in fast fibers. In the pyrophosphate gel pattern of human single fibers, there are at least four myosin isozymes, about the same number as in rabbit single fibers. However, in comigration experiments in a pyrophosphate-gel system, we also found mobility differences between human and rabbit isoenzymes.

45
Regulation of Intracellular Motility by Calcium-Calmodulin

John R. Dedman, PhD

Anthony R. Means, PhD

During the past decade, considerable effort has been directed toward an understanding of the structural and molecular basis of motility in eukaryotic cells. The finding of major muscle contractile proteins in all cells has suggested that many forms of cell movement may occur in a manner analogous to muscle contraction. The concept of cell motility includes not only the migration of entire cells, but also the movement of intracytoplasmic components such as chromosomes, centrioles, lysosomes, secretory granules, and various endocytotic and exocytotic vesicles. The regulation of motility and its relationship with other cellular processes has received considerable attention and has been the topic of recent reviews (1–3) and symposia (4–6). Certain fundamental questions have been raised, especially with regard to the similarity between skeletal muscle and nonmuscle motility, including the involvement of motility in cellular functions such as cell division and secretion, and whether these processes have a common denominator. We present in this chapter the similarities between muscle contraction and secretion, and the dynamic role played by Ca^{2+} in coupling these cellular processes.

EXCITATION-CONTRACTION COUPLING

Few biologic systems are understood at both the physiologic and chemical level as well as the process of skeletal muscle contraction. The cause and effect are clear and exaggerated. Release of acetylcholine by the efferent neurons at the myoneural junctions causes a spike potential and depolarization of the sarcolemma. This depolarization extends through the membranous transverse tubular system and sarcoplasmic reticulum (SR), which surrounds the myofibrillar units. Calcium is liberated from the SR, increasing the free Ca^{2+} levels from 0.1 to 10 μM. The increased Ca^{2+} then binds to troponin, which, in turn, allows the head piece of myosin to interact with actin (the major component of the thin filament). This interaction activates the myosin adenosine triphosphatase (AT-Pase), hydrolyzes adenosine triphosphate (ATP), and promotes shortening of the myofibril (and muscle). Thus, excitation-contraction coupling is complete. Relaxation is essentially the reverse process initiated by sarcolemmal repolarization and active transport of Ca^{2+} from troponin into the SR. As described, Ca^{2+} is the essential factor in this series of events, and troponin acts as the intracellular receptor. Troponin is a tight complex of 3 distinct proteins, troponin-T (binds to tropomyosin), troponin-I (required for ATPase inhibitor), and troponin-C (binds Ca^{2+}). All 3 subunits are necessary for the proper regulation of muscle actomyosin ATPase. Hence, troponin-C (TnC) acts as the Ca^{2+} transducer in the modulation of actin-myosin interaction, ATPase activity, and muscle contraction.

STIMULUS-SECRETION COUPLING

Exocytosis is postulated to be a multiphasic process involving intracellular synthesis of the exportable substance, packaging and intracellular transport of the substance to the cell periphery, and finally, membrane fusion and extracellular discharge. The regulation of secretion may occur at any one of these steps.

One of the better understood mechanisms of secretion is the synthesis and release of insulin from the pancreatic beta cell. The major physiologic initiator of insulin release is D-glucose (10 to 20 mM). Insulin secretion from the perfused rat pancreas in response to glucose is biphasic. The immediate response of the beta cell is to release stored hormone (within 1 minute); secretion then declines within 5 minutes. Continued exposure to glucose (10 minutes) causes a second, more prolonged period of hormone release (7, 8). The first phase of secretion is puromycin independent; the second is partially blocked by the drug, indicating insulinogenesis. In fact, a number of studies have shown that glucose initiates the formation of proinsulin, which is transported (by an energy-requiring process) to the Golgi complex (9–11). There, the C-peptide is enzymatically removed by a specific protease. The newly synthesized insulin is packaged into granules that are surrounded by membranous sacs derived from the Golgi apparatus. Ultrastructural studies show that, after glucose stimulation, the granules move to the plasma membrane, fuse with the plasma membrane, and liberate hormone into the extracellular space (12). Both phases of secretion are Ca^{2+} dependent. However, Ca^{2+} (unlike puromycin or glucose) has no effect on the incorporation of radioactive amino acids into de novo synthesized insulin.

Experiments demonstrating the requirement for Ca^{2+} in the secretory process were pioneered by Douglas and Rubin (13). They demonstrated that acetylcholine-induced catecholamine release from the perfused cat adrenal gland was dependent on the presence of Ca^{2+} in the perfusate. Realizing the similarity with muscle contraction (excitation-contraction coupling), the process was coined "stimulus-secretion coupling." This original concept has provided the basis for the experimental approach regarding the mechanism of secretion. The requirement for Ca^{2+} applies to the release of secretory substances from a wide variety of tissues.

Using electrophysiologic techniques, Dean and Matthews (14) found that glucose stimulation of beta cells produced electrical changes in the membranes. Depletion of Ca^{2+} prevented changes in the electrical activity, and increased Ca^{2+} increased the amplitude of the membrane potential amplitude (15). Furthermore, D-600, a Ca^{2+} antagonist, blocked electrical activity (16), Ca^{2+} uptake, and insulin release (17). These results suggest a voltage-dependent channel for Ca^{2+} (with entry of Ca^{2+} following a spike potential) that is necessary for initiating the intracellular secretory process.

Davis and Lazarus (18) have demonstrated an absolute requirement for Ca^{2+} in insulin secretion. The rate of release was stimulated 6-fold by 2 μM Ca^{2+}; ATP further augmented the rate of release. These findings further describe the similarity between muscle contraction and secretion. Parallels can be drawn between muscle contraction and the secretory process. Nonmuscle cells contain the contractile elements actin, myosin, tropomyosin, and a smooth endoplasmic reticulum analogous to the Ca^{2+}-chelating SR.

CYTOSKELETON AND SECRETION

Non-muscle cell actin is found as 6-nm microfilaments that are distributed, often in parallel arrays, under the plasma membrane and often extend down microprojections. The microfilaments can often form highly organized bundles as large as 1 μm in diameter and may contain a number of associated proteins (myosin, tropomyosin, filamin, α-actinin) (see reference 1). Cells also contain a cytoplasmic microtubular complex composed of polymers of 6S-tubulin dimers. The involvement of the microfilament-microtubular system in the release of insulin was first suggested by Lacy and colleagues (11). They found that colchicine, a drug that depolymerizes microtubules, inhibited glucose-induced insulin secretion. Similarly, Allison (19) reported that vinblastine (also a micro-tubule destabilizer) as well as deuterium oxide (a microtubule-stabilizing agent) inhibited both phases of glucose-induced insulin secretion. Malaisse-Lagae and associates (20) have reported a decreased rate of insulin release from the pancreas of spiny mice (*Acomys cahirinus*), animals with one-fourth the normal level of microtubules.

Pipeleers and coworkers (21) have suggested that insulin secretion may be regulated by the degree of tubulin polymerization. They found that the polymerized fraction and total tubulin decreased in islets of fasted rats; both were restored to normal levels by glucose feeding. Additional studies (22) demonstrated that glucose increased tubulin synthesis 2- to 3-fold, reversing a 75% decrease in synthesis caused by fasting. In contrast, administration of cytochalasin B, which disrupts microfilaments, enhances glucose-induced insulin release (23). This agent does inhibit the release of amylase from the parotid gland (24), histamine from mast cells (25), adrenocorticotropic hormone from the adrenohypophysis (26), and vasopressin from the neurohypophysis (17).

Collectively, these findings suggests that the microfilament and microtubular systems are involved in the normal functioning of the secretory process. Microtubules could provide a structural lattice that defines and orients the directional flow of the secretory granules, and the microfilaments could provide the motile force for granule movement. The model would then require that

Ca^{2+} be involved in the regulation of these cytoskeletal elements during the secretory process.

CALMODULIN

Although smooth and non-muscle cells contain many of the contractile elements found in muscle, the troponin complex (TnT:TnC:TnI) is not present. This suggests that the molecular arrangement and regulation of smooth and non-muscle actomyosin are different from those of muscle. A protein structurally similar to TnC is present in virtually all eukaryotic cells at concentrations ranging from 1 to 10 μM and is referred to as calmodulin (27–29). This heat-stable protein represents the major high affinity Ca^{2+}-binding protein in non-muscle tissue. Each mole of calmodulin binds 4 moles of Ca^{2+} (Kd, approximately 0.4 μM) and this interaction is not affected by high Mg^{2+} levels (30). The binding of Ca^{2+} to calmodulin causes significant intramolecular changes that are necessary for its interaction with other proteins.

Calmodulin consists of 148 amino acids (Mr ~ 17,000), which is 11 residues shorter than skeletal muscle TnC. However, the remaining regions of the sequences align with approximately 50% direct homology and 70% homology in the Ca^{2+}-binding site regions (31, 32). Antibodies to calmodulin have been produced and purified by antigen-affinity chromatography (33). The antibodies specifically inhibit the activation of phosphodiesterase and specifically immunoprecipitate labeled calmodulin (34). Using indirect immunofluorescence, it has been shown that calmodulin is associated with the actin-containing stress fibers of interphase cells (33) and with the mitotic apparatus of dividing cells (34, 35).

To date, calmodulin has been shown to mediate the Ca^{2+} regulation of a number of fundamental intracellular enzyme systems. These enzymes include cyclic nucleotide phosphodiesterase, brain adenylate cyclase, human erythrocyte membrane Ca,Mg-ATPase, myosin light chain kinase, and skeletal muscle phosphorylase kinase (27–29). It has also been shown to be the Ca^{2+}-binding component that regulates Ca^{2+} transport in skeletal microsomes and the Ca^{2+}-dependent phosphorylation in membranes isolated from a variety of tissues (1). Thus, calmodulin, which is the predominant Ca^{2+}-binding protein in smooth and non-muscle cells, is involved in the regulation of such fundamental biological processes as cyclic nucleotide and glycogen metabolism, motility, karyokinesis, and Ca^{2+} transport. The protein is considered to be ubiquitous in eukaryotes, and the primary structure has been strictly conserved through the animal and plant kingdoms. These facts reflect the important role calmodulin plays as an intracellular Ca^{2+} receptor.

REGULATION OF CELLULAR CALCIUM

Calcium is unevenly distributed within cells, as well as across the various membranes. Assessment of the intracellular distribution of Ca is a complex problem because although total cellular Ca concentration is high (approximately 1 mM), it exists in several states. Experiments using $^{45}Ca^{2+}$ exchange have revealed non-exchangeable and exchangeable forms of the cation. Much of the non-exchangeable Ca is in the mineralized precipitated state, such as hydroxylapatite, and is metabolically inaccessible. The exchangeable Ca itself exists in several diffusible states, including complexed and ionized forms. The complexed Ca can be further categorized by high and low affinity binding to intracellular components, e.g., proteins, phospholipids, and metabolites.

Using the photoprotein aequorin and Ca-sensitive dyes such as Arsenazo III, the free, intracellular, cytoplasmic Ca^{2+} has been determined to be approximately 0.1 μM. Because extracellular Ca^{2+} concentrations are approximately 1 mM, there is an estimated 1,000-fold gradient between the extracellular and intracellular concentrations. This gradient is maintained by several mechanisms. Calcium-specific ATPase actively transport Ca from the cytoplasm to the extracellular spaces or sequester this cation intracellularly. These Ca^{2+} "pumps" are located in the plasma membrane, mitochondria, and smooth endoplasmic reticulum. It has been recently shown that a purified cytosolic factor (calmodulin) activates the plasma membrane Ca,Mg-ATPase (27–29).

Blitz and associates (36) have shown that SR and the endoplasmic reticulum of non-muscle cells possess a number of biochemical similarities. Furthermore, Ca^{2+} uptake has been demonstrated in microsome fractions prepared from a number of cell types: in vitro transport studies have been done in platelets, renal cells, fibroblasts, hepatocytes, parotid cells, brain cells, and adipocytes (see reference 1 for review). Even though these studies vary widely in methodology, they have a number of similarities that generally characterize non-muscle microsomal uptake. Transport is Mg-ATP dependent, markedly sustained by oxalate, inhibited by La^{3+}, and reversed by the Ca ionophore A23187. The microsomes contain an associated Ca-stimulated ATPase and membrane proteins that are phosphorylated.

This type of Ca transport system is readily discernible from mitochondrial transport by its insensitivity to ruthenium, azide, and oligomycin. All of these features are also characteristic of SR Ca-uptake systems. Hence, an analogy can be drawn between SR Ca sequestration and non-muscle endoplasmic reticulum Ca uptake. However, non-muscle cells probably use mitochondria as their major means of rapid Ca sequestration from the cytoplasm. Several studies have shown that intracellular Ca transport in non-muscle cells is inhibited 85% to 90% in the presence of specific mitochondrial inhibitors (37–39). These results indicate that mitochondria have a greater ability to suquester Ca, both with respect to initial rate and capacity, than do the endoplasmic reticulum and plasma membrane systems together. However, the plasma membrane pump is responsible for extruding the Ca that continually enters the cells. Otherwise, the capacity of the endoplasmic reticulum in mitochondria would eventually be exceeded. Collectively, these experiments demonstrate that energy-requiring (ATP) Ca extrusion is important in maintaining Ca homeostasis and that calmodulin is involved in this cellular process.

REGULATION OF MICROFILAMENTS

As mentioned, actomyosin has been found in a variety of non-muscle cells and tissues. The myosin molecule is composed of one pair of heavy chains (MW, 200,000 daltons) and a combination of two pairs of light chains (MW, 17,000 to 20,000 daltons). At one end of the heavy chain, the polypeptide chain is globular; this portion contains the actin-binding properties and the ATPase activity. The light chains are associated with the globular region and are proposed to regulate actin-binding and ATPase activities. One pair of light chains may be phosphorylated to different degrees.

Actin activation of the myosin MG-ATPase of non-muscle myosin occurs only after phosphorylation of the light chains (3). Sobieszek (40) and Sobieszek and Small (41) have convincingly demonstrated a direct relationship between Ca concentration and the degree of light chain phosphorylation and ATPase activation. Lebowitz and Cooke (42) have demonstrated that the degree of light chain phosphorylation is directly correlated with development of tension. These studies demonstrate that tissues other than striated muscle are regulated via myosin rather than via the troponin-tropomyosin complex. Pires and Perry (43) found Ca-dependent light chain specific protein kinase in striated muscle. During purification of this kinase, Yazawa and Yagi (44) revealed that it was composed of a catalytic subunit and a Ca-binding regulatory subunit (Mr $\sim$ 20,000). Yagi and colleagues (45) later identified this regulatory subunit as calmodulin. These findings have recently been confirmed in the regulation of smooth muscle myosin ATPase (46, 47) and hamster kidney BHK-22 cells (48).

The contraction-relaxation cycle in non-muscle tissues is regulated by changes in cellular Ca mediated by calmodulin activation of the light chain kinase. In the presence of ATP, the light chains are phosphorylated, the myosin ATPase is actin activated, and tension is developed. The process can be reversed by decreasing the cellular Ca concentration. The myosin light chains are then dephosphorylated by light chain phosphatase. This reversable cascade of events is initially and primarily controlled by changes in the intracellular Ca and may represent the force involved in the movement and release of intracellular secretory granules.

MICROTUBULE ASSEMBLY/DISASSEMBLY

Biochemically, microtubules are primarily composed of dimeric 6S-tubulin subunits (MW 110,000 daltons), which exist in a steady state of equilibrium with the polymer [n(6S) $\leftrightarrows$ (6S)$_n$]. Hence, agents that stabilize the polymerized state (D$_2$O and glycerol) shift this equilibrium to the right, whereas agents that make the dimers unavailable for assembly (vinblastine and colchicine) cause disassembly. Weisenberg (49) found that under the proper conditions, i.e., optimal concentrations of guanosine triphosphate (GTP), Mg^{2+}, ethyleneglycol tetraacetate, (EGTA), buffer, pH 7.0, and 37°C, tubulin and the microtubule-associated proteins (MAPs) will assemble in vitro. Weisenberg (49) and Haga and colleagues (50) reported that in crude extracts, micromolar concentrations of Ca prevented tubulin assembly. In contrast, purified microtubules lose this property, demonstrating half-maximal inhibition of assembly at 0.5 to 1.0 mM Ca.

The fact that tubulin and microtubules are purified from crude systems due to their ability to assemble suggests that agents promoting disassembly of microtubules are selected against and agents important in assembly are selected for during the purification procedures. This suggested that the component which mediated the calcium effect on microtubules during the assembly/disassembly procedure was being purified out of the microtubule preparations. Welsh et al[51] demonstrated that calmodulin was localized to the mitotic spindle, suggesting that calmodulin may be involved in the assembly/disassembly process of microtubules.

Marcum and coworkers (52) extended these studies to the assembly/disassembly process of microtubule proteins isolated from rat brain. In vitro microtubule polymerization was initiated by the addition of GTP at 37° C and monitored by the change in absorbance at 320 nm. In the presence of 0.4 μM Ca, purified microtubule protein demonstrated a rapid rate of polymerization and reached a stable plateau after 10 minutes. Addition of calmodulin to the assembly assay (after removal of free Ca by EGTA) did not appreciably alter either the rate or the degree of microtubule polymerization. Increasing the free Ca^{2+} concentration to 11 μM caused a 15% reduction in the extent of polymerization; however, addition of 11 μM Ca as well as calmodulin resulted in the total inhibition of microtubule assembly. Thus, the Ca-calmodulin complex prevented the assembly of microtubules in vitro. It was shown in a similar manner that Ca-calmodulin could rapidly depolymerize fully polymerized microtubules.

These data offer the possibility that calmodulin may play a physiologic role in the control of microtubule assembly/disassembly process. Thus, one would expect that when a secretory cell is stimulated, (e.g., the beta cell by glucose), there is membrane depolarization and an influx of extracellular Ca, which increases the cytosolic Ca to approximately 10 μM. This Ca saturates the binding sites of calmodulin, which in turn activates both the motile forces of actin and myosin (via light chain kinase) and causes a controlled depolymerization of microtubules.

CONCLUSIONS

We have attempted to demonstrate the correlations among muscle contraction, secretion, and intracellular Ca transients. Of course a number of experiments remain to be completed. It is necessary to localize calmodulin, tubulin, actin, and light chain kinase in muscle and secretory cells such as the beta cell before and during glucose stimulation. This immunochemical information should indicate the special relationship of the cytoskeleton with muscle contraction and the formation, movement, and expulsion of the secretory granules. On a chemical level, it is necessary to isolate Ca-dependent ATPases and elucidate the Ca pump properties. Finally, these findings need to be correlated with the permissive effects of cyclic adenosine monophosphate known to occur during muscle contraction and in the secretory process. As we have described, both processes are highly complex and involve a number of subcellular systems that are not well understood. The one common denominator of all the systems is Ca^{2+}, and the only ubiquitous Ca^{2+} receptor is calmodulin. Future efforts should be directed toward elucidating the precise roles of Ca^{2+}-calmodulin in each of the individual reactions.

ACKNOWLEDGMENTS

The authors' research cited in this chapter was supported by grants, GM25557 (Dr. Dedman) and HD-07503 (Dr. Means) from the National Institutes of Health. Dr. Dedman is a Research and Career Development awardee (AM-00609).

We express our indebtness to Ms. Suzanne Kavanagh for preparing the final manuscript.

REFERENCES

1. Dedman JR, Brinkley BR, Means AR: Regulation of microfilaments and microtubules by calcium and cyclic AMP. Adv Cyclic Nucleotide Res 11:131–174, 1979

2. Hitchock SE: Regulation of motility in non-muscle cells. J Cell Biol 74:1–15, 1977

3. Korn ED: Biochemistry of actomyosin dependent cell motility (a review). Proc Natl Acad Sci USA 75:588–599, 1978

4. Carafoli E, Clementi F, Drabikowski W, Margerth A (eds): *Calcium Transport in Contraction and Secretion.* North-Holland Publishing Co, Amsterdam, 1975

5. Goldman RE, Pollard T, Rosenbaum J (eds): Cell motility. Cold Spring Harbor Conference on Cell Proliferation, 1976

6. Wasserman RH, Corrinadino RA, Carafoli E, et al (eds): *Calcium binding Proteins and Calcium Function.* Elsevier/North-Holland, New York, 1977

7. Curry DL, Bennett LL, Grodsky GM. Dynamics of insulin secretion by the perfused rat pancreas. Endocrinology 83:572–584, 1968

8. Curry DL, Bennett LL, Grodsky GM: Requirement for Ca^{2+} ion in insulin secretion by the perfused rat pancreas. Am J Physiol 214:174–178, 1968

9. Lacy PE: Electron microscopy of the beta cell of the pancreas. Am J Med 31:851–859, 1961

10. Lacy PE: Beta cell secretion-from the standpoint of a pathobiologist. Diabetes 19:895–905, 1970

11. Lacy PE, Howell SL, Young DA, et al: New hypothesis of insulin secretion. Nature 219:1177–1179, 1968

12. Orci LM, Amerhdt R, Malaisse-Lagae F, et al: Insulin release by emiocytosis: demonstration with freeze-etching technique. Science 179:82–84, 1973

13. Douglas WW, Rubin RP: The role of Ca^{2+} in the secretory response of the adrenal medulla to acetylcholine. J Physiol (Lond) 159:40–57, 1961

14. Dean PM, Matthews EK: Glucose-induced electrical activity in pancreatic islet cells. J Physiol (Lond) 210:255–264, 1970

15. Dean PN, Matthews EK: Electrical activity in pancreatic islet cells: effects of ions. J Physiol (Lond) 210:265–275, 1970

16. Matthews EK: Calcium and stimulus-secretion coupling in pancreatic islet cells. In *Calcium Transport in Contraction and Secretion.* Edited by Carafoli E, Clementi F, Drabikowski W, Margreth A. American Elsevier Publishing Co., New York, 1975, pp 203–210

17. Malaisse WJ, Herchuely A, Levt J, et al: Insulin release and the movements of calcium in pancreatic islets. In *Calcium Transport in Contraction and Secretion.* Edited by Carafoli E, Clementi F, Drabikowski W, Margreth A. American Elsevier Publishing Co., New York, 1975, pp 211–226

18. Davis B, Lazarus NR: An in vitro system for studying insulin release caused by secretory granules-plasma membrane interaction: definition of the system. J Physiol (Lond) 256:709–729, 1976

19. Allison AC: The role of microfilaments and microtubules in cell movement, endocytosis and exotyosis. Ciba Found Symp pp 14:109–148, 1973

20. Malaisse-Lagae F, Ravazzola M, Amherdt M, et al: An apparent abnormality of the β-cell microtubular system in spiny mice (*Acomys cahirinus*). Diabetologia 11:71–76, 1975

21. Pipeleers DG, Pipeleers-Marichal MA, Kipnis DM: Microtubule assembly and the intracellular transport of secretory granules in pancreatic islets. Science 191:88–90, 1976

22. Pipeleers DG, Pipeleers-Marichal MA, Kipnis DM: Regulation of tubulin synthesis in islets of Langerhans. Proc Natl Acad Sci USA 73:3188–3191, 1976

23. Orci L, Gabby KH, Malaisse WJ: Pancreatic beta-cell web: its possible role in insulin secretion. Science 175:1128–1130, 1971

24. Butcher FR, Goldman RH: Effect of cytochalasin B and colchicine on the stimulation of γ-amylase release from rat parotid tissue slices. Biochem Biophys Res Commun 48:23–29, 1972

25. Orr TSC, Hall DE, Allison AC: Role of contractile microfilaments in the release of histamine from mast cells. Nature 236:350–351, 1972

26. Kraicer J, Milligan JV: Effect of colchicine on in vitro ACTH release induced by high K^+ and by hypothalamus-stalk-median eminence extract. Endocrinology 89:408–412, 1971

27. Wang JH, Waisman DM: Calmodulin and its role in the second-messenger system. Curr Top Cell Regul 15:47–107, 1979

28. Cheung WY: Calmodulin plays a pivotal role in cellular regulation. Science 207:19–27, 1980

29. Means AR, Dedman JR: Calmodulin: an intracellular calcium receptor. Nature 285:73–77, 1980

30. Dedman JR, Potter JD, Jackson RL, et al: Physiochemical properties of rat testis Ca^{2+}-dependent regulator protein of cyclic nucleotide phosphodiesterase. J Biol Chem 252:8415–8422, 1977

31. Dedman JR, Jackson RL, Schreiber WE, et al: Sequence homology of the Ca^{2+}-dependent regulator of cyclic nucleotide phosphodiesterase from rat testis with other Ca^{2+}-binding proteins. J Biol Chem 253:343–346, 1978

32. Watterson DM, Scharief F, Vanaman TC: The complete amino acid sequence of the Ca^{2+}-dependent modulator protein (Calmodulin) of bovine brain. J Biol Chem 255:962–971, 1980

33. Dedman JR, Welsh MJ, Means AR: Ca^{2+}-dependent regulator: production and characterization of a monospecific antibody. J Biol Chem 253:7515–7521, 1978

34. Chafouleas JG, Dedman JR, Means AR: Calmodulin: development and application of a sensitive radioimmunoassay. J Biol Chem 254:10262–10267, 1979

35. Andersen B, Osborn M, Weber K: Specific visualization of the distribution of the calcium dependent regulatory protein of cyclic nucleotide phosphodiesterase (modulator protein) in tissue culture cells by immunofluorescence microscopy: mitosis and intercellular bridge. Eur J Cell Biol 17:354–364, 1978

36. Blitz AL, Fine RE, Toselli PA: Evidence that coated vesicles isolated from brain are calcium-sequestering organelles resembling sarcoplasmic reticulum. J Cell Biol 75:135–147, 1977

37. Rose B, Loewenstein WR: Calcium ion distribution in cytoplasm visualized by aequorin: diffusion in cytosol restricted by energized sequestering. Science 190:1204–1206, 1975

38. Ash GR, Bygrave FL: Ruthenium red as a probe in assessing the potential of mitochondria to control intracellular calcium in liver. FEBS Lett 78:166–168, 1977

39. Baker PF, Hodgkin AL, Ridgway EB: Depolarization and calcium entry in squid giant axons. J Physiol (Lond) 208:709–755, 1971

40. Sobieszek A: Calcium linked phosphorylation of light chain of vertebrate smooth muscle. Eur J Biochem 73:477–483, 1977

41. Sobieszek A, Small JV: Regulation of the actin-myosin interaction in vertebrate smooth muscle: activation via a myosin light chain kinase and the effect of tropomysin. J Mol Biol 112:559–576, 1977

42. Lebowitz EA, Cooke R: Contractile properties of actomyosin from human blood platelets. J Biol Chem 253:5443–5447, 1978

43. Pires EMV, Perry SV: Purification and properties of myosin light chain kinase from fast skeletal muscle. Biochem J 167:137–146, 1977

44. Yazawa M, Yagi K: A calcium binding subunit of myosin light chain kinase. J Biochem (Tokyo) 82:287–289, 1977

45. Yagi K, Yazawa M, Kakiuchi S, Ohshima M, Uenishi K: Identification of an activator protein for myosin light chain kinase as a calcium-dependent modulator protein. J Biol Chem 253:1338–1340, 1978

46. Dabrowska R, Aromatori D, Sherry JMF, et al: Composition of the myosin light chain kinase from chicken gizzard. Biochem Biophys Res Commun 78:1263–1272, 1977

47. Dabrowska R, Sherry JMF, Aromatori DK, et al: Modulator protein as a component of the myosin light chain kinase in chicken gizzard. Biochemistry 17:253–258, 1978

48. Yerna M-J, Dabrowska R, Hartshorne DJ, et al: Calcium-sensitive regulation of actin-myosin interactions in baby hamster kidney (BHK-21) cells. Proc Natl Acad Sci USA 76:184–188, 1979

49. Weisenberg RC: Microtubule formation in vitro in solutions containing low calcium concentrations. Science 177:1104–1105, 1972

50. Haga T, Abe T, Kurakawa M: Polymerization and depolymerization of microtubules in vitro as studied by flow birefringence. FEBS Lett 39:291–295, 1974

51. Welsh MJ, Dedman JR, Brinkley BR, Means AR: Calcium-dependent regulator protein: localization in the mitotic apparatus of eukaryotic cells. Proc Natl Acad Sci USA 75:1867–1871, 1978

52. Marcum JM, Dedman JR, Brinkley BR, et al: Control of microtubule assembly-disassembly by Ca^{2+}-dependent regulator protein. Proc Natl Acad Sci USA 75:3771–3775, 1978

DISCUSSION

Dr. Michael Bárány: Is there enough calmodulin in skeletal muscle to account for all the enzymes that require calmodulin for activity? I also wish to ask another question. Generally, we assume that during excitation calcium is released from the sarcoplasmic reticulum (SR) and must diffuse from the SR to troponin-C. If we introduce into the sarcoplasm a very high-affinity calcium-binding protein like calmodulin, then a major delay in the attachment of calcium to troponin-C must be considered. Do you think this is likely?

Dr. Anthony Means: These are both very difficult questions to answer, but I will try. To the first question, yes, calmodulin is present in skeletal muscle in sufficient concentrations to justify its various multifunctional roles. Troponin-C represents about 1% to 1.5% of the total protein in skeletal muscle, whereas calmodulin represents about 0.5%. Because of the affinity constants for the two proteins, you could predict that calmodulin could bind about as much calcium as would troponin C. This is particularly true in slow-twitch skeletal muscle but may be somewhat less so in fast-twitch skeletal muscle. The second question is much more difficult; I have no specific answer, because we have not investigated this very important problem. What I can do is reveal to you the suggestion that has been put in the literature by Dr. Jacque Demaille (*Biochemistry*, 1979) dealing with cardiac muscle. In his opinion, calmodulin is only important in the transport of calcium into the SR. He maintains that a calmodulin-dependent kinase is localized in SR that phosphorylates phospholamban in the presence of calmodulin and that this phosphorylation is important for the movement of calcium into the SR. He says nothing about the movement the other way, which is the direction that you are talking about. To my knowledge, there is no information available to answer your question directly.

Dr. John Gergely: In this context, may I ask what is known about the kinetics of the calcium binding and the release from calmodulin?

Dr. Anthony Means: Very little. I was talking with Dr. Prendergast about that earlier. It is known that if you prepare a heat-treated extract from any tissue, add saturating amounts of calcium and a trace amount of ^{45}Ca, and immediately put it onto an ion-exchange column, you can monitor calmodulin via ion-exchange chromatography by the presence of ^{45}Ca, so the metal exchange kinetics must be very rapid.

Dr. Charles Rebouche: Do you know what the role of the trimethyl lysine residue in calmodulin is and whether it is absolutely necessary for its physiologic function?

Dr. Anthony Means: We have speculated that it may be important. In one paper that has just recently appeared (*Proc Natl Acad Sci USA*), Dr. Waterson says that if you synthesize calmodulin in a cell-free system there is no trimethyl lysine. He further maintains that this does not affect the calcium-binding properties of the protein. Whether this may affect the ability of the calcium-calmodulin complex to bind to other proteins remains to be determined, but it is potentially a very important regulatory process.

Dr. Helen Blau: You mentioned that calmodulin is a component of phosphorylase kinase. Is it homologous to troponin-C or calmodulin, or is it yet another distinct calcium-binding protein?

Dr. Anthony Means: This is entirely homologous with calmodulin. Drs. Perry and Cohen have sequenced this molecule and it is identical to calmodulin isolated from any other cell.

46
Malignant Hyperthermia: The Pathogenesis of Abnormal Caffeine Contracture

Donald S. Wood, PhD

Joseph H. Willner, MD

Giovanni Salviati, MD

Clinical and laboratory studies of malignant hyperthermia (MH) are, for the most part, found in journals associated with anesthesiology. Because these studies are not generally familiar, we briefly review observations that led to the concept that MH reactions develop from an inborn error of skeletal muscle metabolism, before discussing our own studies. Extensive discussions of the etiology of this syndrome and of a porcine animal model may be found in two international symposia on MH (1, 2).

GENERAL PERSPECTIVES

Pathognomonic signs of the MH syndrome are an increase in body temperature (hyperthermia, hyperpyrexia), hyperkalemia, and lactic acidosis. Signs that usually precede the increase in body temperature are skeletal muscle rigidity and tachycardia. Cyanosis and myoglobinuria may also occur. The mortality is approximately 70% (3, 4).

Clinical observation and family histories have established that the MH syndrome is pharmocogenetic, requiring an inherited predisposition (autosomal dominant) and a "trigger" event. So far, the only identified "triggers" are inhalational anesthetics such as halothane. Depolarizing muscle relaxants such as succinylcholine are also strongly implicated (4). Malignant hyperthermia reactions in the absence of anesthetics have been reported (5). The "trigger" in these cases is unknown but is postulated to relate to physical or emotional stress.

597

Reports of increased serum creatine phosphokinase (CPK) and abnormal in vitro muscle contracture in response to caffeine in survivors of MH reactions suggested that the genetic error causing susceptibility to MH reactions was expressed in skeletal muscle (6, 7). Subsequent studies of skeletal muscle morphology (8), physiology (9, 10), and serum CPK (11) have extended and confirmed these observations. Nonetheless, this subclinical myopathy remains difficult to define or classify satisfactorily. Abnormalities either are nonspecific (e.g., increased serum CPK level) or lack proof of specificity (e.g., abnormal in vitro muscle contracture).

The only abnormality considered diagnostic for susceptibility to MH reactions is abnormal skeletal muscle contracture in response to caffeine, halothane, succinylcholine, or some combination of these agents (9, 10, 12, 13). However, the muscle preparation used and the results from the contracture studies are controversial. For example, one laboratory reported that halothane elicited contracture in skeletal muscle from virtually all persons who had survived MH reactions but not in control subjects (10). At another center for studies of MH, however, halothane was found to be relatively ineffective at eliciting contracture (9). Reports that succinylcholine-induced contractures are diagnostic for MH are also confined to one laboratory (12); other investigators have been unable to obtain contracture by this approach (9, 10, 13).

The discrepancies between laboratories are unexplained, but could be technical and related to the muscle preparation used. The in vitro muscle preparation used is essentially unique to studies of MH. It consists of a 100- to 300-mg piece of tissue cut at both ends. Maximal forces generated by these preparations are usually less than 0.5 kg/cm^2; intact single fibers or fiber bundles typically develop forces greater than 2.0 kg/cm^2 (14). There are virtually no studies of the basic properties of the cut-end fiber bundles, which makes it difficult to decide between possible explanations of why discrepancies in data occur between different laboratories.

Gallant and associates (15) found that in intact fibers from the porcine animal model for MH, halothane caused depolarization of surface membranes and was without effect in normal muscle. Whether or not these findings in porcine MH are applicable to the human syndrome remains to be determined. Nonetheless, they clearly indicate the need for similar analysis of the electrophysiologic properties of the cut-end preparations. Differences in electrophysiologic properties in these preparations may explain why succinylcholine, a depolarizing muscle relaxant, is found to elicit contracture in one laboratory but not in others.

Interpretation of contracture data is somewhat more straightforward in the case of caffeine. Its site of action is well established to be the sarcoplasmic reticulum (SR), and the effectiveness of caffeine in eliciting contracture does not depend on surface membrane polarity. The possibility of abnormal SR function in MH was first suggested by Kalow and colleagues (7), who reported that isolated SR vesicles accumulated less Ca than normal when exposed to halothane. Subsequent studies of isolated SR vesicles, however, produced conflicting results. Dhalla and coworkers (16) found increased rates of Ca uptake and less Ca release by halothane than normal. Isaacs and Heffron (17) reported generally depressed Ca uptake rates in the absence and presence of halothane. Methods of analysis and vesicle fractions differed in these studies, however, and speculations that differences were "disease related" have not been substantiated.

Our studies of caffeine contracture in single, chemically skinned fiber preparations were initiated to determine whether abnormal caffeine contracture occurred because of abnormal SR function and, if so, whether the abnormality in SR function and caffeine contracture varied between survivors of apparently similar MH reactions.

MATERIALS AND METHODS

Biopsies

Twenty-six control biopsy specimens were obtained from 21 subjects. Biopsy sites were the vastus lateralis (n = 8), gastrocnemius (n = 9), external intercostal (n = 6), and pectoralis (n = 3) muscles. (The number of specimens exceeds 21 because 5 subjects provided 2 biopsy specimens each.)

Control subjects were men and women 17 to 56 years of age without neuromuscular disease and with no family history of the MH syndrome. Six were volunteers, and 3 underwent biopsy procedures after radical mastectomy. The other 12 underwent biopsy for diagnostic reasons. Electromyograms were normal, as were serum enzyme and electrolyte concentrations. Muscle was normal on routine biochemical, morphologic, and histochemical examination.

Our study population consisted of 12 unrelated subjects who had survived MH reactions triggered during anesthesia. The reaction in each case included hyperthermia, skeletal muscle stiffness, and acidosis. Sites of biopsy were vastus lateralis (n = 9) and gastrocnemius (n = 3).

Chemically Skinned Fibers

Biopsy specimens weighing 30 to 50 mg were tied to wooden sticks before excision to maintain fibers at resting length. After excision, they were placed in ice-chilled skinning solution in the operating room and kept at 5° C for 24 hours (18, 19). Exposure of intact mammalian skeletal muscle fibers to "skinning" solution containing 170 mM potassium propionate, 5 mM ethyleneglycol-*bis*-beta(aminoethylether) *N,N'*-tetraacetic acid (EGTA), 2 mM magnesium adenosine triphosphate (Mg-ATP), and 10 mM imidazole at pH 7.00 causes time-dependent changes in morphology and biochemistry that are essentially complete by 24 hours.

After approximately 1 hour, the surface membrane no longer retards the movement of ions into the fiber interior. Measurement of changes in isometric tension show that the fiber responds immediately to changes in bath Ca, ATP, Mg, and EGTA (18, 19). Distinct morphologic changes in surface membranes can be seen after 4 hours (20). The soluble myoplasmic constituents (phosphorylase, lactic dehydrogenase, and glycogen) range between 55% (glycogen) and 95% (phosphorylase) of intact fiber values after 4 hours (Wood DS, DiMauro S: unpublished data).

At 24 hours, distinct holes or gaps are seen in the surface membranes. Mitochondria are swollen, and their internal structure is disrupted; myofilament structures and SR appear similar to those in intact muscle (20). Biochemical analysis shows virtually complete loss of glycogen, lactic dehydrogenase, and phosphorylase (Wood DS, DiMauro S: unpublished data). At this time, the preparation is transferred to solutions of the same ionic composition as skinning solution but made up in 50% (vol/vol) glycerol/H_2O, and stored unfrozen at $-12°$ C. Physiologically, morphologically, and biochemically the preparation appears stable for many weeks under these storage conditions (19–22).

Electron microscopic examination, freeze-fracture analysis, and ^{45}Ca-uptake studies indicate that SR structure is retained and Ca is accumulated at rates comparable to those of isolated SR vesicles (20, 22, 23). Thin sections of chemically skinned fibers show that SR "feet" are absent except for thin, indistinct filamentous structures that bridge the triad gap with the same spacing as the SR feet of control fibers (20).

Data interpretation is based, in part, on the following general characteristics of the skinned fiber preparation: (*a*) soluble myoplasmic proteins and ions are lacking; (*b*) selective permeability of the surface membranes is lost, allowing direct experimental control over solutions within the myofilament space, (*c*) SR structure and function remain essentially intact, as do myofilament structure and function. Experimental procedures and methods are described in detail in other publications from this laboratory (19, 21).

RESULTS

Caffeine Contracture

Caffeine induced a transient, sustained, or oscillating contracture in single skinned fibers from control and MH muscle (Fig. 1). Sustained contractures were observed more often in fibers from MH biopsy specimens than control specimens. Maximal amplitudes of transient caffeine (20 mM) contractures (not shown) relative to the maximal tension (P_0) the fiber could attain when activated by saturating Ca (10^{-5} M) were: MH, $81 \pm 2\%$ of P_0 (n = 92); control, $82 \pm 2\%$ of P_0 (n = 110). Sustained contractures were invariably of low amplitude, typically 20% or less of the maximal amplitude of the transient contractures and never greater than 50%. Ninety-five per cent of the MH fibers that developed sustained contractures did so only at low caffeine concentrations (less than 5 mM); higher caffeine concentrations elicited transient contractures. Because sustained contractures were found in both MH and control muscle, it is unlikely they represent a disease-related phenomenon. The basis for these contractures, however, is unknown.

In control skinned fibers, the lowest concentration of caffeine that elicits tension (caffeine threshold) depends on the Ca accumulated by the SR before the caffeine challenge (21). We compared the effect of Ca load on caffeine thresholds in MH fibers and control fibers (Fig. 2). As in control fibers, the caffeine threshold in MH fibers shifted to lower caffeine concentrations as the free Ca concentration in the load solution was increased from pCa 7.00 to pCa

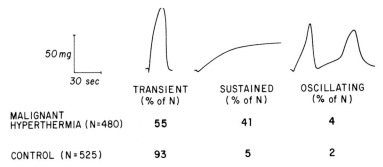

	TRANSIENT (% of N)	SUSTAINED (% of N)	OSCILLATING (% of N)
MALIGNANT HYPERTHERMIA (N=480)	55	41	4
CONTROL (N=525)	93	5	2

Fig. 1. Types of caffeine tension in skinned fibers. Caffeine tensions were obtained by first exposing a skinned fiber to a solution containing 170 mM potassium propionate, 2.0 mM Mg-ATP, 5 mM Ca-EGTA/EGTA, and 10 mM imidizole at pH 7.00 at 20° C. The free Ca level was calculated by solving the multiple equilibria equations for Ca, Mg, ATP, and EGTA using a computer program. After a 30-second exposure to a solution containing free Ca levels of pCa 7.0, 6.6, or 6.4, the fiber was rinsed twice in a similar saline solution that lacked Ca and EGTA, then challenged with caffeine. All caffeine contractures in muscle specimens from control subjects and from patients with malignant hyperthermia were typical of those illustrated. N = number of tensions measured.

6.4, where pCa is the negative logarithm of the Ca concentration in molar units). For each load condition, however, there was a population of MH fibers that had a lower caffeine threshold than any control fiber.

To determine whether enhanced caffeine threshold was common to muscle from all survivors of MH reactions, we analyzed caffeine thresholds after 30-second incubation at pCa 6.6. This condition was chosen because caffeine thresholds for skinned fibers were comparable to thresholds reported for the cut-end fiber bundles used in other studies of MH.

Figure 3 compares caffeine threshold data for individual fibers from each MH biopsy specimen against the range and distribution of caffeine thresholds obtained in control muscle. Each MH biopsy specimen had fibers that developed

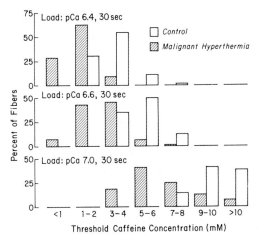

Fig. 2. Caffeine threshold dependence on Ca in load solution. The lowest concentration of caffeine that elicited tension was determined after each of 3 different load conditions in 140 fibers from patients with malignant hyperthermia (MH) and 185 fibers from control subjects. As the Ca available to the fiber was increased, the caffeine concentration necessary to release the Ca accumulated during 30 seconds decreased for both MH and control fibers.

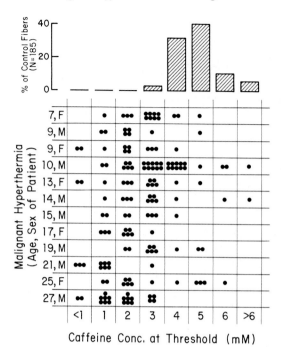

Fig. 3. Caffeine thresholds in fibers from control subjects and from patients with hyperthermia (MH). Caffeine thresholds for each fiber tested (solid circles) in each MH biopsy specimen were compared to the range and distribution of caffeine thresholds in control fibers (histogram). Identical experimental conditions were used for all fibers in this study: Ca uptake by the sarcoplasmic reticulum was measured after a 30-second exposure to a solution of pCa 6.6 (for other components of the solution, see legend to Figure 1. N = number of control fibers.

tension at lower concentrations of caffeine than any control fiber. These data suggest that the abnormality causing enhanced caffeine contracture reported in cut-end multifiber bundles is present in skinned fibers.

Because caffeine elicits tension indirectly, by releasing SR Ca into the myofilament space where it binds to troponin C and activates the contractile apparatus, reduced caffeine thresholds could develop if the contractile apparatus were more than normally sensitive to Ca activation. We therefore measured Ca activation of the contractile apparatus directly by analyzing steady-state tensions at fixed concentrations of free Ca (0.1 to 10 μM, buffered with 5 mM EGTA). No differences in the relationship between Ca concentration and tension were observed between control and MH fibers (Fig. 4). Mean $\pm$ SEM maximal Ca-activated tensions were also comparable: MH, 1.83 $\pm$ 0.05 kg/cm^2 (n = 103); control, 1.85 $\pm$ 0.04 kg/cm^2 (n = 163). These results exclude abnormal contractile protein function and implicate abnormal SR function as the basis for altered caffeine sensitivity in MH muscle.

Calcium Regulation by Sarcoplasmic Reticulum

In SR vesicles from normal muscle, the effectiveness of caffeine in releasing Ca depends, in part, on the Ca load within the SR (24); the greater the Ca load, the greater the fraction of Ca released by a fixed concentration of caffeine. The data shown in Figure 2 indicate that for both MH and control skinned fibers, increasing SR Ca load by incubating fibers in solutions containing increased concentrations of Ca produced a decrease in the threshold caffeine concentration. Thus, one explanation for why, under equivalent experimental conditions, many MH fibers had lower-than-normal caffeine thresholds (Fig. 3) was that during the load period the SR accumulated more Ca than any control fiber.

To test this possibility, rates of oxalate-supported Ca uptake were measured in skinned fibers using a technique involving light scattering that was developed in our laboratories (22). The method consists of positioning a single fiber at right angles to a beam of white light. Part of the incident light is scattered by the fiber and the 90° scattering component is collected by a fiber-optic light quide and directed onto a photodiode. The photodiode signal is amplified, filtered, and displayed on a linear strip chart recorder.

In a saline medium containing Ca and Mg-ATP, the addition of oxalate causes skinned fibers to become visibly darker (25). Calcium oxalate precipitates in the lumen of the SR (20, 22, 26), and the amount of light scattered at 90° increases (22). When ^{45}Ca was included in the loading saline, it was determined that the increase in light scattering was proportional to the increase in Ca concentration within the fiber (22). Thus, light scattering provides a means for determining both rates and steady-state capacities of SR Ca loading.

Rates of oxalate-supported Ca uptake were measured in human skinned fibers in a solution containing 170 mM potassium propionate, 2.5 mM Mg-ATP, 2.5 mM ATP (Na, K salt), 5 mM Ca-EGTA/EGTA (pCa 6.4), 5 mM oxalate, and 10 mM imidazole at pH 7.00. For control skinned fibers (n = 124), rates of Ca uptake fell into two populations: relatively fast (2.07 mmol Ca accumulated/liter fiber/min on average), and relatively slow (0.68 mmol Ca accumulated/liter fiber/min on average). Skinned fibers from MH muscle (n = 34) had Ca uptake rates that ranged from 0.5 mmol Ca accumulated/liter fiber/min to 3.0 mmol Ca accumulated/liter fiber/min; no rate fell outside the range of control values. Two recent observations, however, led us to reexamine the question of SR Ca uptake in MH fibers.

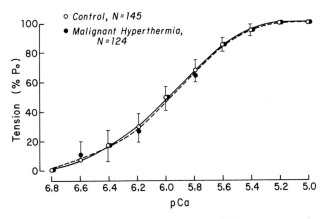

Fig. 4. Relationship between Ca concentration and force generation. Fibers were pretreated with the nonionic detergent, Brij-58, which destroys the ability of the sarcoplasmic reticulum to accumulate Ca, but is without effect on the contractile apparatus (18). Steady-state isometric tensions were measured as described by Wood and colleagues (18). Tensions were normalized to the maximal tension (Po). N = number of fibers.

The first observation was that the adenosine 3', 5' monophosphate (cAMP) content of MH muscle was significantly increased (27, and chapter 34 this volume). The second was that skinned fibers retain adenyl cyclase activity and metabolize cAMP (28, and chapter 34 this volume). It is known that cAMP stimulates Ca uptake into SR vesicles isolated from slow-twitch skeletal muscle (30). In one study, cAMP did not stimulate Ca uptake into SR vesicles isolated from fast-twitch skeletal muscle (30). Bornet and associates (30), however, reported that cAMP-stimulated Ca uptake in fast-twitch muscle microsomes, and Fabiato and Fabiato (31) found that 5 μM cAMP caused an SR-dependent relaxation of tension in skinned fibers from fast-twitch cat muscle.

In chemically skinned control human skeletal muscle, we observed with light-scattering measurements that rates of oxalate-supported Ca uptake were depressed by exogenous Ca-activator independent phosphodiesterase (PDE) and increased by exogenous cAMP (1 to 2 μM) in some fibers, but not in others. Responsiveness to cAMP and PDE was confined exclusively to the skinned fiber population that had relatively slow Ca-uptake rates in the absence of added cAMP. The SR Ca uptake in skinned fibers with initially fast uptake rates (i.e., greater than 1.5 mM Ca accumulated/liter fiber/min) did not respond to either cAMP or PDE.

In chemically skinned MH fibers, however, preparations with initial uptake rates as high as 3.00 mmol Ca accumulated/liter fiber/min were responsive to PDE: rates in the presence of PDE were reduced to as low as 0.5 mmol Ca/liter fiber/min. Figure 5 is a histogram comparing the initial Ca-uptake rates of

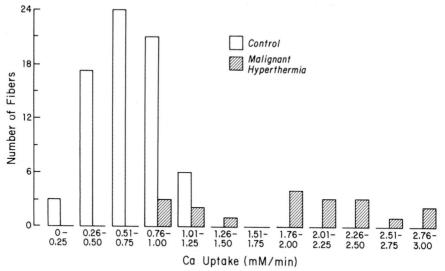

Fig. 5. Histogram of Ca uptake in cAMP-sensitive fibers. The Ca uptake was measured with light scattering as described in text and by Sorenson and associates (22). The histogram shows initial rates of oxalate-supported Ca uptake. After determination of initial rate, cAMP (1 to 2 μM) or phosphodiesterase (PDE) was added and the effect was observed. The histogram shows initial Ca uptake only for fibers that responded to cAMP or PDE. Optical measurement of the light-scattering signal was converted to mmol Ca accumulated/liter fiber/min (mM Ca/min) using a calibration factor determined in separate experiments with [45]Ca, as described by Sorenson and colleagues (22).

control fibers found to be responsive to cAMP or PDE to initial rates in MH fibers. In this comparison, a difference in initial rates of Ca uptake between MH and control fibers is apparent. Because no control fiber with an initial Ca-uptake rate greater than 1.50 mmol Ca/liter fiber/min responded to cAMP or PDE, whereas MH fibers with initial rates as high as 3.00 mmol Ca/liter fiber/min did respond to PDE, the data indicate an abnormality in cAMP regulation of Ca uptake in MH fibers.

DISCUSSION

Chemically skinned single fiber preparations from 12 persons who survived MH reactions developed tension at lower concentrations of caffeine than identically treated normal muscle (Figs. 2, 3). Although caffeine elicits tension by causing SR to release stores of Ca (24), an apparent enhancement of caffeine sensitivity could be caused by increased responsiveness of contractile proteins to Ca rather than altered function of SR. However, maximal tension and the relationship between Ca concentration and tension were virtually identical in MH and normal fibers (Fig. 4). Therefore, abnormalities of caffeine-stimulated Ca-release in MH fibers occurred because of alterations in SR function.

The nature of the SR disorder that causes increased caffeine sensitivity in MH is not known. In biochemical studies, the dose-effectiveness of caffeine is related to the Sr load: the greater the Ca load within SR vesicles, the lower the concentration of caffeine required to elicit Ca release. In Duchenne dystrophy, for example, Ca uptake into isolated SR vesicles is less than normal (32, 33) and the tension response to caffeine in intact (34) and skinnned (35) fibers is also less than normal. In the cut-end muscle preparations from MH muscle, therefore, enhanced caffeine sensitivity could reflect an SR that contains more Ca than normal. In skinned fibers, after equivalent periods of Ca uptake, the SR of MH fibers may accumulate more Ca than normal, and decreased caffeine thresholds could reflect this property of SR.

Measurements of Ca uptake into microsomal vesicles isolated from human MH muscle have been made, but results were inconsistent. Depressed rates, enhanced rates, and no change in Ca-uptake rates have all been reported (reviewed in 36). Differences in vesicle fractions, methods, and results from these studies do not allow any firm conclusion to be drawn about SR function in MH muscle.

We recently found increased cAMP levels in MH muscle apparently due to inceased activity of adenylate cyclase (chapter 38 this volume). Abnormally increased cAMP could lead to enhanced SR Ca load: in both cardiac and slow-twitch mammalian skeletal muscle, a cAMP-dependent protein kinase catalyzes phosphorylation of a protein (phospholamban) in SR membranes, which enhances the rate of Ca accumulation by SR (29, 37). In fast-twitch skeletal muscle, the role of cAMP in SR Ca uptake is controversial (30).

Cyclic-AMP is produced by chemically skinned fibers through retention of membrane-bound adenylate cyclase (28), suggesting possible stimulation of SR Ca uptake by endogenous cAMP-controlled systems. Using a light-scattering technique for measuring oxalate-supported Ca uptake, we identified a population of fibers in control human skeletal muscle whose Ca uptake was responsive to cAMP. Comparing initial Ca-uptake rates in fibers later shown to respond to either PDE or cAMP added to the saline solution revealed that initial rates of Ca accumulation were greater in cAMP-sensitive MH fibers than in any cAMP-sensitive control fibers.

Figure 6 summarizes known or postulated sites of action of caffeine and cAMP on SR. Associated with SR membranes, and apparently retained in skinned fibers (28, and Willner JH, Wood DS, and Salviati G: unpublished data) are PDE, cAMP-dependent protein kinase, phospholamban, and protein phosphaphatase. Stimulation of the Ca pump by cAMP-mediated functions would lead to increased Ca load of the SR. This, in turn, would be expected to lead to increased Ca release by caffeine, which is postulated to act either by depressing Ca pump activity (24) or by increasing passive Ca permeability of SR membranes (38). Both mechanisms would lead to a net efflux of SR Ca along its concentration gradient.

Although these speculations provide one explanation for a relationship between the biochemical abnormality of increased cAMP content and the physiologic abnormality of enhanced caffeine sensitivity, there are other pos-

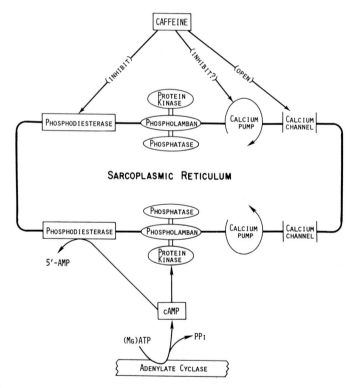

Fig. 6. Diagram of sarcoplasmic reticulum and sites of cAMP and caffeine interaction. Adenylate cyclase is a membrane-bound enzyme primarily associated with the sarcolemma (see chapter 34 of this volume). Elements of the sarcolemma remain in chemically skinned fibers (20) and these preparations synthesize cAMP when exposed to solutions containing Mg-ATP (see chapter 34). For further discussion, see text.

sibilities, e.g., abnormalities subsequent to cAMP production or alterations in caffeine binding to SR membranes. Also, there is the problem of fiber-type involvement in the disease process. Control fibers that did not respond to cAMP or PDE were observed to have Ca-uptake rates as high as those of any MH fiber. In isolated SR vesicle preparations from human muscle, which unavoidably contain both fast and slow fibers, it is possible that variability in results arises from a combination of factors: different proportions of fast and slow fibers, and lack of control for cAMP regulation.

CONCLUSION

Identical caffeine contracture abnormalities were found in chemically skinned single fiber preparations obtained from biopsy specimens of 12 unrelated persons who had survived MH reactions. Because skinned fibers lack functional sarcolemma and mitochondria, and contractile protein function was determined to be normal in MH fibers, abnormal caffeine contracture must develop from alterations in SR function. Our results also indicate a disorder in either cAMP metabolism or function leading to abnormally enhanced Ca uptake in some MH fibers. Abnormal caffeine contracture caused by abnormal SR function may be one consequence of pathologic changes in cAMP-regulated functions in MH muscle.

ACKNOWLEDGMENTS

We thank Dr. Martha M Sorenson and Dr. John P Reuben for their advice and encouragement; Geraldine Plynton, for her excellent technical assistance; and Dr. Ronald Brisman, for obtaining many of the biopsy specimens used in this study. Most especially we owe a debt of gratitude to the patients who, after surviving an MH reaction, were willing to return to the operating room and donate a muscle biopsy specimen for the purposes of research into this disorder. These studies were supported by grants from the Muscular Dystrophy Association and the National Institutes of Health (NS 11766). Donald S. Wood was supported by a senior investigatorship from the New York Heart Association.

REFERENCES

1. Gordon RA, Britt BA, Kalow W (eds) *International Symposium on Malignant Hyperthermia.* Charles C Thomas, Springfield, IL, 1973

2. Aldrete JA, Britt BA (eds): *Second International Symposium on Malignant Hyperthermia.* Grune and Stratton, New York, 1977

3. Britt BA, Kwong FHF, Endrenyi L: The clinical and laboratory features of malignant hyperthermia management: a review. In *Malignant Hyperthermia: Current Concepts.* Edited by Henschel ED. Appleton-Century-Crofts, New York, 1977, pp 8–45

4. Britt BA, Kwong FHF, Endrenyi L: Management of malignant-hyperthermia susceptible patients: a review. In *Malignant Hyperthermia: Current Concepts.* Edited by Henschel ED. Appleton-Century-Crofts, New York, 1977, pp 67–77

5. Wingard DW, Gatz EE: Some observations on stress-susceptible patients. In *Second International Symposium on Malignant Hyperthermia*. Edited by Aldrete JA, Britt BA. Grune and Stratton, New York, 1977, pp 363–372

6. Isaacs H, Barlow MB: Malignant hyperpyrexia during anesthesia: possible association with subclinical myopathy. Br Med J 1:275–277, 1970

7. Kalow W, Britt BA, Terreau ME, Haist C: Metabolic error of muscle metabolism after recovery from malignant hyperthermia. Lancet 2:895–898, 1970

8. Harriman DGF, Sumner DW, Ellis FR: Malignant hyperpyrexia myopathy. Q J Med 168:639–664, 1973

9. Kalow W, Britt BA, Richter A: The caffeine test of isolated human muscle in relation to malignant hyperthermia. Can Anaesth Soc J 24:678–694, 1977

10. Ellis FR, Cain PA, Harriman DGF: Multifactorial inheritance of malignant hyperthermia susceptibility. In *Second International Symposium on Malignant Hyperthermia*. Edited by Aldrete JA, Britt BA. Grune and Stratton, New York, 1977, pp 329–338

11. Britt BA, Endrenyi L, Peters PL, et al: Screening of malignant hyperthermia susceptible families by creatine phosphokinase measurement and other clinical investigations. Can Anaesth Soc J 23:263–284, 1976

12. Moulds RFW, Denborough MA: Biochemical basis of malignant hyperpyrexia. Br Med J 2:241–244, 1974

13. Halsall PJ, Ellis FR: A screening test for the malignant hyperpyrexia phenotype using suxamethonium-induced contracture of muscle treated with caffeine, and its inhibition by dantrolene. Br J Anaesth 51:753–755, 1979

14. Close RI: Dynamic properties of mammalian skeletal muscles. Physiol Rev 52:129–197, 1972

15. Gallant EM, Godt RE, Gronert GA: Role of plasma membrane defect of skeletal muscle in malignant hyperthermia. Muscle Nerve 2:491–494, 1979

16. Dhalla NS, Sulakhe PV, Clinch NF, et al: Influence of fluothane on calcium accumulation by the heavy microsomal fraction of human skeletal muscle: comparison with a patient with malignant hyperpyrexia. Biochem Med 6:333–343, 1972

17. Isaacs H, Heffron JJA: Morphological and biochemical defects in muscles of human carriers of the malignant hyperthermia syndrome. Br J Anaesth 47:475–481, 1975

18. Wood DS, Zollman J, Reuben JP, Brandt PW: Human skeletal muscle: properties of the "chemically skinned" fiber. Science 187:1075–1076, 1975

19. Reuben JP, Wood DS, Eastwood AB: Adaptation of single fiber techniques for the study of human muscle. In *Pathogenesis of the Human Muscular Dystrophies*. Edited by Rowland LP. Excerpta Medica, Amsterdam, 1977, pp 259–269

20. Eastwood AB, Wood DS, Block KL, Sorenson MM: Chemically skinned mammalian skeletal muscle. I. The structure of skinned rabbit psoas. Tissue Cell 11:553–566, 1979

21. Wood DS: Human skeletal muscle: analysis of Ca^{++} regulation in skinned fibers using caffeine. Exp Neurol 58:218–230, 1978

22. Sorenson MM, Reuben JP, Eastwood AB, et al: Functional heterogeneity of the sarcoplasmic reticulum within sarcomeres of skinned muscle fibers. J Membr Biol 53:1–17, 1980

23. Eastwood AB, Bock KR: Morphology of chemically skinned mammalian skeletal muscle: freeze-fracture of skinned rabbit psoas (abstract). J Cell Biol 82:391, 1979

24. Weber A: The mechanism of the action of caffeine on sarcoplasmic reticulum. J Gen Physiol 52:760–772, 1968

25. Orentlicher M, Reuben JP, Grundfest H, Brandt PW: Calcium binding and tension development in detergent-treated muscle fibers. J Gen Physiol 63:168–186, 1974

26. Costantin LL, Franzini-Armstrong C, Podolsky RJ: Localization of calcium accumulating structures in striated muscle fibers. Science 147:158–159, 1965

27. Willner JH, Cerri CJ, Wood DS: Malignant hyperthermia: abnormal cyclic AMP metabolism in skeletal muscle (abstract). Neurology (NY) 29:257, 1979

28. Wood DS, Willner JH, Salviati G, DiMauro S, Cerri C: Cyclic AMP metabolism and function in chemically skinned mammalian skeletal muscle (abstract). Fed Proc 39:2176, 1980

29. Kirchberg MA, Tada M: Effects of adenosine 3',5'-monophosphate-dependent protein kinase on sarcoplasmic reticulum isolated from cardiac and slow and fast contracting muscles. J Biol Chem 251:725–729, 1976

30. Bornet EP, Entman ML, Van Winkle WB, et al: Cyclic AMP modulation of calcium accumulation by sarcoplasmic reticulum from fast skeletal muscle. Biochim Biophys Acta 463:188–193, 1977

31. Fabiato A, Fabiato F: Cyclic AMP-induced enhancement of calcium accumulation by the sarcoplasmic reticulum with no modification of the sensitivity of the myofilaments to calcium in skinned fibers from a fast skeletal muscle. Biochim Biophys Acta 539:253–260, 1978

32. Sugita H, Okimoto K, Ebashi S, Okinaka S: Biochemical alterations in progressive muscular dystrophy: with special reference to sarcoplasmic reticulum. In *Exploratory Concepts in Muscular Dystrophy and Related Disorders*. Edited by Milhorat AT. Excerpta Medica, Amsterdam, 1967, pp 321–326

33. Samaha FJ, Gergely J: Ca^{++} uptake and ATPase of human sarcoplasmic reticulum. J Clin Invest 44:1425–1431, 1965

34. Gruener R, Stern LZ, Baumbach N: Caffeine-modulated acetylcholine sensitivity in denervated rat and diseased human muscle. Life Sci 17:1557–1566, 1975

35. Wood DS, Sorenson MM, Eastwood AB, et al. Duchenne dystrophy: abnormal generation of tension and Ca^{++} regulation in single skinned fibers. Neurology (NY) 28:447–457, 1978

36. Gronert GA, Heffron JA, Taylor ST: Skeletal muscle sarcoplasmic reticulum in procine malignant hyperthermia. Eur J Pharmacol 58:179–197, 1979

37. Tada M, Ohmori F, Yamada M, Abe H: Mechanism of the stimulation of Ca^{2+}-dependent ATPase of cardiac sarcoplasmic reticulum by adenosine 3',5'-monophosphate-dependent protein kinase: role of the 22,000-dalton protein. J Biol Chem 254:319–326, 1979

38. Johnson PN, Inesi G: Anesthetics on fragmented sarcoplasmic reticulum. J Pharmacol Exp Ther 169:308–314, 1969

DISCUSSION

Dr. Frank Sreter: During the past 4 or 5 years we have obtained biopsy specimens from about 50 cases of malignant hyperthermia (MH). Our approach was quite different from yours, and I would like to emphasize that the fiber type distribution is very important. We now use a cryostat serial section method in which, in the same serial section, we can check the fiber type distribution and also determine the calcium uptake. We always found a decreased calcium uptake in the sections received from MH patients. With your method, can you distinguish between type 2A and type 2B fibers, or do you just take a single fiber randomly? There is a rather large difference between the two.

Dr. Donald Wood: We have not distinguished between fiber types in skinned fibers. We are, however, trying to develop a method for fiber typing these preparations, and I believe this is a necessary step. In your case, finding a reduced calcium uptake presents another problem, because as you well know, enhanced, reduced, and no change in calcium-uptake rates have all been reported. I do not know what the causes or differences are among various laboratories. It would be worthwhile to agree on a single method for calcium-uptake studies in this disorder.

Dr. Frank Sreter: Do your fiber populations correspond to types 2A and 2B?

Dr. Donald Wood: They could, but we do not know this for certain.

Dr. Helen Blau: Have you or has anyone looked at calmodulin in these fibers; i.e., its distribution, quantity, or affinity for Ca?

Dr. Donald Wood: No.

Dr. Peter Griffiths: What was the time scale of the calcium uptake by the sarcoplasmic reticulum? Are we talking about milliseconds or seconds?

Dr. Donald Wood: Initial uptake rates using oxalate were maintained constant over several minutes.

Dr. Shirley Bryant: I would like to comment on some studies with the porcine model of MH I made with Dr. Ian Anderson. With a voltage clamp technique, we found that, in general, the affected fibers had a much smaller mechanical threshold, i.e., a mechanical threshold very near the resting potential. I understand that Dr. Gallant from Mayo has similar results using the potassium method to determine the mechanical threshold.

47

Interaction of Pumiliotoxin-B with Calcium Sites in the Sarcoplasmic Reticulum and Nerve Terminal of Normal and Dystrophic Muscle

Edson X. Albuquerque, MD, PhD

Jordan E. Warnick, PhD

Roque Tamburini, PhD

Frederick C. Kauffman, PhD

John W. Daly, PhD

Pumiliotoxin-B (PTX-B) is one of the active toxins obtained from the skin secretions of the Panamanian poison frog *Dendrobates pumilio* (1). The structure of this novel indolizidine alkaloid toxin is 8-hydroxy-8-methyl-6-(6'7'-dihydroxy-2'5'-dimethyl-4'-octenylidene)-1-azabicyclo [4.3.0] nonane, $C_{19}H_{33}NO_3$ (2) and is shown in Figure 1. Initial studies with the toxin have revealed a rather novel effect on membranes of the nerve terminal and sarcoplasmic reticulum (SR) of skeletal muscle: as the result of its action, the directly evoked twitch was markedly potentiated but not blocked (3, 4). PTX-B caused no membrane depolarization, and the effect on both the nerve terminal and skeletal muscles was Ca dependent. The toxin also inhibited Ca-dependent adenosine triphosphatase (Ca-ATPase) contained in isolated vesicles of SR from mammalian and amphibian skeletal muscles (3). An agent with such action can

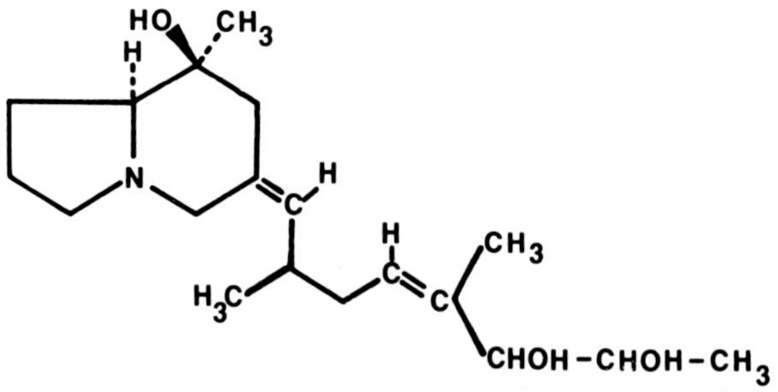

Fig. 1. Structure of pumiliotoxin-B, an indolizidene alkaloid of molecular weight 323.26 daltons.

be of major importance to understanding the nature of excitation-secretion and excitation-contraction coupling in nerve and muscle.

Because we and others had suggested previously that a major problem in inherited muscular dystrophy of chickens may be a Ca-dependent defect primarily at the SR and nerve terminal (5–8), we examined the effects of PTX-B on nerve and muscle membranes of normal and dystrophic chickens as well as on Ca-ATPase in SR isolated from skeletal muscle. A differential response of normal and dystrophic muscles to PTX-B was observed: normal but not dystrophic muscles were affected by PTX-B, suggesting that avian muscular dystrophy is associated with a qualitative change in the mechanism of Ca translocation.

METHODS

Animals and Preparations

Electrophysiologic and contractile studies were carried out at room temperature (21 to 23° C) on sciatic sartorius and semitendinosus muscles of the frog (Rana pipiens) and on posterior latissimus dorsi (PLD) muscles of the normal (line 412) dystrophic (line 413) chickens from 1 to 6 weeks ex ovo. Twitch experiments were done in either the entire muscle or in bundles of 10 to 15 muscle fibers. The contraction time of the twitch is defined as the time for the tension to rise from the baseline to peak, and the half-relaxation time is the time from peak to a point on the falling phase of the twitch equal to one-half the twitch amplitude. Conventional microelectrode techniques were used for intracellular and extracellular recordings (9, 10). A method essentially similar to that described by Katz and Miledi (11–13) was used for studies involving focal depolarizations of the nerve terminal.

Isolation of Sarcoplasmic Reticulum

Vesicles of the SR from frog and rat hindlimb muscles and pectoral muscles of chickens were prepared according to the method of Froehlich and Taylor (14). Briefly, 6 to 8 g of muscle were homogenized for approximately 2 minutes at a setting of 9 in a Polytron blender (Brinkmann). The homogenate was subjected to differential centrifugation as described by the authors except that the initial mixture was not filtered through cheesecloth and the starting supernatant material was centrifuged 2 rather than 3 times at 10,000 g. Dithiothreitol (10 μM) was included in all media used for the isolation of the vesicles.

Measurement of Ca-ATPase

The Ca-ATPase activity was determined using a colorimetric method for the measurement of inorganic phosphate (15). Isolated vesicles equivalent to approximately 0.8 μg of protein were incubated with ATP in the presence and absence of Ca in 100 μl of reagent consisting of 20 mM imidazole HCl (pH 7.0), 100 mM KCl, 2 mM ATP, 1 mM $MgCl_2$, 0.1 mM ethyleneglycol-bis-(β-amino-ethyl ether)N,N'-tetraacetic acid (EGTA), and either 50 or 70 μM Ca. All incubations were performed at 30° C. The assay was linear with time for at least 60 minutes and with tissue varying up to at least 40 μg of SR protein. When ADP was measured fluorometrically, results were identical to those obtained with inorganic phosphate (16). Protein was determined according to the method of Lowry and coworkers (17).

Solutions and Drugs

The physiologic solutions for chicken muscles (7) and for frog muscles (18) were prepared as described elsewhere. All drugs were stored as refrigerated stock solutions until just before use. Tetrodotoxin (3.0 × 10^{-4} M) and D-tubocurarine (10^{-3} M) as the chloride salt (Sigma Chemical Co., St. Louis, MO) were dissolved in double-distilled water. PTX-B was obtained as pure toxin from *Dendrobates pumilio* (2), dissolved in absolute ethanol at a concentration of 6 × 10^{-3} M, and stored at −20° C.

INTERACTION OF PUMILIOTOXIN-B WITH CALCIUM SITES

Amphibian and Mammalian Skeletal Muscles

Effect on Muscle Contraction and Caffeine Contracture

Isometric contractions of the frog sartorius muscles evoked by direct and indirect stimulations at 0.2 Hz were potentiated and prolonged in the presence of PTX-B. Figure 2 shows a concentration-dependent potentiation of both indirectly and directly elicited muscle contractions. At concentrations from 0.5 to 30 μM, PTX-B potentiated the muscle contractions to values between 110% and 340% of control. Although one might expect the toxin to cause muscle contracture in a similar way to that induced by millimolar concentrations of caffeine (19, 20, 21), the baseline muscle tension was unaltered even at the highest concentrations of PTX-B examined (30 μM). Potentiation of muscle tension was coupled with spontaneous contractions at this concentration. The potentiation of both indirectly and directly elicited muscle contraction suggests that this toxin acts by mechanisms unrelated to membrane depolarization. As shown in Figure 3, 1.5 μM PTX-B did not cause membrane depolarization or

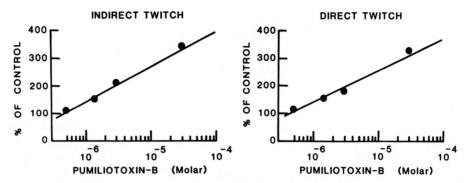

Fig. 2. Dose-response relationship for maximal potentiation of evoked contractions by pumiliotoxin-B in whole frog sartorius muscle. Each point is the mean of 3 to 5 preparations. Maximal potentiation occurred 1 to 3 minutes after addition of the toxin.

alter either the amplitude or the frequency of spontaneous miniature endplate potentials. Furthermore, PTX-B did not affect the extrajunctional input resistance (Fig. 3) even though the specific resistance of a unit area was increased approximately 20% over control values ($P > 0.05$).

To define more clearly the time course of PTX-B action on the contractile mechanism, we examined the influence of the toxin on bundles of 10 to 15 muscle fibers dissected from frog semitendinosus muscles. Within 7 seconds

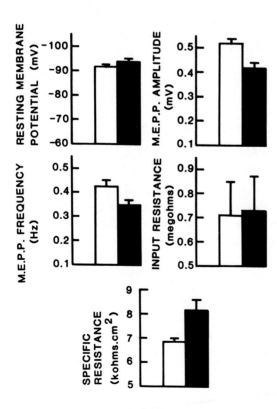

Fig. 3. Effect of 1.5 µM pumiliotoxin-B on various properties of the nerve and sartorius muscle of the frog. Recordings were made before (open bars) and between 30 and 60 minutes after exposure to the toxin. Each value is the mean ± SEM for 15 to 54 fibers of 3 to 8 muscles. M.E.P.P. = miniature endplate potential.

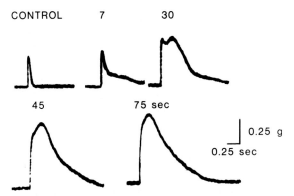

Fig. 4. Effect of 1.5 μM pumiliotoxin-B on the directly elicited twitch in bundles of frog semitendinosus muscles. Each bundle consisted of 10 to 14 fibers. Within 7 seconds after addition of toxin to the bath, the amplitude and duration of the directly elicited contraction was potentiated and prolonged. α-Bungarotoxin (5 μg/ml) was present for 30 minutes before the beginning of the experiment.

after the toxin was added to the experimental chamber, the directly elicited muscle contraction (elicited at 0.2 Hz) was potentiated and prolonged (Fig. 4). The maximal potentiation of muscle contraction occurred after 2 to 4 minutes, and the single contraction subsequently became so large that its amplitude reached values equal to or greater than the peak amplitude of the tetanic tension (Fig. 5). In fact, except for the plateau and decay phase of both responses, the single contraction resembled a tetanic contraction.

The initial effect of PTX-B on the muscle contraction was characterized by a marked potentiation of the single twitch and by a double exponential relaxation phase (Fig. 4). As time progressed, the double exponential relaxation disappeared and the single contraction was further prolonged, i.e., the relaxation phase reverted to a single exponential function. This potentiation of muscle twitch could be reduced significantly by higher rates of stimulation.

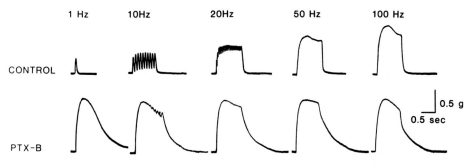

Fig. 5. Effect of 1.5 μM pumiliotoxin-B (PTX-B) on twitch and tetanus characteristics in bundles of fibers from frog semitendinosus muscles. α-Bungarotoxin (5 μg/ml) was present for 30 minutes before the start of the experiments. Note the potentiation and prolongation of the single contractions elicited at 1 Hz, the degree of fusion at low frequencies of stimulation, and the development of after-contractions in tetanic responses.

Increases in frequency from 0.2 to 2 Hz maintained for 2 or 3 minutes resulted in depression of the amplitude of the single twitch; however, the potentiation still remained larger in amplitude and duration than that of control twitches.

The effect of PTX-B on tetanic responses of bundles of semitendinosus fibers is also illustrated in Figure 5. As with the single muscle twitch, PTX-B markedly potentiated the directly evoked tetanic responses at 10 and 20 Hz. In fact, the contractions were nearly fused where the muscle was stimulated at 10 Hz, 5 minutes after exposure to the toxin. That is, in contrast to the responses of the control muscle, which remained clearly visible at 10 Hz, the tetanic tension obtained at 10, 20, and 50 Hz in the presence of the toxin approached that of the control response at 100 Hz.

Thus, the primary actions of PTX-B can be summarized as follows: (*a*) potentiation of the twitch; (*b*) tetanic fusion at lower-than-normal rates of stimulation; (*c*) marked prolongation of the relaxation phase after tetanus with complex decay at stimulation frequencies of 20, 50, and 100 Hz. The failure of the tension to return to baseline within 100 msec of the end of stimulation suggests that the toxin may affect not only the process of Ca release from the SR, but also its reuptake into the SR. It should be mentioned that initial studies done in skinned and glycerinated single fibers revealed a lack of direct action of the toxin on the contractile elements themselves, allowing us to conclude that the action of the toxin on contractile properties of skeletal muscle fibers is related primarily to its direct action on the sarcolemmal membrane or the SR (3).

Several possible actions of the toxin on the sarcolemmal membrane might result in potentiation of twitch. First, the toxin might induce significant increases in Na permeability, which in turn could potentiate the twitch, as with other toxins such as batrachotoxin and veratridine. This potentiation would be transient and have little or no effect on tetanic tension. Such is obviously not the case with PTX-B. Direct measurement of resting membrane and action potentials revealed that the toxin does not affect Na permeability, as revealed by the lack of effect on membrane potential (Fig. 3) and on characteristics of the action potential. Second possibility is that the toxin might alter K conductance and prolong the muscle action potential by a mechanism similar to that of histrionicotoxin (22), phencyclidine (23), and tetraethylammonium (24). Measurement of the decay phase of the action potential as well as of delayed rectification, which is a qualitative indicator of K conductance, disclosed no significant effect of the toxin at 1.5 μM. Thus, the toxin's effects do not appear to be dependent on changes in Na or K conductances. Although an effect on Cl$^-$ conductance is possible, the most plausible explanation is that PTX-B either mobilizes Ca from the sarcoplasmic stores and/or prevents its reuptake, as revealed by the marked potentiation and prolongation of the twitch.

The following experiments suggest that the action of the toxin is related to the mobilization of Ca from the SR rather than an increase in Ca conductance across the sarcolemmal membrane, as suggested for other agents (19). In the absence of external Ca plus 1 mM EGTA, the toxin did not potentiate the single muscle twitch but did prolong contraction time. This argues strongly that PTX-B produces its potentiating action on muscle twitch by causing the release of Ca from the SR rather than increasing Ca conductance across the sarcolemmal membrane of the fast-twitch muscle. Although the latter possibility may play a significant role in excitation-contraction coupling, there is yet no evidence to link depolarization to an increase in Ca conductance and the potentiation of the twitch (19). Furthermore, when the external Ca concentration was increased 5-fold, the potentiation of both directly and indirectly elicited contractions by PTX-B was only delayed. With increasing rates of nerve or muscle stimulation, there was an increase in the blockade of the twitch (3).

Another observation that supports the conclusion that the toxin reacts with Ca sites and affects Ca reuptake is shown in Figure 6. When the muscle was exposed to 20 mM caffeine, a significant contracture of the muscle occurred, and this is primarily related to the removal of Ca^{2+} from the SR to the contractile apparatus (19). This effect of caffeine is not significantly altered by blocking Na conductance with tetrodotoxin (TTX) (Fig. 6), an effect that has been seen previously (19). However, when the preparation was preincubated with TTX, which would ensure complete blockade of Na conductance, treated with 1.5 μM PTX-B, and then subsequently exposed to caffeine, a significant potentiation of the caffeine-induced contracture was observed. Caffeine treatment in the presence of PTX-B probably released amounts of Ca from the SR identical to control amounts. Thus, potentiation of the caffeine-induced contracture by PTX-B appears to be related to its blockade of Ca-ATPase and the reuptake of Ca.

Effect on Ca-ATPase
A direct action of PTX-B on Ca-ATPase was observed in vesicles of SR isolated from frog sartorius muscle and rat hindlimb muscles (Table 1). At 30 μM, PTX-B inhibited Ca-ATPase by 41% in the frog preparation and by 32% in preparations from rats. This action of PTX-B apparently cannot be ascribed to an effect on Na,K-ATPase, because experiments with ouabain indicated that vesicles used in these experiments contained little, if any, of this activity. It would appear that approximately 10-fold higher concentrations of PTX-B are required for significant inhibition of the enzyme as compared to the concentrations needed to potentiate and prolong muscle contraction. Such differences may reflect differing sensitivities of the enzyme in situ and in isolated SR membranes.

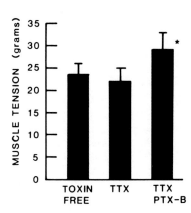

Fig. 6. Potentiation of 20 mM caffeine-induced contracture in frog sartorius muscles by 1.5 μM pumiliotoxin-B (PTX-B). Tetrodotoxin (TTX) (1.0 μM) was present to prevent any involvement of sodium conductance in the response to pumiliotoxin-B. Values are given as the mean ± SEM for 4 to 6 muscles.

Table 1. Effect of PTX-B on Ca-ATPase from Frog and Rat Sarcoplasmic Reticulum[a]

| Source | Ca-ATPase Activity (nmol/mg protein/hr) | | % Inhibition |
	Control	PTX-B (30 µM)	
Frog	1,919 ± 27	1,143 ± 47[b]	41
Rat	2,868 ± 17	2,007 ± 42[b]	32

[a] Each value is the mean ± SEM of triplicate samples. Incubations were carried out in the presence of 70 µM $CaCl_2$. PTX-B, pumiliotoxin-B; Ca-ATPase, calcium-dependent adenosine triphosphatase.

[b] $p < 0.01$.

We also examined the effect of the toxin on Ca-stimulated respiration in mitochondria isolated from rat liver to determine the specificity of PTX-B for Ca-dependent processes. In contrast to the inhibition observed with Ca-ATPase of the SR (Fig. 7), PTX-B did not inhibit Ca-stimulated respiration of mitochondria even at high concentrations (60 µM). Thus, the toxin appears to be relatively specific for the SR Ca-ATPase.

Effect on Evoked Transmitter Release

Although PTX-B did not affect spontaneous transmitter release, the toxin did alter evoked release (4). Thus, the toxin probably reacts with the active sites where Ca is released during the process of evoked transmitter release (25). Exposure of a curarized preparation of either rat or frog skeletal muscle to 1.5 µM PTX-B resulted in repetitive evoked endplate potentials (EPPs) in response to single stimuli (Fig. 8). The EPPs were facilitated to such an extent that the threshold for the particular fiber was reached and an action potential was elicited. Figures 8 and 9 illustrate the effect of PTX-B on the amplitude of the multiple and evoked EPPs. As shown in Figure 9, the potentiation of the second, third, and fourth EPPs was highly dependent on Ca, suggesting that PTX-B also mobilizes Ca involved in the process of evoked transmitter release. The mobilized ion may interact with acetylcholine at the inner membrane surface of the nerve terminal such that large amounts of transmitter are released. The

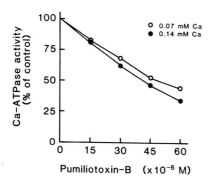

Fig. 7. Dose-response relationship of the effect of pumiliotoxin-B on the sarcoplasmic calcium-dependent adenosine triphosphatase (Ca-AT-Pase) of frog sartorius muscle in the presence of two concentrations of calcium. Each point is the mean of replicates of muscles from 6 frogs.

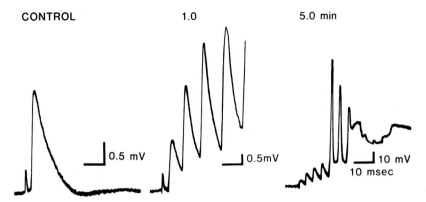

Fig. 8. Effect of 1.5 μM pumiliotoxin-B on evoked release of transmitter in a frog sartorius muscle partially curarized with 1.5 μM D-tubocurarine in the presence of low external calcium (0.45 mM). Single shocks to the nerve normally evoked one endplate potential; in the presence of toxin, repetitive endplate potentials appeared, some of which summated, reached threshold, and gave rise to action potentials. Note the increase in endplate potential amplitude in each train of endplate potentials. Time shown is after the addition of toxin.

mechanism by which PTX-B releases large quantities of the transmitter is, of course, unknown at this time.

We have consistently observed that the repetitive EPPs occur as a result of repetitive electrical activity present at the nerve terminal but not in the axon. The amplitudes of the nerve terminal spikes by the second, third, and fourth multiply evoked EPPs were reduced markedly, suggesting participation of Na conductance in the action of the toxin. Therefore, to eliminate a possible

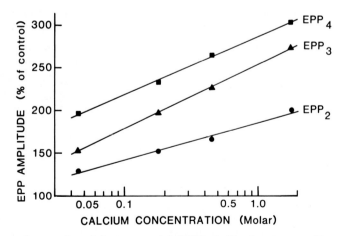

Fig. 9. Dependency of endplate potential (EPP) facilitation by pumiliotoxin-B on the external calcium concentration in frog sartorius muscles. A log-linear relationship between the second, third, and fourth EPPs evoked repetitively by single shocks to the nerve in the presence of 1.5 μM pumiliotoxin-B is apparent at various calcium concentrations. Other conditions as in Figure 8.

involvement of monovalent cations in the potentiation of the EPP by PTX-B, experiments were done in which membrane excitability was blocked by adding 3 μM TTX to the solution bathing the muscle. In these experiments (data not shown), PTX-B markedly shifted the sigmoidal relationship between evoked EPP amplitude and current intensity to the left, i.e., to lower currents, without changing the maximal amplitude of the EPP. This observation suggests that potentiation of EPPs was probably induced by a reaction of PTX-B on the Ca receptor located on the nerve terminal membrane.

The action of the toxin on the nerve terminal may be similar to that on the SR, where PTX-B inhibits Ca-ATPase and appears to enhance evoked release of Ca. The decremental and repetitive action potentials produced by PTX-B could still involve a marked increase in Ca conductance associated with a Na-Ca exchange, because the Na channel present at the nerve terminal is insensitive to the blocking effect of TTX (12). The marked increase in the amount of free Ca seen may result from PTX-B displacing Ca from receptor sites and from an increase in Ca conductance along the nerve terminal membrane. In fact, a log-linear relationship between Ca concentration and amplitude of EPPs was seen in the presence of 1.5 μM PTX-B (Fig. 9), suggesting that PTX-B increases the amplitude of the evoked EPPs by displacing more Ca from the active sites, an effect that could be potentiated by increasing the external Ca concentration as seen in Figure 9.

If one assumes that the toxin blocks Ca-ATPase, one has to accept the proposition that the local presynaptic concentration of Ca would also be increased if the external Ca concentration were increased. Thus, we conclude that PTX-B reacts presynaptically with sites on the nerve terminal membrane and perhaps with the endoplasmic reticulum (26, 27), and postsynaptically in the SR where Ca is bound. PTX-B also inhibits Ca-ATPase, presumably in the presynaptic endoplasmic reticulum as well as postsynaptically in the SR.

Studies in normal and dystrophic chickens disclosed some features that underscore the utility of using PTX-B as a tool for studying mechanisms involving Ca interaction in the SR and nerve terminal. As described earlier (5–8, 28), dystrophic muscles may have an abnormal process of Ca translocation at the SR and motor nerve terminal. This release could be related to a decrease in binding sites located at the SR as well as to other phenomena involving Ca translocation between intracellular compartments. Accordingly, the effect of PTX-B on muscles of normal and dystrophic chickens from 1 to 6 weeks ex ovo was examined.

Avian Skeletal Muscle

Effect on Muscle Contraction and Tetanus

When the posterior latissimus dorsi (PLD) muscles of 9-day-old normal (line 412) and dystrophic (line 413) chickens were exposed to 1.5 μM PTX-B, a major difference was noted between the two types of muscle. The normal muscle showed a pattern of potentiation of the contraction by PTX-B that was qualitatively similar to that seen in rat and frog muscles (Fig. 10; see also Figs. 4, 5), but the muscles from dystrophic animals were unaffected. The contraction noted in normal muscle in the presence of PTX-B showed a typical double

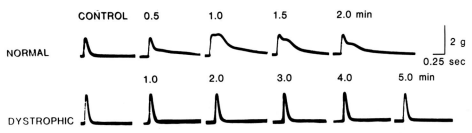

Fig. 10. Effect of 1.5 µM pumiliotoxin-B on the directly evoked twitch of posterior latissimus dorsi muscle from normal (line 412) and dystrophic (line 413) chickens at day 9 ex ovo. Note the potentiation and prolongation of the evoked response in normal but not dystrophic muscle. Time shown is after the addition of toxin.

exponential decay 0.5 minute after exposure to the toxin. This process was complete within 5 minutes, when the single contraction increased nearly 10-fold in duration and the amplitude was enhanced nearly 2-fold (data not shown).

These results are in sharp contrast to the toxin's action on dystrophic muscle, in which neither potentiation nor prolongation of contraction was seen. Figure 10 shows this difference and the time course of the transformation of the single twitch from a small potential to a prolonged and enhanced single contraction in normal muscle. The contrast between normal and dystrophic muscles was also seen when the preparation was exposed to PTX-B and subjected to different rates of tetanic stimulation from 1 to 40 Hz (Fig. 11). After exposure to 1.5 µM PTX-B, tetanic fusion was apparent in normal muscle at 10 Hz; the relaxation phase was significantly prolonged and was transformed into components of fast and much slower relaxation. Tetanic potentiation in the presence of PTX-B was significantly greater than that seen at equivalent tetanic stimulation in the absence of toxin, except that the smallest potentiation was seen at 40 Hz. In contrast, dystrophic muscles treated with PTX-B showed neither prolongation nor potentiation of the single twitch (see also Fig. 10), and the tetanic stimulation at 10 and 20 Hz resembled the pattern observed in control muscle much more than in normal muscle. A striking exception was that the relaxation phase was prolonged immensely. Thus, the dystrophic muscle was still sensitive to PTX-B at this concentration, but the response developed was significantly reduced when compared to that observed in the normal muscle.

Effect on Ca-ATPase
Differences between normal and dystrophic muscles were also observed with Ca-ATPase in SR of the pectoral muscle of normal and dystrophic chickens (5 to 6 weeks ex ovo). Basal activity of Ca-ATPase was essentially the same in preparations isolated from normal and dystrophic animals (Fig. 12). Addition of 30 µM PTX-B to the incubation mixture reduced the activity in normal muscle by 65% but did not inhibit the activity in SR from the dystrophic chicken. The activity of both preparations was stimulated by the addition of 50 µM Ca, but PTX-B inhibited only the activity from the normal chicken. It is noteworthy that 50 µM Ca increased the Ca-ATPase activity from dystrophic birds to a greater extent than that from normal birds. Thus, during the process

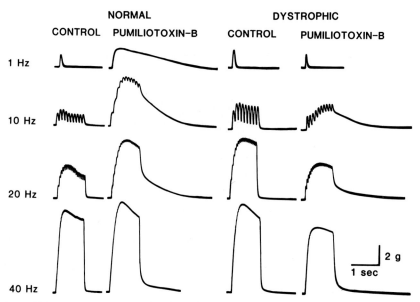

Fig. 11. Effect of 1.5 μM pumiliotoxin-B on the twitch and tetanus tension of posterior latissimus dorsi muscles from normal (line 412) and dystrophic (line 413) chickens at day 9 ex ovo. Records in toxin were obtained between 10 and 15 minutes after addition of the toxin. Note the increased amplitude and prolongation of twitch in normal but not dystrophic muscle after addition of toxin. The tetanic tension increased in normal muscle at all frequencies of stimulation, and after-contraction is evident in the decay phase at termination of the stimulation. In dystrophic muscle the after-contraction was present, but the twitch and tetanus decreased in amplitude on this and other occasions.

of muscular dystrophy in chickens, the Ca-ATPase of the SR becomes markedly insensitive to the effects of PTX-B.

These findings strongly support previous work demonstrating that the ability of Ca-ATPase and SR to release and store Ca in dystrophic muscles is significantly different from that of normal muscles. Characterization of the binding sites of the toxin could conceivably shed light on the nature of the defect in Ca release or storage that appears related to the dystrophic process. In addition, it appears likely that the present differences seen with PTX-B may represent only part of a major alteration in Ca mechanisms whereby levels, binding, and reuptake of Ca in the animals are affected.

Effect on Evoked Transmitter Release

When applied to skeletal muscles of normal chickens, PTX-B affected evoked transmitter release in a way similar to that observed in other species such as the rat and frog (compare Fig. 13 with Fig. 8). In contrast, the nerve terminal of the dystrophic muscle was practically insensitive to the effects of 1.5 to 6.0 μM PTX-B (see Fig. 13). Data in this figure clearly show that PTX-B, although it evoked multiple EPPs (which were facilitated in the normal muscle), did not significantly alter the response of the dystrophic muscle. In contrast, 50-Hz stimulation in curarized normal and dystrophic muscle always resulted in a depression of the EPP amplitude (Fig. 13, Fig. 14).

The failure of PTX-B to enhance EPP frequency or amplitude in dystrophic muscle is clearly related to the inability of the nerve terminal to mobilize Ca in sufficient quantities to generate multiple EPP activity. Thus, the nerve terminal of the dystrophic animals appears to be affected by the disease process, which most likely involves mobilization of Ca and alteration in its storage process (7, and experiments in progress). Although we postulate a primary defect in Ca translocation, our results could also reflect differences in the ability of the toxin to penetrate the synaptic region of the dystrophic muscle as well as SR. Initial studies indicate that PTX-B is a highly lipophilic toxin that easily diffuses into the internal compartments of the nerve as well as the myoplasm in a matter of seconds. It is therefore difficult to argue that the toxin's access in the dystrophic muscle, which is undergoing degeneration, is restricted by diffusion barriers. Work with radiolabeled toxin is needed to clarify this point.

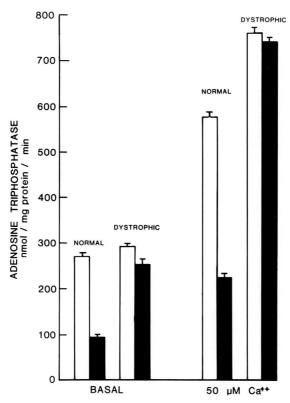

Fig. 12. Activity of calcium-activated adenosine triphosphatase from sarcoplasmic reticulum of pectoral muscles isolated from normal and dystrophic chickens. Open bars are means obtained in the absence of drug; solid bars are values observed in the presence of 30 μM pumiliotoxin-B. Each value represents the mean ± SEM of 3 replicate samples. All incubations were carried out in the presence of 0.1 mM ethyleneglycol-bis-(β-aminoethyl ether)N,N′-tetraacetic acid.

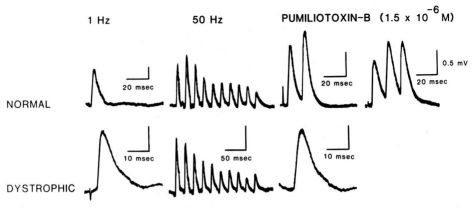

Fig. 13. Effect of 1.5 μM pumiliotoxin-B on evoked release of transmitter in surface fibers of posterior latissimus dorsi muscles from normal (line 412) and dystrophic (line 413) chickens. Single (1 Hz) and tetanic (50 Hz) responses to neural stimulation were first evoked during the course of examining the quantal nature of transmitter. Note the decrease in endplate potential amplitude during the tetanus. Subsequently, each muscle was exposed to pumiliotoxin-B for as long as 2 hours. Only the normal muscle responded with doublet and triplet responses to single shocks applied to the nerve.

In conclusion, PTX-B causes a significant increase in the amplitude and duration of the single muscle contraction in frog, rat, and normal chicken muscles. In the presence of PTX-B, the tetanic tension induced during high-frequency stimulation was potentiated and fusion tension occurred at lower-than-normal rates of stimulation. In addition, the decay phase or relaxation of the muscle after tetanic stimulation was markedly prolonged and the decay showed several different components or decay rates. The toxin produced increases in evoked release of transmitter and multiple EPP discharge after a single nerve shock. Furthermore, the toxin blocked Ca-ATPase. In the normal

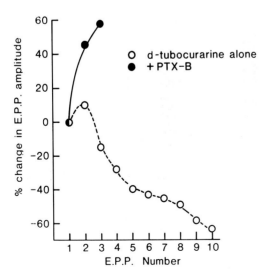

Fig. 14. Facilitation and inhibition of endplate potential (E.P.P.) amplitude in posterior latissimus dorsi muscles from normal (line 412) chickens at 5 to 6 weeks ex ovo. In response to 50-Hz stimulation of the nerve in the presence of 1.2 μM D-tubocurarine chloride, there was an initial facilitation and a profound depression of amplitude. After 1.5 μM pumiliotoxin-B (PTX-B), multiple (2 or 3) endplate potentials were generated in response to single shocks to the nerve. These potentials always were facilitated. Although 50-Hz stimulation of dystrophic muscle also resulted in depression, the toxin never evoked multiple responses. Data are from figure 13.

chicken PLD muscles, the toxin had a qualitatively similar effect on the muscle twitch and tetanus as compared with the frog. However, when the dystrophic PLD muscle was exposed to 1.5 μM PTX-B, no effect on single muscle twitch was recorded and only slight prolongation of the decay phase after attainment of tetanus was observed. The presynaptic effect of the toxin was similar to that seen in the frog, but PTX-B had no effect on the nerve ending of dystrophic chicken skeletal muscle. Finally, PTX-B blocked the Ca-ATPase of normal chicken muscle but not that of dystrophic chicken muscle seen at concentrations of 30 μM. Because PTX-B did not affect Na, K, or Cl^- conductances, the action of the toxin on the presynaptic nerve terminal may be explained by removal and competitive displacement of Ca from its active sites. Thus, PTX-B has proved to be a valuable toxin for reaction with Ca sites at the SR and displacement of the Ca^{2+}.

ACKNOWLEDGMENTS

This work was supported by United States Public Health Service grants NS-12063 and NS-14728, Army Research Office Grant No. DAAG 29-78-G-9293, and by the Muscular Dystrophy Association of America. R. Tamburini was a visiting professor from U.N.E.S.P. in Botucatu, Sao Paulo, Brazil. He was supported by the Conselho Nacional de Desenvolvimento Cientifico e Tecnologico (CNPq), Brazil. The authors are most indebted to Ms. Mabel Alice Zelle for the computer programming and analysis and technical help.

REFERENCES

1. Daly JW, Myers CW: Toxicity of Panamanian poison frogs (*Dendrobates*): some biological and chemical aspects. Science 156:970–973, 1967

2. Daly JW, Tokuyama T, Fujiwara T, Highet RJ, Karle IL: A new class of indolizidine alkaloids from the poison frog, *Dendrobates tricolor*. X-ray analysis of 8-hydroxy-8-methyl-6-(6'7'-dihydroxy-2'5'-dimethyl-4'-octenylidene)-1-azabicyclo[4.3.0]nonane. J Am Chem Soc 102:830–836, 1980

3. Albuquerque EX, Warnick JE, Maleque MA, et al: The pharmacology of pumiliotoxin-B. I. Interaction with calcium sites in the sarcoplasmic reticulum of skeletal muscle. Mol Pharmacol, in press, 1981

4. Warnick JE, Albuquerque EX, Daly JW, et al: The pharmacology of pumiliotoxin-B. II. Interaction with calcium sites in the motor nerve terminal. Mol Pharmacol, in press, 1981

5. Albuquerque EX, Warnick JE: Electrophysiological observations in normal and dystrophic chicken muscles. Science 172:1260–1263, 1971

6. Cosmos E: Intracellular distribution of calcium in developing breast muscle of normal and dystrophic chickens. J Cell Biol 23:241–252, 1964

7. Warnick JE, Albuquerque EX: Changes in genetic expression, development, and the effects of chronic penicillamine treatment on the electrical properties of the posterior latissimus dorsi muscles in two lines of normal and dystrophic chickens. Exp Neurol 63:135–162, 1979

8. Samaha FJ: In *Pathogenesis of Human Muscular Dystrophies*. Edited by Rowland LP. Excerpta Medica, Amsterdam, 1977, pp 633–640

9. Albuquerque EX, McIsaac RJ: Fast and slow mammalian muscles after denervation. Exp Neurol 26:1833–202, 1970

10. Fatt P, Katz B: An analysis of the end-plate potential with an intracellular microelectrode. J Physiol (Lond) 115:320–370, 1951

11. Katz B, Miledi R: Release of ACh from nerve terminal by electric pulses of variable strength and duration. Nature 207:1097–1098, 1965

12. Katz B, Miledi R: Tetrodotoxin and neuromuscular transmission. Proc R Soc Lond [B] 167:8–22, 1967

13. Katz B, Miledi R: The release of acetylcholine from nerve endings by graded electric pulses. Proc R Soc Lond [B] 167:23–28, 1967

14. Froehlich JF, Taylor EW: Transient state kinetic studies of sarcoplasmic reticulum adenosine triphosphatase. J Biol Chem 250:2013–2021, 1975

15. Lowry OH, Lopez JA: In *Methods of Enzymology*, vol III. Edited by Colowick SP, Kaplan NO. 1957, pp 845–849

16. Lowry OH, Passonneau JV: In *A Flexible System of Enzymatic Analysis*. Academic Press, New York, 1972, pp 147–149

17. Lowry OH, Rosenbrough NJ, Farr AL, Randall RJ: Protein measurement with the folin-phenol reagent. J Biol Chem 193:265–275, 1951

18. Albuquerque EX, Warnick JE, Sansone FM, Daly JW: The pharmacology of batrachotoxin. V. A comparative study of membrane properties and the effect of batrachotoxin on sartorius muscles of the frogs *Phyllobates aurotaenia* and *Rana pipiens*. J Pharmacol Exp Ther 184:315–329, 1973

19. Endo M: Calcium release from the sarcoplasmic reticulum. Physiol Rev 57:71–108, 1977

20. Tada M, Yamamoto T, Tonomura Y: Molecular mechanisms of active Ca transport by sarcoplasmic recticulum. Physiol Rev 58:1–79, 1978

21. Warnick JE, Albuquerque EX, Sansone FM: The pharmacology of batrachotoxin. I. Effects on the contractile mechanism and on neuromuscular transmission of mammalian skeletal muscle. J Pharmacol Exp Ther 176:497–510, 1971

22. Albuquerque EX, Adler M, Spivak CE, Aguayo L: Mechanism of nicotinic channel activation and blockade. Ann NY Acad Sci 358:204–238, 1980

23. Albuquerque EX, Tsai M-C, Aronstam RS, et al: Phencyclidine interactions with the ionic channel of the acetylcholine receptor and electrogenic membrane. Proc Natl Acad Sci 77:1224–1228, 1980

24. Armstrong CM: Interaction of tetraethylammonium ion derivatives with the potassium channels of giant axons. J Gen Physiol 58:413–437, 1971

25. Katz B, Miledi R: The role of calcium in neuromuscular transmission. J Physiol (Lond) 195:481–492, 1968

26. Gray EG: In *Synapses*. Edited by Cottrell GA, Usherwood PNR. Academic Press, New York, 1977, pp 6–18.

27. McGraw CF, Somlyo AV, Blaustein MP: Localization of calcium in presynaptic nerve terminals. An ultrastructural and electron microprobe analysis. J Cell Biol 85:228–241, 1980

28. Desmedt JE, Hainaut K: In *Pathogenesis of Human Muscular Dystrophies*. Edited by Rowland LP. Excerpta Medica, Amsterdam, 1977, pp 221–230

Part VI
ALTERATIONS IN METABOLIC REGULATIONS

According to more recent studies, γ-butyrobetaine hydroxylase (EC 1.14.11.1) does not have the same tissue distribution in all species. This enzyme is present in kidney of hamster, rabbit, cat, and Rhesus monkey, but not in kidney of dog, guinea pig, or mouse (24). In humans, we found that the three enzymes subserving γ-butyrobetaine synthesis from ε-N-trimethyllysine were present in all tissues studied (liver, brain, skeletal muscle, heart, and kidney) (12, 25). By contrast, γ-butyrobetaine hydroxylase was present in liver, brain, and kidney but was absent from human heart and skeletal muscle (12, 25). Thus, human skeletal muscle and heart also must depend on carnitine biosynthesis in other tissues and/or on the diet for a supply of this essential nutrient.

We found that hepatic γ-butyrobetaine hydroxylase activity in humans is related to the age of the subject (Fig. 1) (25). Activity is relatively low during the first year of life, gradually increases during childhood, and reaches the adult level in the teens. The increase in activity (y) with age of subject (x) fits the mathematical model $y = ax^b$ (a, 0.139; b, 0.287; r, 0.95; $P < 0.001$). By contrast, hepatic ε-N-trimethyllysine β-hydroxylase activity is not age dependent. Sufficient data are not available to assess age dependence of γ-butyrobetaine hydroxylase in other human tissues. Because it is not clear what proportions of a child's requirement for carnitine are met by diet, hepatic biosynthesis, and biosynthesis by other tissues, the significance of the relatively low hepatic γ-butyrobetaine hydroxylase activity in early life cannot be assessed.

ROLE OF THE KIDNEY

In the rat, intravenously administered ε-N-trimethyllysine is taken up primarily by the kidney (26). There it is converted to γ-butyrobetaine, which then travels

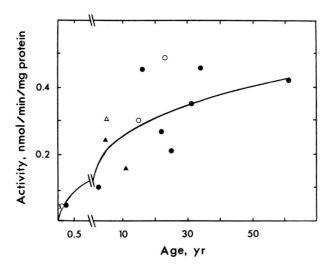

Fig. 1. Dependence of hepatic γ-butyrobetaine hydroxylase activity on age of subject. Male subjects are denoted by closed symbols; female subjects, by open symbols. Circles represent normal control subjects; triangles, patients with systemic carnitine deficiency. The line is a regression of the experimental points fitting the equation $y = ax^b$ (a, 0.139; b, 0.287; r, 0.95; $P < 0.001$).

to the liver for hydroxylation. In nephrectomized rats very little ε-N-trimethyllysine is taken up by the remaining tissues. In humans, as in the rat, intravenously administered ε-N-trimethyllysine is taken up primarily by the kidney, but the fate of γ-butyrobetaine formed in this tissue is altered by the presence of renal γ-butyrobetaine hydroxylase (27). We administered [*methyl*-³H]ε-N-trimethyllysine intravenously to 3 adult males and monitored radioactivity in blood and pooled urine specimens at selected intervals for 48 hours (27). Metabolites were separated by ion-exchange chromatography (Fig. 2). In humans, the ratio of labeled carnitine to labeled γ-butyrobetaine in urine was significantly greater than unity at all time intervals (Table 1). In parallel experiments in rats we found the opposite. At early time intervals after administration of labeled precursor, the urinary excretion of labeled γ-butyrobetaine greatly exceeded that of labeled carnitine.

In humans, the specific activity of carnitine in urine was greater than that in serum at all time intervals (Fig. 3). By contrast, in the rat, the specific activity of carnitine was always higher in serum than in urine. From these results we concluded that in humans intravenous ε-N-trimethyllysine was taken up primarily by the kidney and converted to carnitine. At least part of the newly

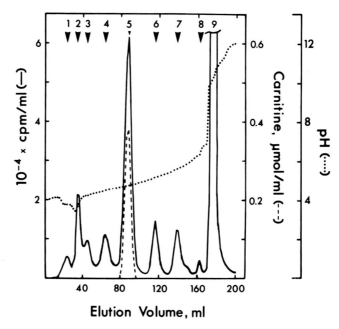

Fig. 2. Separation of metabolites of [*methyl*-³H]ε-*N*-trimethyllysine by ion-exchange chromatography. A column (0.9 × 50 cm) of AG50W-X8 cation-exchange resin (Bio-Rad Laboratories) was equilibrated with 0.25 N (in sodium ions) sodium citrate (pH 4.08) at 50° C. After application of sample (deproteinized and saponified urine or serum), the column was eluted with a linear gradient of 125 ml each of 0.25 N (in sodium ions) sodium citrate (pH 4.08) and 0.25 N NaOH. Two-milliliter fractions were collected, and 1 ml of each was counted. The elution profile shown is 10 ml of a 2 → 6 hour (after administration of precursor) urine specimen of a child with systemic carnitine deficiency. See references 3 and 27 for further procedural details.

Table 1. Ratio of [*methyl*-³H]L-Carnitine to [*methyl*-³H]γ-Butyrobetaine in Urine after Intravenous Administration of [*methyl*-³H]ε-N-Trimethyllysine[a]

| Subjects | Collection Period (hours) | | | | |
	0–2	*2–6*	*6–12*	*12–24*	*24–48*
Normal					
1	2.76	2.50	3.06	3.94	5.41
2	3.90	1.55	2.90	4.19	3.66
3	2.49	2.58	3.46	3.68	8.08
Rats					
1	0.007	0.183			
2	0.004	0.389	3.69		
3	0.004	0.290	0.781	1.35	

[a] One mCi of [*methyl*-³H] ε-N-trimethyllysine (specific activity, 87.9 Ci/mol) was administered to each human subject; 0.1 mCi, to each rat. Urine was collected and analyzed as described in the legend to Figure 2 and in reference 27.

synthesized carnitine entered directly into the tubular lumen, either by secretion or by passive diffusion down a concentration gradient. Carnitine was then efficiently reabsorbed for distribution to other tissues. γ-Butyrobetaine, the end-product of ε-N-trimethyllysine metabolism in rat kidney, probably was handled in a similar manner. Carnitine and γ-butyrobetaine share a common transport mechanism in all systems studied (28, 30). The relatively high excretion of labeled γ-butyrobetaine compared to that of labeled carnitine by the rat kidney suggests that after synthesis by the kidney, some of this compound also enters directly into the tubular lumen. Finally, in the rat the lower specific activity of carnitine in urine compared to serum probably reflects entry of unlabeled carnitine from the kidney into the renal tubular lumen, where it

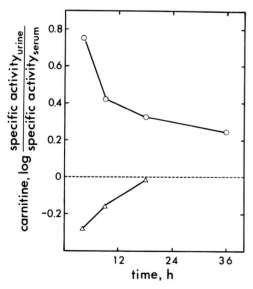

Fig. 3. Ratio of urinary carnitine specific activity to serum carnitine specific activity in rats and humans after intravenous injection of [*methyl*-³-H]ε-N-trimethylly-sine. Values represent the log of the ratio obtained by dividing the average urine carnitine specific activity at each collection period by the average of the serum carnitine specific activity at the start and end of each collection period. Values are plotted at the midpoint of each collection period. Symbols represent the average of determinations in fluids of 3 adult men (circles) and 2 rats (triangles). Values are plotted on a log scale to emphasize that for both humans and rats the ratios converge to unity with time.

mixes with labeled carnitine filtered from the blood, reducing the specific activity of filtered carnitine.

Although the mechanisms described in the preceeding paragraphs are valid for circulating ε-N-trimethyllysine, caution must be exercised in interpreting these conclusions in relation to normal in vivo metabolism. ε-N-Trimethyllysine concentration in the blood is very low, of the order of 0.1 nmol/ml (31). It is not reabsorbed by the kidney (32) and is not taken up readily by tissues (26, 33). In the study cited above, 66% to 84% of the administered dose (average total dose, 142 nmol/kg of body weight) was excreted unchanged in the urine by 48 hours after injection (27). Thus, the amount of circulating ε-N-trimethyllysine available for carnitine biosynthesis is quite low. On the other hand, when ε-N-trimethyllysine is released from proteins by hydrolysis in a given tissue, all or most of it may be converted to γ-butyrobetaine in the same tissue. γ-Butyrobetaine formed in skeletal muscle or heart could then travel via the circulation to kidney or liver for hydroxylation. These tissues internalize γ-butyrobetaine readily compared with ε-N-trimethyllysine (33). Physiologically, this mechanism would conserve carbon chains available for carnitine biosynthesis, because ε-N-trimethyllysine released from tissues would be readily excreted. In humans the kidney probably plays an important role in maintenance of body carnitine stores, because it can synthesize this compound and also efficiently reabsorb it from the tubular lumen.

CARNITINE BIOSYNTHESIS IN PRIMARY SYSTEMIC CARNITINE DEFICIENCY

In Vitro Studies

Low tissue and serum carnitine levels in primary systemic carnitine deficiency suggested a defect in carnitine biosynthesis. Methods for measurement of the four enzymes subserving carnitine biosynthesis from ε-N-trimethyllysine have been established (17, 19, 20, 25). We applied these to liver biopsy specimens from 3 patients with this disease and to a series of control specimens (tissues obtained at autopsy) (34). In 2 patients activity of ε-N-trimethyllysine β-hydroxylase was within the normal range, but in 1 patient the activity of this enzyme was slightly below normal (Table 2). The activities of hepatic β-hydroxy-ε-N-trimethyllysine aldolase and γ-trimethylaminobutyraldehyde dehydrogenase were normal or above normal in all patients. Several "normal ranges" for γ-butyrobetaine hydroxylase activity are listed in Table 2, corresponding to hepatic activity in infants, a child, and adults (15 or more years of age). The activities in 2 patients, 4 and 5 years of age, were high for their age, and activity in 1 patient, an 11-year-old boy, was above the value for the control child but below the normal adult range. Activities of γ-butyrobetaine hydroxylase in these patients are plotted in Figure 1 to show their relationship to the mathematical model established for the control subjects.

From this study, we concluded that all enzymes subserving carnitine biosynthesis from ε-N-trimethyllysine were present and normally active in livers of patients with primary systemic carnitine deficiency. Assessment of the capacity of patient's livers to methylate lysine (the first reaction in the pathway of carnitine biosynthesis) must await development of a suitable assay procedure.

Table 2. Activity of Hepatic Carnitine Biosynthetic Enzymes in Systemic Carnitine Deficiency[a]

Enzyme	Patients			Adult Controls[b]	Infant Controls[b]	Child Control
	1	2	3			
ε-N-Trimethyllysine β-Hydroxylase[c]	43.9	62.2	21.2	45.6 ± 15.5 (28.6–77.9) n = 7	34.2 ± 7.8 (26.2–44.8) n = 3	191
β-Hydroxy-ε-N-trimethyllysine aldolase[d]	111	74.9	76.3	38.7 ± 48.0 (5.8–143) n = 6		
γ-Trimethylaminobutyraldehyde dehydrogenase[d]	34,500	71,000	64,000	46,800 ± 9,200 (36,500–66,300) n = 7	25,700 n = 1	63,900
γ-Butyrobetaine hydroxylase	157	303	243	369 ± 95 (209–488) n = 8	43.3 ± 2.6 (41–47) n = 3	102

[a] Procedures for preparation of tissue homogenates and subcellular fractions and measurement of enzyme activities are described in references 25 and 34. All enzyme activities are given as pmol of product formed per min per mg of protein.
[b] Data are given as Mean ± SD, range, and number of determinations.
[c] Activity was measured in washed mitochondrial fractions.
[d] Activity was measured in 105,000-g supernatant fractions.

In Vivo Studies

The in vitro studies described did not provide information on regulation of the biosynthetic pathway by, for example, hormonal influences or chemical inhibition, processes that might be altered in this disease. Furthermore, the in vitro studies did not test the integrity of the biosynthetic pathway in tissues other than liver. Therefore, we designed in vivo studies to test more rigorously the hypothesis that primary systemic carnitine deficiency results from defective carnitine biosynthesis. For these studies [*methyl*-^{3}H]ε-N-trimethyllysine, rather than labeled lysine, was the precursor of choice. Studies in rats have shown that the amount of a tracer dose of ε-N-trimethyllysine consigned to carnitine biosynthesis is 50 times greater than that for the same dose of lysine (7), and also, ε-N-trimethyllysine has a much shorter biologic half-life than lysine.

One mCi of [*methyl*-^{3}H]ε-N-trimethyllysine (88.7 Ci/mol) was administered intravenously to 2 children (Patient 1, a 7-year-old girl weighing 22 kg; Patient 2, a 5-year-old boy weighing 22 kg) with primary systemic carnitine deficiency, and 3 adult male control subjects 21, 33, and 36 years of age weighing 76, 77, and 85 kg, respectively). Blood samples of 6 to 20 ml and pooled urine specimens were collected at 2, 6, 12, 24, and 48 hours. The labeled precursor and its metabolites were separated by ion-exchange column chromatography using two systems for elution (Fig. 2 and reference 25). Nine metabolites were separated. Six of these were identified by thin-layer, paper, and column chromatography with reference compounds (27). With the exception of carnitine in Patient 1, none of the metabolites was excreted in significantly different amounts by patients compared to control subjects (Table 3). No metabolite seen in patients' urine was absent from control urine, and vice versa. Intermediates in the biosynthetic pathway, i.e., β-hydroxy-ε-N-trimethyllysine and γ-butyrobetaine, were not excreted in greater-than-normal amounts and did not appear increased in serum. Thus, there was no apparent block in the biosynthetic

Table 3. Urinary Excretion of Radioactive Metabolites after Intravenous Administration of [*methyl*-^{3}H] ε-N-Trimethyl-L-lysine[a]

Peak No.[b]	Compound	Control Subjects Mean	Control Subjects Range	Patients A	Patients B
1	?				
2	α-Keto-ε-N-trimethylaminohexanoate	4.33	3.51–5.46	4.74	3.32
3	?				
4	α-N-Acetyl-ε-N-trimethyllysine	3.03	2.14–3.88	2.12	2.16
5	L-Carnitine	5.27	4.43–5.95	24.2	5.62
6	γ-Butyrobetaine	1.68	1.23–2.02	2.62	0.79
7	γ-Trimethylaminopentanoate	1.89	1.40–2.27	1.74	1.80
8	?	0.87	0.58–1.10	1.05	0.55
9A	β-Hydroxy-ε-N-trimethyllysine	4.97	3.88–6.26	6.65	7.30
9B	ε-N-trimethyllysine	758	658–841	792	743

[a] Urine specimens were prepared and chromatographed as described in the legend to Figure 2 and in reference 25. Data are given as μCi of radioactivity excreted per 48 hours.

[b] From Figure 2.

pathway. Furthermore, because there was no abnormal excretion or accumulation in serum of any metabolite, it is unlikely that primary systemic carnitine deficiency results from abnormal catabolism of carnitine.

Patient 1 excreted considerably more labeled carnitine than Patient 2 or the control subjects. This relationship held true even after the data were normalized for differences in precursor dosage per kilogram of body weight. During the first 24 hours of the study, Patient 1, Patient 2, and control subjects excreted 8.50, 4.17, and 3.76 $\pm$ 0.50 μCi (mean $\pm$ SD) of [$methyl$-^{3}H]carnitine, respectively. When normalized, the values become 2.70, 1.33, and 4.25 $\pm$ 0.40 μCi, respectively. However, during the second 24 hours, Patient 1 excreted 15.7 μCi, but Patient 2 excreted only 1.45 μCi and control subjects excreted only 1.40 $\pm$ 0.13 μCi (normalized values, 5.00, 0.46, and 1.58 $\pm$ 0.07 μCi, respectively). Thus, the large increase in labeled carnitine excretion by Patient 1 can be accounted for entirely during the second 24 hours of the study.

A similar pattern was observed in the excretion of total carnitine. During the first 24 hours, Patient 1, Patient 2, and control subjects excreted 3.54, 1.24, and 6.05 $\pm$ 1.70 μmol/kg of body weight, respectively. During the second 24 hours, however, the total carnitine excretion was 34.3, 1.15, and 5.89 $\pm$ 1.69 μmol/kg of body weight, respectively.

The marked increase in both labeled and total carnitine excretion in Patient 1 during the second day of the study is probably related to the increase in serum carnitine concentration of this subject at 24 and 48 hours. At 2, 6, and 12 hours this patient's serum carnitine concentration was 22.7, 20.5, and 20.0 nmol/ml, respectively. However, at 24 and 48 hours the levels were 41.4 and 43.3 nmol/ml, well above her estimated renal threshold of 28 nmol/ml (35). By contrast, the highest serum carnitine concentration measured in Patient 2 was 24.3 nmol/ml (at 12 hours), which was well below his estimated renal threshold for carnitine excretion of 28 nmol/ml.

The specific activity of carnitine in serum peaked at 6 hours in Patient 1 and control subjects, but in Patient 2 it increased sharply at 2 hours, decreased slightly, and then gradually increased to a maximum at 48 hours (Fig. 4). In urine, the specific activity peaked at 2 to 6 hours in both patients and control subjects (Fig. 4). The ratio of carnitine specific activities in urine versus serum was always greater than 1 in both patients and control subjects.

The results of these studies are consistent with normal biosynthesis of carnitine from ε-N-trimethyllysine in primary systemic carnitine deficiency. The lack of accumulation of intermediates and the presence of appreciable amounts of labeled carnitine in both urine and serum, and the relatively high specific activity of carnitine in the patients' body fluids compared with controls' all point to a normal or increased rate of carnitine biosynthesis in patients with this disease.

Our studies have not excluded the possibility of a defect in lysine methylation in systemic carnitine deficiency. As yet, there is no suitable procedure to measure this reaction in vitro. Technical considerations preclude study of lysine methylation in humans in vivo.

As mentioned previously, in mammals, ε-N-trimethyllysine residues destined for carnitine biosynthesis are probably derived from methylation of lysine residues in proteins (16). A generalized defect in protein methylation would

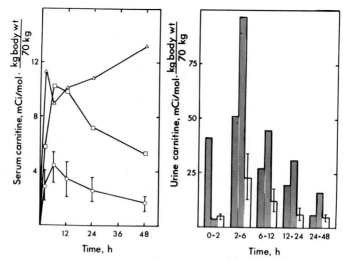

Fig. 4. Specific activity of carnitine in urine and serum after administration of [*methyl*-³H]ε-N-trimethyllysine to control subjects and patients with systemic carnitine deficiency. After 1 mCi of [*methyl*-³H]ε-N-trimethyllysine was given intravenously, blood and urine were collected at the indicated times. Carnitine was separated by ion-exchange chromatography (see Fig. 2) and quantified. All data were normalized for differences in precursor dosage per kilogram of body weight, using the factor (mCi/mol) (kg of body weight) (70 kg)⁻¹. *Left.* Patient 1 is denoted by squares; Patient 2, by triangles; control subjects, by circles. *Right.* Patient 1, diagonal hatching; Patient 2, vertical hatching; control subjects, no hatching. In both panels, bars represent the range of control values.

probably cause widespread metabolic disturbances. On the other hand, if methylation of a single protein were defective, ε-N-trimethyllysine residues from other proteins would still be available for carnitine biosynthesis. It is improbable, based on the incorporation of ε-N-trimethyllysine residues from asialofetuin into carnitine (16), that a single protein, or a group of specific proteins, exclusively provides these residues for carnitine biosynthesis. A deficiency of S-adenosylmethionine could result from absent or defective methionine adenosyltransferase, or lack of methionine. Two cases of human methionine adenosyltransferase deficiency have been described (36, 37). The affected children were clinically normal, except for methioninemia, and did not show the common symptoms of systemic carnitine deficiency. In homocystinuria, caused by decreased 5-methyltetrahydrofolate-dependent homocysteine methylation, serum methionine is decreased (38). However, primary systemic carnitine deficiency is not associated with homocystinuria. Finally, systemic carnitine deficiency may be related to a deficiency of lysine, the ultimate precursor of the carbon chain of carnitine. In rats fed lysine-deficient, essentially carnitine-free diets, heart and skeletal muscle carnitine levels decreased to approximately one-third below normal, but the liver carnitine level increased (39), contrary to what occurs in human systemic carnitine deficiency. From the above arguments, it seems unlikely that defective methylation of lysine could be responsible for the clinical syndrome of primary systemic carnitine deficiency. However, clear proof of this supposition must await further delineation of the pathway by which ε-N-trimethyllysine is formed in vivo and development of a suitable procedure for measuring the rate of this process in vitro.

ACKNOWLEDGMENTS

The authors wish to thank Ms. Jane Tlougan for technical assistance and Ms. Linda Bremner for preparation of this manuscript. This work was supported by a Research Center Grant from the Muscular Dystrophy Association and by NIH grants AM 27451 and NS 06277.

REFERENCES

1. Wolf G, Berger CRA: Studies on the biosynthesis and turnover of carnitine. Arch Biochem Biophys 92:360–365, 1961
2. Bremer J: Carnitine precursors in the rat. Biochim Biophys Acta 57:327–335, 1962
3. Horne DW, Tanphaichitr V, Broquist HP: Role of lysine in carnitine biosynthesis in *Neurospora crassa*. J Biol Chem 246:4373–4375, 1971
4. Paik WK, Kim S: Protein methylation: chemical, enzymological and biological significance. Adv Enzymol 42:227–286, 1975
5. Tanphaichitr V, Horne DW, Broquist HP: Lysine, a precursor of carnitine in the rat. J Biol Chem 245:6364–6366, 1971
6. Horne DW, Broquist HP: Role of lysine and ε-N-trimethyllysine in carnitine biosynthesis. I. Studies in *Neurospora crassa*. J Biol Chem 248:2170–2175, 1973
7. Tanphaichitr V, Broquist HP: Role of lysine and ε-N-trimethyllysine in carnitine biosynthesis. II. Studies in the rat. J Biol Chem 248:2176–2181, 1973
8. Cox RA, Hoppel CL: Biosynthesis of carnitine and 4-N-trimethylaminobutyrate from lysine. Biochem J 136:1075–1082, 1973
9. Cox RA, Hoppel CL: Biosynthesis of carnitine and 4-N-trimethylaminobutyrate from 6-N-trimethyllysine. Biochem J 136:1083–1090, 1973
10. Rebouche CJ, Broquist HP: Carnitine biosynthesis in *Neurospora crassa*: enzymatic conversion of lysine to ε-N-trimethyllysine. J Bacteriol 126:1207–1214, 1976
11. Borum PR, Broquist HP: Purification of S-adenosylmethionine: ε-N-L-lysine methyltransferase: the first enzyme in carnitine biosynthesis. J Biol Chem 252:5651–5655, 1977
12. Rebouche CJ: Comparative aspects of carnitine biosynthesis in microorganisms and mammals with attention to carnitine biosynthesis in man. In *Carnitine Biosynthesis, Metabolism and Functions*. Edited by Frenkel RA, McGarry JD. Academic Press, New York, 1980, pp 57–67
13. Paik WK, Kim S: Protein methylation. Science 174:114–119, 1971
14. Paik WK, Kim S: Solubilization and partial purification of protein methylase III from calf thymus nuclei. J Biol Chem 245:6010–6015, 1970
15. Durban E, Nochumson S, Kim S, et al: Cytochrome c-specific protein-lysine methyltransferase from *Neurospora crassa*: purification, characterization, and substrate requirements. J Biol Chem 253:1427–1435, 1978
16. LaBadie J, Dunn WA, Aronson NN, Jr: Hepatic synthesis of carnitine from protein-bound trimethyllysine. Lysosomal digestion of methyllysine-labeled asialo-fetuin. Biochem J 160:85–95, 1976
17. Hulse JD, Ellis SR, Henderson LM: Carnitine biosynthesis: β-Hydroxylation of trimethyllysine by an α-ketoglutarate-dependent mitochondrial dioxygenase. J Biol Chem 253:1654–1659, 1978

18. Hochalter JB, Henderson LM: Carnitine biosynthesis: the formation of glycine from carbons 1 and 2 of 6-N-trimethyl-L-lysine. Biochem Biophys Res Commun 70:364–366, 1976

19. Hulse JD, Henderson LM: Carnitine biosynthesis: purification of 4-N-trimethylaminobutyral-dehyde dehydrogenase from beef liver. J Biol Chem 255:1146–1151, 1980

20. Lindstedt G, Lindstedt S: Cofactor requirements of γ-butyrobetaine hydroxylase from rat liver. J Biol Chem 245:4178–4186, 1970

21. Haigler HT, Broquist HP: Carnitine synthesis in rat tissue slices. Biochem Biophys Res Commun 56:676–681, 1974

22. Tanphaichitr V, Broquist HP: Site of carnitine biosynthesis in the rat. J Nutr 104:1669–1673, 1974

23. Cox RA, Hoppel CL: Carnitine and trimethylaminobutyrate synthesis in rat tissues. Biochem J 142:699–701, 1974

24. Englard S, Carnicero HH: γ-Butyrobetaine hydroxylation to carnitine in mammalian kidney. Arch Biochem Biophys 190:361–364, 1978

25. Rebouche CJ, Engel AG: Tissue distribution of carnitine biosynthetic enzymes in man. Biochim Biophys Acta 630:22–29, 1980

26. Carter AL, Frenkel RA: The role of the kidney in the biosynthesis of carnitine in the rat. J Biol Chem 254:10670–10674, 1979

27. Rebouche CJ, Engel AG: Significance of renal γ-butyrobetaine hydroxylase for carnitine biosynthesis in man. J Biol Chem 255:8700–8705, 1980

28. Rebouche CJ: Carnitine movement across muscle cell membranes: studies in isolated rat muscle. Biochim Biophys Acta 471:145–155, 1977

29. Christiansen RZ, Bremer J: Active transport of butyrobetaine and carnitine into isolated liver cells. Biochim Biophys Acta 448:562–577, 1976

30. Bohmer T, Eiklid K, Jonsen J: Carnitine uptake into human heart cells in culture. Biochem Biophys Acta 465:627–633, 1977

31. Kakimoto Y, Akazawa S: Isolation and identification of N^G,N^G- and N^G, N'^G-dimethyl-arginine, N^ϵ-mono-, di-, and trimethyllysine, and glucosylgalactosyl- and galactosyl-δ-hydroxylysine from human urine. J Biol Chem 245:5751–5758, 1970

32. Hempel K, Lower R, Owczarek J, et al: Influence of N-methylation in basic amino acids on their transport in kidney. In *Amino Acid Transport and Uric Acid Transport*. Edited by Silbernagl S, Lang F, Greger R, G Thieme Publishers, Stuttgart, 1976, pp 63–70

33. Zaspel BJ, Sheridan KJ, Henderson LM: Transport and metabolism of carnitine precursors in various organs of rat. Biochim Biophys Acta 631:192–202, 1980

34. Rebouche CJ, Engel AG: In vitro analysis of hepatic carnitine biosynthesis in human systemic carnitine deficiency. Clin Chim Acta 106:295–300, 1980

35. Engel AG, Rebouche CJ, Wilson DM, et al: Abnormal renal reabsorption of carnitine in systemic carnitine deficiency (SCD) (abstract). Neurology (Minneap) 30:368–369, 1980

36. Gaull GE, Tallan HH: Methionine adenosyltransferase deficiency: new enzymatic defect association with hypermethioninemia. Science 186:59–60, 1974

37. Finkelstein JD, Kyle WE, Martin JJ: Abnormal methionine adenosyltransferase in hyperme-thioninemia. Biochem Biophys Res Commun 66:1491–1497, 1975

38. Mudd SH, Levy HL: Disorders of transsulfuration. In *The Metabolic Basis of Inherited Disease*, 4th ed. Edited by Stanbury JB, Wyngaarden JB, Fredrickson DS. McGraw-Hill, New York, 1978, pp 458–503

39. Tanphaichitr V, Broquist HP: Lysine deficiency in the rat: concomitant impairment in carnitine biosynthesis. J Nutr 103:80–87, 1973

DISCUSSION

Dr. David Brown: Is there any possibility that your studies in this biosynthetic pathway are complicated by failure of the substrate that you administer, trimethyllysine, to penetrate into the tissues where biosynthesis can occur normally? In other words, is it possible that by using labeled trimethyllysine you are really not investigating adequately the very thing that you are trying to do? If the substrate does not enter the tissues, the demonstration of a defect in carnitine biosynthesis may not be possible.

Dr. Charles Rebouche: We know from our initial studies and from studies in rats that trimethyllysine is taken up by the kidney. We believe this is where most of the labeled carnitine was formed in our in vivo studies. The liver contains all of the enzymes necessary for carnitine biosynthesis. Historically, it has been believed that this is the primary organ for carnitine biosynthesis. We obviated the argument you raised by measuring the activities of the 4 enzymes that subserve carnitine biosynthesis in the liver. There was no defect in these enzymes in primary systemic carnitine deficiency.

Dr. Alfred Goldberg: Is there any disorder of amino acid metabolism in these patients? There have been claims that the branched-chain amino acids require carnitine for their oxidation. These amino acids, and leucine in particular, seem to have a special role in regulating protein balance in muscle.

Dr. Charles Rebouche: In a related study on the renal handling of carnitine, we measured the amino acids in urine of these patients, and they were normal.

Dr. Alfred Goldberg: Concentrations in urine really do not reflect very much at all. It would be valuable in certain experimental studies to get the amino acid pattern of the blood of such patients, especially arterial-venous differences across muscle. This information would be very important for several metabolic questions now being investigated in our own and other laboratories.

Dr. Charles Rebouche: Your point is well taken.

Dr. Fredericus Hommes: Is there any evidence that there is a specific protein or a protein pool made to generate carnitine?

Dr. Charles Rebouche: There is no evidence for that. In fact, if methylation occurs via the protein route, it is probably a nonspecific reaction. Some experiments were reported in 1976 in which asialofetuin that had been methylated in the lysine residues was infused into rat liver. These methylated lysine residues produced carnitine in that system.

Dr. Jarvis Seegmiller: Under conditions of saturation used in in vitro assays, one can find full activity for certain enzymes because there has been a mutation that has affected only the affinity constant, the K_m. Did you look at both high and low substrate concentrations when you were looking at each of these enzymes?

Dr. Charles Rebouche: No, we did not. The substrate concentrations we used (except for the aldehyde dehydrogenase assay) were rather low with respect to the K_m values of the respective enzymes. For the dehydrogenase assay, the substrate concentration we used measured mainly the nonspecific aldehyde dehydrogenase. There has been a report of an aldehyde dehydrogenase that is specific for trimethylaminobutyraldehyde and has a much lower K_m, but we did not measure that.

49
Pathogenetic Mechanisms in Human Carnitine Deficiency Syndromes

Andrew G. Engel, MD

Charles J. Rebouche, PhD

RECOGNITION AND CLASSIFICATION

The discovery in 1973 of a human lipid storage myopathy caused by carnitine deficiency (1) hinged on the fact that by then carnitine was known to facilitate the intramitochondrial oxidation of long-chain fatty acids (2, 3). After 1973, carnitine deficiency was often suspected when pathologic muscle specimens revealed excess lipid, and many, but not all, cases of lipid storage myopathy were shown to be associated with muscle carnitine deficiency. In 1975, observations in a patient with lipid storage myopathy, recurrent episodes of metabolic encephalopathy, fluctuating hepatomegaly, and low carnitine content in muscle, liver, and serum gave rise to the concept of "systemic" carnitine deficiency (4). Since then, carnitine depletion also has been observed in acquired disorders, as in cirrhosis associated with cachexia (5) and chronic renal failure treated by hemodialysis (6). In addition, low muscle carnitine levels have been reported in other metabolic disorders in which the primary abnormality, although undefined, was unlikely to be carnitine deficiency (7–10).

On the basis of these findings, the carnitine deficiency states have been tentatively classified as primary or secondary, and as predominantly myopathic or systemic (11). This classification is still not entirely satisfactory for the following reasons: (*a*) Some patients with muscle symptoms alone demonstrate some of the chemical features of systemic carnitine deficiency (12–14). (*b*) Some patients with systemic symptoms have normal serum or liver carnitine levels at the time of death (15). (*c*) The classification is based on symptoms and tissue and serum carnitine levels, but liver carnitine levels have been determined in only a few cases. The serum carnitine level in itself is not an adequate indicator

643

of tissue carnitine content. (*d*) Some studies report only the free but not the total (free plus acyl) carnitine level. In some disorders, low free but normal total muscle carnitine levels can occur, as in a case of mitochondria-lipid-glycogen disease (8). An altered distribution of carnitine between its free and esterified forms does not indicate carnitine "deficiency."

POSSIBLE CAUSES

According to current knowledge, carnitine biosynthesis in animals proceeds from protein-bound lysine (carbon chain) and methionine (methyl groups) (16, 17). In humans, several tissues (muscle, heart, liver, kidney, and brain) have all of the enzymes required for the formation of the penultimate product, γ-butyrobetaine; but of these tissues, only kidney and liver have significant γ-butyrobetaine hydroxylase activity, which is required for converting γ-buty-robetaine to carnitine (18, and chapter 48 of this volume). Small amounts of this enzyme are present in brain, but none can be found in skeletal or cardiac muscle. Therefore, any contribution to carnitine synthesis by skeletal and cardiac muscle requires the release of preformed γ-butyrobetaine into the circulation and efficient uptake of this compound by liver and kidney.

Carnitine synthesized by liver and kidney is stored in these tissues or is released into the circulation, except for a small amount made by kidney, which is excreted into urine (19, and chapter 48 this volume). Carnitine uptake by most tissues occurs against a concentration gradient, and uptake by skeletal muscle has been shown to be an active transport process (20, 21). One can estimate that the total carnitine content of a 70-kg adult is approximately 100 mmol. Nearly 98% of this amount is in skeletal and cardiac muscle. Liver and kidney account for 1.6%; extracellular fluid, for less than 1% of the total body store (22). The daily urinary carnitine excretion varies within wide limits (23), but only a very small percentage of the filtered load is excreted by the kidney (24, 25). Fecal carnitine excretion is probably not significant in the normal state.

On the basis of the above information, carnitine deficiency in humans could arise from impaired biosynthesis, impaired active transport into cells, excessive release from cells, excessive loss from body fluids, and excessive catabolism. The last cause is purely speculative, because a significant pathway of carnitine catabolism has not been identified.

PRIMARY MYOPATHIC CARNITINE DEFICIENCY

First Reported Case

The first reported patient with primary myopathic carnitine deficiency had slight muscle weakness all her life. At 19 years of age she developed severe generalized muscle weakness and moderate increases in levels of serum enzymes of muscle origin (26). At the height of her illness she also had slight hepatic enlargement and abnormal liver function tests. A muscle biopsy specimen revealed excess lipid, with type 1 fibers more severely affected than other histochemical fiber types. Ultrastructural studies showed mitochondria with indistinct cristae and electron-dense inclusions. This patient's muscle weakness responded dramatically to prednisone. Subsequent metabolic studies established that the patient could utilize fat as well as carbohydrate for basal metabolism and form ketone bodies appropriately on fasting or when ingesting a ketogenic diet. These findings suggested that the metabolic disturbance resided in muscle rather than liver (27). Oxidation by muscle of citric acid cycle substrates and β-hydroxybutyrate was normal. Activities of long-chain fatty acyl-Coenzyme A synthetase and carnitine palmityl-transferase were higher than normal. Oxidation of long-chain fatty acids by homogenates of the patient's muscle was impaired when no carnitine was added to the reaction mixture; but in the presence of added carnitine, the rate of oxidation was within the normal range. This suggested that the patient's muscle lacked carnitine, and this was confirmed by direct assay. Serum carnitine levels in this patient were in the low normal to normal range, but the liver carnitine level was normal (27). The muscle acylcarnitine level was negligible. This patient has experienced a prolonged remission while taking 25 to 50 mg of prednisone and 2 to 4 g of DL-carnitine per day, and now has only mild weakness of cervical, facial, and selected pectoral girdle muscles. However, her muscle carnitine level has remained essentially unchanged.

Spectrum of 'Myopathic' Carnitine Deficiency

Since 1973, 10 additional cases of the more restricted myopathic form of carnitine deficiency have been reported (12, 13, 28–35). Features common to those observed in the first case were muscle carnitine deficiency, excess lipid in muscle, and muscle weakness; 1 patient experienced weakness and fatigability only on exertion (34). Muscle weakness was first noted between 18 months and 38 years of age. Serum enzymes of muscle origin were increased in 8 of 10 cases.

Clinical and biochemical heterogeneity has been noted in this group. The oldest patient developed a peripheral neuropathy; excess lipid was noted in her Schwann cells and leukocytes (28).

Myocardiopathy was detected in 2 patients. This was asymptomatic in an 8-year-old boy (29), but another male child died of congestive heart failure at 3 years of age (33). The cardiac carnitine content in the fatal case was only slightly decreased.

The serum carnitine level was normal in 7 cases but was decreased in 3 others (12, 13, 32). In 1 of these patients the decrease was noted after pregnancy (12).

Liver carnitine content was determined in the first case only and was normal (27). Depressed long-chain fatty acid oxidation by muscle homogenates corrected by carnitine was demonstrated in the first case (1). Similar results were obtained in an unpublished case of myopathic carnitine deficiency (DiDonato S: personal communication). In another patient, not included in this group, such studies revealed a carnitine-resistant depression of fatty acid oxidation (see *Secondary Carnitine Deficiency Syndromes*).

Recurrent myoglobinuria has been observed in 2 patients. One case was reported in an abstract (35); the other case was studied by R.H.T. Edwards (personal communcation).

Prednisone therapy was used in 4 patients (26, 29, 31, 35). Two responded favorably (26, 29), 1 did not respond (35), and 1 did not respond to prednisone alone but improved clinically when propranolol was also administered (32). Carnitine replacement therapy was tried in 7 patients (12, 13, 28, 31, 33, 34, 36); 5 improved clinically (12, 27, 30, 32, 35), but 2 did not (13, 33). Muscle carnitine content was not significantly altered by the replacement therapy (12, 13, 27, 30). Both parents of 1 patient and at least 1 parent of 2 other patients (30, 33) had moderately reduced muscle carnitine levels; 1 patient had a similarly affected sibling (35). This strongly suggests autosomal recessive inheritance.

The low muscle levels but normal serum levels in 7 patients in this group imply impaired active transport of carnitine into muscle and possibly, in some cases, into Schwann cells, leukocytes, and cardiac muscles. However, liver carnitine levels and the effects of carnitine on fatty acid oxidation by muscle homogenates were determined in the first case only (1, 27), and one cannot surmise what these studies might have shown had they been done in the other patients. Thus, the grouping of these patients is somewhat arbitrary, and it is conceivable that "myopathic carnitine deficiency" includes more than one nosologic entity.

PRIMARY SYSTEMIC CARNITINE DEFICIENCY

First Reported Case

The first case, reported by Karpati and coworkers (4), was that of an 11-year-old boy who had always been a weak and clumsy child. He had had acute episodes of encephalopathy at 3.5 and 9 years of age associated with hepatic enlargement and dysfunction. Hypoglycemia was documented during the first episode. The muscle weakness became progressive at 11 years of age. At this time, muscle, serum, and liver carnitine levels were markedly depressed. There was excess lipid in muscle, but not liver. Forearm perfusion studies revealed impaired oxidation of long-chain fatty acids and greatly increased ultilization of glucose (6 times higher than the highest control value). There was also short-chain dicarboxylic aciduria, presumably due to increased omega-oxidation of long-chain fatty acids. The patient's weakness responded remarkably well to carnitine replacement therapy. His serum carnitine level returned to normal, but the muscle and liver carnitine contents remained unchanged.

Spectrum of the Deficiency

Eleven additional cases of systemic carnitine deficiency have been reported in detail since 1975 (15, 25, 36–41). The hallmarks of the syndrome are recurrent episodes of acute encephalopathy, progressive muscle weakness, and excess lipid in muscle and other tissues at one stage of illness or death. Muscle carnitine levels were reduced in all cases. Cardiac carnitine content was decreased in 4 cases in which it was measured (15, 38, 41). Serum carnitine, measured in 9 patients, was reduced in 7 (4, 15, 38–41), but was normal or higher than normal in 2 patients when they were terminally ill (15, 41). Liver carnitine content, determined in 8 cases, was reduced markedly in 5 (4, 15, 25, 36, 40) and slightly in 2 (39). In 2 patients investigated by us, the serum carnitine fluctuated from very low to low normal values on repeated determinations during a period of a few days (26). The kidney carnitine level, measured in 2 patients, was normal (39).

The age of onset of the disease ranged from 8 months to 17 years. In 6 patients, one or more episodes of encephalopathy preceded recognition of the disease by months or years (15, 25, 38, 40); in 4 patients, weakness preceded the encephalopathy (4, 36, 39, 41); in 2 patients weakness was noted shortly after recovery from encephalopathy (37, 39). The 7-year-old sister of a patient who died in an acute attack at 15 years of age was asymptomatic but had low serum and muscle carnitine levels. The parents were unaffected (41), suggesting autosomal recessive inheritance.

The muscle weakness was generally greater proximally than distally, at times also involved the facial and cervical muscles, and was associated with decreased muscle bulk. Typically there was more excess lipid in type 1 than type 2 fibers.

Eight of the 12 patients died during the course of acute attacks (15, 36–39, 41). The age at death ranged from 7 to 28 years. Autopsy studies in 5 fatal cases (15, 36, 38, 41) revealed marked accumulation of fat in muscle and liver and a lesser lipid increase in kidney and heart. One patient had cardiac symptoms and died of congestive heart failure (38). Another patient had a transient episode of renal insufficiency during life (36). In 2 patients progression of the disease was accelerated by pregnancy (36, 38).

Three patients with systemic carnitine deficiency have been treated with carnitine. One of these showed improved muscle strength without change in tissue carnitine levels, even though his serum level returned to normal during therapy (4). One patient died despite replacement therapy (38). One patient showed no change in strength and remained intolerant of fasting after several months of treatment (40).

Encephalopathic Attacks

All patients had multiple episodes of acute encephalopathy. The initial symptom was usually vomiting followed by deepening stupor, confusion, and coma. In 8 cases hypoglycemia was observed during at least one of the acute attacks (4, 15, 25, 37–40). All patients had evidence of hepatic dysfunction during some of the acute episodes. Liver enlargement was noted in all cases. Increased serum levels of hepatic enzymes were observed in 6 cases (15, 25, 36, 38–40). Increased prothrombin time was noted in 2 cases (38, 40) and mild hyperammonemia was documented in 3 (15, 25, 40). Metabolic acidosis (ketonuria and low serum pH or bicarbonate level) was found in 6 patients during the acute attacks (25, 36–38, 41). A high serum lactic acid level was reported in 1 case (37). An excess of short-chain urinary dicarboxylic acids was found in 2 cases (4, 40). In at least 6 patients the attacks followed, or were provoked by, caloric deprivation (25, 36–38, 40).

The acute encephalopathic episodes of systemic carnitine deficiency resemble attacks of Reye's syndrome (42–44). Similarities include hypoglycemia, hypoprothrombinemia, hyperammonemia, increased serum levels of hepatic enzymes, and excess lipid in hepatocytes during the attacks. However, in patients with typical attacks of Reye's syndrome, serum or tissue levels of carnitine were either normal or only slightly depressed (40, 43, 45). On the other hand, the similarities between the acute attacks of systemic carnitine deficiency and Reye's syndrome suggest that impaired fatty acid oxidation represents a common pathway in the pathogenesis of both disorders.

The encephalopathic episodes of systemic carnitine deficiency can also mimic those caused by urea cycle defects (46), ketotic hypoalaninemic hypoglycemia of childhood (47), fructose-1, 6-diphosphatase deficiency (48), phosphoenolpyruvate carboxykinase deficiency (49), and some of the organic acidurias (50).

The reason for the recurrent crises in systemic carnitine deficiency is not clearly understood, but caloric deprivation is probably an important provocative factor. Fasting calls for increased utilization of fatty acids and increased gluconeogenesis. Utilization of fatty acids by the tissues is limited by the carnitine deficiency, and hepatic gluconeogenesis is probably inadequate because it requires energy derived from the oxidation of fatty acids. The already higher-than-normal utilization of glucose by peripheral tissues, the impaired gluconeogenesis, and the lack of dietary carbohydrate probably lead to rapid depletion of available glycogen stores and hypoglycemia.

Accelerated utilization of branched-chain amino acids is also likely to occur (51), but these give rise to branched-chain keto acids which, in turn, may require carnitine for their complete oxidation (52, 53). Accumulation of these compounds, and also of dicarboxylic acids derived from accelerated omega-oxidation of fatty acids, and of lactic acid from accelerated glycogenolysis, could result in metabolic acidosis. The encephalopathy could be a consequence of the hypoglycemia, the metabolic acidosis, the abnormal accumulation of a toxic metabolite, or a combination of these factors.

Etiology

In a series of studies, we have investigated the etiology of primary systemic carnitine deficiency. The low serum, muscle, and liver carnitine levels suggested a defect in biosynthesis (4). However, in livers of 3 patients the activities of each of the biosynthetic enzymes responsible for the conversion of ε-N-trimethyllysine to carnitine were preserved (19, 54). Furthermore, intravenously administered labeled ε-N-trimethyllysine was readily converted to labeled carnitine in the 2 patients in whom this test was performed (19, 55). These studies do not exclude a possible defect in the protein methylation of lysine to ε-N-trimethyllysine, but a defect of this type would be unlikely to occur without other evidence of a severe metabolic disturbance (55).

We also tested the hypothesis that primary systemic carnitine deficiency could be due to a renal carnitine leak (25). Renal tubular reabsorption rates, reabsorptive maxima, and apparent renal plasma thresholds for carnitine were determined in 2 children with primary systemic carnitine deficiency and in 7 control subjects. In the 2 patients, these values were well below those observed in the 7 control subjects, but 1 control subject, a healthy 20-year-old woman with a normal muscle carnitine level, also exhibited a renal carnitine leak (Fig.

1). Tubular secretion of short-chain acylcarnitines was noted in patients and controls at high free plasma carnitine levels.

From this study, we concluded that there was evidence for impaired transport of carnitine across the renal epithelial cell membrane, but this in itself could not account for carnitine depletion of tissues. Therefore, an additional factor, namely abnormal transport of carnitine (decreased uptake or increased release) by other tissues, needs to be postulated to account for the pathogenesis of the disease. According to this scheme, muscle and liver carnitine levels would be depressed because of a transport abnormality involving these tissues. A lowered renal plasma excretory threshold for carnitine would tend to lower the plasma carnitine level, which would further decrease the uptake and/or enhance the efflux of carnitine from the tissues. In addition, a renal carnitine leak would offset compensatory increases in biosynthesis and could lead to an abnormal

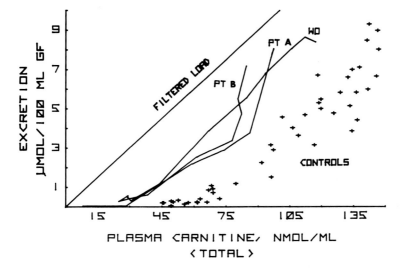

Fig. 1. Excretion of total carnitine per 100 ml of glomerular filtrate versus total plasma carnitine level in 2 patients with systemic carnitine deficiency and in 7 control subjects. In the patients and in 1 control subject (WO) the excretion exceeds that in the remaining control subjects at every plasma carnitine level. Observed points in the patients and WO are connected by lines; individual points are plotted for the remaining control subjects. An upsweep in the excretion curve occurred at high plasma carnitine levels in the 2 patients. A similar upsweep was also observed in 5 of 7 control subjects. Most of this upsweep was accounted for by an augmented excretion of short-chain acylcarnitine compounds at high plasma free carnitine levels. This may be due to increased secretion or production of acylcarnitine by the renal tubules at high plasma free carnitine levels, competitive inhibition of acylcarnitine reabsorption by high free carnitine concentration in the tubular lumen, or both. Augmented acylcarnitine excretion occurred at lower free plasma carnitine levels in the patients than in the control subjects. This may indicate that the reabsorption of both acylcarnitine and free carnitine is impaired in the patients and/ or that tubular secretion of acylcarnitine occurs more readily in the patients than in the control subjects. Intercepts of the curves with the abscissa indicate the apparent renal plasma threshold for carnitine excretion. The curves for the patients and WO approach the abscissa at lower levels of plasma carnitine than the curves for the remaining control subjects.

loss of carnitine from the body when there is mobilization of carnitine from the tissues. An extension of this hypothesis explains myopathic carnitine deficiency in terms of impaired transport involving muscle but not liver or renal cells. An additional implication is related to the fact that carnitine and γ-butyrobetaine compete for a common transport site (20). Therefore, biosynthesis of carnitine might be hindered in systemic carnitine deficiency because γ-butyrobetaine synthesized in muscle would not be readily taken up by liver and kidney for conversion to carnitine. However, it is not known how much of the γ-butyrobetaine made by muscle is used by liver and kidney for carnitine synthesis in the normal state.

SECONDARY CARNITINE DEFICIENCY SYNDROMES

Muscle Deficiency Associated with Other Metabolic Abnormality

Heterogeneous clinical syndromes have been reported with excess lipid and low carnitine levels in muscle. In each case there were associated clinical or laboratory features which suggested that the carnitine deficiency was secondary to another, unidentified, metabolic abnormality. The mechanism and significance of the carnitine deficiency in these cases will remain obscure until the underlying biochemical lesions are clearly defined.

An 11-year-old boy described by Smyth and colleagues (7) had calcification of basal ganglia, seizures, high-tone hearing loss, increased spinal fluid protein, muscle weakness, exertional lactic acidemia, frequent vomiting, but no acute episodes of encephalopathy. Carnitine treatment improved the patient's growth rate, strength, and tendency to vomit. Serum and liver carnitine levels were not assayed before treatment and muscle carnitine was not determined after treatment.

A patient studied by Konigsberger and coworkers (personal communication) had a neurodegenerative disease associated with seizures, growth retardation, lactic acidosis, and episodic cortical blindness. The muscle carnitine level was moderately low, but the serum carnitine level was normal. The oxidation of palmitate, pyruvate, β-hydroxybutyrate, and glucose by muscle homogenates was reduced, which suggests a secondary defect in carnitine metabolism. Carnitine replacement therapy was ineffective.

A 51-year-old woman described by Whitaker and coworkers (9) had progressive muscle weakness, liver dysfunction, structurally abnormal liver mitochondria, and carnitine deficiency in quadriceps but not in biceps muscle. The serum carnitine level was normal. Liver carnitine was not determined. Muscle homogenates oxidized palmitate, β-hydroxybutyrate, and pyruvate at a reduced rate. Prednisone therapy improved the patient's weakness and restored the carnitine content of the quadriceps muscle to normal.

A young adult woman with progressive muscle weakness and muscle carnitine deficiency was studied by Willner and associates (10). The serum carnitine level was normal; the liver carnitine level was not measured. There were no features to suggest a systemic metabolic disturbance, and the patient resembled the first reported case of muscle carnitine deficiency (1). Muscle homogenates oxidized long-chain fatty acids at a reduced rate but, unlike the first reported case, this could not be corrected by the addition of carnitine. Furthermore, the uptake of carnitine by muscle strips in vitro was not significantly different from that found in control subjects. The muscle carnitine deficiency was considered to be secondary to a defect of β-oxidation in muscle. The mechanism by which this reduced the muscle carnitine level was not explained. This case indicates that the syndrome of "myopathic" carnitine deficiency is biochemically heterogeneous.

Carnitine Deficiency in Acquired Disorders

Chronic Renal Failure Treated by Hemodialysis
Muscle carnitine deficiency has been observed in the course of chronic hemodialysis by Bohmer and coworkers (6). The deficiency could not be fully accounted for by carnitine removed by hemodialysis, but the uremic state might have adversely affected the mechanism of carnitine transport into the tissues. The authors suggest that the cardiomyopathy occasionally observed in patients undergoing hemodialysis could be due to carnitine deficiency.

Cirrhosis with Cachexia
Carnitine deficiency in serum and tissues has been observed in cachectic, cirrhotic patients by Rudman and colleagues (5). They attribute this to the combined effects of decreased normal liver mass and low dietary intake of carnitine and its precursors. They also suggest that carnitine deficiency might play a role in the pathogenesis of hepatic coma, but patients with urea cycle defects also have episodes of encephalopathy without carnitine deficiency.

Chronic Severe Myopathies
Decreased muscle carnitine levels have been reported in patients with advanced Duchenne and Becker dystrophy by Borum and colleagues (56). Studies in our laboratory have shown slightly reduced mean carnitine values in Duchenne dystrophy (37). Borum and associates suggest that the low carnitine values in dystrophic muscle are a nonspecific result of severe muscle damage.

Decreased Plasma Carnitine Content, Tissue Levels Not Determined
Decreased plasma carnitine levels have been observed in children with kwashiorkor (57). Decreased plasma and urine carnitine values have been reported in myxedema, hypopituitarism, and adrenal insufficiency (58, 59). Finally, a progressive decrease in the serum carnitine level occurs during pregnancy (12, 60). Tissue carnitine levels have not been examined in these states.

Diphtheritic Cardiomyopathy
Diphtheritic cardiomyopathy in the guinea pig is associated with fatty degeneration and carnitine deficiency of the heart (61). Human diphtheritic cardiom-

yopathy is presumably also associated with carnitine deficiency. The exact mechanism of the carnitine deficiency has not been determined.

UNSOLVED PROBLEMS

Even this brief survey of the human carnitine deficiency syndromes reveals a number of unsolved problems. The first of these pertains to the fact that most studies of carnitine metabolism were done in laboratory animals and are not necessarily applicable to carnitine metabolism in humans. For example, in humans, kidney and brain as well as liver have all of the enzymes required for carnitine biosynthesis, whereas heart and muscle lack only the final enzyme, γ-butyrobetaine hydroxylase (18, and chapter 48 of this volume). Thus, carnitine precursors between ϵ-N-trimethyllysine and γ-butyrobetaine, which are formed in cardiac and skeletal muscle, might be carried by the circulation to the organs that can complete the biosynthesis. This could be functionally important if human liver and kidney had sufficiently active transport mechanisms for the uptake of the precursors and especially γ-butyrobetaine. However, nothing is known of the direction and significance of the precursor traffic between the human tissues involved in carnitine synthesis; the uptake of carnitine precursors by human organs has not been investigated; the relative significance of liver and kidney in carnitine biosynthesis in humans has not yet been assessed; and the rates of carnitine synthesis, turnover and half-life for the entire organism and for the critical organs have not been determined.

With regard to primary systemic carnitine deficiency, the reason for the intermittent character of the acute episodes is not understood, and the exact biochemical reason for the encephalopathy is unknown. The development of metabolic acidosis during the acute episodes is only partially understood, and the excessive formation of ketone bodies in some cases despite the impaired oxidation of long-chain fatty acids has not been thoroughly investigated. Uptake and release of carnitine by critical organs has not been studied in primary systemic carnitine deficiency. Finally, the reason why some patients respond to replacement therapy with no change in their tissue carnitine levels is unexplained.

Muscle carnitine deficiency itself represents a heterogeneous group of disorders. In some patients it may be secondary to a defective transport of carnitine into muscle, but there is no direct proof of this. In other patients the muscle carnitine deficiency might be secondary to a yet undefined metabolic defect. The reason for the clinical response of some patients to replacement therapy without a change in tissue carnitine levels is again unexplained.

It is clear that a careful study of patients suspected of suffering from either systemic or muscle carnitine deficiency should include (a) assays of free as well as short-chain and long-chain acylcarnitines in muscle, liver, and serum, (b) determinations of the rates of long-chain fatty acid oxidation by muscle homogenates, and (c) the determination of the effects of carnitine on these rates.

The significance of the decreased serum carnitine levels in malnutrition, pregnancy, and various endocrinopathies is obscure. Tissue carnitine levels and the factors that regulate the serum level (synthesis, excretion and tissue uptake) have not been studied in these states.

ACKNOWLEDGMENT

Work in the authors' laboratory was supported by a Research Center Grant from the Muscular Dystrophy Association and by National Institutes of Health Research Grants NS 6277 and AM 27451. We thank Ms. Linda Bremner for preparation of this manuscript.

REFERENCES

1. Engel AG, Angelini C: Carnitine deficiency of skeletal muscle associated with lipid storage myopathy: a new syndrome. Science 173:899–902, 1973

2. Fritz IB: The metabolic consequences of the effects of carnitine on long-chain fatty acid oxidation. In *Cellular Compartmentalization and Control of Fatty Acid Metabolism.* Edited by Bremer J, Gran FC. Academic Press, New York, 1967, pp 39–63

3. Bremer J: Factors influencing the carnitine-dependent oxidation of fatty acids. In *Cellular Compartmentalization and Control of Fatty Acid Metabolism.* Edited by Bremer J, Gran FC. Academic Press, New York, 1967, pp 65–88

4. Karpati G, Carpenter S, Engel AG, et al: The syndrome of systemic carnitine deficiency: clinical, morphologic, biochemical and pathophysiologic features. Neurology (Minneap) 25:16–24, 1975

5. Rudman D, Sewell CW, Ansley JD: Deficiency of carnitine in cachectic cirrhotic patients. J Clin Invest 60:716–723, 1977

6. Bohmer T, Bergrem H, Eiklid K: Carnitine deficiency induced during intermittent haemodialysis for renal failure. Lancet 1:126–128, 1978

7. Smyth DPL, Lake BD, MacDermot J, et al: Inborn error of carnitine metabolism ("carnitine deficiency") in man. Lancet 1:1198–1199, 1975

8. DiDonato S, Cornelio F, Balestrini B, et al: Mitochondria-lipid-glycogen myopathy, hyperlacticacidemia and carnitine deficiency. Neurology (Minneap) 28:1110–1116, 1978

9. Whitaker JN, DiMauro S, Solomon S, et al: Corticosteroid responsive skeletal muscle disease associated with partial carnitine deficiency: studies of liver and metabolic alterations. Am J Med 63:805–815, 1977

10. Willner JH, DiMauro S, Eastwood A, et al: Muscle carnitine deficiency: genetic heterogeneity. J Neurol Sci 41:235–246, 1979

11. Engel AG: Possible causes and effects of carnitine deficiency in man. In *Carnitine Biosynthesis, Metabolism and Functions.* Edited by Frenkel RA, McGary JD. Academic Press, New York, 1980, pp 271–284

12. Angelini C, Govoni E, Bragaglia MM, et al: Carnitine deficiency: acute postmortem crisis. Ann Neurol 4:558–561, 1978

13. Carroll JE, Brooke MH, DeVivo DC, et al: Carnitine "deficiency": lack of response to carnitine therapy. Neurology (Minneap) 30:618–626, 1980

14. Carroll JE, DeVivo DC, Brooke MH, et al: Fasting as a provocative test in neuromuscular diseases. Metabolism 28:683–687, 1967

15. Ware AJ, Burton CW, McGarry JD, et al: Systemic carnitine deficiency: report of a fatal case with multisystem manifestations. J Pediatr 93:959–964, 1978

16. Tanphaichitr V, Broquist HP: Role of lysine and ϵ-N-trimethyllysine in carnitine biosynthesis. II. Studies in rat. J Biol Chem 248:2176–2181, 1973

17. LaBadie J, Dunn WA, Aronson NN, Jr: Hepatic synthesis of carnitine from protein-bound trimethyllysine: lysosomal digestion of methyllysine-labeled asialo-fetuin. Biochem J 160:85–95, 1976

18. Rebouche CJ, Engel AG: Tissue distribution of carnitine biosynthetic enzymes in man. Biochim Biophys Acta 630:22–29, 1980

19. Rebouche CJ, Engel AG: Significance of renal γ-butyrobetaine hydroxylase for carnitine biosynthesis in man. J Biol Chem (in press)

20. Rebouche CJ: Carnitine movement across muscle cell membranes: studies in isolated rat muscle. Biochim Biophys Acta 471:145–155, 1977

21. Willner JH, Gisburg S, DiMauro S: Active transport of carnitine into skeletal muscle. Neurology (Minneap) 28:721–724, 1978

22. Rebouche CJ: Comparative aspects of carnitine biosynthesis in microorganisms and mammals with attention to carnitine biosynthesis in man. in *Carnitine Biosynthesis, Metabolism and Functions.* Edited by Frenkel RA, McGarry JD. Academic Press, New York, 1980, pp 57–72

23. Cederblad G, Lindstedt S: Excretion of L-carnitine in man. Clin Chim Acta 33:117–123, 1971

24. Frolich J, Seccombe DW, Hahn P, et al: Effects of fasting and esterified carnitine levels in human serum and urine: correlation with serum levels of free fatty acids and β-hydroxybutyrate. Metabolism 27:555–561, 1978

25. Engel AG, Rebouche CJ, Wilson DM, et al: Primary systemic carnitine deficiency. II. Renal handling of carnitine. Neurology (Minneap) (in press)

26. Engel AG, Siekert RG: Lipid storage myopathy responsive to prednisone. Arch Neurol 27:174–181, 1972

27. Engel AG, Angelini C, Nelson RA: Identification of carnitine deficiency as a cause of human lipid storage myopathy. In *Exploratory Concepts in Muscular Dystrophy. II.* Edited by Milhorat AT. Excerpta Medica Int Congr Ser 333:601–617, 1975

28. Markesbery WR, McQuillen MP, Procopis PG, et al: Muscle carnitine deficiency: association with lipid myopathy, vacuolar neuropathy, and vacuolated leukocytes. Arch Neurol 31:320–324, 1974

29. VanDyke DH, Griggs RC, Markesbery W, DiMauro S: Hereditary carnitine deficiency of muscle. Neurology (Minneap) 25:154–159, 1975

30. Angelini C, Lucke S, Cantarutti F: Carnitine deficiency of skeletal muscle: report of a treated case. Neurology (Minneap) 26:633–637, 1976

31. Isaacs H, Heffron JJA, Badenhorst M, et al: Weakness associated with the pathological presence of lipid in skeletal muscle: a detailed study of a patient with carnitine deficiency. J Neurol Neurosurg Psychiatry 39:1114–1123, 1976

32. Scarlato G, Albizatti MG, Bassi S, et al: A case of lipid storage myopathy with carnitine deficiency: biochemical and electromyographic correlations. Eur Neurol 16:222–229, 1977

33. Hart ZH, Chang CH, DiMauro S, et al: Muscle carnitine deficiency and fatal cardiomyopathy. Neurology (Minneap) 28:147–151, 1978

34. Jerusalem F, Engel AG, Sengupta CH, et al: Carnitin-Mangel-Myopathie. Episodische belastungsabhanginge Myalgien und Schwache. Dtsch Med Wochenschr 105:469–473, 1980

35. Engel WK, Prockop LD, Askanas V, et al: Nearly-fatal lipid-laden myopathy with myoglobinuria and myodeficiency of carnitine: prednisone failure but dramatic improvement with carnitine, and cultured muscle cell dependence on carnitine (abstract). Neurology (Minneap) 30:368, 1980

36. Boudin G, Mikol J, Guillard A, et al: Fatal systemic carnitine deficiency with lipid storage in skeletal muscle, heart, liver and kidney. J Neurol Sci 30:313–325, 1976

37. Engel AG, Banker BQ, Eiben RM: Carnitine deficiency: clinical, morphological and biochemical observations in a fatal case. J Neurol Neurosurg Psychiatry 40:313–322, 1977

38. Cornelio F, DiDonato S, Peluchetti D, et al: Fatal cases of lipid storage myopathy with carnitine deficiency. J Neurol Neurosurg Psychiatry 40:170–178, 1977

39. Scarlato G, Pellegrini G, Cerri C, et al: The syndrome of carnitine deficiency: morphological and metabolic correlations in two cases. Can J Neurol Sci 5:205–213, 1978

40. Glasgow AM, Eng G, Engel AG: Systemic carnitine deficiency simulating recurrent Reye syndrome. J Pediatr 96:889–891, 1980

41. Scholte HR, Meijer AEFH, Van Wijngaarden GK, et al: Familial carnitine deficiency: a fatal case and subclinical state in a sister. J Neurol Sci 42:87–101, 1979

42. DeVivo DC, Keating JP: Reye's syndrome. Adv Pediatr 22:175–229, 1976

43. Haymond MW, Karl IE, Keating JP, DeVivo DC: Metabolic response to hypertonic glucose administration in Reye syndrome. Ann Neurol: 3:207–215, 1978

44. Trauner D, Sweetman L, Holm J, et al: Biochemical correlates of illness and recovery in Reye's syndrome. Ann Neurol 2:238–241, 1977

45. Willner JH, Chutorian AM, DiMauro S: Tissue carnitine levels in Reye syndrome. Ann Neurol 4:468–469, 1980

46. Shih VE: Urea cycle disorders and other congenital hyperammonemic syndromes. in *The Metabolic Basis of Inherited Disorders*, 4th ed. Edited by Stanbury JB, Wyngaarden JB, Fredrickson DS. McGraw Hill, New York, 1978, pp 362–386

47. Pagliara AS, Karl IE, Haymond MW, et al: Hypoglycemia in infancy and childhood. Part II. J Pediatr 82:558–577, 1973

48. Pagliara AS, Karl IE, Keating JP, et al: Hepatic fructose-1,6-diphosphatase deficiency. J Clin Invest 51:2115–2123, 1972

49. Hommes FA, Bendien K, Elema JD, et al: Two cases of phosphoenolpyruvate carboxykinase deficiency. Acta Paediatr Scand 65:233–240, 1976

50. Dancis J, Levitz M: Abnormalities of branched chain amino acid metabolism. In *The Metabolic Basis of Inherited Disorders*, 4th ed. Edited by Stanbury JB, Wyngaarden JB, Fredrickson DS. McGraw Hill, New York, 1978, pp 397–410

51. Felig P: Amino acid metabolism in man. Annu Rev Biochem 44:933–955, 1975

52. Bieber LL, Choi YR: Isolation and identification of aliphatic short-chain acylcarnitines from beef heart: possible role for carnitine in branched-chain amino acid metabolism. Proc Natl Acad Sci USA 74:2795–2798, 1977

53. Van Hinsbergh WV: Veerkamp JH, Engelen PJM, et al: Effect of L-carnitine on the oxidation of leucine and valine by rat skeletal muscle. Biochem Med 20:115–124, 1978

54. Rebouche CJ, Engel AG: In vitro analysis of hepatic carnitine biosynthesis in human systemic carnitine deficiency. Clin Chim Acta (in press)

55. Rebouche CJ, Engel AG: Primary systemic carnitine deficiency. I. Carnitine biosynthesis. Neurology (Minneap) (in press)

56. Borum PG, Broquist HP, Roelofs RI: Muscle carnitine levels in neuromuscular disease. J Neurol Sci 34:279–286, 1977

57. Khan L, Bamji MS: Plasma carnitine levels in children with protein-calorie malnutrition before and after rehabilitation. Clin Chim Acta 75:163–166, 1977

58. Maebashi M, Kawamura N, Sato M, et al: Urinary excretion of carnitine in patients with hyperthyroidism and hypothyroidism: augmentation by thyroid hormone. Metabolism 26:351–356, 1977

59. Maebashi M, Kawamura N, Sato M, et al: Urinary excretion of carnitine and serum concentrations of carnitine and lipids in patients with hypofunctional endocrine diseases: involvement of adrenocorticoid and thyroid hormones in ACTH-induced augmentation of carnitine and lipid metabolism. Metabolism 26:357–361, 1977

60. Scholte HR, Jennekens FGI: Low carnitine levels in serum of pregnant women. N Engl J Med 299:1079–1080, 1978

61. Wittels B, Bressler R: Biochemical lesion of diphtheria toxin in heart. J Clin Invest 43:630–637, 1964

DISCUSSION

Dr. H. W. Swick: In systemic carnitine deficiency, at the time of the episodic acute encephalopathy, is there evidence of some precipitant stress, preceding infection, or change in diet similar to what occurs in Reye's syndrome and in the urea cycle defects?

Dr. Andrew Engel: Frequently, the patient has had a respiratory infection, stopped eating, then started to vomit, became stuporous, and then comatose. One can induce this syndrome by starving the patient even after recovery from the acute episode. It is important to prevent caloric deprivation in these patients.

Dr. Michel Fardeau: Did you observe in normal control or pathologic conditions some variations in the serum carnitine level in relation to muscle exercise or fatigue?

Dr. Andrew Engel: We have not. Dr. Felix Jerusalem has studied a patient with carnitine deficiency who had symptoms resembling McArdle's disease. Perhaps he would like to comment.

Dr. Felix Jerusalem: We did not study the relationship of serum carnitine to exercise.

Dr. Andrew Engel: In our studies, control and patient serum carnitine values were all measured in the resting state.

Dr. Stefano DiDonato: I would like to make a brief comment on the problem of systemic carnitine deficiency. We have recently been studying the effect of carnitine on the metabolism of normal cultured fibroblasts; the major effects seen were those of a decrease in the oxidation of pyruvate labeled in the C-2 molecule and an increase in the oxidation of palmitate-1-^{14}C. For the oxidation of pyruvate, labeled in C-2, the decrease in this oxidation is accompanied by quantitative formation of acetylcarnitine. We looked at cultured fibroblasts from carnitine-deficient patients; we have looked at 4 patients, 2 with muscle carnitine deficiency and 2 with systemic carnitine deficiency. The effects of carnitine seen in the patients with muscle carnitine deficiency were comparable to those observed in normal controls, whereas no effect of externally added carnitine was seen in patients with systemic carnitine deficiency. This may be related to a defect of carnitine receptors in cultured cells from systemic carnitine deficient patients and it would fit with the observation made by Dr. Engel that a defect exists in tubular reabsorption of carnitine; this disease may be due to a generalized defect of carnitine receptors, that is expressed in the kidney tubule, too.

50
Carnitine Palmityltransferase (CPT) Deficiency: A Review

Salvatore DiMauro, MD

Carlo Trevisan, MD

In this review of carnitine palmityltransferase (CPT) deficiency, we will consider the clinical presentation and laboratory abnormalities, the functional consequences and postulated pathogenic mechanism of myoglobinuria, and a variety of biochemical problems.

Before discussing any aspect of the disease, however, it may be useful to review the normal metabolic pathway involved in the oxidation of long-chain fatty acids. These become available to muscle from exogenous and endogenous sources. Exogenous sources consist of plasma free fatty acids, which are complexed to albumin or the more abundant plasma triglycerides, mostly in the form of very low density lipoproteins (VLDL). Fatty acids are liberated from VLDL by a triglyceride lipase known as lipoprotein lipase, which appears to be located on the endothelial lining of capillaries (1, 2). Lipoprotein lipase is released into the circulation by heparin, is inhibited by salt, and requires a specific serum apolipoprotein for full activation (2).

Endogenous sources of free fatty acids consist of lipid droplets; these triglyceride depots are normally present in muscle in close proximity to mitochondria. The presence of intracellular triglycerides that can be mobilized with exercise (3–5) indicates that both synthetic and degradative pathways are present in muscle. However, the relative importance of intracellular compared to extracellular sources of fatty acids at rest and during exercise remains to be clarified. The intracellular triglyceride lipase of muscle has not been studied as extensively as the presumably extracellular lipoprotein lipase or the hormone-sensitive, cyclic adenosine monophosphate–dependent intracellular lipase of adipose tissue (6), and its physiologic control is virtually unknown. Irrespective of their origin, intracellular long-chain fatty acids are activated to palmityl coenzyme A (CoA) at the expense of adenosine triphosphate by a thiokinase (palmityl CoA synthetase or ligase). In both animal muscle (7) and human muscle (Trevisan C: unpublished data), the thiokinase appears to be predominantly or exclusively bound to the outer mitochondrial membrane.

The inner mitochondrial membrane is impermeable to palmityl CoA. Carnitine palmityltransferase I, which is loosely bound to the outer face of the inner mitochondrial membrane (8, 9), catalyzes the formation of palmitylcarnitine. As carnitine esters, long-chain fatty acids can cross the inner mitochondrial membrane barrier. It has recently been proposed that this transport may occur by a process of exchange diffusion facilitated by a carnitine-acylcarnitine translocase (10–12). Once inside the mitochondrion, palmitylcarnitine is again converted to palmityl CoA by a second form of CPT (CPT II), which appears to be tightly bound to the inner face of the inner mitochondrial membrane. Palmityl CoA can then undergo β-oxidation.

Carnitine palmityltransferase deficiency was discovered in 1973 in 2 brothers with recurrent myoglobinuria (13). The diagnosis at admission was "probable McArdle disease," but unlike most patients with phosphorylase or phosphofructokinase deficiency, these young men did not complain of cramps or intolerance to short intense exercise, and myoglobinuria was precipitated by prolonged rather than strenuous activity. Glycogen storage disease was excluded by the normal increase in venous lactate concentration after ischemic exercise, normal muscle biopsy, and normal activities of phosphorylase and phosphofructokinase in muscle extracts.

The need for studies of lipid metabolism in these patients was suggested by two considerations. First, a clinical syndrome so similar to McArdle disease and yet not involving glycogen metabolism could well be due to impaired utilization of the other major fuel for muscle contraction, namely, lipid. Second, a similar syndrome of recurrent myoglobinuria due to impaired utilization of long-chain fatty acids had been described a few years earlier in identical twin girls; a defect of muscle CPT had been postulated but not documented (14). In a prophetically accurate editorial appearing with that article, Bressler envisioned defects of carnitine and of each of the twin CPT enzymes as possible causes of myopathy (15). We found that carnitine concentration, and the activities of palmityl CoA synthetase and of the short-chain acyl carnitine transferase (carnitine acetyl transferase) were essentially normal in muscle extracts from the brothers, but CPT activity, whether measured by a colorimetric assay or by more sensitive radioactive assays, was markedly decreased both in muscle homogenates and in crude mitochondrial preparations (13, 16).

We then asked the patients to fast for a few days while at complete rest: by 72 hours, there was a sharp increase in serum creatine phosphokinase, and myoglobin was detected in plasma and urine (16). Ketone body production during fasting was decreased or delayed in these patients, suggesting that the enzyme defect may affect the liver as well (16).

Since 1973, many more patients with CPT deficiency have been identified; Figure 1 summarizes the clinical features of 21 cases, 16 of which have been reported (13, 16–27). The clinical presentation is relatively homogeneous and consists of recurrent episodes of muscle necrosis and myoglobinuria. Unlike patients with muscle phosphorylase or phosphofructokinase deficiency, patients with CPT deficiency do not have painful cramps on exercise, although they

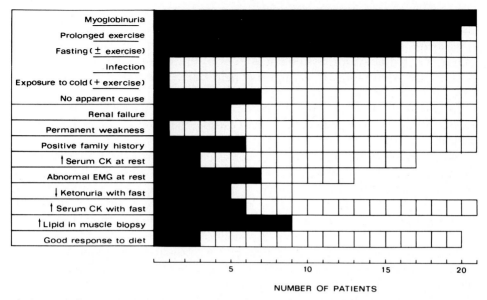

Fig. 1. Graphic representation of clinical and laboratory findings in 21 patients with carnitine palmityltransferase deficiency. Sixteen patients have been reported (13, 16–27); the others have been studied at Columbia-Presbyterian Medical Center, but not described in detail. Each block represents 1 patient; filled blocks indicate positive symptoms or signs. CK, creatine kinase; EMG, electromyogram.

may experience a feeling of "tightness" or "stiffness" of their muscles before episodes of myoglobinuria. Lack of cramps, which act as warning signals in patients with glycogenoses, probably explains the numerous episodes of myoglobinuria in CPT deficiency: 8 of the 21 patients had had 5 or more attacks.

The main precipitating factors are prolonged exercise, not necessarily of great intensity, fasting, or a combination of the two circumstances. Anxiety and lack of sleep may play a role: 2 students noticed that some attacks occurred before final examinations. Exposure to cold was considered to be a precipitating factor in a man who fell into a mountain lake (19), but he had also been hiking for several hours before reaching his unintentional icy destination. Mild infections or viral illnesses may precipitate myoglobinuria, as was evident in 1 patient who had led a sedentary life because of congenital neurologic deficits (26). In some patients, however, no precipitating factor can be identified, as illustrated by an airline pilot who had episodes of myoglobinuria after transatlantic flights during which he was confined in the cockpit and did not fast.

Unlike McArdle disease (28), myoglobinuria occurred in childhood in a few cases. In most patients, however, the first attacks occur during adolescence, and the diagnosis is usually made in young men 15 to 30 years of age. Considering the frequent episodes of myoglobinuria, it is surprising that renal failure occurred only in 5 of the 21 patients. Fixed weakness, which is seen in approximately 25% of patients with McArdle disease (28), is not a feature of CPT deficiency, outside the acute episodes of myoglobinuria. Among the 21 patients there were 3 sets of siblings. Parents were clinically unaffected, and we found intermediate levels of CPT activity in the leukocytes of the mother of our first 2 patients (29). Transmission is probably autosomal recessive but the overwhelming prevalence of men (so far, only 1 affected woman has been described) (19, Case 3) is difficult to explain solely on the basis of different gender-related activities. Systematic studies of muscle or leukocytes from both parents and asymptomatic siblings will help clarify the mode of transmission, but these have not yet been reported.

Although there is no specific therapy, in several patients a diet rich in carbohydrates has been beneficial in reducing the number of myoglobinuric attacks.

No laboratory test is specifically or consistently abnormal in CPT deficiency. Serum creatine kinase (CK) is usually normal between episodes of myoglobinuria, and electromyography showed nonspecific "myopathic" features in only 3 patients (18–20). The hypertriglyceridemia that we had observed in the first 2 patients and considered secondary to the defective utilization of free fatty acids by muscle was found in only 2 patients (19, 21).

Thus, hypertriglyceridemia is neither an obligatory consequence of the metabolic defect nor a useful diagnostic clue. The effects of prolonged fasting also vary in different patients: decreased or delayed ketonemia and increased serum CK were each seen in approximately half of the patients tested (Figure 1). Muscle biopsy specimens may be completely normal, as they were in the first 2 patients (13, 16), or show variable increase in the number of lipid droplets (17, 19, 22, 23, 26, 30). In the same patient, the degree of lipid storage may vary considerably from time to time (17, 26) and from muscle to muscle (26).

The enzyme defect has been documented in several tissues besides muscle. Decreased activity in leukocytes was found in the first 2 patients (29) and has been confirmed in 2 more (Fig. 2) (26, 27). The activity was also lower than normal in platelets (27), in transformed lymphoblasts (31), and in fibroblast (21, 27) and muscle (32) cultures. Indirect evidence that the activity of liver CPT may also be decreased had come from studies showing impaired ketonemia in some fasting patients. In 1 of these patients (Fig. 2), the enzyme defect has

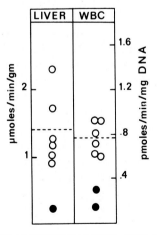

CPT ACTIVITY IN LIVER AND WBC

Fig. 2. Scatter plots of carnitine palmityltransferase (CPT) activity determined by isotope exchange in liver biopsy specimens and leukocytes (WBC) from control subjects and from 2 patients with muscle CPT deficiency. For methodologic details, see Bertorini and coworkers (26). Dotted lines represent mean control values.

been documented by liver biopsy (26): CPT activity was approximately one fourth of the lowest control value. Higher residual activities may explain the normal ketonemic response to fasting in other patients.

Current knowledge about the metabolic requirements of muscle during exercise explains the circumstances leading to myoglobinuria in patients with CPT deficiency. For heavy exercise (at work intensities close to the maximal O_2 uptake), energy is derived almost exclusively from glycogen metabolism, and glycogen depletion appears to coincide with exhaustion (33). During prolonged exercise of moderate intensity, there is a gradual shift from carbohydrate to lipid metabolism. Muscle glycogen and blood glucose are predominantly utilized for approximately 40 minutes. As exercise is prolonged, fatty acids become increasingly important; after about 4 hours, they are the main source of energy (33).

Glycogen metabolism is normal in patients with CPT deficiency, and so is their capacity for intense exercise of short duration. With prolonged activity, however, an "energy crisis" (34) occurs as their dependence on long-chain fatty acids increases. Fasting worsens the situation, probably because it reduces not only the concentration of muscle glycogen but also the availability of blood glucose, thus increasing the dependence of muscle on lipid metabolism. The inadequate production of ketone bodies during fasting in many of these patients deprives muscle of still another alternative fuel. These pathogenic mechanisms have been confirmed by several physiologic investigations. The respiratory quotient (RQ) was abnormally high in 1 patient both at rest and during exercise (27), in keeping with the increased dependence on carbohydrate. This critical need for carbohydrate "fuel" was also shown by the severe intolerance to exercise shown by the same patient after his muscle glycogen had been intentionally depleted by a combination of ketogenic diet and exercise (27). Direct demonstration of the impaired utilization of long-chain fatty acids was provided by studies of radioactive CO_2 excretion after infusion of labeled palmitate (27). Prolonged exercise caused an excessive increase in serum CK in 1 patient (20, 35) and prolonged fasting caused both serum CK increase and decreased production of ketone bodies.

Although CPT deficiency appears to be a well-documented genetic cause of recurrent myoglobinuria, several biochemical questions remain to be defined. When CPT is measured in muscle extracts by radioisotope assays such as the "isotope-exchange" reaction (36), the activity in patients, although distinctly less than that in control subjects, is not zero; in our series, it varied between 7% and 21% of the normal mean (Fig. 3). If the enzyme defect is not complete, does it affect mainly CPT I, CPT II, or both to the same extent? A related question is whether CPT I and II are two functionally and structurally different isoenzymes or one and the same enzyme with different localization on the two sides of the inner mitochondrial membrane.

CPT I was purified to apparent homogeneity and CPT II was partially purified from beef liver mitochondria (37). The CPT I was extracted from a mitochondrial fraction with the non-ionic detergent Tween-20, precipitated with ammonium acetate, and adsorbed on a calcium phosphate gel. The CPT II was obtained in fractions that did not adsorb to a calcium phosphate gel (37).

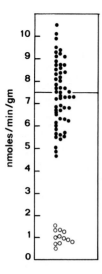

Fig. 3. Scatter plot of carnitine palmityltransferase (CPT) activity determined by isotope exchange in muscle biopsy specimens from 57 control subjects and 12 patients with CPT deficiency. The horizontal line represents the mean control value.

The two enzymes had several different characteristics (38, 39):

1. The reaction from palmitylcarnitine to palmityl CoA was catalyzed reversibly by CPT I, but proceeded only in the direction of palmityl CoA with CPT II.

2. CPT II, but not CPT I, required preincubation with coenzyme A (CoASH) for full activity, and was inhibited by miristoyl- and decanoyl-carnitine.

3. The range of fatty acid chain length specificity was narrower for CPT II than for CPT I. Although these findings seemed to suggest the existence of two different CPT enzymes, the properties of solubilized enzymes might have been changed by the purification procedure and might not have accurately reflected those of the native, membrane-bound enzymes (37, 40).

To obviate this problem, Solberg (40) suggested an ingenious procedure to distinguish the two enzyme activities in intact liver mitochondria. He exploited the fact that intact mitochondria are impermeable to CoASH. After removal of all external CoASH by addition of tetrathionate (which itself does not penetrate the mitochondria), only the endogenous pool of CoASH is left; this is accessible only to CPT II, which alone will be active under these conditions. A limitation of this method is that CPT I activity is not studied directly, but by difference of CPT II from "total" CPT activity measured without tetrathionate and in the presence of exogenous CoASH. A second limitation is the difficulty of isolating structurally intact mitochondria, particularly from skeletal muscle. A few studies in tissues of CPT patients have attempted to clarify whether the genetic defect involves CPT I, CPT II, or both. All 3 possibilities have been reported to occur in 5 different patients; this is not impossible, but it may reflect more the pitfalls of the methods used than the genetic heterogeneity of CPT deficiency.

Polarographic studies of isolated muscle mitochondria in 1 patient (13) showed that oxidation of palmitylcarnitine was not impaired, indirectly suggesting that CPT I was predominantly affected. Similar studies, also suggesting CPT I deficiency, have been briefly reported by Hostetler and associates (41) in another patient. Patten and colleagues (24) measured total CPT and CPT II by the method of Solberg (40) in isolated muscle mitochondria from a third patient, and concluded that the major deficiency was of CPT II activity. However, the method described for the isolation of mitochondria raises questions about mitochondrial integrity. Scholte and coworkers (25) also suggested a selective defect of CPT II in their patient, on the basis of a normal "forward reaction" (from palmityl CoA to palmitylcarnitine) and abnormal kinetics of the isotope exchange reaction in extracts of frozen muscle. However, their assumption that the "forward reaction" only measures CPT I activity is contradicted by data in rat liver mitochondria (42). Layzer and associates (27) isolated mitochondria from cultured fibroblasts rather than muscle, and separated CPT I and II by releasing the loosely bound CPT I with digitonin. They found the same degree of enzyme deficiency in the two fractions and suggested that the two enzymes may be identical, or at least share a subunit under common genetic control.

Another potentially useful approach to this question is the use of specific inhibitors for CPT I or II, several of which have been described (39, 42–44). A practical advantage of this approach is that it may allow characterization of the residual CPT activity in frozen muscle biopsy specimens, because the specificity of CPT I inhibition by malonyl CoA (42) and 2-tetradecylglycidic acid (44) does not seem to be dependent on mitochondrial integrity. Another possible source of error in studies of residual CPT activity is due to the presence of the medium-chain acyl carnitine transferase (carnitine octanoyl transferase, COT). As reported for human liver (45), we found in human muscle that the activity of COT is much higher than that of CPT, and it is even higher than normal in patients with CPT deficiency (26). Because the fatty acyl chain length specificity of COT may not be very narrow, what we consider "residual" CPT activity in muscle of patients may in fact be a "tail" of COT activity. This possibility should be excluded before attempting to attribute the residual activity to CPT I or II.

In summary, our knowledge of CPT deficiency at the molecular level is incomplete, but studies of this genetic error may help clarify the structural and functional relationship of CPT I and II in normal tissues.

ACKNOWLEDGMENTS

Some of the work described was supported by Center Grant NS-11766-06 from the National Institutes of Neurological and Communicative Diseases and Stroke, a grant from the Muscular Dystrophy Association, and Grant AM-25599-01 from the National Institute of Arthritis, Metabolism and Digestive Diseases.

Dr. Trevisan is the recipient of a postdoctoral fellowship from the Muscular Dystrophy Association.

REFERENCES

1. Schotz MC, Twu J-S, Pedersen ME, et al: Antibodies to lipoprotein lipase: application to perfused heart. Biochim Biophys Acta 489:214–224, 1977

2. Severson DL: Regulation of lipid metabolism in adipose tissue and heart. Can J Physiol Pharmacol 57:923–937, 1979

3. Froberg SO, Mossfeldt F: Effect of prolonged strenuous exercise on the concentration of triglycerides, phospholipids and glycogen in muscle of man. Acta Physiol Scand 82:167–171, 1971

4. Essen B: Intramuscular substrate utilization during prolonged exercise. Ann NY Acad Sci 301:30–44, 1977

5. Essen B, Hagenfeldt L, Kaijser L: Utilization of blood-borne and intramuscular substrates during continuous and intermittent exercise in man. J Physiol (Lond) 265:489–506, 1977

6. Steinberg D: Interconvertible enzymes in adipose tissue regulated by cyclic AMP-dependent protein kinase. Adv Cyclic Nucleotide Res 7:157–198, 1976

7. Aas M: Organ and subcellular distribution of fatty acid activating enzymes in the rat. Biochim Biophys Acta 231:32–47, 1971

8. Hoppel CL, Tomec RJ: Carnitine palmityltransferase: location of two enzymatic activities in rat liver mitochondria. J Biol Chem 247:832–841, 1972

9. Brosnan JT, Kopec B, Fritz IB: The localization of carnitine palmitoyltransferase on the inner membrane of bovine liver mitochondria. J Biol Chem 248:4075–4082, 1973

10. Pande SV: A mitochondrial carnitine acylcarnitine translocase system. Proc Natl Acad Sci USA 72:883–887, 1975

11. Pande SV, Parvin R: Characterization of carnitine acylcarnitine translocase system of heart mitochondria. J Biol Chem 251:6683–6691, 1976

12. Parvin R, Pande SV: Carnitine-acylcarnitine translocase. J Biol Chem 253:1944–1946, 1978

13. DiMauro S, Melis-DiMauro PM: Muscle carnitine palmityltransferase deficiency and myoglobinuria. Science 182:929–931, 1973

14. Engel WK, Vickna, Glueck J, Levy RI: A skeletal muscle disorder associated with intermittent symptoms and a possible defect in lipid metabolism. N Engl J Med 282:697–704, 1970

15. Bressler R: Carnitine and the twins. N Engl J Med 282:745–746, 1970

16. Bank WJ, DiMauro S, Bonilla E, et al: A disorder of muscle lipid metabolism and myoglobinuria. N Engl J Med 292:443–449, 1975

17. Cumming WJK, Hardy M, Hudgson P, Walls J: Carnitine-palmityltransferase deficiency. J Neurol Sci 30:247–258, 1976

18. Herman J, Nadler HL: Recurrent myoglobinuria and muscle carnitine palmityltransferase deficiency. J Pediatr 91:247–250, 1977

19. Brownell AKW, Severson DL, Thompson CD, Fletcher T: Cold-induced rhabdomyolysis in carnitine palmityltransferase deficiency. Can J Neurol Sci 6:367–370, 1978

20. Carroll JE, Brooke MH, DeVivo DC, et al: Biochemical and physiologic consequences of carnitine palmityltransferase deficiency. Muscle Nerve 1:103–110, 1978

21. DiDonato S, Cornelio F, Pacini L, et al: Muscle carnitine-palmityltransferase deficiency: report of a case with enzyme deficiency in cultured fibroblasts. Ann Neurol 4:465–467, 1978

22. Hostetler KY, Hoppel CL, Romine JS, et al: Partial deficiency of muscle carnitine palmityl transferase with normal ketone production. N Engl J Med 298:553–557, 1978

23. Reza MJ, Kar NG, Pearson CM, et al: Recurrent myoglobinuria due to muscle carnitine palmityltransferase deficiency. Ann Intern Med 88:610–615, 1978

24. Patten BM, Wood JM, Harati Y, et al: Familial recurrent rhabdomyolysis due to carnitine palmityltransferase deficiency. Am J Med 67:167–171, 1979

25. Scholte HR, Jennekens FGI, Bouvy JJBJ: Carnitine palmityltransferase II deficiency with normal carnitine palmityltransferase I in skeletal muscle and leukocytes. J Neurol Sci 40:39–51, 1979

26. Bertorini T, Yeh YY, Trevisan C, et al: Carnitine palmityltransferase deficiency: myoglobinuria and respiratory failure. Neurology (NY) 30:263–271, 1980

27. Layzer RB, Havel RJ, McIlroy MB: Partial deficiency of carnitine palmityltransferase. Neurology (NY) 30:627–633, 1980

28. DiMauro S: Metabolic myopathies. In *Handbook of Clinical Neurology*, vol 41, part II. Edited by Vinker PJ, Bruyn GW. North Holland Publishing Co., Amsterdam, 1979, pp 175–234

29. DiMauro S, Eastwood AB: Disorders of glycogen and lipid metabolism. Adv Neurol 17:123–142, 1977

30. Engel AG, Santa T, Stonnington HH, et al: Morphometric study of skeletal muscle ultrastructure. Muscle Nerve 2:229–237, 1979

31. Hostetler KY, Yazaki PJ: Deficiency of carnitine palmitoyltransferase in transformed lymphoblasts from a patient having a deficiency of carnitine palmitoyltransferase in skeletal muscle. Biochem Biophys Res Commun 94:270–277, 1980

32. Miranda A, Trevisan C, Shanske S, et al: The expression of genetic enzyme defects in muscle cultures: now you see it, now you don't (abstract). Neurology (NY) 30:367, 1980

33. Felig P, Wahren J: Fuel homeostasis in exercise. N Engl J Med 293:1078–1084, 1975

34. Warshaw JB: An energy crisis in muscle. N Engl J Med 292:476–477, 1975

35. Brooke MH, Carroll JE, Davis JE, Hagberg JM: The prolonged exercise test. Neurology (NY) 29:636–643, 1979

36. Norum K: Palmityl-CoA: carnitine palmityltransferase. Biochim Biophys Acta 89:95–108, 1964

37. Kopec B, Fritz IB: Properties of a purified carnitine palmitoyltransferase, and evidence for the existence of other carnitine acyltransferases. Can J Biochem 49:941–948, 1971

38. Koepc B, Fritz IB: Comparison of properties of carnitine palmitoyltransferase I with those of carnitine palmitoyltransferase II, and preparation of antibodies to carnitine palmitoyltransferases. J Biol Chem 248:4069–4074, 1973

39. Fritz IB, Kopec B, Brosnan JT: Localization of carnitine palmitoyltransferase on inner membranes of mitochondria, and their possible role in the regulation of fatty acyl group translocation. In *Regulation of Hepatic Metabolism*. Edited by Lundquist F, Tygstrup N. Academic Press, New York, 1974, pp 482–497

40. Solberg HE: Acyl group specificity of mitochondrial pools of carnitine acyltransferases. Biochim Biophys Acta 360:101–112, 1974

41. Hostetler KY, Hoppel CL, Romine JS, et al: Lipid myopathy with recurrent myoglobinuria due to carnitine palmitoyltransferase A deficiency in skeletal muscle mitochondria (abstract). Clin Res 25:496A, 1977

42. McGarry JD, Leatherman GF, Foster DW: Carnitine palmitoyltransferase I: the site of inhibition of hepatic fatty acid oxidation by malonyl-CoA. J Biol Chem 253:4128–4136, 1978

43. Chase JFA, Tubbs PK: Specific inhibition of mitochondrial fatty acid oxidation of 2-bromopalmitate and its coenzyme A and carnitine esters. Biochem J 129:55–65, 1972

44. Tutwiler GF, Ryzlak MT: Inhibition of mitochondrial carnitine palmitoyltransferase by 2-tetradecylglycidic acid. Life Sci 26:393–397, 1980

45. Solberg HE: Different carnitine acyltransferases in calf liver. Biochim Biophys Acta 280:442–433, 1972

DISCUSSION

Dr. Corrado Angelini: Is myoglobinuria the only symptom by which we can pick up this patient? We had a family in which the brother was affected by myoglobinuria and had muscle, liver, and platelet carnitine palmityltransferase (CPT) deficiency and his sister (probably the second affected woman) had no symptoms except occasional increases in transaminases. Although essentially asymptomatic, she had total CPT deficiency in muscle. Unlike her brother, she had normal ability to produce ketone bodies. Judging by the CPT activity in platelets, the parents seem to have intermediate levels of the enzyme. I wonder whether the preponderance of men is due to the fact that we study only patients that have myoglobinuria.

Dr. Salvatore DiMauro: Well, you did identify your patient because he had myoglobinuria. You are right that we have measured CPT activity only in patients who had recurrent myoglobinuria. It is possible that, as we screen more patients, we may find some with different clinical features. The findings in the family you described are very interesting, particularly the fact that the sister seemed to have the enzyme defect but was not symptomatic. This suggests that the other factors, e.g., hormonal factors, might be responsible for whether or not the myoglobinuria occurs.

Dr. Donald Wood: Has ATP actually been measured and shown to be decreased in these patients?

Dr. Salvatore DiMauro: No, ATP has not been measured in any of these patients. In patients with CPT deficiency, there is an additional problem in looking for decreases of ATP or creatine phosphate, and that is *when* to study these compounds. The only way to do this would be to submit the patients to prolonged, carefully controlled exercise, fasting, or the two conditions together. However, that might cause muscle necrosis, which would complicate the determinations. It is easier to do such studies in McArdle's disease, which is probably what prompted your question. As you know, a decrease in ATP or creatine phosphate was never documented in McArdle's disease after ischemic exercise or during contractures. I am sure Dr. Edwards will discuss this later.

51
Definitive Assays for Glycogen Debranching Enzyme in Human Fibroblasts

Barbara I. Brown, PhD

David H. Brown, PhD

The subject matter of this paper was selected because it relates to alterations in metabolic regulation, carrier detection, the use of cultured cells, and muscle involvement. No attempt will be made to review the field of glycogen storage diseases. Table 1 shows the various enzyme deficiencies and the distribution of the types of glycogen storage disease for which tissue samples have been studied in Saint Louis during the past three decades. Two of the common forms of glycogen storage disease (Types I and VI) do not result in significant aberrations in muscle metabolism. Progress made in the treatment of Type I disease, also known as von Gierke's disease, by nocturnal nasogastric infusion has been reviewed recently by Greene and colleagues (1), Fernandes (2), and associates and Stacey (3). Fructose diphosphatase deficiency (see chapter 52) appears in this table because liver samples from such patients were analyzed to ascertain whether glucose-6-phosphatase or fructose diphosphatase deficiency was the primary cause of the hepatomegaly, hypoglycemia, and hyperlactic acidemia manifested by these patients.

Table 1 includes the number of families known to have more than one affected member and the sex of the affected persons. Most available evidence suggests that the glycogenoses are inherited as autosomal recessive traits, although there is a clearly documented sex-linked deficiency of hepatic phosphorylase kinase, as well as a report of dominant inheritance of McArdle's syndrome in one affected family (4). Moreover, it has also been noted that the number of affected children in families at risk is greater than expected, perhaps due to the small number of sibships considered and the preponderance of small-sized families in the sampling (5).

The glycogenoses affecting muscle are Types II, III, and V. Type V, also known as "McArdle's disease," is due to a deficiency of myophosphorylase,

Table 1. Distribution of Glycogen Storage Disease Studied in St. Louis (1951–1979)

Type	Enzyme Deficiency	Number Affected			Families with >1 Affected Patient
		Total	M	F	
I	Glucose-6-phosphatase	97	58	39	29
II	α-Glucosidase (lysosomal)				
	Infantile type	51	34	17	17
	Adult type	12	9	3	3
III	Glycogen debranching enzyme				15
	Liver and muscle	56	27	29	
	Liver only	12	6	6	
	Muscle status unknown	16	7	9	
IV	Glycogen branching enzyme	15	9	6	3
V	Glycogen phosphorylase (muscle only)	10	6	4	
VI	Reduced phosphorylase activity or other factors (liver)	97	76	21	21
	Fructose-1,6-diphosphatase (liver)	8	4	4	2
	Total	374	236	138	90

which leads to muscular pain, stiffness, and weakness after exercise, and failure to form lactic acid during ischemic exercise. Similar symptoms are found in another and even rarer syndrome, that due to phosphofructokinase deficiency. Of interest in McArdle's disease have been the reports of reappearance of phosphorylase activity in regenerating and cultured muscle cells from patients (6) and the subsequent demonstration that this activity was due to increased levels of fetal and liver isozymes of phosphorylase, not to true skeletal muscle phosphorylase (7, 8).

Type II glycogen storage disease had been known as a clinical entity ("Pompe's disease") for three decades before Hers (9) showed in the early 1960s that an α-glucosidase, active at acid pH, was deficient in the tissues of affected infants. The recognition of the lysosomal nature of the deficiency led Hers to the concept of inborn lysosomal disease (9). In time, a highly variable degree of phenotypic expression among patients was noted, leading eventually to a classification of "infantile," "juvenile," and "adult" forms of Type II disease, depending on the age of the affected patients when studied. We found more than a 10-fold difference in glycogen content of various individual skeletal muscles from an 11-year-old child who died of the disease, with no evidence of acid α-glucosidase activity in any of these muscle samples. Beratis and associates (10) have suggested recently that the infantile form is due to the synthesis of a catalytically inactive enzyme, and that the traces of activity reported in some adult patients are due to a markedly diminished amount of enzyme. These authors have also reported the purification of an isozyme with reduced catalytic activity toward glycogen (11).

Our studies of the lysosomal pathway have been focused on the rate at which glycogen is degraded hydrolytically in fibroblasts. An overall rate of catabolism of 2 to 4 nmol/hr/mg of total cellular protein was measured (12). This is less than 1% of the rate at which the lysosomal enzyme can act to degrade glycogen in vitro. Subsequent studies have suggested that the rate-limiting step in the degradation of glycogen by this pathway may be the rate at which autophagic vacuoles are formed and/or that at which the internalized polysaccharide moves into secondary lysosomes within which hydrolysis occurs when α-glucosidase is present (13).

We shall turn now to a detailed discussion of assay methods for the debranching enzyme that is deficient in Type III glycogen storage disease. Of the cases reported in Table 1, 22.5% had a deficiency of the debranching enzyme. In some cases the deficiency was generalized, affecting both liver and muscle. Less frequently, enzyme activity was absent in the liver but was retained in the muscle. In 16 cases, no muscle tissue was available for study, nor had siblings been classified previously.

Table 2 shows two of the common analytical methods for the assay of the debranching enzyme. The first, the limit dextrin assay, involves measuring the amount of glucose formed from a phosphorylase limit dextrin corrected for the glucose formed by nonspecific glucosidase action on glycogen. The ^{14}C-glucose incorporation method depends on the limited reversibility of the hydrolytic activity. Under the conditions we used, the incorporation was 0.6% of the hydrolytic action of the purified enzyme. The ^{14}C-glucose incorporation assay can be used successfully in liver and muscle to predict whether or not a patient is deficient in debranching enzyme, and the ratio of the two activities for these tissues is similar to that of the purified enzyme. However, after both false positives and false negatives were obtained with cultured skin fibroblasts in our laboratory, the ^{14}C-glucose incorporation method was abandoned. Efforts to make this method discriminatory were unsuccessful. The relatively high ratio of ^{14}C-glucose incorporation to limit dextrin assay units in fibroblasts (Table 2)

Table 2. Analytical Methods for Assay of the Glycogen Debranching Enzyme

	Enzyme Activity at 30°C, pH 6.5 (nmol/min/mg protein)			
	Pure Rabbit Muscle Enzyme	Human Liver	Human Muscle	Skin Fibroblasts
Limit dextrin (LD) assay LD $\xrightarrow{\text{debrancher}}$ glucose^a (from outer α-1,6 bonded units)	8,000	4.64	3.22	0.32
^{14}C-Glucose incorporation^b ^{14}C-Glucose + glycogen $\rightarrow$ ^{14}C-Glycogen (containing covalently linked ^{14}C-glucose)	48	0.027	0.022	0.0078
$\dfrac{^{14}\text{C-glucose incorporation}}{\text{(LD-glycogen) assay}}$ %	0.60	0.57	0.70	2.44

^{a} After subtracting the glucose formed by nonspecific glucosidase action on α-1,4-bonded glucose units of glycogen. 1% Polysaccharide; 50 mM sodium maleate.
^{b} 5% Rabbit liver glycogen; 1.8 mM U-^{14}C-glucose (7.7 × 10^3 dpm/nmol); 50 mM sodium maleate.

suggests either that glucose may be incorporated into bonds other than α-1,6 branch points in glycogen, or that the cells contain other enzymes capable of incorporating glucose into glycogen.

Table 3 shows the glucose yield from added polysaccharide for fibroblasts from various sources. The first column of data for glycogen as a substrate shows little difference in the rates for control fibroblasts, cultured amniotic cells, heterozygotes for Type III, or Type III fibroblasts themselves. The differences among these groups lie in their capacity to form glucose from a limit dextrin, calculated in the final column as the net difference between the rates for the two substrates. Three conclusions can be drawn from these data: (a) the presence of activity in cultured amniotic cells allows for prenatal diagnosis; (b) the intermediate value in the small series of heterozygotes suggests that they can be detected; (c) essentially zero activity for Type III fibroblasts allows for diagnosis of the disease without an open biopsy procedure, although the test does not indicate whether the deficiency is generalized or confined to the liver.

One problem with the assay is the lack of general availability of the phosphorylase limit dextrin substrate. For that reason, a more universally usable, simple test has been developed (Table 4). If cultured fibroblasts are exposed to glucose-free medium for 16 to 24 hours, the polysaccharide content of control cells decreases to very low levels, with a persistence of the normal glycogen structure as measured by how much glucose-1-phosphate can be formed from the endogenous polysaccharide by phosphorylase free of the debranching enzyme. Some commercially available samples of phosphorylase B have been found to be suitable for this purpose. In general, fibroblasts are maintained in 10% fetal calf serum (frequently, heat treated), but in the experiments without glucose, dialyzed serum is required. In contrast to the results obtained with control cells, Type III fibroblasts show a persistence of polysaccharide and a decrease in the yield of glucose-1-phosphate from the polysaccharide that remains, showing that the accumulated endogenous material approached the structure of a phosphorylase limit dextrin.

Table 5 shows the remarkable persistence of polysaccharide in two different Type III glycogen storage disease cell lines exposed to glucose-free medium

Table 3. Glucose Yield from Added Polysaccharide[a]

	Glucose Yield (nmol/min/mg protein)		
Fibroblasts	Glycogen	Phosphorylase Limit Dextrin of Glycogen	Net Difference (Limit Dextrin − Glycogen)
Controls (n = 25)	0.41–1.10	0.80–1.85	0.40–0.99
Control cultured amniotic cells (n = 10)	0.34–0.85	1.14–1.80	0.42–1.05
Heterozygotes for GSD Type III (n = 6)	0.62–1.17	0.90–1.44	0.22–0.41
GSD Type III (n = 20)	0.65–0.88	0.59–0.89	0–0.05

[a] Fibroblasts were cultured in Earle's minimal essential medium with 10% fetal calf serum before harvest. Aliquots of sonicates were incubated with 2% polysaccharide in 40 mM maleate (pH 6.5) at 37°C. Reactions were terminated by heating in boiling water for 1 minute. n, Number of cell lines analyzed; GSD, glycogen storage disease.

Table 4. Effect of Overnight Exposure of Cultured Fibroblasts to Glucose-Free Medium[a] on Glycogen Content and Structure

	With Glucose		Without Glucose	
Source of Fibroblasts	Glycogen (μm/mg)	G-1-P (%)	Glycogen (μm/mg)	G-1-P (%)
Control	0.30	25.3	0.06	28.6
	0.36	26.8	0.06	24.3
	0.44	29.1	0.08	27.0
	0.48	28.7	0.14	26.1
	0.53	27.9	0.16	22.7
Type III GSD	0.60	22.6	0.47	11.3
	0.62	23.3	0.53	7.3
	0.68	23.4	0.55	11.1
	1.15	22.4	0.84	2.9
Type IV GSD	0.89	39.9	0.12	35.1
	1.48	37.2	0.42	33.7

[a] Fibroblasts were cultured in Earle's minimal essential medium containing 10% dialyzed fetal calf serum, with and without glucose (5.5 μmol/ml).
Abbreviations: G-1-P, glucose 1-phosphate formed from endogenous polysaccharide by phosphorylase free of the debranching enzyme; GSD, glycogen storage disease.

for as long as 3 days. Cell line A had a yield of 5% glucose-1-phosphate at 24 hours, and the value was similar at the later harvestings. Under these conditions, at 72 hours, approximately one-third of the fibroblasts had detached, as judged by the recovery of protein from the remaining adherent cells.

Table 6 contains data for Type III fibroblasts grouped as to the kind of patient from whom the cultures were derived. Fibroblasts from Type IIIA disease, i.e., patients with a generalized deficiency of the debranching enzyme, retained 79% of their starting polysaccharide, whereas fibroblasts from patients

Table 5. Effect of Prolonged Exposure to Glucose-Free Medium on Glycogen Content of Fibroblasts from Patients with Type III Glycogen Storage Disease

	Glycogen Contents (μm/mg)		G-1-P[a] (%)
Hours	Cell A	Cell B	Cell B
24	0.93	0.71	10.6
48	0.72	0.53	9.5
72	0.66	0.52	8.8

[a] Glucose-1-phosphate formed from endogenous polysaccharide by phosphorylase free of the debranching enzyme.

Table 6. Effect of Overnight Exposure of Cultured Fibroblasts to Glucose-Free Medium[a] on Glycogen Content and Structure

Source of Fibroblasts	With Glucose		Without Glucose	
	Glycogen ($\mu m/mg$)	G-1-P (%)	Glycogen ($\mu m/mg$)	G-1-P (%)
Type IIIA GSD	0.60	22.6	0.47	11.3
No debranching enzyme in liver or	0.62	23.3	0.53	7.3
muscle	0.68	23.4	0.55	11.1
	1.15	22.4	0.84	2.9
Type IIIB GSD	0.62	15.9	0.30	5.3
Debrancher deficient in liver but	0.81	24.9	0.47	10.4
present in muscle	0.90	27.0	0.51	17.8
	1.13	25.0	0.77	11.2
Type III GSD	0.55	18.8	0.34	6.2
Debrancher deficient in liver,	0.58	19.4	0.26	8.1
unknown in muscle	0.65	20.1	0.58	11.8
	0.74	24.7	0.56	10.0

[a] Fibroblasts were cultured in Earle's minimal essential medium containing 10% dialyzed fetal calf serum with and without glucose (5.5 $\mu mol/ml$).
Abbreviations: G-1-P, glucose-1-phosphate formed from endogenous polysaccharide by phosphorylase free of the debranching enzyme; GSD, glycogen storage disease.

with persistence of enzyme activity in the muscle retained an average of 58%. In both instances, the polysaccharide remaining had short outer chains. Although the series was small, one is tempted to predict that in instances in which status of the muscle is unknown, as shown in the third group in Table 6, the first two cell lines might have been derived from patients with Type IIIB disease; the last two, from patients with Type IIIA disease. It will be of interest to expand the series to test the validity of the hypothesis using this simple procedure, and we would welcome viable cultures from other documented cases.

ACKNOWLEDGMENTS

The work described in this paper was supported in part by research grants HD 12184 and GM 04761 from the National Institutes of Health. We thank Deborah Sprinkle, Alice Rickard, and Sally Janes for expert technical assistance.

REFERENCES

1. Greene HL, Slonim AE, Burr IM: Type I glycogen storage disease: a metabolic basis for advances in treatment. Pediatr 26:63–92, 1979

2. Fernandes J: Hepatic glycogenosis: diagnosis and management. In *Inherited Disorders of Carbohydrate Metabolism*. Edited by Burman D, Holten JB, Pennock CA. University Park Press, Baltimore, 1980, pp 297–312

3. Stacey TE, Macnab A, Strang LB: Recent work on treatment of Type I glycogen storage disease. In *Inherited Disorders of Carbohydrate Metabolism*. Edited by Burman D, Holten JB, Pennock CA. University Park Press, Baltimore, 1980, pp 315–325

4. Chiu LA, Musat TL: Dominant inheritance of McArdle's syndrome. Arch Neurol 33:636–641, 1976

5. Brown BI, Brown DH: Disorders of glycogen metabolism. In *Practice of Medicine*, vol. VIII. Harper & Row, Hagerstown, 1979, Chapter 9, pp 1–18

6. Roelofs RI, Engel WK, Chauvin PB: Histochemical phosphorylase activity in regenerating muscle fibers from myophosphorylase deficient patients. Science 177:795–797, 1972

7. Sato K, Imai F, Hatayama I, et al: Characterization of glycogen phosphorylase enzymes present in cultured skeletal muscle from patients with McArdle's disease. Biochem Biophys Res Commun 78:663–668, 1977

8. DiMauro S, Arnold S, Miranda A, et al: McArdle disease: the mystery of reappearing phosphorylase activity in muscle culture: a fetal isoenzyme. Ann Neurol 3:60–66, 1978

9. Hers HG: The concept of inborn lysosomal disease. In *Lysosomes and Storage Diseases*. Edited by Hers HG, Van Hoof F. Academic Press, New York, 1973, pp 147–171, 197–216

10. Beratis NG, LaBadie GU, Hirschhorn K: Characterization of the molecular defect in infantile and adult acid α-glucosidase deficiency fibroblasts. J Clin Invest 62:1264–1274, 1978

11. Beratis NH, LaBadie GU, Hirschhorn K: An isozyme of acid α-glucosidase with reduced catalytic activity for glycogen. Am J Hum Genet 32:137–149, 1980

12. Brown DH, Waindle LM, Brown BI: The apparent activity in vivo of the lysosomal pathway of glycogen catabolism in cultured human skin fibroblasts from patients with Type III glycogen storage disease. J Biol Chem 253:5005–5011, 1978

13. Brown DH, Brown BI, Waindle LM: Studies on the lysosomal degradation of glycogen in cultured human skin fibroblasts. American Chemical Society Symposium, 176th National Meeting: *Mechanisms of Saccharide Polymerization and Depolymerization*. Edited by Marshall JJ. Academic Press, New York, 1980, pp 187–208

DISCUSSION

Dr. Salvatore DiMauro: There is no evidence for tissue-specific isoenzymes of the debranching enzyme. In fact, in most patients, the enzyme defect seems to be expressed in all tissues. Do you care to speculate about what the genetic basis may be in those cases in which the enzyme defect seems to be expressed in muscle but not liver?

Dr. Barbara Brown: That is an interesting problem, but we have no information to contribute.

52
Muscle Fructose 1,6-Diphosphatase Deficiency and Atypical Core Disease

Carl M. Pearson, MD*

Nirmal C. Kar, PhD

Since the first description of central core disease in 5 members from 3 generations of the same family by Shy and Magee (1) in 1956, more than 30 other cases have been reported. Histologically, muscle fibers contain "cores" of abnormal myofibrils in otherwise normal fibers, and cores usually lack oxidative enzymes and phosphorylase. The pathogenesis of central core disease remains unknown; no specific biochemical defect has yet been found.

In this report we describe a young woman with a atypical central core disease in whom an abnormality of muscle fructose 1,6-diphosphatase (FDPase) was also noted.

The patient, a 25-year-old white woman, was first seen in 1977 at UCLA complaining of diffuse muscular weakness since birth. She had not walked until 2 years of age and was relatively poor at sports, but had developed normally otherwise. Motor examination revealed proximal muscle weakness in both upper and lower extremities and neck; the distal muscle groups were normal. The patient's father is well at 56 years of age, and the mother has emphysema. The patient's 23-year-old brother is normal. There was no other neuromuscular disease in the family.

The following laboratory studies were normal: creatinine, blood urea nitrogen, electrolytes, bicarbonate, lactate, fasting blood sugar, and serum aldolase. Serum creatine phosphokinase was slightly increased.

METHODS

Portions of biopsy specimen from the patient's right quadriceps muscle were rapidly frozen to $-170°$ C in 2-methylbutane chilled by liquid nitrogen for

675

* Deceased.

histologic and histochemical studies (2) using hematoxylin and eosin, azure B, oil red 0, Gomori trichrome, periodic acid-Schiff (PAS), and myofibrillar adenosine triphosphatase (ATPase) (pH 9.3) after preincubation at pH 4.3, phosphorylase, nicotinamide adenine dinucleotide tetrazolium reductase, and succinate dehydrogenase. The remaining muscle was used for biochemical studies.

Portions of muscle were homogenized either in 9 volumes of deionized water or in 9 volumes of 50 mM Tris-HCl (pH 8.0) containing 5 mM ethylenediamine tetra-acetic acid. The homogenate was centrifuged at 1,000 g for 10 minutes at 2° C, and the supernatant was collected. The aqueous homogenate was used to estimate phosphorylase, adenylate deaminase, and FDPase. The assays of phosphorylase, phosphohexoseisomerase, phosphofructokinase, aldolase, pyruvate kinase, lactate dehydrogenase, adenylate deaminase, citrate synthetase, and carnitine acetyltransferase were done by standard methods. The FDPase and protein content were assayed as described previously (3).

RESULTS

Histochemistry

Cryostat and paraffin sections showed mild distortion of the fasicular architecture but no endomysial connective tissue proliferation. Transversely oriented cryostat sections demonstrated no inflammation or necrosis but variation in fiber size with some atrophic angular fibers and type I fiber predominance. The core structures assumed two distinct forms and could be differentiated on the basis of size and PAS, phosphorylase, and dehydrogenase reactivity. A few fibers contained both forms, whereas 13% of the fibers contained two or more smaller core structures. The more prevalent smaller cores were 4.1 μm in minimal diameter, were linear or ellipsoid, and were strongly PAS positive. In contrast, the larger well-formed cores measured approximately 13.3 μm in diameter. A detailed account of pathologic findings will be reported elsewhere (Kar NAC, Pearson CM, Verity MA: unpublished data).

Biochemistry

The levels of phosphorylase, phosphohexoseisomerase, phosphofructokinase, aldolase, pyruvate kinase, lactate dehydrogenase, adenylate deaminase, citrate synthetase, and carnitine acetyltransferase in the patient's muscle were similar to those in control muscle (Table 1). The data on muscle FDPase are shown in Table 2. The FDPase activity in the patient's muscle was markedly decreased to 8.8% of that in control muscle and 14.9% of that in disease control muscle characterized by type I fiber predominance due to multiple etiologies. Among muscle specimens from disease control subjects, there was generally a correlation between the number of type II fibers present and the level of muscle FDPase activity. No evidence of enzyme inhibition was observed when equal portions of muscle homogenate from the patient were added to that control preparation.

Table 1. Enzyme Levels in Human Skeletal Muscle[a]

Enzyme	Patient	Control Subjects (mean ± SD, n = 5)
Phosphorylase	0.62	0.77 ± 0.18
Phosphohexoseisomerase	1.94	2.88 ± 0.93
Phosphofructokinase	0.15	0.20 ± 0.07
Aldolase	0.59	0.61 ± 0.17
Pyruvate kinase	2.70	3.05 ± 0.87
Lactate dehydrogenase	2.44	3.15 ± 1.16
Adenylate deaminase	1.89	2.73 ± 1.23
Citrate synthetase	0.22	0.22 ± 0.10
Carnitine acetyltransferase	0.04	0.03 ± 0.01

[a] Activities of phosphorylase and adenylate deaminase are expressed as μmol/mg of noncollagen protein/min. Activities of all other enzymes are given as μmol/mg protein/min in 1,000 g supernatant.

DISCUSSION

The patient described in this report represents an atypical form of central core disease notably because of the small size, occasional multicore pattern in a single fiber, negative myofibrillar ATPase, and abortive changes in many fibers, suggesting an early or evolving phase in which there was microfocal accentuation of PAS and dehydrogenase reaction product. Although a single central core has been the rule within individual fibers in central core disease, multiple cores have been seen in other cases. In addition to central core disease, cores may be associated with other diseases of muscle (Table 3). In liver and kidney, FDPase, pyruvate carboxylase, phosphoenolpyruvate carboxykinase, and glucose-6-phosphatase comprise the 4 unidirectional enzymes involved in the conversion of pyruvate to glucose in the gluconeogenetic pathway. Although pyruvate carboxylase is presumed to be the rate-limiting step, FDPase may also be important,

Table 2. Levels of Fructose 1,6-Diphosphatase (FDPase) in Human Skeletal Muscle

Subjects	Type I Fibers (%)	FDPase Activity[a]
Patient	91.9	9.1
Controls (n = 12)	—	103.0 ± 29.9[b]
Disease controls		
Nonprogressive myopathy	98.7	38.8
Neurogenic disease	88.2	46.7
Spinal muscular atrophy	78.5	73.1
Progressive muscular atrophy	63.8	97.0
Kugelberg-Welander variant	56.4	50.6

[a] Activity is given as nmol of inorganic phosphate released/mg of noncollagen protein/10 min.

[b] Mean ± SD.

Table 3. Clinicopathologic Conditions Associated with Core or Multicore Structures

Condition	Reference
Tenotomy	Shafiq et al. (4)
Nemaline myopathy	Afifi et al. (5)
	Karpati et al. (6)
Malignant hyperpyrexia	Denborough et al. (7)
	Eng et al. (8)
	Moulds and Denborough (9)
Multicore disease	Engel et al. (10)
Type III glycogenosis	Pellisier et al. (11)
Arthrogryposis multiplex congenita	Cohen et al. (12)
Fructose 1,6-diphosphatase deficiency	This case

as a deficiency of FDPase activity in liver is known to cause severe hypoglycemia and lactic acidosis in infants (13).

The finding of FDPase activity in muscle (14, 15), however, was unexpected, because this tissue is not considered to play a significant role in gluconeogenesis. Based on levels of FDPase and phosphofructokinase in muscles from various animals, Newsholme and Crabtree (16) have hypothesized that FDPase in muscle provides a cycle between fructose 6-phosphate and fructose 1,6-diphosphate when the muscle is at rest. This cycle increases the sensitivity of fructose 6-phosphate phosphorylation to changes in the concentration of adenosine monophosphate (AMP). An increase in AMP concentration in muscle during conditions of heavy muscular exercise will activate phosphofructokinase with a concomitant inhibition of FDPase and will ensure that the restriction of the rate of glycolysis at the stage of fructose 6-phosphate phosphorylation is reduced to a minimum. The finding of a normal level of muscle FDPase in patients with hepatic FDPase deficiency has demonstrated that FDPase of muscle is a distinctly different enzyme (17, 18). This is in agreement with the reported differences in amino acid content (19) and immunologic properties (20) between rabbit muscle FDPase and liver FDPase analogous to the phosphorylase enzyme that exists in distinct molecular forms in human muscle and liver.

Biochemical studies of relevant muscle enzymes demonstrated a marked deficiency of FDPase but normal activities of several other glycolytic and mitochondrial enzymes. In this patient the defect in muscle FDPase appears, therefore, to be unique. The hepatic FDPase is presumably normal, because the patient never had any clinical symptoms of liver disease. Because FDPase is present almost exclusively in type II muscle fibers (20), the disappearance of type II fibers found in this biopsy specimen may account for the decreased enzyme activity found biochemically. This argument appears to be ruled out by our finding of reduced but still considerable amounts of FDPase activity in biopsy specimens showing type I fiber predominance from different disease etiologies. However, the relationship between core formation in type I fibers, type II fiber disappearance, and FDPase deficiency in core disease is unclear; whether this represents an isolated case of FDPase deficiency or, at least, one of the basic metabolic defects in central core disease(s), remains to be seen.

ACKNOWLEDGMENT

This work was supported in part by a Center Grant from the Muscular Dystrophy Association.

REFERENCES

1. Shy GM, Magee KR: A new congenital non-progressive myopathy. Brain 79:610–621, 1956
2. Dubowitz V, Brooke MH: Muscle biopsy: a modern approach. WB Saunders, Philadelphia, 1973, pp 20–33
3. Kar NC, Pearson CM: Fructose 1,6-diphosphatase in normal and diseased human muscle. Clin Chim Acta 38:252–254, 1972
4. Shafiq SA, Gorycki MA, Asiedu SA, Milhorat AT: Tenotomy: effect on the fine structure of the soleus of the rat. Arch Neurol 20:625–633, 1969
5. Afifi AH, Smith JW, Zellweger H: Congenital nonprogressive myopathy-central core disease and nemaline myopathy in one family. Neurology (Minneap) 15:371–381, 1965
6. Karpati G, Carpenter S, Anderman F: A new concept of childhood nemaline myopathy. Arch Neurol 24:291–304, 1971
7. Denborough MA, Dennett X, Anderson R: Central core disease and malignant hyperpyrexia. Br Med J 1:272–273, 1973
8. Eng GD, Epstein BS, Engel WK, et al: Malignant hyperthermia and central core disease in a child with congenital dislocating hips. Arch Neurol 35:189–197, 1978
9. Moulds RFW, Denborough MA: Myopathies and malignant hyperpyrexia. Br Med J 3:520, 1974
10. Engel AG, Gomez MR, Groover RO: Multicore disease: a recently recognized congenital myopathy associated with multifocal degeneration of muscle fibers. Mayo Clinic Proc 46:666–681, 1971
11. Pellissier JF, de Barsey T, Faugere MC, Rebuffel P: Type III glycogenesis with multicore structures. Muscle Nerve 2:124–132, 1979
12. Cohen ME, Duffner PK, Heffner RF: Central core disease in one of identical twins. J Neurol Neurosurg Psychiatry 41:659–663, 1978
13. Baker L, Winegrad AI: Fasting hypoglycemia and metabolic acidosis associated with deficiency of hepatic fructose 1,6-diphosphatase activity. Lancet 1:13–16, 1970
14. Fernando J, Enser M, Pontremoli S, Horecker BL: Purification and properties of rabbit muscle fructose 1,6-diphosphatase. Arch Biochem Biophys 126:599–606, 1968
15. Krebs HA, Woodford M: Fructose 1,6-diphosphatase in striated muscle. Biochem J 94:436–444, 1965
16. Newsholme EA, Crabtree B: The role of fructose 1,6-diphosphatase in the regulation of glycolysis in skeletal muscle. FEBS Lett 7:195–198, 1970
17. Melancon SB, Khachadurian AK, Nadler HL, Brown BI: Metabolic and biochemical studies in fructose 1,6-diphosphatase deficiency. J Pediatr 82:650–657, 1973
18. Pagliara AS, Karl AE, Keating JP, et al: Hepatic fructose 1,6-diphosphatase deficiency: a cause of lactic acidosis and hypoglycemia in infancy. J Clin Invest 51:2115–2123, 1972
19. Fernando J, Pontremoli S, Horecker BL: Fructose 1,6-diphosphatase from rabbit muscle. II. Amino acid composition and activation by sulfhydryl compounds. Arch Biochem Biophys 129:370–376, 1969
20. Opie LH, Newsholme EA: The activities of fructose 1,6-diphosphatase, phosphofructokinase and phosphoenolpyruvate carboxykinase in white muscle and red muscle. Biochem J 103:391–399, 1967
21. Enser M, Spiro S, Horecker BL: Immunological studies of liver, kidney and muscle fructose 1,6-diphosphatases. Arch Biochem Biophys 129:377–383, 1969

DISCUSSION

Dr. Corrado Angelini: This is a very interesting case, and the report of this enzyme defect in muscle is intriguing. A number of things must be asked regarding the primary pathogenetic significance of this defect. First, it would be nice to know whether the parents have a 50% enzyme defect in muscle; this should prove that it is not a secondary enzyme defect. Also, if AMP is involved in the pathogenesis of muscle dysfunction, you could try in vitro glycolysis and add AMP to overcome the defect.

Dr. Carl Pearson: We have looked at the parents and the brother and they seem to be normal. With regard to your other comment, Dr. Angelini, we have not done anything about that as yet.

Dr. Michael Bárány: Looking with ^{31}P NMR at human muscle biopsy specimens for the MDA Clinic of the University of Illinois in Chicago, we once found a muscle in which all the phosphate was in the form of fructose-1,6-diphosphate; there was really nothing else in it. Did you measure fructose-1,6-diphosphate in this muscle? If you did, what was its concentration?

Dr. Carl Pearson: The fructose-1,6-diphosphate was essentially normal. We also took equal quantities of the patient's muscle and normal muscle to see whether their inhibitory factor(s) were present in a homogenate of the muscle. There did not seem to be any present.

Dr. Michael Bárány: I would still like to make a theoretical comment. The reverse reaction, the transformation of fructose-1,6-diphosphate to fructose-1-phosphate requires the absence of AMP. In a muscle that produces only a little lactic acid, the synthesis of ATP is slow. If you cannot produce ATP through the glycolytic pathway, then the 2 ADP $\rightleftharpoons$ ATP + AMP reaction goes on in the muscle; thus, we have a lot of AMP so that the fructose-1,6-diphosphatase should be inactive. This means that the reduced glycolysis in your muscle does not support the idea that the fructose-1,6-diphosphatase is affected.

Dr. Carl Pearson: Well, these postulates were made a number of years ago on normal muscle. I just wonder whether the AMP is getting to the right place and doing its work in this sort of situation.

Dr. Michael Bárány: I do not think there is any compartment for fructose-1,6-diphosphatase and AMP in the muscle; these materials are soluble in the sarcoplasm.

Dr. Carl Pearson: I do not think we can resolve this further.

Dr. John Gergely: Maybe this question is related to Dr. Bárány's. Did I understand you to suggest that the absence of the enzyme would make it impossible to accelerate glycolysis?

Dr. Carl Pearson: Glycolysis was impossible to accelerate to a great extent. It accelerates modestly, but only about 25% of what one would normally expect.

Dr. Andrew Engel: Dr. W. King Engel, you looked at central core and phosphorylase deficiencies or the notion that they may be related. You might have done some studies on glycogen analysis. Could you comment?

Dr. W. King Engel: We did not look at this enzyme. However, even though explanations do not come readily to the floor for the enzyme defect, the explanations of how this might affect overall muscle metabolism may come years later. The important thing is to find out the extent of the defect in central core disease, because it may relate not only to central core disease, but also to malignant hyperthermia. Establishing the defect is very important; we can worry about its pathogenic mechanism later.

53
The Use of Protease Inhibitors to Investigate Pathways of Protein Breakdown in Muscle

Peter Libby, MD

Alfred L. Goldberg, PhD

In skeletal muscle, as in other cells, protein breakdown appears to be a carefully regulated process that helps determine both overall mass of the tissue and the level of specific tissue proteins (1). Consequently, there has been appreciable interest in the possibility that a failure in the regulation or selectivity of intracellular protein breakdown may contribute to the pathogenesis of muscular dystrophy, various forms of muscle atrophy, and other neuromuscular disorders, such as myasthenia gravis. There is now strong evidence that an acceleration of protein breakdown contributes to the muscle atrophy that occurs after denervation, hyperthyroidism, or in certain inherited forms of muscular dystrophy (2–5). Furthermore, evidence from several laboratories indicates that the impairment of neuromuscular transmission in myasthenia gravis results from a decrease in the number of acetylcholine receptors on the muscle membrane due to an accelerated rate of destruction of this protein (6–8).

The recognition of the significance of muscle protein catabolism in these pathologic states and also in the overall regulation of gluconeogenesis and fasting (9) has led many investigators to attempt to define the mechanism of this process. Despite appreciable progress in clarifying the factors normally regulating proteolysis, the degradative pathway(s) for protein in muscle remain quite controversial (10). Muscle contains many proteases, some associated with lysosomes, and others apparently found in the cytoplasm (11, 12). Enzymes of both categories can hydrolyze contractile proteins in cell-free extracts, and activities of proteases of either class have been reported to increase under conditions that provoke muscular atrophy (11–16). Such observations have led some to postulate a primary role for lysosomal enzymes in protein breakdown

683

in the intact tissue (17, 18) and others to the opposite conclusion (14, 19, 20). The recent recognition that much of the apparently nonlysosomal protease activity in muscle extracts is not found within myocytes but within associated mast cells has increased the confusion about the mechanism of protein breakdown in muscle (11, 21–24). On the other hand, the recent demonstration of novel adenosine triphosphate (ATP)-dependent proteolytic systems in reticulocytes and other cells (10, 25, 26) emphasizes the possibility that the physiologically important degradative system in muscle has not yet been identified, and this problem will require appreciable sophistication to be resolved.

One approach to clarifying the function of these various enzymes in intact muscle involves the use of inhibitors of proteases or of lysosomal function (27–29). This paper will summarize some of the results of our own studies using such inhibitors. The results of these studies suggest that *both* lysosomal and nonlysosomal pathways play important roles in catabolism of various types of muscle proteins. In addition to their interest as reagents in cell biology, selective inhibitors of proteins breakdown in muscle might represent a new approach to the treatment of neuromuscular diseases.

CHOICE OF APPROPRIATE INHIBITORS

The general design of our experiments was to measure the rate of protein breakdown in muscle tissue exposed to a known inhibitor of proteases. A decrease in proteolysis would suggest that this process involves an enzyme or enzymes sensitive to that agent. The ideal inhibitor for use in such experiments should have the following properties:

1. The inhibitors should readily enter the cell and whatever subcellular compartment(s) may be involved in the process under study (e.g. the lysosome).
2. The inhibitor should inhibit selectively specific enzymes or a discrete cellular function (e.g., the entry of protein substrates into a degradative organelle).
3. The inhibitor should not affect other cell processes or produce any toxic effect. This point is of obvious importance if protease inhibitors might eventually be used therapeutically. In addition, possible toxic effects must be considered when inhibitors are used to investigate intracellular pathways. For example, such an agent could block proteolysis by a mechanism other than protease inhibition if it interfered with protein synthesis or ATP production (1).

In practice, the protease inhibitors available are far from ideal in their selectivity. Furthermore, although it is often easy to demonstrate inhibition of a particular process, it is very difficult or impossible to be certain that an agent has no other effects. Similar problems are associated with most other inhibitors widely used in cell biology. In fact, recognition of undesired effects of inhibitors generally increases as a function of the length of time and care with which the agent has been studied, as with actinomycin D and cytocholasin B.

In the case of protease inhibitors capable of entering cells, until the past decade, the agents available appeared to be so toxic to cells or organisms as to preclude their use as probes for definition of the enzymes involved in intracellular proteolysis (e.g., diisopropylfluorophosphate or the chloromethyl ketone derivatives). In the late 1960s, Umezawa and his colleagues at the Institute for Microbial Chemistry in Tokyo, Japan isolated and characterized a series of novel inhibitors of various proteases. These agents are produced by Actinomycetes and are peptide aldehyde derivatives (30). These compounds appear to have structures resembling those of the natural substrate moiety of the respective transition state of the enzyme-substrate complex and bind tightly to the enzyme active site. Concentrations of the agents less than 1 μM inhibit susceptible proteases very effectively by this mechanism. Furthermore, these agents seemed even at relatively high doses not to produce toxic effects in animals (31).

Unfortunately, most of these agents do not inhibit a single proteolytic activity (see later). The one exception is pepstatin, which is believed to inhibit only one lysosomal protease, cathepsin D, but this inhibitor appears not to be able to enter cells readily. Thus, none of these inhibitors has all of the properties of the ideal inhibitor. Nonetheless, careful interpretation of experiments using these agents has increased our knowledge of the pathways for protein breakdown in muscle and other cells.

EFFECTS OF PEPTIDE ALDEHYDES ON MUSCLE PROTEOLYSIS

To determine rates of breakdown of cell protein in isolated rat muscles, we measured the release of the amino acid tyrosine from cell protein. Skeletal muscle neither synthesizes this amino acid nor degrades it to other compounds. Therefore, in this tissue, tyrosine can be generated only by proteolysis, and its release from cell protein can be used to evaluate overall protein balance in isolated muscle (32). This approach and analogous ones in perfused heart or hindlimb muscles have proved very useful for evaluating the effects of hormones, food supply, and other conditions on rates of protein synthesis and breakdown.

In muscle obtained from normal rats and incubated in vitro with leupeptin, chymostatin, or antipain, protein breakdown proceeded significantly more slowly than in contralateral muscle incubated without these agents (Table 1, 23, 29). Antipain was a less potent inhibitor of protein breakdown than was leupeptin, possibly because it enters the muscle more slowly (Table 1, 10). Leupeptin and chymostatin also reduced proteolysis in muscles undergoing atrophy due to denervation and in muscles from mice with hereditary muscular dystrophy (Table 1). These effects were evident within 1 hour of the addition of leupeptin or chymostatin. In related studies, Hopgood and coworkers (33) and our own group (34) have shown that leupeptin and antipain are also capable of inhibiting protein catabolism in isolated hepatocytes, where they inhibit the breakdown of more long-lived cellular components without affecting the rapid degradation of short-lived protein or abnormal polypeptides. As discussed below, this selectivity suggests the existence of discrete proteolytic systems for the breakdown of these classes of cell proteins (Fig. 1).

Concentrations of leupeptin and chymostatin that effectively reduced protein

Table 1. Effects of Protease Inhibitors on Protein Breakdown[a] in Normal and Diseased Rodent Muscle

	Protein Breakdown (% control rate)		
Muscles Tested	Leupeptin (25 μM)	Chymostatin (20 μM)	Antipain (50 μM)
Normal rat muscles			
EDL[b]	46	63	42
Soleus	64	63	60
Denervated rat muscles			
EDL	63	54	
Soleus	46	77	
Muscles from dystrophic mice[c]			
EDL	66	73	
Plantaris	76	81	

[a] Rates of protein breakdown in isolated rat muscles were determined during incubation in vitro in Krebs-Ringer bicarbonate buffer in the presence of cycloheximide (29).
[b] Extensor digitorum longus.
[c] The dystrophic mice were of the C57B16Jdy^2 strain from Jackson Laboratories.

breakdown did not affect rates of protein synthesis (23, 29). This finding and others indicated that these agents were not toxic to the tissue. Therefore, these compounds probably interfered with proteolysis by inhibiting one or more cell proteases.

Leupeptin, chymostatin, and antipain all inhibit cathepsin B (and perhaps the related enzyme cathepsin L) and the calcium-activated protease found in muscle (23, 30, 35). In addition, chymostatin inhibits the protease that has an alkaline pH optimum found in muscle but is believed to be located in mast cells (see above).

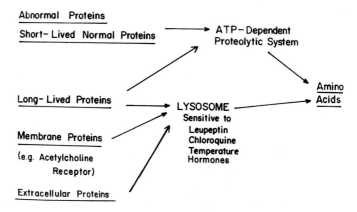

Fig. 1. Pathway for protein degradation in mammalian cells. This figure summarizes current beliefs about the physiologic roles of lysosomal and nonlysosomal proteolytic enzymes. The exact roles of the calcium-activated protease and the system responsible for degrading the contractile apparatus in muscle remain to be clarified.

To prove that leupeptin and chymostatin actually entered cells and inhibited a protease, we measured cathepsin B activity in homogenates of muscles that had been exposed to these agents, and then washed the tissue extensively. Both leupeptin and chymostatin inhibited this enzyme as well as overall proteolysis (23, 29). Therefore, inhibition of this lysosomal protease appears to be a likely mechanism for leupeptin's actions on proteolysis. (However, these results do not exclude a role for the calcium-activated protease or other unknown nonlysosomal enzymes as the site of leupeptin's action.)

Inhibition of Muscle Atrophy by Leupeptin

The studies described above measured the effects of various protease inhibitors in explants of striated muscle incubated for brief periods of a few hours. Fetal mouse hearts can be maintained in culture for as long as several days. Hearts incubated under these conditions continue to contract spontaneously. Therefore, this preparation allowed us to determine whether leupeptin produced toxic effects during more prolonged exposure to tissues. These hearts also undergo rapid atrophy, when cultured in vitro, probably because they pump against no pressure gradient (i.e., there is no afterload). These experiments therefore also enabled us to test whether inhibition of proteolysis would slow the atrophy of these cultured hearts. Incubation with leupeptin for 48 hours did not reduce the rate of protein synthesis, decrease ATP levels, or cause release of lactate dehydrogenase from fetal hearts. However, this agent inhibited protein breakdown by as much as 50%. As a consequence, hearts incubated with leupeptin for 48 hours contained approximately 20% more protein than control hearts (36). The demonstration that a protease inhibitor may retard atrophy of a muscle is clear evidence for the physiologic importance of protein breakdown in vivo. Furthermore, Stracher and colleagues (37) have also reported that treatment of chicken with a mixture of leupeptin and pepstatin can reduce denervation atrophy in vivo. More recent results from several groups suggest that leupeptin can also slow the atrophy of dystrophic muscles from mice or chickens (Stracher A: personal communication; Hudecki MS: personal communication).

THE BREAKDOWN OF THE ACETYLCHOLINE RECEPTOR OCCURS IN LYSOSOMES

The demonstration that leupeptin, chymostatin, and antipain inhibit overall protein breakdown in muscle led us to investigate whether they might affect differentially the breakdown of specific cell components, such as membrane receptors. One purpose of these studies was to try to clarify the role of the lysosome in degrading the acetylcholine receptor (AChR), a well-characterized surface glycoprotein. In addition to its biologic interest, the turnover of this protein is of particular medical import, and inhibitors of its degradation might represent a useful approach to the treatment of myasthenia gravis.

Like adult striated muscle fibers, embryonic chick myotubes grown in culture contain AChRs on their surface, although they are not localized at neuromuscular junctions in these non-innervated cells. As discussed elsewhere in this volume, techniques using the specific ligand α-bungarotoxin permit convenient measurement of the number of AChRs on the cell surface, the rates of incorporation of new receptors into the plasma membrane, and the rate of receptor internalization and degradation (6, 38, 39). On the basis of electron microscopic autoradiography, Devreotes and Fambrough (40) had suggested a lysosomal site for degradation of AChRs in myotubes. Therefore, it was of interest to study the effects of these protease inhibitors on the breakdown of the AChR, an intrinsic membrane glycoprotein, as well as on average protein in these same cultured muscle cells.

Leupeptin (20 μM) almost completely inhibited breakdown of the AChR-bungarotoxin complex (Table 2). Antipain and chymostatin also slowed this process, although to a lesser extent (Table 2). The effects of leupeptin and chymostatin were not additive; therefore, these agents probably act on the same enzyme or pathway (41). We also examined the effects of chloroquine on this process. This commonly used antimalarial drug is a weak base that readily crosses cell membranes in its nonionized form. The agent becomes protonated in the acidic milieu of the lysome and cannot readily exit in this polar form. The drug therefore accumulates at high levels within this organelle. Poole and coworkers (42, 43) and others showed that chloroquine inhibits the hydrolysis of certain cell proteins, presumably by interfering with lysosomal function(s). In fact, in cells treated with chloroquine, intralysosomal pH increases and lysosomal morphology is highly abnormal (42).

In chick myotubes, this agent inhibited the breakdown of the AChR almost completely (Table 2). Like leupeptin, chloroquine did not appreciably decrease the synthesis of new receptors or their incorporation into the surface membrane. These agents would therefore be expected to lead to an increase in the number of surface receptors. However, no such effect was observed. The explanation of the apparent contradiction was that the undegraded receptors did not remain on the cell surface. Instead, the internalization of the receptors appeared to

Table 2. Effects of Protease Inhibitors on Overall Protein Degradation and Degradation of the Acetylcholine Receptor (AChR) in Chick Myotubes[a]

	Rate of Degradation (% control rate)	
Protease Inhibitor	AChR	Cell Proteins
Control	100	100
Leupeptin (20 μM)	10	87
Antipain (20 μM)	22	87
Chymostatin (20 μM)	52	90
Chloroquine (10 μM)	15	78

[a] The degradation of acetylcholine receptors was measured with ^{125}I-α-bungaratoxin. The breakdown of average cell proteins was evaluated after labeling with radioactive leucine or phenylalanine as described previously.

continue at control rates in the presence of chloroquine or leupeptin, and the undegraded AChR accumulated intracellularly (41). Ultrastructural and cell fractionation observations suggested that these internalized but undegraded receptors were associated with endocytic vesicles. In the presence of these inhibitors, "coated vesicles" that probably bear the AChR accumulate intracellularly, apparently because they fail to fuse with the abnormal lysosomes (41, and Bursztajn S, Libby P: unpublished observations). These findings are of biological interest in that they suggest a pathway for the turnover of this membrane glycoprotein. However, these results also indicate that such inhibitors will probably not prove useful for treatment of myasthenia gravis, because the additional AChRs are intracellular and cannot function in neuromuscular transmission.

Multiple Pathways of Protein Degradation

It is noteworthy that in the myotubes, leupeptin and chloroquine inhibited the breakdown of average cell protein much less effectively than they inhibted degradation of the AChR (Table 2). For example, leupeptin (20 μm) reduced catabolism of the AChR by approximately 90% but inhibited overall proteolysis in the same cells by only 13%. Thus, the lysosome is required for breakdown of this intrinsic membrane protein, but does not seem essential for breakdown of the bulk of cell protein. In other words, muscle cells use both lysosomal and nonlysosomal enzymes for degradation of different cell components. The lysosome seems to play a special role in the catabolism of extracellular and membrane proteins (Fig. 1).

This conclusion has been confirmed in related studies (Lockwood T, Goldberg AL: in preparation), in which we followed simultaneously in cultured chick myotubes and fibroblasts the degradation of membrane glycoproteins and the remaining soluble proteins. The inhibitors of lysosomal function selectively decreased breakdown of membrane-associated glycoproteins (labeled with ^{3}H-fucose) without affecting the hydrolysis of the bulk of cell proteins. Thus in these rapidly growing embryonic cells, the lysosome seems to play a more restricted role than in nongrowing cells or in atrophying muscles.

The proteolytic system actually involved in the degradation of most proteins in the muscle cells thus remains to be identified. Because this process can be inhibited by agents that block production of ATP, the responsible enzyme(s) may be similar to the nonlysosomal ATP-dependent proteolytic systems found in reticulocytes, liver, and *Escherichia coli* (25, 26, 44, 45).

PROBLEMS IN THERAPEUTIC USE OF THESE AGENTS

The foregoing summary illustrates the utility of protease inhibitors as tools for learning more about pathways of intracellular protein breakdown, and many additional studies are in progress that build on this and related work. Our experiments with fetal mouse hearts clearly emphasize the importance of protein breakdown in the process of muscle atrophy and indicate the lack of toxicity of certain protease inhibitors on isolated organs.

Because these agents can retard atrophy of muscles in experimental situations and can inhibit the breakdown of AChRs, there has been growing interest in their use in the treatment of denervation atrophy and human muscular dystrophy. Of particular promise are the observations that treatment of intact animals with a mixture of protease inhibitors can retard muscle wasting in animals with hereditary dystrophy or denervated limbs and in some cases decrease the concentration of muscle enzymes in the blood (37, 46). However, not all of the studies of the in vivo effects of these agents have shown beneficial effects (47). Therefore, in our opinion, further detailed investigations of the pharmacology and toxicology of these agents should be pursued. The synthesis of various derivatives of these compounds or of additional protease inhibitors could be of particular value. Unfortunately, the agents currently available have many possible drawbacks that may prevent their therapeutic usefulness in these and other situations.

As mentioned previously, the undegraded receptors that accumulate in inhibitor-treated myotubes are not found on the surface membrane where they function physiologically, but instead build up in an inappropriate intracellular location. If other surface components also accumulate intracellularly, then cellular architecture and function may be adversely affected by such treatments.

Another potential impediment to the clinical use of leupeptin and related inhibitors is their effects on extracellular serine proteases. The enzymes involved in blood coagulation, fibrinolysis, and the complement, kinin, angiotensin, and other pathways are mainly serine proteases, resembling trypsin in their specificity and mode of action. Some of these enzymes are inhibited by leupeptin, chymostatin, and antipain (30, 48). It is also possible that these agents affect other proteolytic processes important in intact organisms (e.g., those involved in the maturation of secreted proteins or in digestion of food). Perhaps inhibition of protein breakdown in muscle could seriously affect energy homeostasis of the organism, because the mobilization of protein reserves in muscle is an important initial step in gluconeogenesis (9, 49). The possible effects of leupeptin and related compounds on such homeostatic systems obviously merit further study, especially because limited proteolysis is important in many diverse regulatory mechanisms in intact organisms. Investigation of these issues will have to precede testing of the use of these inhibitors in the treatment of muscular wasting.

In any case, we believe their use has increased knowledge of the pathways of protein breakdown in muscle. We hope these findings will stimulate future investigations of the effects of these agents in vivo and catalyze efforts to find additional more selective inhibitors of intracellular protein degradation that might not have these drawbacks.

REFERENCES

1. Goldberg AL, St. John AC: Intracellular protein degradation in mammalian and bacterial cells II. Annu Rev Biochem 45:747–803, 1976
2. Goldberg AL: Protein turnover in skeletal muscle II: Effects of denervation and cortisone on protein catabolism in skeletal muscle. J Biol Chem 244:3223–3229, 1969

3. Rourke AW: Myosin in developing normal and dystrophic chicken pectoralis. J Cell Physiol 86:343–352, 1975

4. Goldspink DF, Goldspink G: Age related changes in protein turnover and ribonucleic acid of the diaphragm muscle of normal and dystrophic hamsters. Biochem J 162:191–194, 1977

5. Goldberg AL, Griffin GE, Dice JF: Regulation of protein turnover in normal and dystrophic muscle. In *Pathogenesis of human muscular dystrophies.* Edited by Rowland LP. Excerpta Medica, Amsterdam, 1977, pp 376–385

6. Fambrough DM, Drachman DB, Satyamurti S: Neuromuscular junction in myasthenia gravis: decreased acetylcholine receptors. Science 182:293–295, 1973

7. Heinemann S, Bevan S, Kulberg R, et al: Modulation of acetylcholine receptor by antibody against the receptor. Proc Natl Acad Sci USA 74:3090–3094, 1977

8. Drachman DB: Myasthenia gravis. N Engl J Med 298:136–142 and 186–193, 1978

9. Goldberg AL, Tischler M, DeMartino G, et al: Hormonal regulation of protein degradation and synthesis in skeletal muscle. Fed Proc 39:31–36, 1980

10. Libby P, Goldberg AL: The control and mechanism of protein breakdown in striated muscle: studies with selective inhibitors. In *Degradative Processes in Heart and Skeletal Muscle.* Edited by Wildenthal K. Elsevier Press, Amsterdam, 1980, pp 201–222

11. Pennington RJT: Proteinases of muscle. In *Proteinases in Mammalian Cells and Tissues.* Edited by Barrett AJ. North-Holland and Biomedical Press, Amsterdam, 1977, pp 516–543

12. Bird JWC, Carter JH, Triemer RE, et al: Protinases in cardiac muscle. Fed Proc 39:20–25, 1980

13. Weinstock IM, Iodice AA: Acid hydrolase activity in muscular dystrophy and denervation atrophy. In *Lysosomes in Biology and Pathology.* Edited by Dingle JT, Fell HB. American Elsevier, New York, 1969, p 450

14. Mayer M, Amin R, Shafrir E: Rat myofibrillar protease: enzyme properties and adaptive changes in conditions of muscle protein degradation. Arch Biochem Biophys 161:20–25, 1974

15. Lockshin RA, Colon AD, Dorsey AM: Control of muscle proteolysis in insects. Fed Proc 39:48–52, 1980

16. Kar NL, Pearson CM: Muscular dystrophy and activation of proteinases. Muscle Nerve 1:308–315, 1978

17. Bird JWC: *Lysosomes in Biology and Pathology.* North Holland Publishing Co., Amsterdam, 1975, pp 75–109

18. Schwartz WN, Bird JWC: Degradation of myofibrillar proteins by cathepsin B' and D. Biochem J 167:811–820, 1977

19. Dayton WR, Goll DE, Zeece MG, et al: A Ca^{++}-activated protease possibly involved in myofibrillar protein turnover. Purification from porcine muscle. Biochemistry 15:2150–2158, 1976

20. Dahlmann B, Reinauer H: Purification and some properties of an alkaline proteinase from rat skeletal muscle. Biochem J 171:803–810, 1978

21. Woodbury RG, Gruzenski GM, Lagunoff D: Immunofluorescent localization of a serine protease in rat small intestine. Proc Natl Acad Sci USA 75:2785–2789, 1978

22. Woodbury RG, Everitt M, Sanada Y, et al: A major serine protease in rat skeletal muscle: evidence of its mast cell origin. Proc Natl Acad Sci USA 75:5311–5313, 1978

23. Libby P, Goldberg AL: Effects of chymostatin and other proteinase inhibitors on protein breakdown and proteolytic activities in muscle. Biochem J 188:213–220, 1980

24. Clark MG, Beinlich CJ, McKee EE, et al: Relationship between alkaline proteolytic activity and protein degradation in rat heart. Fed Proc 39:26–30, 1980

25. Etlinger J, Goldberg AL: A soluble ATP-dependent proteolytic system responsible for the degradation of abnormal proteins in reticulocytes. Proc Nat Acad Sci USA 74:54–58, 1977

26. Hershko A, Heller H, Ganoth D, et al: Mode of degradation of abnormal globin chains in rabbit reticulocytes. In *Protein Turnover and Lysosomal Function.* Edited by Segal HL, Doyle DJ. Academic Press, New York, 1978, pp 149–169

27. Wildenthal K, Wakeland JR, Morton PC, et al: Inhibition of protein degradation in mouse hearts by agents that cause lysosomal dysfunction. Circ Res 42:787–792, 1978

28. McGowan EB, Shafiq SA, Stracher A: Exp Neurol 50:649, 1976

29. Libby P, Goldberg AL: Leupeptin, a protease inhibitor, decreases protein degradation in normal and diseased muscles. Science 199:534–536, 1978

30. Umezawa H: Structures and activities of protease inhibitors of microbial origin. In *Methods in Enzymology* 45:678–695, 1976

31. Aoyagi T, Miyata S, Nanbo M, et al: Biological Activities of Leupeptins. J Antibiot 22:558, 1969

32. Fulks R, Li JB, Goldberg AL: Effects of insulin, glucose, and amino acids on protein turnover in rat diaphragm. J Biol Chem 250:290–298, 1975

33. Hopgood MF, Clark MG, Ballard FJ: Inhibition of protein degradation in isolated rat hepatocytes. Biochem J 164:399, 1977

34. Neff NT, DeMartino GN, Goldberg AL: The effect of protease inhibitors and decreased temperature on the degradation of different classes of proteins in cultured hepatocytes. J Cell Physiol 101:439–458, 1979

35. Toyo-Oka T, Shimizu T, Masaki T: Inhibition of proteolytic activity of calcium activated neutral protease by leupeptin and antipain. Biochem Biophys Res Commun 82:484–491, 1978

36. Libby P, Ingwall JS, Goldberg AL: Reduction of protein degradation and atrophy in cultured fetal muscle hearts by leupeptin. Am J Physiol 237:E35–39, 1979

37. Stracher A, McGowan EB, Shafiq SA: Muscular dystrophy: inhibition of degeneration in vivo with protease inhibitors. Science 200:50–51, 1978

38. Brockes JP, Berk DK, Hall ZW: The biochemical properties and regulation of acetylcholine receptors in normal and denervative muscles. Cold Spring Harbor Symp Quant Biol 40:253–262, 1976

39. Devreotes PN, Fambrough DM: Acetylcholine receptor turnover in membranes of developing muscle fibers. J Cell Biol 65:335–358, 1975

40. Devreotes PN, Fambrough DN. Turnover of acetylcholine receptors in skeletal muscle. Cold Spring Harbor Symp Quant Biol 40:237–251, 1976

41. Libby P, Bursztajn S, Goldberg AL: Degradation of the acetylcholine receptor in cultured muscle cells: selective inhibitors and the fate of undegraded receptors. Cell 19:481–491, 1980

42. Poole B, Okhuma S, Warburton M: Some aspects of the intracellular breakdown of exogenous and endogenous proteins. In *Protein Turnover and Lysosome Function*. Edited by Segal HL, Doyle DJ. Academic Press, New York, 1978, pp 43–58

43. Goldstein JL, Brunschede GY, Brown MS: Inhibition of the proteolytic degradation of low density lipoprotein in human fibroblasts by chloroquine, Concanavalin A, and Triton WR 1339. J Biol Chem 250:7854–7862, 1975

44. Murakami K, Voellmy R, Goldberg AL: Protein degradation is stimulated by ATP in extracts of *Escherichia coli*. J Biol Chem 254:8194–8200, 1979

45. DeMartion GN, Goldberg AL: Identification and partial purification of an ATP-stimulated alkaline protease in rat liver. J Biol Chem 254:3712–3715, 1979

46. Chelmicka-Schorr EF, Arnason BGW, Astrom KE, et al: Treatment of mouse muscular dystrophy with the protease inhibitor pepstain. J Neuropathol Exp Neurol 37:263–268, 1978

47. Enomoto A, Bradley WG: Therapeutic trials in muscular dystrophy. Studies of microbial proteinase inhibitors in murine dystrophy. Arch Neurol 34:771–773, 1977

48. Okamura K, Fujii S: Isolation and characterization of different forms of Clr̄, a subunit of the first component of human complement. Biochim Biophys Acta 534:258–266, 1978

49. Goldberg AL, Chang TW: Regulation and significance of amino acid metabolism in skeletal muscle. Fed Proc 37:2301–2307, 1978

DISCUSSION

Dr. Alfred Stracher: I want to present some of our results on the use of leupeptin in vivo. This first slide shows some of the results that we obtained when leupeptin was injected in vivo directly into denervated chicken muscle. In the control situation, there is about 40% loss in muscle weight compared to a 4% to 5% loss with leupeptin treatment. The same is true in the denervated rat. The inhibition of muscle atrophy is corroborated on the next slide. One can see that there is about a 25% decrease in fiber diameter in the denervated animals, whereas in the treated animals there is about a 3% to 4% loss in fiber diameter. More recently, we have been studying the use of leupeptin in vivo in the dystrophic mouse. The next slide shows typical 5-month-old mouse dystrophic gastrocnemius muscle and dystrophic mouse muscle treated intraperitoneally with leupeptin for 4 months, starting at 2 weeks of age. Histochemical studies of this muscle show a normal pattern, and we have maintained this pattern in dystrophic mice for as long as 8 months. In addition, the clinical symptoms of hindleg paralysis have been almost uniformly alleviated in these mice.

Dr. Alfred Goldberg: Those data are very interesting and promising. They are consistent with the in vitro data that I have described. In our experience, there is no reason to believe that pepstatin can enter muscle and have any effect on protein degradation despite repeated attempts to obtain such effects. However, we are convinced that leupeptin would have the consequences you have described, which further demonstrates the possible therapeutic value of these protease inhibitors.

Dr. John Bird: You have certainly given very strong supportive evidence for lysosomal involvement in the degradation of proteins with a long turnover time, the myofibrillar proteins. I want to ask you a question on your ATP-dependent enzyme, the 480K enzyme. Will this enzyme degrade the myofibrillar proteins in addition to the other cytosol proteins?

Dr. Alfred Goldberg: We have no information one way or the other. Its properties have not been extensively studied. There are obviously many important questions to resolve.

Dr. John Bird: Do you think it is a serine protease?

Dr. Alfred Goldberg: It is a serine protease.

Dr. Susan Benoff-Rind: Is there any evidence of a skeletal muscle state in which the primary defect is in the ATP-dependent system, so that relative degradation occurs in apparently normal structural proteins?

Dr. Alfred Goldberg: Neither in muscle nor in any other cell have we been able to quantify the amount of the cytoplasmic pathway in a meaningful way, so the question cannot be answered as yet. We cannot say at the moment whether it is under endocrine control (e.g., by insulin), as is the lysomal apparatus. As the biochemistry of that pathway is defined further, we hope to investigate its relevance to human disease.

Dr. Hyun Dju Kim: What happens to your ATP-dependent system when reticulocytes develop in red blood cells?

Dr. Alfred Goldberg: That is a very interesting question. In cell extracts, we have problems finding ATP-stimulated proteolysis when the reticulocytes develop into erythrocytes, which has been also the experience of Dr. Etlinger.

However, we can show that it exists in such cells by physiologic methods. If we take adult red cells and cause an oxidizing injury (such as with phenylhydrazine or nitrite) to produce methemoglobin, we would show a marked stimulation of proteolysis, which occurs by an ATP-dependent pathway. We think it exists for the lifespan of the red cell and helps protect it against various injuries to proteins, such as from free radicals or oxidizing influences.

Dr. Barry Festoff: I have two questions. Have you noticed that the ATP-dependent 480K protein system is secreted from your organ culture systems (fetal heart or any other)? The second question is, do you know whether there is a plasminogen dependency for protein breakdown in that system?

Dr. Alfred Goldberg: We have never looked and do not think it possible to find this activity if it is secreted. The biochemistry is very difficult. The enzyme is very labile. We are just not ready to ask that question. We are sure plasminogen is not involved.

Dr. R.A. Pieter Kark: Could you tell us how abnormal proteins might be recognized by the ATP-dependent system?

Dr. Alfred Goldberg: I wish I could. In fact, I do not really know what an abnormal protein is. All we can say is that various perturbations and various mutations lead to proteins whose half-lives are much shorter than the normal gene products. There is an important point of general interest that should be emphasized. Many normal proteins have very short half-lives (i.e., of the order of minutes or hours); others have very long half-lives (e.g., a matter of days), so the question you are really asking is not just "what is an abnormal protein?" but "what are the differences in protein conformation that distinguish short-lived from long-lived proteins?" We have spent a lot of time thinking about that issue without definitive answers.

Dr. Ivan Diamond: We know that the receptor is internalized and degraded, and you report that you can inhibit this response. We also know that the receptor can be phosphorylated and dephosphorylated. Is there any evidence that covalent modification of membrane proteins, or any other proteins for that matter, makes them more or less available for internalization or proteolytic degradation?

Dr. Alfred Goldberg: Well, in terms of membrane proteins, the main point that I did not get a chance to discuss is that the degradation of membrane receptors can be blocked with leupeptin or chloroquine, but internalization continues. The internalization seems to be the rate-limiting step. As a result, we get intracellular accumulation of these receptors. In the process of receptor degradation or in the breakdown of soluble proteins there is no evidence for ATP-dependent phosphorylation. This possibility is very attractive, because a lot of the short-lived proteins in liver undergo such a modification. ATP-dependent phosphorylation is the sort of simple-minded explanation of the ATP requirement for proteolysis that we have been assuming. However, we cannot support this model. For the abnormal protein, we believe ATP is affecting the proteolytic enzyme. However, a very complex ATP-dependent modification that involves a peptide conjugation reaction has been suggested by Hershko, Rose, and coworkers. Models analogous to yours for degradation of soluble proteins have been suggested many times without clear evidence for supporting them. I think such models are still viable and attractive, especially in terms of the cAMP-dependent phosphorylations or the insulin-dependent phosphorylations of proteins which do not lead to changes in enzymatic properties but may affect half-lives.

54
Nuclear Magnetic Resonance Studies of Muscle

Michael Bárány, MD, PhD

Joseph M. Chalovich, PhD

C. Tyler Burt, PhD

Thomas Glonek, PhD

Application of nuclear magnetic resonance (NMR) to the analysis of intact muscle was initiated in 1973 by Moon and Richards (1), who recorded the ^{31}P NMR spectrum of whole blood. Since then, many papers have appeared on studies of cellular metabolism by NMR (2, 3).

Among the nuclides used, ^{31}P has an advantage in that it is not only the common isotope of elemental phosphorus, but it is present at nearly 100% natural abundance. In living cells, phosphorus is present in relatively few compounds, and their individual resonances can be readily resolved by existing spectrometers. The application of ^{31}P NMR to muscle is especially favorable, because the breakdown of phosphocreatine (PCr) and adenosine triphosphate (ATP) are correlated with contraction, and a decrease in high-energy phosphates is associated with several muscle diseases. In fact, the techniques developed for ^{31}P NMR of muscle (4, 5) formed the basis for study of other tissues by this method. In this paper we summarize our results on ^{31}P NMR of normal and diseased muscle, including the detection of phosphodiesters that are markers for muscular dystrophies (6).

Another nuclide with great potential in investigations of intact tissue is ^{13}C. Although this isotope is present in all organic molecules, its natural abundance is only 1.1%; ^{13}C NMR analysis of biologic molecules is therefore limited by the resulting low sensitivity. Recently, we were able to record ^{13}C NMR spectra of intact muscle, and our preliminary results are reported in this paper.

^{31}P NMR OF MUSCLE

Concentration of Phosphate Metabolites

The simplest analytical method for measuring the concentration of phosphorus-containing metabolites in muscle is ^{31}P spectroscopy. With appropriate calibrations, the integral of the phosphate signals was used for determination of ATP, PCr, inorganic phosphate (Pi), and sugar phosphate contents of muscles from frog (5, 7), toad (5), normal and dystrophic chickens (7), and normal and diseased humans (6, 8–10). The NMR data agreed reasonably well with chemical measurements (5, 7, 8). Because ^{31}P NMR enables the simultaneous determination of the phosphate compounds in a single muscle sample, the time necessary for a complete analysis is greatly reduced.

We used this technique to measure the phosphate profiles in a large variety of normal and diseased human muscle biopsy specimens (9). The concentrations of phosphates were expressed per 173 mg of noncollagenous protein (the protein content in 1.0 g of normal human muscle) to compensate for the nonspecific loss of phosphate metabolites due to the wasting of muscle tissue in certain diseases. Both ATP and PCr were significantly decreased in Duchenne muscular dystrophy (DMD) and myotonic dystrophy (MyD) but were only slightly diminished in neurogenic, inflammatory, and primary muscle diseases. In both DMD and MyD, a decrease in nicotinamide adenine dinucleotide content was demonstrated. In contrast, sugar phosphate concentrations were increased in all disorders, especially in inflammatory diseases.

^{31}P NMR is a nondestructive method of analysis. Using this method, we have determined that resting frog muscle contains very little Pi and even less sugar phosphate; on the other hand, its PCr content is higher than that measured chemically (7, 9). Thus, in our laboratory, a 10-minute signal-averaged spectrum from a freshly dissected frog muscle revealed 28 mM PCr and <1 mM Pi in the muscle water. This indicates that in a resting skeletal muscle the Pi is built into high-energy phosphates and that the glycolytic cycle is essentially idle.

Time-Course Data

By measuring the ^{31}P NMR spectrum of intact muscle at various times, the changes in the concentration of phosphate metabolites can be observed. Figure 1 shows ^{31}P NMR spectra of freshly dissected barnacle muscles 10 minutes and 127 minutes after the muscles were placed into a 10-mm NMR tube. The relative concentration of each metabolite was determined by integrating the spectra, and the total concentration of phosphate metabolites was determined by a chemical phosphate analysis. Phosphoarginine (P-arginine), the predominant peak of both spectra, comprised 58% and 33% of the total phosphates after 10 and 127 minutes, respectively. These percentage values correspond, respectively, to 22.5 and 12.9 mM P-arginine in the muscle water. Furthermore, the loss of 9.6 mmol of P-arginine per L of muscle was accompanied by a gain of 5.0 mmol of Pi and 4.4 mmol of sugar phosphates. On the other hand, the ATP concentration remained constant at 3.6 mM from 10 to 127 minutes.

Figure 2 compares changes in concentrations of phosphate metabolites in normal human quadriceps muscle versus a quadriceps muscle from a patient with nemaline rod myopathy under anaerobic conditions as a function of time.

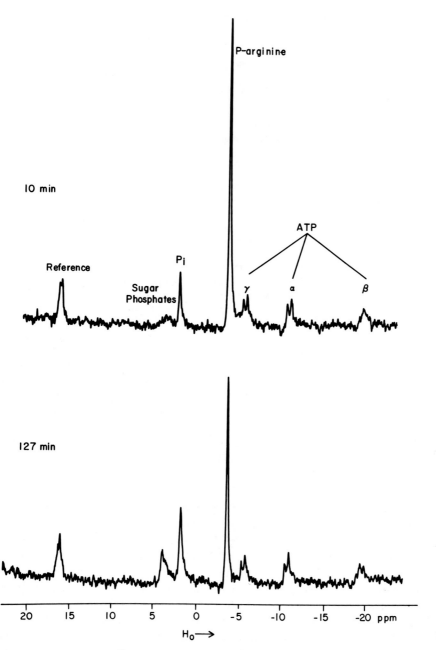

Fig. 1. Proton-decoupled ^{31}P NMR spectra of intact barnacle muscles. The conditions of data acquisition were the same as those previously described (5). Each spectrum is from a 20-minute accumulation of NMR data. The upper spectrum is from the first 20-minute block of data, and the lower spectrum is from the last block of data collected from the same barnacle muscle. The muscle was kept in the NMR tube under anaerobic conditions at 31°C for the duration of the experiment. The times shown on the spectra represent the midpoint of data acquisition. The reference compound was methylene-diphosphonic acid. The chemical shift scale is relative to 85% orthophosphoric acid, and downfield shifts are shown as positive, following the recommendation of IUPAC. H_0 is the magnetic field, and the arrow shows the direction of its increase. The γ, α, and β denote the 3 phosphates of adenosine triphosphate (ATP); Pi, inorganic phosphate.

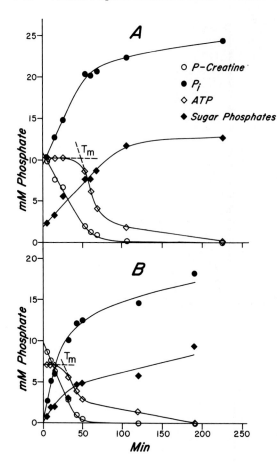

Fig. 2. Time dependence of human muscle phosphate concentrations. **(A)** Normal quadriceps. The maintenance time (T_m) is the point at which adenosine triphosphate (ATP) begins to decrease. **(B)** Quadriceps from nemaline rod myopathy. (Reprinted with permission from Burt CT, Glonek T, Bárány M: Analysis of living tissue by phosphorus-31 magnetic resonance. Science 195:145–149, 1977. Copyright 1977 by the American Association for the Advancement of Science.)

In the normal muscle (Part A), PCr is initially present at a concentration of 10 mM, but decreases linearly to a concentration of 2.3 mM within approximately 50 minutes. In the diseased muscle (Part B), PCr is degraded more rapidly. Furthermore, the rate of increase of Pi is faster in the diseased than in the normal muscle. Finally, ATP remains constant for 48 minutes in the normal muscle but only for 24 minutes in the diseased muscle (compare values for maintenance time). These data indicate changes in the ATPase and creatine phosphotransferase activity of the diseased muscle that may be caused either by alteration of the amount of available enzyme and substrate, or by a change in the environment of the enzyme.

Myosin ATPase in Intact Muscle

Under anaerobic conditions, ^{31}P NMR may be used to measure the ATPase activity of myosin in muscle. This is based on the following equations:

$$\text{ATP} \xrightarrow{\text{myosin}} \text{ADP} + \text{Pi} \tag{1}$$

$$\text{ADP} + \text{PCr} \xrightarrow{\text{creatine phosphotransferase}} \text{ATP} + \text{Cr} \tag{2}$$

$$\text{PCr} = \text{Cr} + \text{Pi} \tag{3}$$

Because the equilibrium in reaction 2 is shifted far to the right (12) under anaerobic conditions and before the onset of glycolysis, the initial breakdown of PCr should be equal to the breakdown of ATP. Indeed, in various muscles we found a decrease in PCr and a stoichiometric increase in Pi while ATP remained constant, in agreement with the above scheme (13). In muscle, several ATPases may contribute to the observed hydrolysis of PCr. The Na,K-ATPase activity was eliminated by finding no difference between oubain-treated and untreated muscles (13). The amount of ATPase in sarcoplasmic reticulum is small, and this ATPase is not activated in resting muscle; therefore, the rate of decrease of PCr should represent mainly the myosin ATPase in the intact muscle.

From the decay curves of PCr in ^{31}P NMR spectra, we calculated the steady-state rate constant for the subfragment-1 moiety of myosin in intact muscles and compared these values with constants from in vitro studies. The results in Table 1 show that the rate constants for myosin ATPase in intact resting muscle vary from 7 to 10 times less than the in vitro values. This difference would be even greater if the contribution of the sarcoplasmic reticulum ATPase were subtracted from the total ATPase. Accordingly, one may postulate that an inhibitor of myosin ATPase may exist in vivo.

Dawson and colleagues (7) developed methods for stimulating muscles in the field of superconducting magnets and recording the tension of muscles while at the same time accumulating their ^{31}P NMR spectra. At 4° C, they measured a rate of 1.6 μmol of PCr hydrolyzed per second per g of toad muscle, and a value one-third of this in the sartorius. Their values correspond to rate constants of 5.72 and 1.91 sec^{-1}, respectively, for subfragment-1 ATPase in contracting muscle. These values are 1,500 to 5,000 times higher than the rate constant in resting frog muscle at 4° C, which is 0.0012 sec^{-1} (Table 1). Accordingly, the transformation of myosin ATPase from rest to contraction involves a 1,500- to 5,000-fold activation in frog muscle. This value is considerably higher than any value measured in any in vitro system.

Table 1. Activity of Myosin ATPase in Resting Muscle and In Vitro[a]

Sample	Steady-State Rate Constant of Subfragment-1 (sec^{-1})	Reference
Frog muscle, 28° C	0.0089	Bárány and Burt (13)
Frog muscle, 4° C	0.0012	Cohen and Burt (14)
Rat muscle, 20° C	0.0078	Hoult et al. (4)
Human muscle, 28° C	0.0092	Bárány and Burt (13)
Frog myosin, 25° C	0.0620	Bárány M (unpublished data)
Frog myosin, 0–2° C	0.0040	Ferenczi et al. (15)
Frog subfragment-1, 0–2° C	0.0110	Ferenczi et al. (15)
Rabbit myosin, 25° C	0.0600	Schliselfeld (16)
Rabbit subfragment-1, 20° C	0.0600	Bagshaw and Trentham (17)
Rabbit subfragment-1, 3° C	0.0150	Sleep and Taylor (18)

[a] The subfragment-1 content of muscle was taken as 0.28 μmol/g of muscle.

Creatine Phosphotransferase in Intact Muscle

Brown and colleagues (19) measured creatine phosphotransferase activities in skeletal and cardiac muscle by saturation transfer ^{31}P NMR. In the case of the frog gastrocnemius, the rate of phosphate transfer from PCr to ADP was 0.85 μmol/sec/g of muscle at 4° C, which is within the same range as the breakdown of PCr by these muscles under similar conditions (19). This example shows the potential of spin magnetization transfer techniques, which can measure reaction rates directly, with a time resolution on the order of 1 second. These techniques represent a new approach to studying enzyme kinetics in vivo.

Determination of Intracellular pH

At physiologic pH values, the chemical shifts of ATP, inorganic orthophosphate, and the sugar phosphates vary with the hydrogen ion concentration. By comparing the chemical shift of one of these metabolites in the muscle to that in a solution whose composition is similar to that of myoplasm, a value may be assigned to the internal pH. Model studies have shown that the titration curve of Pi is unaffected by KCl or $MgCl_2$, whereas ATP and sugar phosphates do vary with changes in these salts (4, 5). Therefore, the chemical shift of the Pi peak in the muscle can be used to calculate the intracellular pH. In freshly dissected muscles, the pH values are above 7. Specifically, they are 7.2 to 7.5 in frog (5, 7); 7.1 in rat (4); 7.2 in human; 7.3 in the barnacle (unpublished results). During development of rigor under anaerobic conditions, the pH of frog muscle was reduced to 6 to 6.5 (5). From such pH changes, the quantity of lactic acid produced in frog muscle was estimated (20).

The noninvasive measurement of pH by ^{31}P NMR was also applied to follow the extent of ischemia in heart. It was reported that the intracellular pH decreased from 7.4 to 5.7 during total ischemia, and the pH returned rapidly to its initial value with reperfusion (2).

The Phosphodiesters

^{31}P NMR studies of intact muscles have revealed that phosphodiesters comprise a significant fraction of the total observable phosphate metabolites (5, 7, 11, 21, 22). Figure 3 shows ^{31}P spectra from intact frog gastrocnemius, rabbit soleus, rabbit heart, and dystrophic chicken pectoralis. The phosphodiesters give rise to the group of signals indicated by the arrows in the figure, which occur at approximately 0 ppm in the ^{31}P spectrum. We extracted the phosphodiester compounds from the muscles with perchloric acid. These compounds were purified by barium and alcoholic fractionations and by column and paper chromatography. Two pure compounds were isolated. One, which resonates at −0.13 ppm, was identified (22) as sn-glycerol 3-phosphorylcholine (GPC):

$$\begin{array}{l} CH_2OH \\ | \\ CHOH \quad\quad O- \\ | \quad\quad\quad\quad | \\ CH_2-O-P-O-CH_2-CH_2-N^+(CH_3)_3 \\ \quad\quad\quad\quad \| \\ \quad\quad\quad\quad O \end{array}$$

Because GPC is a derivative of lecithin, a constituent of muscle membranes, it is reasonable to assume that alterations in GPC metabolism reflect changes in dystrophic membranes. Indeed, Kunze (26) demonstrated a decreased lecithin and an increased lysolecithin content in DMD muscles. An increased lecithinase activity was found in muscles of hereditary dystrophic mice (27), as predicted from Kunze's observation. On the other hand, the lysolecithinase activities of normal and dystrophic mouse muscles were the same; this speaks against the theory that a decrease in lysolecithinase accounts for the decreased GPC in DMD (6, 10). Alternatively, the rate of GPC production may be controlled by a GPC phosphodiesterase. However, the ultimate answer must come from the study of human muscles.

L-Serine Ethanolamine Phosphate

SEP is the characteristic diester of avian, reptilian, fish, and amphibian muscles, and it is not found in mammalian muscles (3, 6, 23). Rosenberg and Ennor (28) reported high levels of SEP in the chicken kidney and intestinal mucosa as well.

Because SEP occurs in the pectoralis muscle of hereditary dystrophic chickens but not in the normal chicken pectoralis (5, 6, 10, 23–25), its study may lead to a better understanding of the nature of chicken dystrophy. ^{31}P NMR readily detects (Fig. 3) and quantifies SEP. Thus, we measured 2 to 2.5 μmol of SEP per g of dystrophic pectoralis (6, 23), which is in the same range as the ATP content of this muscle. However, the pectoralis muscle from normal chicken contained less than 10 nmol of SEP per g (this low concentration was estimated in the extract of 40 g of normal muscle, which was concentrated to 2 ml). Similarly, fatty deposits from heart, liver, and the neck area of these chickens contained less than 10 nmol of SEP/g of tissue. This indicates that SEP accumulation in dystrophic muscle is not due to fatty infiltration. The concentration of SEP in dystrophic and normal chicken blood was determined in perchloric acid extracts of 20-ml blood samples after 10-fold concentration. No SEP signal was detected in any type of blood. This suggested that SEP is not transported from another organ (e.g., kidney) to the muscle through the blood, a conclusion verified by uptake studies with radioactive SEP (29).

^{31}P NMR monitoring of dystrophic chicken muscles showed that SEP is not absolutely specific for the pectoralis, but is also present in the slow anterior latissimus dorsi (ALD) muscle (6, 10). Moreover, SEP resonances were also observed in the ALD of normal chicken. On the other hand, an SEP signal was not detected in the fast posterior latissimus dorsi (PLD) muscle of either the dystrophic or normal chicken. Inasmuch as fast muscle develops from slow muscle, the presence of SEP in the dystrophic pectoralis (a fast muscle) indicates a possible developmental alteration in the dystrophic muscle. That muscular dystrophy may represent a failure of the muscle to develop beyond the immature state had been proposed earlier (30).

The cause of accumulation of SEP in dystrophic muscle is the presence of an enzyme system capable of synthesizing SEP according to the following reaction: L-serine + cytidine diphosphate ethanolamine → L-serine ethanolamine phosphate + cytidine monophosphate. The SEP synthase activity is localized to the microsomal fraction. Dystrophic chicken muscle microsomes also contain SEP diesterase, which hydrolyzes SEP: L-serine ethanolamine phosphate → L-serine + ethanolamine phosphate.

Both of these enzymic activities have been described in chicken kidneys and intestinal mucosae (31, 32). The activity of SEP-metabolizing enzymes is much higher in dystrophic muscle microsomes than in the normal microsomes. Thus, SEP synthase is not detectable in normal muscle, whereas SEP diesterase is decreased approximately 13-fold in normal muscle compared to dystrophic muscle (6). Because dystrophic chicken muscle accumulates SEP in vivo, there must be a special mechanism that prevents the degradation of SEP. One may postulate regulation either by a specific SEP phosphodiesterase inhibitor or by compartmentalization of the synthetic and/or degradative enzyme.

The SEP-metabolizing enzymes undergo a characteristic change during the development of the chicken (29). Neither normal nor dystrophic pectoralis microsomes have detectable SEP synthase activity between 1 and 3 weeks ex ovo. Eventually, the synthase activity is manifested in dystrophic microsomes, reaching a constant level at approximately 5 weeks ex ovo. Synthase activity never appears in normal microsomes.

Normal tissue undergoes an age-related change in SEP diesterase activity. At 1 to 3 weeks ex ovo, microsomes from normal and dystrophic pectoralis muscles have a high diesterase activity. There is no major change in the activity of dystrophic microsomes through 24 weeks ex ovo. The diesterase activity of normal muscles decreases approximately 8-fold between the period of 3 to 5 weeks ex ovo. This pattern of enzymic changes also supports the idea of altered muscle maturation in dystrophy.

The role of SEP in tissue metabolism is not known. It has been suggested that in reptilian and amphibian brain, SEP is a donor of serine and O-phosphoryl-ethanolamine for phospholipid synthesis (33, 34). We tested this theory in both dystrophic and normal ALD muscles by comparing the turnover of serine moieties of SEP and phosphatidylserine. The turnover was slower in SEP than in phosphatidylserine, suggesting that SEP is not a precursor of serine phospholipid synthesis (29).

^{13}C NMR OF MUSCLE

Although ^{13}C is present in low natural abundance, modern spectrometers make it possible to obtain spectra of proteins, lipids, and low molecular weight organic substances in intact muscle. Fung (35) was the first to report the proton-decoupled ^{13}C spectra of mouse muscle at 25.2 MHz. He observed 3 peaks centered around 30, 130, and 175 ppm (from tetramethylsilane) and assigned them to aliphatic, aromatic, and carbonyl carbons. He also showed that the methylene peaks (30 ppm) can be observed even in dehydrated muscle, indicating that these groups must be relatively mobile.

We recorded proton-decoupled and proton-coupled ^{13}C spectra of intact chicken muscle in 20-mm tubes at 45.26 MHz (Fig. 5). We had to accumulate data for approximately 21 hours to generate each of these spectra. Based on literature data (36, 27), the various peaks from right to left were assigned to the alkyls (14 to 48 ppm), amines and α-carbons (50 to 60 ppm), alcohols (61 to 70

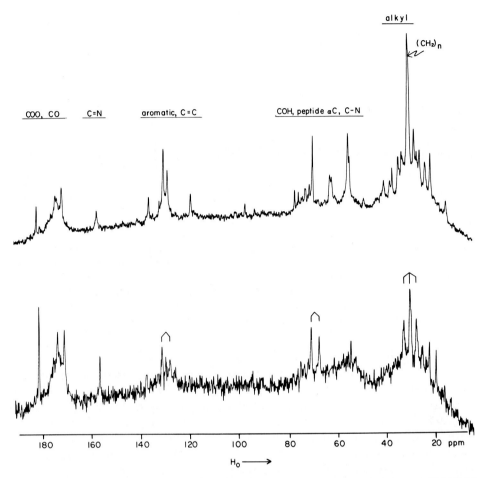

Fig. 5. High-resolution proton-decoupled (upper) and proton-coupled (lower) ^{13}C NMR spectra of intact chicken pectoralis muscle. The freshly dissected muscle was placed into 20-mm tubes without any solvent, and the spectra were recorded on a Bruker CXP-180 spectrometer at 45.26 MHz. The number of scans recorded were 14,990 for decoupled and 14,706 for the coupled spectrum. Spectrometer conditions: sweep width, 11,000 Hz; dwell time, 45 μsec; 4 K data point; pulse repetition rate, 5 sec; filter band width, 11,000 Hz; pulse width, 9.8 μsec; line broadening, 1 Hz; spinning rate, 30 Hz. The temperature of the muscle in the coupled spectrum was ambient (30° C); however, for the decoupled spectrum, it was considerably higher because of the heat generated by the decoupler. The chemical shift scale is relative to tetramethylsilane. H_0 is the magnetic field, and the arrow shows the direction of its increase.

ppm), aromatic and allyls (118 to 140 ppm), guanidinos (157 ppm), and carbonyl (170 to 190 ppm) regions.

To identify the resonances, we recorded spectra of standard compounds as well as spectra of various subfractions of muscle.

Figure 6 shows the spectrum of phosphatidylcholine-cholesterol vesicles. As in the muscle spectrum, one finds resonances from the alkyl, amine, allyl, and carbonyl regions. The peak at 14.1 ppm is derived from the methyl group of

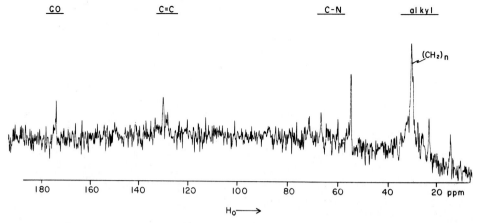

Fig. 6. Proton-decoupled ^{13}C NMR spectrtum of phosphatidylcholine-cholesterol vesicles. Phosphatidylcholine and cholesterol were mixed in a molar ratio of 10 : 3, evaporated, and freeze dried. Vesicles were formed by sonication in 10% D_2O, 0.15 M KCl, 10 mM KPi (pH 7.0), and 2 mM ethylenediamine tetra-acetic acid saturated with N_2. The concentration of phosphatidylcholine in the vesicles was 20 mM. The number of scans recorded was 1066; for other conditions, see the legend to Figure 5.

cholesterol at the C-18 position. The other cholesterol resonances exist as minor components in the alkyl and allyl regions. This statement is based on experiments in which spectra were taken from vesicles prepared from phosphatidylcholine alone; these spectra were virtually identical to the spectrum of Figure 6 with the exception of the 14.1 ppm peak. The most characteristic resonance, at 54.5 ppm, is due to the N-methyl groups of the choline moiety. Other predominant resonances are from the methylene carbons of the fatty acid chains at 30.1 ppm, the unsaturated carbons at 130 ppm, and the carbonyl carbons of the ester linkages at 173.9 ppm.

Because microsomes contain a rather large amount of phosphatidylcholine, we recorded the spectrum of muscle microsomes (Fig. 7). The major peaks correspond to those in phospholipid vesicles (Fig. 6). Because the specific resonance of vesicles is derived from choline, at 54.8 ppm, we calculated the ratio of the choline resonance area to that of the alkyl, allyl, and carbonyl regions in both the vesicles and the microsomes. The ratios were 0.15, 0.93, and 2.10 for the vesicles and 0.09, 0.34, and 0.58 for the microsomes, respectively. This suggests that proteins and phospholipids contribute to the ^{13}C NMR spectrum of microsomes.

At another extreme, we recorded the spectra of a dialyzed 100,000-g supernatant from chicken muscle homogenate, which can be considered a protein mixture free of lipids (Fig. 8). This spectrum shows several sharp resonances not seen in the microsomal preparations, e.g., in the aliphatic region at 26.4, 32.6, 36.2, and 68.8 ppm due to the amino acid β-carbons, and at 120.1, 136.5, and 149.6 ppm, due to the aromatic amino acid carbons. Based on literature data (36), the peak at 53.8 ppm is attributed to the α-carbons of the protein backbone. The peptide C=O is responsible for the increased area in the carbonyl region.

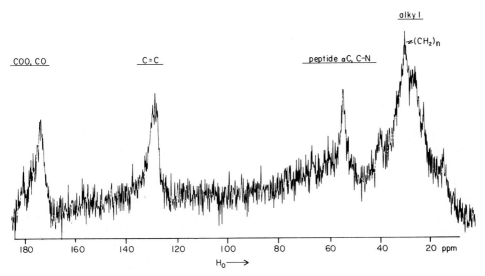

Fig. 7. Proton decoupled ^{13}C NMR spectrum of chicken muscle microsomes, with approximately 150 mg of protein per ml in 10% D_2O, 0.15 M KCl, and 10 mM KPi (pH 7.0). The number of scans recorded was 8,192.

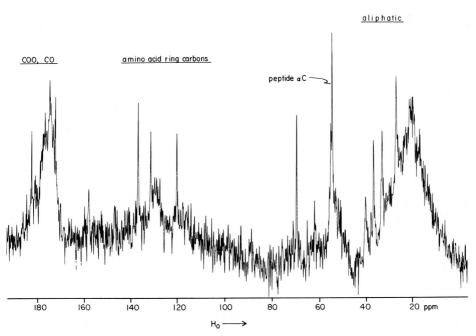

Fig. 8. Proton-decoupled ^{13}C NMR spectrum of the 100,000-g supernatant of chicken muscle homogenate. Before spectroscopy, the supernatant was exhaustively dialyzed against distilled water to remove soluble organic nonprotein carbon compounds. After freeze drying, a solution of approximately 400 mg of protein per ml in 10% D_2O, 0.15 M KCl, and 10 mM KPi (pH 7.0) was prepared. The number of scans recorded was 1,300.

709

To take into account the soluble organic molecules of muscle, we prepared a percholoric acid extract from a muscle left at room temperature overnight (conditions imitating those of Figure 5). After neutralization with KOH and centrifugation to remove perchlorate, the ^{31}C spectrum was recorded. The major resonance was presumably from the lactic acid that accumulated in muscle with rigor. The characteristic peaks were at 68.7 ppm from its alcoholic group and at 182.4 ppm from its carboxylic group. Pronounced resonances were also observed from creatine: at 53.6 ppm, its nitrogen-bound carbon; at 157.2 ppm, its guanidino residue.

Based on the information obtained from the described model spectra (Fig. 6–8), we made a tentative assignment of the major resonances in the proton-decoupled spectrum of intact muscle (Fig. 5, upper part). The proton-coupled spectrum of the same muscle (Fig. 5, lower part) helped in making these assignments. The alkyl region of the upper spectrum in Figure 5 has contributions from aliphatic carbons of fatty acids and amino acid residues. The major resonance at 29.8 ppm in the decoupled spectrum is probably due to the methylene carbon atoms of the fatty acid chains. This is supported in the lower proton-coupled spectrum where this resonance appears as a triplet, which is consistent with a carbon with two bound protons. The carbon-hydrogen coupling constant is 119 Hz, which is similar to a literature value of 125 Hz for similar C–H bonds (38).

The resonance centered at 54.2 ppm has contributions from the N-methyl groups of choline in phospholipids, N-methyl groups of creatine in the sarcoplasm, and the α-carbon in the backbone. In the coupled spectrum, this gives rise to a complicated pattern that cannot be resolved.

The resonance at 68.7 ppm in the decoupled spectrum is from the alcoholic C atom of lactic acid. As expected, this gives rise to a doublet in the proton-coupled spectrum. The C–H coupling constant is 143 Hz, which agrees very closely with the literature value of 140 Hz for similar CH bonds (38).

The resonance at 129.8 ppm is from unsaturated carbon atoms derived from fatty acids, tyrosine, and phenylalanine residues. In the proton-coupled spectrum, this appears as a doublet, which is consistent with the assignment of $CH=CH$ (J_{CH} = 146; literature J_{CH} = 156).

The resonance at 157.6 ppm is probably from the guanidino carbon of creatine; this gives rise to a singlet in the coupled spectrum because no proton is bound to the C atom.

The resonances between 171.9 and 176.4 ppm in the decoupled spectra are described in the literature as those derived from peptide $C=O$, esterified carbons in phospholipids, and glutamyl and asparaginyl side chains.

The last sharp peak at 182.4 ppm in the decoupled spectrum and its counterpart at 182.5 ppm in the coupled spectrum are probably due to a carboxylic acid present in lactic acid, creatine, or other metabolites (e.g., citric acid), or to glutamic and aspartic acid in the side chains.

It was of interest to record a spectrum of a chicken smooth muscle, the gizzard (Fig. 9). The most striking feature of this decoupled spectrum is the missing $(CH_2)_n$ resonance at 29.8 ppm, which is the predominant peak of skeletal muscle spectra. In accordance, one does not see major peaks in the choline or allyl region. In contrast, the carbonyl region is very pronounced. On

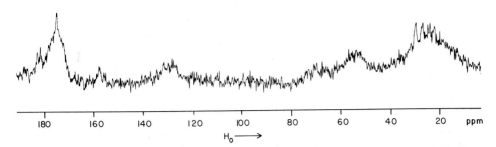

Fig. 9. Proton-decoupled ^{13}C NMR spectrum of intact chicken gizzard muscle. The number of scans recorded was 6,094.

the whole, this spectrum resembles that of a pure protein rather than that of a protein-phospholipid mixture. This is understandable because smooth muscle is known to have a greatly reduced sarcoplasmic reticulum, the structure that contains most of the phospholipids in muscle.

The example of gizzard shows that ^{31}C NMR can differentiate between skeletal and smooth muscle. It is hoped that with a further improvement of the technique more subtle differences may be resolved among various muscles, including diseased muscles.

ACKNOWLEDGMENTS

This work was supported by the Muscular Dystrophy Association, and by National Institutes of Health Grant NS-12172. We are grateful to Dr. Daniel Fiat and Mr. William Valentine for their help in using the Bruker CXP-180 Spectrometer; Dr. Andrew G Engel, for the biopsy specimens of Duchenne muscle; Dr. Edward E Bittar, for the barnacle muscles; and Ms. Barbara A Rogowski, for typing the manuscript. We also wish to thank Marilyn Uhl-Tauginas for the fine illustrations.

REFERENCES

1. Moon RB, Richards JB: Determination of intracellular pH by ^{31}P magnetic resonance. J Biol Chem 248:7276–7278, 1973

2. Radda GK, Seeley PJ: Recent studies on cellular metabolism by nuclear magnetic resonance. Annu Rev Physiol 41:749–769, 1979

3. Burt CT, Cohen SM, Bárány M: Analysis of intact tissues with ^{31}P NMR. Annu Rev Biophys Bioeng 8:1–25, 1979

4. Hoult DI, Busby SJW, Gadian DG, et al: Observation of tissue metabolites using ^{31}P nuclear magnetic resonance. Nature 252:285–287, 1974.

5. Burt CT, Glonek T, Bárány M: Analysis of phosphate metabolites, the intracellular pH, and

the state of adenosine triphosphate in intact muscle by phosphorus nuclear magnetic resonance. J Biol Chem 251:2584–2591, 1976

6. Chalovich JM, Burt CT, Danon MJ, et al: Phosphodiesters in muscular dystrophies. Ann NY Acad Sci 317:649–668, 1979

7. Dawson MJ, Gadian DG, Wilkie DR: Contraction and recovery of living muscles studied by ^{31}P nuclear magnetic resonance. J Physiol (Lond) 267:703–735, 1977

8. Bárány M, Burt CT, Labotka RJ, et al: ^{31}P NMR of diseased muscle. In *Pathogenesis of Human Muscular Dystrophies*. Edited by Rowland LP. Excerpta Medica, Amsterdam, 1977, pp 337–340

9. Glonek T, Burt CT, Labotka RJ, et al: Phosphorus-31 nuclear magnetic resonance spectroscopic analysis of intact tissue. Benjamin Goldberg Symposium on Engineering in Health Sciences, University of Illinois Medical Center, Chicago, 1977, pp 214–235

10. Burt CT, Chalovich JM, Danon MJ, et al: Phosphorus nuclear magnetic resonance of diseased muscle. In *Frontiers of Biological Energetics*. Edited by Dutton PL, Leigh JS, Scarpa A. Academic Press, New York, 1978, pp 1371–1378

11. Burt CT, Glonek T, Bárány M: Analysis of living tissue by phosphorus-31 magnetic resonance. Science 195:145–149, 1977

12. Carlson FD, Wilkie DR (eds): *Muscle Physiology*. Prentice-Hall, Englewood Cliffs, NJ, 1974, pp 90–94

13. Bárány M, Burt CT: The adenosine triphosphatase activity of myosin in intact muscle (abstract). Fed Proc 38:338, 1979

14. Cohen SM, Burt CT: [31]P nuclear magnetic relaxation studies of phosphocreatine in intact muscle: determination of intracellular free magnesium. Proc Natl Acad Sci USA 74:4271–4275, 1977

15. Ferenczi MA, Homsher E, Trentham DR, et al: Preparation and characterization of frog muscle myosin subfragment 1 and actin. Biochem J 171:155–163, 1978

16. Schliselfeld LH: Steady-state studies of the actin-activated adenosine-triphosphate activity of myosin. Biochim Biophys Acta 445:234–245, 1976

17. Bagshaw CR, Trentham DR: The characterization of myosin-product complexes and of product-release steps during the magnesium ion–dependent adenosine triphosphatase reaction. Biochem J 141:331–349, 1974

18. Sleep JA, Taylor EW: Intermediate states of actomyosin adenosine triphosphatase. Biochemistry 15:5813–5817, 1976

19. Brown TR, Gadian DG, Garlick PB, et al: Creatine kinase activities in skeletal and cardiac muscle measured by saturation transfer NMR. In *Frontiers of Biological Energetics*. Edited by Dutton PL, Leigh JS, Scarpa A. Academic Press, New York, 1978, pp 1341–1349

20. Dawson MJ, Gadian DG, Wilkie DR: Muscular fatigue investigated by phosphorus nuclear magnetic resonance. Nature 274:861–866, 1978

21. Burt CT, Glonek T, Bárány M: Phosphorus-31 nuclear magnetic resonance detection of unexpected phosphodiesters in muscle. Biochemistry 15:4850–4853, 1976

22. Seeley PJ, Busby SJW, Gadian DG, et al: A new approach to metabolite compartmentation in muscle. Biochem Soc Trans 4:62–64, 1976

23. Chalovich JM, Burt CT, Cohen SM, et al: Identification of an unknown ^{31}P nuclear magnetic resonance from dystrophic chicken as L-serine ethanolamine phosphodiester. Arch Biochem Biophys 182:683–689, 1977

24. Peterson DW, Lilyblade AL, Lyon J: Serine-ethanolamine-phosphate, taurine and free amino acids of muscle in hereditary muscular dystrophy of the chicken. Proc Soc Exp Biol Med 113:798–802, 1963

25. Wilson BW, Peterson DW, Lilyblade AL: Free amino acids of developing skeletal musculature of normal and genetically dystrophic chickens. Proc Soc Exp Biol Med 119:104–108, 1965

26. Kunze D: Lipids: composition and metabolism in human dystrophy. In *Pathogenesis of Human Muscular Dystrophies*. Edited by Rowland LP. Excerpta Medica, Amsterdam, 1977, pp 404–414

27. Kwok CT, Austin L: Phospholipid composition and metabolism in mouse muscular dystrophy. Biochem J 176:15–22, 1978

28. Rosenberg H, Ennor AH: Preliminary observations on the distributions and biosynthesis of serine ethanolamine phosphodiester. J Biochem (Tokyo) 50:81–84, 1961

29. Chalovich JM, Bárány M: Serine ethanolamine phosphate in avian muscular dystrophy: mechanism of accumulation in dystrophic muscle and relationship to phospholipid synthesis. Arch Biochem Biophys 199:615–625, 1980

30. Peterson DW, Hamilton WH, Lilyblade AL: Composition of hypertrophic and atrophic muscles in genetic muscular dystrophy of the chicken. Proc Soc Exp Biol Med 127:300–305, 1968

31. Allen AK, Rosenberg H: The mechanism of action and some properties of serine ethanolamine phosphate synthetase. Biochim Biophys Acta 151:504–519, 1968

32. Hagerman DD, Rosenberg H, Ennor AH, et al: The isolation and properties of chicken kidney serine ethanolamine phosphate phosphodiesterase. J Biol Chem 240:1108–1112, 1965

33. Procellati G, Di Jeso F, Malcovati M: The conversion of L-serine ethanolamine phosphate and L-threonine ethanolamine phosphate to microsomal phospholipid in brain tissue. Life Sci 5:769–774, 1966

34. Procellati G, Di Jeso F, Malcovati M, Biasion MG: The conversion of the ethanolamine phosphate moiety of L-serine ethanolamine phosphate to microsomal phospholipid in brain tissue. Life Sci 5:1791–1799, 1966

35. Fung BM: Carbon-13 and proton magnetic resonance of mouse muscle. Biophys J 19:315–319, 1977

36. Gurd FRN, Keim P: The prospects for carbon-13 nuclear magnetic resonance studies in enzymology. Methods Enzymol 27:836–911, 1973

37. Godici PE, Landsberger FR: The dynamic structure of lipid membranes: ^{31}C nuclear magnetic resonance study using spin labels. Biochemistry 13:362–368, 1974

38. Levy GC, Nelson GL (eds): *Carbon-13 Nuclear Magnetic Resonance for Organic Chemists.* Wiley-Interscience, New York, 1972, p 28

DISCUSSION

Dr. Robert Barchi: Presumably, the reason why you see a sharp phosphorus resonance peak from your glycerol phosphorylcholine and not from a diacyl glycerol phosphorylcholine is because of the slow rotational movement of the latter under normal membrane conditions. Do you think there is any possibility that this peak that you see in the ^{13}C NMR is actually from phosphatidylcholine molecules that for one reason or another either are more in the hydrophilic environment or are more freely mobile in dystrophic muscle and hence give you a sharp spectrum?

Dr. Michael Bárány: All we can say is that the long fatty acid side chains are very mobile and therefore give rise to a sharp resonance at 30.1 ppm. This peak does not really differentiate between methylene carbons of phosphatidyl-choline and phosphatidylethanolamine, or anything else.

Dr. Frederick Samaha: Can you tell the difference between a fast-twitch and a slow-twitch muscle? The gizzard shows a dramatic difference, but can you pick up the difference in the diminished sarcoplasmic reticulum between slow and fast muscle?

Dr. Michael Bárány: We did not study slow- and fast-twitch muscles as yet.

Dr. John Gergely: I have two questions. Have you looked at muscles of carriers? If the disappearance of one of the peaks is so characteristic of Duchenne muscular dystrophy, one might well find the same in the mothers. The other question concerns ^{13}C NMR. Does the diacyl peak that you see correspond to that fraction of the chains that are mobile, or do you pick up all the chains? Do you think that the differences between striated and smooth muscle are due to differences in the fraction of mobile chains, or are they due to differences in the total membrane fraction?

Dr. Michael Bárány: Concerning your second question, we see only the mobile chains. Concerning your first question, if you will send us muscles from carriers, we will be glad to look into their glycerol phosphocholine content.

Dr. Jarvis Seegmiller: About a year ago I heard Dr. Chance present a lecture in which he put a whole mouse into the tube and showed that the ATP dropped off as the oxygen supply was turned off and increased when oxygen was turned on. This suggests the great value that this technology might have if it could be applied to intact persons rather than a muscle biopsy specimen. I would be interested in your comment on how near we are to such a technology.

Dr. Michael Bárány: You will be pleased to learn that about a month ago I heard a lecture in which a slide showed that a living man underwent NMR analysis, so this really is the modern trend. Currently at the NIH and in England great progress is being made toward use of NMR for detection of all kinds of pathologic states such as those which may exist in brain, lung, or bone. Certainly, the time is not too far when a ^{31}P NMR spectra will be recorded in patients without a muscle biopsy.

55
Energy Metabolism in Human Myopathy

R. H. T. Edwards, PhD, FRCP

C. M. Wiles, PhD, MRCP

K. Gohil

S. Krywawych, BS

D. A. Jones, Phd

Energy is required for many cell functions in muscle in addition to the obvious ones of generating force and heat. New techniques have been described to investigate energy exchange by biochemical analysis of needle biopsy samples of human muscle (1, 2) and by measurement of metabolic heat production (1, 3). In addition, by studying patients with defined abnormalities of energy exchange, it is possible to gain insights into the factors that may limit muscle performance in patients with less well defined conditions. The purpose of this paper is to show how specific abnormalities in the rates of either energy utilization or production result in characteristic changes in muscle performance.

Detailed physiologic and biochemical studies are presented in patients who fall into four distinct categories: those with either an increased (hyperthyroid) or a decreased (hypothyroid) metabolic rate; those with a specific defect in glycolysis (myophosphorylase deficiency); and a patient with a muscle mitochondrial lesion that prevents the oxidative metabolism of pyruvate. The first part of this paper will be a brief description of this patient; we will then compare and contrast the functional and metabolic features of this patient with those of the other patients.

MUSCLE MITOCHONDRIAL ABNORMALITY

Patient MF is a 20-year-old man with markedly impaired exercise tolerance. He is able to walk only 100 yards before feeling exhausted. His symptoms first became troublesome at approximately 11 years of age and since then have become progressively worse. A muscle biopsy specimen revealed some fibers

715

with an increased density of mitochondrial staining in the subsarcolemmal regions, and electron microscopy demonstrated accumulations of rather large mitochondria and glycogen in the periphery of these fibers. When exercising on a bicycle ergometer the patient was capable of only minimal amounts of work which, nevertheless, produced the symptoms of respiratory distress, exhaustion, and muscle pain (Fig. 1). Details of the cardiorespiratory response to exercise are given in Table 1.

The plasma lactate concentration at rest was usually slightly increased; with exercise it rose rapidly (Fig. 1, Table 2) and was slow to return to the resting level. β-hydroxybutyrate concentration decreased on exercise; pyruvate increased, but not to the same extent as lactate (Table 2).

Mitochondrial Function

Studies of mitochondrial oxidative metabolism were carried out by Dr. J. Morgan-Hughes and colleagues on isolated mitochondria obtained from a specimen of the quadriceps muscle obtained by open biopsy. Details of the techniques have been published elsewhere (4, 5).

Typical polarographic traces of mitochondrial oxygen utilization using different substrates are shown in Figure 2. Trace A shows the absence of observable oxygen uptake with pyruvate and malate as substrates. Addition of succinate brought about a marked enhancement of oxygen utilization, indicating that the respiratory chain between CoQ/cytochrome b and cytochrome oxidase was intact. The mitochondria were coupled (Trace B) and showed good respiratory control ratios.

In parallel with these studies, an investigation of mitochondrial oxidative

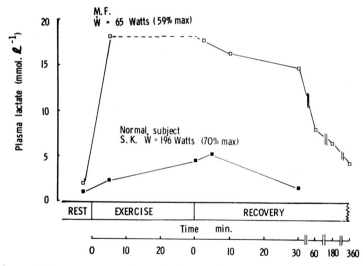

Fig. 1. Plasma lactate concentrations during and after exercise in Patient MF (open squares), who had abnormal mitochondria, and in Subject SK (closed squares), a normal subject of similar age. Patient MF was able to sustain the exercise for only 5 minutes despite the low work rate; note his large increase in lactate and its slow recovery. W = work rate.

Table 1. Physiologic Measurements in the Sixth Minute of Maximal Exercise

| | Patient MF[a] | Normal Men[b] | |
		Untrained (n = 4)	Trained (n = 5)
Work rate (kpm/min)	400	1,200 ± 82	1,840 ± 39.8
Heart rate (beats/min)	183	181 ± 3.4	188 ± 2.0
Oxygen intake (ml/min STPD)	542	3,065 ± 220	4,148 ± 122
Respiratory exchange ratio	3.33	1.17 ± 0.04	1.06 ± 0.03
Pulmonary ventilation (L/min BTPS)	102.0	106.4 ± 3.2	124.4 ± 7.2
Mixed expired P_{CO_2} (mm Hg)	15	29 ± 2.0	31 ± 1.0
Blood lactate (mmol/L)	18.0	12.2 ± 0.75	10.0 ± 0.44

[a] This patient had mitochondrial myopathy.

[b] Data from Edwards, et al. (5).

metabolism was carried out using material from needle biopsy samples. The activity of key enzymes in the mitochondrial oxidative pathways can be determined spectrophotometrically by following the reduction or oxidation of added cytochrome c. The studies confirmed that mitochondrial oxidative metabolism was abnormal and pointed to a deficiency of the pyruvate-plus-malate cytochrome c reductase activity (Table 3). It is of interest that there was an apparent cellular adaptation to impaired oxidation, in that the cytochrome oxidase and succinate cytochrome c reductase activities were higher than those in a normal subject or other patients with muscle pain on exertion (in whom no abnormality of mitochondrial structure or function was detected).

The precise site of the mitochondrial lesion has not been settled. It could be a defect in the pyruvate translocase, a defect in the pyruvate dehydrogenase complex itself, or a defect located between reduced nicotinamide adenine dinucleotide dehydrogenase and the CoQ/cytochrome b complex. What is clear, however, is that the patient's muscles cannot oxidize pyruvate, and this is responsible for the striking lactacidosis with exercise.

Table 2. Plasma Organic Acids before and at the End of Maximal Exercise

| Organic Acid (mmol/L plasma) | At Rest before Exercise | | After Exercise | |
	Patient MF[a]	Normal Subjects[b]	Patient MF[a]	Normal Subjects[b]
Lactic[c]	3.35	0.15 ± 0.14	37.50	15.00 ± 1.0
Pyruvic	0.13	0.10 ± 0.011	0.34	0.60 ± 0.08
α-Hydroxybutyric	0.18	0.02 ± 0.002	0.08	0.03 ± 0.01
β-Hydroxybutyric	0.39	0.03 ± 0.002	0.08	0.09 ± 0.03
Citric	0.22	0.10 ± 0.004	0.20	0.12 ± 0.003

[a] This patient had mitochondrial myopathy

[b] Data are given as mean ± SEM for 6 subjects.

[c] Note the very high plasma lactic acid level at the end of exercise. With the exception of those shown above, all organic acids were normal both at rest and after exercise.

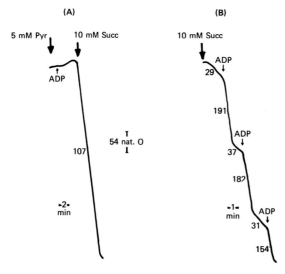

Fig. 2. Polarographic traces of oxygen utilization by isolated mitochondria obtained from an open muscle biopsy specimen from Patient MF, who had mitochondrial myopathy. For detailed explanation, see text. **(A)** There was no oxygen uptake in the presence of pyruvate (Pyr) and malate; addition of adenosine diphosphate (ADP) had no effect. **(B)** In the presence of succinate (Succ), respiration was stimulated by additions of ADP.

Similar clinical symptoms, although not necessarily because of the same mitochondrial lesion, have been reported in a patient with cytochrome b deficiency (4).

COMPARISONS AMONG GROUPS OF PATIENTS

Isometric Force and Endurance

None of the patients was significantly weak, as judged by the maximal voluntary contractice force of the quadriceps when related to body weight (6). However, there were interesting differences in the abilities of the various patient groups to sustain equivalent (submaximal) isometric contractions.

Table 3. Mitochondrial Enzyme Activities in Needle Biopsy Samples of Human Quadriceps Muscle

	Enzyme Activity[a]		
	(P + M)CR	SCR	Cyt Ox
Patient MF (mitochondrial myopathy)	0	16.4	105
Normal man	1.2	4.7	37
Patients with muscle pain			
1	0.39	2.3	15.2
2	0.24	1.44	6.1
3	0.63	1.28	8.7
4	0.28	1.05	4.9

Abbreviations: (P + M)CR, pyruvate, malate cytochrome c reductase; SCR, succinate cytochrome c reductase; Cyt Ox, cytochrome c oxidase.

[a] Activities are given as μmol of cytochrome c oxidized or reduced per g of muscle per minute at 37° C.

Under ischemic conditions hypothyroid patients were able to sustain sub-maximal contractions for similar (one patient) or longer (4 patients) periods than could normal subjects (Fig. 3). In contrast, one hyperthyroid patient could maintain a contraction for less than half the normal duration. This difference has been found to be associated with differing rates of ATP turnover (7). The hypothyroid patients had low rates of turnover and therefore could maintain force very efficiently, whereas the hyperthyroid patient had a high rate of ATP turnover and could maintain the contraction only at a higher energetic cost (Fig. 3).

Despite having a very restricted aerobic exercise capacity, Patient MF (with a mitochondrial lesion) could sustain a submaximal isometric contraction under ischemic conditions for just as long as the normal subjects and also had an ATP turnover rate indistinguishable from normal (Fig. 3).

Patients with myophosphorylase deficiency had reduced endurance but, unlike the hyperthyroid patient, had a somewhat reduced average rate of ATP turnover during prolonged contractions (Fig. 3), although there is evidence (8) that energy turnover rate is normal in the first few seconds of contraction.

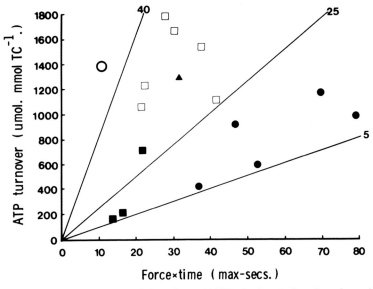

Fig. 3. Turnover of adenosine triphosphate (ATP) during ischemic submaximal quad-riceps contractions sustained to fatigue in normal subjects (open squares) and patients with four types of metabolic myopathy: hyperthyroidism (open circle); hypothyroidism (closed circles); myophosphorylase deficiency (closed squares); and mitochondrial ab-normality (closed triangle). The overall energy expenditure is expressed as the interval of force × time on the abscissa. The total ATP turnover, expressed as μmol per mmol of total creatine (TC), is given on the ordinate. Note that the hyperthyroid patient had a higher-than-normal energy turnover associated with reduced endurance, whereas the hypothyroid patients sustained equivalent force × time for a lower total ATP turnover. The patient with the mitochondrial lesion and the patients with myophosphorylase deficiency had nearly normal maintenance of economy of force, but endurance was reduced in patients with myophosphorylase deficiency. Isopleths are the ATP turnover rates calculated from the indicated rates during maximal voluntary contractions.

The varius energetic reactions occurring during a fatiguing contraction are given in Table 4, and the differences in metabolite levels for normal subjects and the patient with the mitochondrial lesion in resting and fatigued muscle are shown in Figure 4.

All patients were able to utilize the muscle phosphoryl creatine (PC), so the ability to use the available energy did not limit endurance. In myophosphorylase-deficient patients, however, the glycolytic pathway is inoperative; in these patients the available energy store is much lower than that of normal subjects and other groups of patients.

The results suggest that endurance, or the point at which fatigue occurs, is determined by a metabolic event. Either the level of some substrate falls below, or the level of some product rises above, a critical value. This would account for the decreased endurance of the hyperthyroid patient, because with a high rate of ATP turnover the end point is reached more rapidly than normal. Conversely, with hypothyroid patients, the slow ATP turnover allows force to be maintained for longer than usual before the critical metabolite level is reached. With the mitochondrial myopathy, contractions under ischemic conditions are no different from those of normal muscle. Patients with myophosphorylase deficiency, because the reserves of energy available for muscle contractions are limited, reach the critical metabolite level sooner than normal. The results from these latter patients indicate that it is not lactate or hydrogen ion accumulation that limits contraction.

Excitation and Muscle Energy Supply

It has previously been shown that repetitive supramaximal nerve stimulation under ischemic conditions in myophorphorylase deficiency is associated with unusually rapid fading of the action potential (9, 10). A systematic way of demonstrating this phenomenon is shown in Figure 5. For nearly 60 seconds, the ulnar nerve was submaximally stimulated (20 Hz) at the wrist under conditions of local ischemia. Recordings from the adductor pollicis revealed

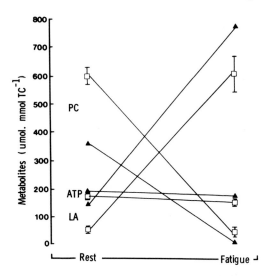

Fig. 4. Changes in quadriceps muscle metabolites during ischemic submaximal isometric contractions. Open squares denote mean ± SEM endurance at 53% maximal voluntary contraction (MVC) for 59 seconds in 6 normal subjects. Closed triangles indicate endurance at 50% MVC for 65 seconds in Patient MF, who had abnormal mitochondria.

Table 4. Energy Metabolism in Human Skeletal Muscle

Anaerobic metabolism
  $ATP \rightarrow ADP + P_i + energy$
  Phosphoryl creatine $+ ADP \rightleftharpoons ATP +$ creatine
  Glycogen (glycosyl units) $\rightarrow$ lactate $+ ATP$
Aerobic metabolism
  Muscle glycogen (glycosyl units)
  Blood-borne $\begin{cases} Glucose \\ Free\ fatty\ acids \end{cases}$ $+ ADP + P_i + O_2 \rightarrow CO_2 + H_2O + ATP$

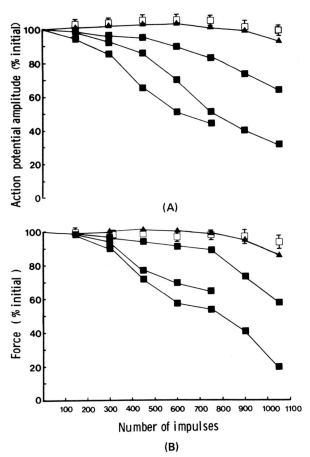

(A)

(B)

Fig. 5. Force fatigue and failure of excitation during electrical stimulation at 20 Hz with local ischemia of the adductor pollicis muscle in 5 normal subjects (open squares, mean ± SEM), 3 patients with myophosphorylase deficiency (closed squares), and 1 patient with abnormal mitochondria (closed triangles). **(A)** Action potential amplitude, expressed as a percentage of the initial value in rested muscle. **(B)** Force plotted as a function of the number of impulses delivered to the ulnar nerve at the wrist. Note that there was no loss of amplitude or force in normal subjects or in the patient with mitochondrial abnormality. Force fatigue was striking in patients with impaired glycolysis and was associated with progressive decrement in the amplitude of the muscle action potential.

721

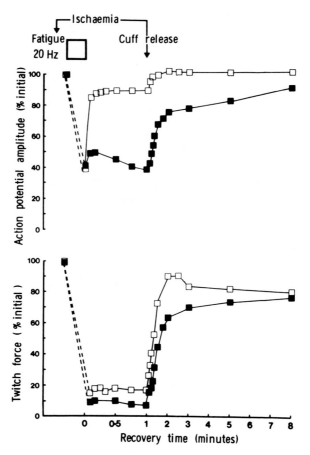

Fig. 6. Twitch and action potential amplitude during recovery from ischemic fatigue in the adductor pollicis in a 30-year-old normal man (open squares) and an 18-year-old male patient with myophosphorylase deficiency (closed squares). After an ischemic contraction continued to the same degree of fatigue by stimulation at 20 Hz, there was a striking reduction in the amplitude of the action potential and twitch force. With continuing ischemia there was a rapid recovery of the amplitude of the action potential in the normal subject, but no recovery in the patient with myophosphorylase deficiency until the circulation was restored.

that the amplitude of the evoked muscle action potential decreased and that there was no loss of isometric contraction force in normal subjects or the patient with a mitochondrial myopathy. In patients with myophosphorylase deficiency, the premature loss of force was always accompanied by fading of the action potential.

An extension of this experimental approach is illustrated in Figure 6. Substantial decreases in the action potential amplitude and in the force of contraction (twitch force) were produced in normal subjects and myophosphorylase-deficient patients (Fig. 5). With continuing ischemia at rest, there was substantial recovery of the amplitude of the action potential in the normal subject (seen also in several other unpublished studies of ischemic recovery from fatigue), but no recovery of contraction force, indicating impairment of excitation-contraction coupling (see later). In a patient with myophosphorylase deficiency there was no anaerobic recovery of the action potential amplitude.

The fading of the action potential with repetitive nerve stimulation and the lack of recovery until circulatory oxygen supply was restored in the myophosphorylase-deficient patients suggests that energy supplied by glycolysis is important for maintaining the electrical properties of the muscle membrane during sustained ischemic contractions.

Intermittent Isometric Contractions

Patients were asked to make 30% maximal voluntary quadriceps contractions (MVC) every 2 seconds for 40 seconds in every minute with the circulation to the leg unobstructed. Normal subjects were able to continue this exercise for 20 minutes without experiencing any discomfort, whereas the patients with myophosphorylase deficiency and the patient with a mitochondrial lesion felt discomfort and pain early in the series of contractions (Fig. 7A). In the patient with the mitochondrial abnormality, the discomfort continued to increase, and

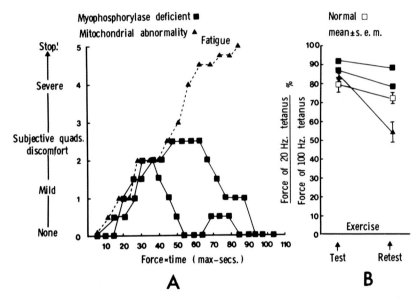

Fig. 7. Quadriceps muscle (quads.) discomfort and fatigue during repeated 30% maximal voluntary contractions every 2 seconds for 40 seconds in each minute in normal subjects and in patients with metabolic myopathies. **(A)** Abscissa indicates integrated force × time as a measure of total energy expenditure; ordinate gives a subjective scale of discomfort. During the experiment, normal subjects experienced no discomfort or fatigue. Note that the patient with the mitochondrial abnormality showed a progressive increase in discomfort sufficient to terminate the study, whereas 2 patients with myophosphorylase deficiency showed a temporary increase of discomfort in the muscle followed by relief associated with continuing submaximal activity. **(B)** The ratio of the force generated at 20 Hz to that generated at 100 Hz (ordinate) before and after the study. (See also Figure 8.)

after approximately 15 minutes it reached a level at which the patient was forced to stop. The myophosphorylase-deficient patients experienced discomfort in the early stages of the exercise, but showed a characteristic "second wind" (11): the discomfort lessened and they were able to continue the exercise for the full 20 minutes.

With the circulation to the muscle intact, the myophosphorylase-deficient patients were able to utilize blood-borne substrates for oxidative metabolism and thus overcome the consequences of their glycolytic enzyme deficiency. In contrast, the patient with the mitochondrial lesion was unable to oxidize pyruvate and therefore could not obtain the full benefit of either the muscle glycogen stores or blood-borne glucose. Even with the circulation intact, his muscles were working under conditions that were essentially anaerobic.

Excitation-Contraction Coupling

As described previously, with the circulation intact, normal subjects can sustain a series of contractions at 30% MVC without discomfort and without any impairment of muscle contractility, as judged by the response to electrical stimulation. However, if the force of contraction is increased to 60% MVC or if the contractions are performed with the circulation occluded, then not only do these subjects experience discomfort, but they also experience an interesting type of fatigue that is slow to recover and is probably due to a failure in excitation-contraction coupling.

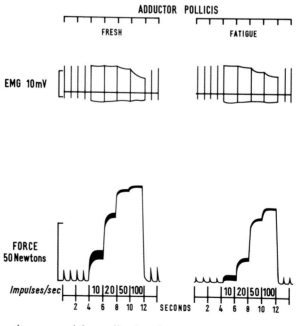

Fig. 8. Evoked action potential amplitude (above) and force (below) of the adductor pollicis muscle stimulated via the ulnar nerve at various frequencies. Records on the left are from rested muscle; records on the right are from muscle after fatiguing contractions under ischemic conditions.

Figure 8 shows traces of force and evoked action potential amplitude from a normal subject both when the muscle was fresh and after the 10-minute aerobic recovery period that followed a series of fatiguing contractions under ischemic conditions. The amplitude of the action potential was fully recovered, and the force obtained by stimulating at 100 Hz, was reduced by approximately 20%. Most striking, however, was the loss of force seen with stimulation at 10 and 20 Hz. At 20 Hz the force was reduced to much less than half that obtained in the fresh muscle, so the ratio of force at 20 Hz to that at 100 Hz changed from approximately 0.7 to 0.3 in the fatigued muscle. After severe exercise, this form of fatigue may take as long as 24 hours to recover, and it has been suggested that it is a consequence of a reduced quantity of activator released with each muscle action potential (12).

After repetitive contractions at 30% MVC, patients with myophosphorylase deficiency showed no abnormal change in the ratio of force produced by stimulation at 20 and 100 Hz (Fig. 7b). The patient with the mitochondrial myopathy, however, showed a large decrease in the ratio (Fig. 7b) similar to that which a normal subject might show if the contractions were carried out under ischemic conditions. This reemphasizes the fact that the patients' muscles are functioning under conditions that are essentially anaerobic.

CONCLUSIONS

We studied muscle function and energy metabolism in patients with thyroid disease, in patients with myophosphorylase deficiency, and in a patient with mitochondrial lesion whose muscles were unable to utilize pyruvate.

Although the range of abnormalities of energy metabolism was wide and in many cases the ensuing disability was severe, none of the patients was weak when judged by the strength of brief voluntary or stimulated contractions. Only with prolonged or repeated contractions did abnormalities and differences between the various patient groups become evident.

Differences in endurance between the hypothyroid and hyperthyroid patients were related to the rates of ATP turnover; the hypothyroid patients were able to sustain isometric contractions more efficiently than the hyperthyroid patient and normal subjects.

Patients with myophosphorylase deficiency and the patient with the mitochondrial lesion differed in their response to exercise. With the circulation to the muscle occluded, the patient with the mitochondrial lesion fared as well as the normal subjects, whereas the myophosphorylase-deficient patients had reduced endurance, probably as the result of premature failure of the muscle action potential. Conversely, during repeated contractions with the muscle circulation intact, it was the patient with the mitochondrial myopathy who showed a reduced capacity, whereas the myophosphorylase-deficient patients could make use of blood-borne substrates in place of their unusable muscle glycogen.

Our observations indicate that there is no single consequence of impaired energy supply; rather, the functional abnormality will differ according to the specific site of the metabolic defect. The underlying cause of the failure of muscle force may also vary. The results from patients with myophosphorylase deficiency and the patient with the mitochondrial myopathy make it clear that failure of muscle membrane excitability and of excitation-contraction coupling are important factors that must be considered in assessing the cause of weakness or impaired endurance in patients.

ACKNOWLEDGMENTS

Support from The Wellcome Trust, Birth Defects Group, and Muscular Dystrophy Group of Great Britain is gratefully acknowledged.

REFERENCES

1. Edwards RHT: Energy metabolism in normal and dystrophic human muscle. In *Pathogenesis of Human Muscular Dystrophy.* Edited by Rowland LP. Excerpta Medica, Amsterdam, 1977, pp 415–428

2. Edwards RHT, Young A, Wiles M: Needle biopsy of skeletal muscle in the diagnosis of myopathy and the clinical study of muscle function and repair. N Engl J Med 302:261–271, 1980

3. Edwards RHT, Wiles CM: Energy exchange in human skeletal muscle during isometric contractions. Circ Res (in press) 1980

4. Morgan-Hughes JA, Darveniza P, Kahn SN, et al: A mitochondrial myopathy characterized by a deficiency in reducible cytochrome c. Brain 100:617–640, 1977

5. Edwards RHT, Jones NL, Oppenheimer EA, et al: Interrelation of responses during progressive exercise in trained and untrained subjects. Q J Exp Physiol 54:394–403, 1969

6. Edwards RHT, Young A, Hosking GP, et al: Human skeletal muscle function: description of tests and normal values. Clin Sci Mol Med 52:283–290, 1977

7. Wiles CM, Young A, Jones DA, et al: Muscle relaxation rate and energy turnover in hyper- and hypothyroid patients. Clin Sci 57:375–384, 1979

8. Wiles CM, Edwards RHT: Energy turnover and fatigue in human muscle. Clin Sci 57:1P–2P, 1979

9. Dyken M, Smith DM, Peake RL: An electromyographic diagnostic screening test in McArdle's disease and a case report. Neurology (Minneap) 17:45–50, 1967

10. Brandt NJ, Buchthal F, Ebbsen F, et al: Post-tetanic mechanical tension and evoked action potentials in McArdle's disease. J Neurol Neurosurg Psychiatry 40:920–925, 1977

11. Pernow BB, Havel RJ, Jennings DB: The second wind phenomenon in McArdle's syndrome. Acta Med Scand 472 (Suppl):294–307, 1967

12. Edwards RHT, Hill DK, Jones DA, et al: Fatigue of long duration in human skeletal muscle after exercise. J Physiol (Lond) 272:769–778, 1977

DISCUSSION

Dr. Robert Barchi: There is an interesting question to be dealt with here in terms of the relationship between cellular energy, ATP, and fatigue in these systems. With myophosphorylase deficiency, you see normal ATP after exercise and marked reduction in creatine phosphate. Based on this, you conclude that the reason for contraction failure cannot be energy depletion, because the ATP level is normal. During the past 5 or 6 years, however, Dr. David Wilson's group has shown fairly clearly that the important factor is the phosphorylation potential, which is the ratio between ATP and ADP times Pi. It is really the amount of energy that you can obtain from hydrolysis of the gamma phosphate from ATP. With the decrease in creatine phosphate and normal ATP, one would suspect that Pi is going up. Under the conditions of normal ATP and elevated inorganic phosphate, the phosphorylation potential goes down, such that even in the face of a normal ATP level, the free energy that is obtained from hydrolysis of each ATP molecule can be unacceptably small. Thus, you can be in a situation of energy "depletion" for those enzyme reactions requiring ATP, despite the fact that the actual ATP concentration is normal.

Dr. Richard Edwards: I agree that may well be the situation at the end of contraction in the normal subjects and in the patients with hypothyroidism, but in the case of the patients with myophosphorylase deficiency, the creatine phosphate level was much higher. I do not think that you could conclude, on the basis of that evidence, that the phosphorylation potential was as low as it was in the normal and hypothyroid subjects.

Dr. Klaus Wrogeman: I have a question regarding your mitochondrial patient. Is the defect expressed in any tissue other than muscle? Is it expressed in fibroblasts, and is there any family history or any other information that might indicate that it is a genetically determined condition?

Dr. Richard Edwards: There was no family history. Fibroblasts show a deficiency of pyruvate dehydrogenase. The liver shows evidence of impairment in the cytochrome system, which might possibly explain the slow clearance of lactate. We are more than suspicious, from electrocardiographic changes during exercise that his heart is also involved. It appears that he has multisystem involvement. However, it has not affected his mental capacity, for he is a university graduate student and working very well with his brain.

Dr. Earl Homsher: To back up Dr. Edwards' reply to Dr. Barchi, if you tetanize a frog muscle so that the isometric force falls to practically nothing, you could say it is really fatigued, and the creatine phosphate is low. If you then perform a potassium depolarization of that muscle fiber, it will develop a normal isometric force, which clearly indicates that, even though you might have what you would call low energy charge, it still is quite capable of developing force. Thus, as Dr. Edwards has indicated, this has to indicate that there is a defect somewhere before the cross-bridge site.

Dr. Alfred L. Goldberg: I am not clear on the electrical stimulation. You are stimulating presynaptically. Does anyone know for certain whether there is a glycogen phosphorylase deficiency in the motor neuron also?

Dr. Richard Edwards: I think that various people have raised that possibility. I have no information on that myself.

Dr. Andrew G. Engel: Dr. King Engel, have you looked at that?

Dr. W. King Engel: It is very hard to biopsy the spinal cord.

Dr. Andrew G. Engel: Dr. Rowland, do you have anything to add to that?

Dr. Lewis P. Rowland: There is certainly no clinical suggestion of a neural defect except for Dr. McComas' experiment.

Dr. Alfred L. Goldberg: In your experiment, if you stimulate postsynaptically under those conditions, do you get excitation-contraction?

Dr. Richard Edwards: I should say that excitation is very difficult to study postsynaptically. It has recently been achieved by Hill, McDonnell, and Morton (J Physiol (Lond) 1980) and I have had my adductor pollicis directly stimulated. It involves the discharge of a single bireb shock of about 1,000 to 1,500 V and it feels as though you have been kicked by a mustang! We have not done it in patients. It is possible to demonstate under conditions of fatigue, such as we have just described, impaired neuromuscular transmission in normal subjects.

Dr. Lewis P. Rowland: That sounds like the kind of experiment you want to do with your head and an NMR machine. The question I wanted to ask has to do with our frustration about phosphorylase deficiency. We have recognized the enzymatic defect but we cannot explain the symptoms of the disease or demonstrate the presumed fall in ATP. When you describe fatigue in that state, was there contracture of muscle, and if not, why not? In either case, how do you explain the lack of change in ATP?

Dr. Richard Edwards: In the case of the contractions in which we had biopsies, these were sustained half-maximal voluntary contractions of the quadriceps muscle made until fatigue, as defined as a failure to generate the required force. At that stage, the phosphorylase-deficient patients had some discomfort in their muscles, but they were not in a state of contracture such as they might possibly be driven into by other circumstances. Frankly, we try to avoid producing contractures. The other circumstance in which there is a risk of producing a contracture is electrical stimulation. A note of warning is needed, because electrical stimulation did result in contracture of the adductor pollicis that lasted for several days in some of the phosphorylase-deficient patients. We use electrical stimulation with very great care and do not allow contraction to go on to marked fatigue. I think that the reason why our phosphorylase-deficient patients did not develop appreciable contracture with voluntary contactions was because of the presynaptic or sarcolemmal excitation failure.

Part VII

GENETIC CONTROL OF PROTEIN SYNTHESIS

Overview

Henry F. Epstein, MD

The problem of genetic control of protein synthesis is central to the understanding and the ultimate clinical resolution of muscular dystrophy and other inherited muscle diseases. We now recognize that the striking differences between the anatomy, biochemistry, and physiology of specialized, differentiated cells such as skeletal muscle fibers and other kinds of cells are due to the synthesis of specific proteins. In turn, these differences in protein synthesis represent both qualitative and quantitative changes in the expression of many genes. During vertebrate skeletal muscle differentiation, specific genes may be switched on uniquely, so that only one specific type of muscle fiber will synthesize a special protein. Examples include special forms of myosin heavy and light chains, α-actin, creatine kinase M, and aldolase A_4 (1–9). Other genes may be switched off so that the muscle fiber no longer synthesizes less specific forms of these proteins. The disappearance of embryonic forms of myosin subunits, the β and γ forms of actin, aldolase C, and creatine kinase B are due in part to turned-off genes (1–9). Certain genes may be expressed throughout muscle cell differentiation, but the amount of the ultimate gene product, a specific protein, changes. The difference in glyceraldehyde-3-phosphate dehydrogenase levels between various kinds of skeletal muscle appears to be due to quantitative changes in the expression of the same gene (Schwartz RJ: personal communication).

What are the mechanisms underlying these changes in gene expression and the resulting differences in the synthesis of specific proteins? We do not have final answers today, but we do have well-formed hypotheses and, more importantly, methods to test them. It is such hypotheses and methods that this session will discuss. I will outline the general approaches and ideas as an introduction to the papers that follow.

Most of our hypotheses concerning the genetic control of protein synthesis were originally formulated from experiments in bacteria. In these simple organisms, the flow of information from the gene to protein is deoxyribonucleic acid (DNA) $\rightarrow$ messenger ribonucleic acid (mRNA) $\rightarrow$ polypeptide (10). Control of this process is principally at the DNA $\rightarrow$ mRNA step. In the now classic operon model of Jacob and Monod (Fig. 1), the reading of specific genes (DNA sequences) into mRNA messages is regulated by the action of regulatory macromolecules (e.g., the repressor protein) on a regulatory gene (e.g., the

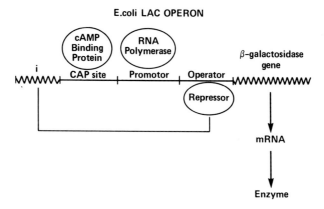

Fig. 1. Model of Jacob-Monod operon. Some deoxyribonucleic acid (DNA) sequences serve to control the expression of coding sequences or structural genes. This control occurs by the interaction of regulatory proteins with regulatory DNA sequences to permit or prevent synthesis of messenger ribonucleic acid (mRNA) from coding sequences. cAMP, cyclic adenosine monophosphate.

DNA sequence called operator) (11). The binding of repressor to operator prevents the reading of the specific gene DNA (the z gene coding for β-galactosidase) because the responsible enzyme, RNA polymerase, cannot move from its special recognition site, the promotor DNA sequence, down the chromosome. Only when a specific inducer (e.g., allolactose) binds to the repressor, and the repressor then falls off the operator DNA sequence, can reading of specific DNA take place. This whole process can be modulated by more general metabolites such as cyclic adenosine monophosphate.

In other regulatory systems within bacteria, this motif is modified in various ways, but two entities are always present: specific regulatory macromolecules, usually proteins, that can diffuse on or off specific regulatory DNA sequences to control the flow of genetic information. One can reasonably speculate on parallels between this bacterial model and hormone action and differentiation

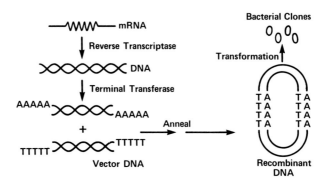

Fig. 2. Flow diagram of specific gene cloning using modern recombinant deoxyribonucleic acid (DNA) techniques. This technique permits the purification and amplification of specific animal genes and the manufacture of specific gene probes. mRNA, messenger ribonucleic acid.

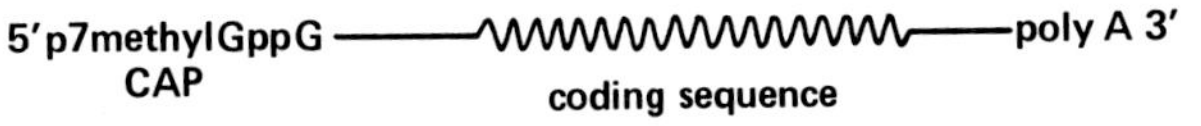

5′ p7methylGppG ———————— ᴡᴡᴡᴡᴡᴡᴡᴡᴡᴡᴡ ————— poly A 3′
        CAP   coding sequence

Fig. 3. Animal mRNA, structure of active messenger ribonucleic acid (mRNA). Note 5′ cap and 3′ poly A.

in animal cells. This model was worked out by the methods of classic molecular genetics. In this approach, one finds mutants with specific effects and biochemically characterizes the consequent alterations in the activity, structure, and synthesis of proteins. This approach is being followed in the work on nematode muscle from Dr. Waterston's and our laboratories (see chapters 56 and 57 of this volume).

There is yet another approach to the genetic control of protein synthesis, the "new" molecular genetics (Fig. 2). This approach includes the isolation and purification of a specific mRNA, its "reverse transcription" into a cDNA, the recombination of this cDNA into a special infectious vector, and the cloning of the recombinant DNA in bacterial cells (12–16). The cloned cDNA can then be used as a probe to isolate and characterize the actual genes or homologous DNA and RNA molecules from either the native or other sources (17–21).

Several important surprises have been discovered by this battery of methods. Mature mRNA in higher organisms has the region actually coding for polypeptide synthesis flanked by noncoding sequences (21, 22). At the 5′ end, the mRNA is capped by 7 methylGppGp or 7 methylGppAp, as shown in Figure 3 (3). A tail of polyA is placed upon the 3′ end (24, 25). We do not know the function of these maturation processes, but they appear to be nearly ubiquitous in animal cells. Even more surprising is the common finding of noncoding sequences interspersed between the coding sequences in the actual genomic DNA (Fig. 4) (21, 22, 26, 27). These intervening noncoding sequences are transcribed into RNA along with the coding sequences; however, specific splicing of the RNA leads to the linking of the coding sequences and removal of the internal noncoding sequences (28). Many hypotheses have been presented as to the function of these intervening sequences; no single hypothesis has been established as generally applicable (29).

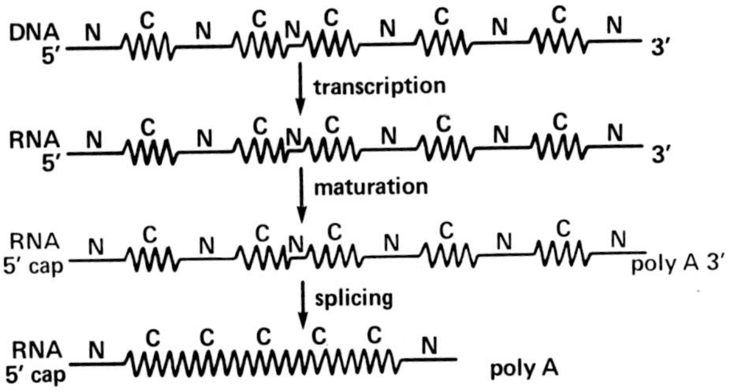

Fig. 4. Synthesis and maturation of messenger ribonucleic acid (mRNA). The gene is split into coding and noncoding regions. The RNA transcript is spliced to place all coding sequences together and matured by capping (cap) and polyadenylation (poly A) into active mRNA.

This new molecular genetic approach and its application to muscle-specific genes are discussed in chapters 58 and 59. The combination of the classic and new molecular genetics in particular experimental and human situations may provide both functional and structural insights into genetic control mechanisms for protein synthesis.

Several recent hypotheses regarding animal cell regulation are worth noting with respect to muscle development. The switching-off or down-regulation of genes may be due to modification of their specific DNA sequences. The most likely candidate is the enzymatic methylation of deoxycytosine to produce 5 methyldeoxycytosine (30, 31). The activation of a gene may involve the binding of specific chromosomal proteins to the gene's DNA. Two candidates are HMG proteins 14 and 17 (32, 33). Related genes such as immunoglobins and hemoglobins appear to be clustered (21, 22, 32, 34, 35). One might speculate about the isozymes of contractile proteins. How these mechanisms function and relate to muscle cell development are promising specific aims of current research.

ACKNOWLEDGMENTS

Henry F Epstein is a Research Career Development Awardee of the National Institute of Health. He is a member of the Jerry Lewis Neuromuscular Disease Research Center of the Muscular Dystrophy Association at Baylor College of Medicine.

REFERENCES

1. Whalen RG, Schwartz K, Bouveret P, et al: Contractile protein isozymes in muscle development: identification of an embryonic form of myosin heavy chain. Proc Natl Acad Sci USA 76:5197–5201, 1979

2. Frank G, Weeds AG: The amino acid sequence of the alkali light chains of rabbit skeletal-muscle myosin. Eur J Biochem 44:317–334, 1974

3. Weeds AG: Light chains from slow-twitch muscle myosin. Eur J Biochem 66:157–173, 1976

4. Rubinstein NA, Pepe FA, Holtzer H: Myosin types during the development of embryonic chicken fast and slow muscles. Proc Natl Acad Sci USA 74:4524–4527, 1977

5. Whalen RG, Butler-Browne GS, Sell S, et al: Transitions in contractile protein isozymes during muscle cell differentiation. Biochemie 61:625–632, 1979

6. Garrels JI, Gibson W: Identification and characterization of multiple forms of actin. Cell 9:793–805, 1976

7. Caravatti M, Perriard J-C, Eppenberger HM: Developmental regulation of creatine kinase isoenzymes in myogenic cell cultures from chicken: biosynthesis of creatine kinase subunits M and B. J Biol Chem 254:1388–1394, 1979

8. Perriard J-C: Developmental regulation of creatine kinase isoenzymes in myogenic cell cultures from chicken: levels of mRNA for creatine kinase subunits M and B. J Biol Chem 254:7036–7041,

9. Lebherz HG: Ontogeny and regulation of fructose diphosphate aldolase isoenzymes in "red" and "white" skeletal muscles of the chick. J Biol Chem 250:5976–5981, 1975

10. Brenner S, Jacob F, Meselson M: An unstable intermediate carrying information from genes to ribosomes for protein synthesis. Nature 190:576–581, 1961

11. Jacob F, Monod J: Genetic regulatory mechanisms in the synthesis of proteins. J Mol Biol 3:318–356, 1961

12. Darnell JE, Jelinek WR, Molloy GR: Biogenesis of mRNA: genetic regulation in mammalian cells. Science 181:1215–1221, 1973

13. Jackson DA, Symons RH, Berg P: Biochemical methods for inserting new genetic information into DNA of simian virus 40: circular SV40 DNA molecules containing lamda phage genes and the galactose operon of *Escherichia coli*. Proc Natl Acad Sci USA 69:2904–2909, 1972

14. Lobban PE, Kaiser AD: Enzymatic end-to-end joining of DNA molecules. J Mol Biol 78:453–471, 1973

15. Morrow JF, Cohen SN, Chang ACY, et al: Replication and transcription of eukaryotic DNA in *Escherichia coli*. Proc Natl Acad Sci USA 71:1743–1747, 1974

16. Ross J, Aviv H, Scolnick E, et al: In vitro synthesis of DNA complementary to purified rabbit globin mRNA. Proc Natl Acad Sci USA 69:264–268, 1972

17. Packman S, Aviv H, Ross J, et al: A comparison of globin genes in duck reticulocytes and liver cells. Biochem Biophys Res Commun 44:813–819, 1972

18. Sullivan D, Palacios R, Stavnezer J, et al: Synthesis of a deoxyribonucleic acid sequence complementary to ovalbumin messenger ribonucleic acid and quantification of ovalbumin genes. J Biol Chem 248:7530–7539, 1973

19. Grunstein M, Hogness DS: Colony hybridization: a method for the isolation of cloned DNAs that contain a specific gene. Proc Natl Acad Sci USA 72:3961–3965, 1975

20. Kindle KL, Firtel RA: Identification and analysis of *Dictyostelium* actin genes, a family of moderately repeated genes. Cell 15:763–778, 1978

21. Jeffrey AJ, Flavell RA: A physical map of the DNA regions flanking the rabbit β-globin gene. Cell 12:429–439, 1977

22. Rabbits TH: Evidence for splicing of interrupted immunoglobulin variable and constant region sequences in nuclear RNA. Nature 275:291–296, 1978

23. Shatkin AJ: Capping of eukaryotic mRNAs. Cell 9:645–653, 1976

24. Kates J: Transcription of the vaccinia virus genome and the occurrence of polyriboadenylic acid sequences in messenger RNA. Cold Spring Harbor Symp Quant Biol 35:743–752, 1970

25. Edmonds M, Vaughan MH, Nakazato H: Polyadenylic acid sequences in the heterogeneous nuclear RNA and rapidly-labeled polyribosomal RNA of Hela cells: possible evidence of a precursor relationship. Proc Natl Acad Sci USA 68:1336–1340, 1971

26. Berget SM, Moore C, Sharp PA: Spliced segments at the 5′ terminus of adenovirus 2 late mRNA. Proc Natl Acad Sci USA 74:3171–3175, 1977

27. Aloni Y, Dhar R, Laub O, et al: Novel mechanism for RNA maturation: the leader sequences of simian virus 40 mRNA are not transcribed adjacent to the coding sequences. Proc Natl Acad Sci USA 74:3686–3690, 1977

28. Darnell JE Jr: Implications of RNA-RNA splicing in evolution of eukaryotic cells. Science 202:1257–1260, 1978

29. Crick F: Split genes and RNA splicing. Science 204:264–271, 1979

30. Scarano E: The control of gene function in cell differentiation and in embryogenesis. Adv Cytopharmacol 1:18–24, 1971

31. Van der Ploeg LHT, Flavell RA: DNA methylation in the human αδβ-globin locus in erythroid and nonerythroid tissues. Cell 19:947–958, 1980

32. Weisbrod S, Groudine M, Weintraub H: Interaction of HMG 14 and 17 with actively transcribed genes. Cell 19:289–301, 1980

33. Stalder J, Groudine M, Dodgson JB, et al: Hb switching in chickens. Cell 19:973–980, 1980

34. Flavell RA, Kooter JM, DeBoer E, et al: Analysis of the β-δ-globin gene loci in normal and Hb Lepore DNA: direct determination of gene linkage and disturbance. Cell 15:25–41, 1978

35. Mears JG, Ramirez F, Leibowitz D, et al: Organization of human δ and β-globin genes in cellular DNA and the presence of intragenic inserts. Cell 15:15–23, 1978

56
Gene Regulation in Muscle Development

Henry F. Epstein, MD

John M. Mackenzie, Jr., PhD

The development of muscle cells is associated with the apppearance of highly organized arrays of thick and thin filaments and specialized membranes. These structures are necessary for the acquisition of the excitatory and contractile functions of muscle. Underlying these anatomic and physiologic transformations are changes in the control of synthesis of specific proteins. All of these developmental events must be regulated by interactions between genes, gene actions, and gene products. At present, we are trying to understand the logic of this genetic network that directs muscle development.

We already understand from studies in bacteria that genes may have characteristically different functions. Structural genes code for enzymes, other proteins, and special nucleic acids such as transfer ribonucleic acid (RNA) and ribosomal RNA species. Some structural genes have regulatory functions in that the proteins or nucleic acids encoded interact with specific deoxyribonucleic acid (DNA) sequences to control expression of other genes (1). The third class of genes includes the specific DNA sequences that are recognized by regulatory macromolecules, DNA replication enzymes, or RNA transcription enzymes.

To understand the molecular logic of muscle development, we have pursued a combined approach of biochemical, genetic, and ultrastructural studies of muscle mutants of the nematode, *Caenorhabditis elegans* (2, 3). Specifically, we have applied this methodologic combination to the properties and synthesis of a single nematode polypeptide, the myosin B heavy chain. This polypeptide self-associates to form only homodimers, myosin B molecules (4). Myosin B is synthesized only in the 95 body-wall muscle cells of the nematode (5). The myosin B heavy chains are encoded by the *unc-54* I gene. The amount of myosin B synthesized is coordinately regulated with respect to the synthesis of separately coded myosin A, and this coordinate synthesis appears to be regulated by or dependent on the *unc-52* II gene (6, 7). The assembly of myosins A and B into body-wall thick filaments of proper dimensions is regulated by paramyosin, a protein chemically and genetically distinct from myosin, encoded by *unc-15* (8–10).

ORGANIZATION OF HEAVY CHAINS

The Two Myosin Molecules

The organization of myosin heavy chains into two major kinds of myosin molecule was demonstrated by three lines of evidence: chromatographic, peptide mapping, and immunochemical. Hydroxyapatite chromatography resolved two major populations of myosin, myosins A and B. One class, myosin B, was affected by *unc-54* I mutants; for example, it was absent in the E190 strain and altered in the E675 strain. The two chromatographic species exhibited different CNBr-cleaved peptides that were separable by polyacrylamide gel electrophoresis. These peptides were derived from the heavy chains, suggesting that different structural genes code for the heavy chains and that one of the structural genes is *unc-54* I. (11–13).

Immunologic differences were also found between the two myosins. Under conditions of quantitative precipitation, antibodies specific to the myosin B heavy chain interact only with myosin molecules composed of only myosin B heavy chain. No hybrid myosin molecules containing one of each kind of heavy chain were detected. Thus, myosin B is composed of heavy chains encoded by *unc-54* I only. Myosin A is composed of heavy chains coded by one or more structural genes distinct from *unc-54*.

Location of Myosin B

The initial report describing *unc-54* mutants indicated that the altered heavy chain in the E675 mutant appeared only in dissected body walls (2). The body-wall muscles were also specifically affected by this and other *unc-54* mutants (2, 12, 13). The hypothesis that myosin B containing the *unc-54*-encoded heavy chains is located only in body-wall muscle cells was confirmed by immunocytochemistry (5). Using specific antimyosin B and the peroxidase-antiperoxidase technique, myosin B was identified in all sarcomeres of all body-wall muscle cells (Fig. 1B). No reaction with antimyosin B was detected in the pharynx or gut. In contrast, antimyosin reacted with both of these structures as well as all of the body-wall muscles (Fig. 1A).

SYNTHESIS OF HEAVY CHAINS

Coordinate Synthesis

During larval development, there is an exponential increase in nematode body mass and total protein. Increases in myosin heavy chain content parallel the more general growth (15). When the different forms of myosin and myosin heavy chain are examined during this period, the body wall–specific myosin B heavy chains as measured by radioactivity in specific bands in polyacrylamide gels or the intact myosin B quantitatively precipitated by specific antibody accumulate at a more rapid rate than do the other myosins (Fig. 2). As determined by short-term incorporation of myosin B relative to the other

A

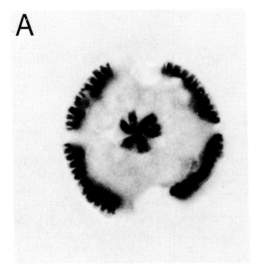

B

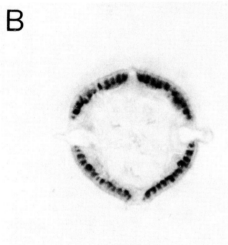

Fig. 1. Antibody localization of myosin B. Peroxidase-antiperoxidase labeling of antibody-antigen complexes. **(A)** Reaction of nematode anterior cross section with specific antimyosin IgG. **(B)** Reaction with specific antimyosin B IgG. (Reprinted with permission from Mackenzie JM, Schachat FH, Epstein HF: Immunocytochemical localization of two myosins within the same muscle cells in *Caenorhabditis elegans.* Cell 15:413–419, 1978. Copyright 1978, MIT Press.)

myosins, synthesis is relatively constant during this period. The synthetic fraction of myosin B to total myosin is approximately equal to the final accumulated fraction, 0.64, suggesting that the relative rates of synthesis are primarily responsible for the relative rates of accumulation. The same result was obtained in wild-type strains and in structurally altered myosin mutants that were paralyzed and had severely disrupted myofibrillar structure.

Structural alteration of the myosin molecule or of the myofibrillar lattice per se do not lead to enhanced degradation of myosin over wild-type rates in nematode body-wall muscle cells during larval development (15).

Some regulatory mechanism or mechanisms must operate within the nematode body-wall muscle cells to coordinate the synthesis of these two myosins. Could we find specific mutations affecting this regulation?

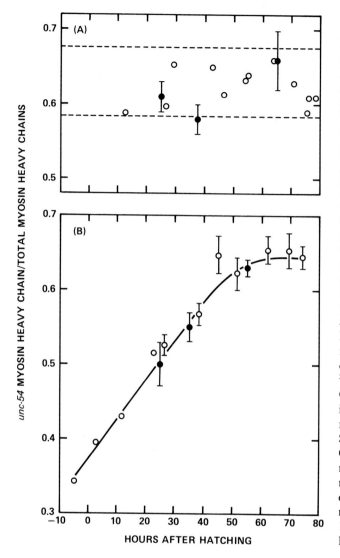

Fig. 2. Coordinate synthesis of myosins A and B. **(A)** Pulse studies. Developing nematodes were incubated for 2 hours on lawns of ^{35}S-SO$_4$-labeled *Escherichia coli*. Open circles represent fractions of myosin heavy chain B to total myosin heavy determined by densitometry of radioautographs of 4.5% sodium dodecyl sulfate-polyacrylamide gels. Closed circles represent myosin B precipitated by specific antimyosin B IgG as a fraction of total myosin precipitated by specific antimyosin. **(B)** Accumulation studies. Developing nematodes were grown continuously on lawns of ^{35}S-SO$_4$-labeled *E. coli*. Open and closed circles, as in A. (Reprinted with permission from Garcea RL, Schachat F, Epstein HF: Coordinate synthesis of two myosins in wild-type and mutant nematode muscle during larval development. Cell 15:421–428, 1978. Copyright 1978, MIT Press.)

Regulation by *Unc-52*

One group of mutants was found that moved normally and possessed normal body-wall muscle structure early in development, but became progressively more paralyzed and structurally abnormal later in development. The responsible mutations were mapped to the *unc-52* II locus (6). These *unc-52* mutants exhibit retardation or arrest of myofibrillar growth after constructing the first larval sarcomeres in each body-wall muscle cell. Biochemical studies indicated that total myosin heavy chains failed to accumulate normally. By adulthood, a 2-fold specific decrease in body-wall muscle myosin heavy chains was noted in the mutants relative to wild-type strains. The defect in accumulation was reflected in 10-, 5-, and 2-hour incorporation experiments, suggesting that decreased rates of synthesis were likely to be responsible for the abnormally low accumulation (7).

Doubly homozygous mutants of *unc-52* mutants with the structurally altered E675 myosin mutant of the *unc-54* I gene suggested that the effect was even more specific. The E675 alteration affects the electrophoretic properties only of myosin B heavy chains that are specific to the body-wall muscle; it does not alter the relative rates of accumulation or synthesis of these chains (7). In the double homozygotes, there was decreased synthesis specifically of the *unc-54*-encoded B chains at 203 kdal versus A chains at 210 kdal or pharyngeal myosin heavy chains at 206 kilodaltons (Fig. 3). Furthermore, early in development, when *unc-52* mutants were phenotypically normal, no effect on myosin B heavy chain synthesis was detected. By 36 hours of development, significant changes in B chain synthesis were associated with detectable structural retardation. By adulthood, the rate of myosin B heavy chain synthesis was one half of normal, reflecting the severe decrement in myofibrillar construction and paralysis apparent at this stage.

Interestingly, this progressive molecular defect must be based on the action of mutant *unc-52* genes on chromosome II upon the expression of the *unc-54* gene on chromosome I. At present, the most reasonable explanation is that *unc-52* codes for some nucleic acid or polypeptide that diffuses within the muscle cell to regulate or enhance the production of myosin B heavy chains at some point in protein biosynthesis. More experiments are required to elucidate the mechanism of this interaction (7).

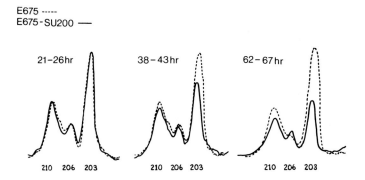

E675 -----
E675-SU200 ——

21–26hr   38–43hr   62–67hr

210 206 203   210 206 203   210 206 203

Fig. 3. Genetic alteration of coordinate synthesis of myosins A and B during development. Nematodes of either strain were incubated for the 5-hour periods shown on lawns of radiolabeled *Escherichia coli*. Tracings are densitometries of radioautographs of sodium dodecyl sulfate-polyacrylamide gels of homogenized nematodes. (Reprinted with permission from Zengel JM, Epstein HF: Mutants altering coordinate synthesis of specific myosins during nematode muscle development. 210 refers to the 210,000 M_r myosin A heavy chain; 206 refers t the 206,000 M_r myosin C heavy chain, and 203 refers to the 203,000 M_r myosin B heavy chain that is specifically present in E675. Proc Natl Acad Sci USA 77:852–856, 1980.)

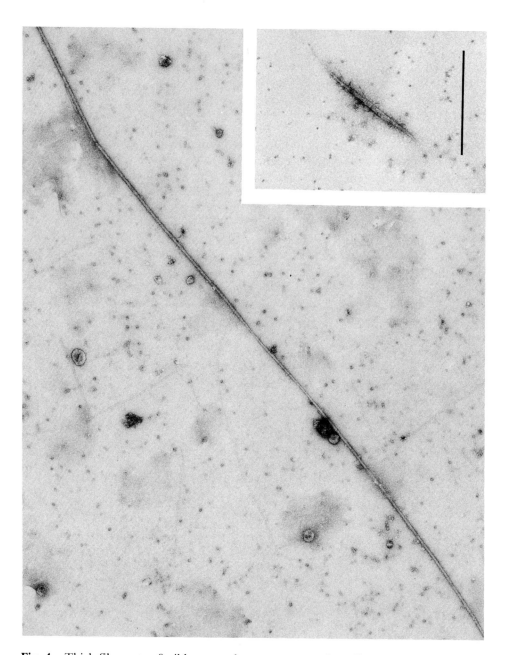

Fig. 4. Thick filaments of wild-type and mutant nematodes. Filaments were isolated in an identical manner from N2 wild-type nematodes (larger micrograph) and E1214 *unc-15* mutant nematodes lacking paramyosin (inset). Filaments were negatively stained with uranyl acetate. The bar represents 1 μm. Note thin filaments in background of N2 thick filament for comparison.

MYOSIN ASSEMBLY

The thick filaments of all muscles contain myosin, whose central role in contraction is clearly understood (16). Invertebrate muscles of many varieties contain paramyosin, a coiled-coil, rodlike protein similar to but distinct from tropomyosin and light meromyosin. Paramyosin is now believed to be located in the core of invertebrate thick filaments, and myosin is at the surface (17). Suggested physiological functions of paramyosin have included regulation of actomyosin interaction and determination of thick filament length (17–20). Invertebrate muscle thick filaments may have significantly larger lengths and diameters than their vertebrate counterparts; both dimensions correlate with paramyosin content (20).

Nematode body-wall muscles contain paramyosin within thick filaments approximately 9.7 μm in length and 250 nm in diameter (Mackenzie JM, Epstein HF: unpublished results). Isolated filaments exhibit a 2:1 molar ratio of paramyosin to myosin heavy chains consistent with the native lengths. In contrast to the very long filaments of wild-type strains, E1214, an *unc-15* I mutant with no detectable paramyosin (10), produces short filaments of increased diameter (Fig. 4). These bipolar filaments have a mean length of 1.53 μm. In situ, paramyosin appears necessary for the proper assembly of myosin molecules and other protein components of the thick filaments. The exact nature of the normal myosin-paramyosin interaction disrupted in these mutants is under study.

CONCLUSIONS

We have begun to decipher the logic of gene regulation during muscle development in the nematode *Caenorhabditis elegans*. One primary level of control is the switching on or off of the specific expression of a gene and the synthesis of its encoded protein. An example of this kind of regulation in the nematode is the unique expression of the *unc-54* gene in body-wall muscle cells and the appearance of myosin B only in these cells.

A second important regulatory mechanism is modulation of specific gene expression and the quantitative increase or decrease of the synthesis of its encoded protein. The *unc-52* gene appears necessary for full quantitative expression of the *unc-54* gene in larval development. *Unc-52* mutants exhibit decreased synthesis of myosin B in nematode body-wall muscle cells late in development and during adulthood. It is important that this developmentally associated decrease in myosin B synthesis produces a mutant animal with progressive paralysis and myopathy. It is certainly worth reflecting on such a mechanism, a defect in modulation of synthesis of a specific muscle protein, with respect to human muscular dystrophy.

A third regulatory mechanism is dependent on the interaction of specific gene products in the sarcoplasm to produce the physiologic myofibrillar architecture. Paramyosin, the core protein of nematode thick filaments, can be considered to regulate myosin assembly. The absence of paramyosin from body-wall muscle, as in the E1214 mutant of *unc-15*, leads to the assembly of abnormally short and wide myosin-containing filaments.

Clearly, we have uncovered only a tiny window to the hierarchy of genetic control of specific muscle protein synthesis and action in the nematode. Even with this limited view, a reasonable conclusion is that regulation of even a single class of molecules, the myosin B of nematode body-wall muscle cells, occurs at multiple levels from the nucleus to the sarcoplasm and sarcomere. The extent and overall coordination of this regulatory network in muscle is the focus of our current work.

ACKNOWLEDGMENTS

We thank Sue Allen, Lois Bolton, and Irving Ortiz for their contributions to the experimental work presented here. Henry F Epstein is a Research Career Development Awardee of the (NIH), and John M Mackenzie, Jr. is a Muscular Dystrophy Association (MDA) Research Fellow. The research was supported by the Jerry Lewis Neuromuscular Disease Research Center of the MDA at Baylor and grants from the National Institute on Aging and NICHD.

REFERENCES

1. Jacob F, Monod J: Genetic regulatory mechanisms in the synthesis of proteins. J Mol Biol 3:318–356, 1961

2. Epstein HF, Waterston RH, Brenner S: A mutant affecting the heavy chains of myosin in *Caenorhabditis elegans*. J Mol Biol 90:291–300, 1974

3. Zengel JM, Epstein HF: Identification of genetic elements associated with muscle structure in the nematode *Caenorhabditis elegans*. Cell Motility 1:73–97, 1980

4. Schachat F, Garcea RL, Epstein HF: Myosins exist as homodimers of heavy chains: demonstration with specific antibody purified by nematode mutant myosin affinity chromatography. Cell 15:405–411, 1978

5. Mackenzie JM, Schachat F, Epstein HF: Immunocytochemical localization of two myosins within the same muscle cells in *Caenorhabditis elegans*. Cell 15:413–419, 1978

6. Mackenzie JM, Garcea RL, Zengel JM, et al: Muscle development in *Caenorhabditis elegans*: mutants exhibiting retarded sarcomere construction. Cell 15:751–762, 1978

7. Zengel JM, Epstein, HF: Mutants altering coordinate synthesis of specific myosins during nematode muscle development. Proc Natl Acad Sci USA 77:852–856, 1980

8. Waterston RH, Epstein HF, Brenner S: Paramyosin of *Caenorhabditis elegans*. J Mol Biol 90:285–290, 1974

9. Harris HE, Epstein HF: Myosin and paramyosin of *Caenorhabditis elegans*: biochemical and structural properties of wild-type and mutant proteins. Cell 10:709–719, 1977

10. Waterston RH, Fishpool RM, Epstein HF: Mutants affecting paramyosin in *Caenorhabditis elegans*. J Mol Biol 117:825–842

11. Epstein HF, Schachat FH, Wolff JA: Molecular genetics of nematode myosin. In *Pathogenesis of Human Muscular Dystrophies*. Edited by Rowland LP Jr, Excerpta Medica, Amsterdam, 1977, pp 460–467

12. Schachat FH, Harris HE, Epstein HF: Two homogeneous myosins in body-wall muscle of *Caenorhabditis elegans*. Cell 10:721–728, 1977

13. MacLeod AR, Waterston RH, Fishpool RM, et al: Identification of the structural gene for a myosin heavy chain in *Caenorhabditis elegans*. J Mol Biol 114:133–140, 1977

14. MacLeod AR, Waterston RH, Brenner S: An internal deletion mutant of a myosin heavy chain in *Caenorhabditis elegans*. Proc Natl Acad Sci USA 74:5336–5340, 1977

15. Garcea RL, Schachat F, Epstein HF: Coordinate synthesis of two myosins in wild-type and mutant nematode muscle during larval development. Cell 15:421–428, 1978

16. Koretz JF, Hunt T, Taylor EW: Studies on mechanism of myosin and actomyosin ATPase. Cold Spring Harbor Symp Quant Biol 37:179–184, 1973

17. Szent-Györgyi AG, Cohen C, Kendrick-Jones J: Paramyosin and the filaments of "catch" muscles. I. Native filaments: isolation and characterization. J Mol Biol 56:239–250, 1971

18. Epstein HF, Aronow B, Harris HE: Interaction of myosin and paramyosin. J Supramolec Struct 3:354–360, 1975

19. Epstein HF, Aronow B, Harris HE: Myosin-paramyosin cofilaments: enzymatic interactions with F-actin. Proc Natl Acad Sci USA 73:3015–3019, 1976

20. Levine RJC, Elfvin M, Dewey MM, et al: Paramyosin in invertebrate muscles. II. Content in relation to structure and function. J Cell Biol 71:273–279, 1976

DISCUSSION

Dr. Susan Benoff-Rind: Do you have any mutant that is more pleiotropic that would affect not just the heavy chain, but multiple contractile elements?

Dr. Henry Epstein: To date, we have not found anything that can affect several genes. Of course, total protein synthesis is down and you could call that pleiotropic, but I think that is easily explained in terms of secondary effects. A mutation in myosin, for example, does not seem to affect the role of synthesis of other proteins.

Dr. Wilfried Mommaerts: Is it possible that the noncoding parts of the DNA coincide in part with the numerous genes that we know are there, as shown by the Gurdon experiment, but are kept suppressed as a part of differentiation and development?

Dr. Henry Epstein: It is possible, but it is my impression that these intermediate sequences rather quickly lead to nonsense, i.e., to sequences that will lead to the cessation of protein synthesis. The indications are that what you describe is probably not the case, but I do not know that we can absolutely rule that out.

Dr. Robert Wydro: Do you have any evidence that the *unc-52* mutant is really affecting the transcription, or could the effect occur at the posttranscriptional level?

Dr. Henry Epstein: It could occur at any level from the nucleus to the cytoplasm.

57
Mutations Affecting Myosin Heavy Chain Accumulation and Function in the Nematode *Caenorhabditis elegans*

R. H. Waterston, MD, PhD

D. G. Moerman, PhD

D. Baillie, PhD

T. R. Lane, PhD

The small nematode *Caenorhabditis elegans* is the subject of intensive investigation into the genetic specification of muscle structure and function (1–3). Many mutations affecting muscle structure have been identified, and more than 20 genes have been defined by complementation and recombinational analysis. Biochemical and genetic studies have proved that one of these loci, *unc-54* I, is the structural gene for a 210,000-dalton myosin heavy chain in the body-wall musculature (4–6). Specific mutations in this gene could help us to understand the role of the myosin heavy chain in the assembly and contraction of muscle. Additional myosin heavy chains, the products of other genes, are present in the body wall and pharyngeal musculature (4). Alterations in the tissue-specific expression of this family of genes might be useful in studying gene regulation.

The classic genetic approaches of reversion and intracistronic recombinational analysis can be applied to these problems in *C. elegans* because of the ease of handling the large number of animals necessary for systematic application of these methods, and because of the strong phenotype associated with most *unc-*

54 mutations. Reversion analysis can reveal intragenic suppressors of a variety of types and could be especially powerful in the study of the genetic specification of muscle where many gene interactions may be involved (7). We have, in other work, described allele-specific generalized suppressors in *C. elegans* that are likely to be informational suppressors (8, 9). Riddle and Brenner (10) reverted *unc-54* mutants and uncovered a gene-specific suppressor, *sup-3V*. Part of our current work has been directed toward understanding the molecular basis for *sup-3* action on *unc-54* mutants. We have also carried out reversion analysis on *unc-22* mutants and, surprisingly, have found new alleles of *unc-54* that suppress *unc-22* expression. In addition, a genetic intracistronic map of the *unc-54* gene has been constructed, and we have begun to position these new alleles on this map.

PREVIOUS WORK

Before relating the results growing out of these genetic approaches, some of the previously published analyses of the *unc-54* mutations will be summarized. The chemical analysis of the *unc-54* mutants has been complicated by the presence of multiple myosin heavy chain isozymes. However, cleavage of total nematode myosin at cysteinyl residues by cyanylation produces a small number of relatively large peptides that can be analyzed by gel electrophoresis (6). Two of these peptides have been shown to be unique products of *unc-54* myosin heavy chain and have been used to identify 3 distinct types of *unc-54* mutations. Most isolates examined, e.g., *e190*, are designated as null alleles, because neither of the two *unc-54*-specific peptides are found in cyanylation digests of myosins prepared from animals homozygous for these mutations. The yield of total myosin is reduced, and no lower molecular weight myosins have been detected in gel electrophoresis of total protein from such homozygotes. Phenotypically, these animals are very slow moving and are almost totally paralyzed. The body wall musculature of this set is obviously disorganized and, as expected, the number of thick filaments is reduced. The molecular basis of this set had not been established, but several different molecular mechanisms could account for complete absence of gene product, such as premature chain termination, deficiencies, or degradation of unstable polypeptides.

Of the remaining isolates, all but one of the described mutations result in the production of the *unc-54* myosin heavy chain of the wild-type molecular weight at approximately normal levels. Both of the *unc-54*-specific peptides are present in cyanylation digests of myosins from animals homozygous for these mutations (e.g., *e1152*). The homozygous animals are paralyzed; their body wall muscle structure is disorganized and the number of thick filaments is reduced, as in the null alleles. However, some variability in the extent of paralysis is apparent between alleles in this set: some move better than null alleles, and others show complete paralysis and lethality as homozygotes. Most of these alleles are codominant with the wild-type allele such that, for example, *e1152/+* animals are intermediate in paralysis and in muscle structure. Two alleles, *e1301* and *e1157*, are temperature sensitive. These features taken together indicate that this set of mutations may be missense mutations resulting in the production of an abnormal heavy chain that fails to assemble into normal thick filaments.

The remaining allele, *e675*, contains a shortened *unc-54* heavy chain (4). The *unc-54* unique cyanylation peptides are smaller in *e675* (6). End labeling of the cyanylation peptides with ^{14}C-cyanide followed by partial CNBr cleavage demonstrates that the *e675* mutation is a deficiency resulting in the loss of approximately 10,000 daltons from the heavy chain in a region 40,000 to 50,000 daltons from the carboxyl terminus (5). This shortened myosin is stable, but like the putative missense alleles, it fails to form normal thick filaments, and *e675* homozygotes move only slowly (11). An unexplained feature of its phenotype is a slight, but nearly constant, twitching of the body-wall musculature.

The *e675* deficiency provides a ready entry into cloning of the *unc-54* gene. A. R. MacLeod (personal communication) has prepared complementary deoxyribonucleic acid (cDNA) to a partially purified myosin messenger ribonucleic acid (mRNA) and inserted this into plasmids. Because the deficiency in *e675* results in a smaller *unc-54* restriction fragment than that of wild-type strains, MacLeod was able to use this to identify a cDNA plasmid containing a myosin sequence. This probe may be used to identify the genomic *unc-54* sequence in libraries of *C. elegans* DNA.

Sup-3 MUTATIONS

Riddle and Brenner (10) treated several strains homozygous for *unc-54* null mutations with mutagens and selected animals with improved movement. By appropriate genetic crosses, they were able to show that many of these revertants still contain the original *unc-54* mutation as well as a second mutation in a gene designated *sup-3 V*. In cross-suppression tests, *sup-3* mutations partially suppressed all *unc-54* null alleles and more weakly suppressed the putative missense class and *e675*. In addition, *sup-3* suppressed *unc-15(e73)*, a presumed missense allele of the paramyosin gene (12) and *unc-87(e843)*, another mutation affecting muscle structure (2). However, it failed to suppress mutations in a variety of other genes. Riddle and Brenner (10) also noted an improved organization of thick filaments into A bands in *unc-54; sup-3* animals and postulated that *sup-3* might alter the regulation of one of the non-*unc-54* myosin genes.

To test this hypothesis, we examined the myosin heavy chains using polyacrylamide gel electrophoresis. Initially, we were able to show that *sup-3* did not result in the restoration of *unc-54* protein, as determined by the continued absence of the *unc-54*-specific polypeptides in myosin prepared from *unc-54(e190), sup-3(31407)* strains. The presence of multiple myosins and the question of how to normalize any results quantifying the myosins initially frustrated further efforts.

More recently, substantially better resolution of the myosin heavy chains has been obtained using 4% polyacrylamide gels with a tris borate buffer system rather than the tris glycine system previously used (13, 14). This better resolution has been important in allowing us to analyze the specific myosins, and these results are summarized in the following section. We also applied these gels to the analysis of *sup-3* action, as discussed later.

Myosin Heavy Chain Isozymes

When purified wild type myosin is run into polyacrylamide gels using the tris glycine system, 2 bands are resolved in the heavy chain region of the gel: a major one of molecular weight 210,000 daltons, and a minor one of 206,000 daltons (4). Dissection experiments and genetic analysis show that the 210,000-dalton band contains the *unc-54* heavy chain and a second body-wall isozyme. The pharyngeal musculature also possesses, in approximately equal amounts, a 210,000-dalton band that is not a product of *unc-54* and a 206,000-dalton band (4).

The tris borate system can resolve these 4 different heavy chains as illustrated in Figure 1. The large amount of the *unc-54* species obscures band 1 in wild-type strains, but bands 2, 3, and 4 are visible (Fig. 2a). In myosin from *unc-54(e190)* homozygotes, where no *unc-54* myosin is present, 3 bands are still resolved (Fig. 2b) (6). Bands 3 and 4 are relatively more abundant; in addition, there is band 1 of a slightly slower mobility than the *unc-54* band 2. Thus, the presence of 4 bands in the wild type can be inferred, and 4 bands can be resolved in mixtures of *e190* and wild-type myosins. Four bands are also present in myosins from *unc-54* alleles suppressed by the informational suppressor *sup-7 X* (9).

The comparison of the wild-type and *e190* myosins show that band 2 is the product of the *unc-54* gene. To establish the relationship of the 3 bands in *e190* with those previously identified in the tris glycine system, we ran *e190* myosin on a tris borate gel buffer system, cut out the lane, and reran it at 90° into a second gel using either the tris borate or tris glycine system in the second dimension (Fig. 3). Each of the bands ran true when rerun into the tris borate system (Fig. 3b), but their relative mobilities differed in the tris glycine system, such that bands 1 and 3 overlapped at 210,000 daltons and band 4 ran slightly ahead. Band 4 thus corresponds to the previously identified 206,000-dalton

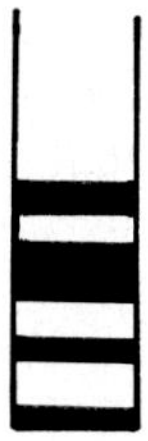

4% gel	band	gene	location	prior molecular weight assignment by tris gel system
	1	?	body wall	210,000
	2	unc-54	body wall	210,000
	3	?	pharynx	210,000
	4	?	pharynx	206,000

Fig. 1. The 4 electrophoretically distinct myosin heavy chain isozymes in wild-type strains of *Caenorhabditis elegans*. The diagram at the left is a schematic representation of the 4 bands present in the region of the myosin heavy chain as they would appear on an idealized 4% polyacrylamide gel using a tris borate buffer system (13). Current knowledge about these bands is summarized in the remainder of the figure. (See text for details.)

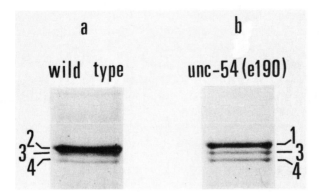

Fig. 2. Myosin heavy chains from wild-type and *unc-54(e190)* mutant *Caenorhabditis elegans*. Segments of tris borate gels containing myosin heavy chains from **(a)** wild-type and **(b)** *unc-54(e190)* strains are shown. Animals of the appropriate genotype were grown and extracted as outlined in Table 1 and run on a 4% polyacrylamide gel using a tris borate gel buffer system (13). Ten-centimeter slab gels were prepared, run at 17.5 mamp per gel until 1.5 hours after the dye front ran off the bottom of the gel. Gels were stained with 0.2% Coomassie blue in 50% methanol and 7% acetic acid, and were destained with 20% methanol and 7% acetic acid. The two bottom bands, labeled 4 in each case, have the same mobilities in the two stains, as does band 3. The major band of the wild type has a mobility intermediate between bands 1 and 3 of *unc-54(e190)*.

pharyngeal protein. Band 3 has been tentatively assigned as the second pharyngeal myosin, based on its relative abundance and its slightly reduced mobility relative to band 1 in the tris glycine system, something previously noted for the upper pharyngeal band in dissection experiments (Waterston RH: unpublished data). Band 1 is thus likely to be derived at least in part, from the body-wall musculature. How many genes code for these proteins is unknown, because their mobilities could reflect posttranslational modifications rather than primary sequence differences; alternatively, several gene products could comigrate in band 1, 3, or 4. Further improvements in the gels might reveal other bands. Preliminary experiments using partial proteolysis in gels do indicate that all 3 bands in *e190* are related and thus are all likely to be myosins (15).

Abundance of Band 1 Myosin

The improved resolution achieved with the tris borate gels has enabled us to examine the effect of *sup-3* on the levels of the individual myosin bands. The strategy has involved preparing a crude but quantitative actomyosin extract from strains with and without *sup-3* and determining the relative amounts of each myosin band by densitometry. Comparison of traces of myosins from *unc-54(e190)* with those from *unc-54(e190); sup-3(e1407)* and of myosins from *unc-54(e675)* with *unc-54(e675); sup-3(e1407)* (Fig. 4) indicate that band 1 is specifically increased in strains containing *sup-3*. Using synchronized populations of third-stage larvae to eliminate possible age-related differences, we have quantified this increase, normalizing the results in each case to the fastest migrating band.

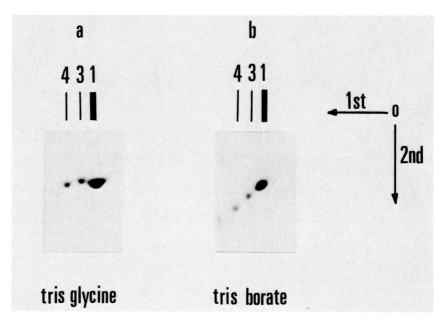

Fig. 3. Mobilities of bands 1, 3, and 4 on tris glycine gels. To establish the relationship of the 3 myosin bands of *unc-54(e190)* resolved in the tris borate gel system with bands previously identified in tris glycine gels, samples of *unc-54(e190)* protein were run on the tris borate system as described in the legend to Figure 2. The gels were then removed. Without staining, strips of the gel containing the myosin region were cut out, equilibrated for 10 minutes with appropriate sample buffers, and placed on the sample wells at 90° to the original direction of migration as indicated diagramatically. When the sample was rerun on gels with the tris borate system **(b)** the expected diagonal of spots was obtained. However, when the sample was rerun on gels using the tris glycine system **(a)**, bands 3 and 4 were retarded in their migration relative to band 1 such that bands 1 and 3 have similar mobilities as measured by the trailing edge of the spots. The greater relative mobility of band 4 identifies it as the 206,000-dalton band of the pharynx.

Table 1 shows the results from densitometry of the myosin heavy chain bands from strains of the genotype listed. The amounts of the upper bands in each case have been normalized to the amount in the lower band to permit pooling of data and cross comparisons. To obtain the data, eggs from each strain were prepared by hypochlorite treatment of adults and placed on fresh plates at 20° C for 42 to 46 hours (16). At this time, most animals were third-stage larvae, as determined by vulval and gonad morphology. Care was taken to ensure that growths of different strains were closely matched. The worms were collected over sucrose and frozen (17). The worms were subsequently broken open with a French press at 10,000 psi, washed with a low-salt buffer solution, and extracted with 0.5 M KSCN (6) (0.5 M potassium thiocyanate, 50 mM sodium sulfite, 50 mM Tris pH 8.0, 1 mM ethyleneglycol tetra-acetate, 2 mM $MgCl_2$, 1 mM phenylmethyl-sulfonyl fluoride, 10 mM 2-mercaptoethanol, and 5 mM ATP). The KSCN was used to extract the myosin because a more complete and reproducible extraction of all myosins was achieved than with 0.6 M NaCl. This modified actomyosin extract was applied to 4% polyacrylamide tris borate gels and run as described in Figure 2. The gels were scanned using a Gilford spectrophotometer, and the areas under the peaks were determined with a Zeiss MOP3 Digital Image Analyzer System. The ratio of the peaks was calculated from 5 wells for each sample and averaged. Three or 4 separate determinations were done for each strain; data are given as the average, with the range in parentheses.

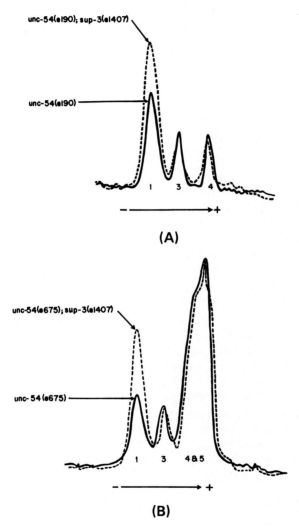

Fig. 4. Densitometer traces are shown of the bands of *unc-54* strains in normal genetic backgrounds (solid line) and with *sup-3(e1407)* (dashed line). **(A)** The null allele *unc-54(e190)* was used, and the traces were normalized to band 4, which is well resolved from band 3 and 1. **(B)** Strains containing *unc-54(e675)*, normalized to the peak from bands 4 and 5. Band 5 is the product of the *unc-54* gene but is shifted in mobility by the deficiency of the *e675* mutation. In this gel system, the lower pharyngeal band is poorly resolved from the *e675* band and is seen only as a slight shoulder. In both *unc-54(e190)* and *unc-54(e675)*, the presence of *sup-3(e1407)* results in a significant increase of band 1 relative to other myosins.

Table 1. The Effect of *sup-3 (el407)* on the Relative Abundance of Myosin Heavy Chain Bands in *unc-54* Mutants

Genotype	Ratio of Bands	
	1:4	3:4
unc-54 (el90)	3.0	1.1
	(2.9–3.2)	(1.0–1.2)
unc-54 (el90); sup-3 (el407)	4.6	1.2
	(4.2–4.8)	(1.2–1.3)
	1:4 + 5	3:4 + 5
unc-54 (e675)	0.22	0.11
	(0.20–0.25)	(0.09–0.12)
unc-54 (e675); sup-3 (el407)	.51	0.17
	(0.41–0.59)	(0.13–0.19)

In the case of *e190*, band 1 shows an approximate 1.7-fold increase relative to the pharyngeal band 4. Band 3 is not significantly altered relative to band 4. In the case of *e675*, the normalization is to a sum of band 4, and the mutationally altered *unc-54* myosin (designated band 5). Band 1 shows a relative increase of approximately 2.2-fold. Thus, *sup-3* appears to increase specifically the relative abundance of the band 1 or the minor body-wall myosin isozyme(s) by approximately 2-fold.

The normalization to either the pharyngeal band 4 or to the *e675* myosin plus band 4 suffers from uncertainties. The ratio of body-wall musculature to pharyngeal musculature changes with age and perhaps with animal size. Although populations of the same age have been compared, *sup-3* may secondarily alter this ratio. The *e675* myosin is a better standard in the sense that it is derived from the same cells as band 1, and it has been shown that this altered chain is stable (11). However, the action of *sup-3* on the stability of the *e675*-shortened myosin has not yet been evaluated. We have therefore compared the amounts of myosin relative to total protein and to other muscle proteins; these measurements consistently indicate that *sup-3* strains have more myosin (data not shown). We have begun to look at L1 larvae and late L4 larvae; again, *sup-3* appears to increase the amount of band 1 myosin, but as yet the data are incomplete.

Basis for *Sup-3* Action

The increase in the relative abundance of a minor body-wall band 1 myosin in *sup-3* mutants satisfactorily explains the suppression of the *unc-54* mutants. The suppression of the *unc-15(e73)* missense mutation in paramyosin is more difficult to account for, but perhaps a minor body myosin interacts more favorably with the mutant paramyosin molecule. In fact, one might be able to use suppressibility by *sup-3* as a criterion for determining whether a particular mutation affects primarily thick filament proteins. For instance, an *unc-87* I allele is suppressible and an *unc-52* II allele is not (10).

The mechanism by which *sup-3* affects this relative increase in band 1 is uncertain. It could act by increasing synthesis at either the translational or the transcriptional level. Alternatively, *sup-3* could increase the stability of either protein or its mRNA. Among the many possible mechanisms, two are particularly interesting. The *sup-3* gene might code for a specific repressor of the minor body-wall myosin gene. Thus, mutations in the gene would eliminate repressor function, allowing full expression of this second myosin gene. Alternatively, the *sup-3* gene could be the second myosin gene itself, and the amount of the second myosin could be increased either by mutations in the control region or by tandem duplication. Various arguments can be made for or against either hypothesis based on various genetic experiments, but at present, none is conclusive. Further experiments are in progress to establish the mechanism of action of the *sup-3* mutations.

MISSENSE ALLELES OF *unc-54* I AS SUPPRESSORS OF *unc-22* IV

As part of our studies of other genes affecting muscle structure, we have searched for intergenic suppressors of mutations of several genes. A particularly intriguing result has been obtained in reversion studies of *unc-22* IV (1, 2, 18). Animals homozygous for mutations in this locus exhibit a fine twitching in the body-wall muscle cells, and show varying degrees of disorganization of the myofilament lattice, depending on the allele being carried in the strain (2). Most mutant *unc-22* worms are slower and thinner than the wild type, but despite the twitching and the muscle disorganization they retain considerable capacity for movement. Nonetheless, reversion of the *unc-22* phenotype has been possible and all have been due to mutations in the *unc-54* gene. These suppressors of *unc-22* twitchers are unlike previously described mutations in *unc-54* in that muscle structure is substantially normal.

Isolation and Mapping of *unc-22* Revertants

Three different strains homozygous for different *unc-22* alleles have been treated with 0.05 M ethylmethane sulfonate, and F1 progeny were examined for "revertants," i.e., animals lacking the twitching phenotype (1). Although 2 strains yielded no revertants in more than 10^5 events each, the third strain, homozygous for *unc-22(s12)*, yielded 6 revertants in 8×10^5 tested chromosomes. Homozygous revertant strains were obtained in all cases. Subsequent genetic manipulations showed that the *unc-22(s12)* mutation is still present in each of these revertants, and that a second intergenic suppressor mutation is dominantly suppressing the expression of the *s12* mutation. In addition, 5 of the suppressor mutations impart a slowness and stiffness to worms that are homozygous for the suppressor mutation, whether or not *s12* is present. Worms homozygous for the sixth mutation (*s75*) resemble wild type worms in movement.

Using the slow, stiff phenotype, one of the suppressors, *s74*, has been mapped to linkage group I approximately 23 map units from *dpy-5*. Because the *unc-54* gene is a similar map distance from *dpy-5*, complementation tests were performed with *unc-54(e190)*. The *s74/e190* animals resemble, but are marginally slower than, *s74* homozygotes, indicating that *s74* is an *unc-54* allele. Recombinational analysis has confirmed this assignment (see later). Complementation tests of the other suppressor mutations with *s74* indicates that all 6 are *unc-54* alleles.

Phenotype and Muscle Structure of the Novel *unc-54* Mutations

To facilitate further study, all of the suppressor mutations were obtained in a wild-type background. These new mutant strains differ in their ability to move, and unlike previously described *unc-54* alleles, are normal in size. The *s75* homozygotes are similar to the wild type in movement, whereas *s74*, *s76*, and *s77* strains are slow and stiff. Finally, *s78* and *s95* are almost totally paralyzed. The ability of animals of these strains to lay eggs is correlated with their movement. Surprisingly, the structure of the body-wall musculature of these mutant strains is nearly normal. The *s74* allele has abundant thick filaments in a sarcomere organization similar to wild type (Fig. 5). On close inspection, however, the A bands in *s74* are not as sharply defined, and filament packing is slightly altered compared to wild type. In contrast, the null allele, *e190*, and the temperature sensitive allele, *e1301*, at the restrictive temperature (25° C), show a dramatic reduction in the thick filament number, and the residual thick filaments do not form an ordered array (4, 6). The muscle structure of the *s95* homozygotes, despite their severe paralysis, is similar to that of the *s74* mutant. The muscle structure of the *s95* homozygotes, despite their more severe paralysis is similar to that of the *s74* mutant.

Interpretation of the *unc-54* Suppressors and Intracistronic Mapping

Reversion analysis of *unc-22(s12)* has revealed a new set of mutations in the *unc-54* gene in which structure is minimally affected, and movement is variably affected depending on the specific allele. Since the *unc-54* gene product, is a multifunctional protein, the identification of alleles with different phenotypes at this locus is not unexpected (19, 20). As yet, however, we do not know which region of the molecule contains the suppressor mutations and is thus responsible for generating this new phenotype. It is tempting to speculate that this new class lies in the heavy meromyosin region, altering the ability of the myosin molecule to generate tension in a controlled fashion. However, control of the generation of tension may be a complex process in the nematode, where at least part of the regulation is imparted by the thick filament (21, 22). Our speculations would be more informed if we knew the basis of the *unc-22* phenotype. Biochemical studies of the enzyme activity of the myosin would be informative; these are difficult in *C. elegans*, but they must be done.

A different approach to the problem offered by *C. elegans* is a genetic one. An intracistronic map of the *unc-54* gene has been constructed using the null alleles and the *e675* mutation (Waterston RH: unpublished data). The gene so far has been divided into 11 regions, and a map with even better resolution is

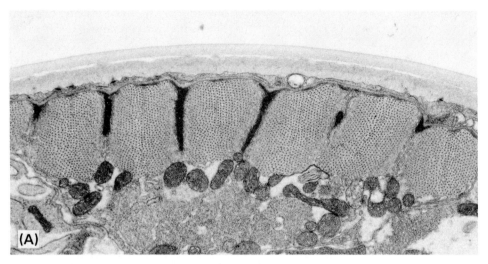

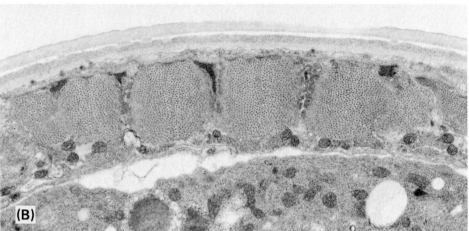

Fig. 5. These two electron micrographs of transverse sections through the body-wall musculature compare **(A)** wild type and **(B)** *unc-54(s74)*. In both strains similar numbers of thick filaments are present, assembled into repeating A bands adjacent to the hypodermis and cuticle, shown on the left of each micrograph. Other muscle structures also appear similar between the two strains. The intermittent dense bodies are more prominent in the wild type in this particular section, but overall, no difference was noted. However, the *s74* muscle does show some slight abnormalities. The boundaries of the A bands are more irregular than in the wild type, a difference more easily appreciated with polarized light microscopy. In addition, packing of the thick filaments within the A band is not as regular in *s74* as in the wild type. (Original magnification ×18,000.)

possible. Two of the missense alleles affecting structure and two of the *unc-22* suppressor alleles are currently being mapped to determine their relative locations. Both of the alleles affecting structure, *e1301* and e1152, map to the right of the deficiency *e675*. The suppressor alleles, *s74* and *s95*, also map in the right of *e675* and to the right of *e1420* as well, placing them in the rightmost region of the map with *st60*. These results are intriguing, but until the genetic map can be interpreted in physical terms, the results remain ambiguous.

CONCLUSIONS

The application of reversion analysis to the study of *unc-54* and *unc-22* mutants has revealed new mutations not identified in normal forward mutagenesis procedures. The absence of a discernible phenotype of the *sup-3* mutations precludes its identification in wild-type background. The relative rarity of the new *unc-54* alleles, occurring at about one-hundredth the frequency of null alleles, would make them difficult to find in normal mutagenesis of wild type.

By combining reversion analysis and the information available from the fine-structure genetic map, it may be possible to dissect genetically the functions of the myosin molecule both in thick filament assembly and in the controlled generation of tension. The ability to isolate mutations affecting accumulation of a specific myosin indicates the feasibility of using reversion analysis to identify mutations affecting regulation of myosin synthesis. Perhaps one might even alter tissue specific expression of one of the myosins. By being able to combine these genetic approaches with the approaches offered by molecular cloning, the nematode *C. elegans* provides a chance to understand the myosin heavy chain in depth.

ACKNOWLEDGMENTS

We thank Santiago Plurad for the electron microscopy; Raja Rosenbluth and Clara Salamanca for technical assistance; and Sharon Musgrove for preparing the manuscript. This work was supported in part by grants to RH Waterston from U.S. Public Health Service grant GM 23883; a Jerry Lewis Neuromuscular Research Center Grant to Washington University; and grants to DL Baillie from the Muscular Dystrophy Association of Canada and the National Science and Engineering Research Council of Canada. RH Waterston is an Established Investigator of the American Heart Association. DG Moerman is a fellow of the Medical Research Council of Canada.

REFERENCES

1. Brenner S: The genetics of *Caenorhabditis elegans*. Genetics 77:71–94, 1974
2. Waterston RH, Thomson JN, Brenner S: Mutants affecting muscle structure in *Caenorhabditis elegans*. Dev Biol 77:271–302, 1980.
3. Zengel JM, Epstein HF: Identification of genetic elements associated with the muscle structure in the nematode *Caenorhabditis elegans*. Cell Motility 1:73–97, 1980.
4. Epstein HF, Waterston RH, Brenner S: A mutant affecting the heavy chain of myosin in *C. elegans*. J Mol Biol 90:291–300, 1974
5. MacLeod AR, Waterston RH, Brenner S: An internal deletion mutant of a myosin heavy chain in *Caenorhabditis elegans*. Proc Natl Acad Sci USA 74:5336–5340, 1977

6. MacLeod AR, Waterston RH, Fishpool RM: Identification of the structural gene for a myosin heavy chain in *Caenorhabditis elegans*. J Mol Biol 114:133–140, 1977

7. Hartman P, Roth JR: Mechanisms of suppression. In Adv Genet 17:1–105, 1973

8. Waterston RH, Brenner S: A suppressor mutation in the nematode acting on specific alleles of many genes. Nature 275:715–719, 1978

9. Waterston RH: A second informational suppressor *sup-7 X* in Caenorhabditis elegans. Genetics (in press) 1981

10. Riddle DL, Brenner S: Indirect suppression in *Caenorhabditis elegans*. Genetics 89:299–314, 1978

11. Schachat F, Harris HE, Epstein HF: Two homogeneous myosins in body-wall muscle of *Caenorhabditis elegans*. Cell 10:721–728, 1977

12. Waterston RH, Fishpool RM, Brenner S: Mutants affecting paramyosin in *Caenorhabditis elegans*. J Mol Biol 117:679–697, 1977

13. Chua NH, Bennoun P: Thykaloid membrane polypeptides of *Chlamydomonas reinhardtii*: wild-type and mutant strains deficient in photosystem II reaction center. Proc Natl Acad Sci USA 72:2175–2179, 1975

14. Laemmli UK: Cleavage of structural proteins during the assembly of the head at bacteriophage T4. Nature 227:680–685, 1970

15. Cleveland DW, Fischer SG, Kirschner MC, et al: Peptide mapping by limited proteolysis in sodium dodecyl sulfate and analysis by gel electrophoresis. J Biol Chem 252:1102–1106, 1977

16. Johnson K, Hirsh D: Patterns of proteins synthesized during development of *Caenorhabditis elegans*. Dev Biol 70:241–248, 1979

17. Sulston J, Brenner S: The DNA of *Caenorhabditis elegans*. Genetics 77:95–104, 1974

18. Moerman DG, Baillie DL: Genetic organization in *Caenorhabditis elegans*: fine-structure analysis of the *unc-22* gene. Genetics 91:95–103, 1979

19. Huxley HE: The mechanism of muscular contraction. Science 164:1356-1366, 1969

20. Lowey S, Slayter HS, Weeds AG, et al: Substructure of the myosin molecule. I. Subfragments of myosin by enzymatic degradation. J Mol Biol 42:1–29, 1969

21. Lehman W, Svent-Gyorgi AG: Regulation of molluscan contractor. J Gen Physiol 66:1–30, 1975

22. Harris HE, Tso MW, Epstein HF: Actin and myosin linked calcium regulation in the nematode *C. elegans*: biochemical and structural properties of native filaments and purified proteins. Biochemistry 16:859–865, 1977

DISCUSSION

Dr. Susan Benoff-Rind: In your reversion analysis, have you ever come across a suppressor that is due to a gene duplication rather than an effect on a second gene or within the first gene itself?

Dr. Richard Waterston: Duplication of the original mutant gene?

Dr. Susan Benoff-Rind: No, duplication, e.g., of your myosin A genes, so that you would be producing twice the amount of A.

Dr. Richard Waterston: Well, that could be what the *sup-3* is. It is a possibility we will look into. Dr. Anderson, who is working with the *unc-54* gene, has been able to generate duplications in that case.

Dr. Kate Barany: What are the molecular weights of bands 1, 2, 3 and 4? Did you separate them, and did you do an amino acid analysis? What are the differences in the amino acid composition of the various bands?

Dr. Richard Waterston: We have not done that much. The molecular weights are all around 200,000 daltons. The band 4 on Laemmli gels was shown by Dr. Epstein to be about 206,000 daltons. Bands 1, 2, and 3 comigrated in the Laemmli gel system at 210,000 daltons.

Dr. John Gergely: Would you clarify the second example you gave? You had a mutant which showed some abnormality that improved in the second mutant, right?

Dr. Richard Waterston: In the case of the *unc-22*, right.

Dr. John Gergely: You suggested that in this reversing mutation the structure is not changed, but the function is defective.

Dr. Richard Waterston: Yes.

Dr. John Gergely: But superimposed on the first one there is improvement.

Dr. Richard Waterson: The mutations in *unc-22* cause the animals to twitch very obviously and almost continuously. It is a fine, continuous twitching. When the new *unc-54* mutation is induced, the double mutant no longer twitches. I do not mean to imply that it is restored to normal motility. The muscle structure improves, but the animal is still slow. One could interpret that as saying that the *unc-54* mutation is "epistatic" to the *unc-22*.

Dr. Anthony Martonosi: What are the electrical properties of these mutants that do not move, but have apparently normal myosin structure?

Dr. Richard Waterson: When we analyze the mutation in the *unc-54* gene alone, we have removed it from the original mutant background and have it in a genetic background that should otherwise be identical to the wild type. We know that *unc-54* is the structural gene for the myosin heavy chain. As far as we know, that is the only mutation this animal has, yet its muscles do not contract normally. In the double mutant there might be what I would call "upstream" defects in the process of excitation-contraction coupling that are masked by the properties of this new mutation in *unc-54*. In other words, if the myosin cannot contract, then it does not matter whether there is a defect in the sarcoplasmic reticulum.

Dr. Anthony Martonosi: Can one be absolutely certain that the *unc-54* mutation affects only myosin? Alternatively, the rearrangement in myosin-related filament structure could cause disorganization of the membrane systems related to excitation-contraction coupling. Membrane assembly during the development of these cells could be somehow interrelated with the assembly of the myosin filaments.

Dr. Richard Waterston: I believe that these mutations are single mutations because we have done fine-structure recombinational analysis and found recombinants within this gene at appropriate frequencies.

58

Cloning and Analysis of Expression of Muscle-Specific Genes

D. Yaffe, PhD

U. Nudel, PhD

M. Shani, PhD

D. Katcoff, MSc

Y. Carmon, MSc

D. Zevin-Sonkin, MSc

The application of recombinant deoxyribonucleic acid (DNA) techniques to the study of development and cell differentiation has enabled physiologic and biochemical studies to be correlated with investigations on gene structure and expression at the nucleic acid level. The present communication describes the isolation and characterization of recombinant plasmids containing sequences that hybridize with actin and with myosin heavy and light chain messenger ribonucleic acids (mRNAs), and the isolation of recombinant bacteriophages containing sequences of 8 different actin genes, 3 myosin heavy chain genes, and 1 myosin light chain gene.

RESULTS

Cloning of DNA Complementary to Actin mRNA

In an earlier study, we investigated the hybridization of DNA complementary to muscle RNA with RNA extracted from cultures consisting of proliferating myoblasts and from differentiated cultures containing multinucleated fibers. This study showed that muscle RNA contains sequences that are abundant in muscle but are absent from or very rare in RNA extracted from proliferating myoblasts (1). In the reticulocyte cell-free system, such RNA directed the synthesis of myosin, actin, tropomyosin, and other muscle-specific proteins.

Our experimental approach was therefore to use total muscle polyadenylated RNA as a template for the synthesis of double-stranded DNA, which was then cloned in bacterial plasmids.

The DNA complementary to polyadenylated muscle RNA was made double stranded and inserted into the Pst1 site of plasmid pBR322, using conventional methods (in collaboration with A.-M. Frischauf and H. Lehrach) (2). This plasmid contains a gene for resistance to tetracycline (Tet[+]) and a gene for resistance to ampicillin (Amp[-]). Because the double-stranded cDNA was inserted into a Pst1 site located in the β-lactamase gene, plasmids containing an insert conferred resistance to tetracycline but not to ampicillin when introduced into a suitable host by transformation. The Tet[+]/Amp[-] colonies were isolated and screened for those carrying sequences that hybridized strongly to cDNA prepared on muscle polyadenylated RNA template but not to cDNA prepared on RNA extracted from liver or from cultures of proliferating myoblasts. These colonies were isolated and further characterized.

Four plasmid clones, designated p254, p649, p749, and p106 (containing inserts of 350, 225, 630, and 270 nucleotides, respectively), hybridized strongly with DNA complementary to RNA enriched for muscle actin mRNA, but not with cDNA enriched for myosin light-chain sequences. Immobilized DNA of each of the 4 plasmids was hybridized to rat skeletal muscle mRNA, and the hybridizable RNA was isolated. In each case, RNA selected in this way directed the synthesis of actin in the reticulocyte lysate cell-free system (2). Hybridization of labeled plasmids with size-fractionated RNA blotted on DBM-cellulose paper showed that plasmids p749, p254, and p649 contained inserts that hybridized with muscle as well as with nonmuscle actin mRNA (Fig. 1). However, plasmid

Time (hr)

0   36   72

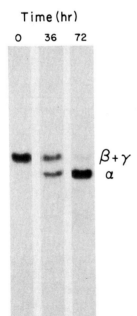

β+γ

α

Fig. 1. Hybridization of labeled plasmid 749 to size-fractionated RNA extracted from L8 cells. Cultures of the myogenic cell line L8[19] grown in medium that stimulates cell proliferation without fusion were switched to fusion-permissive medium. At the indicated times (0, 36, and 72 hours after the switch to the fusion-permissive medium), RNA was extracted from the cultures. Polyadenylated RNA was prepared and size fractionated on 1% agarose gels containing 5 mM methylmercury hydroxide. The RNA was then blotted onto DBM paper, hybridized to nick-translated plasmid 749 DNA, and fluorographed. Cell fusion started approximately 30 hours after the change of medium. The mRNA coding for alpha actin migrated faster than the mRNA coding for beta and gamma actins suggesting an estimated difference in size of approximately 500 nucleotides (3, 4). Only nonmuscle actin mRNA was detected in proliferating myoblasts (0 hour). After cell fusion (72 hours), the label was predominantly in the alpha actin mRNA region. Plasmid 106 hybridizes only to the lower band (2).

p106 contained an insert that hybridized specifically with the muscle alpha actin mRNA. A more detailed examination showed that plasmid p106 hybridized only with skeletal muscle and cardiac actin mRNAs, and not with smooth (stomach) muscle actin mRNA. However, this plasmid hybridized strongly with skeletal muscle actin mRNAs from other mammalian species (rabbit and dog), but not with chick muscle actin mRNA. Plasmid p749 hybridized with all of the mRNA preparations tested.

In collaboration with A.-M. Frischauf and H. Lehrach, we also found that plasmid p749, which cross-hybridized with nonmuscle actin mRNA, contains the nucleic acid sequences coding for skeletal muscle alpha actin of the region from amino acid 171 to approximately the C terminal. Based on partial sequencing and estimated sizes of DNA fragments produced by restriction enzymes, we had previously estimated that the insert of plasmid p749 extended from amino acid 162 to approximately the C terminal (2). Plasmid p106, which hybridizes specifically with alpha actin, contains sequences coding for a poly-adenylated tail of 42 residues and 230 nucleotides of the untranslated 3' end of the actin mRNA (22).

The results of the hybridization experiments and the DNA sequencing indicate that the DNA coding for the translated part of the actin mRNA is conserved and is similar enough to cross-hybridize with mRNA from nonmuscle actins (beta and gamma actins). However, the untranslated 3' end of the mRNA is different in muscle and nonmuscle actins; as a consequence, plasmid p106 can be used as a specific probe for the muscle alpha actin mRNA. The results also indicate that the muscle actin genes diverged from the nonmuscle actin genes very early in the evolution of higher organisms.

Cloning of DNA Complementary to Myosin Heavy Chain and Light Chain mRNAs

Myosin, the largest known protein involved in muscle contraction, has a molecular weight (MW) of 480 kilodaltons (kd). It is composed of 2 heavy chains, each of MW 200 kd, and 3 or 4 light chains of MW 15 to 30 kd. Three different forms of skeletal muscle myosin have been reported to appear at different stages during development, and additional forms were described as nonmuscle myosins (5–12). It was of interest to measure quantitatively the expression of myosin genes during differentiation, to find out how many myosin genes exist and to study the structural and evolutionary relationships between the myosin genes.

Using an approach similar to that used for the construction of plasmids containing actin sequences, we obtained a plasmid, designated p103, containing an insert of 330 base pairs (bp). The RNA from rat muscle, isolated by hybridization to plasmid p103, coded for myosin light chain 2 in a reticulocyte cell-free system (2). Hybridization of this probe with size-fractionated RNA extracted from various sources showed that RNA sequences hybridizable to this plasmid are present in skeletal muscle and in differentiated cultures, but are undetectable in RNA from proliferating myoblasts and from nonmuscle tissues. The RNA that hybridizes with this plasmid has an estimated size of 800 nucleotides, which fits the expected size of mRNA coding for a protein with

MW on the order of 17 kd (2). Sequence analysis (in collaboration with J. Calvo unpublished data) has shown that the insert in plasmid p103 contains 213 nucleotides coding for 71 amino acids at the C-terminal end of myosin light chain 2 plus 61 nucleotides within the 3′ untranslated region.

The estimated size of mRNA coding for myosin heavy chain is more than 6 kb. It was therefore assumed that double-stranded cDNA made on a myosin heavy chain mRNA template has a reasonable probability of containing 2 or more restriction sites, which would be useful for ligation into a plasmid. Because myosin mRNA is abundant in muscle RNA, double-stranded cDNA was synthesized on total polyadenylated RNA extracted from muscle. The double-stranded DNA was digested with restriction enzyme Pst1, and the products were ligated with Pst1-cut plasmid pBR322. After transformation of bacteria and selection of colonies containing recombinant plasmids (Tet$^+$/Amp$^-$), the colonies were screened by hybridization with labeled cDNA made on muscle RNA template. Clones showing strong hybridization were selected for further characterization. Using this approach, we constructed a plasmid designated p82, which contained a 225-bp insert. Labeled plasmid p82 hybridizes specifically to size-fractionated RNA from muscle tissue and differentiated myogenic cultures, forming a single radioactive band (3). The estimated size of the

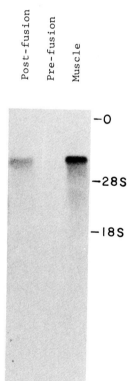

1   2   3

Fig. 2. Hybridization of labeled plasmid 82 DNA with size-fractionated RNA. The RNA was extracted from **(1)** differentiated L8 cultures containing multinucleated fibers; **(2)** proliferating L8 mononucleated myoblasts; **(3)** rat skeletal muscle, and was fractionated on a 1% methylmercury hydroxide agarose gel and transferred to DBM paper. The paper-bound RNA was hybridized with ^{32}P-labeled plasmid 82 and autoradiographed. The zero indicates the position of the origin; 28S and 18S indicate the positions of 28S and 18S rRNA, respectively. (Reprinted with permission from Nudel U, Katcoff D, Carmon Y, et al: Identification of recombinant phages containing sequences from different rat myosin heavy chain genes. Nucleic Acids Res 8:2133–2146, 1980.)

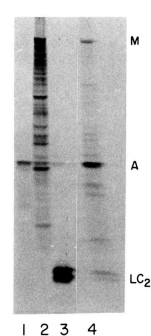

M

A

LC$_2$

1 2 3 4

Fig. 3. Sodium dodecyl sulfate(SDS)-polyacrylamide gel electrophoresis of translation products of RNA selected by hybridization to plasmid DNA. The RNA preparations, selected by hybridization of muscle polyadenylated RNA to plasmid DNA linked to cellulose, were translated in the reticulocyte cell-free system. The products were analyzed by 10 to 20% polyacrylamide-SDS gel electrophoresis. The RNA was selected by hybridization to (1) plasmid 749 (containing actin mRNA sequences); (2) plasmid 82; (3) plasmid 103 (myosin light chain 2 mRNA). Track 4 contains cell-free translation products of unfractionated rat skeletal muscle polyadenylated RNA. The letters M, A, and LC$_2$ indicate the positions of myosin heavy chain, actin, and myosin light chain 2 markers, respectively. (Reprinted withe permission from Nudel U, Katcoff D, Carmon Y, et al: Identification of recombinant phages containing sequences from different rat myosin heavy chain genes. Nucleic Acids Res 8:2133–2146, 1980.)

hybridizable RNA is approximately 7,000 nucleotides, which fits the expected size of myosin mRNA (Fig. 2).

To identify the RNA that hybridized to this clone, plasmid p82 DNA was isolated, bound to DBM cellulose, and hybridized to muscle mRNA as described previously. The hybridized RNA was eluted and translated in a cell-free system; the products were analyzed by sodium dodecyl sulfate(SDS)-polyacrylamide gel electrophoresis. The eluted RNA directed the synthesis of a heterogeneous population of polypeptides that appeared as many bands on SDS polyacrylamide gels. The largest and most prominent band comigrated with a myosin heavy chain marker (Fig. 3).

To determine the identity of the largest band, the cell-free system products were coelectrophoresed with muscle myosin heavy chain. The unlabeled marker together with the largest radioactive band were cut out and subjected to partial proteolysis with V8 protease and electrophoresis. The partial proteolysis peptide pattern of the radioactive product was almost identical to that of the myosin marker (Fig. 4, tracks 3 and 4). To determine whether the smaller products were incomplete polypeptides formed during translation of the large myosin mRNA, the entire acrylamide track containing the undigested products of the cell-free system (Fig. 3) was cut out of the SDS gel and laid horizontally on another SDS polyacrylamide gel, digested with V8 protease, and electrophoresed. As shown in Figure 4 (track 5), the major digestion products along the gel were of identical size and therefore appeared as horizontal bands across the gel. These peptides were identical to those obtained by partial proteolysis of the myosin marker. No such bands were formed in control experiments in which the products of the cell-free system directed by total polyadenylated muscle RNA were treated in an identical way (Fig. 4, track 6). The results thus show

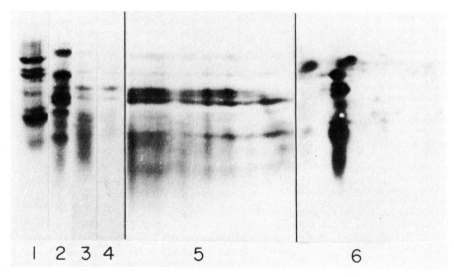

Fig. 4. Sodium dodecyl sulfate(SDS)-polyacrylamide gel electrophoresis of products of partial proteolysis. The following regions were excised from SDS-polyacrylamide gels, digested with *Staphylococcus aureus* V8 protease, and electrophoresed on a 15% SDS-polyacrylamide gel: **(1)** cell-free system (CFS) translation products of skeletal muscle RNA comigrating with actin marker; **(2)** ^{35}S-methionine-labeled myosin heavy chain isolated from differentiated L8 cultures; **(3)** myosin heavy chain isolated from rat skeletal muscle (stained with Coomassie blue); **(4)** the largest radioactive band (comigrating with myosin marker) cut out of SDS gel containing products of CFS directed by muscle RNA that hybridized to immobilized plasmid 82; **(5)** the entire track of CFS products of RNA hybridizing to immobilized recombinant plasmid 82 (see Fig. 3, track 2); **(6)** the entire track of CFS products of unfractionated polyadenylated skeletal muscle RNA. (Reprinted with permission from Nudel U, Katcoff D, Carmon Y, et al: Identification of recombinant phages containing sequences from different rat myosin heavy chain genes. Nucleic Acids Res 8:2133–2146, 1980.)

that all major products of the cell-free system directed by the RNA that hybridized to plasmid p82 were fragments of a single protein. The multiple peptides were apparently formed by early quitting of the nascent polypeptides during translation in the cell-free system.

Bacteriophages Containing Inserts of Myosin and Actin Genes

The labeled recombinant plasmids were used as probes to screen a library of lambda recombinant phages containing inserts of rat genomic DNA. Approximately 400,000 recombinant phages (about two genome equivalents) were screened. Fifteen clones that hybridized to labeled plasmid 749 DNA were isolated. Analysis of these phages by digestion with restriction enzymes together with electron microscopic examination of the heteroduplexes formed between them showed that at least 8 different genes containing actin sequences were represented among the 15 cloned phages. The detailed structure of these genes and the question of which actins they code for are currently under investigation.

Screening the rat genomic library with labeled plasmid 82 (myosin heavy chain) yielded 6 phages that hybridized to this plasmid. Digestion with restriction enzymes and hybridization analysis of the isolated clones indicated that they had originated from 3 different myosin genes. Three clones (CMH1, CMH3, and CMH4) had the same restriction and hybridization pattern; 2 others were identical (CMH2, CMH5), and 1 was unique (CMH3) (3). To confirm that the different genomic clones originated from different genes, DNA molecules from recombinant phages CMH1 and CMH3 were hybridized, and the heteroduplexes were analyzed by electron microscopy.

Figures 5 and 6 show the existence of several homologous regions interrupted by regions of nonhomology. The differences in size of the two strands formed in the nonhomologous regions strongly suggest the existence of intervening

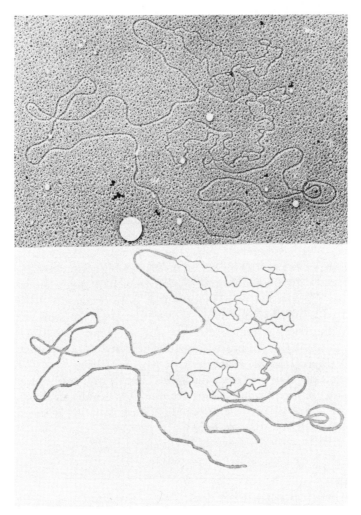

Fig. 5. Electron micrograph of heteroduplex between the recombinant phages CMH1 and CMH3. The DNA molecules from recombinant phages CMH1 and CMH3 were hybridized. Heteroduplexes were mounted for electron microscopy by the formamide procedure (13). (Reprinted with permission from Nudel U, Katcoff D, Caron Y, et al: Identification of recombinant phages containing sequences from different rat myosin heavy chain genes. Nucleic Acids Res 8:2133–2146, 1980.)

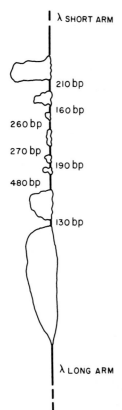

Fig. 6. Schematic representation of the heteroduplexes formed between recombinant phages CMH1 and CMH3. Heteroduplexes were photographed, and the homologous (hybridized) and non-homologous (loops) regions were measured. The numbers of base pairs are the average measurements of 10 different heteroduplexes.

sequences in these regions. The two arms of the big loop close to the lambda long arm (Fig. 6) are probably nonhomologous flanking regions of the two genes. Electron microscopic examination of R loops formed by hybridization of CMH1 DNA with muscle RNA showed that this phage contains approximately two-thirds of the coding sequence of the myosin gene. The CMH3 seems to contain one-third of the coding region (unpublished data obtained in collaboration with Y. Shaul and M. Finer).

Using labeled plasmid 103 (myosin light chain 2) as a probe, we have so far isolated one recombinant phage clone containing a 15-kb insert of rat genomic DNA. The structure of the region of this clone containing the myosin light chain 2 sequences is being investigated.

DISCUSSION

The work presented here, although it is in its early stages, has yielded several interesting results. Despite the great similarity between the various actins, cloning of sequences of the untranslated 3' ends of the mRNA molecules provide probes that hybridize specifically with striated muscle alpha actin mRNA. The cross-hybridization of these probes with mRNA for skeletal muscle actin of different mammalian species suggests that these probes may be used to identify the corresponding genes in human DNA. Cross-hybridization with other species has also been found with probes for myosin heavy chain (plasmid 82) and myosin light chain (plasmid 103).

The investigation also substantiated the notion derived from studies at the protein level of the complexity of the genetic system that codes for the synthesis of contracile proteins. This study demonstrates the existence of at least 8 different genes containing sequences that hybridize with actin mRNA and 3 genes that hybridize with myosin mRNA. Hybridization of the recombinant plasmids with fractionated genomic DNA digested with restriction enzymes (Southern technique) strongly suggests the existence of more actin and myosin genes (unpublished observations). Further studies on these genes may provide important information on their evolution, organization, and control of expression.

One of the advantages of the experimental approach described here is that it is in great part a "test tube genetics" study. It reduces very much the continuous dependence on and contact with the object animal. This, of course, is important for studying human diseases. Using a similar approach, it was possible to map and analyze in great detail the molecular structure of the globin genes and to pinpoint to the DNA level the defects involved in thalassemia (14–16). Furthermore, by combining recombinant DNA techniques with somatic cell hybridization techniques (17–20), it might be possible to map the DNA sequence of the entire X chromosomes on which many genes determining hereditary diseases are located. This, in turn, would facilitate identification and isolation of the gene that determines Duchenne muscular dystrophy. If it is a structural gene coding for a protein, then perhaps it will be feasible to isolate by selective hybridization the homologous mRNA and identify the protein it codes for by cell-free system translation (2, 3). Using a similar approach, it might be possible to construct a plasmid that would serve as a sensitive diagnostic probe to determine on a small sample of DNA or RNA the genetic constitution of the donor with regard to this disease.

ACKNOWLEDGMENTS

We wish to thank Ms. Zehava Levy, Ms. Michaella Miller, and Ms. Ora Saxel for excellent technical help. Ms. Malvine Baer provided editorial assistance. We thank Dr. Joseph Calvo for his helpful comments on the manuscript and Dr. J Bonner and Dr. TD Sargent for the rat genomic DNA library. The work was supported by the Muscular Dystrophy Association, New York; the National Institutes of Health under grant NIGMS 2 R01 GM 22767, and the United States–Israel Binational Science Foundation, Jerusalem.

REFERENCES

1. Zevin-Sonkin D, Yaffe D: Accumulation of muscle-specific RNA sequences during myogenesis. Dev Biol 74:326–334, 1980

2. Katcoff D, Nudel U, Zevin-Sonkin D, et al: Construction of recombinant plasmids containing rat muscle actin and myosin light chain DNA sequences. Proc Natl Acad Sci USA 77:960–964, 1980

3. Nudel U, Katcoff D, Carmon Y, et al: Identification of recombinant phages containing sequences from different rat myosin heavy chain genes. Nucleic Acids Res 8:2133–2146, 1980

4. Hunter T, Garrels JI: Characterization of the mRNAs for alpha-, beta-, and gamma-actin. Cell 12:767–781, 1977

5. Gauthier GF, Lowey S, Hobbs A: Fast and slow myosin in developing muscle fibers. Nature 274:25–29, 1978

6. Dalla Libera L, Sartore S, Schiaffino S: Comparative analysis of chicken arterial and ventricular myosins. Biochim Biophys Acta 581:283–294, 1979

7. Kuczmarski ER, Rosenbaum JL: Chick brain actin and myosin. J Cell Biol 80:341–355, 1979

8. Bhatnagar GM, Freedberg IM: Contractile proteins in epidermis: isolation and properties of guinea pig epidermal myosin. Biochim Biophys Acta 581:295–306, 1979

9. Whalen RG, Schwartz K, Bouveret P, et al: Contractile protein isozymes in muscle development: identification of an embryonic form of myosin heavy chain. Proc Natl Acad Sci USA 76:5197–5201, 1979

10. Hoh FJY, Yeoh GPS, Thomas MAW, Higginbottom L: Structural differences in the heavy chain of rat ventricular myosin isoenzymes. FEBS Lett 97:330–334, 1979

11. Rubinstein NA, Holtzer H: Fast and slow muscle in tissue culture synthesize only fast myosin. Nature 280:323–325, 1979

12. Yablonka Z, Yaffe D: Synthesis of myosin light chains and accumulation of translatable mRNA coding for light chain-like polypeptides, in differentiating muscle cultures. Differentiation 8:133–143, 1977

13. Davis R, Simon M, Davidson N: Electron microscope heteroduplex methods for mapping regions of base sequence homology in nucleic acids. In *Methods in Enzymology*, vol 21. Edited by Grossman L, Moldave K. Academic Press, New York, 1971, pp 413–428

14. Embury SH, Lebo RV, Dozy AM, Wai Kan Y: Organization of the alpha globin genes in the Chinese alpha thalassemia syndrome. J Clin Invest 64:1307–1310, 1979

15. Orkin SH, Old J, Lazarus H, et al: The molecular basis of alpha thalassemia: frequent occurrence of dysfunctional alpha loci among non-Asians with Hb H disease. Cell 17:33–42, 1979

16. Lauer J, Che Kun Shen J, Maniatis T: The chromosomal arrangement of human alpha-like globin genes: sequence homology and alpha globin gene deletions. Cell 20:119–130, 1980

17. Gusella J, Varsanyi-Breiner A, Fa Ten Kao, et al: Precise localization of human beta globin gene complex on chromosome II. Proc Natl Acad Sci USA 76:5239–5243, 1979

18. Owerbach D, Rutter WJ, Martial JA, et al: Genes for growth hormone, chorionic somatotropin and growth hormone-like gene on chromosome 17 in humans. Science 209:289–292, 1980

19. Lin PF, Slate DL, Lawyer FC, Ruddle FH: Assignment of the murine interferon sensitivity and cytoplasmic superoxide dismutase genes to chrommome 16. Science 209:285–287, 1980

20. Gusella J, Keys C, Varsany-Breiner A, et al: Isolation and localization of DNA segments from specific human chromosomes. Proc Natl Acad Sci USA 77:2829–2833, 1980

21. Yaffe D, Sascel O: Amyogenic cell line with altered serum requirements for differentiation. Differentiation 7:159–166, 1977

22. Shani M, Nudel U, Zevin-Sonkin D, et al: Skeletal muscle actin mRNA. Characterization of the 3′ untranslated region. Nucl Acids Res, in press

DISCUSSION

Dr. Allen D. Roses: To use these techniques in human diseases, will we have to know what protein we are looking for first?

Dr. David Yaffe: It makes it much easier, but a difference in RNA or DNA between normal and diseased tissue is enough. For example, I suggest we should start to think about mapping the X chromosome. It is visible already, and there are so many genetic diseases located in this chromosome. The collaborative work of many laboratories could accomplish this in a few years. After this chromosome is mapped, you know where to look for what.

Dr. Alan Emery: Just a technical question: what decides whether you use a plasmid or a phage?

Dr. David Yaffe: The size of the insert. A phage can contain a much bigger piece of DNA. If you want to insert a small DNA fragment, e.g., several hundred base pairs, you take a plasmid. If you want to insert 15 to 20 kilobase pairs, you take a phage.

Dr. Robert Wydro: When you were screening for your genomic clones for actin, which probe did you screen with, plasmid 749 or plasmid 106?

Dr. David Yaffe: We screened with both of them. So far, we have found clones that hybridize with plasmid 749. We have some clones that probably also hybridize with plasmid 106, but this investigation is not yet finished.

Dr. Robert Wydro: All of the 9 you have isolated?

Dr. David Yaffe: Yes, we screened all of them with plasmid 749. We have some hybridization problems with plasmid 106, but I do not want to speculate on these yet. However, we should find those which hybridize with this clone, because they must exist somewhere.

Dr. Margaret Thompson: We might not have to look at the whole X chromosome to find where the Duchenne and Becker genes are located and what their products are. The Becker locus is probably fairly close to HPRT near the end of the long arm, and evidence from X-autosome translocation females suggests that the Duchenne gene is in band 21 of the short arm, so we might be able to concentrate on those smaller areas.

Dr. David Yaffe: It makes it much easier because you can start with cloning the HPRT gene and then, as it is called in the jargon, "walk along the chromosome," i.e., take clones to the right and to the left until you reach the right place. Theoretically, this can be done, but it is a lot of work.

Dr. Alfred Goldberg: Would you say a little bit more about the 9 actin genes that you are talking about?

Dr. David Yaffe: I said all that I know.

59
Cloning of Muscle α Actin Copy DNA

Robert J. Schwartz, PhD

Jay A. Haron, BS

Katrina N. Rothblum, BS

Achilles Dugaiczyk, PhD

Differentiation of embryonic skeletal muscle in culture follows a succession of developmental phases including the proliferation of myoblasts, the fusion of mononucleated cells, and the formation of functional myofibrillar fibers (1). Specific increases in the content of several myofibrillar proteins such as actin, heavy chain myosin, and tropomyosin provide suggestive evidence that myoblast differentiation is caused by selective gene expression. Of these proteins, actin was once thought to be highly conserved protein in all cell types, although multiple forms have recently been found (2–8). The first actin described, α actin, is a major constituent of the contractile apparatus of skeletal muscle. Two other types of actins, designated β and γ, appear to be ubiquitous cytoskeletal proteins found in all nonmuscle tissue. Multiple forms of actin have been resolved by 2-dimensional gel electrophoresis of chick and mammalian proteins (4–6). Amino acid sequence differences between the actins contribute to their isoelectric focusing heterogeneity and prove that the actins are products of different genes (2, 3). Recent experiments have shown that actin represents a middle repetitive class of genes in lower eukaryotes (8), insects (9), and vertebrates (10).

According to current concepts, changes in morphogenesis and cell differentiation may be caused by selective gene expression. The increased accumulation of one gene product versus the other polymorphic forms appears to be a key regulatory event in muscle development. α Actin, the most acidic form, is found only in muscle tissue and appears to be induced during myogenesis. The appearance of α actin is paralled by an increase in total translatable actin messenger ribonucleic acid (mRNA) (11), and accounts for 8% of the total mRNA in differentiated muscle (10). Concomitant with the increase in α actin, a reduction and an eventual inhibition of β and γ actin synthesis occurs during terminal muscle differentiation. Because no cell type other than skeletal muscle expresses α actin, the appearance of α actin can be used as a specific marker for monitoring muscle cell differentiation.

Recently, we have described the isolation, partial purification, and characterization of α actin mRNA (10). Conventional techniques of RNA purification were used to prepare an actin-enriched mRNA. Because translation and hybridization analysis demonstrated that this actin mRNA was at most 50% pure, the purification was completed by molecular cloning (12). Double-stranded deoxyribonucleic acid (DNA) was synthesized from an RNA fraction enriched in actin mRNA, annealed to the bacterial plasmid pBR322, and used to transform *Escherichia coli* strain RR1. Several recombinant DNA clones containing actin complementary DNA (cDNA) were identified by hybridization to highly enriched actin mRNA and by positive translation product analysis. A full-length actin clone pAC269 was used stringent hybridization conditions to quantify the induction of α actin mRNA during myogenesis in culture.

Because α actin is specifically expressed in muscle, a hybridization probe to α actin would serve to analyze the early gene expression in muscle development. We have shown that several conventional techniques of mRNA purification yield a partial purification of α actin mRNA from chick breast muscle (10). Substantial purification of actin mRNA was accomplished by selective isolation of polyadenalate [poly(A)] containing RNA by affinity chromatography on oligo deoxythymidylate (dT) cellulose and a combination of sizing techniques. As shown in Figure 1, total muscle poly(A) containing RNA electrophoresed on denaturing gels is enriched in 2 major RNA species, band I (molecular weight, 5.2×10^5) and band II (molecular weight, 4.6×10^5, slot C).

The RNA was sequentially fractionated by sucrose gradients and Sepharose 4B chromatography and was finally electrophoresed on disulfide cross-linked

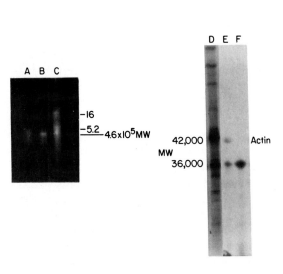

Fig. 1. Electrophoretic analysis of actin-enriched RNA and in vitro translation products. The RNA samples (*left panel*), including band I actin-enriched RNA (slot A), band II RNA (slot B), and total poly(A) containing RNA (slot C), were electrophoresed on denaturing 2% agarose gels (13). Poly(A) RNA (slot D), actin-enriched RNA (slot E), and band II RNA (slot F) were translated in an mRNA-dependent reticulocyte lysate (*right panel*). Products that had incorporated ^{35}S-methionine were electrophoresed on sodium dodecyl sulfate 10% polyacrylamide gel and autoradiographed on x-ray film. (Reprinted with permission from Schwartz RJ, Haron JA, Rothblum KN, Dugaiczyk A: Regulation of muscle differentiation: cloning of sequences from α actin mRNA. (12).)

Table 1. Purification of Actin mRNA Measured by Translational Activity[a]

Source of Poly(A) RNA	Total ^{35}S-Methionine[b] Incorporation (cpm/μg RNA)	Radioactivity bound[c] to DNAse Agarose (cpm/μg RNA)	% Incorporated into Actin
Oviduct	240,000	5,400	2
Reticulocyte	193,900	3,500	2
Muscle	218,000	22,200	10
Sucrose gradient	350,000	67,400	19
Sepharose 4B	400,000	185,600	46
Preparative polyacryl-amide gels	360,000	184,000	51
Hybridized to pAC269 DNA-cellulose	470,000	422,000	90

[a] Reprinted with permission from Schwartz R, Rothblum K: Regulation of muscle differentiation: isolation and purification of chick actin messenger ribonucleic acid and quantitation with complementary deoxyribonucleic acid probes. Biochemistry (10). 19:2506–2514, 1980.

[b] Total incorporation of acid-precipitable ^{35}S-methionine in a 60-μl translation assay.

[c] Radioactivity eluted from 100 μl of packed DNAse agarose beads with 3 M guanidine-HCl as described in *Methods* and by Schwartz and Rothblum (10).

polyacrylamide gels. Unfortunately, these conventional methods of RNA purification could not completely purify actin mRNA identified as band I (Fig. 1, slot A) away from RNA species of lower molecular weight, identified as band II (Fig. 1, slot B). The isolated RNA species were translated in the mRNA-dependent reticulocyte lysate (Fig. 1, slots D, E, and F). Actin mRNA purification was monitored by binding of the translation products to DNase agarose (Table 1) and by autoradiography on sodium dodecyl sulfate polyacrylamide gel.

Globular actin (G-actin) has the unique property of inhibiting DNase activity by binding rapidly to form a 1:1 stable complex between the two proteins. This highly specific interaction was used to identify in vitro synthesized actin (10). Analysis of band I–directed translation products showed that approximately 50% of the incorporated ^{35}S-methionine resided with actin, the remainder was shared with a 36,000 MW polypeptide (Fig. 1, slot E, and Table 1). The translation product of band II RNA revealed that 95% of the incorporated label migrated with the 36,000 MW polypeptide, whose identity has been preliminarily identified as glyceraldehyde-3-phosphate dehydrogenase (Fig. 1, slot F).

AMPLIFICATION OF CHIMERIC PLASMIDS

Because it was clear that actin mRNA was not a pure species, and because conventional methods of RNA purification had been exhausted, we decided to complete the purification and isolate the coding actin DNA sequence at the same time by molecular cloning. To this end, double-stranded DNA was synthesized from an enriched actin mRNA preparation of a 15S to 18S sucrose gradient size cut of poly(A) containing RNA with avian myoblastosis virus (AMV) reverse transcriptase (10). In 2 different experiments, cDNA yields of 15% and 20% of the input actin mRNA preparations were obtained as calculated from the incorporation of ^{3}H-labeled deoxycytidine triphosphate into the first strand.

The hairpin loop of the double-stranded cDNA was cut with S_1 nuclease, and approximately 15 to 20 deoxycytidine (dC) residues were then added to the 3' termini of double-stranded cDNA by using terminyl deoxynucleotidyl transferase. The bacterial plasmid pBR322 was cleaved with *Pst* I at the single site. The linearized plasmid was then tailed with 15 deoxyguanosine (dG) residues. Equimolar amounts of double-stranded DNA and the plasmid DNA were annealed and used to transform *E. coli* RR1. Four hundred clones that were sensitive to ampicillin but resistant to tetracycline were obtained from 0.3 μg of double-stranded cDNA and 1.2 μg of the plasmid DNA.

For screening of clones carrying actin gene sequences, clones were replica plated 2 times and transferred directly to nitrocellulose filters. The filters were processed for hybridization by in situ lysis (14) and were treated with Denhardt's solution (15, 16). To select colonies that contained actin recombinant DNA, we used the relative purity of band I RNA (~50% actin mRNA and ~50% band II RNA) and band II RNA (codes for 36,000 MW product) for the synthesis of ^{32}P-cDNA as hybridization probes. We were able to select the clones containing actin by the difference in the number of radioactive colonies. We screened 400 tetracycline-resistant colonies and picked 25 colonies that contained putative actin sequences.

Preliminary restriction endonuclease cleavage analysis with several enzymes allowed us to determine the size of inserted actin DNA in one actin recombinant DNA clone, pAC269 (Fig. 2). The DNA was initially digested with *Bam* HI and divided into 4 aliquots, 3 of which were digested with a second endonuclease. The complete restriction map of pBR322 as presented by Sutcliffe (18) was used to verify our results and to determine the exact size of the fragments. As shown in Figure 2, the digestion with *Bam* HI and *Pst* I released 3 fragments. The largest fragment, 3.2 kilobases (kb), contained parental plasmid DNA. The second fragment of 1.75 kb contained a 0.6-kb portion of actin DNA and a 1.15-kb fragment of the parental pBR322 because of an unreconstituted *Pst* I site in the inserted actin DNA. The 0.8-kb fragment was caused by a single recovered *Pst* I site and a single internal *Bam* HI site centrally located in the actin insert. Double digestion of *Bam* HI and *Hind* III showed that *Hind* III does not cut the actin insert, but releases fragments of 1.45 kb and 0.3 kb. *Eco* RI cuts close to the *Hind* III site within pBR322 DNA and produces 2 small fragments of 1.35 kb and 0.35 kb plus a large fragment of 4 kb. *Bam* HI alone causes a release of a 1.75-kb fragment that contains approximately 0.6 kb of actin DNA sequences. The partial restriction endonuclease cleavage map of pAC269 shows that 1,400 base pairs (bp) of actin DNA were inserted in the recombinant plasmid and provides sufficient orientation to determine the insert size by the technique of RNA looping.

Electron microscopy was used to analyze R loops formed between *Eco* RI linearized pAC269 DNA and muscle poly(A) containing RNA. Almost all the DNA molecules observed possessed an R loop structure when hybridization was

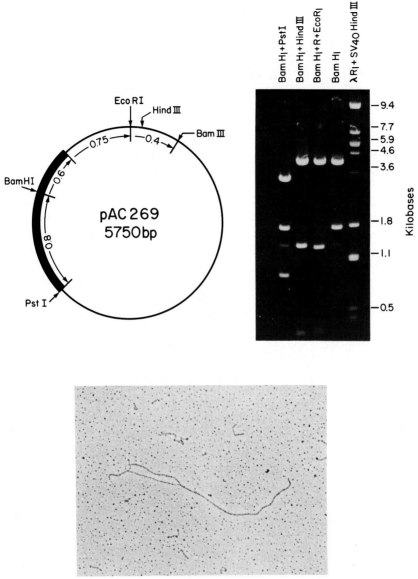

Fig. 2. A partial restriction map of pAC269. The map (*left*) shows the inserted actin DNA fragment and its orientation, in heavy black, in the pBR322 plasmid DNA. The cleavage sites of *Bam* HI, *Pst* I, *Hind* III, and *Eco* RI in pAC269 (*right*) are indicated. The R loop of pAC269 and actin mRNA was performed by Dr. Myles Mace Jr. under the conditions described by Chow and colleagues (17). The orientation of the R loop in the micrograph is described in *Results*. (Reprinted with permission from Schwartz RJ, Haron JA, Rothblum KN, Dugaiczyk A: Regulation of muscle differentiation: cloning of sequences from α action mRNA. (12).)

performed according to the method of Chow and co-workers (17) in mRNA excess. On close examination of R loops with linearized pAC269, only one protruding RNA tail of heterogeneous length could be detected that was always oriented toward the short arm of the asymetrically split DNA (bottom of Figure 2). Therefore, we conclude that this RNA tail represents the 3′ poly(A) sequence of the mRNA and allows us to orient the insert within the plasmid. The overall length of the actin insert by R looping is 1,400 bases, essentially identical to 1,360 bp determined by endonuclease mapping, with additional 3,450 bases and 800 bases of plasmid DNA flanking the insert DNA region.

The pAC269 probably contains sequences to the entire length of actin mRNA. Our data estimated by both restriction digest and R looping indicate that a sizable and continuous actin-specific gene sequence was present in pAC269 that contained 1,400 ± 50 bp. The size of α actin mRNA determined under denaturing conditions is 1,575 bases (10) and is comparable to the size estimated from the L8 rat myoblast line (7). If the poly(A) stretch of 100 nucleotides is excluded, then the α actin clone is approximately 95% of the full length of the transcribed nucleotides. Skeletal muscle actin has been shown to contain 374 amino acids, indicating a coding region of the message of approximately 1,120 bases in length. Therefore, 350 additional transcribed nucleotides in the mRNA must be in the noncoding regions. Interestingly, the other nonmuscle β and γ actin mRNA contain a much larger noncoding region of approximately 1,000 nucleotides (2). The significance of such extraordinarily large untranslated regions in the β and γ actin mRNAs is currently not known.

POSITIVE CONFIRMATION OF THE ACTIN INSERT BY HYBRIDIZATION TO DNA CELLULOSE

To confirm the identity of pAC269 as actin cDNA, we used a positive proof in which cloned plasmid DNA was covalently linked to cellulose and was used to isolate mRNA by affinity chromatography. Purified plasmid DNA was immobilized onto diazobenzyloxymethyl cellulose (19). Poly(A) containing RNA from chick breast muscle was hybridized to an excess of pAC269 cellulose, and the bound RNA was eluted. We recovered 5% to 10% of the input poly(A) containing RNA.

Figure 3 compares the electrophoretic mobility of the translated protein directed by the RNA preparation bound to cellulose with that of authentic chicken skeletal actin. The single translation product has the same migration as actin. Further comparison of the translation product and pure actin was possible by fragmentation with a cyanylation reagent. Because skeletal actin has 5 cysteinyl residues at positions 10, 217, 256, 284, and 373, cleavage of the actin at some of these positions by dithiodinitrocyanobenzoic acid (TNB-CN) treatment should give rise to many fragments observed on sodium dodecyl sulfate 12% polyacrylamide slab gel (Fig. 3). If actin is completely or partially cleaved by TNB-CN treatment, as many as 20 kinds of actin fragments may be produced. In comparison, both the autoradiograph of the cyanylated translated product and actin had exactly the same number of fragments (17), molecular weights, and relative contents (Fig. 3, slots c and d).

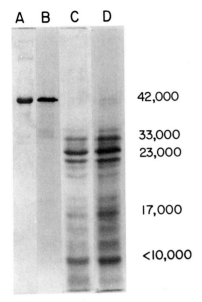

A   B   C   D

42,000

33,000
23,000

17,000

<10,000

Fig. 3. Electrophoresis of translation products of RNA selected by hybridization to pAC269 DNA. Total poly(A) containing muscle RNA was hybridized to pAC269 cellulose as described by Schwartz and associates (12). Hybridized RNA was eluted, translated, and then electrophoresed on a sodium dodecyl sulfate 12% polyacrylamide slab gel. Numbers at right indicate molecular weights. Slot A: authentic chick muscle actin stained with Coomassie blue. Slot B: autoradiograh of the translation product. Slot C: stained cyanylation fingerprint of chick muscle actin. Slot D: autoradiograph of the cyanylation fingerprint of the translation product. (Reprinted with permission from Schwartz RJ, Haron JA, Rothblum KN, Dugaiczyk A: Regulation of muscle differentiation: cloning of sequences from α actin mRNA. (12).)

The actins α, β, and γ are products of different genes and are separable from each other by 2-dimensional gel electrophoresis. Because we showed that actin DNA cross hybridizes to the repeated family of actin DNA sequences in the chicken genome (10), it was reasonable to assume that the α actin clone pAC269 would contain sufficient homology to isolate β and γ actin mRNAs by affinity chromatography. The translation products of the RNA bound to pAC269 were examined directly by 2-dimensional gel electrophoresis (Fig. 4A). Acidic conditions (pH 3 to 6) were necessary to ensure resolution of actin within the isoelectric focusing gel.

Inspection of autoradiographs of 2-dimensional slab gels for the hybridized RNA–directed products resolved a single spot with a molecular weight of 42,000 daltons focused within a pH range of 5.4 to 5.5 (Fig. 4A). This autoradiographic spot comigrated with skeletal actin standard and corresponds to the α form of actin. Poly(A)-containing RNA isolated from 14-day embryonic chick brain was hybridized to pAC269 DNA. The bound RNA was translated, and the radioactive products were separated by 2-dimensional gel electrophoresis and autoradiographed (Fig. 4B). Essentially all the radioactive material resided in 2 spots that comigrated with β and γ actin. When affinity-purified α actin mRNA from Fig. 4A was mixed with β and γ mRNA and translated in the mRNA-dependent reticulocyte lysate, 3 radioactive spots were found to comigrate with α, β, and γ actins.

It should be emphasized that the localization of actin on a 2-dimensional gel is characteristic. Using the high-resolution 2-dimensional gel system of O'Farrell (20), we separated the 3 major actins, which were translation products of mRNA selectively hybridized to pAC269 DNA (Fig. 4). The fingerprints of cyanylated peptides of the translation product were identical to those of fragments of authentic skeletal actin (Fig. 3). Furthermore, the translation products effectively bound to DNAase agarose, an additional proof of the biologic function of the

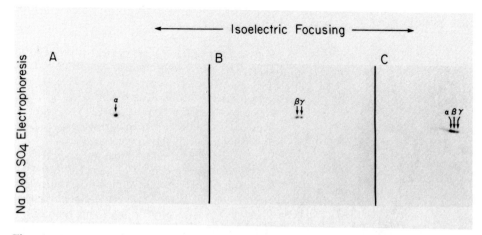

Fig. 4. Two-dimensional sodium dodecyl sulfate gel electrophoresis of translation products of RNA hybridized to pAC269 DNA-cellulose. **(A)** The RNA fraction was prepared and translated as described by Schwartz and coworkers (12). **(B)** The RNA preparations selected by hybridization of embryonic brain poly(A)-containing RNA of pAC269 were translated in the mRNA-dependent reticulocyte lysate. **(C)** Both muscle RNA and brain RNA, which were selectively hybridized to pAC269 DNA-cellulose, were mixed and translated in the reticulocyte lysate. The products were analyzed by 2-dimensional gel electrophoresis. The identification of α actin was by alignment of the radioactive spot with the stained nonradioactive actin from muscle. (Reprinted with permission from Schwartz RJ, Haron JA, Rothblum KN, Dugaiczyk A: Regulation of muscle differentiation: cloning of sequences from α actin mRNA. (12).)

synthesized actin. These results strongly support the conclusion that pAC269 is complementary to actin mRNA.

MEASUREMENT OF α ACTIN mRNA IN MYOGENESIS

The end point of myogenesis provides a well-defined morphologic marker of cell differentiation that is complemented by changes in the levels of contractile proteins, muscle-specific enzymes, and mRNA population (21–23). Therefore, the availability of a clone DNA probe to α actin specific for muscle differentiation would facilitate our analysis of the mechanism underlying the induction of muscle gene transcription. However, because of the large preexisting population of β and γ actin mRNAs in the prefusion myoblasts, it has been difficult to analyze separately the regulation of the α actin gene in muscle culture. To develop a more stringent hybridization assay for the measurement of α actin mRNA, it was necessary first to examine the homology and sequence divergence of the muscle actin gene sequence in comparison to those of nonmuscle actin species.

The homology of β and γ actin mRNAs to α actin mRNA was preliminarily compared by saturation hybridization of complementary single-stranded ^{3}H-pAC269 DNA. Figure 5 (panel A) shows the saturation hybridization of pAC269 DNA with excess muscle total RNA. Complete saturation of the α actin DNA probe was observed within an RNA-to-DNA ratio of 100 to 1. Brain RNA isolated from 14-day chick embryos, which contains β and γ actin mRNA, required a ratio of 500 to 1 to reach a maximal 70% protection for the α actin DNA probe from S_1 nuclease digestion. Brain RNA has a slight enrichment in β rather than γ actin. In experiments using gizzard RNA, which is enriched in smooth muscle actin (24), similar results were also obtained (data not shown). These data suggest that a maximum of 470 nucleotides of the 1,570 transcribed nucleotides in the α actin structural gene sequence are nonhomologous to the combined β and γ mRNA. Differences in nucleotide sequence in the noncoding region of the actins might provide the overall 30% nonhomology between α actin mRNA and the other actin species.

The thermal stability properties were examined using the denaturation chracteristics of hybrids formed between RNA and ^{3}H-pAC269 DNA. The temperature at which 50% of the hybridized sequences are separated (Tm) has proved to be a useful parameter in relating the degree of complementarity between hybridized nucleic acid species. The fidelity of cloned pAC269 DNA, the α actin structural gene sequence, was ascertained by examining the thermal melting of the α actin DNA:mRNA duplex hybridized with an excess of muscle RNA. The Tm was 93° C and occurred with a sharp transition, indicating that accurate base pairing was present in the pAC269 DNA:actin mRNA hybrid (Fig. 5B). Thermal properties of brain β and γ actin mRNA:pAC269 DNA hybrids revealed a broad multiphasic melt curve in which hybrids began to denature at temperatures as low as 70° C. An overall Tm of 81° C was assessed for the nonmuscle actin mRNA:muscle actin DNA hybrids. In general, changes in Tm values parallel the differences in amino acid sequences observed for the corresponding polypeptide chain, such as those of globin chains (25). Several laboratories have shown that the change in Tm is related to the number of nucleotide differences (sequence divergence) between nonidentical hybridizing sequences (26–28). The reduction in Tm has been variously estimated at 1.6 to 3.4° C for each 1% sequence divergence. Therefore, the data suggest that of the 70% homology that exists between a α actin mRNA and β and γ actin

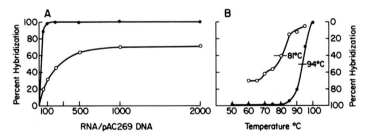

Fig. 5. Homology of pAC269 DNA sequences with β and γ actin mRNAs. **(A)** RNA excess hybridizations were performed with total muscle RNA (closed circles) and total embryonic brain RNA (open circles) using single-stranded complementary ^{3}H-pAC269 DNA. **(B)** ^{3}H-pAC269 DNA:RNA hybrids were incubated for 5 minutes at each temperature and then digested with S_1 nuclease. The line through each melt curve is the Tm point, i.e., the temperature at which 50% of the hybrids are separated. (Reprinted with permission from Schwartz RJ, Haron JA, Rothblum KN, Dugaiczyk A: Regulation of muscle differentiation: cloning of sequences from α actin mRNA (12).

mRNAs, there is probably a minimum of 3.8% and a maximum of 8.1% sequence devergence between actin mRNA species.

The difference observed in thermal melts between skeletal and cytoplasmic actin mRNAs to pAC269 DNA have allowed us to develop a stringent hybridization assay to quantify α actin mRNA specifically during muscle development. We found that hybridization of pAC269 DNA to actin mRNA at 78° C in aqueous medium could discriminate α actin from the other actin mRNA species. These conditions have been shown to be sufficient to prevent cross reaction between β and γ globin cDNA and their mRNA (25). Because prolonged incubation at this temperature results in extensive breakdown of RNA, we did not attempt to exploit the specificity achieved in the aqueous hybridization system. Instead, we used formamide to reduce the high thermal requirement for stringent hybridization under conditions of 50% formamide, 0.4 M NaCl and 65° C.

Total RNA was isolated from 12-day embryonic chick thigh muscle cultures staged according to the criteria of Moss and colleagues (29). The concentration of α actin mRNA was determined by comparing the kinetics of the hybridization of each RNA sample with that of total poly(A)-containing RNA from 3-week-old chick breast muscle (Fig. 6). The data were plotted as the inverse of the fraction of single-stranded plasmid cDNA versus the concentration of RNA × time (CrT) according to the method of Wetmur and Davidson (30) and Bishop (31). The absolute concentration of actin mRNA in the unknown sample can be determined by comparing the slope of an unknown sample to that of an RNA standard. All slopes were determined by a linear regression program. Three-week-old chick breast muscle poly(A)-containing RNA was assumed to contain 8% α actin mRNA (10).

Figure 6 is a graphic representation of hybridization data used to determine the accumulation of α actin mRNA in myogenic cultures. Table 2 provides the slopes of each curve and the calculated α actin mRNA content per diploid nucleus. Under the culture conditions used, myogenic cells attached to the

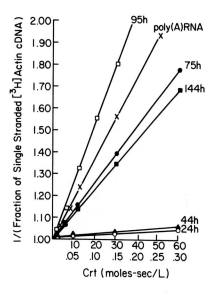

Fig. 6. Hybridization of α actin pAC269 DNA to total myoblast RNA. ^{3}H-cDNA isolated from the plasmid pAC269 was used to quantify α actin mRNA sequences in total myoblast RNA. This figure and Table 2 show how the hybridization data were used to obtain the percentage of α actin mRNA present in each RNA sample. The results are for total myoblast RNA prepared from 20, 44, 75, 95, and 144 hours in culture and for poly(A) RNA from 3-week-old chick breast muscle, which served as a standard. Single-stranded ^{3}H-labeled actin cDNA was hybridized to each RNA sample under the conditions of "DNA excess" and hybrids were detected after treatment with S_1 nuclease. The slope obtained from each of these hybridization curves is proportional to actin mRNA concentration. Crt, concentration of RNA × time.

Table 2. Hybridization of pAC269 DNA to myoblast RNA.

	Slope $(L\,Mol^{-1}S^{-1})$A	αActin mRNA[B] (% of Total RNA)	pg RNA/Diploid Nucleus	αActin mRNA/ Diploid Nucleus
Standard[C]	5.41	9.0	—	—
Myoblast Culture				
20h	.0002	.0003	11	40
45h	.0003	.0005	19	110
75h	.0209	.0348	29	11,700
95h	.0411	.0685	37	29,300
144h	.0132	.00243	52	14,700

A Slopes were determined by linear regression for each of the RNA samples

B % α actin mRNA

$$= \frac{\text{Slope of the Sample}}{\text{Slope of the Standard}} \times (\% \text{ Actin mRNA in standard})$$

$$= \frac{\text{Slope of the Sample 9\%}}{5.41}$$

C The standard RNA solution is breast muscle poly (A) RNA which contains 9% Actin mRNA

culture dish and underwent DNA synthesis and replication throughout the first 30 to 40 hours in culture. The α actin mRNA content was estimated at 130 molecules per cell during replication. This value is probably an overestimate of the α actin mRNA content in prefusion myoblasts because of the use of primary cultures. After withdrawal from the cell cycle, myoblasts proceeded to orient for fusion; this occurred on a large scale after approximately 45 hours in culture. At the beginning of fusion there was no increase in α actin mRNA in comparison to prefusion values. For the most part, fusion was complete by 90 to 100 hours in culture.

A substantial increase in α actin mRNA was found at 75 hours, a midfusion time point; the maximal value of 36,000 molecules of α actin mRNA per nucleus was reached after 95 hours in culture. By 6 days, cultures contained fully differentiated myotubes that were observed to contract spontaneously. At this stage of terminal differentiation, the content of α actin mRNA was reduced to a maintenance level of 8,000 molecules per nucleus. Although not described here, the levels of β and γ actin mRNA, the nonmuscle types, were considerably reduced during myoblast differentiation and disappeared; α actin mRNA become the only expressed actin gene in mature muscle fibers.

The development and characterization of specific recombinant DNA clones will help us to understand the mechanisms involved in the regulation of the actin genes during myogenesis. Hybridization data using a full-length α actin DNA clone pAC269 showed that, after the cessation of cell replication and the onset of myoblast fusion, α actin mRNA selectively accumulated. The increase of 36,000 molecules of actin mRNA per nucleus within a period of 50 hours strongly suggests direct transcriptional regulation of the α actin gene. However, regulation at posttranscriptional sites such as nuclear RNA processing and mRNA stability may also provide important roles in controlling α actin mRNA content. Because pulse-chase measurements are the most effective technique for analyzing molecules after synthesis, it is possible through their use to establish transcription rates, decay rates, intermediates in decay, and the stability of the final products of the transient molecules. We are now proceeding with pulse-chase analyses to determine the metabolism of the α actin gene product during muscle cell differentiation.

ACKNOWLEDGMENTS

We wish to thank Earl Scharff III and Olivia Dennison for excellent technical assistance. This work was supported by United States Public Health Service (USPHS) Grant NS-15050 and by a grant from the Muscular Dystrophy Association of America. R Schwartz is a recipient of a USPHS Research Career Development Award.

REFERENCES

1. Herrmann H, Heywood SM, Marchok A: Reconstruction of muscle development as a sequence of macromolecular syntheses. Curr Top Dev 5:181–234, 1970
2. Elzinga G, Lu RC: Comparative amino acid sequence studies on actins. In *Contractile Systems in Non-Muscle Tissues*. Edited by Perry SV, Margreth A, Adelstein RS. Elsevier North Holland Biomedical Press, Amsterdam, 1976, pp 29–37
3. Vandekerchove J, Weber K: Mammalian cytoplasmic actins are the products of at least two genes and differ in primary structure in at least 25 identified positions from skeletal muscle actins. Proc Natl Acad Sci USA 75:1106–1110, 1978
4. Garrels J, Gibson W: Identification and characterization of multiple forms of actin. Cell 9:793–805, 1976
5. Gruenstein E, Rich A, Weihing RR: Actin associated with membranes from 3T3 mouse fibroblasts and HeLa cells. J Cell Biol 64:223–234, 1975
6. Whalen R, Butler-Browne GS, Gros F: Protein synthesis and actin heterogeneity in calf muscle cells in culture. Proc Natl Acad Sci USA 73:2018–2022, 1976
7. Hunter T, Garrels JI: Characterization of the mRNAs for α, β and γ-actin. Cell 12:767–781, 1977
8. Kindle KL, Firtel RA: Identification and analyses of dictyostellium actin genes, a family of moderately repeated genes. Cell 15:763–778, 1978
9. Tobin SL, Zulauf E, Sanchez F, et al: Multiple actin-related sequences in the *Drosophila melanogaster* genome. Cell 19:121–131, 1980
10. Schwartz R, Rothblum K: Regulations of muscle differentiation: isolation and purification of chick actin messenger ribonucleic acid and quantitation with complementary deoxyribonucleic acid probes. Biochemistry 19:2506–2514, 1980
11. Paterson BM, Roberts BE, Yaffe D: Determination of actin messenger RNA in cultures of differentiating embryonic chick skeletal muscle. Proc Natl Acad Sci USA 71:4467–4471, 1974
12. Schwartz RJ, Haron JA, Rothblum KN, Dugaicyzk A: Regulation of muscle differentiation: cloning of sequences from α actin mRNA. Biochemistry 19:5883–5890, 1980
13. Bailey JM, Davidson N: Methylmercury as a reversible denaturing agent for agarose gel electrophoresis. Anal Biochem 70:75–85, 1976

14. Grunstein M, Hogness DS: Colony hybridization: a method for the isolation of cloned DNAs that contain a specific gene. Proc Natl Acad Sci USA 72:3961–3965, 1975

15. Denhardt D: A membrane-filter technique for the detection of complementary DNA. Biochem Biophys Res Commun 23:641–646, 1966

16. Botchan M, Topp W, Sambrook J: The arrangement of simian virus 40 sequences in the DNA of transformed cells. Cell 9:269–288, 1976

17. Chow L, Roberts JM, Lewis JB, Broker TR: A map of cytoplasmic RNA transcripts from lytic adenovirus type 2 determination of RNA:DNA hybrids. Cell 11:819–836, 1977

18. Sutcliffe JG: pBR322 restriction map derived from the DNA sequence: accurate DNA size marker up to 4361. Nucleic Acid Res 5:2721–2728, 1978

19. Noyes BE, Stark GR: Nucleic acid hybridization using DNA covalently coupled to cellulose. Cell 5:301–310, 1975

20. O'Farrell PH: High resolution two-dimensional electrophoresis of proteins. J Biol Chem 250:4007–4021, 1975

21. Buckingham ME: Muscle protein synthesis and its control during the differentiation of skeletal muscle in vitro. In *Biochemistry of Cell Differentiation*. Edited by Paul J. Int Rev Biochem 15:209–332, 1978

22. Colbert DA, Coleman JR: Transcriptional expression of non-repetitive DNA during normal and BudR-mediated inhibition of myogenesis in culture. Exp Cell Res 109:31–42, 1977

23. Paterson BM, Bishop JO: Changes in the mRNA population of chick myoblasts during myogenesis in vitro. Cell 12:751–765, 1977

24. Saborio JL, Segura M, Flores M, et al: Differential expression of gizzard actin genes during chick embryogenesis. J Biol Chem 254:11119–11125, 1979

25. Benz EJ, Geist CE, Steggles AW, et al: Hemoglobin switching in sheep and goats: preparation and characterization of complementary DNAs specific for the α-, β- and γ globin messenger RNAs of sheep. J Biol Chem 252:1908–1916, 1977

26. Laird CD, McConaughy BL, McCarthy BJ: Rate of fixation of nucleotide substitutions in evolution. Nature 224:149–154, 1969

27. Leder P, Aviv H, Gielen J, Ikawa Y, Packman S, Swan D, Ross J: Regulated expression of mammalian genes: globin and immunoglobulin as model system. Cold Spring Harbor Symp Quant Biol 38:753, 1973

28. Ullman JS, McCarthy BJ: The relationship between mismatched base pairs and the thermal stability of DNA duplexes. Biochim Biophys Acta 294:405–415, 1973

29. Moss M, Asch B, Schwartz R: Differentiation of actin-containing filaments during chick skeletal myogenesis. Exp Cell Res 121:167–178, 1979

30. Wetmur JG, Davidson N: Kinetics of renaturation of DNA. J Mol Biol 31:349–370, 1968

31. Bishop JO: DNA-RNA hybridization. Acta Endocrinol 168 (Suppl):247–276, 1972

DISCUSSION

Dr. Sergio Pena: Dr. Yaffe has already referred to the possibility of using these clones for clinical studies, and you showed very nicely that for a highly conserved protein you can use your chick clones to work on rabbit and other animals. Do you expect that this will turn out to be a general phenomenon, or do you think that for less conserved proteins the chicken clones will not be as useful? Will we have to develop a human clone? In this light, have you done the same work with glyceraldehyde-3-phosphate dehydrogenase?

Dr. Robert Schwartz: If you had genes with highly conserved amino acid sequences, it is conceivable that these clones would be useful for human diseases.

In answer to your second question, yes, we have done experiments with glyceraldehyde-3-phosphate dehydrogenase; it has a 50% homology to the mammalian gene sequence and can be useful in quantifying mRNA sequences in mammalian species.

Dr. Susan Benoff-Rind: Have you looked for the intracellular localization of the small amount of message that is present before fusion?

Dr. Robert Schwartz: No, but we will.

Dr. Stanley Appel: Let me set a theoretical framework for you. We heard the question raised as to whether you can use this sort of analysis for studying disease, specifically Duchenne muscular dystrophy. The point was made that we might need to know the protein gene product before we could use these techniques. Is it not possible that one could stay strictly at the mRNA level and determine the differences in message populations between a group of cells from an affected patient, especially in a sex-linked disorder, and a group of cells from a non-affected parent? These could be contrasted with the appropriate copy DNAs. It might even be possible to assess such differences in a fibroblast population or after amniocentesis. We might thus be able to get the information and help solve the defect without ever knowing the gene product.

Dr. Robert Schwartz: Absolutely. You can map the chromosome if you have the manpower to do those experiments. It may be possible to find a chromosomal map difference because of various chromosomal DNA rearrangements, or a mutation difference in structure by complete restriction digests, e.g., of a clone bank to an X-chromosomal gene clone bank. You can look for differences in restriction digest pattern between a dystrophic or Duchenne X-linked chromosome. It would be possible to isolate the DNA in a lambda clone, amplify it, link the DNA to a matrix, pull out mRNA, if it is transcribed, and then identify the translated protein product. I see nothing wrong with what you propose; it is a much more straightforward way to approach the problem.

Part VIII

ASPECTS OF CARRIER DETECTION

60

Altered Mononuclear Cell Spreading and Microtubules in Duchenne Muscular Dystrophy Patients and Carriers

Jerry W. Shay, PhD

Leigh E. Thomas, BS

John W. Fuseler, PhD

Because we still have little information about the primary metabolic defect in Duchenne muscular dystrophy (DMD), carrier detection and genetic counseling have become increasingly important in prevention of the disease. In general, female carriers do not show any clinical manifestations of the disease, which has resulted in efforts to develop new techniques that may help to identify carriers.

More than 20 years ago, Ebashi and colleagues (1) and Dreyfus and associates (2) reported that creatine phosphokinase (CPK) activity was increased in the serum of some female carriers (1, 2). Subsequently, this test became recognized as the most effective means of identifying carriers. However, this test has been estimated to identify only 50% to 80% of definite carriers. For the purpose of this study, obligate or definite carriers were defined as persons with at least one affected son and an affected brother or some other affected male relative on the maternal side, such as an uncle, cousin, or nephew (3). From a practical standpoint, if one knows that an individual is a definite carrier by pedigree analysis, then demonstrating increased CPK activity only helps verify the reliability of the assay. However, the CPK assay does not identify all definite carriers, so other techniques need to be developed to improve the percentage of carriers detected.

New techniques for carrier detection require validation by several approaches. An obligate or definite carrier is defined by genetic criteria from a retrospective analysis of pedigree. However, for genetic counseling, one tries to determine prospectively whether someone is a definite carrier by using a combination of in vitro assays and pedigree analysis. In such situations, the validity of any test depends on the rate of false-negative and false-positive results. The false-negative rate can be determined by applying the assay to the analysis of definite carriers, but the false-positive rate depends on the analysis of many more subjects, some normal and some with related neuromuscular disorders.

In this study, we report 2 potential carrier detection techniques based on mononuclear cell spreading and alterations in microtubules. Our preliminary results indicate that we may be able to identify some carriers who have normal CPK levels. In light of the controversy surrounding other carrier detection techniques, we urge caution in interpreting the data until more subjects are studied.

MATERIALS AND METHODS

Blood Samples

Fifteen milliliters of blood were drawn by venipuncture using a 20-gauge needle and a 20-ml sterile disposable syringe, with 10 units of heparin added for each 1 ml of whole blood (Weddel Pharmaceuticals, Ltd., London). Of this sample, 15 ml were added to a separate sterile tube to be used for CPK assay and differential white blood cell count. The remaining 10 ml were placed in a sterile 50-ml conical polyethylene centrifuge tube with a screw cap (Corning) for the Ficoll-Hypaque gradient.

Ficoll-Hypaque Gradient

Mononuclear cells (lymphocytes and monocytes) were isolated from the heparinized whole blood at room temperature using a Ficoll-Hypaque gradient. The 10 ml of heparinized blood were diluted 1:4 with RPMI-1640 culture medium (Microbiological Associates). Penicillin G (100 U/ml) and streptomycin sulfate (100 mg/ml) (Gibco) were added (hereafter, this medium is referred to as RPMI-PS). The diluted blood sample was carefully layered onto 10 ml of sterile Ficoll-Hypaque (9% Ficoll, 34% Hypaque; solution density, 1.078 at 25° C) contained in another sterile 50-ml conical centrifuge tube (Hypaque sodium 50%, diatrizoate sodium; Ficoll-400, Sigma). This gradient was centrifuged at 500 g for 20 minutes at room temperature. The mononuclear layer was carefully removed from the diluted plasma:Ficoll-Hypaque interface with a sterile Pasteur pipette and placed in a fresh sterile 50-ml centrifuge tube.

After the mononuclear cells were removed from the interface, they were diluted 1:3 with fresh RPMI-PS medium and centrifuged at 500 g for 15 minutes at room temperature. The supernatant was discarded, and the pellet was carefully suspended in 1.0 ml of RPMI-PS. This cell suspension was layered onto 3.0 ml of sterile, heat-inactivated human AB-positive plasma contained in a sterile 15-ml polystyrene conical centrifuge tube (Corning). This gradient was centrifuged for 10 minutes at 200 g to separate the blood platelets suspended in the plasma-RPMI supernatant. The mononuclear cells formed a pellet that was resuspended in 1.0 ml of RPMI-PS and centrifuged again at 200 g for 10 minutes at room temperature. The supernatant was discarded, and the cells were washed twice more in the same manner before final resuspension in 1.0 ml of RPMI-1640, which included 20% human AB-positive plasma and 1% antimicrobial drugs. With this method, we recovered approximately 90% of the mononuclear cells. A mean of 10.4×10^6 cells were obtained from 10 ml of whole blood. These cells were plated on plastic tissue culture dishes with or without coverslips (Corning) for further use. The mononuclear cells were allowed to remain in culture for 5 to 7 days with 1 change of medium on day 2. At least 2 coverslips for each patient were then processed for immunofluorescence and spreading counts.

Immunofluorescence Studies

The coverslips with attached mononuclear cells were rinsed in phosphate-buffered saline (PBS), fixed in 3% ultrapure formaldehyde (Tousimis) in PBS for 20 minutes, and then extracted in acetone at $-20°$ C for 7 minutes. The cells were incubated with either of 2 tubulin antibodies: affinity-purified rabbit anti-tubulin serum provided by BR Brinkley, which as been characterized previously (4) and a nonaffinity purified rabbit anti-tubulin serum provided by JA Connolly, which has also been characterized previously (5). The tubulin antiserum provided by Brinkley was used undiluted, whereas the tubulin antiserum provided by Connolly was used diluted 1:20 in PBS. In both instances, the cells were incubated for 45 to 60 minutes at $37°$ C and 100% humidity, followed by several rinses in PBS, and then incubated in fluorescein-conjugated goat anti-rabbit IgG (Meloy) diluted 1:10 with PBS for 30 minutes. The cells were rinsed several times in PBS and finally mounted on glass slides in a drop of glycerol:PBS 9:1 vol/vol at pH 9.5 to 10.0. The slides were coded and then examined and scored in a Zeiss universal fluorescence microscope so that the observer was unaware of the nature of each slide.

CPK Activity

The CPK activity was determined in heparinized plasma. The assay was in kit form (Bio-Dynamics/BMC). The substrate for CPK control was a nonhuman matrix (Sigma), and controls were included in each set of assays. Creatine phosphate and adenosine diphosphate were used as substrates, and substrate conditions were optimal. A faster reaction rate in this so-called "reverse reaction" made the test more sensitive, allowing us to use smaller sample volumes. The assay did not require sample blanks. The sensitivity of the test was important because in female carriers of DMD, the CPK activity is often only slightly increased. Creatine phosphokinase is a sulfhydryl enzyme and is rapidly inactivated in serum. Reactivation with glutathione in this assay was an important consideration, because samples were stored frozen for approximately 1 week at

$-20°$ C until used. Adenosine monophosphate was added to inhibit myokinase activity, which caused interference. This system was also free of sulfates that influence kinetic rates. For studies of plasma, heparin is the anticoagulant of choice because it does not have the inhibitory effect of certain other antico-agulants. The CPK activity was monitored on a Beckman model 25 spectropho-tometer at 340 nm and 30° C constant temperature. The data were then corrected to 25° C so they could be reported in international units per liter. A minimum of 6 readings 1 minute apart were obtained for each sample. The normal range of CPK values in this study was not adjusted for age and sex.

RESULTS

The main objective of this study was to determine, in experiments scored blind, whether the mononuclear cell spreading and microtubule counts of obligate carriers with normal CPK levels more closely resembled those of patients with DMD or normal subjects. The preliminary results (Table 1) are based on a relatively small sample size and should be considered tentative until more data are accumulated, especially because information on false positives is not adequately addressed in this article.

The average CPK value for our 38 control subjects was 35 mU/ml (26 adults, 35.1 mU/ml; 12 children, 31.6 mU/ml); for 29 patients with DMD, 1,223 mU/ml; for 6 obligate carriers, 97.5 mU/ml; and for 35 probable and possible carriers, 28.5 mU/ml. Mononuclear cells maintained in culture medium for 6 days are shown for a normal subject in Figure 1 and for a patient with DMD in Figure 2. Most of the cells in these figures are monocytes, as determined by an esterase stain. As observed in the phase contrast microscope, most of the cells in Figure 1 are relatively flat, whereas the cells in Figure 2 are hemispheric (see arrows). Approximately 61% of cells from the 38 normal subjects spread very flat, whereas only 34% of those from the 29 patients with DMD were flat (Table 1). This difference between patients with DMD and control subjects is significant at $P = 0.002$ by the Mann-Whitney U test. After 6 days in culture,

Table 1 Frequency of Cytoplasmic Microtubule Complexes in Mononuclear Cells

Sample Size	Normal Controls (n = 38)	Carriers (Obligate, Probable Possible) (n = 41)	DMD (n = 29)
CPK, mU/ml	35	40	1,223
Flat mononuclear cells, %	61	41	34
+CMTC %	74	20	16
I CMTC %	9	55	27
−CMTC %	17	25	56

CMTC +, Full cytoplasmic microtubule complex. In each case, at least 200 cells were counted. A cell was considered positive only if numerous microtubules radiated to the cell surface.

Abbreviations: DMD, Duchenne muscular dystrophy; CPK, creatine phosphokinase; CMTC, cyto-plasmic microtubule complex (+, full complement of cytoplasmic microtubule complex; −, diminished microtubules; I, intermediate between + and −.)

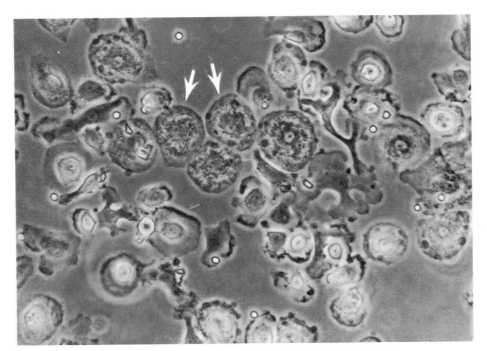

Fig. 1. Mononuclear cells from a normal subject as observed in the phase contrast microscope. After 5 to 7 days in culture, most of the cells are relatively flat (arrows). Compare with Figure 2.

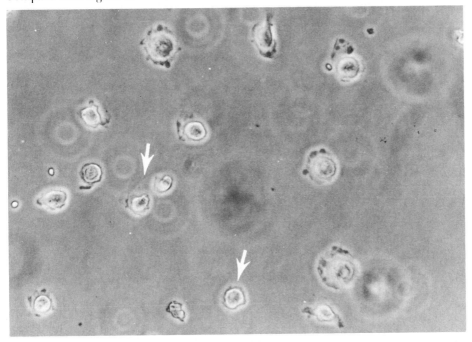

Fig. 2. Mononuclear cells from a patient with Duchenne muscular dystrophy as observed in the phase contrast microscope. After 5 to 7 days in culture, most of the cells are hemispheric (arrows).

an average of 41% of mononuclear cells from all carriers (obligate, probable, and possible) were flat (Table 1), whereas 26.5% of cells from obligate carriers were flat. The difference between obligate carriers and normal subjects was significant at $P = 0.002$, and the difference between the remaining carriers (possible and probable) and control subjects was significant at $P = 0.01$.

The raw data on the percentage of flat mononuclear cells in patients with DMD, control subjects, and carriers is illustrated in Figure 3. The numbers within the boxes represent each subject's CPK value expressed in mU/ml. The mean ± SD percentage of spreading i.e., flat, mononuclear cells for normal persons was 61.1 ± 9.8%; for patients with DMD, 33.9 ± 14.6%; for all carriers, 41.4 ± 15.6%. Initial inspection of the data suggest that there is a significant difference between patients with DMD and control subjects, and that the carriers' data are randomly distributed. It should be pointed out that of all carriers' specimens examined for spreading, only 6 were from obligate carriers,

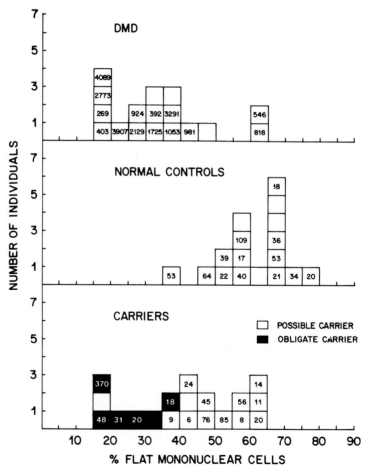

Fig. 3. Comparative mononuclear cell spreading data for patients with Duchenne muscular dystrophy (DMD), normal control subjects, and carriers of DMD. The numbers within the boxes represent the average of each subject's creatine phosphokinase values, expressed in mU/ml.

and the mean ± SD percentage of spreading for this group was 26.5 ± 7.9%. Many of the other carriers tested were possible carriers (i.e., sisters of patients with DMD, whose chance of being a carrier was only 50%) and some of these subjects were probably normal (many had normal CPK values). However, if we assume that anyone at 50% or greater risk of being a carrier of DMD has mononuclear cells with a spreading value 2 SD below the average for normal persons (41.5%), our data indicate that all of our obligate carriers fall within this category. Most of these obligate carriers had normal CPK values.

Cell spreading values for at least 2 other subjects at risk fell below this range. One had a normal CPK value and would have been considered normal by currently used techniques. Only one of our normal control subjects had less than 40% flat mononuclear cells; however this person had slightly increased CPK activity. There is no way to be sure that persons at risk are actually carriers, but it does seem interesting that mononuclear cells from all of our obligate carriers spread poorly. Obviously, many more obligate carriers and persons at risk of being carriers must be studied with these techniques. We certainly are not suggesting that this spreading assay is a replacement for CPK tests, but we do suggest that it might be an easily accomplished aid in genetic counseling. Our data indicate that there is not a clear relationship between CPK and spreading: some obligate carriers had normal CPK values, but 1 had a greatly increased level. All, however, had spreading values 2 SD below normal.

We decided to test the spreading assay by another technique. In view of our previous observations on microtubules in avian dystrophy, we stained these mononuclear cells with a tubulin antiserum and looked for differences in cytoplasmic microtubule complexes (CMTC) with the fluorescence microscope (6). In these experiments all coverslips were scored blind so that the observer was not aware of the nature of each slide. For practical purposes, we subdivided the cells into 3 categories, as illustrated in Figure 4. A cell was considered "positive" (+CMTC) if numerous microtubules radiated to the cell surface and most cells were quite flat (Fig. 4A). A cell was considered "negative" (−CMTC) if there were few elongated, intact microtubules (Fig. 4B). These cells were either flat or round and contained small dot-like areas of tubulin or were completely diminished in microtubules. A more difficult category is the one illustrated in Figure 4C, which we termed "intermediate" (I CMTC). This type of cell was not very common in control subjects or patients with DMD, but appeared frequently in carriers. These cells were usually more hemispheric than the cells illustrated in Figure 4A and appeared to protrude off the substrate into the culture medium. As illustrated in Figure 4B, we often observed both areas where microtubules radiated to the cell surface and areas with diminished microtubules.

The average results for 15 subjects are shown in Table 1. Clearly, the percentage of +CMTC cells was much higher in normal subjects (74%) than carriers (20%) or patients with DMD (16%). The percentage of −CMTC cells indicated that in normal subjects and carriers, 17% and 25% of the cells, respectively, had diminished microtubules; in patients with DMD, microtubules were diminished in 56% of the cells. As with the cell-spreading assay, we again urge caution in interpreting these results, because they are based on a relatively small sample size.

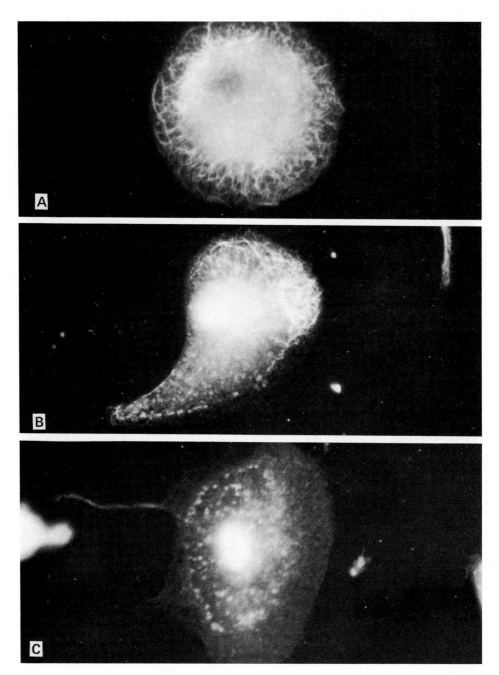

Fig. 4. Mononuclear cells stained with a tubulin antiserum and observed in the flourescence microscope. **(A)** This cell is considered to be "positive" (microtubules radiate out to the cell margins). **(B)** This cell is considered to be "intermediate": it has some areas with intact microtubules and some areas with diminished microtubules. **(C)** This cell is considered to be "negative," i.e., it contains mostly diminished microtubules.

796

To test this microtubule assay in a typical genetic counseling situation, we examined the pedigrees of 2 families with a history of DMD (Fig. 5). In the top pedigree, Subject I,1 has 3 sons with DMD, but no other known male relative with DMD. This subject is considered a probable carrier for DMD, but has a normal CPK value (20 mU/ml). The microtubule assay showed that Subject I,1 has a large number of I CMTC, and her daughter (Subject II,1) has almost an identical pattern of CMTC. Subject II,1, however, has an increased CPK level and, based on family pedigree and CPK analysis, would probably be considered to be at high risk of being a carrier of DMD. All 3 sons with DMD in this family (Subjects II,2; II,3; II,4) had greatly diminished CMTC values.

The pedigree of the other family we examined is illustrated at the bottom of Figure 5. In this family, Subject II,1 had 2 sons (Subjects III,2 and III,3) with DMD and, like the at-risk carrier in the top pedigree, would be considered a probable carrier. Three items concerning microtubules are of interest in this family. First, Subject II,1's mother (I,1) was still living and had a completely normal CMTC value. This, in fact, might suggest that the dystrophic gene is not present in somatic cells from Subject I,1 but is present in those of Subject II,1. Another interpretation is that this assay may not be valid in older persons; the number of control subjects studied is inadequate to be sure. Second, Subject II,1 had a high percentage of I CMTC cells and a normal CPK value. Finally,

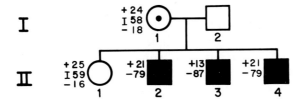

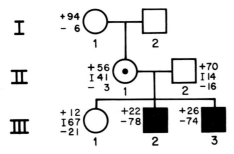

Fig. 5. Two families with patients with Duchenne muscular dystrophy studied for the percentage of mononuclear cells with various types of microtubule profiles. The numbers to the left of each individual represent the percentage of each type of cell illustrated in Figure 4 (+, positive for radiating microtubules; −, negative for microtubules; I, intermediate, with some areas of intact microtubules and some areas of diminished microtubules).

her daughter (III,1) also had a normal CPK value, but a large percentage of I CMTC cells, as did the other carriers we had studied. Based on these assays, we cannot be sure that Subject III,1 is a carrier of DMD, but we feel confident in stating that the microtubules in her cultured mononuclear cells are quite different from those of known normal persons we have studied.

DISCUSSION

The preliminary results of this study suggest that there are striking differences in mononuclear cell spreading between patients with DMD and normal control subjects. In addition, the microtubules in DMD mononuclear cells appear to be greatly diminished when compared to those of control cells. These differences in microtubules may be related to an inherent abnormality in the ability of DMD mononuclear cells to spread. However, the results of this study are consistent with numerous reports of systemic membrane defects in blood cells and muscle tissue of patients with DMD. In addition to these differences between patients with DMD and normal control subjects, we have also observed that cells from most at-risk carriers display intermediate levels of spreading and microtubules. Even though these observations were made with a very small sample of obligate carriers, it should be pointed out that all of the obligate carriers we studied had a profile of mononuclear cell spreading more closely resembling that of patients with DMD than that of normal subjects. The obvious value of this spreading assay is to help identify carriers of DMD when CPK values are normal. In this study, all but one of the obligate carriers had relatively low (i.e., normal) CPK values, but all of these carriers had mononuclear cells that spread poorly (i.e., 2 SD or more below the average for the normal control subjects).

In conclusion, based on these limited initial results, we believe that additional studies are warranted to test the validity of these carrier detection techniques more adequately. Obviously, more obligate carriers need to be studied to determine the false-negative rate, and more normal subjects need to be studied to determine the false-positive rate before such techniques can be applied to genetic counseling.

ACKNOWLEDGMENTS

This work was supported by a grant to Jerry W Shay from the Muscular Dystrophy Association. The help and valuable discussions with Dr. Feit and Dr. Faria are sincerely appreciated.

REFERENCES

1. Ebashi S, Toyokura Y, Momoi H, et al: High creatine phosphokinase activity of sera of progressive muscular dystrophy patients. J Biochem (Tokyo) 46:103–104, 1959

2. Dreyfus JC, Schapira G, Demos J: Étude de la creatine-kinase serique chez les myopathes et leur familles. Rev Fr Etud Clin Biol 5:384–388, 1960

3. Dubowitz V: Carrier detection and genetic counseling in Duchenne dystrophy. Dev Med Child Neurol 17:352–356, 1975

4. Brinkley BR, Fistel SH, Marcum JM, et al: Microtubules in cultured cells: indirect immunofluorescent staining with tubulin antibody. Int Rev Cytol 63:59–95, 1980

5. Connolly JA, Kalnins VI, Cleveland DW, et al: Intracellular localization of the high molecular weight microtubule accessory protein by indirect immunofluorescence. J Cell Biol 76:781–786, 1978

6. Shay JW, Fuseler JW: Diminished microtubules in fibroblast cells derived from inherited dystrophic muscle explant. Nature 278:178–180, 1979.

DISCUSSION

Dr. Henry Epstein: If your tentative conclusions are generally valid, what are the functional consequences of the severe defects in microtubules that you have reported in platelets, mononuclear cells, and leukocytes of patients with Duchenne muscular dystrophy (DMD) or carriers?

Dr. Jerry Shay: We have looked at fibroblasts and muscle from patients with DMD; in no instance have we ever found any differences in microtubules. The microtubule differences are not present in any cells subjected to trypsinization; that is a most important point. In addition, there does not seem to be a structural defect in microtubules obtained from dystrophic cells. The altered microtubules might, in fact, be a secondary effect; we are not saying that it represents a primary defect in microtubules. One could speculate, however, that a membrane leakage problem in DMD that leads to increased intracellular calcium could induce the microtubule profiles that we see. Did I answer your question?

Dr. Henry Epstein: Well, in part. Are you saying that these alterations in microtubules, secondary or not, have no functional consequences in those cells?

Dr. Jerry Shay: I cannot say for sure. As far as I know, there are no immunologic problems in patients with DMD.

Dr. Jarvis Seegmiller: Have you looked yet in permanent lymphoblast lines established from peripheral lymphocytes of affected patients by Epstein-Barr virus transformation to see whether this kind of defect persists in permanent cell culture?

Dr. Jerry Shay: We have not looked at virus-transformed lymphocytes for these microtubule alterations but would be glad to if you would send them to us.

Dr. Jarvis Seegmiller: We have been using permanent lymphoblast lines transformed by Epstein-Barr virus for detailed biochemical studies of a number of other human hereditary diseases and have devised a way of shipping blood samples so that the lymphocytes remain viable for several days. Perhaps the same procedure could be used for shipping lymphocytes to your laboratory for testing, if further studies warrant extension of your test. How many probable and positive obligate heterozygotes have you tested, and what were the results?

Dr. Jerry Shay: We looked at 7 obligate carriers and 42 carriers altogether. We pooled the data for probable and possible carriers. You have to recognize in the histogram I showed of the carriers, that many of those subjects were only at 50% risk of being a carrier (they are sisters of patients with DMD). Some of them have normal CK activity, so probably some are perfectly normal. Pooling our data that way makes the data on the carriers look worse statistically. We try to put our data in the worse possible light by placing anybody who is at 50% risk or more in one pool versus obligate carriers identified by pedigree analysis.

With regard to the inclusions, they have been seen in normal individuals. Dr. Malech has reported that lymphocytes from people who have had viral infections have an increased number of these inclusions. It has also been observed by Dr. Heinkart, I believe, that lymphocytes with the Fc receptor have an increased number of these inclusions. Some normal persons have a lot of them and some do not. We do not understand what the inclusions are, but some of the membrane-bound inclusions appear to contain tubulin. The structures we observed in the fluorescence microscope are within an appropriate size range to be these inclusions. In addition, tubular structures in these inclusions are about 240 Å across and you can count the subunits in them. They have the right number of subunits to be microtubules.

Dr. Fred Roisen: Are you familiar with the work of Drs. Folkman and Moscona (1978) who used poly(2-hydroxyethyl methacrylate) to vary substrate adhesiveness? I believe you could use their techniques to enhance the differences among your various test groups and thus achieve a significantly increased sensitivity. We have had success with neuroblastoma cells, i.e., we have been able to cause additional spreading. I also have a question concerning whether the defect is in the loss of tubulin subunits in their assembly. Have you been able to alter the shape of these dystrophic cells and cause them to elongate or increase their spreading by adding either dibutylryl cAMP to enhance microtubule assembly or by putting them in a high level of exogenous calcium to disrupt further their intact microtubules?

Dr. Jerry Shay: We have done some of those experiments, but the results are tentative because of the limited number we have looked at. When we add exogenous dibutyryl cAMP, the Duchenne cells spread back out. When we add exogenous calcium they tend to get more round. We know that high levels of calcium in vitro depolymerize microtubules, and these tubulin assembly reactions are usually accomplished in the presence of ethyleneglycol tetra-acetic acid (EGTA). In some of our other studies in which we have added EGTA to dystrophic cells, it seems to cause them to spread flatter.

Dr. Alfred Stracher: We also have studied platelets from patients with DMD. We have compared some of the physiologic functioning of DMD platelets and their secretion-aggregation properties with those from normal individuals and have found no differences. I would suggest, as has Dr. Epstein, such a derangement in microtubular structure would profoundly affect secretion and aggregation. Since we have not seen this, I would like to get your comments on this result.

Dr. Jerry Shay: We have not examined the platelets in all of our patients with DMD, and it is entirely possible that our observations do not reflect the condition of the cells in vivo. All our cells are cultured in medium containing AB-positive serum, and these observations on microtubules may be cell culture–induced artifacts.

Dr. Klaus Wrogemann: These changes in shape that you see remind me very much of reversible changes in shape that one can see in cultured macrophages with E-type prostaglandins. It would be very interesting to see whether you could produce such changes in your cells with prostaglandins, or whether you could prevent the differences between carriers and controls by inhibitors of prostaglandin synthesis.

Dr. Jerry Shay: We have not looked at E-type prostaglandins. That is a good point.

61
Capping in Carrier Detection

Hanns-Dieter F. Gruemer, MD

Barbara M. Goldsmith, BS

Walter E. Nance, MD, PhD

Nathan A. Pickard, PhD

Edward R. Isaacs, MD

Edwin C. Myer, MD

The hypothesis that Duchenne and other muscular dystrophies may be the manifestations of generalized cell membrane defects has triggered the interest of many investigators. Rowland has recently reviewed the evidence for, as well as the limitations of, the membrane hypothesis (1).

Our suggestion to apply the lymphocyte capping test as a cell-surface marker or as an indicator for a cell surface-associated abnormality in patients with muscular dystrophy originated with the observation that injections of imipramine and serotonin into rats led to a considerable increase of creatine kinase (CK) activity in serum (2). It was subsequently found that in isolated lymphocytes these drugs almost completely inhibited the cell surface aggregation of membrane proteins into a single polar cap (3).

Membrane proteins of some cells, when cross-linked with certain ligands, have the ability to aggregate. B lymphocytes demonstrate aggregation on cross-linking with antibodies to cell surface immunoglobulins (SIg); T lymphocytes, with the lectin concanavalin A (Con A). After stimulation with anti-immunoglobulins, the surface proteins of B lymphocytes pass from an initially uniform pattern through stages of clustering and patching to the final aggregation as a single polar cap on the cell surface before shedding, or endocytosis, of the fluorescent-labeled protein aggregate takes place. Con A stimulated aggregation which primarily involves T lymphocytes, appears to proceed directly from the uniform pattern to the capping stage.

Our original proposal of a membrane or membrane-associated defect in lymphocytes of persons affected with Duchenne muscular dystrophy (DMD), as well as of carriers, was based on the observation of diminished capping by 2 ligands with selectivities for different sites. Satisfactory results require the use of polyvalent anti-human immunoglobulin because of greater sensitivity in carrier detection than is obtained with Con A. We have evaluated 117 simultaneous comparisons of both techniques. We will describe our findings and summarize our experience with 111 female relatives of patients with DMD.

METHODS

We have recently provided a detailed account of our capping procedure (5), which differs substantially from those used in many research laboratories (6, 7). In brief, blood is collected in sodium heparin vacutainers; the plasma is

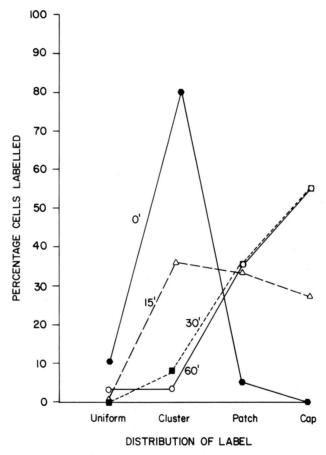

Fig. 1. Effect of incubation time on capping at 37° C. While kept below 4° C, most cells are in the uniform or clustered distributions; within minutes after warming to 37° C, the ligand-receptor complexes redistribute such that within 30 minutes at least 48% of the cells are in the capped state. With continued exposure to 37° C, there is no further increase in capping; in fact, counting at 60 minutes of incubation becomes difficult to perform as endocytosis and shedding result in fewer cells being labeled.

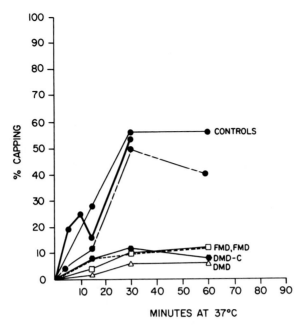

Fig. 2. The effect of incubation time at 37° C on the capping process in 3 normal control subjects, 3 patients with muscular dystrophy, and 1 carrier of mucular dystrophy. FMD denotes facioscapulohumeral muscular dystrophy; DMD, Duchenne muscular dystrophy; DMD-C, the carrier status of DMD.

separated by centrifugation and the cells are resuspended in Seligmann's balanced salt solution, containing ethylenediamine tetra-acetate to complex metals. Ficoll-Paque is layered beneath the cell suspension; after centrifugation, the mononuclear leukocyte layer is carefully aspirated. The residual cells are lysed with distilled water. After the cells have been washed 3 times in Seligmann's balanced salt solution, they are labeled at 2 to 4° C with fluorescein isothio-cyanate-conjugated polyvalent anti-human immunoglobulin from goat, washed again several times, and finally incubated at 37° C for 30 minutes. Figures 1 and 2 demonstrate that this incubation time is optimal under our experimental conditions. A wet-mount slide of the cell suspension is prepared for viewing under the microscope, and 50 cells are identified according to their pattern within 20 minutes at most. We use a low-intensity fluorescence microscope with a footswitch that allows us to alternate rapidly between fluorescence and tungsten light to distinguish between the cells to be counted and those to be disregarded. The proficiency in cell pattern recognition largely determines the success of this method for patient and carrier identification.

An aliquot of the washed cell suspension is used for labeling with fluorescein-conjugated Con A at concentrations that are somewhat inhibitory to the aggregation of cell-surface proteins. The interpretation of capping patterns is easier with Con A stimulation than with a polyvalent antibody stimulation, but unfortunately, Con A is not quite so reliable for carrier detection in individual cases (see later)

RESULTS

In a retrospective study, we analyzed the findings in our patients with sex-linked DMD and in their relatives, in whom we performed capping studies both by the surface immunoglobulin (SIg) procedure and the Con A test. To establish whether the 2 methods agree, we divided our population into 4 groups as shown in Figure 3. Group A consists of 12 patients with Duchenne-type dystrophy with low capping. The next two groups, B and C, are female relatives of the afflicted subjects; group B contains 40 female relatives who had decreased capping and group C includes 25 female relatives with normal capping. Group D included 40 normal control subjects, including fathers and other apparently

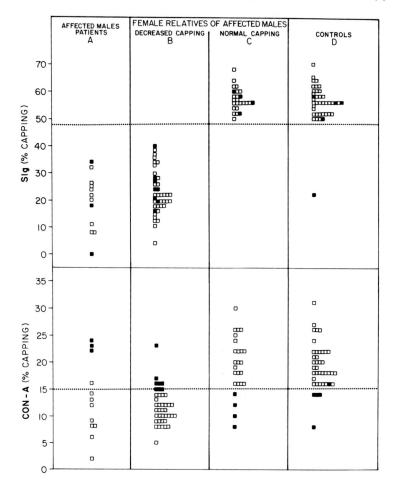

□ SIg + CON-A AGREE
■ SIg + CON-A DISAGREE

Fig. 3. Comparison between capping results by the surface immunoglobulin (SIg) technique with polyvalent anti-human immunoglobulin from goat and those by the concanavalin A (CON A) procedure in the lymphocytes of 117 subjects. Open squares symbolize agreement between the SIg and CON A techniques; closed squares show disparity.

healthy adult male relatives of the patients with DMD, as well as some young female employees. The upper part of Figure 3 demonstrates the capping results by the SIg technique. Groups A and B, with capping results of less than 48%, are well separated from groups C and D, with normal capping of more than 48%. The results of Con A-induced capping are demonstrated in the lower part of Figure 3. Although there is some overlap among these groups, statistical analysis by Student's t test demonstrates a significant difference between the mean of group D (19.4%) and the means of groups A or B (11.6 and 11.7%), respectively ($P < 0.005$). That is, the capping results with Con A support the findings with the SIg technique.

We have evaluated the results of the capping test of 111 female relatives within 45 kindreds that included 1 or more patients affected with DMD (Table 1). The study revealed that the number of female carriers in our population (maternal grandmothers, mothers, sisters, and maternal aunts of affected patients) exceeded that predicted from the Haldane assumption.

DISCUSSION

Under our experimental conditions, the optimal incubation time for whole goat anti-human polyvalent immunoglobulins that stimulated capping at 37° C is close to 30 minutes. Ho and coworkers (8), under similar conditions, found 15 minutes to be the optimal incubation time. Both of these incubation periods are somewhat longer than the 5-minute time reported by Hauser and associates (6), who used fragments of rabbit-derived anti-immunoglobulins with F(ab')$_2$ reagents and polyvalent rabbit anti-human immunoglobulin. Alexander (9, 10) recently reported that goat IgG has a lower affinity for Fc receptors than does rabbit IgG, and observed that cell-separating gels, e.g., Ficoll-Paque, alters the affinity of lymphocyte Fc receptors to immunoglobulins. Thus, differences in affinity to cell-surface receptors, and therewith in cross-linkage, might have a bearing on the kinetics of the capping process itself.

Because our surface immunoglobulin procedure is potentially not specific for B lymphocytes, a disadvantage balanced by its applicability in routine use, we included experiments with Con A, which preferentially caps thymus-derived lymphocytes (11). Despite the fact that Con A capping permits an overlap between the normal and the abnormal range and causes a greater experimental variability than does the SIg technique, the Con A procedure is helpful in confirming the results of the SIg method in Duchenne-type dystrophy. Ho and coworkers (8) demonstrated independently the usefulness of the Con A procedure in conjunction with the SIg technique in 19 patients with DMD, 13 mother carriers, and 52 normal control subjects. Similar results were obtained in 19 families by Bader and colleagues (12).

Elaborating on their previous studies of dystrophic chickens, Shay and associates (13 and chapter 60, this book) observed a diminished complex of microtubules in platelets and leukocytes of afflicted subjects and obligate carriers of Duchenne-type dystrophy as compared to normal control subjects. If confirmed, the findings are consistent with our original hypothesis of a membrane or membrane-associated defect in leukocytes.

Table 1. Comparison of Capping Results to Carrier Status as Predicted by the Haldane Hypothesis versus a No-Mutation Assumption[a]

Subjects	No.	Capping			% of Population with Carrier Status Predicted	
		Normal	Decreased	% Decreased	Haldane Hypothesis	Assuming No Mutation
Maternal grandmothers						
Total	12	1	11	92	33 (R)	100 (A)
Mothers						
Obligate carrier	15	0	15	100	100	100
Simplex	30	8	22	73	<67 (A)	100 (A)
Total	45	8	37	82	67 (R)	100 (A)
Daughters of						
Obligate carrier mothers	6	3	3	50	50 —	50 (A)
Simplex mothers	34	18	16	47	<33 (A)	50 (A)
Total	40	21	19	48	33 (R)	50 (A)
Sisters of mothers						
Total	16	8	8	50	17 (R)	50 (A)

[a] An obligate carrier as defined here is a mother with 2 or more affected sons or 1 affected son and at least 1 other known affected male in the kindred; a simplex mother refers to a woman with 1 affected son in a kindred and no other affected males. (A) denotes acceptance of the null hypothesis of no difference between observed and expected frequencies; (R) denotes rejection of the null hypothesis by the Chi square test (p < 0.05) for the Haldane and no mutation assumption.

Roses and coworkers (14) have repeatedly emphasized that studies with serum lactate dehydrogenase isozyme-5 activity measurements (14) as well as with endogenous phosphorylation of peak II activity in red cells have disclosed an excess of carriers for the DMD trait. More recently, we have also noted a low mutation rate by the capping technique (15). Table 1 summarizes our findings in 111 female relatives of patients with DMD. All 15 obligatory carriers demonstrated decreased capping. In simplex families 73% of the mothers showed decreased capping compared to the less than 67% expected under the Haldane hypothesis, which states that the genes of a genetic lethal that are lost must be replaced by new mutations if the pool of defective genes is to remain stable. The carrier frequency shown in Table 1 has been estimated under the assumption that the mutation rate in males equals the rate in females, whereas the percentage given under the extreme postulate of "no mutation" makes no such assumption.

If lymphocyte capping is used to detect carriers, the actual percentage of carriers we have observed is generally close to the percentages given in the "no mutation" column of Table 1, with the exception of the mothers of simplex cases. Our population suffers from an ascertainment bias for kindreds with a single affected son. However, this bias should not influence the observed frequency of carriers in other categories of female relatives in the table. Our earlier estimate of an 8-fold higher mutation rate in males than in females, when applying Haldane's equation (16), might have to be revised in the light of the high percentage of carriers in maternal grandmothers. Further studies will show whether this trend continues. At face value, our present data suggest that relatively few cases of DMD appear to be new mutations, an observation that is at variance with the conventional assumption that one-third of these cases should be mutational in origin.

ACKNOWLEDGMENTS

This work was supported by a grant from the Muscular Dystrophy Association.

REFERENCES

1. Rowland LP: Biochemistry of muscle membranes in Duchenne muscular dystrophy. Muscle Nerve 3:3–20, 1980

2. Silverman LM, Gruemer H-D: Sarcolemmal membrane changes related to enzyme release in the imipramine/serotonin experimental animal model. Clin Chem 22:1710–1714, 1976

3. Verrill HL, Gruemer H-D, Pickard NA: Studies into the mechanisms of cellular enzyme release. I. Alterations in membrane fluidity and permeability. Clin Chem 23:2219–2225, 1977

4. Pickard NA, Gruemer H-D, Verrill HL, et al: Systemic membrane defect in the proximal muscular dystrophies. N Engl J Med 299:841–846, 1978

5. Goldsmith BM, Gruemer H-D, Hawley RJ, et al: The contribution of assays for lymphocyte capping and creative kinase to detection of the Becker-type dystrophy trait. Clin Chem 26:754–759, 1980

6. Hauser SL, Weiner HL, Bresman MJ, et al: Lymphocyte capping in muscular dystrophy. Neurology (NY) 29:1419–1421, 1979

7. Stern CMM, Kahan MC, Dubowitz V: Lymphocyte capping in Duchenne muscular dystrophy. Lancet 1:300, 1979

8. Ho AD, Stojakowits S, Reiter B, et al: Capping of lymphocytes in patients and carriers of Duchenne muscular dystrophy. Klin Wochenschr 58:377–381, 1980

9. Alexander EL, Sanders SK: F(ab')$_2$ reagents are not required if goat, rather than rabbit, antibodies are used to detect human surface immunoglobulins. J Immunol 119:1084–1088, 1977

10. Alexander EL, Titus JA, Segal DM: Quantitation of Fc receptors and surface immunoglobulin is affected by cell isolation procedures using Plasmagel and Ficoll-Hypaque. J Immunol Methods 22:263–272, 1978

11. Schreiner GF, Unanue ER: Membrane and cytoplasmic changes in B lymphocytes. Adv Immunol 24:37–167, 1976

12. Bader PI, Creason MT, Bender CJ: Capping studies in carrier detection of the X-linked muscular dystrophies (abstract). J Clin Res 28:487A, 1980

13. Shay JW, Fuseler JW: Diminished microtubules in fibroblast cells derived from inherited muscular dystrophic muscle explants. Nature 278:178–180, 1979

14. Roses AD, Roses MJ, Nicholson GA, et al: Lactate dehydrogenase isoenzyme 5 in detecting carriers of Duchenne muscular dystrophy. Neurology (Minneap) 27:414–421, 1977

15. Roses AD, Appel SH: Erythrocyte spectrin peak II phosphorylation in Duchenne muscular dystrophy. J Neurol Sci 29:185–193, 1976

16. Haldane JBS: The rate of spontaneous mutation of a human gene. J Genet 31:317–326, 1935

62

Lymphocyte Capping in the Muscular Dystrophies: A Review

Stephen L. Hauser, MD

Kenneth A. Ault, MD

Michael J. Bresnan, MD

Howard L. Weiner, MD

Although the pathogenesis of the muscular dystrophies remains unknown, some data support the concept of a defect in muscle membrane (1). This has prompted investigators to search for evidence of a more generalized membrane abnormality. In the erythrocyte, surface membrane alterations have been reported in some electron microscopic studies (2–5) but not in others (6, 7). Increased red blood cell fragility has been suggested (8), but in vivo erythrocyte survival is normal (9). Recent studies have focused on the mechanisms of cellular capping as a model of membrane function, and capping techniques have now been applied to the muscular dystrophies.

CAPPING

Capping refers to the membrane changes that follow the binding of various ligands to cell-surface glycoprotein receptors. Under proper conditions, bound receptors rapidly redistribute along the cell surface membrane, aggregating into patches and finally into a single polar cap that is then expelled or endocytosed. Capping has been studied most intensively in the lymphocyte, but has also been observed in the red blood cell, fibroblast, and even in protozoan cells and may reflect a fundamental mechanism whereby cells interact with and respond to the external environment. For the lymphocyte, capping of surface receptors is related to cell motility, differentiation, and clonal expansion and may be important in the activation of the immune response. Although a variety of surface receptors on the human lymphocyte may undergo capping, the

811

redistribution after the cross-linking of surface immunoglobulin and of the concanavalin A binding site have been best characterized.

Immunoglobulin Capping

Human B cells are characterized by the presence of IgD and IgM on their cell surface. After the cross-linkage of surface immunoglobulin by fluorescein-labeled anti-immunoglobulin, B-cell capping is observed. Capping is energy-dependent, is associated with a change in cell shape and with stimulation of motility, and is complete by 5 minutes at 37° C. With longer incubation, caps are either ingested or shed, and new immunoglobulin gradually reappears on the cell surface.

Considerable evidence suggests that immunoglobulin cap formation requires a reversible interaction with the cytoplasmic skeleton, perhaps involving a contractile event. Capping is abolished by inhibition of the microfilament apparatus (10–11) or by an increase in intracellular calcium (12, 13). Local anesthetics, believed to disrupt interactions between the surface membrane and contractile proteins (14, 15), also inhibit immunoglobulin capping. Cytoplasmic actin (16) and myosin (17) accumulate under the surface cap, and the cross-linked surface immunoglobulin is bound to cytoplasmic actin (18).

Concanavalin A Capping

Lymphocyte capping induced by the plant lectin concanavalin A (con A) differs in several respects from the surface immunoglobulin cap. Con A caps primarily (although not exclusively) T cells. Capping proceeds slowly, requiring approximately 30 minutes of incubation at 37° C for completion. Participation of the microfilament system is not well established. Although some cytoplasmic actin and myosin are located under the con A cap (19, 20), the accumulation is less than that under the immunoglobulin cap (17). Whereas immunoglobulin capping precedes and can be dissociated from cell motility (21), con A capping requires simultaneous cell movement. As cytoplasmic streaming and cell movement begin, the bound con A gradually redistributes along the trailing edge of the membrane. Schreiner and Unanue (11) have postulated that con A capping reflects the passive backward flow of bound surface receptors as a consequence of cytoplasmic streaming. However, because con A is a multivalent ligand that may bind to and aggregate a variety of surface receptors, including surface immunoglobulin, there may well be more than one potential mechanism involved in cap formation.

CAPPING IN THE MUSCULAR DYSTROPHIES

Initial Report

In 1978, Pickard and colleagues (22) reported that lymphocytes from patients with muscular dystrophy had reduced capping after incubation with anti-immunoglobulin antibody. In addition, asymptomatic carriers displayed a similar reduction in immunoglobulin capping activity. Decreased percentages of capped B cells were seen in Duchenne, Becker, facioscapulohumeral, limb-girdle, and "congenital" dystrophy, but not in myotonic dystrophy. A total of 100 affected patients and suspected carriers were studied; all had reduced capping, and there was no overlap between their data and data for normal control subjects or patients with other neuorological diseases. Although the data were not presented in detail, con A capping was found to be similarly reduced in a smaller group of 22 dystrophic patients and carriers.

Subsequent Studies

Our patients population (23) was selected from patients and families attending the Muscular Dystrophy Clinic of Boston Children's Hospital Medical Center. Seven patients with Duchenne muscular dystrophy (DMD) and 2 with limb-girdle dystrophy were studied. Nine probable carriers (all with increased creatinine phosphokinase activity on at least one determination) were also investigated. Initial studies were performed using our laboratory's routine capping protocol. Lymphocytes were separated by standard techniques and labeled with fluoresceinated F(ab')$_2$ fragments of rabbit antihuman IgD and IgM. The washed, labeled cells were incubated for 5 minutes at 37° C and fixed. Cells were visually scored for fluorescence. A cell was defined as capped if fluorescent label occupied one-half or less of its circumference. All specimens were coded and read blindly by 2 different observers.

We found no differences among patients, carriers, and control subjects in either the percentage of labeled lymphocytes or the percentage of cells that were capped after incubation at 37° C for 15 minutes (Fig. 1). This was true whether the lymphocytes were prepared with or without monocyte depletion. Most cells from all samples aggregated immunofluorescence into surface caps. Even the lymphocytes that did not satisfy the criteria for capping (and thus were identified as cap-negative) demonstrated partial redistribution of surface label.

In an attempt to duplicate more closely the assay conditions of Pickard and

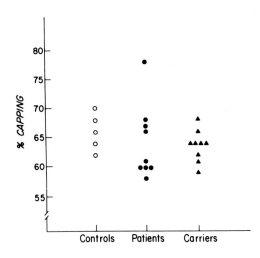

Fig. 1. Mean ± SEM percentage of labeled cells showing capping in control subjects (65.6 ± 1.5), patients (63.4 ± 0.9), and carriers (64.3 ± 2.1). (Reprinted with permission from Hauser SL, Weiner HL, Bresnan MJ, et al: Lymphocytes capping in muscular dystrophy. Neurology (NY) 29:1419–1421, 1979.)

coworkers (22), we incubated labeled lymphocytes for 30 minutes at 37° C. After this longer incubation, there was a marked decrease in the number of cells retaining label. This was consistent with our prior experience (24) that immunoglobulin caps are rapidly ingested or shed at 37° C. Nevertheless, of the relatively few cells retaining label at 30 minutes, most were capped and there were no differences among the groups studied. Finally, when lymphocytes were labeled with a polyspecific antihuman immunoglobulin, as was done by Pickard and associates, a larger fraction of cells retained label, and it was apparent that B cells were not exclusively identified. Even with this less specific fluorescent label, capping was observed after incubation for either 5 or 30 minutes and occurred to the same extent in patients, carriers, and control subjects.

In a parallel series of experiments, we investigated lymphocyte capping in 2 animal forms of muscular dystrophy. Lymphocytes were prepared from the spleens of dystrophic mice (129 dy/dy, Jackson Labs, Bar Harbor, ME) and cardiomyopathic hamsters (courtesy of Dr. F. Hamburger, Biorsch Institute, Cambridge, MA) and were labeled with polyspecific rabbit antimouse immunoglobulin or rabbit antihamster immunoglobulin. In neither instance was B-cell capping deficient when compared to that of normal animals.

The discrepancy between our data and those of Pickard and associates is not easily explained. Pickard and colleagues reported a lymphocyte preparation of more than 95% purity after Ficoll-Hypaque separation without prior monocyte depletion; in our hands, similar techniques yield a mixed lymphocyte-monocyte suspension of lesser purity. Monocytes will bind but not cap fluoresceinated immunoglobulin (24), will retain immunoflourescence after long incubation periods, and may be confused with lymphocytes under the light microscope (25). Second, although it has been reported that whole goat, as opposed to rabbit, antihuman immunoglobulin has a low affinity for the human Fc receptor (26), in our experience, use of $F(ab')_2$ fragments provides cleaner and more easily interpretable staining patterns and eliminates the potential problem of null cell (lymphocytes without conventional T- or B-cell surface markers) labeling via surface Fc receptors. Null cells do not cap after binding immunoglobulin via the Fc receptor. We consistently find that caps present at 5 minutes are lost by 30 minutes of incubation. It is possible that the cells retaining label at 30 minutes include a large number of null cells and/or monocytes and that, as reported by Pickard and colleagues, the decrease in capping percentages observed in patients and carriers is due to an increase in the ratio of these cells to conventional B lymphocytes. However, when we attempted to duplicate Pickard and associates' experimental conditions exactly, we still found no abnormalities in capping activity. Pickard and colleagues' associated finding of defective con A capping is not explained by any of the above mechanisms. Both studies were carried out "blind" and thus were not subject to observer bias.

Studies by Other Investigators

Four other groups have now documented their experience with lymphocyte capping in the muscular dystrophies. Three have failed to identify differences among patients, carriers, and control subjects. Stern and associates (27), using

Table 1. Lymphocyte Capping in the Muscular Dystrophies

Reference	No. of Patients	No. of Carriers	Fluoresceinated Reagent Used	Incubation (min)	Results
Pickard et al. (22)	61 (DMD, Becker, FSH, LG)	39 (DMD, Becker)	Anti-human Ig	30	Capping in all patients and carriers < that in controls
	12	10	Con A	30	
Hauser et al. (23)	9 (DMD, LG)	7 (DMD)	F(ab')₂ Anti-human IgM and IgD	5, 30	No differences among patients, carriers, controls
			Anti-human Ig	5, 30	
Stern et al. (27)	27 (DMD, LG)	21 (DMD)	Anti-human Ig	45	No differences among patients, carriers, controls
			Anti-human IgG	45	
			Anti-human IgD	45	
			Con A	45	
Bader (30)	26 (LG; Old Amish Schwartz kindred)	43 (16 Parents, 27 Sibs)	Anti-human Ig G,M,A.	30	Decreased capping in all patients and many (but not all) carriers
			Con A	30	
Sands and Harris (28)	3 (DMD)	13 (4 Obligate, 9 Possible)	F (ab')₂ Anti-human Ig	7	Decreased capping in 1/3 patients and 1/13 carriers only; others, normal
Sybert et al. (29)	—	4 (DMD)	F (ab')₂ Anti-human Ig M,D	5	No differences among patients, carriers, controls; no change with monocyte depletion
			Anti-human Ig	5, 30	

Abbreviations: DMD, Duchenne muscular dystrophy; FSH, fascioscapulohumeral; LG, limb-girdle.

815

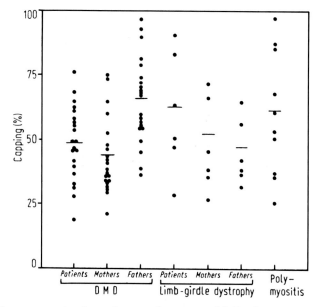

Fig. 2. Lymphocyte capping in patients and parents with Duchenne muscular dystrophy (DMD) and limb-girdle dystrophy and in patients with polymyositis. (Reprinted with permission from Stern CMM, Kahan MC, Dubowitz V: Lymphocyte capping in Duchenne muscular dystrophy (letter). Lancet 1:1300, 1979.)

a variety of fluoresceinated ligands including polyvalent antihuman immuno-globulin, class-specific immunoglobulin, and Con A, reported no consistent differences in the capping behavior of Duchenne and limb-girdle patients compared with control subjects (Fig. 2). Sands and Harris (28) described decreased capping in only one of 3 patients with DMD and in none of 4 obligate carriers. Sybert and associates (29), studying 4 carriers of DMD, also reported normal capping under a variety of conditions including short (5-minute) versus long (30-minute) incubation times, differing monocyte concentrations, and use of polyvalent whole immunoglobulin versus class-specific F(ab')$_2$ fragments. On the other hand, Bader (30) found diminished capping in Amish kindred with limb-girdle dystrophy as well as in their parents and unaffected siblings. These studies are summarized in Table 1.

In a related series of experiments, Newman (31) investigated con A capping on the surface of in vitro cultured fibroblasts and found no qualitative differences between patients with DMD (n = 6) and control subjects.

CONCLUSIONS

An association between muscular dystrophy and a major abnormality of lymphocyte capping remains unproved. Several considerations might argue against such an association. First, the various muscular dystrophies are clinically and genetically distinct, and it would be surprising if these disparate syndromes should share an identical functional membrane abnormality. Second, the finding that asymptomatic carriers and affected patients are equally impaired in cap formation is unexpected; in disease states characterized by recessive transmission, one usually expects the heterozygous state to display activity intermediate between normal and disease states. Third, if immunoglobulin capping is important to the activation of the B-cell immune response, then capping abnormalities might correlate with defective humoral immunity. Muscular dystrophy is not associated with an immune deficiency state. Fourth, if the mechanisms of immunoglobulin and con A capping are fundamentally different, it is surprising that the same abnormality should be found with both ligands.

Nevertheless, it is possible that a difference in reagents or technique is responsible for the different results obtained by various investigators, and it might be appropriate to arrange an exchange of materials and coded specimens to determine the role of lymphocyte capping in the study of muscular dystrophy.

REFERENCES

1. Mokri B, Engle AG: Duchenne dystrophy: electron microscopic findings pointing to a basic or early abnormality in the plasma membrane of the muscle fiber. Neurology (Minneap) 25:1111–1120, 1975

2. Lumb EJ, Emory AEH: Erythrocyte deformation in Duchenne muscular dystrophy. Br Med J 23:467–468, 1975

3. Matheson DW, Howland JL: Erythrocyte deformation in human muscular dystrophy. Science 184:165–166, 1973

4. Miller SE, Roses AD, Appel SH: Scanning electron microscopy studies in muscular dystrophy. Arch Neurol 33:172–174, 1976

5. Wakayama Y, Hodson A, Pleasure D, et al: Alteration in erythrocyte membrane structure in Duchenne muscular dystrophy. Ann Neurol 4:253–256, 1978

6. Matheson DW, Engel WK, Derrer EC: Erythrocyte shape in Duchenne muscular dystrophy. Neurology (Minneap) 26:1182–1183, 1976

7. Miale TD, Frias JL, Lawson DL: Erythrocytes in human muscular dystrophy. Science 187:453–454, 1975.

8. Fisher ER, Silvestri E, Vester JW, et al: Increased erythrocyte osmotic fragility in pseudohypertrophic muscular dystrophy. JAMA 236:955, 1976

9. Adornato BT, Corash L, Engel WK: Erythrocyte survival in Duchenne muscular dystrophy. Neurology (Minneap) 27:1093–1094, 1977

10. Taylor RB, Duffus WPH, Raff MC, et al: Redistribution of lymphocyte surface immunoglobulin molecules induced by anti-immunoglobulin antibody. Nature 233:225–229, 1971

11. Schreiner GF, Unanue ER: Membrane and cytoplasmic changes in B lymphocytes induced by ligand-surface immunoglobulin interaction. Adv Immunol 24:37–165, 1976

12. Schreiner GF, Unanue ER: Calcium sensitive modulation of Ig capping: evidence supporting a cytoplasmic control of ligand-receptor complexes. J Exp Med 143:15–31, 1976

13. Braun J, Fujiwara K, Pollard TD, et al: Two distinct mechanisms for redistribution of lymphocyte surface macromolecules. II. Contrasting effects of local anesthetics and calcium ionophore. J Cell Biol 79:419–426, 1978

14. Poste G, Papahadiopoulos D, Jacobson K, et al: Local anaesthetics increase susceptibility of untransformed cells to agglutination by Con A. Nature (Lond) 253:552–554, 1975

15. Schreiner GF, Unanue ER: The disruption of immunoglobulin caps by local anesthetics. Clin Immunol Immunopathol 6:264–269, 1976

16. Gabbiani G, Chaponnier C, Zumbe A, et al: Actin and tubulin co-cap with surface immunoglobulins in murine B lymphocytes. Nature 269:695–697, 1977

17. Braun J, Fujiwara K, Pollard TD, et al: Two distinct mechanisms for redistribution of lymphocyte surface macromolecules. I. Relationship to cytoplasmic myosin. J Cell Biol 79:409–418, 1978

18. Flanagan J, Koch GLE: Cross-linked surface Ig attaches to actin. Nature 273:278–281, 1978

19. Toh BH, Hard GC: Actin co-caps with concanavalin A receptors. Nature 269:695–697, 1977

20. Condeelis J: Isolation of concanavalin A caps during various stages of formation and their association with actin and myosin. J Cell Biol 80:751–758, 1979

21. Schreiner Gf, Unanue ER: The modulation of spontaneous and anti-Ig-stimulated motility of lymphocytes by cyclic nucleotides and adrenergic and cholinergic agents. J Immunol 114:802–808, 1975

22. Pickard NA, Gruemer HD, Verrill HC, et al: Systemic membrane defect in the proximal muscular dystrophies. N Engl J Med 299:841–846, 1978

23. Hauser SL, Weiner HL, Bresnan MJ, et al: Lymphocyte capping in muscular dystrophy. Neurology (NY) 29:1419–1421, 1979

24. Ault KA, Unanue ER: Comparison of the two types of immunoglobulin-bearing lymphocytes in human blood with regard to capping and motility. Clin Immunol Immunopathol 7:394–404, 1977

25. Reinherz EL, Moretta L, Roper M, et al: Human T-lymphocyte subpopulations defined by Fc receptors and monoclonal antibodies. J Exp Med 151:969–974, 1980

26. Alexander EL, Sanders SK: F(ab')$_2$ reagents are not required if goat, rather than rabbit, antibodies are used to detect human surface immunoglobulin. J Immunol 119:1084–1088, 1977

27. Stern CMM, Kahan MC, Dubowitz V: Lymphocyte capping in Duchenne muscular dystrophy (letter). Lancet 1:1300, 1979

28. Sands ME, Harris R: Lymphocyte capping and carrier detection in Duchenne muscular dystrophy (letter). Lancet 2:698, 1979

29. Sybert VP, Setran KN, Kadin ME: Lymphocyte capping in carriers of Duchenne muscular dystrophy (letter). N Engl J Med 301:724–725, 1979

30. Bader PI: Lymphocyte capping in Duchenne muscular dystrophy (letter). Lancet 2:306, 1979

31. Newman GC: Fluoroscein-conjugated concanavalin A staining of Duchenne muscular dystrophy skin fibroblasts (abstract). Neurology (NY) 30:401, 1980

DISCUSSION

Dr. Sergio Pena: We have looked at capping in 10 fibroblast strains from patients with Duchenne muscular dystrophy (DMD) using concanavalin A (con A)-peroxidase; there is no difference from normal. We also evaluated the cytoskeleton in these cultured fibroblasts with antitubulin, antiactin, antimyosin, and antifibronectin; again, there were no differences from normal. It looks like a lot of the abnormalities are not reproduced in cell cultures and are variably present in blood cells. I wonder whether what we are seeing is simply the result of a noxious procedure during isolation of these blood cells, e.g., excessive use of *g* forces. All of the results reported by Dr. Shay and Dr. Gruemer are negative in the sense that the cells are behaving, in a way, like damaged cells. With regard to Dr. Shay's results, of course, it would be impossible for patients with DMD to have such defects in their platelets or white cells in vivo (if they did, they would have a coagulation disorder or immune deficiency). So it would be interesting to see whether the DMD defect just causes the membrane to be more fragile to damage by isolation procedures. This could explain some of the defects described and also their lack of reproducibility in different laboratories.

Dr. Hanns-Dieter Gruemer: It is very difficult to respond; certainly, everything you have said is possible. I would only like to mention the findings by Neuman in fibroblasts: he did not see any qualitative difference, but did see some quantitative difference using con A. However, those experiments were rather difficult to interpret, and one would really have to see the published analysis.

Dr. Daniel Drachman: We sent to Dr. Meyers, of the Medical College of Virginia, some lymphocytes from 12 patients with DMD, 2 carriers, and 4 controls. In a coded double-blind study, we made every effort to fool Dr. Gruemer, even using duplicate coded samples from a single patient. Of 16 blood samples from 12 different patients with DMD, 15 were correctly identified by the immuno-globulin method; 5 of 7 were correctly identified by the con A method. Two samples were rejected as being uninterpretable. Of the 4 control samples, 3 were correctly identified by the immunoglobulin method, and 2 of 2 were correctly identified by the con A method. One of 2 definite carriers was correctly identified by both methods.

Dr. Alan Emery: Dr. Gruemer and Dr. Piccard very kindly let us have the precise details of their methodology. One of my colleagues, Dr. Alberto Horenstein, has repeated their methodology in minute detail and confirms that there is reduced capping in DMD. However, he has also found that it is significantly correlated with age and also with serum creatine kinase (CK) levels. In other words, as the disease progresses and the CK decreases, the reduction in capping becomes more obvious. Therefore, I have some doubt as to whether such a technique would be valuable in carrier detection.

Dr. Hanns-Dieter Gruemer: We have not found such a correlation with age or with CK.

Dr. Jerry Shay: Seeing that the cytoskeleton seems to be related to the capping phenomenon, I wonder whether either of you incubated your lymphocytes in cytochalasin B or an antimitotic agent such as colchicine to see what effect this would have on normal versus dystrophic capping with immunoglobulin and con A.

Dr. Hanns-Dieter Gruemer: We have done about 10 preliminary studies with colchicine in normal subjects and found an increase in capping with con A. In patients with DMD we did not find such an increase when the increase in the normal subjects was significant; it was not significant by the Run test in the patient with DMD. With cytochalasin B, capping was reduced in the normals to the same degree as in the patients with DMD.

Dr. Stephen Hauser: The effects of the cytochalasins on capping activity has been known for some time. Cytochalasin B is a very sensitive inhibitor of con A capping and less sensitive inhibitor of the immunoglobulin capping. Cyto-chalasin D is reported to be a more potent inhibitor of the immunoglobulin cap. Colchicine increases the rate of con A capping and, to a lesser extent, of immunoglobulin capping.

Dr. Richard Armstrong: We have studied a small group of 4 patients and 11 carriers, trying to reproduce Dr. Gruemer's technique. Overall, there appears to be a significant difference in capping between the patients with DMD and our normal control subjects, but the overlap of values would preclude its use as a clinical test.

Dr. Allen Roses: Dr. Hauser, I noticed that your cell medium lacks calcium. I would like to ask you and others who have not been able to obtain the same results, whether you use calcium-free medium?

Dr. Stephen Hauser: We used a calcium-containing medium, Hanks' balanced salt solution (BSS) supplemented with HEPES buffer. I do not recall the exact calcium concentration of that medium.

Dr. Allen Roses: It was 10 mM. Does calcium have an effect on capping?

Dr. Richard Armstrong: We examined that in several patients but could see no difference whether or not the medium contained calcium. We also compared Hanks' BSS with Seligman's solution; it made no difference.

Dr. Alan Emery: There is some evidence from Schneider's laboratory that when normal lymphocytes are exposed to the ionophore A23187, which increases calcium influx and raises intracellular calcium, the lymphocyte capping is reduced, thus mimicking the phenomenon seen in dystrophic lymphocytes.

63
Carrier Detection in Duchenne Muscular Dystrophy: A Critical Assessment

Peter S. Harper, MA, MD, FRCP

The relatively high incidence of Duchenne muscular dystrophy (DMD) (1), the severe burden that the disease imposes, and the possibility of transmission by healthy female relatives arising from its X-linked recessive inheritance are all factors that combine to make the accurate detection of heterozygous carriers one of the major aims in the prevention of this disorder. Indeed, carrier detection in this condition is perhaps the single most important problem in the field of genetic counseling for mendelian disorders and is of direct practical relevance to pediatricians, medical geneticists, and obstetricians quite apart from those working primarily in the field of muscle disease.

For many years, tests have been available which help in the identification of carriers, the most frequently used being an increased level of serum creatine kinase (CK) (2–8). Every year large numbers of women undergo carrier testing and are given genetic counseling based largely on the results of these tests; for many of them this advice is critical in determining whether they will or will not embark on childbearing.

Despite this, there is genereal agreement that our current methods of carrier detection are far from perfect, and that it is impossible for many potential carriers to be identified unequivocally as carriers or as normal. There is also widespread concern that even the tests that are established are often not used efficiently, and that some women may be seriously misinformed as a result. Numerous new approaches have been advocated to improve carrier detection, but results are frequently conflicting and difficult to reproduce. Hopes that all problems would be resolved by the identification of a single primary molecular defect have still not been fulfilled and show no immediate signs of being so.

The purpose of this review is to examine three questions:

1. What methods have been proposed for carrier detection in DMD and how far can they be considered reliable enough to use in clinical practice?

821

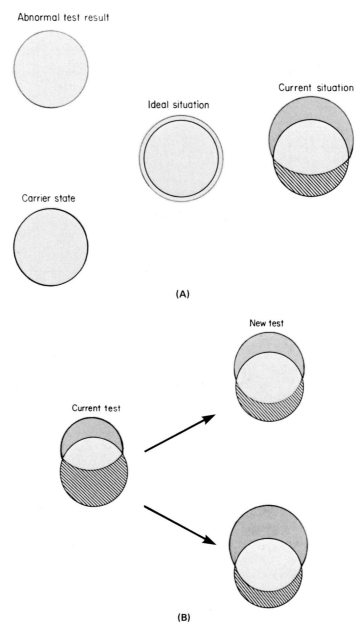

Fig. 1. Basic aims of tests of carrier detection in Duchenne muscular dystrophy. **(A)** The perfect test (left) would identify precisely the carrier population. In practice, the available tests (right), such as the creatine kinase level, have significant false-positive and false-negative rates. **(B)** Tests claimed to be superior to established methods are usually judged on the extra carriers detected, and it may be assumed that the false-positive rate is little affected (above right). If this is not so (lower right), the disadvantage of the increased false-positive rate may outweigh the advantage of fewer false negatives. **(C)** The use of multiple tests may allow a higher proportion of carriers to be detected, but as in B, no true assessment of the value of the combination can be made without information on the extra false negatives. See text for further details.

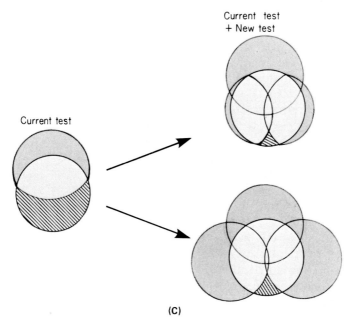

Fig. 1. (Continued)

2. Given the imperfect situation existing at present, how can we make the best use from the information we do have in the identification of carriers?
3. What approaches might prove helpful in the future?

Before discussing in detail the various tests that have been used in DMD carrier detection, it is important to examine our general aims and our approach to the assessment of any proposed test. Figure 1 summarizes the main points, which are obvious but have, nonetheless, been frequently overlooked when a new proposed test has been advocated.

In the ideal situation (Fig. 1A), the group defined by showing abnormality in the proposed test should correspond completely with the population requiring identification, i.e., women heterozygous for the DMD gene. There should be no false positives or false negatives. It is obvious that no current test fulfills these criteria, nor does any come close to doing so. However, we do have methods that provide a partial solution, CK level being the best documented; these are represented by the "current situation" in Figure 1A. The false-positive rate is relatively low, but the false-negative rate (carriers who cannot be conclusively identified by the test) is much higher.

When new tests are proposed, they may be considered either as a superior alternative to the established test or as supplementary to it. Figure 1B shows the first situation. A new test must be judged not only on the proportion of known carriers that it identifies, but also on the proportion of normal persons misidentified (false positives). It is often assumed that a new test that identifies a greater proportion of carriers is necessarily a "superior" test, but this is only so if the number of false positives remains little changed. If not, the new test may well be far from superior in practice.

Figure 1C shows the situation for new tests that are proposed to supplement or complement existing procedures. Again, it is often claimed that the combined use of such tests will enable a higher proportion of carriers to be identified; this may be so, but such an increase is of no practical value unless one has corresponding information on the extra number of false positives resulting from the additional tests.

In practice, few new tests have been critically evaluated in this way. Obligatory carriers on genetic grounds have often not been distinguished from potential carriers, and the quantitative genetic risk for persons in the latter group may not have been defined, making the proportion of false negatives difficult to assess. Identifying the proportion of false positives is even harder, because prospective follow-up of births to such persons is required, as is the use of normal control subjects; if potential carriers have been told that the test result is abnormal, few are likely to risk childbearing.

The problems of carrier detection are not entirely methodologic. There are genuine biologic difficulties that combine to hinder satisfactory carrier detection; some of these are listed in Table 1. The most obvious problem is our ignorance of the primary biochemical abnormality in the disease; if this were known, the greater part of this chapter would be irrelevant. Not only does this mean that the available tests measure secondary phenomena, but it also means that no one of them can be regarded as necessarily more definitive than another. Thus, a new test whose results conflict with others cannot be rejected out of hand but must be examined on its merits.

A second natural difficulty is the X-linked nature of the disease, with X-chromosome inactivation resulting in much greater variability of phenotype in the heterozygote than is seen with autosomal disorders. In one way this helps in carrier detection, because some heterozygotes are symptomatic or show definite clinical abnormalities; at the other extreme, however, it means that a proportion of carriers are likely to remain undetectable by any methods except for those utilizing cloned cells to identify a double population, or those based on deoxyribonucleic acid (DNA) rather than related to the gene product.

APPROACHES TO CARRIER DETECTION

Having outlined some of the general problems and pitfalls, one can now turn to the various methods that have been attempted and used in carrier detection for DMD. Table 2 groups the major ones; it is convenient, though arbitrary, to consider them under three headings: test related to abnormality of muscle structure or function; tests on cell types other than muscle, and tests on factors present in serum.

TESTS RELATED TO MUSCLE STRUCTURE OR FUNCTION

The simplest and most obvious test in this group is clinical examination for muscle weakness and wasting. It has long been recognized that a small number of heterozygous women may be symptomatic (9) and that approximately 10%

Table 1. Problems in Carrier Detection of Duchenne Muscular Dystrophy

Natural
    X-linked (variability due to X inactivation)
    Primary defect unknown
    Not *obviously* expressed outside muscle, or in culture
    No homologous animal model
Methodologic
    Obligatory and potential carriers not clearly distinguished
    Genetic risks of potential carriers not quantitatively assessed
    New proposed tests not compared with established tests on some patients
    Inadequate controls and assessment of false positives
    Too hasty application of research investigations in service use

of carriers show unequivocal muscle weakness (10). It is certainly important to examine potential carriers carefully for such weakness. In practice, however, almost all "manifesting carriers" show unequivocally increased CK levels and there is little doubt as to their carrier status. The interpretation of minimal degrees of weakness is another matter. It has been suggested that a high proportion of carriers, including many potential carriers not abnormal by CK testing, show minor abnormalities on manual muscle testing (11), but this remains to be validated.

Paradoxically, it is heterozygous women with the most overt muscle disease who are most likely to be misidentified, simply because they may be believed to

Table 2. Approaches to Carrier Detection in Duchenne Muscular Dystrophy

Studies primarily related to muscle
    Clinical examination
    Muscle biopsy
        Light microscopy
        Electron microscopy
        Biochemical changes
    Electromyography
    Electrocardiography
Studies on other cell types
    Red blood cell membrane abnormalities
        Protein phosphorylation
        Morphologic changes
        Biophysical changes
    Lymphocyte capping
Studies on serum
    Creatine kinase (+isoenzymes)
    Aldolase
    Lactic dehydrogenase
    Pyruvate kinase
    Myoglobin
    Hemopexin

have a myopathy quite distinct from DMD, especially if no affected males are known or if a proper family history has not been taken. If the diagnosis of autosomal recessive limb girdle dystrophy is made, the woman may be falsely reassured regarding the risk to her offspring.

Muscle Histology

Histologic abnormalities in biopsy specimens of muscle are regularly seen in women with clinical abnormalities. More systematic studies of light microscopic changes have shown that histologic changes also occur in definite carriers without clinical abnormalities. Emery (12) found some degree of abnormality in 7 of 9 definite carriers, the most severe changes occurring in those with clinical features. Swollen and hyaline fibers, variation in fiber size, and increased number of nuclei were the main features noted. However, of the 3 whose CK levels were normal, 2 showed normal muscle histologic features and the remaining 1 had only minimal changes. Pearce and colleagues (13) studied 8 definite carriers. All had increased CK levels and all had some histologic abnormalities, but only one-third had diagnostic changes, the others having changes that were also seen in normal persons.

These and other early studies, while demonstrating the existence of histologic abnormalities in carriers, also showed the drawbacks of this approach: the uncertainty of defining the limits of normal, and the tendency for those whose other test results (such as CK level) are normal to have normal or near normal histologic features as well. The same problems were encountered with histochemical studies (14) in which an increased proportion of abnormal type 1 fibers was the main finding, and in electron microscopic examinations. Afifi and associates (15) studied 5 definite carriers and reviewed electron microscopic changes in a total of 25 (it is not clear that all were definite carriers). In 21 cases abnormalities were found, with changes in the Z line being especially marked; however, 18 of these would have been detected by increased CK level or other means.

Again, the question arises as to whether all of the abnormalities seen on electron microscopy are really related to the carrier state. This worry is increased when abnormal electron microscopic findings are claimed to exist in *all* of a series of 19 mothers of children with DMD, at least some of whom are likely not to be carriers (16). Absence of genetic and CK data and of normal control data makes reports such as this impossible to assess.

Uncertainty of interpretation, together with the traumatic nature of open muscle biopsy, have prevented the histological approach from being generally accepted as having a useful role in carrier detection of DMD outside a few centers with special interest. However, this situation is likely to change given the availability of needle biopsy (17, 18) and the application of quantitative light and electron microscopic techniques. A more satisfactory body of information is now available on normal female volunteers, and a recent study (19) of data from 13 definite and 49 possible carriers has shown that quantification of a number of parameters, including fiber diameter, proportions of fiber types, and numbers of internal nuclei allows some carriers to be identified as clearly abnormal in whom simple qualitative visual inspection would not have given an unequivocal result. Nonetheless, 4 of the 13 definite carriers were still normal by all criteria, so the problem of interpreting the normal result still remains.

Electron microscopic analysis of intracellular and intranuclear calcium is an interesting development. An extensive study (20) has shown increased intracellular calcium to be a consistent and early feature in patients with DMD. Analysis of nuclear calcium in both affected males and carriers has shown all of 9 definite carriers so far examined to have increased nuclear calcium:phosphorus ratios, with increased values being found for morphologically normal as well as for abnormal fibers (21, 22). Whether this will prove to be both sensitive and free from false-positive results will depend on study of considerably more normal persons as well as carriers.

Should all potential carriers now be submitted to needle biopsy as well as measurement of CK, and should definite histologic abnormalities override favorable odds coming from genetic and CK information? It is still too early to give a definite answer to this question, but my opinion is that muscle biopsy should be used only by the few centers that have experience both in taking satisfactory needle samples and in interpreting the results in terms of a large series of known carriers and normal persons.

Biochemical Studies of Muscle

Few biochemical tests of muscle biopsy specimens have yet reached the stage of being considered seriously as methods of carrier detection. Most biochemical studies of dystrophic muscle have been aimed at finding a reproducible abnormality in muscle from affected males. Until such a reproducible change is found, it seems premature to rely on changes found in carriers as providing a test for carrier detection. Such studies of muscle biochemistry comprise a large part of basic research in this field and are not discussed here. Changes in muscle enzymes are considered later with serum assays of these enzymes, but one test that requires mention is the measurement of muscle protein synthesis by incorporation of amino acids into isolated muscle polyribosomes. Ionasescu and colleagues (23, 24) have found this to be increased in both patients with and carriers of DMD. A total of 63 female relatives were studied, of whom 11 were definite carriers; unfortunately, results for definite and possible carriers were not given separately, nor were precise risks given for the possible carriers. Other groups have not yet confirmed this work. Although changes have been reported in cultured muscle in patients with DMD (25), as well as in cultured fibroblasts (26), this technique cannot be considered to be a practical means for carrier detection.

Electromyography

At present, electromyography appears to be "in limbo" with regard to carrier detection in DMD. Van den Bosch (27) initially reported that it was helpful in discriminating carriers from noncarriers. After some negative or equivocal reports (28, 29), a thorough quantitative study by Gardner-Medwin and colleagues (30, 31) showed that a combination of mean action potential duration, number of phases per potential, and proportion of polyphasic potentials could identify two thirds of definite carriers. Many of these had "normal" CK levels, so more than 90% of definite carriers would have been identified by both approaches.

Moosa and coworkers (32) performed a smaller study using a less time-consuming, automated technique and again found that the procedure detected definite carriers with normal CK levels. In view of these reports, it is perhaps surprising that this approach has not been studied more extensively and that it is no longer used in centers that produced apparently promising results. Whether this is due to difficulties in reproducibility or whether the technique is simply too tedious to perform on an extensive scale is difficult to say.

Electrocardiography

Clinical cardiac involvement is frequent in advanced DMD and electrocardiographic (ECG) changes are common at an earlier age, but gross changes are rare in carriers. Emery (33) found that the mean value of the sum of the amplitudes of R and S waves in lead V1 was significantly increased in 50 obligatory carriers, but the difference was insufficient to detect carriers. Lane and associates (34) recently showed that, using the sum of R and S in V1 and the ratio $\log_e$ R/S in V2, a series of probabilities can be assigned for a particular result indicating the carrier state; these values are not correlated with CK level. It thus seems possible that this technique, like electromyography, may find use as an auxiliary method of carrier detection, and it certainly deserves further study with this in view.

Hausmanowa-Petrusewicz and coworkers (35) have advocated an exercise ECG for detecting abnormalities in a high proportion of carriers, but whether these changes genuinely reflect the carrier state is uncertain.

CELL TYPE OTHER THAN MUSCLE

Realization that the primary genetic defect of many mendelian disorders is to be found in a wide variety of cell types, and that the tissue most affected clinically may not be the one most suitable or easy for identifying the primary abnormality has led many investigators to look outside muscle for the basic defect in DMD. Red and white blood cells and cultured fibroblasts have been the main targets of study. Although most investigations have been aimed at finding a consistent abnormality in affected males, results on definite or possible carriers have often been reported along with those on patients. A worrisome feature about many of these reports has been the emphasis on the practical application of any abnormality to carrier detection before the consistency of the results has been thoroughly validated even in affected males. One suspects that pressure from grant-giving agencies naturally concerned in finding an improved test of carrier detection or a method of prenatal diagnosis might have contributed to this overhasty approach.

Because most of these studies have been concerned only secondarily with carrier detection, they will be considered briefly here. It should be clearly understood that most of the reservations expressed concern the conclusions about carriers rather than affected persons.

The Red Blood Cell

Roses and colleagues (36–38) initially found abnormalities of protein phosphorylation in red blood cell (RBC) membranes of patients with DMD, as part of a study on myotonic dystrophy. Later confirmation of this as a specific finding in its own right justifiably produced both excitement and controversy, because this was the first indication that a cell type other than muscle might show a definite biochemical abnormality. The fact that the changes in carriers of DMD were as great as those in affected males was obviously important, but also disconcerting, because one might have expected a lesser degree of abnormality in carriers. The situation became even more difficult when it became clear that many potential carriers, notably mothers of isolated cases, showed more abnormal results than would have been expected either from results of CK testing or from accepted genetic theory (39) for a genetically lethal X-linked disease. One had to accept either that conventional methods were resulting in the false reassurance of many women who were carriers, or that the new test was falsely identifying as carriers many who were not. It should be said that Roses and colleagues explicitly did *not* regard their methods as a practical means for detecting carriers, because the methods were complex and the data varied over a considerable range. Nevertheless, it was clear that both positions could not be correct.

Unfortunately, the situation is still not fully resolved. The membrane changes, principally an increase in band 2 phosphorylation (spectrin), have not yet been identified as a specific and reproducible defect. Attempts by other groups to do this have also produced conflicting results (40–42). The current status of studies using more specific techniques is reviewed by Roses and associates (38, and chapter 33 of this volume), who emphasize the importance of accurately standardized methods of analysis. Thus, this work remains as before: it is a valuable, original, and pioneering attempt to isolate a biochemical defect in DMD outside muscle, not a current approach to carrier detection. In fact, prospective studies (43, 44) and reanalysis of genetic data (45, 46) (see later) suggest that results based on older CK studies are not grossly misleading. In contrast to some other X-linked disorders such as hemophilia (47) and the Lesch-Nyhan syndrome (48), nearly one third of cases of DMD result from a new mutation and are not transmitted by a carrier mother.

While the significance of the biochemical changes in the RBC were being debated, other workers identified abnormalities in RBC shape and deformability (49–51). Increased numbers of stomatocytes and echinocytes were found in scanning electron micrographs of RBCs from both patients with and carriers of DMD; reduced deformability of RBCs aspirated into micropipettes was also found (52).

Again, the current status of this work is extremely uncertain; conditions of study and methods of preparation have been found to yield considerable differences in the data obtained. It seems likely that Duchenne RBCs do behave abnormally in vitro, probably as a result of a membrane defect, but the lack of specificity and consistency makes this approach unsuitable for diagnosis of the affected male, let alone the potential carrier.

A recent development in this work has been measurement of the elastic shear modules of individual RBCs by micropipette aspiration (53). As with related tests, both potential and definite carriers, as well as affected males with DMD, showed an increased elastic shear modulus. Interestingly, there was no suggestion of a bimodal RBC population in carriers.

The Lymphocyte

While controversy was surrounding the RBC, studies on lymphocytes were reported that appeared, at first sight, to lead to similar conclusions. Unfortunately, however, these tests were never carried out in the same series of patients. Verrill and colleagues (54, 55) and Pickard and associates (56) reported a marked decrease in the capping response of lymphocytes from patients with DMD. The 25 patients were clearly separated from normal subjects, and the same was true of most carriers. However, closer examination makes the data less clear. Surprisingly, 16 mothers of isolated cases of DMD were all said to have normal CK levels, and 9 of these had abnormal lymphocyte capping. Three of the 7 mothers with normal lymphocyte capping had a relative with a low capping response. A further complication was that patients with other muscular dystrophies (including facioscapulohumeral dystrophy and limb girdle dystrophy, but not myotonic dystrophy) had abnormal capping.

Subsequent reports on lymphocyte capping have on the one hand shown abnormalities in other disorders such as Huntington's chorea (57) and on the other hand have failed to reproduce the original findings in DMD (58). I am aware of several false-positive results with serious clinical implications. Again, a worrisome feature of this work has been the over-hasty attempt to use an interesting and potentially valuable research tool as a clinical service before its accuracy was validated.

The cultured skin fibroblast has so far not proved helpful in identifying the primary biochemical defect in DMD, nor have consistent abnormalities been found in the fibroblasts from carriers. An initial report of an altered pattern of cell growth in patients (59) has not been confirmed (60). The protein composition of the fibroblast cell membrane appears to be considerably more complex than that of the RBC and is currently under investigation (38). Once a primary defect is identified, the fibroblast would be an excellent target for carrier detection based on cloning methods similar to those used in other inherited metabolic disorders. Cultured amniotic cells might allow prenatal diagnosis. Whether such an abnormality will actually be discovered by using the fibroblast is an entirely different matter.

It is worth noting that none of the proposed abnormalities in DMD cells outside muscle have shown any hint of bimodality in carriers, whereas the clinical and histologic changes in muscle of carriers are patchy, despite the multinucleate nature of muscle. This suggests that the various extramuscular abnormalities are, if they really exist, some way from the primary defect. They could even be secondary to changes in circulating factors such as serum enzymes.

MUSCLE-RELATED ENZYMES

Among the various enzymes that are of major importance in muscle but are also detectable in serum, CK has proved to be the most helpful in DMD carrier detection and is considered separately later. A number of other enzymes have also been examined for their potential to be more sensitive in detecting the carrier state or to serve as adjuncts to CK testing.

Aldolase activity is usually markedly increased in affected males and was studied along with CK in early investigations of carriers (2). In general, it shows less significant and less consistent increases in serum concentration.

Analysis of lactic dehydrogenase (LDH) from muscle and blood, and particularly its isoenzyme electrophoretic pattern, has been claimed to be helpful. Emery (61) found a consistently decreased level of LDH-5 in muscle biopsy specimens from known carriers. Similar findings were reported by Johnston and colleagues (62), although the numbers of subjects were small. Emery found no changes in serum levels of LDH in his carriers. However, Johnston and associates (62) found female relatives (not definite carriers) who showed increased levels of LDH and of hydroxybutyrate dehydrogenase but normal CK levels; they suggested that combined use of these enzymes would allow more efficient carrier detection. The current situation remains debatable. Roses and associates (63) found increased serum levels of LDH-5 in a number of potential carriers with normal CK levels but Burt and Emery (64) showed no advantage of this measurement over CK.

Isoenzymes of CK have also been studied in the hope that a specific pattern would be helpful in the recognition of carriers (65–67). The pattern in affected males is certainly distinctive, resembling that seen in fetal muscle, but there is no evidence that such isoenzyme studies are more helpful than total CK analysis in carrier detection.

Pyruvate kinase (PK) is the other enzyme that has received considerable attention; again, the argument has been that abnormal serum levels may occur in carriers who would not be identified using CK alone, and that combined use of CK and PK will identify a higher proportion of carriers. This was the original finding of Alberts and Samaha (68); unfortunately, subsequent reports have been conflicting. Seay and colleagues (69) found no advantage in the combined use of CK and PK; Yamuna and coworkers (70) found that PK was less sensitive than CK. Although other recent reports (71, 72) have again suggested that PK and CK together are more useful than either alone, the case is far from proved. The current conclusion must be that measurement of no other serum enzyme has any advantage over a carefully performed CK study (see later) in the testing of potential carriers and in the evaluation of their risks.

Two non-enzymic serum factors should be mentioned briefly. Myoglobin, derived from muscle and found in serum in a variety of muscle disorders, was found by Adornato and associates (73) in the serum of 14 of 18 patients with

DMD and in 10 of 16 known carriers, 4 of whom had normal CK levels. The same investigators (74) also found increased levels of hemopexin, a heme-binding serum glycoprotein, in a proportion of potential carriers with normal CK levels. Whether these findings will be reproducible remains to be seen.

Creatine Kinase

An increased serum level of CK was the first significant biochemical abnormality to be discovered in carriers of DMD (2–8) and remains the mainstay of current carrier detection (75–78). This reflects both the inadequacy of other methods that have been proposed and the fact that, although CK testing is far from perfect, we know a great deal about its limitations and deficiencies.

It thus becomes all the more important to examine how CK can be used to maximal effectiveness. Not only is this of immediate practical importance in genetic counseling of potential carriers, but it allows more accurate evaluation of any proposed new test in terms of extra carriers identified as well as those likely to be misidentified.

The first and most obvious point is the use of accurate and reproducible methods. It might seem unnecessary to stress this point, but a recent quality control study in the United Kingdom (79) showed alarming differences in the results of identical samples analyzed in different laboratories. Paradoxically, this may in part be the result of the analysis being too easy and being available in most general hospitals. Samples to be studied for the DMD carrier state are often mixed in with more numerous samples to be studied for cardiac disease, for which the emphasis may be more on speed than accuracy. However, the laboratories cannot be assigned all of the blame, because delay in analysis, exposure to bright light, and temperature fluctuations may all seriously invalidate a sample before it ever reaches the laboratory (80). Exercise is another factor that must be considered as a cause of variability of CK levels. It increases the CK level in both carriers and normal persons, but these changes are not reproducible enough for aiding carrier detection (81).

Even with reliable laboratory procedures, a result may be of little use unless an accurately determined normal range is available. Probably only a minority of laboratories have actually constructed their own normal range based on data from healthy women; even fewer have studied a comparable series of obligatory carriers. Yet these are the basic starting points for any reliable system of carrier detection.

Special problems exist in the normal ranges for childhood and for pregnant women. The CK levels in umbilical cord blood and during the first few days of life are extremely variable and are often markedly increased (82). This variability makes even diagnosis of an affected male unwise, let alone the carrier state. From infancy until the menarche, most studies (83, 84), with one exception (85), suggest that normal levels are slightly but significantly higher than those of adult women. It has been suggested that in carriers of DMD the increase is even greater and is more consistent in premenarchal girls then in adults (75, 86). If this is confirmed, it would provide a strong case for testing potential carriers during childhood. Because there are no obligatory carriers for DMD during childhood, the evidence remains indirect, based on the proportion of carriers expected in a sibship, and it is by no means clear whether those with slightly increased CK levels in childhood will later be carriers. My current policy is not to test before puberty unless specifically requested and then to regard the results as provisional unless they are grossly abnormal.

Pregnancy results in a dramatic decrease in the CK level of normal women (83, 84), so that the mean for the nonpregnant adult corresponds to the ninety-fifth percentile for pregnancy. The decrease appears to occur early and is well established by the sixteenth week, so hemodilution is unlikely to be responsible. The practical effect of this change is to make it most unwise to rely on a normal result during pregnancy. This emphasizes the importance of completing carrier testing and genetic counseling before a pregnancy occurs. Otherwise, a woman whose chance of being a carrier is later proved to be very low might needlessly undergo amniocentesis for fetal sexing or even termination of pregnancy.

All studies of serum CK in carriers for DMD have shown a considerable overlap between normal and carrier ranges. Approximately 30% of known carriers have levels below the ninety-fifth percentile of normal persons, so it makes little sense to think in terms of "normal" or "abnormal" except for the relatively small number whose level is grossly increased. The use of specific odds or likelihood ratios for individual levels of CK, which have been well established for more than 10 years (8, 76), allows sensitive discrimination between values within the normal range, and also avoids the illogical situation of assigning totally different risks to those with results marginally outside and marginally within the normal range. It is often not appreciated that a result within the normal range defined by the ninety-fifth percentile may give odds in favor of that person being a carrier if the actual level of CK is taken into consideration. Table 3, part A, gives a practical example.

Table 3. Potential Pitfalls in Using Creatine Kinase to Determine Carrier Risk

Subject	Prior Genetic Risk	CK Level (IU/L)	Odds of Being a Carrier from CK Result[a]	Final Risk Estimate
		A. NOT ALL "NORMAL" RESULTS ARE THE SAME[b]		
A	1/2	94	1.7 :1	63%
B	1/2	35	0.12:1	11%
		B. THE GENETIC RISK AS WELL AS THE CK LEVEL MUST DETERMINE THE FINAL RISK[c]		
A	1/2	120	10:1	91%
B	1/20	120	10:1	34%
C	1/2,000	120	10:1	0.5%

[a] These odds are based on data of the author and colleagues (78). The normal range for adult female volunteers is <100 IU/L.

[b] Subjects A and B are unmarried daughters of an obligatory carrier for Duchenne muscular dystrophy (DMD). Both have CK levels within the normal range, but using specific odds, the final risk for each is very different. Had their results simply been regarded as "normal," the two would have been given identical risks.

[c] All 3 subjects have a CK level outside the normal range. For Subject A with a high prior risk, the test provided very strong evidence of being a carrier. For Subject B, who might be a moderately close relative, the test has increased the chances of being a carrier, but it is still more likely that she is not. For Subject C, detected through a population screening study, the final chance is still overwhelmingly against her being a carrier, despite the high CK level.

Despite the theoretical and practical validation of this approach, it is disturbing to find how often it is ignored or misapplied. Two recent examples of this deserve attention. The quality control survey already cited (79) added a question on the interpretation of CK results; replies produced risk estimates varying from less than 10% to 100% for the same sample, a variability that could not be explained by differences in laboratory analyses. Even more disturbing is the result of a questionnaire to clinical geneticists asking for risk of the carrier state in several simple pedigrees of DMD (87). Only 7 of 18 respondents gave correct risk estimates.

Perhaps the most common and most serious error is to interpret the results of carrier detection as being directly equivalent to the risk for an individual being a carrier without reference to the genetic risks. Pedigree data may be misinterpreted or entirely ignored, and the result is almost invariably an overestimate of the final risk given to the potential carrier. Table 3, part B, makes the obvious, but nonetheless important point that the same CK result will give very different final risks depending on the genetic situation. For the person at high genetic risk, the result is to make it overwhelmingly likely that she is a carrier. This is far from being so in the second case, who might well be a moderately distant relative. In the person drawn from the general population, the risk of being a carrier on this evidence is minimal. A lesson is to be learned here for the testing of persons at low risk. There is a real danger of falsely labeling such persons as carriers, an error that will increase the more distant the relationship (and, hence, the lower the risk). This may, in part, explain the excessive number of carriers identified by extensive carrier testing in the studies of Roses and colleagues (88, 89). The extreme situation is that of population screening for carriers (90), in which it should be obvious that serum CK level is a totally unsuitable test, regardless of the merits or demerits of screening for *affected* persons (91).

Most studies of the use of CK for carrier detection in DMD have concentrated on providing accurate information to persons requiring genetic counseling. There has been little evidence as to how an entire population of potential carriers can be satisfactorily resolved into those who are likely to be carriers and those who are not. Evidence on this point from Wales is shown in Figure 2 and confirms that most potential carriers can be assigned to either a very high or a very low risk category, provided that all available information is used. The use of the computer program PEDIG (92, 93) is helpful for large kindreds with considerable negative information, but in most instances the risks can be worked out by hand.

If the risks predicted by the correct use of CK testing are valid, the number of subsequent affected children born into families given low risks after CK testing should be small, and evidence is now becoming available that this is the case. In the study of Dennis and coworkers (43) none of the 19 males among the 44 children born to 46 mothers considered to have a low risk was affected. By contrast, the high-risk group of 25 women bore no sons at all.

Similar evidence comes from studies of new cases of DMD born into populations in which systematic family testing has been carried out. Studies from Australia (94), Canada (44), and England (Gardner-Medwin D: personal communication) have all suggested a decrease in incidence. However, these data must be treated with reserve, because in the two series in which they could be distinguished, the incidence of initial cases in a family decreased as much as the incidence of subsequent cases, something that cannot be attributed to carrier detection and may suggest underascertainment. A thorough study in Scotland (95) showed no decrease in the incidence of new cases of DMD.

Data from Wales, collected by the author and his colleagues are shown in Table 4 and support a decreased incidence of new cases of DMD that appears to be confined to second or subsequent cases. A much longer prospective study will be required, however, before this can be accurately assessed. The prevention of initial cases remains entirely unresolved, as does the prevention of the small but tragic number of cases in which a second affected male has been born before diagnosis of the initial case. Whether neonatal screening of males for this latter group is justified is a matter of considerable debate. What is quite clear is that neonatal screening by CK for the carrier state is not feasible.

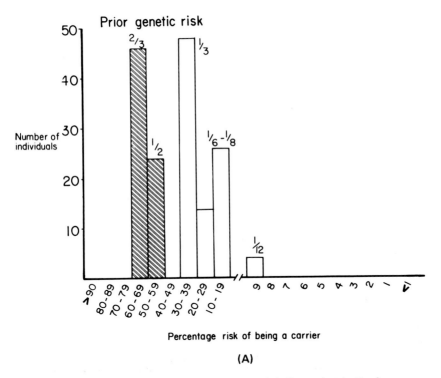

(A)

Fig. 2. The combined use of biochemical and genetic information in Duchenne muscular dystrophy (DMD) carrier detection. Data are for 161 potential carriers from established DMD families in Wales. **(A)** Distribution of prior risks (persons with prior risk less than $\frac{1}{12}$ were not tested. **(B)** Distribution of risks of same group based on prior risk and CK of the individual test (odds based on CK range of Sibert et al [78]). **(C)** Distribution of risks when all information is taken into account, including all genetic data and CK results of all members tested. Although CK data for a single person has partially resolved the group, the use of all information provides much clearer resolution into groups at high risk and at low risk of being a carrier and decreases the number with an indeterminate risk.

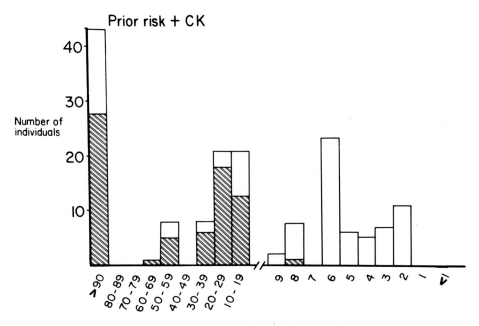

(B)

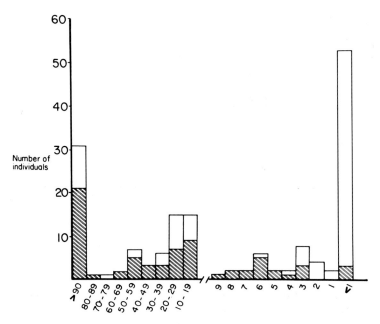

(C)

Fig. 2. (Continued)

Table 4. Incidence of Duchenne Muscular
Dystrophy in Wales

Year of Birth	New Cases		
	Total	1st in Family	2nd or more
1955–1959	18	7	11
1960–1964	28	17	11
1965–1969	24	15	9
1970–1974	15	11	4
1975–1979[a]			1

[a] Data for this period are relevant only for second or subsequent cases; all male births at significant risk in known families were tested within the first 6 months of life.

The conclusions to be drawn from this review so far are essentially that CK is a reasonably reliable, though far from perfect, test for carrier detection in DMD, provided that it is used properly. Most of the newer tests claimed to be superior to CK have not been satisfactorily validated by comparison with risks estimated by genetic and CK data, nor by prospective study of subsequent births to such persons. It seems more likely that persons will be falsely identified as carriers by these tests than that they will be falsely given a low risk by CK testing.

There is no clear indication that the combined use of CK testing with other methods will more accurately assign risks to carriers. The study of ECG abnormalities and the occurrence of histologic changes in muscle biopsy specimens are two approaches that deserve close consideration as auxiliary tests but they will require further evaluation before they can be used with confidence as a basis for genetic counseling.

FUTURE DEVELOPMENTS

Two fundamental changes might be expected to lead to significantly improved carrier detection for DMD: identification of the abnormal or deficient primary gene product, and identification of the abnormality in the DNA of the gene itself. The first target has appeared to be feasible for many years, but is still far from being achieved. Until recently, the second would have been considered unrealistic, but rapid advances in recombinant DNA techniques may result in it being reached before the first.

A number of techniques of carrier detection already mentioned have been undertaken primarily as a means of approaching the basic defect. Abnormalities in RBC membrane protein phosphorylation and in lymphocyte capping are cases in point. Both, however, have proved to be less specific and more variable than was originally believed. The fact that comparable abnormalities have been claimed to exist in a variety of other diseases makes it unlikely that these abnormalities are close to the abnormality of the primary gene product. The value of these studies has been to show that a generalized membrane defect appears to exist, and that expression of gene action is not confined to muscle, something that was already apparent at a clinical level from central nervous system involvement in patients with DMD.

The possibility of using the gene itself, rather than the gene product, in the identification of carriers has recently attracted considerable interest. Two main approaches might be expected to be fruitful. (*a*) Accurate mapping of the DMD gene might allow prediction of its transmission by the inheritance of neighboring polymorphic marker systems. (*b*) Analysis of the DNA of the gene itself might identify an abnormality detectable in the heterozygote.

The first approach is essentially an extension of the use of genetic linkage techniques, which have already found limited practical application in the prediction of myotonic dystrophy. The X-linked nature of DMD itself narrows the field to be searched, but unfortunately, there is a dearth of marker genes on the X chromosome. Whereas the locus for Becker muscular dystrophy is linked to that for deutan color blindness (96), that for DMD is not (97), nor is there linkage with the Xg blood group (99) or with glucose-6-phosphate dehydrogenase (GGPD) (98). However, information on the possible location of the DMD gene has come from study of affected females with chromosomal defects.

Lindenbaum and associates (100) have described a girl with the clinical picture of DMD who had a chromosome rearrangement involving an X chromosome and chromosome one. Banding studies suggested the short arm (sites Xp 1106 or Xp 2107) as a likely location for the gene. The short arm site has also been suggested by 2 other similar patients studied by Canki and colleagues (101).

The possibility of more accurate localization of the DMD gene has been brought nearer by the finding that polymorphic DNA sequences exists on many chromosomes which are so closely related to the locus for a structural gene that crossing-over is never a practical problem. The use of recombinant DNA techniques has allowed this approach to be used diagnostically in thalassemias and hemoglobinopathies (102, 103); X-chromosome specific sequences are currently under study. Obviously an approximate chromosomal location is of help in suggesting the area of the X chromosome on which to concentrate. If this approach proves to be fruitful, it should be applicable to both carrier detection and prenatal dignosis, because the DNA of any accessible cell type could be used, and because X-chromosome inactivation and its resulting variability in gene expression in the heterozygote would not affect techniques based on DNA analysis.

There is also a possibility that the use of recombinant DNA techniques might actually identify an abnormality, such as a small deletion of genetic material, which could itself be used directly in carrier detection. The thalassemias have already provided examples of a comparable situation with practical diagnostic applications (104). It may also be that heterogeneity exists at the molecular level, and it remains to be proved that a single genetic locus is responsible for DMD (105). Heterogeneity has been suggested on clinical grounds according to the presence or absence of mental retardation (106–108).

CONCLUSION

Despite the many tests advocated for identifying carriers for DMD, most have proved to be of no value or remain inadequately validated. None has yet proved superior to the use of CK, although new histologic techniques for the study of muscle specimens obtained by needle biopsy may prove helpful. Creatine kinase itself has proved an effective test, but one that has been greatly misused. When combined with other available information, most potential carriers can be assigned a very high or very low risk and such prospective evidence as exists does not suggest that these risks are seriously misleading. Further advances may well have to await identification of the gene product or of the DNA itself. When this occurs, the entire subject of carrier detection in DMD should appear much simpler and more satisfactory than it does at present.

ACKNOWLEDGMENT

The support of the Muscular Dystrophy Group of Great Britain and the Muscular Dystrophy Association of America is gratefully acknowledged.

REFERENCES

1. Emery AEH: Genetic considerations in the X-linked muscular dystrophies. In *Pathogenesis of Human Muscular Dystrophies*. Edited by Rowland LP. Excerpta Medica, Amsterdam, 1977, pp 43–52

2. Schapira F, Dreyfuss JC, Schapira G, et al: Étude de l'aldolase et de la créatine kinase du sérum chez les meres de myopathes. Rev Fr Etud Clin Biol 5:990–994, 1960

3. Richterich R, Rosin S, Aebi U, et al: Progressive muscular dystrophy. V. The identification of the carrier state in the Duchenne type by serum creatine kinase determination. Am J Hum Genet 15:133–154, 1963

4. Griffiths PD: Serum levels of creatine phosphokinase. J Clin Pathol 17:56–57, 1964

5. Pearce JMS, Pennington RJ, Walton JN: Serum enzyme studies in muscle disease. 1. Variations in serum creatine kinase activity in normal individuals. J Neurol Neurosurg Psychiatry 27:1–4, 1964

6. Pearce JMS, Pennington RJ, Walton JN: Serum enzyme studies in muscle disease. II. Serum creatine kinase activity in muscular dystrophy and in other myopathic and neuropathic disorders. J Neurol Neurosurg Psychiatry 27:96–99, 1964

7. Pearce JMS, Pennington RJ, Walton JN: Serum enzyme studies in muscle disease. III. Serum creatine kinase activity in relatives of patients with the Duchenne type of muscular dystrophy. J Neurol Neurosurg Psychiatry 27:181–185, 1964

8. Wilson KM, Evans KA, Carter CO: Creatine kinase levels in women who carry genes for three types of muscular dystrophy. Br Med J 1:750–753, 1965

9. Dubowitz V: Myopathic changes in a muscular dystrophy carrier. J Neurol Neurosurg Psychiatry 26:322–325, 1963

10. Moser H, Emery AEH: The manifesting carrier in Duchenne muscular dystrophy. Clin Genet 5:271–284, 1974

11. Roses MS, Nicholson MT, Kircher CS, et al: Evaluation and detection of Duchenne's and Beeker's muscular dystrophy carriers by manual muscle testing. Neurology (Minneap) 27:20–25, 1977

12. Emery AEH: Muscle histology in carriers of Duchenne muscular dystrophy. J Med Genet 2:1–7, 1965

13. Pearce GW, Pearce JMS, Walton JN: The Duchenne type muscular dystrophy: histopathological studies in the carrier state. Brain 89:109–120, 1966

14. Morris CJ, Raybould JA: Histochemically demonstrable fibre abnormalities in normal skeletal muscle and in muscle from carriers of Duchenne muscular dystrophy. J Neurol Neurosurg Psychiatry 34:348–353, 1971

15. Afifi AK, Bergman RA, Zellweger H: A possible role for electron microscopy in detection of carriers of Duchenne muscular dystrophy. J Neurol Neurosurg Psychiatry 36:643–650, 1973

16. Fisher ER, Wissinger HA, Gerneth JA, et al: Ultrastructural changes in skeletal muscle of muscular dystrophy carriers. Arch Pathol 94:456–460, 1972

17. Edwards RHT, Maunder CA, Lewis PD, et al: Percutaneous needle biopsy in the diagnosis of muscle disease. Lancet 2:1070–1071, 1973

18. Edwards R, Young A, Wiles M: Needle biopsy of skeletal muscle in the diagnosis of myopathy and the clinical study of muscle function and repair. N Engl J Med 302:261–271, 1980

19. Maunder-Sewry CA, Dubowitz V: Needle muscle biopsy for carrier detection in Duchenne muscular dystrophy. 1. Light microscopy—histology, histochemistry and quantitation. J Neurol Sci. In press 1981

20. Bodensteiner JB, Engel AG: Intracellular calcium accumulation in Duchenne dystrophy and other myopathies: a study of 567,000 muscle fibres in 114 biopsies. Neurology (NY) 28:439–446, 1978

21. Maunder-Sewry CA, Dubowitz V: Myonuclear calcium in carriers of Duchenne muscular dystrophy: an x-ray microanalysis study. J Neurol Sci 42:337–347, 1979

22. Maunder-Sewry CA, Dubowitz V: Intranuclear calcium in carriers of Duchenne muscular dystrophy. In Muscular Dystrophy Research. Advances and New Trends. Edited by Angelini C, Darieli GA, Fontanari D. Excerpta Medica Int. Congress Series 527, 1980, pp 14–22

23. Ionasescu V, Zellweger H, Conway TW: A new approach for carrier detection in Duchenne muscular dystrophy: protein synthesis of muscle polyribosomes in vitro. Neurology (Minneap) 21:703–709, 1971

24. Ionasescu V, Zellweger H, Shirk P, et al: Identification of carriers of Duchenne muscular dystrophy by muscle protein synthesis. Neurology (Minneap) 23:497–502, 1973

25. Ionasescu V, Zellweger H, Ionasescu R: Protein synthesis in muscle cultures from patients with Duchenne muscular dystrophy. Acta Neurol Scand 54:241–247, 1976

26. Boule M, Vanasse M, Brakier-Gineras L: Decrease in the rate of protein synthesis by polysomes from cultured fibroblasts of patients and carriers with Duchenne muscular dystrophy. Can J Neurol Science 6:355–358, 1979

27. Bosch J van den: Investigations of the carrier state in the Duchenne type dystrophy. In Research in Muscular Dystrophy. Pitman, London, 1963, pp 23–33

28. Davey MR, Woolf AL: The electromyographic detection of carriers of muscular dystrophy. Electroenceph Clin Neurophysiol 17:705, 1964

29. Emery AEH, Teasdall RD, Coombes EN: Electromyographic studies in carriers of Duchenne muscular dystrophy. Bull Johns Hopkins Hosp 118:439–443, 1966

30. Gardner-Medwin D: Studies of the carrier state in the Duchenne type of muscular dystrophy. 2. Quantitative electromyography as a method of carrier detection. J Neurol Neurosurg Psychiatry 31:124–134, 1968

31. Gardner-Medwin D, Pennington RJ, Walton JN: The detection of carriers of X-linked muscular dystrophy genes: a review of some methods studied in Newcastle Upon Tyne. J Neurol Sci 13:459–474, 1971

32. Moosa A, Brown BH, Dubowitz V: Quantitative electromyography: carrier detection in Duchenne type muscular dystrophy using a new automatic technique. J Neurol Neurosurg Psychiatry 35:841–844, 1972

33. Emery AEH: Abnormalities of the electrocardiogram in female carriers of Duchenne muscular dystrophy. Br Med J 2:418–420, 1969

34. Lane RJM, Gardner-Medwin DM, Roses AD: Electrocardiographic abnormalities in carriers of Duchenne muscular dystrophy. Neurology 30:497–501, 1980

35. Hausmanowa-Petrusewicz I, Niebroj-Dobosz I, Borkowska J, et al: Carrier detection in Duchenne dystrophy. In *Pathogenesis of Human Muscular Dystrophies*. Edited by Rowland LP. Excerpta Medica, Amsterdam, 1977, pp 32–41

36. Roses AD, Appel SH: Erythrocyte spectrin peak II phosphorylation in Duchenne muscular dystrophy. J Neurol Sci 29:185–193, 1976

37. Roses AD, Herbstreith M, Metcalf B, et al: Increased phosphorylated components of erythrocyte membrane spectrin band II with reference to Duchenne muscular dystrophy. J Neurol Sci 30:167–178, 1976

38. Roses AD, Hartwig GB, Mabry M, et al: Red blood cell and fibroblast membranes in Duchenne and myotonic muscular dystrophy. Muscle Nerve 3:36–54, 1980

39. Haldane JBS: The rate of spontaneous mutation of a human gene. J Genet 31:317–326, 1935

40. Fischer S, Tortolero M, Piau JP, et al: Protein kinase and adenylate cyclase of erythrocyte membrane from patients with Duchenne muscular dystrophy. Clin Chim Acta 88:437–440, 1978

41. Kobayashi T, Mawatari S, Kuroiwa Y: Lipids and proteins of erythrocyte membrane in Duchenne muscular dystrophy. Clin Chim Acta 85:259–266, 1978

42. Vickers JD, McComas AJ, Rathbone MP: Alterations of membrane phosphorylation in erythrocyte membranes from patients with Duchenne muscular dystrophy. J Can Sci Neurol 5:437–442, 1978

43. Dennis NR, Evans K, Clayton B, et al: Use of creatine kinase for detecting severe X-linked muscular dystrophy carriers. Br Med J 2:577–579, 1976

44. Hutton EM, Thompson MW: Carrier detection and genetic counselling in Duchenne muscular dystrophy: a follow up study. Can Med Assoc J 115:749–752, 1976

45. Davie AM, Emery AEH: Estimation of proportion of new mutants among cases of Duchenne muscular dystrophy. J Med Genet 15:339–345, 1978

46. Yasuda N, Kondo K: No sex difference in mutation rates of Duchenne muscular dystrophy. J Med Genet 17:106–111, 1980

47. Graham J: Genotype assignment in the haemophilias. Clin Hematol 8:115–145, 1979

48. Francke V, Felsenstein J, Gartler SM, et al: The occurrence of new mutants in the X-linked recessive Lesch Nyhan disease. Am J Hum Genet 28:123–136, 1976

49. Matheson AW, Howland JL: Erythrocyte deformation in human muscular dystrophy. Science 184:165–166, 1974

50. Miller SE, Roses AD, Appel SH: Scanning electron microscopy and studies in muscular dystrophy. Arch Neurol 33:172–174, 1976

51. Grassi E, Lucci B, Marchini C, et al: Deformed erythrocytes in muscular dystrophies. Neurology (NY) 28:842–844, 1978

52. Percy AK, Miller ME: Reduced deformability of erythrocyte membranes from patients with Duchenne muscular dystrophy. Nature 258:147–148, 1975

53. Missirlis YF, Goldsmith CH, Chan GHS, et al: Increased resistance to deformation of the membrane of erythrocytes in human muscular dystrophy. In press 1980

54. Verrill HL, Pickard NA, Gruemer HD: Diminished cap formation in lymphocytes from patients and carriers of Duchenne muscular dystrophy. Clin Chem 23:2341–2343, 1977

55. Verrill HL, Pickard NA, Gruemer HD: Mechanisms of cellular enzyme release. 1. Alteration in membrane fluidity and permeability. Clin Chem 23:2219–2225, 1977

56. Pickard NA, Gruemer HD, Verrill HL, et al: Systemic membrane defect in the proximal muscular dystrophies. N Engl J Med 299:841–846, 1978

57. Noronha ABC, Roos RP, Antel JP, et al: Concanavalin A-induced lymphocyte capping in Huntington's disease. Adv Neurol 23:419–428, 1979

58. Hauser S, Weiner H, Ault K, et al: Lymphocyte capping in Duchenne muscular dystrophy. N Engl J Med 300:861, 1979

59. Wyatt PR, Cox DM: Duchenne's muscular dystrophy: studies in cultured fibroblasts. Lancet 1:172–174, 1977

60. Cullen MJ, Parsons R: Inclusion bodies in muscular dystrophy. Lancet 2:929, 1977

61. Emery AEH: The electrophoretic pattern of lactic dehydrogenase in carriers and patients with Duchenne muscular dystrophy. Nature 201:1044–1045, 1964

62. Johnston HA, Wilkinson JH, Withycombe WA, et al: Alpha-hydroxybutyrate dehydrogenase activity in sex-linked muscular dystrophy. J Clin Pathol 19:250–256, 1966

63. Roses AD, Roses MJ, Nicholson GA, et al: Lactate dehydrogenase isoenzyme 5 in detecting carriers of Duchenne muscular dystrophy. Neurology (Minneap) 27:414–421, 1977

64. Burt D, Emery AEH: Serum LDH-S in carriers of Duchenne muscular dystrophy. Neurology (NY) 29:239–241, 1979

65. Pearson CM, Kar NC: Isoenzymes: general considerations and alterations in human and animal myopathies. Ann NY Acad Sci 138:293, 1966

66. Yasmineh WG, Ibrahim GA, Abbasnzhad M, et al: Isoenzyme distribution of creatine kinase and lactate dehydrogenase in serum and skeletal muscle in Duchenne muscular dystrophy, collagen disease and other muscular disorders. Clin Chem 24:1985–1989, 1978

67. Tzvetanova E: Serum creatine kinase isoenzymes in progressive muscular dystrophy. Enzyme 23:238–245, 1978

68. Alberts MC, Samaha FJ: Serum pyruvate kinase in muscle disease and carrier states. Neurology (Minneap) 24:462–464, 1974

69. Seay AR, Ziter FA, Wu LH, et al: Serum creatine phosphokinase and pyruvate kinase in neuromuscular disorders and Duchenne dystrophy carriers. Neurology (NY) 28:1047–1050, 1978

70. Yamuna S, Valmiknathan K, Burt D, et al: Serum pyruvate kinase in carriers of Duchenne muscular dystrophy. Clin Chim Acta 79:277–279, 1977

71. Zatz M, Shapiro LJ, Campion DS, et al: Serum pyruvate kinase (PK) and creatine-phosphokinase (CPK) in progressive muscular dystrophies. J Neurol Sci 36:349–362, 1978

72. Percy ME, Murphy I, Oss C, et al: Serum creatine kinase and pyruvate kinase in Duchenne muscular dystrophy carrier detection. Muscle Nerve 2:329–339, 1979

73. Adornato BT, Kagen LJ, Engel WK: Myoglobinaemia in Duchenne muscular dystrophy patients and carriers: a new adjunct to carrier detection. Lancet 2:499–501, 1978

74. Adornato BT, Engel WK, Foidart-Desalle M: Elevations of hemopexin levels in neuromuscular disease. Arch Neurol 35:577–580, 1978

75. Thompson MW, Murphy EG, McAlpine PJ: An assessment of the creatine kinase test in the detection of carriers of Duchenne muscular dystrophy. J Pediatr 71:82–93, 1967

76. Emery AEH: Genetic counselling in X-linked muscular dystrophy. J Neurol Sci 8:579–587, 1969

77. Gale AN, Murphy EA: The use of serum creatine phosphokinase in genetic counselling for Duchenne muscular dystrophy. 1. Analysis of results from 29 studies. J Chronic Dis 31:101–109, 1978

78. Sibert JR, Harper PS, Thompson RJ, et al: Carrier detection in Duchenne muscular dystrophy: evidence from a study of obligatory carriers and mothers of isolated cases. Arch Dis Child 54:534–537, 1979

79. Bullock DG, McSweeney FM, Whitehead TP, et al: Serum creatine kinase activity and carrier status for Duchenne muscular dystrophy. Lancet 2:1370, 1979

80. Thomson WHS: The biochemical identification of the carrier state in X-linked recessive (Duchenne) muscular dystrophy. Clin Chim Acta 26:207–221, 1969

81. Hodgson P, Gardner-Medwin D, Pennington R, et al: Studies of the carrier state in the Duchenne type of muscular dystrophy. 1. Effect of exercise on serum creatine kinase activity. J Neurol Neurosurg Psychiatry 30:416–419, 1967

82. Gilboa N, Swanson JR: Serum creatine phosphokinase in normal newborns. Arch Dis Child 51:283–285, 1976

83. Smith I, Elton RA, Thomson WHS: Carrier detection in X-linked recessive (Duchenne) muscular dystrophy: serum creatine phosphokinase values in premenarchal, menstruating, postmenopausal and pregnant normal women. Clin Chim Acta 98:207–216, 1979

84. Bundey S, Crawley JM, Edwards JH, et al: Serum creatine kinase levels in pubertal, mature, pregnant and postmenopausal women. J Med Genet 16:117–121, 1979

85. Satapathy RK, Skinner R: Serum creatine kinase levels in normal females. J Med Genet 16:49–51, 1979

86. Nicholson GA, Gardner-Medwin D, Pennington RJT, et al: Carrier detection in Duchenne muscular dystrophy: assessment of the effect of age on detection rate with serum-creatine-kinase-activity. Lancet 1:692–694, 1979

87. Bundey S: Calculation of genetic risks in Duchenne muscular dystrophy by genetics in the United Kingdom. J Med Genet 15:249–253, 1978

88. Roses AD, Roses MJ, Miller SE, et al: Carrier detection in Duchenne muscular dystrophy. N Engl J Med 294:193–198, 1976

89. Roses AD, Roses MJ, Metcalf BS, et al: Pedigree testing in Duchenne muscular dystrophy. Ann Neurol 2:271–278, 1977

90. Zellweger H, Antonik A: Newborn screening for Duchenne muscular dystrophy. Pediatrics 55:30–34, 1975

91. Gardner-Medwin D, Bundey S, Green S: Early diagnosis of Duchenne muscular dystrophy. Lancet 2:1102, 1978

92. Heuch I, Li FHF: A computer program for calculation of genotype probabilities using phenotype information. Clin Genet 3:501–504, 1972

93. Conneally PM, Heuch I: A computer program to determine genetic risks: a simplified version of PEDIG. Am J Hum Genet 26:773–775, 1974

94. Hurse PV, Kakulas BA: Genetic counselling in inherited muscle disease in Western Australia. Excerpta Medica Int Congr Series 334:88, 1974

95. Brooks, AP, Emery AEH: The incidence of Duchenne muscular dystrophy in the South East of Scotland. Clin Genet 2:290–294, 1977

96. Skinner R, Smith C, Emery AEH: Linkage between the loci for benign (Beeker type) X-borne muscular dystrophy and deutan colour-blindness. J Med Genet 2:317–320, 1974

97. Emery AEH: Genetic linkage between the loci for colour blindness and Duchenne type muscular dystrophy. J Med Genet 3:92–95, 1966

98. Zatz M, Itskan SB, Sanger R, et al: New linkage data for the X-linked types of muscular dystrophy and G6PO variants, colour blindness and Xg blood groups. J Med Genet 2:321–327, 1974

99. Blyth H, Carter CO, Dubowitz V, et al: Duchenne's muscular dystrophy and the Xg blood groups: a search for linkage. J Med Genet 2:157–160, 1965

100. Lindenbaum RH, Clarke G, Patel C, et al: Muscular dystrophy in an X;1 translocation female suggests that Duchenne locum is on X chromosome short arm. J Med Genet 16:389–392, 1979

101. Canki N, Dutrillaux B, Tivadar I: Dystrophie musculaire de Duchenne chez une petite fille porteuse d'une translocation t (X;3)(p21:q13) de novo. Ann Génet 22:35–39, 1979

102. Kan YW, Dozy AM: Polymorphism of DNA sequence adjacent to human beta-globin structural gene: relationship to sickle mutation. Proc Natl Acad Sci USA 75:5631–5635, 1978

103. Kan YW, Lee KY, Furbetta M, et al: Polymorphism of DNA sequence in the beta globin gene region: application to prenatal diagnosis of β° thalassaemia in Sardinia. N Engl J Med 302:185–188, 1980

104. Weatherall DJ, Clegg JB: Recent developments in the molecular genetics of human haemoglobin. Cell 16:467–479, 1979

105. Pena DJ: Is Duchenne muscular dystrophy a simple genic disorder? Lancet 2:630, 1978

106. Dubowitz V: Intellectual impairment in muscular dystrophy. Arch Dis Child 40:296–301, 1965

107. Dubowitz V: Mental retardation in Duchenne muscular dystrophy. In *Pathogenesis of Human Muscular Dystrophies*. Edited by Rowland LP. Excerpta Medica, Amsterdam, 1977, pp 688–694

108. Emery AE, Skinner R, Holloway S: A study of possible heterogeneity in Duchenne muscular dystrophy. Clin Genet 15:444–449, 1979

DISCUSSION

Dr. Sergio Pena: Do you do 3 CK tests, and what do you do with the woman who has one high result and a series of normal results

Dr. Peter Harper: Because of the variability inherent in the entire system, I always use the mean of 3 tests. I try not to look at the results until we have 3. There is a great temptation, if you get one that is borderline, to go on doing a few more until it comes down, or if you feel the person really is a carrier and you get some normal results, to go on doing a few more until you get a high one. There is great potential for bias here, so we have a standarized approach. All the results I showed were the mean of 3 determinations.

Dr. Corrado Angelini: If you only use CK, how do you identify false negatives? Some normal persons have a high CK level. Second, I think that a panel of tests should be used to detect a spectrum of abnormalities. For example, we use repetitive CK determinations at rest and after exercise, aldolase, and hemopexin. With this approach we have an 80% detection rate.

Dr. Peter Harper: In answer to the first question, I never regard anything as abnormal or normal. I think in terms of odds. I believe a lot of trouble would be avoided if this were done more regularly. By using odds, you can get around the difficult situation of reassuring someone with a result one point below the borderline, but saying to someone with a result one point over the limit, "I'm sorry, but you're a carrier." Odds let you use all the information to best advantage. The odds may be stronger or weaker, for or against, but the question of a sharp division into normal or abnormal does not arise. With regard to other tests, I would be happy to use them if I could be sure that they would not also increase the false-positive rate. This was the point I was trying to make earlier. We still do not have adequate information as to how much these other tests increase the false-positive rate. One can get part of the way by using an extensive series of normal control subjects, but one does not know whether the potential carriers identified as abnormal with the new test are really carriers, because only rarely do you have data on whether they have had children, especially affected children.

Dr. Helen Blau: Perhaps you do this, but it seems worth emphasizing that one way to refine the prior probability of carrier risk is to measure the CK level in family members. Analysis of these values in conjunction with the pedigree, using Bayesian statistics, will give a better estimate of risk.

Dr. Peter Harper: Yes, we do this. In fact, the data I showed were produced using the PEDIG program of Dr. Conneally and included the CK results for all family members as well as the genetic risks for all family members. I think this is an important point. Rather than test 1 person, we calculate the risks, test other family members, and then revise the estimate. It is helpful to test everybody, to obtain the entire body of biochemical and genetic information for the whole kindred, and only then determine the likelihood of the carrier state for various individuals. Sometimes, with a big family, this can get complicated; that is where PEDIG helps.

Dr. Hans-Dieter Greumer: I agree with the difficulties in interpreting CK tests. We have done studies on approximately 250 normal persons involving twins and found that monozygotic twins often have values very close together. One of the great difficulties with this test is to establish a normal range. There is no well-defined reference range, so all one can do is present probabilities that something is normal or abnormal by a Bayesian approach. The techniques are usually relatively reliable if performed in a clinical laboratory.

Dr. Peter Harper: I did not have time to discuss in full the problems of variation of CK with pregnancy, age, and other factors, but these variations are very important. I am interested by what you say about concordance between twins, because this raises another big problem that I did not mention: the question of correlation within families. If, in a family, you find an obligate carrier who has a low CK level and a potential carrier with a comparably low CK level, should this information influence the risks you assign, and if so, how? It is a very difficult problem for which we do not have an answer.

Dr. Jarvis Seegmiller: During the past decade or so, we have been working with another X-linked disorder and been fortunate to identify the abnormal gene product. Some of our findings in this mutation of the X chromosome may be relevant to Duchenne muscular dystrophy (DMD). We were rather surprised when we got all our data together. In 47 families, we found only 5 mothers who were heterozygotes. This number is substantially less than the one-third predicted from the hypotheses that have been discussed here today. The possibility of a similar disparity in mothers of children with DMD will need to be kept in mind in evaluating our carrier detection systems. The one-third new mutations, predicted from theoretical considerations, may not be found in actual assessment. One possible explanation that we proposed to account for this disparity was that the site of mutation is the maternal grandfather's sperm.

Dr. Peter Harper: I entirely agree that for both the Lesch-Nyhan syndrome and for hemophilia there is strong evidence of unequal mutation between the sexes. I do not think that holds for DMD. The practical evidence from CK testing and from prospective studies, quite apart from the genetic considerations, strongly supports a figure of approximately one third of cases being new mutations.

Dr. Jarvis Seegmiller: One other unrelated consideration may belong more properly in your panel discussion. The members of the Muscular Dystrophy Association could provide a nucleus for a valuable pooling of resources in one way that I have not heard discussed that could provide a valuable aid for future research. In cases in which parents elect, after genetic counseling, to terminate a pregnancy carrying a male fetus, special efforts should be made to obtain fetal cells and tissues in a viable state. To this end, the pregnancy should be terminated using prostaglandin rather than saline induction. Various fetal organs, including muscle, could then be minced up in culture media containing glycerol or dimethyl sulfoxide and frozen away in a bank for future culture of cells. Most investigators do not realize that it is not necessary to grow cells out before they can be frozen and then be revived. Even though we cannot identify the affected fetus at this state of our knowledge, the cells could be used for development of diagnostic tests. I am convinced that the progress might be much enhanced if a bank of such normal and mutant tissues were available.

64
Carrier Detection
Panel Discussion

Moderator: *Allen D. Roses, MD*

Panelists: *Alan E. H. Emery, MD*

                  Peter S. Harper, MD

                  Allen D. Roses, MD

                  Margaret W. Thompson, MD

                  Sir John Walton, TD, MD, DSc, SRCP

Dr. Allen Roses: This session represents a major concern for those of us who are interested in the eradication and control of Duchenne muscular dystrophy (DMD). We are here to examine several important questions related to carrier detection and the possible genetic attack on this disease; we will address several questions in relatively controversial areas. I expect, therefore, that more questions will be raised than answered by this discussion, and I hope that the pertinent questions will be clearer at the end of the discussion for the audience as well as for the participants.

We will delineate several avenues of investigation: (*a*) the definition of carrier detection tests that can be used to evaluate individual patients; (*b*) means of detecting carriers that are under study but have not been sufficiently evaluated to serve as tests; (*c*) biochemical or other phenomena that demonstrate significant differences between patients with DMD and control subjects, are not applicable as carrier detection tests, but do have implications for research; and (*d*) genetic concepts derived from seemingly incontrovertible assumptions. Among the most difficult areas are relating biochemical tests and genetic theory to the clinic, and testing certain genetic assumptions.

We have several experts in the audience whom I would like to be able to call upon as the discussion proceeds. To begin our discussion, I will first ask direct questions of each member of the panel. To start in alphabetical order: Dr. Emery, is there any evidence of clinical and genetic heterogeneity in DMD?

Dr. Alan Emery: Before answering that question, I would first like to acknowledge Professor Ebashi and Dr. Sugita, because they have not been mentioned so far in any of our discussions. It was their work, as long ago as 1959, that led to development of the serum creatine kinase (CK) test for detecting carriers.

One of the first problems to consider is the very high incidence of DMD, roughly 1 in 3,000 male births. It is difficult to account for this except by postulating a very high mutation rate. Because this rate would have to be exceptionally high, investigators have sought other explanations for the very high incidence of what is essentially a lethal disease. One possibility, of course, is heterozygous advantage. However, it has been calculated that carriers would have to have at least twice the fertility of normal women to account for the very high incidence, and this is not realistic. The other possibility is genetic heterogeneity, and there may be some evidence for this. Some boys with this disease are very severely mentally handicapped. In our experience, when a boy is sufficiently mentally handicapped to require institutionalization and he has other affected relatives, they, too, are mentally handicapped. This suggested to us some time ago that there might be genetic heterogeneity in this disease.

We recently studied 15 boys who were severely mentally handicapped and an equal number of affected boys who were not mentally handicapped. We found significant differences. In those with severe mental handicap, onset of the disease and confinement to a wheelchair occurred later in life; the decrease in serum CK levels with age was less marked, and urinary excretion of certain amino acids was greater than that in affected boys with normal intelligence (Clin Genet 15:444–449, 1979). Correlations among relatives with regard to age at onset and age at confinement to a wheelchair, reported by Feingold, also support the hypothesis of genetic heterogeneity. There is also recent biochemical evidence of two different patterns of muscle sarcoplasmic reticulum membrane proteins observed by Samaha and Congedo, and erythrocyte membrane spectrin peptides reported by Dr. Roses. In work on DMD, we should bear in mind that this may not be a single disease entity.

Dr. Allen Roses: Dr. Margaret Thompson, would you explain the mathematical treatment of multiple test results to arrive at risk figures?

Dr. Margaret Thompson: Dr. Maire Percy and I recently published our results using CK and pyruvate kinase levels in combination. We have analyzed CK and hemopexin in a similar way, and have added lactate dehydrogenase to the test panel. First, it is necessary to know the distribution of each variable in obligate carriers and in age-matched control subjects tested under similar conditions. Dr. David Andrews has helped us produce an equation that will identify more carriers than can be identified by CK assay alone. By using our 4 tests in combination, we can now distinguish 89% of the heterozygotes from 95% of the control group. We combine the probability that a subject is a carrier, as estimated from biochemical test results, with the probability estimated from pedigree analysis to obtain the final risk figure that is used in genetic counseling.

Dr. Allen Roses: Sir John, how successful has carrier detection been at preventing new cases in DMD in Newcastle? You also have some data concerning age and serum CK in a carrier population. What implications do your data have for the age at which the carriers should be tested?

Dr. John Walton: I would like to begin by making two points. The first is that I agree entirely with Dr. Harper's point of view (see chapter 63) that it is wise to concentrate, at present, on the estimation of serum CK activity and to work out the statistical probability that an individual is a carrier; this is still by far the most reliable method of carrier detection. During the past few years, our program of carrier detection appears to have reduced by approximately one-third the number of new cases of DMD. But contrary to findings of Dr. Harper, there is some evidence in Newcastle of an unexplained reduction in isolated cases: the incidence of first-born affected cases in a family also appears to have been reduced, which cannot have been the result of our carrier detection program.

Even for those of us who consider CK activity to be the most reliable method of carrier detection, we must remember that, however good our statistics, we are dealing, as Dr. Harper said, in terms of odds. Someone may look at a situation, accept the odds as being reasonable, and then be let down by the result. We have seen two failures where women in whom the odds were 1 in 4 ignored that level of risk (which most would regard as unacceptably high) and had affected children. We also had one family in which the prior probability was 1 in 4 for the grandmother, but 1 in 10 for her daughter. She thought these odds were reasonable, but had a child affected by DMD.

Turning to the other question you raised, Lane, Pennington, Gardner-Medwin, and I carried out a series of tests in known carriers that included, among others, age-dependent change in red blood cell shape, serum hemopexin, red blood cell potassium efflux, and spectrin phosphorylation; all were negative. Manual muscle testing, as described by Dr. Roses and colleagues and carried out in a very careful quantitative way, was positive in 11 of 12; however, 2 of 12 control subjects had a false-positive finding with this method. In the scalar electrocardiogram, the RS ratio in V1 and V2 was abnormal in most of the carriers but did not seem to be sufficiently reliable for regular carrier detection.

In a study of CK activity in a large number of young girls from a local school and in volunteer adults, it was clear that 95% of all normal females less than 16 years of age have a CK activity of less than 75 IU/I; for females more than 16 years of age, the normal upper limit appeared to be 60 IU/I. Lane and Nicholson also looked at serial CK measurements in 11 known DMD carriers and found a progressive decrease in activity in most of those serially tested over a period of years. One would expect this from the Lyon hypothesis, because if there is random inactivation of the X chromosome, a proportion of the cells in carrier female muscle will express the effect of the dystrophic gene; then, with increasing age, the nuclei which express that dystrophic gene in the muscle will die off progressively, leaving a greater population of normal nuclei in the affected muscle. Hence, what we did was to look at the age effect by looking at the serum CK activity in known DMD carriers and their daughters. In a series of known carriers with a mean age of 38 years, only 53% had a CK activity outside the normal range. In daughters of known carriers with a mean age of 16 years, each of whom would have a 50% risk on genetic grounds of being a carrier, 45% had increased serum CK activity, suggesting that approximately 90% of the carriers were being detected. However, when one looked at daughters of known carriers less than 16 years of age (mean age, 11 years), there was a detection of 0.61, even greater than the expected 50%.

Of course, there is no way to know whether these young daughters of known carriers are also carriers. But the evidence from this finding strongly suggests that the CK test is much more reliable in girls less than 16 years of age and that the detection rate is likely to be higher in that age group.

Dr. Allen Roses: One of the issues raised is how difficult it is to test an individual, even for CK activity. The application of other tests obviously produces even more problems. Over the years, on the basis of published data, we have raised some questions concerning the genetic hypotheses on which current counseling is based. I would like to ask Dr. Emery to go through the Bayesian statistical approach to counseling. Then I will ask Dr. Mike Conneally, who is a population geneticist in the audience, about alternative explanations for the high mutation rate. After that, we will throw this discussion open to any questions that the audience might have.

Dr. Alan Emery: The technique to which Dr. Roses refers is that usually attributed to the Reverend Bayes, who published this in 1763, so we are really trying to keep up with the literature (!). The method depends on taking into account prior probabilities, i.e., antecedents and conditional probabilities.

For DMD carrier detection, one estimates the probability of a woman having a particular serum CK level given that she is (or is not) a carrier. I would like to emphasize that CK levels are *not* normally distributed among either carriers or controls, and the two distributions overlap. If a suspected carrier has a CK level less than the normal ninety-fifth percentile, you can not assure her that she is not a carrier. Using the Bayesian approach, one can take into account not only the suspected carrier's CK level, but also the CK levels of all her first-degree postpubertal female relatives, and the number of normal brothers and sons she has.

Intuitively, one can imagine that a sporadic case in a family is more likely to represent a new mutation, so that the mother is unlikely to be a carrier if she has a normal CK level and several normal brothers, and if her mother and perhaps sisters also have normal CK levels. By combining all of these data for the family, it is quite possible that the probability of a suspected carrier actually being a carrier may be so small that the likelihood of her having an affected son is less than the risk of amniocentesis. This is an important point, because in such a situation the woman might well wish to decline the offer of prenatal sexing and selective abortion. In counseling a woman at risk of having an affected son, it is essential to take into account as much genetic and biochemical data as possible. This can be achieved using Bayesian statistics.

Dr. Allen Roses: Dr. Conneally, for the sake of argument, let me just say as an optimistic clinical neurologist, that I have trouble believing that DMD differs from other genetic diseases that are biochemically defined. I would like to know what positive data support a high mutation rate; of course, I am saying this strictly for argument! What is the basis for the belief that one third of cases of the disease are due to new mutations, and that these mutations occur in the ova of nonheterozygous women?

Dr. Mike Conneally: Under Haldane's hypothesis, we assume that the frequency of the disease is 3 times the mutation rate: one-third are new mutations in the egg; one-third are new mutations in the egg or sperm that made the mother; and the final one-third are old mutants. Children with DMD do not reproduce, so approximately half the genes are lost each generation. They must be made up some way, because if they were not we would not all be here today talking about DMD.

What are the alternatives to the classic hypothesis that one third of the cases are new mutants? Four come to mind, although I can dismiss some of them. The first is lack of penetrance, a genetic phenomenon in which an individual carries the gene but does not manifest the trait. Thus, there is the possibility in DMD that there are males going around who have the gene without the disorder and therefore reproduce. Obviously, all of their daughters would be carriers. There is absolutely no evidence for this, and I think we can dismiss it, because segregation analyses of families show that half the males are affected. Lack of penetrance would show up in the analysis.

The second way to account for the high mutation rate is the alternative that Dr. Emery just mentioned: genetic heterogeneity. In this situation, multiple independent loci are involved in the trait. This could account for the high mutation rate. In fact, we would have not 3μ, but the sum of 3μ as the frequency of affected males. This, however, could not account for the fact that one third of all affected males would still represent new mutations. Thus, this explanation could not account for the excess number of carrier mothers.

A third explanation would be one which Dr. Emery mentioned: increased fertility in carrier females. The problem is that you would require, as Dr. Emery pointed out, approximately twice the fertility in carrier females to make up for the loss of the gene in affected males. Finally, the most plausible explanation, alluded to by Dr. Seegmiller when he spoke about the Lesch-Nyhan syndrome, may be that mutations occur predominantly in the sperm. In this case, for all affected males, the mothers are carriers, but two thirds of the carrier mothers would be isolated cases. In other words, the grandmother would not be affected. I would make a plea that you look at the sisters of mothers with affected offspring when using new methods of carrier detection. If the hypothesis of predominance of sperm mutations is correct, then approximately two thirds of the sisters should not be carriers. I would stress that recent data from Yasuda in Japan do not agree that there is a differential mutation rate between males and females, because the frequency of affected uncles is not different from that expected.

Dr. Sergio Pena: I would like to review briefly what we are arguing about, what is being called here the "Haldane's hypothesis." It is not Haldane's hypothesis at all, but simply the equilibrium frequency of lethal X-linked disorders. There is no hypothesis to it. Basically, the first data to challenge it were Dr. Roses' data on phosphorylation, and Dr. Roses mentioned himself that phosphorylation was never meant to be a carrier detection test. So the data on phosphorylation could not be used to challenge a classic concept in genetics. The second challenge came from the data on lymphocyte capping, which are not accepted by the panel or, as you know, as a carrier detection test. A third challenge was the data from Lesch-Nyhan syndrome and hemophilia, brought up by Dr. Seegmiller today, but one cannot apply data from one disease to another disease. We are talking about completely different disorders and we should not allow concepts to get mixed up. By the way, the Lesch-Nyhan data have been challenged by Newton Morton on the base of a possible ascertainment bias. So I think we have to stick with the classic studies of C.A.B. Smith and of Newton Morton in the 1950s, who calculated the equilibrium frequency and found it to be exactly as expected, 33%. I do not see any point in discussing the matter further.

Dr. Allen Roses: I did want to not get the concepts of a carrier detection test and other biochemical data mixed up, but I think we already have. We have defined a carrier detection test as one that could be applied to an individual. What we did with the Band 2 phosphorylation data was to apply it to all the carriers in our series and to their matched control subjects. We then analyzed the groups of carriers separately: those who were definite carriers by genetic criteria, those who would be probable carriers by Dr. Thompson's criteria, and possible carriers (mothers with CK activity way above the range of normal). We presumed that all the new mutation mothers in our clinic had to come from the group with normal or low CK levels and were not genetically implicated to be carriers. The Band 2 phosphorylation in that group of women was identical to that of the genetic carrier group. The Band 2 phosphorylation in any individual cannot be used as a carrier detection test. However, the group who could contain, or "should" contain the new mutants had data, biochemical parameters, that we measured paired and prospectively, that were equal to those of definite carriers and significantly different from those of matched controls.

Dr. Sergio Pena: I agree with you, and I remember the details of the paper. Considering the standard errors of the data and the fact that you were not, as you said, identifying individual carriers, the data may be just too soft to challenge classic concepts in genetics.

Dr. Henry Epstein: I would like to make a comment and then ask a couple of related questions. I hope that the statistical arguments presented this afternoon will not impede the attempts of many laboratories all over the world to understand the molecular defect in DMD. Clearly, CK is not. We might then be able to make at least almost precise diagnoses.

I would like to raise a question for the geneticists on the panel or in the audience. It has clearly been established in experimental situations that mutations in genes can affect the phenotypic expression of mutations in another particular gene. For example, there are homozygotes for sickle cell hemoglobin whose cells never sickle. Accordingly, I think it is an open question whether there could be people who are Duchenne genetically but not phenotypically.

I would also like to ask exactly how sure we are that Newcastle, Wales, New York, and Rochester have identical populations of patients with DMD and/or their families. Has there ever been an experiment where one professor of neurology reviews in some blind fashion the neuromuscular patients in another clinic?

Dr. John Walton: I do not think that has been done. Many people who have experience in neuromuscular disease have had the opportunity to visit other centers and to see a selection of their patient population, but I am not aware of anyone having undertaken a formal study. Nevertheless, if ever a disease appears clinically to breed true, it is DMD. In autosomal dominant disorders, like the facioscapulohumeral syndrome, there is immense variability in clinical expression from case to case within the same family. In autosomal recessive disorders, such as some of the biochemically determined myopathies like Pompe's glycogeneosis, there occur within the same sibship, severe and much less severe cases. But in DMD, despite the evidence which Dr. Emery and others have presented to suggest heterogeneity, the clinical pattern breeds very true. On the basis of my experience in visiting many centers throughout the world, I do not believe that I can recognize any significant variation in clinical expression or even biochemical expression of DMD. Going back to your first point, you are absolutely right. Until we identify a basic or fundamental biochemical effect, such as the enzyme defect that Dr. Seegmiller refers to in the Lesch-Nyhan syndrome, then we are studying epiphenomena and are not using anything that gives a clue to the fundamental part of the disease process. Nevertheless, we must make the best possible use of the methods we do have.

Dr. Jarvis Seegmiller: In this matter of genetic heterogeneity, we need to keep in mind the possibility, because we have examples of this in Lesch-Nyhan disease, that the degree of heterogeneity we see at a clinical level may merely represent a genetic heterogeneity in the site of the mutation in the abnormal gene product. Certainly, we find variations in clinical expression, particularly neurologic dysfunction, depending on how severe the enzyme deficit is in Lesch-Nyhan disease. Now, if we were looking only at the epiphenomena of uric acid overproduction, we would probably have included another enzyme defect, that of increased phosphoribosylpyrophosphate synthetase, which is a cause of overproduction of uric acid in some of our gout patients and, surprisingly, maps very close to the gene for hypoxanthine-guanine phosphor-ibosyltransferase and the Lesch-Nyhan disease on the X chromosome. Initially, we might think in terms of variations in severity of the primary abnormal gene product of the mutation, i.e., in the abnormal gene product as a first cause or most simple explanation for the clinical heterogeneity that has been described here.

Dr. Alan Pestronk: I would like to take Dr. Harper's concept of familial variation in the levels of CK a bit further and ask two questions about it. First of all, it is clear that patients with DMD show up to a 5-fold differences in CK level, even taking age into account. Dr. Harper, what might that tell us about the probability that a family member might have an increased CK level?

Dr. Peter Harper: One practical thing must be borne in mind here: with most assays, the degree of accuracy declines very much at the top end of the range. Once one gets up to 5,000 and 10,000, which is what we usually are dealing with, the margin for error is very wide; there is wide variation, in terms of thousands, between results for the same DMD child from week to week. I do not know of any evidence that levels in the child affect carrier results. However, there is strong evidence of a correlation within families of CK values. What we do not know is how to use this correlation. Can we quantify it and somehow use it in the same way as other information? This is something I would dearly like to know.

Dr. Alan Pestronk: Dr. Emery, would not the fact that CK levels tend to correlate within families make it invalid to use the low level of CK in one family member in the determination of the probability that another family member is a carrier? That is, unless the CK level of the second family member deviates significantly from that of the first?

Dr. Alan Emery: There is no doubt that CK levels in sisters of affected boys are correlated, but though this is statistically significant in a large body of data, the actual correlation is relatively small (about 0.3 in our own data) and overshadowed by considerable variations within individuals. For this reason, I would think that information on intrafamilial correlations in CK levels would not be very helpful in the counseling situation.

Dr. David Gardner-Medwin: I want to make two comments. One is about the variability of serum CK levels in children with DMD. During a treatment trial recently, we looked at serum CK activity once a month for 13 months in boys with DMD; there was a 4-fold variation from month to month within cases, which is a very important point.

Next, I would just like to widen the question of preventing DMD a little and look at reasons why one fails by summarizing 55 cases born in our region since 1950 that might have been prevented with perfect carrier tracing and detection. Thirty-one were born because of failure to give or respond to genetic advice; the others were born because of late diagnosis in a previously affected member of the family. Only 3 mothers in the first group had been given genetic advice; these were the 3 Sir John mentioned. Two mothers were at high risk (1 in 4 of having an affected child in each pregnancy); 1, a low risk (1 in 40). The difficulty is not to give effective advice to women once you have got them into the room for counseling; the difficulty is getting to counsel them all. The other 28 cases in the "failure of counseling" group had not been seen by us.

I would also like to remind you of the importance of early diagnosis. In 24 cases the births might have been prevented by earlier diagnosis of an affected brother or cousin (14 by early clinical diagnosis and 24 altogether, if there had been neonatal diagnosis by screening). We have some evidence that the present methods work quite well. We studied CK levels retrospectively in mothers of 30 preventable cases to see what would have been found by prenatal testing. Some of these women were definite carriers, with a risk of 1 of being a carrier; many had a risk of 0.5. Only one had a very low risk based on the pedigree (0.006). After serum CK estimation, none had a risk of less than 1 in 10 of being a carrier, and almost all of them were shown to be virtually definite carriers. We could have prevented virtually all of these cases by the present methods. Devising better methods of carrier detection is not going to make a contribution of any significance to the prevention of the disease. All it will do is help the many unfortunate women who now have infertility imposed on them because they have been assigned too high a risk, even though many are not carriers.

Last, I want to summarize what might and might not be done by better prevention methods to alter the incidence of the disease. One third of cases are mutants, as believed by everyone in this room except one person, and cannot be prevented. One-third are born to mothers who actually are carriers but who have no previous family history to make them suspect that fact. Even if you did total population carrier screening, which would be a very inefficient, inaccurate, and a thoroughly unsupportable method of trying to find carriers, you would not detect more than half of them, so you would still have about half of all cases of DMD that are theoretically not preventable. The remaining one third of cases occur after a previous case in the family. Twenty per cent of all cases might be prevented by better carrier tracing, 13% by screening newborns, or about 8% by earlier diagnosis of cases with early clinical manifestations of the disease.

Dr. Allen Roses: Let me just say something about the philosophy of science, in answer to Dr. Pena's remarks about classic concepts and classic hypotheses. Hypotheses, whether classic or not classic, are simply hypotheses that are meant to be tested. Hypotheses are tested with data, and data can be argued about. I do not see anything sacrosanct about a classic theory, making it immune to data. Our data raise questions concerning the assumptions of the hypothesis on which counseling techniques are based. Whether or not I am alone in the room, as Dr. Gardner-Medwin has suggested, in believing it, I think that part of the reason we are having this discussion is that these assumptions have not been seriously questioned. A hypothesis does not necessarily mean dogma. Science is based on testing hypotheses, with due respect to the generators of those hypotheses.

Dr. Howard Feit: I would like to ask the panel whether the Bayesian statistical analysis has ever been validated in the situation of counseling in DMD.

Dr. Margaret Thompson: Among our definite carriers, only 3 have had male offspring to term, although others have become pregnant and have gone through the amniocentesis program. Two of the three sons were affected. Of 15 sons born to mothers with a carrier risk less than 10%, only 1 was affected. The carrier risks were calculated on the basis of CK assay in combination with Bayesian analysis. Although the numbers are small, this kind of information helps to validate the Bayesian approach.

Dr. Peter Harper: I would like to comment in defense of Dr. Roses' and Dr. Appel's work. Until their work, hardly anyone ever thought about studying nonmuscular cells. The fact that all of the results may not hold up is quite a small point compared with the fact that this work has stimulated a tremendous shift in opinion toward looking at DMD and other dystrophies as generalized diseases. It would have been very sad if that work had not been done, and I think it has had great value.

Dr. Stephen Hauschka: I want to make two points. One is to reply to Dr. Seegmiller about the saving of fetuses at risk for dystrophy. We and Dr.

Konigsberg have been doing this for a couple of years, and we have 4 fetuses at risk. This is a good start, but I am sure many more such fetuses have been electively aborted during this year. Could I see a show of hands from people who have been involved in a situation in which an at-risk fetus has been electively aborted during the past year? How many? You see, we could have a dozen or so by now. That would be terrific. We are prepared to travel anywhere in the country with the proper equipment to collect such fetuses. The tissue will be frozen, stored in several tissue banks, and will be available to anybody who wants them.

My second point concerns the amniocytes from tests being done to determine the sex of fetuses at risk for DMD. There are several reasons not only for studying these, but for saving the amniocytes from all of the genetic counseling studies that are being done. A critical decision for any parent who is counseled is whether, even when informed of the genetic probabilities, they may elect to abort a perfectly normal son or daughter who would not be a carrier. Obviously, it would be extremely valuable to be able to tell the parents whether or not this child has the disease. So we should be saving all of the amniocytes being gathered in these counseling situations. This could be accomplished with the standard freezing techniques for cultured cells. We would be glad to explain these to any labs involved with such amniocytes.

A particularly valuable class of amniocytes that people should be aware of is from cases in which the parents elect to have the amniocentesis, and then elect not to abort, even when informed that the fetus is a male. If the child turns out to have DMD, these aminocytes would be extremely valuable diagnostic tools. Some day, we are going to know the biochemical marker for DMD. We would then be able to look at the amniocytes of unknown fetuses and determine whether they contained the lesion. Such information could prevent incredible anxiety for parents who are now faced with nothing more than probabilities.

Dr. Allen Roses: I think a number of us in this room are holding some of this material. I know Dr. Mitchell Golbus in San Francisco has some; perhaps we might get together and produce some written notations on where this material is and how it can be obtained.

Dr. Jarvis Seegmiller: You may not all be aware of a national repository in New Jersey supported by the National Institute of General Medical Sciences that may well serve these needs. At present, they accept fibroblasts and lymphoblast lines and might well be persuaded to accept the amniotic cells you propose. They routinely perform tests for mycoplasmal contaminants before freezing cells away for storage. They publish a catalogue every year or so listing all of the mutant cells in their repository and make the cells available to any investigator at a modest price. I concur with Dr. Hauschka that this would be a very valuable resource for developing and testing prenatal diagnostic techniques.

Dr. Sergio Pena: I have two comments and one question. I would like to mention a mother who delivered a baby with DMD. She had normal CK levels on 3 testings. Her twin sister, who is apparently clinically identical, and blood group identical (the HLA data are not ready yet) has 3 CK values around 400

IU. With regard to Dr. Gardner-Medwin's data, it worries me a little bit as a geneticist, to talk about "genetic advice not followed." In genetic counseling, we give probabilities and the patient must decide what to do with those probabilities. If you give a probability of 10% and the patient has a son with DMD, that is not an error, it is bad luck. I also have a question for Dr. Emery as to whether the IQ in DMD correlates with the median parental IQ.

Dr. Alan Emery: A great deal of work has been done on the IQ problem. When we reviewed this matter a couple of years ago, we found that in 15 such studies concerning IQ in DMD involving 810 affected boys, on average, about one-third had IQs less than 75. There is a high correlation in IQ in affected siblings. This reduction in IQ in DMD seems to be specific for this disorder and not secondary to lack of educational opportunities, for in patients with spinal muscular atrophy, with the same degree of muscle weakness, intelligence is normal. As I mentioned earlier, affected boys who are severely mentally handicapped and often require institutional care may represent a special group.

Dr. Arthur Buller: I would like to say that the Medical Research Council in the United Kingdom already operates a modest fetal tissue bank (I have since been informed by Sir John Walton that the Muscular Dystrophy Group of Great Britain also has a bank). However, in the United Kingdom there are strict rules concerning the collection and distribution of fetal material, but it is hoped that these will not prejudice the laudable objectives set by Dr. Hauschka.

As I am on my feet, may I make one other observation? As I have been away from my laboratory for the last 2 years and during that time working in administration, I am surprised that no one has mentioned the individual costs of the variety of tests that have been used in carrier detection. By and large, the greater the number of laboratory tests undertaken on a single individual, the greater the cost of the advice that is finally given. We must distinguish clearly between research (the hunt for the biochemical marker) and the provision of the best service that can be given at a particular point in time. I was greatly impressed by Dr. Harper's case, and by the additional precision that could be added to the average CK value of an individual by genetic data and a pencil and paper. Before additional tests are routinely added, the cost-effectiveness of such action needs to be considered.

Dr. Peter Harper: In cost-effective terms, one would need to prevent hardly any cases of DMD to provide an overwhelming cost-effective benefit. It is much more a question of accuracy of detection rather than the economics at the moment. Taking the subject of effective prevention a stage further, one badly needed facility is an accurate and prospective register of DMD carriers. If there was ever a case for a genetic register, DMD provides it. We now have one for Wales and were amazed to find that less than 10% of women at high risk had been adequately tested, even though at the outset of our work we were assured that everyone in the families had been tested. We hope we have overcome that problem.

Dr. Corrado Angelini: Disputing a genetic theory on the basis of biochemical data is certainly difficult. There are other ways to test the Haldane theory to see if whether it applies completely to DMD. Some of the data collected by Dr.

Daniels, a geneticist who works in our group, corroborates Dr. Roses' data. In a large study of numerous families, we have shown that there is an advantage of the heterzygote DMD carrier in their reproduction. With regard to this point, I would like to ask Dr. Walton how he explains that 17 of 28 daughters of known carriers had high CK activity. Does this suggest a possible advantage of the affected X-chromosome of carriers in reproduction? As far as cost benefit of expensive strategies for DMD, we have recently observed a noticeable decline in the incidence of DMD in our region. I think that this proves that working on the prevention of this disease is cost effective.

Dr. John Walton: The impact of a case of DMD on the family and on the community is so immense that any test, unless it is vastly expensive, will pay for itself in no time at all if it is reliable. In answer to the point made by Dr. Angelini, it did look as though among carriers, daughters less than 16 years of age we ascertained much more than the expected 50%. However, statistical analysis showed that the figure identified by CK alone was not significantly different from the expected 50%. What it did suggest is that the test was coming very close to detecting 100% of the young girls who were likely to be carriers, but this must be validated by future information.

I would also add that Dr. Harper is absolutely right in drawing attention to the immense impact of the work of Dr. Roses and Dr. Appel on research into dystrophy and its pathogenesis, because we have been seeking for years for biochemical, morphologic, and other markers that might identify abnormalities in cells other than muscle in patients with DMD. This has opened up a completely new field of research. However, there is a good deal of information (which we do not have time to go into) that supports the classic Haldane hypothesis. What does concern us, Dr. Roses, is that some of the biochemical methods you have used might have been diagnosing false positives; this is a matter of continuing controversy and one that will be resolved only by a great deal more work.

Dr. Victor Dubowitz: I want to comment first on the occasional lack of concordance of CK levels in DMD carriers within a family. Some years ago, I studied a family in which identical twin sisters each had a son with DMD; one mother had consistently increased CK values, and the other had consistently normal CK values; both had histologic changes on biopsy (Dubowitz, 1963, Proc R Soc Med 1963).

I would like to move from that to the point Dr. Harper made about the possibility of other methods in the individual case. During the past few years, we have been doing needle biopsies on carriers and control subjects and various quantitative light and electron microscopic studies. The results of these tests and some of the x-ray microanalysis studies on intranuclear calcium and phosphorus done by Maunder-Sewry, and me are shown in Table 1.

We divided carriers into definite or obligate carriers on genetic grounds (n = 13); presumptive carriers were those in whom CK activity was increased beyond the 95% confidence limits of our normal range (n = 12), and possible carriers were those with CK activity within our normal range. The table shows the percentages that deviated from the range of our normal controls. These were adult female volunteers who underwent biopsy specifically for this study.

Table 1. Percentage of Carriers Showing Abnormality[a]

Carrier Status	CK Activity	Light Microscopy	Electron Microscopy	Microprobe Analysis (Cal + Cal/P ratio)	Combined Biopsy Results (without CK)
Definite (n = 13)	54	69	75	92	92
Presumptive[b] (n = 12)	100	92	42	67	100
Possible (n = 37)	0	78	53	60	81

[a] Outside range of 10 normal female volunteer needle biopsies.
[b] With increased CK levels.

The last column shows the combined results without CK activity, and the proportion that were abnormal by one of the criteria. It shows that the incidence among the possible carriers was higher than expected. We have not done the prior risk calculations for individual cases in this group in relation to this analysis.

Dr. Alan Murray: I would like to second Dr. Hauschka's suggestion. Dr. Seegmiller has suggested that the cell depository in New Jersey be used. I have had some contact with Dr. Green of that facility; he seemed to be interested in getting cells from about 5 patients with DMD to add to what they have. Their financial constraints are such that the number of cells from different patients that they store is directly proportional to the number of requests they get for those cells; they do not have a lot of requests right now.

Dr. Allen Roses: I would like to make one final comment that I think would be somewhat constructive, is cost-effective, and is something that can be done. I would like to make a plea for data relevant to some of the genetic questions. With the help of geneticists, we should design experiments to test the underlying assumptions of the current genetic basis for counseling. Are the mutation rates identical in males and females? Are the mutation rates in males greater than females? Is there heterozygous advantage? For instance, is there any testable evidence for a more heterozygous female being born than normal female, thus affecting the genetic analysis.

No single clinic has the numbers to pursue these questions, but using the data of many clinics may provide statistically useful parameters. Could we design a multicenter study capable of attacking these questions before we know the biochemical defect in DMD? Dr. Russell Lane and I published an abstract in *Clinical Research* last year concerning this question. We would love to get the same type of data from more clinics. In each clinic, one needs to determine all of the families that were ascertained by the first affected DMD son. Eliminate families ascertained initially by the second affected or multiple births or by referral for carrier detection. Determine by pedigree analysis whether the mother is a definite genetic carrier, and set this group aside so as not to prejudice any subsequent analysis. Record the sex ratio of all births in the sibship subsequent to the first affected male and whether or not any subsequent sons are affected, as would be expected in families of women subsequently classified as probable carriers. The sex of any therapeutic abortions should also be noted. It is imperative to document the correct birth order. Subsequent births, rather than the total births, would be used because we have no way to determine the sex ratio in families of genetic heterozygotes who never had an affected son. If all, or nearly all, mothers of affected sons are heterozygotes, then the ratio would be 1:1:2 (1 affected male to 1 normal male to 2 females). If a significant proportion are mothers of an affected male due to a spontaneous new mutation in that generation, then the ratio would be significantly different.

Large numbers in multiple clinics are really necessary to correct the data statistically for sibship size, the effect of multiple affected births in the series, and so on. It costs nothing but time and careful pedigree analysis to do this. Most of the people who run clinics have this material readily at hand. In the 3 clinics already studied, the subsequent birth ratios are precisely 1:1:2. However, we do not have enough data in those 3 clinics to correct for the effect of sibship size or one particular pedigree that had multiple births of 4 affected males. We look forward to receiving data from any clinic director.

I hope our discussion has crystallized some of the important issues in DMD. Perhaps we will soon obtain more data testing the controversial hypotheses.

Part IX

MUSCLE IN CULTURE

65
Development of Fiber Type Specificity in Embryonic Avian Skeletal Muscle

Laura Reeburgh Keller, PhD

Charles P. Emerson, Jr, PhD

Differentiation of embryonic skeletal muscle is evidenced morphologically by fusion of mononucleated myoblasts and formation of multinucleated myotubes. This morphological differentiation is accompanied by the appearance of new proteins and messenger ribonucleic acids (mRNAs). At the time of fusion, synthesis of the protein constituents of the contractile apparatus such as actin, tropomyosins, troponins, and myosin heavy and light chains is activated coordinately, i.e., simultaneously and at equimolar rates (1, 2). However, most of these contractile proteins are represented in the genome by families of closely related genes, and the genes expressed in adult fast-contracting muscles are different from the genes expressed in adult slow muscles. This means that in addition to the developmental program of coordinate expression of the contractile protein genes at fusion, there must be another developmental program to select the appropriate members of these gene families for expression in the fast and slow fiber types.

Although adult fast and slow contracting muscle fibers have been well characterized physiologically and biochemically (3), expression of fiber type characteristics in embryonic fibers is less well understood. Based on studies of contraction speeds, some investigators have concluded that embryonic muscles are slow and that fast fibers develop from originally slow muscle (4). On the other hand, others have detected only the fast myosin light chain isozymes in embryonic muscle and have proposed that slow fibers develop from these muscles, probably in response to later innervation (5, 6). In other work, both fast and slow isozymes of myosin light chains were detected in embryonic muscles initially, and it has been proposed that expression of subsets of isozymes is repressed later to produce the appropriate fiber types (7, 8). Also, evidence has been presented for the expression of unique embryonic isozymes of myosin

863

heavy and light chains in developing muscle (9, 10). Although these earlier studies have resulted in conflicting conclusions about which fiber type specific proteins are initially expressed in embryonic muscle, they clearly show that expression of contractile protein gene families changes as embryonic muscles mature into individual adult fiber types.

Our studies have focused on the mechanisms regulating fiber type differentiation during avian muscle development. Establishment of the appropriate pattern of fiber-specific gene expression could, in theory, be regulated by two general mechanisms. The first such mechanism might involve the successive replacement of embryonic fibers by adult-type fibers formed from fusion of unique stem cell populations with different potentials for synthesis of contractile protein isozymes. Alternatively, changes in contractile protein isozymes could occur within individual embryonic fibers by changes in gene expression. To distinguish between these alternatives, we have studied myosin light chain synthesis and mRNA accumulation in embryonic muscle derived from areas of chick and quail embryos that will give rise to either fast or slow adult muscles. Our results are consistent with a simple model for fiber type differentiation in which the changes in fiber type expression occur within embryonic muscle fibers rather than by the successive differentiation of fiber type specific stem cells during development. We speculate that fiber type specificity develops initially by a generalized muscle program in which synthesis of both fast and slow genes for skeletal muscle contractile proteins is activated at fusion, followed later by the selective repression of transcription or nuclear processing of mRNA for one set of fiber type genes.

INITIAL COEXPRESSION OF FAST AND SLOW MYOSIN LIGHT CHAINS

Synthesis of adult skeletal muscle myosin light chains has been examined in cultures of presumptive fast (breast) and slow (anterior latissimus dorsi, ALD) muscles of chick embryos. A hypothesis that myoblast stem cells that give rise to fast and slow muscles have different stem cell lineages would predict that the muscle formed from myoblasts in either fast or slow muscle regions might be expected to synthesize different fiber type specific isozymes of the contractile proteins. Cultures of embryonic muscle are particularly suited for analysis of gene expression during the early events of muscle differentiation, because myoblasts will differentiate synchronously and in the absence of nerves, which may influence the process of fiber type differentiation. Also, myosin light chains are unambiguous markers for fiber type differentiation, because adult fast and slow muscles have different light chains that are easily resolved by 2-dimensional electrophoresis (11) (Figure 1A,B,C).

Figure 1 (D,E,F) shows 2-dimensional gels of the proteins synthesized by secondary cultures of ALD or breast muscle from day 12 chick embryos. As the figure indicates, differentiated cultures derived from both fast and slow muscles synthesize proteins that comigrate on gels with the 5 myosin light chains of adult skeletal muscle, LC_{1f}, LC_{2f}, LC_{3f}, LC_{1s}, and LC_{2s} (8). Cultures of embryonic quail breast also synthesize all 5 myosin light chains. Undifferentiated cultures of dividing myoblasts do not synthesize any of these light chains (Fig. 2A), and

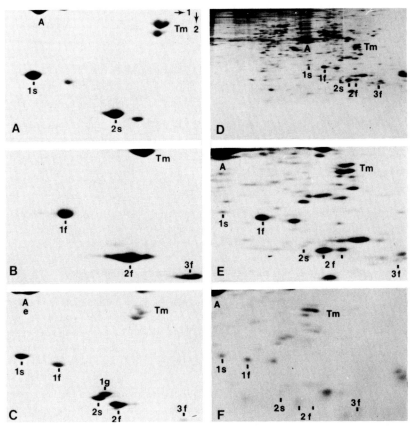

Fig. 1. Two-dimensional gels of **(A)** anterior latissimus dorsi (ALD) actomyosin; **(B)** breast actomyosin; **(C)** Mixture of ALD, breast, and gizzard actomyosin. **(D)** Autoradiograph of ^{35}S-methionine-labeled proteins synthesized during a 1-hour pulse by differentiated chick breast cultures (200,000 trichloroacetic acid-precipitable cpm, 10-day exposure, Kodak SB film). **(E)** Enlargement of the region in D containing myosin light chains. **(F)** Enlargement of the light chain region of an autoradiograph containing proteins synthesized during a 3-hour pulse by ALD cultures (800,000 cpm; 10-day exposure, Kodak SB film). In A, B, and C, the samples were prepared by 3 cycles of high-salt extraction/low-salt precipitation in 0.6 M KCl, 2 mM MgCl$_2$, 0.5 mM K phosphate (pH 7.3). Approximately 25 μg of protein were applied to the gels, which were stained with Coomassie blue 250. Electrophoresis was performed according to the method of O'Farrell (11) using a pH gradient of 7 to 4 ($\rightarrow$1) and sodium dodecyl sulfate gel of 10% to 20% acrylamide ($\downarrow$2). In A, the proteins migrating to the acidic right of LC$_{1s}$ and LC$_{2s}$ represent the 10% contamination of this adult muscle by fast fibers.[12] The less intense spot to the right of LC$_{2f}$ in D is believed to be the phosphorylated form of this light chain. Molecular weights of the myosin light chains, in daltons, are: LC$_{1s}$, 27,000; LC$_{1f}$, 25,000; LC$_{2s}$, 20,000; LC$_{2f}$, 19,000; LC$_{3f}$, 17,000.

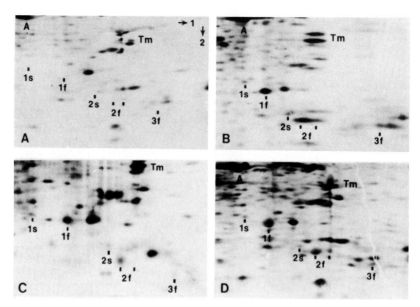

Fig. 2. Two-dimensional gel autoradiographs of total ^{35}S-methionine-labeled proteins synthesized by **(A)** undifferentiated quail myoblasts (100,000 cpm, 32-day exposure, Kodak SB film); **(B)** a single quail myogenic clone (400,000 cpm, 12-day exposure, Kodak XR film); **(C)** cultures differentiated in F12 medium (500,000 cpm, 13-day exposure, Kodak Xr film); **(D)** cultures of day 14 embryonic chick breast, grown in culture for 9 days (500,000 cpm, 32-day exposure, Kodak SB film). Quail myoblasts were used in A because the cultures are uncontaminated by small fibers early after plating. In C, the cells were plated onto medium containing 5% embryo extract and 10% horse serum in minimal essential medium, and fed after 18 to 24 hours with medium containing F12 and PVP (8).

their synthesis is activated with the other adult contractile proteins at myoblast fusion (2). Limited proteolysis peptide mapping confirms that the proteins are myosin light chains (8). LC_{1f} and LC_{2f} are synthesized at 3- to 5-fold higher rates than LC_{1s}, LC_{2s}, and LC_{3f} (Table 1), although all of these proteins are synthesized at very high rates of 10,000 to 40,000 molecules/min/nucleus. These results indicate that myosin light chain expression is not restricted to synthesis of light chains specific to a single fiber type. In fact, all 5 of the fast and slow adult myosin light chains are cosynthesized after myoblast fusion in cultures of myoblasts derived from both presumptive fast and slow muscles.

Clonal analysis has shown that coexpression of fast and slow myosin light chains in culture is not due to a heterogeneous mixture of stem cells with differing potentials for synthesis of contractile protein isozymes. Examination of protein synthesis by myogenic clones (Fig. 2B) (30 individual clones have been analyzed) has demonstrated that all clones synthesize both fast and slow isozymes of the myosin light chains. Therefore, by the criterion of myosin light chain synthesis, individual myoblasts are unrestricted in fiber type expression and synthesize all 5 adult isozymes.

Components in medium such as horse serum (HS) and embryo extract (EE) are required for growth of muscle cells (13). Conceivably, these components could stimulate coexpression of both sets of fiber-specific light chains, or they could favor growth of selected subpopulations or lineages of myoblasts. We have found that myoblasts which differentiate in defined medium completely lacking HS and EE, F12, synthesize both fast and slow light chains (Fig. 2C). Furthermore, the plating efficiency and the extent of muscle colony formation are very similar in clonal cultures of breast and leg muscle grown in media containing differing concentrations of HS and EE (Fig. 3). The plating efficiency of breast clonal cultures was usually slightly lower than that of leg clonal cultures, but both plating efficiencies were within the 10% to 25% usually reported for chick muscle cultures (14). These data suggest that media conditions do not select for the growth of different cell populations in the different media.

Developing muscle is progressively assembled from successive generations of myoblasts (15), and age-dependent differences in clone morphology and media requirements for differentiation of myoblasts have been reported (14). To determine whether myoblasts derived from embryos of different ages change their capacity for synthesis of fiber-specific proteins, the myosin light chains synthesized by cultures of ALD and breast muscles from day 9, day 14, and day 19 embryos have been examined in addition to the day 12 embryos described in studies above (Fig. 2D). We find no differences in the capacity of differentiated myoblasts derived from muscles of different embryonic ages to synthesize the fast and slow myosin light chains in culture. In addition, muscle clones maintained in culture for 2 weeks, mass cultures maintained for 9 days, and cultures examined immediately after myoblast fusion synthesize the fast and slow myosin light chains. Therefore, we conclude that neither embryonic age nor the culture age of cells appears to effect coexpression of the fast and slow myosin light chains.

These results support the conclusion that activation of synthesis of all adult

Table 1. Quantitation of Myosin Light Chain Synthesis in Embryonic Muscle Cultures by Pulse Labeling[a]

	Chicken		Quail
Myosin Light Chain	Day 12 Br	Day 12 ALD	Day 10 Br
LC_{1s}	7.4 ± 1.2	13.6	7.2 ± 2.2
LC_{1f}	32.2 ± 7.2	30.6	31.9 ± 1.0
LC_{2s}	6.6 ± 5.0	17.7	13.8 ± 0.1
LC_{2f}	49.7 ± 5.0	30.6	36.2 ± 2.6
LC_{3f}	4.2 ± 2.7	7.6	3.9 ± 3.0

[a] The absorbance of each light chain on a two-dimensional gel autoradiograph or fluorogram was quantified by scanning densitometry (1), and the sum of the absorbances from the 5 light chains on each autoradiograph were used to determine the percentages shown. Data for quail and chick breast cultures represent the mean ± SD for 2 determinations; the ALD represents a single determination. All light chains contain an average of 6 methionines/molecule, so the relative intensities reflect the amount of protein present. Quantification of LC_{2f} includes both densities of the LC_{2f} spot and the phosphorylated form of the subunit.

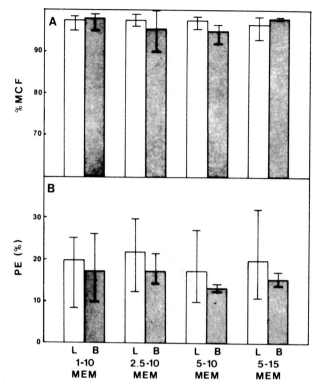

Fig. 3. **(A)** Percentage plating efficiency (%PE), calculated as number of clones counted × 100) number of cells plated. **(B)** Percentage of muscle colony-forming (%MCF) capacity of secondary clonal cultures of day 12 embryonic chick leg (L) and breast (B) grown in minimal essential medium (MEM) supplemented with differing concentrations of horse serum (HS) and embryo extract. (EE). For example, 1–10 MEM contains 1% EE and 10% HS in MEM. %MCF was calculated as (total number of fused colonies × 100) total number of colonies.

fast and slow myosin light chains is part of a generalized program of gene expression during myoblast differentiation, and this program is activated in myoblasts derived from regions of the embryo that give rise to either fast or slow muscles.

DIFFERENTIAL LIGHT CHAIN MESSENGER RNA ACCUMULATION

Accumulation of fiber type specific myosin light chains was next examined in vivo in embryonic muscles of different ages to determine when the switch from coexpression to fiber type expression occurs. The light chains accumulated in ALD and breast muscles of day 12 and day 19 embryos and adult chickens were analyzed by gel electrophoresis of either total muscle homogenates or actomyosin extracts. We have detected both fast and slow myosin light chains in day 12 muscles; however, by this time, the slow ALD muscle has already preferentially accumulated slow type myosin light chains compared to fast breast muscles or muscle cells in culture. By day 19 of embryonic development, 1 day before hatching, these muscles are almost completely differentiated in terms of the light chain isozymes they have accumulated (data not shown). Light chains in fully differentiated adult fiber types are shown in Figure 1A and B. These results indicate that fiber-type light chain patterns in embryonic avian muscle are established by a progressive change from coexpression of fast and slow forms to selective expression of fiber specific proteins. This change in expression is nearly complete by hatching.

Cell-free translation of RNA isolated from embryonic and adult muscles was studied to distinguish whether the switch to fiber specific light chain expression during later embryonic development is regulated transcriptionally by a change in mRNA populations or posttranscriptionally by differential protein turnover or mRNA utilization. Translation of RNAs in a heterologous system generally reflects the relative abundance of RNA species (16). Therefore, we used this approach to determine whether the restriction in accumulation of light chain proteins is mirrored by a loss of specific, functional light chain mRNAs. Our results show that mRNAs coding for all 5 adult fast and slow light chains are present in day 12 ALD and breast muscles (Fig. 4, Table 2). However, by day 19, the ALD muscle is completely differentiated into a slow muscle, as judged by the translation of only slow, light chain mRNAs, whereas the fast breast muscle still contains small amounts of mRNAs coding for LC_{1s} and LC_{2s}. Similar analyses of RNAs isolated from adult muscles indicate that the abundant, translatable mRNA species code only for the appropriate fiber type proteins. These experiments do not directly rule out the possibility that mRNAs are still present but are not translatable in muscle fibers of a specific fiber type; however, the fact that we find similar results using a different translation system, the wheat germ extract (16), and from *in vivo* studies of light chain accumulation supports this interpretation. Therefore, between day 12 and day 19, these muscles have switched from coexpression of both fast and slow fiber type myosin light chains to restricted expression of their characteristic adult proteins, and this switch is regulated by a change in the accumulation of the translatable mRNAs coding for light chain proteins, and not by a posttranslational mechanism.

Table 2. Quantitation of Myosin Light Chain Synthesis in Embryonic and Adult Muscles in Reticulocyte Cell-Free Translations[a]

Myosin Light Chain	Day 12		Day 19		Adult	
	Br	ALD	Br	ALD	Br	ALD
LC_{1s}	21.1	40.5	0.6	31.5	0.1	20.7
LC_{1f}	23.9	14.8	47.5	5.4	26.8	2.7
LC_{2s}	43.7	41.0	5.9	62.8	0.2	67.8
LC_{2f}	11.3	3.7	46.0	0.3	72.9	8.9

[a] See Table 1 legend for methodology. LC_{3f} was not included in quantitation of translated RNAs because a protein with similar electrophoretic mobility that has not yet been identified interfered with densitometry. The entire LC_{1s} spot was included in calculation, although it migrates as a streak or doublet on some gels.

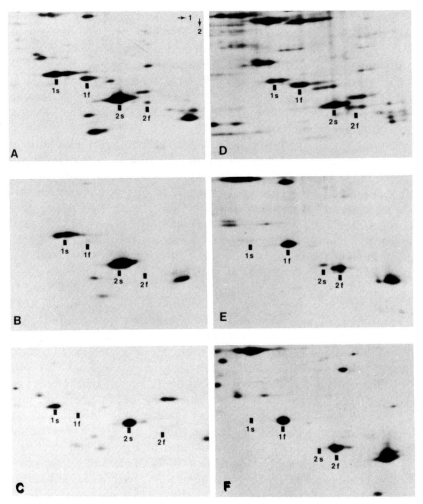

Fig. 4. Light chain regions from fluorograms of 2-dimensional gels of ^{35}S-methionine-labeled reticulocyte translation products using RNA isolated from **(A)** day 12 anterior latissimus dorsi (ALD); **(B)** day 19 ALD; **(C)** adult ALD; **(D)** day 12 breast; **(E)** day 19 breast; **(F)** adult breast muscle. The RNA was extracted from frozen tissue that had been homogenized directly in 1 volume of phenol and 1 volume of buffer containing 0.1 M NaCl, 1 mM MgCl$_2$, 1% sodium dodecyl sulfate, 2% Triton X-100, 1 mg/ml heparin, and 20 mm Tris (pH 7.6) using a Polytron homogenizer (Brinkman Instruments). The reticulocyte translation system was purchased from Bethesda Research Laboratories. After determining the sensitivity of the system to added exogenous RNA, 4 μg of total RNA were added to each reaction. Stimulation was in all cases 2 to 8 times background. A 1-μl aliquot of each translation assay was applied to a 2-dimensional gel, and exposure was varied to make cpm × time equivalent.

DISCUSSION

The accumulation of myosin light chain proteins and mRNAs in differentiating embryonic muscle has been examined to determine the mechanisms that regulate the development of muscle fiber types. Our results are consistent with a simple, 2-step model in which the primary program of muscle differentiation includes activation of synthesis of the entire set of fast and slow adult skeletal muscle myosin light chains at the time of myoblast fusion. Imposed on this initial activation is a secondary control that selectively restricts expression of subsets of light chain genes later during development. Previous kinetics studies have shown that synthesis of these light chains is activated at fusion by the coordinate accumulation of their mRNAs (2). These studies of mRNA in embryonic and adult muscles now demonstrate that the later selection of subsets of light chain genes during fiber type differentiation is regulated by the differential accumulation of mRNAs coding for the fiber type specific proteins.

Our studies have focused on the synthesis and accumulation of adult myosin light chains, but there are fiber type specific forms of the other contractile proteins such as myosin heavy chains, troponins, and tropomyosins in fast and slow adult muscles. Studies using immunologic probes have demonstrated the presence of both fast and slow isozymes of light chains (7), troponins, and tropomyosins (17) in single fibers of developing muscle, suggesting that coexpression of fast and slow isozymes of these other proteins also occurs during the early stages of muscle development. In addition to adult isozymes, a unique myosin heavy and light chain has been described in embryonic mammalian muscles (9, 10). These embryonic isozymes have not been detected in developing avian muscle. At this time, it is not clear whether these are species differences in expression of embryonic forms of contractile proteins. However, it should be noted that chick muscles are virtually mature with respect to fiber types and physiologic function by hatching (12), whereas rat muscles mature more slowly and do not develop fiber types until late in neonatal development (18). Therefore, embryonic isozymes may play a specific physiologic role in the prolonged mammalian muscle development, or such embryonic isozymes could be present at earlier stages of avian development than we have examined. Analysis similar to that presented in this report of changes in accumulation of mRNA for fast and slow (and embryonic) isozymes of the other contractile proteins also will be necessary to confirm whether our model for fiber type differentiation can be generalized to include other fiber type specific skeletal muscle contractile proteins.

Immunochemical studies have shown that changes occur in fiber type contractile proteins when adult muscles are chronically stimulated, and that these switches occur within preexisting muscle fibers rather than by the growth of new fibers (19). Our clonal analysis suggests that fiber types develop by the same mechanism. Myogenic clones derived from chick breast, leg, and ALD and quail breast muscles synthesize both fast and slow myosin light chains. Also, cells grown in different media and cells derived from embryos of different ages synthesize fast and slow myosin light chains. We find no evidence that the myoblasts which fuse into fibers differ in their capacity to synthesize fast and slow light chain isozymes, which suggests that the later synthesis of only subsets of fiber-type light chains occurs by changes in expression within fibers rather than by replacement of old fibers by new lineages of myoblasts with different potentials for fiber type synthesis. Results of both of these very different approaches therefore support the conclusion that the switch from coexpression to fiber-specific expression of contractile protein isozymes occurs by changes in gene expression within individual developing fibers.

In vitro translations of RNA isolated from embryonic and adult muscles indicate that fiber-type specificity is regulated by the accumulation of specific subsets of functional mRNA sequences for myosin light chains. Selective accumulation of functional messenger RNAs may occur by changes in the stability or the translatability of messenger RNAs for one subset of isozymes, or by repression of transcription or nuclear processing of transcripts of selected subsets of fiber specific genes. To distinguish between these molecular mechanisms, it will be necessary to use specific hybridization probes for the different contractile protein mRNAs. The signal that directs differential accumulation of mRNAs is unknown. Nerves are important for maintaining adult muscle fibers and in regulating the switch in fiber types after cross-innervation of adult muscles, and it is probably reasonable to assume that innervation plays a similar role in the development of fiber type expression. However, the requirement for innervation during fiber type development, the signal by which innervation may regulate fiber type gene expression, and the molecular mechanism that coordinates the initial activation of contractile protein synthesis during myoblast differentiation are unknown, and remain important directives for future research.

ACKNOWLEDGMENTS

The authors thank Vicki Bowman and Druen Robinson for their assistance with the myoblast cultures.

This investigation was supported by Predoctoral Training Grant T01 H00430-05 to LR Keller and Grant R01 HDO 7796-07 to CP Emerson from the National Institutes of Health.

REFERENCES

1. Devlin R, Emerson CP: Coordinate regulation of contractile protein synthesis during myoblast differentiation. Cell 13:599–611, 1978

2. Devlin R, Emerson CP: Coordinate accumulation of contractile protein mRNAs during myoblast differentiation. Dev Biol 69:202–216, 1979

3. Close R: Dynamic properties of mammalian skeletal muscle. Physiol Rev 52:129–197, 1972

4. Buller AJ, Eccles JC, Eccles RM: Interactions between motorneurones and muscles in respect of characteristic speed of their responses. J Physiol (Lond) 150:417–439, 1960

5. Rubinstein NA, Holtzer H: Fast and slow muscles in tissue culture synthesize only fast myosin. Nature 280:323–325, 1979

6. Roy R, Sreter F, Sarkar S: Changes in tropomyosin subunits and myosin light chains during development of chicken and rabbit striated muscles. Dev Biol 69:15–30, 1979

7. Gauthier GF, Lowey S, Hobbs AW: Fast and slow myosin in developing muscle fibers. Nature 274:25–29, 1978

8. Keller LR, Emerson CP: Synthesis of adult myosin light chains by embryonic muscle cultures. Proc Natl Acad Sci USA 77:1020–1024, 1980

9. Whalen RG, Butler-Browne GS, Gros F: Identification of a novel form of myosin light chain present in embryonic tissue and cultured muscle cells. J Mol Biol 126:415–431, 1978

10. Whalen RG, Schwartz K, Bouveret P, et al: Contractile protein isozymes in muscle development:

identification of an embryonic form of myosin heavy chain. Proc Natl Acad Sci USA 76:5197–5201, 1979

11. O'Farrell P: High resolution two-dimensional electrophoresis of proteins. J Biol Chem 259:4007–4021, 1975

12. Rubinstein NA, Pepe FA, Holtzer H: Myosin types during the development of embryonic chicken fast and slow muscles. Proc Natl Acad Sci USA 74:4524–4527, 1977

13. Konigsberg IR: Protocol IV: 11-day skeletal muscle. In *Methods in Developmental Biology*. Edited by Wilt F, Wessells NK. Crowell-Collier, New York, 1968, pp 520–521

14. Hauschka SD, White NK: Studies of myogenesis *in vitro*. In *Research in Muscle Development and the Muscle Spindle*. Edited by Banker BQ, Przybylski RJ, Van der Meulein JP, Victor M. Excerpta Medica, Princeton, 1972, pp 53–71

15. Kelly AM, Schotland DL: The evolution of the "checkerboard" in a rat muscle. In *Research in Muscle Development and the Muscle Spindle*. Edited by Banker BQ, Przybylski RJ, Van der Meulein JP, Victor M. Excerpta Medica, Princeton, 1972, pp 32–48

16. Paterson BM, Roberts BE, Yaffe D: Determination of actin messenger RNA in cultures of differentiating embryonic skeletal muscle. Proc Natl Acad Sci USA 71:4467–4471, 1974

17. Dhoot GH, Perry SV: Distribution of polymorphic forms of troponin components and tropomyosin in skeletal muscle. Nature 278:714–718, 1979

18. Rubinstein NA, Kelly AM: Myogenic and neurogenic contributions to the development of fast and slow twitch muscles in rat. Dev Biol 62:473–485, 1978

19. Rubinstein NA, Mabuchi K, Pepe F, et al: Use of type-specific antimyosins to demonstrate the transformation of individual fibers in chronically stimulated rabbit fast muscles. J Cell Biol 79:252–261, 1978

DISCUSSION

Dr. Robert Schwartz: This question is for investigators who have used clone probes. It has been found that the muscle-specific mRNA peaks sometime during fusion and then falls. This is true for the hybridization assay using Dr. Nadal Ginard's myosin heavy chain clone DNA, for my αactin clone, and for Dr. Yaffe's actin clone. Why do your translation assays not demonstrate any decrease in the translation activity of any of these proteins? I also have a comment. The increase in protein product in your translation assay appears to be sequential, not coordinate. You can see an increase in actin and myosin followed by an increase in mRNA content in the translation assay.

Dr. Charles Emerson: With regard to why do we not see a decrease in the synthesis of the proteins or the translatable messengers, I have no answer other than that is what we find in our system. In cell culture, there is a period when the cultures differentiate, the fibers are maintained, and contractile proteins accumulate. With prolonged periods of culture, a degenerative process occurs. If one is talking about the loss of particular components, one must show, e.g., selective loss of just the contractile protein mRNAs. There could be differences among chicken, quail, and rat, but I doubt that there are. It could be some process associated with terminal culture or it could be significant for those systems.

Dr. Robert Schwartz: Would you like to comment on my comment?

Dr. Charles Emerson: I would not like to leave the impression that there is a precise temporal relationship between the accumulation of the messages and the activation of protein synthesis. All we can say from the translation data is that at about the time the synthesis is activated (within, say, 5 to 6 hours), the message accumulates. The precise temporal relationship is sorted out using the clone probes. A short period of translational control, say 4 to 5 hours, may precede the activation of synthesis for any proteins under translational control. The point I would like to stress, however, a point supported by the recent studies of Dr. Yaffe (see chapter 58), is that in the dividing myoblasts the messages are not there by translation assay or by hybridization assay. This means that the primary regulation of the transition from myoblast to differentiated cell is at the level of the accumulation of the message, not translational control of a large amount of stored message.

Dr. James Florini: I was struck by the apparent difference in stoichiometry between the messenger accumulation and the protein accumulations. Is that just because of a difference in the way the data are normalized, or do you think this has to do with preferential translation of one message versus another?

Dr. Charles Emerson: There are differences in the stoichiometry of translation of several of the messages. From the data presented you could not deduce what they are really, because they are not normalized to the number of methionines on a molar basis. However, there are 2- to 3-fold differences between, for instance, light chain 1 and light chain 2. What we do not know is whether those differences reflect some intrinsic property of the translatability of a particular message or the actual level of the mRNA. That will be sorted out with clone probes. The point is that there are not large differences in the translatability of these messengers. Again with regard to translational control, there may be modulation, as with alpha and beta hemoglobin mRNAs, for which messenger concentrations differ slightly to yield the correct stoichiometry of synthesis. In the overall mechanistic sense, such control provides a refinement of a major mechanism of control, which is accumulation of the mRNAs to high but approximately the same level.

Dr. Jerry Shay: Have you ever looked at any of the dystrophic models of muscular dystrophy for activation of these contractile proteins to see whether there were any differences?

Dr. Charles Emerson: No.

Dr. Henry Epstein: With respect to your quantification of 2-dimensional gels, which is an important technique, how did you allow for the fact that you had a great deal of material at the origin that did not move into the gel on focusing? Second, calculating from the ratios of different proteins, did you account for differences in amino acid composition and label? Third, on whose model did you actually establish those predicted values for myofibrillar proteins? That latter point is controversial among many structural molecular biologists.

Dr. Charles Emerson: The stoichiometries were based on one set of data for the myofibrillar proteins; that is different from a control. With regard to quantification of the 2-dimensional gels, we purified labeled proteins from the culture to make an actomyosin preparation, purified myosin from that preparation, and then determined how much of these purified proteins entered the gels.

Under appropriate conditions, we can get 90% to 95% into the gel for quantification with relatively minor variation between gels. As with any technique, there are many variables to worry about with 2-dimensional gels, but you can appropriately control for the problem of proteins that do not migrate. Was there a third question?

Dr. Henry Epstein: Do you correct for amino acid composition when comparing stoichiometries?

Dr. Charles Emerson: Yes. We use methionine labels, and we know the sequence of all of these proteins, so the data are appropriately corrected.

Dr. Henning Schmalbruch: Do you observe fast and slow proteins in culture, or does that require a motor neuron?

Dr. Charles Emerson: We know that we can observe the synthesis of all 5 light chains (3 fast and 2 slow) without neurons present. We have no idea how involvement of the nervous system establishes that specific pattern, although studies in adult animals make it is very clear that the nerves have an important role in maintaining the light chain pattern.

Dr. Hans Eppenberger: Is there any qualitative difference in contraction of myofibrils from the very large myotubes you showed compared to the very thin ones? For example, do you see more contraction in the large, very flat myotubes?

Dr. Charles Emerson: No, but I have not looked at this parameter. These quail cells do not spontaneously contract in culture like the chick cells do.

66
Cloning of Muscle Protein Genes from *Drosophila melanogaster*

Robert V. Storti, PhD

Cellular growth and differentiation are believed to result from the coordinate expression of groups of genes. A characteristic property of muscle cell differentiation is the coordinate synthesis of the myofibrillar proteins, a group of structurally and functionally related proteins that collectively make up myofibrillar structures and are responsible for muscle contraction. The myofibrillar proteins can represent as much as 90% of the cell mass in the adult muscle tissue and are, therefore, easily isolated and well characterized. Muscle cells can also be isolated in relatively pure form; because their development can be studied in cell culture, the muscle cell provides an exceptionally good system for studying coordinate gene expression during differentiation.

Our interests have been concerned with the molecular events that regulate coordinate gene expression during myogenesis in cell culture. We have been particularly interested in the fine structure of muscle protein genes and their function during development. For this reason, we have been studying myogenesis in the fruit fly *Drosophila melanogaster*. Myogenesis in *Drosophila* can be studied in primary cell culture and is very similar to myogenesis in vertebrates (1–3). The small size of the *Drosophila* genome and the large polytene chromosomes of some of its tissue render it a more attractive organism for studies on gene structure and mapping than the more often studied vertebrate systems. In addition, because of the well-defined genetics in *Drosophila*, the potential exists for studying mutations affecting the expression of muscle protein genes.

To exploit this system for the study of muscle genes and to gain some insights into their function, we have recently set out to isolate by recombinant deoxyribonucleic acid (DNA) techniques muscle protein genes for *Drosophila*. A ^{32}P-labeled complementary DNA (cDNA) probe, enriched for myotube messenger ribonucleic acid (mRNA)-specific cDNA sequences, has been used to screen a lambda phage recombinant *Drosophila* genomic DNA library. We report here the isolation and preliminary identification of *Drosophila* genomic DNA clones coding for muscle genes expressed during myogenesis.

MATERIALS AND METHODS

Cell Culture and RNA Extraction

Gastrula-stage embryos of *Drosophila melanogaster*, P2 line of the Oregon-R strain, were collected, washed, and dechorionated. The sterilized gastrulae were homogenized and plated as described previously (1). Twenty hours after plating, myotube cell cultures were rinsed in cold Ringer's solution and lysed in 1.5 ml per 60-mm Petri dish of 0.5% Triton X-100, 100 mM NaCl, 10 mM $MgCl_2$, 30 mM Tris (pH 8.3), and 0.5% fresh diethylpyrocarbonate. The cytoplasmic supernatant from a 1,500-*g* centrifugation was made 150 mM NaAc, 10 mM ethylenediamine tetra-acetate (EDTA), and 0.5% sodium dodecyl sulfate (SDS), digested at room temperature for 1 hour with 500 μg/ml Proteinase K, and extracted with phenol-chloroform (4). The RNA was ethanol precipitated and RNA containing polyadenylation [poly(A)] was separated on oligo (dT) cellulose (4). The RNA from Schneider L-2 cells was isolated as previously described (5).

Synthesis of ^{32}P-cDNA and Conditions of Hybridization

The protocol for synthesis of ^{32}P-cDNA of high specific activity, complementary to mRNA from myotube cells, was similar to that described by Friedman and Rasbash (6), except that unlabeled deoxynucleotides were present at 200 μm and ^{32}P-labeled deoxyadenosine triphosphate and ^{32}P-labeled deoxycytosine triphosphate (specificity activity of both >2,000 Ci/mmol, Amersham) were used carrier free. After incubation at 37° C for 1 hour, the myotube RNA was digested with alkali and the ^{32}P-cDNA was purified by Sephadex G-50 chromatography and ethanol precipitation.

Myotube-specific ^{32}P-cDNA sequences were enriched by exhaustive hybridization to excess RNA (log Cot > 3) from Schneider L-2 cells. Hybridization was carried out in 0.4 M Na_2HPO_4 (pH 7) and 0.2% SDS for 22 hours with a 10^5-fold excess of Schneider cell total RNA. Single-stranded ^{32}P-cDNA was separated from hybrid ^{32}P-cDNA by hydroxyapatite chromatography and collected by ethanol precipitation in the presence of 10 μg/ml carrier transfer RNA (tRNA). In some experiments, the unhybridized, myotube-enriched ^{32}P-cDNA from the first hybridization was further enriched for muscle sequences by a second cycle of hybridization.

Screening of Genomic Library

The *Drosophila* genomic DNA library was constructed and supplied by Dr. Tom Maniatis. This library consists of randomly sheared *Drosophila* DNA fragments of 15 to 20 kilobase pairs (kb) inserted into Charon 4 lambda phage. The library was screened using the in situ plaque hybridization technique (7). Five 100-mm Petri dishes, each containing approximately 2,000 lambda phage plaques, were transferred to nitrocellulose filters and hybridized according to the method of Maniatis and colleagues (8). Input ^{32}P-cDNA was from 5×10^6 to 10^7 cpm. Plaques from the region of the Petri dishes corresponding to a positive on the autoradiograph were picked and rescreened 2 additional times. Positive plaques derived from purified single phage were stored at 5° C in 1.0 ml SM [0.1 M NaCl, 0.05 M Tris HU (pH 7.5), 10 mM Mg SO$_4$, 0.01% gelatin] buffer with chloroform (8).

Hybridization-Selection Translation

DNA was isolated from phage by the method of Blattner that accompanies the Charon phage (19). Briefly, approximately 5 μg of DNA, isolated from 10-ml cultures, was heat denatured, spotted on nitrocellulose filters (10 mm in diameter), and baked for 2 hours at 80° C *in vacuo*. Hybridization was carried out in 100 μl of 65% formamide, 400 mM NaCl, and 10 mM PIPES buffer (pH 6.8) for 2 hours at 45° C (9). Approximately 3 to 5 μg of RNA containing poly (A) extracted from 12- 24-hour embryos were included in each reaction. After hybridization, the filters were washed 2 times in 150 mM NaCl, 15 mM sodium citrate, 0.5% SDS at 55° C, and 2 times in 2 mM EDTA, 10 mM Tris (pH 7.2) at 55° C. The filters were boiled for 1 minute in the presence of 2 mM EDTA at pH 7.0 and 10 μg of calf liver tRNA (9). The RNA was collected by ethanol precipitation and translated in a micrococcal nuclease–treated rabbit reticulocyte lysate cell-free protein-synthesizing system in the presence of 40 μCi of ^{35}S-methionine (10). Electrophoresis of the products in 1- and 2-dimensional polyacrylamide gels has been described (1, 11).

RESULTS

Strategy for Screening Muscle Protein Genes

Myogenic cells from *Drosophila* gastrula-stage embryos preferentially attach to Petri dishes coated with protamine (1). Initially after plating, the relatively pure myogenic cells are mononucleated and have a polygonal shape. From 6 h to 24 hours after plating, more than 80% of these cells fuse to form multinucleated myotubes, each containing an average of 10 to 15 nuclei per cell (Fig. 1). Concomitant with cell fusion there are also dramatic changes in protein synthesis. One of these changes is the appearance of several new abundant proteins whose synthesis can be correlated with the accumulation of new mRNA.

The accumulation of new mRNA was determined by cell-free translation of mRNA isolated from cultures at different times during myogenesis and analyzing the protein products on 2-dimensional gels (unpublished observation). These results suggest that synthesis of new proteins during cell fusion is transcriptionally regulated. Moreover, these abundant myotube mRNAs are not present in unfused myoblast cells. This difference in mRNA population between unfused and fused cells formed the rationale for screening myotube-specific proteins.

An outline describing the rationale and protocol for the preparation of a

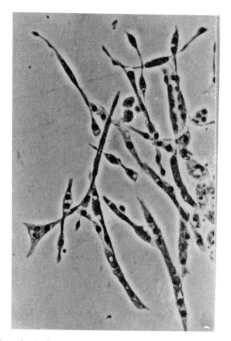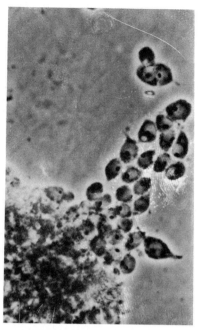

Fig. 1. Primary myogenic cultures of gastrula-stage embryos. **(A)** Four hours after plating (original magnification ×750). **(B)** Cultures 24 hours after plating (original magnification ×600). Cells were stained with hematoxylin.

myotube-specific probe is shown in Figure 2. Poly(A)-containing mRNA from 20-hour myotube cultures was used as a template for making ^{32}P-cDNA. The ^{32}P-cDNA sequences complementary to myotube RNA were enriched for by hybridization to excess amounts of nonmuscle Schneider cell RNA. "Household" cDNA sequences that are common to both cells will form hybrids and be separated by low-salt hydroxyapatite elution. The ^{32}P-cDNA myotube sequences not homologous to Schneider cell RNA will remain single stranded and are eluted by high-salt hydroxyapatite elution. This ^{32}P-cDNA, enriched for myotube sequences only, was used as a probe for screening recombinant DNA clones to identify those clones encoding muscle proteins.

Screening of Genomic DNA Library

The *Drosophila* genomic DNA library constructed by Maniatis was used for the isolation of muscle-specific clones (8). This library consists of randomly sheared embryonic DNA fragments of 15 to 20 kb cloned in Charon 4 lambda phage. Filters containing a sufficient number of plaques to represent an entire *Drosophila* genomic DNA content were screened using the muscle-specific ^{32}P-cDNA probe. Plaques showing positive hybridization on the autoradiograph were rescreened 2 additional times to yield a total of 285 plaque-purified clones homologous to myotube ^{32}P-cDNAs. A representative filter from a final screen is shown in Figure 3.

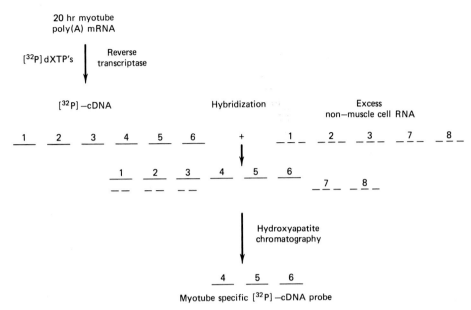

Fig. 2. Strategy for preparing muscle-specific ^{32}P-cDNA probe.

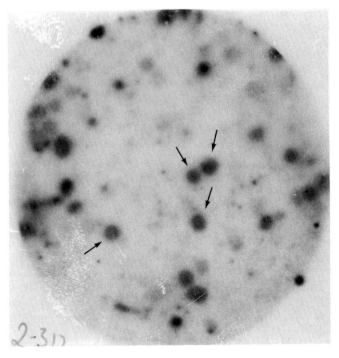

Fig. 3. A representative autoradiograph showing ^{32}P-cDNA hybridization to DNA from plaque purified λ-*Drosophila* recombinant DNA clones transferred to nitrocellulose filter paper. The arrows indicate some of the plaques showing positive hybridization.

881

Identification and Partial Characterization of DNA Clones

Each of the clones showing positive hybridization to the ^{32}P-cDNA probe is currently being analyzed to determine the specific protein sequences encoded. The method of hybridization-selected translation is being used to correlate DNA sequences with mRNA and protein (9). The technique involves denaturing and immobilizing plaque-purified cloned DNA onto nitrocellulose filters and hybridization to muscle mRNA. After hybridization and thorough washing of the filters to remove unhybridized mRNA, the mRNA in hybrid is recovered by heat denaturing and ethanol precipitation and translated in the cell-free protein-synthesizing system from rabbit reticulocyte lysates. The ^{35}S-methionine-labeled protein product is then identified by 1- and 2-dimensional polyacrylamide gel electrophoresis. Each hybrid-selection analysis requires 5 to 10 μg of poly(A) mRNA. To facilitate the analysis, mRNA from 12- to 24-hour *Drosophila* embryos was used in the hybridization reaction instead of mRNA from myotube cultures, because larger quantities of RNA can be extracted from embryos. At this stage of embryogenesis myogenesis is at a maximum in vivo,

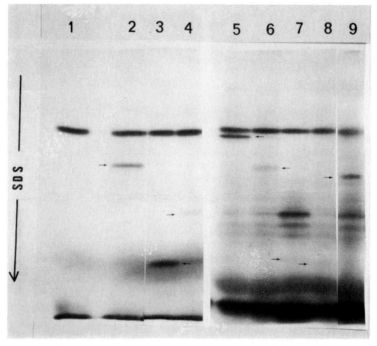

Fig. 4. Fluorogram of the ^{35}S-methionine-labeled polypeptides directed by mRNA hydrid-selection from cloned DNA. Lane 1 is an endogenous translation containing carrier tRNA. Lanes 2 through 8 are hybrid selections of clones Dm 85, Dm 217, Dm 231, actin, Dm 161, Dm 270, Dm 205, and Dm 227, respectively. Each lane contains 4 μl of a 25-μl reaction mixture. Samples in lanes 1–4 were digested with RNAase before electrophoresis. Lanes 5–9 were not digested with RNAase and were electrophoresed on a different gel from that used for samples in lanes 1–4. The actin clone was a gift of Dr. Peter Wensink. Fluorography was for 2 days. The high level of endogenous products in lanes 5–9 is due primarily to the added carrier tRNA (see *Discussion*). Arrows indicate the products of selected mRNAs.

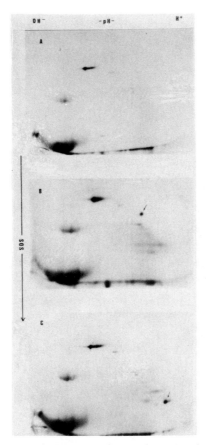

Fig. 5. Fluorogram of 2-dimensional gel electrophoresis of **(A)** Hybrid selection containing blank nitrocellulose filter; **(B)** sample from lane 2 of Figure 4 and **(C)** sample from lane 3 of Figure 4. Samples were not digested with RNAase before electrophoresis. Each gel had 15 µl of a 25-µl reaction mixture. Fluorography was for 2 days.

and cell-free translation of this RNA and gel electrophoresis of the cell-free products show the same distribution of proteins as mRNA of myotube cultures.

Approximately 50 clones have been analyzed by hybrid selection. A representative sample of the protein products encoded by some of these clones electrophoresed in 1-dimensional gels are shown in Figure 4. The proteins encoded by DNA showing specific hybrid selection are indicated by arrows. The additional bands common to each sample in lanes 5–9 result from the added tRNA carrier used in the mRNA precipitation. These bands probably represent aminoacylated tRNA and disappear when the translation samples are treated with RNAase before electrophoresis (lanes 1–4). Figures 5B and C show examples of 2 of the positive hybrid selections (lanes 2 and 3, Fig. 4) electrophoresed in 2-dimensional gels. We have successfully identified by hybrid selection and 1-dimensional gel electrophoresis the proteins encoded by 12 recombinant DNA clones. Five of these clones coelectrophoresed with abundant translation products of embryonic mRNA and mRNA from myotube cells when

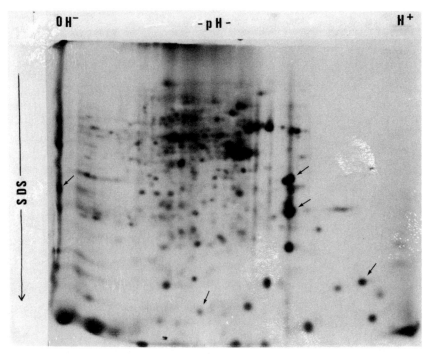

Fig. 6. Fluorogram of ^{35}S-methionine-labeled polypeptides directed by mRNA from 12 to 24-hour embryos and translated in rabbit reticulocyte lysates and electrophoresed in 2-dimensional gels. Fluorography was for 3 days. Arrows indicate protein encoded by cloned DNA.

electrophoresed in 2-dimensional gels. These proteins are identified by arrows in the total translation products of embryo mRNA (Figure 6).

DISCUSSION

The strategy used for isolating muscle-specific recombinant DNA clones is based on the observation that muscle proteins and their mRNAs are synthesized predominantly or exclusively in muscle cells. Although this is probably correct for most muscle proteins, it may not necessarily be true for all. Some myofibrillar proteins, for instance, are now known to occur as isoforms in nonmuscle cells. Some of these proteins are very similar in amino acid sequence and structure to their muscle counterparts (1, 11, 12). Actin, for instance, is involved in myofibrillar structure and function in muscle cells, but it is also found in all nonmuscle tissue. Although these nonmuscle actions are coded for by separate genes, they differ only slightly in amino acid sequence (13, 14). These similarities in amino acid sequence between the actins of different tissues and different organisms also exist at the level of their structural genes. *Dictyostelium* actin genes, for instance, can cross-hybridize with actin genes from *Drosophila* and chick (15, 16). It is, therefore, reasonable to suggest that cDNA complementary to actin mRNA from our muscle cells will have sufficient homology to actin mRNA from the Schneider cells to cross-hybridize. If so, actin-coding sequences would have been removed from our probe used to screen muscle protein coding cloned genomic DNA.

Our results thus far appear to substantiate this possibility. In addition to being the most abundant mRNA in our embryo mRNA preparation, actin has also been shown to be encoded by at least 6 different structural genes (15, 16). This should, therefore, increase the number of genomic DNA clones carrying actin-coding sequences. Both of these considerations should increase the probability of detecting actin-coding sequences in the hybrid-selection assay. In our analysis of approximately 50 clones by hybrid selection, we have not detected a single clone containing actin-coding sequences. These results would suggest that actin cDNA sequences were removed from our ^{32}P-cDNA probe by hybridization to Schneider cell RNA.

Whether isoforms of other muscle proteins exist in nonmuscle cells is unclear. In vertebrates, some but not all isoforms of myofibrillar proteins are found in nonmuscle cells (12). In general, however, these nonmuscle counterparts show less amino acid homology than the muscle and nonmuscle isoforms of actin. Hence, the genes coding for these proteins may be sufficiently different in DNA sequence to show little cross-hybridization. Even less is known about the isoforms of muscle proteins in *Drosophila*. However, the fact that we have identified several clones coding for abundant muscle mRNAs and their protein products suggests that Schneider cells may not contain mRNAs coding for other myofibrillar proteins or that if they do have isoforms of these proteins the mRNAs for these isoproteins are sufficiently different so as not to cross-hybridize.

The hybrid-selection technique has been successful in identifying approximately 20% of the clones tested. This is probably an underestimate of the actual number of clones encoding authentic muscle proteins. For instance, the resolving power of the hybrid-selection technique is probably limited in detecting only the abundant mRNAs and their translation products. The hybridization conditions are not designed for hybridizing rare mRNA sequences, but are constructed to minimize RNA degradation. Moreover, rare mRNA would probably not be translated with sufficient efficiency in vitro to allow detection of their protein products by gel electrophoresis and fluorography.

The identity of our muscle protein clones has been limited thus far to characterizing the encoded proteins by electrophoretic mobility in 1- and 2-dimensional gels. Although these proteins comigrate with abundant proteins coded for by mRNAs of muscle cells, the structural or functional identity of these proteins is still unknown. However, many of the proteins found in *Drosophila* muscle cells grown in culture have very similar electrophoretic mobilities in 2-dimensional gels as the myofibrillar proteins of vertebrates (17, 18). One of our clones, for instance, codes for an abundant protein with the same electrophoretic mobility as vertebrate tropomyosin. However, until the myofibrillar proteins from *Drosophila* have been purified and characterized, their potential homology with vertebrate myofibrillar protein will only prove useful for preliminary identification. We are currently in the process of purifying muscle proteins from *Drosophila*.

Our immediate goal in this work is to gain some insights into the regulation of coordinate gene expression of muscle proteins at the level of DNA structure and function. We are currently determining the number of genes for each of these proteins as well as the chromosomal map position for each of these genes by in situ hybridization. This work, coupled with nucleotide sequence analysis of the coding and noncoding DNA sequences in each clone, may give some indication of common structural features possibly important in regulating their coordinate expression. With muscle-specific DNA sequences, we can also use these clones as probes in analyzing the regulation of specific mRNA metabolism during myogenesis. A long-range goal of this work is to use muscle gene probes to study abnormal muscle development and function. In addition, *Drosophila* offers the opportunity to induce and genetically study muscle abnormalities to complement our biochemical studies and is thus an ideal model system for studying myogenesis.

ACKNOWLEDGMENTS

I would like to thank Dr. Tom Maniatis for providing the *Drosophila* recombinant DNA library. The screening of *Drosophila* clones was done in the laboratory of Dr. Mary Lou Pardue at the Massachusetts Institute of Technology. I would like to express my deep appreciation and thanks to Drs. Pardue, Dietmar Mischke, and Barbara Young for their participation and helpful discussions. The author is also indebted to Dr. Anthony Mahowald for providing *Drosophila* embryos and to Drs. R Ricciardi, B Roberts, and B Paterson for helpful discussion of hybrid-selection translation. I am also indebted for the expert technical assistance of Ms. Alice Szwast. This work was supported in part by a grant from the National Institute of General Medical Sciences, GM27611.

REFERENCES

1. Seecof RL, Unanue RL: Differentiation of embryonic *Drosophila* cells *in vitro*. Exp Cell Res 50:654–660, 1968

2. Storti RV, Horovitch SJ, Scott MP, et al: Myogenesis in primary cell cultures from *Drosophila melanogaster*: Protein synthesis and actin heterogeneity during development. Cell 13:589–598, 1978

3. Bernstein SI, Fyrberg EA, Donady JJ: Isolation and partial characterization of *Drosophila* myoblasts from primary cultures of embryonic cells. J Cell Biol 78:856–865, 1978

4. Spradling AC, Pardue ML, Penman S: Messenger RNA in heat-shocked *Drosophila* cells. J Mol Biol 109:559–571, 1977

5. Scott MP, Storti RV, Pardue ML, et al: Cell-free protein synthesis in lysates of *Drosophila melanogaster* cells. Biochem 18:1588–1598, 1979

6. Friedman EY, Rashbash M: The synthesis of high yields of full-length reverse transcripts of globin mRNA. Nucleic Acid Res 4:3455–3471, 1977

7. Benton WD, Davis RW: Screening of λgt recombinant clones by hybridization to single plaques *in situ*. Science 196:180–182, 1977

8. Maniatis T, Hardison RC, Lacy E, et al: The isolation of structural genes from libraries of eucaryotic DNA. Cell 15:687–701, 1978

9. Ricciardi RP, Miller JS, Roberts BE: Purification and mapping of specific mRNAs by hybridization-selection and cell-free translation. Proc Natl Acad Sci USA 76:4927–4931, 1979

10. Pelham HRB, Jackson RJ: An efficient mRNA-dependent translation system from reticulocyte lysates. Eur J Biochem 67:247–256, 1976

11. Storti RV, Coen DM, Rich A: Tissue-specific forms of actin in the developing chick. Cell 8:521–527, 1976

12. Lazarides E: Actin, α-actinin, and tropomyosin interaction in the structural organization of actin filaments in non-muscle cells. J Cell Biol 68:202–219, 1976

13. Elzinga M, Maron DJ, Adelstein RS: Human heart and platelet actins are products of different genes. Science 191:94–96, 1976

14. Vandederckhave J, Weber K: Mammalian cytoplasmic actins are the products of at least two genes and differ in primary structure in at least 25 identified positions from skeletal muscle actins. Proc Natl Acad Sci USA 75:1106–1110, 1978

15. Tobin SL, Zuluf E, Sanchez F, et al: Multiple actin-related sequences in the *Drosophila melanogaster* genome. Cell 19:121–131, 1980

16. Fyrberg EA, Kindle KL, Davidson N: The actin genes of *Drosophila*: a dispersed multigene family. Cell 19:365–378, 1980

17. Giometti CS, Anderson NG, Anderson NL: Muscle protein analysis. I. High-resolution two-dimensional electrophoresis of skeletal muscle proteins for analysis of small biopsy samples. Clin Chem 25:1877–1884, 1979

18. Devlin RB, Emerson CP: Coordinate accumulation of contractile protein mRNA during myoblast differentiation. Dev Biol 69:202–216, 1979

19. Blattner FR, Williams BG, Blechl AE, et al: Charon phages: safer derivatives of bacteriophage lambda for DNA cloning. Science 196:161–169, 1977

DISCUSSION

Dr. Robert Wydro: I have two questions. First, have you made certain the genomic clones of your 250 isolates are muscle specific?

Dr. Robert Storti: Yes.

Dr. Robert Wydro: We are currently going back and hybridizing these clones to myotube and myoblast RNA to show that they are specific.

Dr. Robert Storti: Do you mean, have we determined whether they are temporally regulated during myogenesis?

Dr. Robert Wydro: Just that they code for muscle-specific RNA.

Dr. Robert Storti: We know that they hybridize to RNA from myogenic clones and code for proteins expressed in muscle cell culture. We also know that at least for some of these clones the encoded proteins appear only in myotubes and not myoblast cells.

Dr. Robert Wydro: My second question is, have you done "Northern's" with these clones to show that you have only one structural sequence cloned in each one of those genomic clones?

Dr. Robert Storti: All we have done is hybridize 5'-labeled RNA to restriction fragments of each of those clones; we get only single fragments that hybridize. This does not mean that we could not have more than one message-coding region on any given fragment, but it looks like they have probably single copied, i.e., it looks like there is only one gene located in each of those 15-kb fragments. We have one clone that suggests that there may be message-coding regions, but we have to do more work on that.

Dr. Joav Prives: Could you comment on the degree of homology between the *Drosophila* muscle-specific proteins and their mammalian or avian counterparts?

Dr. Robert Storti: It is clear that the actins cross-hybridize; in fact, the *Drosophila* actin clone was originally isolated by its cross hybridization to chick and *Dictyostelium* actin mRNA. It is not entirely clear whether the others do. We are in the process of testing this, but we do not know yet. One might expect enough cross homology in contractile proteins to isolate vertebrate genes using *Drosophila* genes and vice versa.

67
Physiology of Myotonic Dystrophy in Culture

Michael Merickel, PhD

Richard Gray

Priscilla Chauvin

Stanley Appel, MD

Myotonic muscular dystrophy (MyD) is an autosomal dominant disorder of humans with clinical expression involving many different organ systems (including skeletal and cardiac), smooth muscle, multiple endocrine tissues, eye, and bone. No clear-cut biochemical defect has emerged from studies of skeletal muscle of tissues such as red blood cells. However, studies of both skeletal muscle and red blood cells have documented the presence of plasma membrane abnormalities. In biopsied MyD muscle fibers, these membrane abnormalities include a decreased resting membrane potential (RP) and an increased tendency to fire repetitive action potentials (APs).

This enhanced tendency to fire repetitive APs is termed myotonia, and it becomes clinically manifest as stiffness and difficulty in relaxing a muscle after voluntary contraction. Electromyographically, myotonia is characterized by repetitive bursts that increase and decrease in frequency (1). Myotonia is not limited to MyD, but may also occur in other inherited human disorders such as myotonia congenita. This latter syndrome is usually much more benign than MyD and is associated with skeletal muscle hypertrophy and weakness with few systemic manifestations. Although the biochemical defect is not known in MyD, the pathophysiology is reasonably well characterized. Human myotonia congenita appears to resemble goat myotonia in that chloride conductance is decreased (2, 3). In human myotonia congenita, potassium conductance may also be decreased (4).

The pathophysiology of myotonia in MyD is not well understood. In biopsied specimens, membrane resistance is not uniformly increased, and an abnormality in chloride conductance does not appear to explain the enhanced excitability. To help define the basis for myotonia in MyD, we have grown normal and

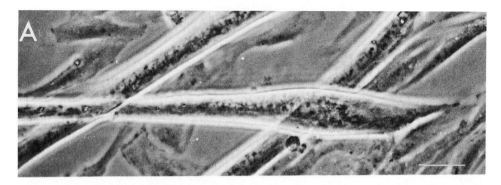

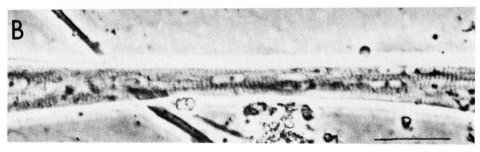

Fig. 1. Photomicrographs of control human myotubes after 3 to 4 weeks in culture, showing variations in morphology. Myotubes had a diameter of 10 to 20 μm, variable length (50 μm to more than 1 mm), and often underwent extensive bifurcation. No differences in morphology or rate of cell fusion were detected in myotubes cultured from biopsy specimens of patients with myotonic dystrophy. **(A)** Low-power phase contrast photomicrograph showing variations in myotube morphology. **(B)** High-power phase contrast photomicrograph of portion of myotube showing striations and peripheral nuclei (with nucleoli).

diseased human muscle in a primary tissue culture system. Tissue culture has many advantages over the intact muscle preparation, but it has the major difficulty that the abnormality underlying the disease may not be faithfully replicated in culture. Nevertheless, such a system may provide a convenient model for exploring pertinent physiologic parameters.

In our studies, muscle biopsy specimens were obtained from the vastus lateralis muscle with the consent of control patients or patients with electro-myographic evidence of myotonia and clinical features of MyD. Cultures were prepared from biopsy specimens by trypsin dissociation (Chauvin P, Appel SH: unpublished data). Well-developed myotubes were grown from both control and MyD biopsy specimens after 3 to 5 weeks in culture (Fig. 1). We have observed no morphologic differences in the rate of development or maturity of control and MyD myotubes by light microscopy.

FUNDAMENTAL ELECTROPHYSIOLOGIC ABNORMALITIES

Initial experiments were designed to determine whether some of the electro-physiologic abnormalities detected in fibers from MyD muscle were also present in MyD myotubes in culture. In biopsied specimens, decreased RP, decreased AP amplitude, and increased excitability have been reported (5, 6, 7, 8). All of these changes have been noted in our studies of MyD cells in culture.

Increased Excitability

One of the most conspicuous differences between control and MyD myotubes in culture was the tendency of MyD myotubes to fire repetitive APs in response to the injection of a single current pulse or a slowly depolarizing current ramp. More than 360 control and 370 MyD myotubes were examined, of which approximately 20% of the MyD and only 2% of the control MyD myotubes fired more than one AP when stimulated by anode break excitation. The increased tendency of MyD myotubes to fire repetitive APs was closely related to the characteristics of the AP afterhyperpolarization. The AP afterpotential of control myotubes was typically hyperpolarizing, whereas the afterpotential of MyD myotubes exhibited considerably more variability (Fig. 2). Many of the MyD myotubes (approximately 50%) exhibited afterpotentials with a depolarizing phase; these are termed depolarizing afterpotentials (DAPs). The MyD myotubes that displayed prominent DAPs typically fired repetitively in response to a slow depolarizing current ramp even if they did not fire repetitively in response to a single current pulse.

Gruener (5) has also shown that intact MyD muscle in particularly sensitive to depolarizing current ramps. The common appearance of DAPs in MyD myotubes is believed to be intimately associated with their repetitive firing behavior. Depolarizing afterpotentials have been observed in a number of nerve and muscle preparations that fire repetitive APs, such as spinal motoneurons (9), and hippocampal neurons (10) are indicative of systems having increased excitability and a tendency toward repetitive firing.

Decreased RP

The RP of MyD myotubes was significantly decreased, by approximately 10 mV, compared to control myotubes (Table 1). Such a decreased RP has also been observed by many other investigators in MyD muscle fibers studied from biopsy specimens (5, 8–10).

Table 1. Mean Resting Potentials of Cultured Human Myotubes[a]

Myotube Source	N_B	N_M	RP (mV)
Control	8	120	-52.8 ± 1.5
MyD	9	181	-42.3 ± 1.8

Abbreviations: N_B, number of biopsies; N_M, number of myotubes; RP, resting membrane potential; MyD, myotonic dystrophy.

[a] The RP data are given as the mean $\pm$ SEM for the number of myotubes shown. The difference between control and MyD RP of 10.5 mV was significant at P < 0.0005.

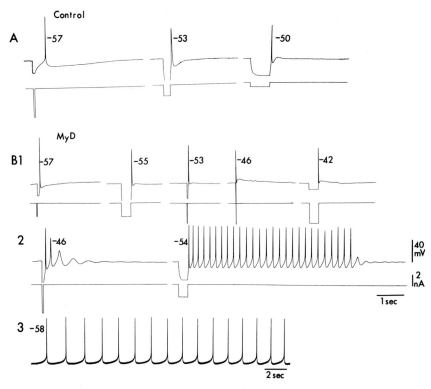

Fig. 2. Comparison of control **(A)** and dystrophic **(B)** activity in response to single anode break stimulus. Control myotubes typically fired a single action potential (AP) followed by an afterhyperpolarization (AHP) of variable magnitude and duration. The activity resulting from stimulating myotubes from patients with myotonic dystrophy (MyD) was much more variable than that observed in control myotubes. Approximately half of the MyD myotubes repetitively fired APs (B3) with no stimulus. (Reprinted with permission hyperpolarizing (B1, frame 1). The remaining MyD myotubes exhibited a depolarizing afterpotential that was either completely depolarizing (B1, frames 4 and 5) or delayed, following a small, short AHP (B1, frames 2 and 3). Approximately 20% of the MyD myotubes investigated fired repetitive APs when stimulated (B2, see text). Sometimes, MyD myotubes repetitively fired APs (B3) with no stimulus. (Reprinted with permission from Merickel M, Gray R, Chauvin P, Appel S: Muscular dystrophy patients: altered membrane electrical properties. PNAS 78:648–652, 1981.)

An explanation for the decreased RP in culture is not clear. Additional experiments have demonstrated that both control and MyD myotubes are more permeable to potassium than to sodium (P_{Na}/P_K of 0.14 ± 0.06). Alteration in the external chloride had no effect on RP or conductance. Although ouabain reduced the RP of control myotubes by only 2 to 4 mV, we still cannot rule out a contribution of the Na-K pump to the decreased RP. In any event, the decreased RP appears to be of secondary importance, because control cells depolarized to the same potentials as MyD cells do not demonstrate enhanced excitability. Thus, the RP permits us to differentiate MyD fibers from control fibers, but does not explain the basis for the enhanced tendency to fire repetitive APs.

Table 2. Mean Action Potential Parameters of Cultured Human Myotubes[a]

Myotube Source	N_B	N_M	AftP (mV)	Ap Amplitude (mV)		Half-Amp Duration (ms)
				Max	Overshoot	
Control	8	66	-5.7 ± 0.6	88.3 ± 3.4	35.5 ± 2.0	9.8 ± 0.9
MyD	9	164	-2.1 ± 0.9	73.4 ± 2.9	28.6 ± 2.2	8.4 ± 0.4
P value			< 0.005	< 0.005	< 0.05	

Abbreviations: N_B, number of biopsies; N_M, number of myotubes; AftP, maximal amplitude of the afterpotential that followed an anode break action potential, measured relative to the resting potential; AP, action potential; Max, maximal AP amplitude; Half Amp Duration, AP, duration measured at one-half the maximal AP amplitude. All AP amplitudes and 0.5-amp durations were measured for APs elicited by anode break stimulation.
[a] Data are given as the mean $\pm$ SEM for the number of myotubes shown. The P values represent the significance of differences between control and MyD means.

Decreased Amplitude of AP and Afterhyperpolarization

Action potential characteristics were examined to obtain an indication of defects in active membrane properties in MyD myotubes. The AP amplitude was significantly decreased, by an average of 14.9 mV (Table 2). A large portion, but not all, of the decrease in AP amplitude in MyD myotubes was due to their decreased RP. The AP overshoot was independent of RP and was decreased by 6.9 mV in MyD myotubes. No significant differences were found in AP half-amplitude duration in MyD and control myotubes.

The amplitude of the AP afterhyperpolarization was also significantly decreased in MyD myotubes (Table 2). In fact, two MyD biopsies had average positive (depolarizing) afterpotentials. The decrease in AP afterhyperpolarization amplitude and frequent presence of positive afterpotentials in MyD myotubes is a reflection of the common appearance of DAPs described in *Increased Excitability*. The decreased afterhyperpolarization amplitude and DAPs in MyD myotubes are apparently not secondary effects of the decreased RP, because depolarizing control myotubes by artificial current injection increases but never decreases the amplitude of the afterhyperpolarization.

Decreased Outward-Going Rectification

Comparison of steady-state curent-voltage (I-V) plots has indicated that MyD myotubes have a decreased long-time-course outward-going rectification compared to control myotubes. This decreased outward-going rectification is most reasonably explained as a decrease in slow-time-course outward potassium current. It is believed that a decreased outward-going potassium current could underlie the reduced AP afterhyperpolarization and common appearance of DAPs in MyD myotubes.

SUMMARY OF ELECTROPHYSIOLOGIC PROPERTIES

These studies have shown that MyD myotubes have abnormalities in many of their fundamental electrophysiolgic properties, including decreased RP of approximately 10 mV; decreased amplitudes of both the AP and the AP afterhyperpolarization; increased tendency to fire repetitive APs in response to a single stimulus or a slowly depolarizing ramp and the common appearance of DAPs; decreased slow outward-going rectification. All of these abnormalities can best be explained by a single membrane defect that reduces a slow outward-going potassium current.

The most important difference between control and MyD myotubes is the increased repetitive firing tendency of MyD myotubes, because the repetitive firing is a direct expression of myotonia, the hallmark of this disease. The increased repetitive firing and decreased AP afterhyperpolarization may thus be more closely related to the primary defect underlying the disease than is the decreased RP. The enhanced excitability is probably related to dynamic membrane properties (particularly those affecting potassium) rather than steady-state membrane properties.

VOLTAGE-CLAMP STUDIES

We have begun to use voltage-clamp techniques to study MyD myotubes. The advantage of voltage clamp is that we can identify and isolate various membrane current processes underlying the MyD abnormalities. Furthermore, abnormalities determined by voltage clamp can be expected to be more closely related to the basic membrane defect underlying MyD than are AP and RP properties; such voltage-clamp measurements of MyD myotubes may therefore be less variable.

Our initial voltage-clamp experiments were designed to examine the slow membrane outward current processes most likely to underlie repetitive firing, DAPs, and the reduced AP afterpotential observed in MyD myotubes. Because of the small size of human myotubes, it is not possible to use the traditional 2-electrode voltage-clamp technique routinely to obtain a large enough sample of the myotubes. The single-electrode voltage-clamp technique is ideally suited to the study of slow membrane currents in small cells such as human myotubes (11, 12).

The most striking difference we have observed between control and MyD myotubes is the rate of activation of the outward current. The outward current in MyD myotubes, particularly those exhibiting prominent DAPs, was activated significantly more slowly than the outward current in control myotubes. To date, we have examined myotubes in biopsy specimens from 3 control subjects and 3 patients with MyD. Figure 3 shows a typical example from a control myotube in which a 90% activation of the outward current required approximately 100 ms, compared to 900 ms for the MyD myotube shown in Figure 4 with the common command potential of +15 mV from a holding potential of −55 mV.

Detailed quantification of the outward current kinetics has not yet been performed. A quantitative estimate of the rate of activation of the outward current was obtained by comparing the outward current measured at 200 ms to the peak outward current for command potentials of −35, −15, and +5 mV from a holding potential of −55 mV (Table 3). The time of 200 ms was chosen for comparison because it represents the time to the peak of the

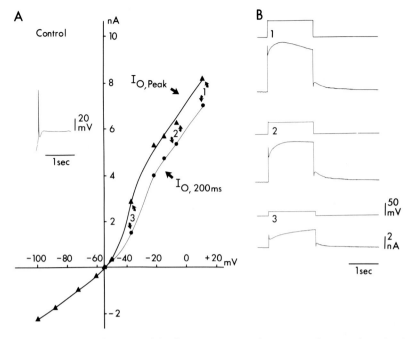

Fig. 3. Development of outward ionic currents (I_0) in a control myotube. **(A)** Current-voltage plot of peak outward current (triangles) and outward current at 200 ms (circles). The peak outward current was measured as the maximal outward current reached during the time course of the voltage command, and the 200-ms current was measured at 200 ms after the start of the command. Numbered points refer to the corresponding transients shown in B. The inset shows an anode break action potential with a distinct afterhyperpolarization. **(B)** Top traces, voltage command; bottom traces, current. Note the rapid rise of the peak outward current with large depolarizing commands.

Table 3. Ratio of Outward Currents in Myotubes Under Voltage Clamp[a]

Biopsy	Command Potential		
	$-35\ mV$	$-15\ mV$	$+20\ mV$
Control			
1	$0.65 \pm 0.05\ (4)$	$0.81 \pm 0.01\ (4)$	$0.89 \qquad (1)$
2	$0.77 \pm 0.04\ (8)$	$0.84 \pm 0.03\ (8)$	$0.83 \pm 0.03\ (7)$
3	$0.94 \qquad (1)$	$0.89 \pm 0.05\ (2)$	$0.88 \pm 0.07\ (2)$
Mean $\pm$ SEM	0.79 ± 0.08	0.85 ± 0.02	0.87 ± 0.02
Myotonic dystrophy			
1	$0.62 \pm 0.00\ (2)$	$0.72 \pm 0.04\ (3)$	$0.93 \pm 0.01\ (3)$
2	$0.70 \pm 0.09\ (4)$	$0.69 \pm 0.04\ (9)$	$0.68 \pm 0.06\ (6)$
3	$0.60 \pm 0.05\ (6)$	$0.53 \pm 0.05\ (9)$	$0.58 \pm 0.08\ (5)$
Mean $\pm$ SEM	0.64 ± 0.03	0.65 ± 0.06	0.73 ± 0.10
	—	$P < 0.025$	—

[a] The ratio was calculated as the current measured at 200 ms divided by the peak outward current (I_{200}/I_{Peak}) for command potentials of -35, -15, and $+20$ mV from a holding potential of -55 mV. The mean $\pm$ SEM values shown were calculated for the number of myotubes indicated in parentheses. There was a significant difference between control and MyD outward current ratios only for command potentials of -15 mV.

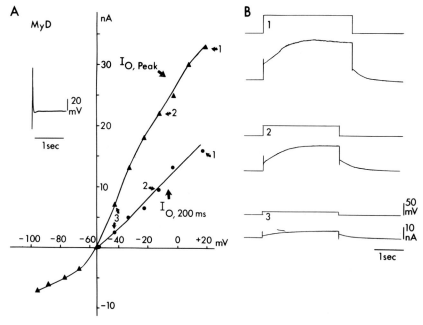

Fig. 4. Development of outward ionic currents (I_0) in a dystrophic myotube. **(A)** Current-voltage plot of peak and 200-ms currents measured in the same manner described in Figure 3. Note the marked difference in currents at these two times compared to control myotubes. The inset shows an anode break action potential with a small afterhyperpolarization. Numbered points refer to corresponding transients in B. **(B)** Note the relatively slow increase in outward current during the voltage command compared to control myotubes.

afterhyperpolarization of most APs, and these currents were considered to be of primary importance in determining the characteristics of the afterhyperpolarization and repetitive firing behavior. Command potentials of -15 mV produced the largest difference between control and MyD myotubes (Table 3). For command potentials of -15 mV, the outward current of control myotubes at 200 ms attained 85% of the peak outward current value, compared to only 65% for MyD myotubes. The decreased outward current ratio in MyD myotubes at 200 ms is a reflection of the delayed activation of MyD outward current, which can be expected to be directly responsible for the reduced AP afterhyperpolarization amplitude, DAPs, and repetitive firing behavior in MyD myotubes.

PATHOPHYSIOLOGY OF MYOTONIA IN MyD

All of the results obtained from our physiologic investigations of MyD myotubes can be best explained by a decreased slow outward-going potassium current. This decrease in slow potassium current could be due either to a decrease in the potassium equilibrium potential (i.e., intracellular potassium concentration) or to a decrease in a potassium conductance pathway. At this point, it is not possible to distinguish between these two possibilities. At any rate, it is clear that MyD myotubes possess definite physiologic abnormalities in vitro and that the presence of innervation is not required for expression of such abnormalities. It is important to note, however, that defects noted in tissue culture may not be identical to defects noted in adult fibers in vivo.

Even though we have suggestive evidence that a potassium current is deficient in MyD myotubes, it is not clear what potassium current is involved. Our previous biochemical data suggested the potential involvement of the calcium-dependent potassium system in MyD (14). Data from the present electrophysiologic studies in human MyD myotubes are in accord with this hypothesis. This system clearly contributes to the regulation of mammalian myotube excitability, because primary cultured rat myotubes possess a calcium-dependent potassium current that contributes to their AP afterhyperpolarization. When this current is blocked, repetitive firing occurs and is similar to the myotonia observed in MyD myotubes (Merickel M, Gray R: unpublished data). The calcium-dependent potassium system has also been shown to influence repetitive firing in a number of nerve and muscle systems in vivo (13, 15, 16). It is anticipated that future experiments using voltage clamp will enable us to characterize the nature of the defective potassium current and its relationship to calcium.

ACKNOWLEDGMENTS

The authors wish to thank Curtis Martin for help with the data analysis and figure preparation, and Vikki Seelig for her excellent assistance with the preparation of the manuscript. These studies were supported by the Muscular Dystrophy Association and the Robert J Kleberg, Jr. and Helen C Kleberg Foundation.

REFERENCES

1. Buchthal F: Diagnostic significance of the myopathic EMG. In *Pathogenesis of Human Muscular Dystrophies*. Edited by Rowland L. Excerpta Medica, Amsterdam, 1977, pp 205–218
2. Lipicky R, Bryant S: Sodium, potassium, and chloride fluxes in intercostal muscle from normal goats and goats with hereditary myotonia. J Gen Physiol 50:89–111, 1966
3. Lipicky R, Bryant S: A biophysical study of the human myotonias. In *New Developments in Electromyography and Clinical Neurophysiology*. Edited by Desmedt J. S. Karger Basel, 1973, pp 451–463
4. Lipicky R: Studies in human myotonic dystrophy. In *Pathogenesis of Human Muscular Dystrophies*. Edited by Rowland L. Excerpta Medica, Amsterdam, 1977, pp 729–738
5. Gruener R: Electrophysiologic properties of intercostal muscle fibers in human neuromuscular diseases. Muscle Nerve 2:165–172, 1979
6. Gruener R: In vitro membrane excitability of diseased human muscle. In *Pathogenesis of Human Muscular Dystrophies*. Edited by Rowland L. Excerpta Medica, Amsterdam, 1977, pp 243–258

7. Hoffman WW, Alston W, Rowe G: A study of neuromuscular junctions in myotonia. Electroencephalogr Clin Neurophysiol 23:521–537, 1966

8. McComas AJ, Mrozek K: The electrical properties of muscle fibre membranes in dystrophica myotonica and myotonia congenita. J Neurol Neurosurg Psychiatry 31:441–447, 1968

9. Calvin W: A third mode of repetitive firing: self-regenerative firing due to large delayed depolarizations. In *Control of Posture amd Locomotion.* Edited by Stein R, Pearson K, Smith R, Redford J. Plenum Press, New York, 1973, pp 173–178

10. Kandel E, Spencer W: Electrophysiology of hippocampal neurons. II. After-potentials and repetitive firing. J. Neurophysiol 24:243–259, 1961

11. Merickel M: Design of a single electrode voltage clamp. J Neurosci Methods 3:87–96, 1980

12. Merickel M, Gray R: Investigation of burst generation by the electrically coupled cyberchron network in the snail *Helisoma* using a single-electrode voltage clamp. J Neurobiol 11:73–102, 1980

13. Meech RW: Calcium-dependent potassium activation in nervous tissues. In *Annual Review of Biophysics and Bioengineering.* Edited by Mullins LJ. Annual Reviews Inc., Palo Alto, 1978, pp 1–18

14. Appel SH, Roses AD: Membranes and myotonia. In *Pathogenesis of Human Muscular Dystrophies.* Edited by Rowland L. Excerpta Medica, Amsterdam, 1977, pp 747–758

15. Fink R, Luttgaü: An evaluation of the membrane constants and the potassium conductance in metabolically exhausted muscle fibers. J Physiol (Lond) 263:215–238, 1976

16. Sanchez JA, Stefani E: Inward calcium current in twitch muscle fibers of the frog. J Physiol (Lond) 283:197–209, 1978

DISCUSSION

Dr. Irwin Konigsberg: Before entertaining questions for Dr. Appel, Dr. Askanas has a summary slide of neuromuscular diseases that have been studied in culture and in which the defect is expressed in culture.

Dr. Valerie Askanas: This table lists various neuromuscular diseases in which culturing of human muscle provided important information.

Table 1. Results of Culturing Human Muscle

Our Laboratory
   Reincarnated biochemical or morphologic defects in muscle fibers
      Acid maltese deficiency—biochemical and morphologic defects (1)
      Ragged-red fibers—mitochondrial morphologic defects (2, 3)
      Nonspecific vacuolar myopathy—morphologic inclusions, increased acid
        phosphatase (2, 4)
      Congenital X-linked fiber hypotrophy with central nuclei—rampant growth,
        impaired maturation, decreased adenylate cyclase (5)
      Adrenomyeloneuropathy—lipid inclusions, excess very long chain (C_{22}–C_{26}) fatty
        acids (6, 7)
      Gyrate atrophy of choroid and retina with muscle tubular aggregates—excessive
        tubules, ornithine toxicity, absent ornithine-aminotransferase (8)
   Other Findings
      Some cases of muscle carnitine deficiency—growth only with excess (10 mM)
        carnitine (9)
      Muscle phosphorylase deficiency—presence of phosphorylase (adult and fetal
        forms of isoenzymes) (10)

Table 1. (Continued)

Duchenne muscular dystrophy—normal growth, development, and morphology (4)

Myotonic atrophy—normal growth and RMP (-55 to -60 mV), R_{in}, firing threshold; no myotonia; trains of normal-amplitude APs in hyperpolarized (-80 mV) fibers (11)

Myotonia congenita—normal growth and RMP; no myotonia (unpublished observations)

Acid maltase deficiency—RMP greater than control, decreased R_{in}, APs elicitable at RMP; as fibers become vacuolated, decreased RMP and R_{in}, and loss of elicitable APs (12)

Laboratory of Armand Miranda
  Reincarnated defects
    Debrancher enzyme deficiency—biochemical and morphologic defects (13)
    Carnitine palmityltransferase deficiency—biochemical defect (13)
Laboratory of Andrew Engel
  Duchenne muscular dystrophy—normal plasmalemma by freeze-fracture studies (14)

Abbreviations: RMP, resting membrane potential; R_{in}, internal resistivity; AP, action potential.

Dr. Irwin Konigsberg: Thank you Dr. Askanas. That was an unabashed attempt to proselytize for the use of cell culture.

Dr. Elis Stanley: Muscle fibers in culture show marked changes in electrophysiologic properties during development. Are the differences between myotonic and normal cultures evident at all stages, or only in mature fibers?

Dr. Stanley Appel: All of these have been looked at consistently between 2 and 4 weeks. There may be some changes, but I think all characteristics appear to hold. In other words, the changes go on not only in control cultures, but also in myotonic cultures. There are not enough to give rise to the differences that we have described here.

Dr. Stephen Thesleff: Several of the differences you described are similar to those seen in chronically denervated rat muscle, which also has anode break excitation and resulting repetitive firing. There it appears the firing is caused by alterations in the kinetics of the sodium channel. I noticed a difference in the rate of rise of your action potentials, compared to your control; have you examined the kinetics of the sodium channel?

Dr. Stanley Appel: Not yet. This is one of the major reasons that we have gone to the voltage clamp. The only reason we are putting more emphasis on potassium until we get final-voltage clamp data, is that we think it would be unlikely that the changes in afterhyperpolarization would be due to sodium. Under no circumstances can we rule out a contribution of the sodium channel.

Dr. Jerry Shay: Have you ever looked at the effects of ethyleneglycol tetraacetate or calcium on these cultures and then looked at them after hyperpolarization? It might be interesting to test that in light of your observations on the effects of calcium.

Dr. Stanley Appel: Dr. Merickel looked at this in terms of the afterhyperpolarization in rat myotubes. It is quite clear that there is an effect, and that is one of the ways you can document the importance of extracellular calcium in the rat system. The human system does not seem to be similarly responsive, but these studies are now underway and can be done a lot more effectively with the voltage clamp.

Dr. Donald Wood: Have you measured sodium and potassium levels in these cultured cells, and do you have any information on the equilibrium potentials for sodium and potassium?

Dr. Stanley Appel: Some studies were done. Dr. Merickel, do you want to comment on this?

Dr. Michael Merickel: Our initial experiments demonstrated a decreased resting potential, which we initially thought might be very important in causing repetitive behavior. First of all, the cells are not significantly permeable to chloride, which has been seen in other tissue culture systems. We did not find any major difference in P_{Na}/P_K, even though there could be subtler differences we did not detect. Additionally, no differences were found in internal potassium concentration, indicating no difference in potassium equilibrium. More experiments, however, are needed to confirm this. We looked at some of the more dynamic aspects such as the repetitive firing behavior seen in myotonic aspects of the disease.

Dr. Fritz Buchthal: One of the characteristic electrophysiologic changes in myotonic dystrophy is that a single stimulus usually does not evoke a myotonic response; you need to give 3 or 4 stimuli at a frequency of about 10 or 20 per second. Have you applied a similar technique in tissue culture?

Dr. Stanley Appel: I do not think the situation at the single-cell level in tissue culture is really comparable.

Dr. Barry Festoff: With regard to calcium activation of potassium permeability, as in studies of pancreatic beta cells, would you predict that the pancreas in these dystrophic patients would release insulin more readily or less readily than normal?

Dr. Stanley Appel: More readily would be the prediction from those studies; in fact, that is what we see. It was surprising to us. We knew the clinical fact, and the data from the basic science literature suggested that this mechanism is presumably the operative one in beta-cell function.

References

1. Askanas V, Engel WK, DiMauro S, et al: Adult-onset acid maltase deficiency. N Engl J Med 294:573–578, 1976
2. Askanas V, Engel WK: Diseased human muscle in tissue culture: a new approach to the pathogenesis of human neuromuscular disorders. In *Pathogenesis of the Human Muscular Dystrophies*. Edited by Rowland LP. American Elsevier Publishing Co., New York, 1977, pp 856–871
3. Askanas V, Engel WK, Britton DE, et al: Reincarnation in cultured muscle of mitochondria abnormalities from two patients with epilepsy and lactic-acidosis. Arch Neurol 35:809–810, 1978

4. Askanas V, Engel WK: Normal and diseased human muscle in tissue culture. In *Handbook of Clinical Neurology*, vol. 40. Edited by Vinken PJ, Bruyan GW. 1979, pp 183–196

5. Askanas V, Engel WK, Reddy NB, et al: X-linked recessive congenital muscle fiber hypotrophy with central nuclei. Arch Neurol 36:604–609, 1979

6. Askanas V, McLaughlin J, Engel WK, Adornato BT: Abnormalities in cultured muscle and peripheral nerve of a patient with adrenomyeloneuropathy. N Engl J Med 301:588–590, 1979

7. McLaughlin J, Askanas V, Engel WK: Adrenomyeloneuropathy: increased accumulation of very-long-chain fatty acid in cultured skeletal muscle. Biochem Biophys Res Commun 92:1202–1207, 1980

8. Askanas V, Valle D, Kaiser-Kupfer MI, et al: Cultured muscle fibers of gyrate atrophy (GA) patients: tubules, ornithine toxicity, and 1-ornithine-2-oxyacid aminotransferase (OAT) deficiency. Neurology (NY) 30:368, 1980

9. Engel WK, Prockop LD, Askanas V, et al: Nearly-fatal lipid-laden myopathy with myoglobinuria and myodeficiency of carnitine: prednisone failure but dramatic improvement with carnitine and cultured muscle dependence on carnitine. Neurology (NY) 30:368, 1980

10. Meinhofer MC, Askanas V, Proux-Daeglen D, et al: Muscle type phosphorylase activity in muscle cells cultured from three patients with myophosphorylase deficiency. Arch Neurol 34:779–781, 1977

11. Tahmoush AJ, Askanas V, Nelson PG, Engel WK: Electrophysiologic properties of aneurally cultured muscle from myotonic atrophy patients compared with controls. Neurology (NY) 30:404, 1980

12. Tahmoush AJ, Askanas V, Engel WK, et al: Adult onset acid maltase deficiency: electrophysiologic properties of aneurally cultured muscle fibers compared with controls. Neurology (NY) 30:401, 1980

13. Miranda A, Trevisau C, Shanske S, et al: The expression of genetic enzyme defects in muscle cultures: now you see it, now you don't. Neurology (NY) 30:367, 1980

14. Osame M, Engel AG, Rebouche CJ, Scott RE: Freeze fracture electron-microscopic (study) analysis of plasma membranes of cultured muscle cells in Duchenne dystrophy. In *Disorders of the Motor Unit*. Edited by Schotland DL. John Wiley & Sons, Inc., New York, 1982, pp. 489

68
Skeletal Muscle Development

Stephen D. Hauschka, PhD

Richard Rutz, PhD

Thomas A. Linkhart, PhD

Christopher H. Clegg

Gary F. Merrill, PhD

Claire M. Haney

Robert W. Lim

A complete understanding of skeletal muscle development will entail descriptions and mechanistic explanations of every cellular change occurring, from the embryonic determination of the first myogenic cells in the mesoderm to the modulation of muscle fiber biochemistry by nerve-muscle interaction and contractile activity in adults. At present, our understanding of the sequence is fragmentary and is restricted primarily to events occurring during terminal differentiation, i.e., the transition of proliferating myoblasts into multinucleated myotubes. Molecular details of the regulation of a few muscle-specific genes during terminal differentiation are beginning to be understood, but little is known concerning the initial signals that cause myoblasts to differentiate. Even less is known concerning the earlier cell lineage processes that give rise to myoblasts.

This paper will summarize recent studies our group has directed toward early as well as terminal phases of muscle development. Our studies have been carried out with chicken, mouse, and human muscle cells; the basic approach has been to break new experimental ground with chicken and mouse myoblasts, and then to follow with analogous experiments using human cells. Our experiments have concentrated on what may be a unique class of determined myogenic cells, the "muscle colony-forming cells" (MCF cells). In most experiments, MCF cells are obtained from single-cell suspensions made directly from skeletal muscle tissue. Our working assumption is that each muscle colony derived from these suspensions represents a single progenitor cell (MCF cell) that had acquired the capacity for extensive in vitro replication and for muscle differentiation *before* its removal from the organism. If this assumption is valid, in vitro colony formation ("clonal analysis") may then be used as a means of assessing quantitative and qualitative fluctuations occurring within MCF cell populations in vivo.

Knowledge concerning MCF cell behavior seems worthwhile because these cells have properties similar to those of stem cells (i.e., the capacity for extensive proliferation as well as for production of progeny that differentiate). Subtle changes in MCF cell population dynamics could thus have major effects on the timing and pattern of subsequent muscle development or on the response of muscle tissue to injury and disease (1, 2).

Experiments directed toward later phases of muscle development have been focused on analyzing factors that regulate the transition of determined myogenic cells from proliferation to terminal differentiation. The major thrust of these studies concerns the mechanism by which specific polypeptide growth factors (mitogens) regulate muscle differentiation. Most such studies involve permanent clonal lines of mouse myoblasts (derived from MCF cells), because these homogeneous cell populations respond rapidly and irreversibly to manipulation of mitogenic components in the culture medium (3–5). As information accrues from mouse myoblast studies, analogous experiments are being attempted with human myoblasts (6). These studies suggest that mitogens regulate terminal muscle differentiation *in a negative sense*. When specific mitogens are present, terminal differentiation is *repressed* and myoblasts proliferate; when mitogens decrease below some threshold level, myoblasts withdraw from the cell cycle and differentiate. While the studies with permanent mouse myogenic cell lines described below appear to represent the most convincing evidence that mitogens regulate the onset of terminal differentiation, earlier reports by many other investigators have contributed to this hypothesis (7–14).

The studies reported below emphasize embryonic muscle development, but these same approaches can be applied to problems of muscle disease and regeneration (1, 2). Recognition and quantification of myogenic stem cell populations (with colony-forming assays) will allow more detailed analysis of the cellular response to muscle injury or disease. An understanding of the molecular mechanisms regulating myoblast proliferation and differentiation is essential to understanding and eventually influencing muscle regeneration.

DEVELOPMENTAL CHANGES IN MCF

Analyses of initial phases of muscle development indicate that MCF cells first appear at an early limb bud stage (the third day of chick development, stage 21, and on about the thirty-third day of human development, horizon XIV) (15, 16). At this stage, MCF cells represent approximately 10% of the total colony-forming cells derived from leg soft tissue regions. During subsequent development, the proportion of MCF cells increases to a maximal steady-state level of about 90% (16, 17). In both species, clonal plating efficiency also increases during this interval from 1% approximately to 25%; thus, the "absolute" number of MCF cells appears to increase from 1 per 1,000 single cells to approximately 225 per 1,000 cells. The extent to which this increase depends on proliferative expansion of a small initial MCF cell population versus recruitment of other cells into the MCF cell class is not known.

The transition from 10% to 90% MCF cells is roughly linear and occurs with equivalent kinetics during comparable stages of chick and human development (17, 18). In the more extensively analyzed and accurately staged case of chick leg development, however, it is possible to detect an intermediate plateau level of about 60% between days 6 and 8 (17). Further experiments suggest that the increase in MCF cells subsequent to the plateau is influenced by innervation (19–21).

In addition to numerical differences in the proportion of MCF cells in both human and chick, younger and older embryos also differ with respect to the types of MCF cells they contain. To summarize results from many different studies, MCF cells from young embryos give rise to muscle clones that exhibit less multinuclearity and require "more complex" growth media than their later counterparts (16, 17, 22–24). Biochemical differences between "early" and "late" muscle colony types have not yet been detected.

With this information in mind we have asked the following questions: Where are early and late MCF cell types located during limb development? Are "early" MCF cells the progenitors of "late" MCF-cells?

Location of MCF Cells

Determination of where MCF cells are located during limb development necessitated perfection of techniques for limb microdissection that would permit precise and reproducible localization of various internal limb regions. Initial attempts at direct manual dissection indicated that this approach lacked such precision and gave almost no resolution of internal limb regions because of the poor optical qualities of thick limb pieces. For these reasons, we devised a technique in which entire limb buds are embedded in a gelatin-growth medium mixture and then sectioned transversely using a vibrator to give a proximodistal series of limb slices. Depending on the embryonic stage and desired resolution, slice thickness may be varied from 30 to 300 μm. When viewed under a dissecting microscope, the flat surfaces of such slices exhibit excellent optical properties, so that regions differing in histologic cell associations are relatively simple to discern (Fig. 1). This resolution permits one to follow developing muscles along their entire lengths. Various regions can be dissected from such sections and either grown as explants or dissociated to the single cell level and subjected to clonal analysis (25, 26). By photographing each section and marking the dissected regions, an accurate reconstruction of the entire limb can be achieved. The technique also offers the opportunity for performing biochemical analyses on adjacent sections so that cellular and biochemical correlations may be made.

Clonal analysis of dissected limb slices was initially applied to chick limbs between stages 21 and 26 to determine the "boundaries" of muscle, cartilage, and connective tissue regions. Figure 1 and Table 1 illustrate data obtained with this approach. The 250-μm section through the tibia-fibula region encompasses the region 1,150 to 1,400 μm from the distal tip of a stage-26 chick

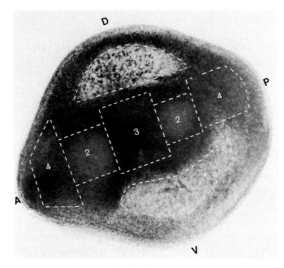

Fig. 1. A 250-μm transverse section through a stage 26 leg bud taken 1,150 to 1,400 μm from the distal tip. Discrete histiotypic regions are discernible within the section. In typical experiments these regions are dissected out along the approximate boundaries indicated and are then dissociated to single cells and subjected to clonal analysis. Such analyses indicate (Table 1) that dorsal and ventral region 1 contain most muscle colony-forming cells; region 2 contains most of the cartilage colony-forming cells, and regions 3 and 4 contain primarily fibroblastic cells. D, dorsal; V, ventral; A, anterior; P, posterior orientations of the section.

embryo. From the data, it is evident that MCF cells are restricted to discrete dorsal and ventral regions; 95% of the clones derived from these regions form myotubes, whereas 0% form cartilage and only 5% appear to be fibroblastic. In the same section, cartilage colony-forming cells are restricted to the prospective tibia and fibula regions, and fibroblast colony-forming cells are found primarily in the anterior and posterior regions. When tissue from the same dorsoventral and anteroposterior locations (but from progressively more distal limb sections) is subjected to clonal analysis, MCF cells are detected almost exclusively within the dorsal and ventral regions. Similarly, cartilage colony-forming cells are restricted to the central region, and fibroblast colony-forming cells are found primarily in the more peripheral anterior and posterior regions.

As a general rule, the proportions of all colony-forming cell types decrease in progressively more distal sections. MCF cells never extend to the most distal tip region, and the proportion of MCF cells attenuates more sharply than that of cartilage and fibroblast colony-forming cells. The most distal extension of MCF cells depends on embryonic stage; for example, MCF cells extend to within 300, 600, 800, and 1,200 μm of the distal tip at stages 23, 25, 27, and 29, respectively (see Table 3).

Detection of MCF Cell Precursors

Previous clonal studies indicated that the earliest period at which MCF cells can be detected is stage 21 (15, 17). Assays of dorsoventral prospective muscle regions from even the most proximal sections of stage-20 limbs detect no MCF cells. It appears then that MCF cells make their initial appearance between stages 20 and 21. This observation raised the question of whether MCF cell precursors were present in limb buds younger than stage 21.

This question was initially examined by preparing 50-μm sections of stage 17 to 21 chick embryo leg buds and culturing these as explants. The cultures were scored daily during the next 7 days for the appearance of multinucleated myotubes. Explants from stage 17 leg buds failed to exhibit myotube formation, whereas those from stage 18 onward formed myotubes in all of the more proximal sections. Results from several experiments are provided in Table 2. These indicate that by stage 18, cells with the capacity for myotube formation are present to within 250 to 300 μm of the distal tip. More refined explant experiments, in which various regions were dissected from each 50-μm section, indicate that most myotube-forming cells are located in the same dorsoventral regions as those containing high proportions of MCF cells during later stages.

Results from the initial explant experiments demonstrated that cells with muscle-forming capacity are present within limb bud stages in which MCF cells cannot be detected by direct clonal analysis. Was it possible that early limbs contained precursors to MCF cells and that the precursor-MCF cell transition was occurring in the explants? This question was approached by growing explants for various periods, and then subjecting them to clonal analysis.

Table 1. Clonal Analysis of Dissected Regions Within Stage 26 Leg Bud Section[a]

| | Colony Types[b] | | | | | |
| | Muscle | | Fibroblast | | Cartilage | |
Region	% Total Colonies	% Cells Seeded	% Total Colonies	% Cells Seeded	% Total Colonies	% Cells Seeded
Dorsal						
1	95	22	5	0.8	0	<0.1
Ventral						
1	94	20	6	1.3	0	<0.1
2	9	0.6	91	6.7	95[c]	1.8
3	12	0.25	88	1.8	0	<0.1
4	11	0.4	89	3.6	0	<0.1

[a] A 250-μm section located 1,150 to 1,400 μm from the distal tip of a stage 26 chick embryo leg was dissected into Regions 1 through 4, as indicated in Figure 1. These regions were dissociated and plated as single cells in medium that potentiated the expression of muscle and fibroblast colony-forming cells or of cartilage colony-forming cells. Clones were permitted to develop for 2 weeks and were then fixed and scored. Muscle colonies contained multinucleated myotubes; fibroblast colonies contained "nondescript" unfused cells; cartilage colonies contained polygonal cells that had secreted a metachromatically staining extracellular matrix.

[b] Muscle was assayed in muscle-conditioned medium (Hams F-10 with 15% horse serum and 3% embryo extract); fibroblasts, in muscle-conditioned medium; cartilage, in fresh medium (Hams F-10 with 15% calf serum).

[c] Because cartilage clones were assayed in a different media and in different dishes, they are not included in the *same* calculation of total percentage clonal differentiation provided for muscle and fibroblast clones.

Table 2. Myotube Formation in Explants of Sections From Early Chick Limb Bud[a]

Distance from Distal Tip (μm)	Stage		
	18	19	21
Tip–50	−	−	−
50–100	−	−	−
100–150	−	−	−
150–200	−	−	−
200–250	+	−	−
250–300	+	+	+
300–350	+	+	+
350–400	+	+	+
400–450		+	+
450–500		+	+
500–550		+	+
550–600			+
600–650			+

[a] Stage 18, 19, and 21 chick embryo limb buds were sectioned at 50 μm and individual slices were grown 1 week in vitro. Explants were scored daily for the appearance of multinucleated myotubes and scored as positive when myotubes appeared.

Although this series of experiments is incomplete, the results clearly indicate that MCF cells arise in stage 18 to 19 explants by the fourth day in vitro. Thus, whatever the environmental requirements for the precursor-MCF cell transition, these conditions appear to exist within the explant cultures. In ongoing experiments, we are attempting to identify the precursor cell type and to determine limiting requirements for MCF cell formation.

Distribution of MCF Cell Types

As summarized above, early MCF cells differ from late MCF cells with respect to clonal morphology and media requirements (16, 17). To determine how MCF cells expressing such qualitative differences are distributed within developing limbs, MCF cells obtained from sequential limb sections such as those described above were analyzed with respect to early and late phenotypes.

Results from an extensive series of such experiments indicate that (a) early limb buds contain exclusively early MCF cells (Table 3, stage 23); (b) limb buds of intermediate age contain late MCF cells in the most proximal limb section, and these cells extend outward in a gradient that decreases toward more distal limb regions (Table 3, stage 27); (c) later limb stages contain late MCF cells in progressively more distal regions, whereas early MCF cells become restricted to the most distal limb regions in which skeletal muscle precursor cells can be detected (Table 3, stage 31) (26).

Table 3. Proximodistal Distribution of Muscle Colony-Forming Cells during Chick Leg Development[a]

Proximal → Distal

STAGE 23 (100-μm SECTIONS)

Section number	8	7	6	5	4	3	2	1
% MCF cells[b]	19	35	30	30	27	11	0	0
% late MCF cells[c]	0	0	0	0	0	0	—	—

STAGE 27 (200-μm SECTIONS)

Section number	11	10	9	8	7	6	5	4	3	2	1
% MCF cells[b]	75	87	81	88	85	84	76	28	0	0	0
% late MCF cells[c]	55	59	57	45	40	31	14	1	—	—	—

STAGE 31 (300-μm) SECTIONS

												Toe Muscles				
Section number	21	20	19	18	17	16	15	14	13	12	11	10	9	8	7	6 to 1
% MCF cells[b]	95	93	97	97	89	85	84	72	23	0	0	94	91	76	30	0
% late MCF cells[c]	97	97	97	98	98	97	97	95	93	—	—	97	94	89	46	—

[a] Stage 23, 27, and 31 chick limb buds were serially sectioned; dorsal and ventral prospective muscle regions were dissected from each section, and these were subjected to clonal analysis.

[b] Percentage of total colonies that formed myotubes when cultured in medium that supports maximal expression of muscle differentiation.

[c] Percentage of the total muscle colonies that exhibited the characteristic late muscle clone phenotype (extensive multinuclearity) (24).

Subclonal Analysis of MCF Cell Types

The proximodistal replacement of early by late MCF cell types during limb development raised the question of whether early MCF cells were the direct progenitors of late MCF cells. One test of this possibility was to determine whether the subclonal progeny of early MCF cells converted to a late MCF cell phenotype during repeated in vitro passages, or whether MCF cell phenotype remained constant.

Experiments performed with early or late MCF subclones isolated from stage 23 to 33 chick embryos gave similar results: subclonal progeny from early MCF colonies produced colonies that were phenotypically early (approximately 30% nuclei in myotubes), whereas those derived from late MCF clones produced clones that were phenotypically late (approximately 60% nuclei in myotubes) (26). Such phenotypic heritability persisted through 4 sequential subclonal passages and for at least 40 in vitro doublings.

These results suggest that early MCF cells are not the direct progenitors of late MCF cells, or at least that an early-to-late transition, if it occurs in vivo, is not supported by in vitro conditions that permit extensive proliferation and differentiation of both early and late myoblast types. Additional evidence arguing against an early-to-late MCF cell transition comes from experiments in which pooled subclone populations of early chick MCF cells were transplanted into quail limb buds followed by clonal analysis after several days of graft development (21). As in our in vitro experiments, no late MCF cells were derived from the early MCF cell grafts; thus, it may be that early and late MCF cell types represent divergent routes in the muscle cell lineage pathways.

MCF Cell Distribution in Human Limb Buds

Due to the infrequent availability of early human limb buds, analogous studies of MCF cell distribution during human limb development are still in their initial stages. Nevertheless, results from the few cases analyzed appear consistent with those from comparable chick embryo stages. Results from the most extensively examined case are reported below.

This experiment involved clonal analysis of the proximodistal distribution of MCF cell types in 300-μm transverse serial sections through arm and leg buds from a 42-day fetus. Prospective muscle regions were dissected from each section, dissociated to single cells, and plated at clonal densities. Quantitative differences in MCF cell distribution were calculated from clonal plating efficiencies and percentage muscle colony formation observed for each section. Qualitative differences between MCF cell types were assessed according to clonal morphology: early human MCF cells form colonies that exhibit low levels of multinuclearity and a preponderance of long, thin, refractile myotubes, whereas late MCF cells form colonies with extensive multinuclearity and wide, flat myotubes (16).

Results from this experiment (Table 4) indicate that MCF cells are distributed in a proximodistal gradient and that late MCF cells are also more prevalent in proximal regions. These gradients occur in both leg and arm sections, but the

Table 4. Proximodistal Distribution of Muscle Colony-Forming Cells in 42-Day Human Embryo Leg and Arm Buds[a]

Proximal → Distal

LOWER LEG (300-μm SECTIONS)

Section number	14	13	12	11	10	9	8	7	6	5	4	3 to 1
% MCF cells[b]	81	66	51	49	46	65	65	50	34	9	38	2
% late MCF cells[c]	98	89	72	58	25	32	17	19	20	16	11	0

ENTIRE ARM (300-μm SECTIONS)

Section number	18	17	16	15	14	13	12	11	10	9	8	7	6	5	4	3 to 1
% MCF cells[b]	77	82	74	77	67	85	86	70	70	66	43	56	36	45	0	0
% late MCF cells[c]	92	91	90	88	79	81	66	68	63	59	38	79	79	50	—	—

[a] Lower leg and upper and lower arm segments from a 42-day therapeutically aborted human fetus were sectioned at 300 μm. Prospective muscle regions were dissected from each section, and these were subjected to clonal analysis in media that support maximal muscle differentiation.

[b] Percent total colonies that contain multinucleated myotubes.

[c] Percent total muscle colonies that exhibit the phenotype characteristic of late MCF cells (i.e. extensive multinuclearity, wide myotubes) (16).

gradual attenuation of late MCF cells in the lower leg region appears to differ from the rather sharp attenuation observed in the arm.

MYOBLAST COMMITMENT TO TERMINAL DIFFERENTIATION

Many in vitro studies have suggested that the terminal step in muscle differentiation (conversion of proliferating myoblasts to nonproliferating, biochemically differentiated, multinucleated myotubes) is regulated by factors that influence myoblast proliferation (6–14). In most such studies, the onset of terminal differentiation could be accelerated by switching cultures from "rich" to "conditioned" or "depleted" media or by lowering or eliminating the serum and/or embryo extract components of the standard growth medium. In response to such changes, myoblasts were reported to commence fusion and to elaborate muscle-specific gene products (e.g., acetylcholine receptor, creatine kinase, myosin) within one or two cell cycle equivalents after the medium switch. Our mouse myoblast system extends and refines these observations by measuring the kinetics of myoblast commitment to terminal differentiation at the single-cell level, by coupling these commitment kinetics directly to alterations in cell cycle parameters, and by demonstrating that a purified polypeptide mitogen, fibroblast growth factor (FGF) (27, 28) is capable of preventing myoblast commitment when added to cells switched to depleted medium.

Onset of Differentiation

Acceleration Due to Medium Conditioning
As mentioned above, the onset of terminal muscle differentiation is regulated by factors that affect cell proliferation. Evidence that this relationship exists in the mouse myoblast system comes from observations that the initiation of myotube formation in clonal cultures is dependent on clonal density (29). Cultures with 500 clones per dish begin fusing on day 4, whereas cultures with 20 clones per dish begin fusing on day 5 or 6. As in analogous experiments with muscle cells from other species (7, 11, 22), this behavior suggests that mouse myoblasts affect the onset of their terminal differentiation by altering their culture medium. This possibility was examined by switching low-density clonal cultures to "conditioned medium" that had been exposed to high density cultures for several days. The results of this experiment are clear cut. Clones fed fresh medium on day 3 do not fuse, whereas clones fed conditioned medium exhibit extensive fusion within 24 hours (Fig. 2). It is also evident that clones fed fresh medium continue to proliferate; e.g., the colony shown in Figure 2b contains about 4 times as many cells as it did 24 hours earlier (Fig. 2a). In contrast, clones fed conditioned medium appear to cease or slow proliferation; the colony shown in Figure 2d contains only about twice as many cells as 24 hours earlier (Fig. 2c).

Delay Due to Addition of Purified Mitogen
To determine whether the decreased proliferation and accelerated fusion observed when clones are switched to conditioned medium is linked to the absence of specific mitogens, clonal cultures were refed with conditioned

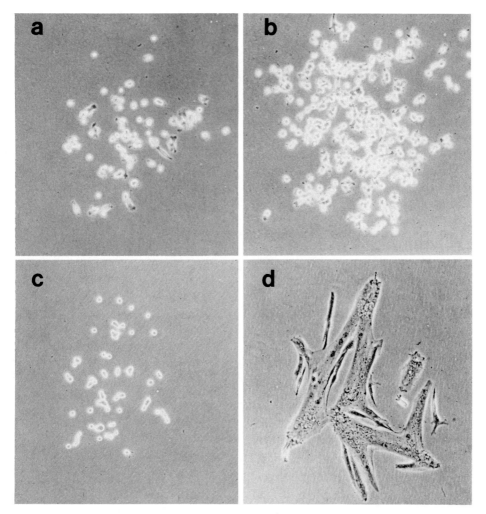

Fig. 2. Phase micrographs of living mouse muscle colonies taken at the time of feeding 3-day clones (a and c) with either mitogen-rich or mitogen-depleted media. Twenty-four hours later, the same clones were rephotographed. Clones refed mitogen-rich medium (b) continue proliferating and do not fuse; clones switched to mitogen-depleted medium (d) cease proliferating and form multinucleated myotubes.

medium containing a number of different purified mitogens. Epidermal growth factor, insulin, nerve growth factor, multiplication-stimulating activity, platelet-derived growth factor, and endothelial cell growth factor had no effect on the onset of fusion, but fibroblast growth factor (FGF) added at a concentration of 10 ng/ml maintained myoblast proliferation and delayed the onset of fusion for 48 hours.

This result suggests that the alteration in conditioned medium most relevant for initiating myoblast differentiation is removal of one or more mitogens. When this deficit is replaced by addition of purified FGF, proliferation continues and terminal differentiation is delayed.

Effect of Mitogen-Depleted Medium

The onset of fusion observed when clonal cultures are switched to mitogen-depleted medium commences approximately 14 hours after the medium switch. By this time, terminal differentiation is clearly occurring within the nascent myotubes; but does commitment (i.e., an *irreversible* change in developmental potential) occur earlier than the onset of myoblast fusion? This question was investigated by switching 3-day clones to mitogen-depleted medium for various durations and then refeeding them with fresh medium. Thirty hours later, the clones were fixed and examined for myotubes. We reasoned that if commitment occurred before the onset of myoblast fusion, then clones refed with fresh medium at times before 14 hours would contain myotubes.

Results from this experiment (Fig. 3) indicate that some myoblasts within each colony become committed to terminal differentiation after only 3 to 4 hours of exposure to mitogen-depleted medium. Exposure to mitogen-rich medium for the following 26 hours does not reverse the process. It is also evident from these experiments that not all of the myoblasts in each clone undergo fusion in response to 4 hours of mitogen depletion. Thus, it appears that clonally related myoblasts differ with respect to their ability to respond to mitogen depletion. What could explain such intraclonal differences? The most likely explanation related to mitogens appeared to be cell cycle asynchrony between myoblasts in each clone, i.e., during brief exposure to mitogen-depletion medium some myoblasts would have been in each phase of the cell cycle. If commitment occurred in only one phase, then only the fraction of myoblasts in that portion of the cell cycle would become committed. The

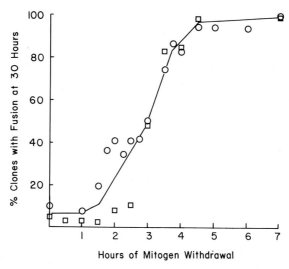

Fig. 3. Clonal density cultures of mouse myoblasts plated in mitogen-rich medium (100/60-mm plate) were rinsed twice with F10 and CaCl$_2$ and fed mitogen-depleted medium on day 3 after plating. At each time point the medium in duplicate plates was replaced with mitogen-rich medium. All plates were fixed at 30 hours, and the percentage of clones with myotubes (containing 3 or more nuclei) was determined. The data points (average from 2 plates each) are from 2 separate experiments.

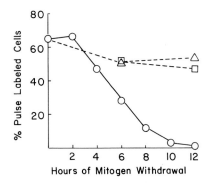

Fig. 4. Clonal density mouse myoblast cultures 3 days after plating were rinsed and fed mitogen-depleted medium (○), mitogen-rich medium (△), or mitogen-depleted medium + 20 ng/ml FGF (□). At 30 minutes before each time point, ^{3}H-thymidine was added in a small volume to one culture plate. After a 30-minute incubation, the plate was rinsed twice in saline and fixed. Autoradiographs were scored for the percentage of cells that had incorporated ^{3}H-thymidine. Twenty clones (500 to 1,000 cells) were estimated for each time point.

relationship between commitment and the cell cycle was then pursued in subsequent experiments.

Kinetics of Commitment

Cell cycle-commitment relationships have been studied by a number of approaches. In an initial experiment, the effect of mitogen deprivation on the myoblast cell cycle was examined by pulse-labeling cells in S phase with ^{3}H-thymidine and collecting mitotic cells after various intervals to assess the percentage of labeled metaphases (3, 30). This study indicated a 12.5-hour doubling time and G_1, S, and G_2 and M phases of 2.0, 7.5, and 3.0 hours, respectively, for myoblasts grown in mitogen-rich medium. When myoblasts were switched to mitogen-depleted medium after ^{3}H-thymidine pulse-labeling, cells labeled in S traversed the remainder of S, G_2, and M with the same kinetics as those maintained in mitogen-rich medium; but in contrast, mitogen-deprived cells failed to progress through a second cell cycle. Presumably, cells that had been in S at the time of the ^{3}H-thymidine pulse completed the cycle they were in and then withdrew from the cycle after entering the next G_1 phase.

To determine the rapidity with which mitogen deprivation affects myoblast proliferation, 3-day clones were switched to mitogen-depleted medium, and the fraction of cells synthesizing DNA (cells in S) was monitored by 30-minute ^{3}H-thymidine pulses and autoradiography. Data presented in Figure 4 indicate that approximately 60% of the myoblast population is initially in S. This percentage persists for the next 2 to 3 hours; thus, cells continue entering S during this interval even though they are in the presence of mitogen-depleted medium. The fraction of myoblasts that can be pulse-labeled then falls off with kinetics that approximate the rate at which cells would be expected to traverse a 7.5-hour S period. By approximately 10 hours after the medium switch, virtually no cells can be pulse labeled; thus, it appears that the entire population has withdrawn from the cell cycle. Are such withdrawn myoblasts committed to terminal differentiation?

Figure 4 also illustrates that myoblasts maintained in either mitogen-rich fresh medium or in mitogen-depleted medium to which 20 ng/ml FGF or 3% chick embryo extract has been added remain in a proliferative state throughout the duration of this experiment. This evidence supports our contention that the withdrawal observed in cultures switched to mitogen-depleted medium alone stems from mitogen deprivation and not from some other alteration during the conditioning process.

To pursue the relationship between withdrawal from the cell cycle and commitment, we hypothesized that an early step in myoblast commitment to terminal differentiation might involve *irreversible withdrawal* from the cell cycle. If this were so, then individual committed cells could be identified by the fact that they would not reenter the cell cycle when exposed to mitogen-rich medium. At various intervals after mitogen deprivation, committed cells could then be detected by refeeding a culture with mitogen-rich medium plus ^{3}H-thymidine. Committed cells should remain unlabeled, whereas cells not yet committed should traverse another cell cycle and become labeled. By allowing 20 to 30 hours after refeeding for cells to become labeled, uncommitted myoblasts that were not in S phase when the mitogen and ^{3}H-thymidine were added would have time to cycle into S phase and become labeled; uncommitted cells that might have become quiescent in response to mitogen depletion would also have time to reenter the cell cycle and become labeled. In the same experiment, the percentage of committed cells after any interval of mitogen deprivation could be assessed by fixing parallel cultures at the time of mitogen readdition and determining the average number of cells per clone. The percentage of committed cells could then be calculated as (the average number of unlabeled cells per clone/the average number of cells per clone at that time of mitogen refeeding) × 100%.

Results from an experiment such as this are presented in Figure 5. They indicate that irreversible withdrawl from the cell cycle commences 3 to 4 hours after mitogen deprivation and increases steadily for the next 8 to 9 hours. By 12 hours, all cells are irreversibly withdrawn. Additional data presented in this figure indicate that when FGF (20 ng/ml) is added to the mitogen-depleted medium with which the cultures were fed, irreversible withdrawal from the cell cycle is prevented. This result again supports the concept that the relevant alteration in mitogen-depleted medium is the lack of one or more specific mitogens and not one of many other alterations that undoubtedly occur during medium conditioning.

If the hypothesis that irreversible withdrawal from the cell cycle is an early expression of myoblast commitment is correct, then withdrawn cells should also express biochemical markers of skeletal muscle differentiation. This correlation was tested by switching parallel cultures to mitogen-depleted conditions for various time intervals, and monitoring one set as described above for irreversible withdrawal from the cell cycle and the other set for the presence of acetylcholine receptor (AChR). Single cells were identified as containing AChR by ^{125}I-α-bungarotoxin binding followed by autoradiography. Thus, at each interval, 2 cultures were refed with mitogen-rich medium: one also received ^{3}H-thymidine

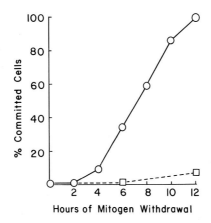

Fig. 5. Clonal density mouse myoblast cultures 3 days after plating were rinsed and fed mitogen-depleted medium (O) or mitogen-depleted medium + 20 ng/ml fibroblast growth factor (FGF) (□). At each time point the medium in one plate was replaced with mitogen-rich fresh medium + ³H-thymidine (0.2 μCi/ml). The cultures were rinsed with saline and fixed at 30 hours after the initial switch to mitogen-depleted medium. The number of unlabeled nuclei per clone (N_C) was determined in autoradiographs (average of 20 clones per time point). The average clone size (N_T) at the time of mitogen refeeding was determined in a parallel series of cultures that were fixed at each time point (average of 20 clones per time point). The percentage of cells committed at increasing times of exposure to mitogen-depleted medium was calculated as the percentage of cells committed = $N_C/N_T \times 100\%$. This experiment was performed with the same cells and at the same time as the experiment in Figure 4.

for 30 hours and was analyzed for withdrawn cells, and the other was analyzed after 30 hours for the presence of AChR by ¹²⁵I-α-bungarotoxin binding. The percentage of irreversibly withdrawn cells after various intervals of mitogen deprivation could then be directly compared to the percentage of cells demonstrating their commitment to terminal differentiation by the elaboration of AChR. When this comparison was made, both cultures exhibited a 2-hour lag, and then irreversibly withdrawn cells and AChR-positive cells increased with equivalent kinetics during the next 6 hours (3). This coincidence supports the hypothesis that irreversibly withdrawn cells are synonymous with committed cells.

When viewed together, results from the various cell cycle experiments suggest that myoblasts commit to terminal differentiation during a restricted phase of the cell cycle. Most such evidence is consistent with commitment occurring in G_1 to cells that enter this compartment after 3 to 4 or more hours of mitogen deprivation. Further discussion of evidence suggesting that commitment occurs in G_1 is provided in reference 3 and will not be reiterated here; however, results from one additional experiment seem relevant.

In this experiment, myoblasts were synchronized by mitotic shake-off and plated directly onto mitogen-rich or mitogen-depleted medium. Cultures of each type were then monitored autoradiographically for irreversibly withdrawn cells, i.e., cells that failed to incorporate ³H-thymidine during the 30-hour interval after plating, and for AChR-positive cells, (i.e., cells that bound ¹²⁵I-α-bungarotoxin 30 hours after plating). The results indicate that essentially all mitotically synchronized cells commit when plated into mitogen-depleted medium and that no cells commit when mitogens are present. Because mitotically synchronized cells complete cytokinesis and enter G_1 within a few minutes of plating, these data are clearly consistent with the hypothesis that myoblasts commit in G_1 when deprived of mitogens.

Gene Expression and Fusion

If, as presented above, irreversible withdrawal from the cell cycle is an early indication of commitment to terminal differentiation, it seemed worthwhile to determine when commitment occurs relative to the first detectable increase in muscle specific-gene products. High-density cultures were thus switched to mitogen-depleted medium and assayed for AChR and myosin heavy chain accumulation at various intervals after the switch. Neither product had increased by 4 hours, but both were significantly above background 8 hours after mitogen deprivation. Because myoblasts begin committing within 4 hours of mitogen removal, this implies that muscle-specific gene expression is well underway within 4 hours of the first detectable commitment event (irreversible withdrawal from the cell cycle).

Assays of myotube formation in similar experiments indicate that fusion does not commence until 12 hours after mitogen withdrawal. Fusion thus follows commitment by at least 8 hours and follows the initial accumulation of muscle-specific gene products by 4 hours.

Bromodeoxyuridine Sensitivity

Bromodeoxyuridine (BUdR) is known to inhibit selectively the terminal differentiation in many developing systems, including skeletal muscle (31–34). Previous studies had confirmed that BUdR inhibits mouse myoblast differentiation, as monitored by fusion and creatine kinase accumulation (35). It was not known, however, whether incorporation of BUdR into a myoblast's DNA would prevent it from withdrawing from the cell cycle in response to mitogen deprivation or whether BUdR interfered with some later event in the mitogen-regulated commitment process.

After determining a minimally toxic BUdR concentration that would inhibit terminal differentiation, muscle cultures were grown for 30 hours in thymidine-free medium containing 5 μM BUdR, switched to mitogen-depleted medium in the continued presence of BUdR, and then monitored at intervals for the percentage of cycling cells by 30-minute ^{3}H-thymidine pulses. Parallel cultures were assayed for commited cells by refeeding with mitogen-rich medium plus ^{3}H-thymidine to detect unlabeled cells after 30 hours.

Results from this experiment were clear cut (36). When deprived of mitogens, BUdR-treated myoblasts withdrew from the cell cycle with kinetics similar to those of untreated controls (Fig. 4). However, when refed with mitogens, BUdR-treated cells reentered the cell cycle. Thus, BUdR inhibits commitment (i.e., irreversible withdrawal from the cell cycle), but does not inhibit the process of withdrawal. This suggests that in response to mitogen deprivation, withdrawal per se is not obligatorily coupled to commitment; rather, a BUdR-sensitive commitment event closely follows withdrawal and renders the process irreversible.

DISCUSSION

The relevance of the studies described here to the behavior of normal muscle cells in vivo deserves consideration. Although many of the studies involve permanent myoblast cell lines, it should be emphasized that early passage, nontransformed mouse myoblasts behave similarly when subjected to mitogen deprivation (3). Furthermore, this behavior is not limited to mouse cells, because human myoblasts also respond to mitogen deprivation by exhibiting an accelerated onset of fusion and creatine kinase synthesis (6). Such accelerated differentiation is also consistent with previous observations in many other systems (7–14).

The responsiveness of various chick and human MCF cells to specific mitogens has not yet been studied, but experiments using crude medium components (various sera types and embryo extract) containing mitogen indicate that early and late MCF cells differ with respect to their media requirements (16). If these requirements prove to be mitogen related, understanding how the levels of various mitogens fluctuate during development might provide clues as to the regulation of various muscle cell populations. What determines the extent to which in vivo myoblasts proliferate versus differentiate? How are muscle satellite cells maintained in a quiescent state without committing to terminal differentiation, and what mitogenic stimuli initiate their reentry into the cell cycle? Further understanding of specific muscle cell types (e.g., early and late MCF cells) as well as the molecular mechanism of how myoblasts are affected by specific mitogens may provide answers to these questions. Such information should be helpful in formulating a rational approach to many types of muscle disease and injury.

ACKNOWLEDGMENTS

The authors thank Christy Lin, Marsha Ose, Elizabeth Witter, Diane Daubert, and Tony Kwan for their expert technical assistance, and are very grateful to Laura Glenn for unstinting secretarial help. They also thank Jeff Chamberlain for many useful discussions. This research was supported by grants from the National Institute of Health and the Muscular Dystrophy Association, Inc.

REFERENCES

1. Hauschka SD: Application of clonal assay methods to the analysis of tissue development and diseased states. In *Regulation of Cell Proliferation and Differentiation*: NIH Symposium on Aging. Edited by Nichols WW, Murphy DG. Plenum Press, New York, 1976, pp 143–164

2. Hauschka SD, Linkhart TA, Clegg C, et al: Clonal analysis of mouse and human muscle. In *Muscle Regeneration*. Edited by Mauro A. Raven Press, New York, 1978, pp 311–322

3. Linkhart TA, Clegg CH, Hauschka SD: Control of mouse myoblast commitment to terminal differentiation by mitogens. J Supramolec Struct (in press)

4. Linkhart T, Clegg C, Hauschka SD: Proliferation and differentiation of mouse myoblasts in vitro: mitogen removal and the commitment for cell fusion (abstract). J Cell Biol 79:25A, 1978

5. Linkhart T, Clegg C, Hauschka SD: Kinetics of mouse myoblast commitment for differentiation and response to purified mitogens (abstract). J Cell Biol 83:24, 1979

6. Zalin RJ, Linkhart TA, Hauschka SD: The synchronous differentiation of fetal human myoblasts cultured *in vitro* at high density. Exp Cell Res (in press)

7. Konigsberg IR: Diffusion-mediated control of myoblast fusion. Dev Biol 26:133–152, 1971

8. Yaffe D, Saxel O: A myogenic cell line with altered serum requirements for differentiation. Differentiation 7:159–166, 1977

9. Buckley PA, Konigsberg IR: Myogenic fusion and the duration of the postmitotic gap (G_1). Dev Biol 37:193–212, 1974

10. Doering JL, Fischman DA: The *in vitro* cell fusion of embryonic chick muscle without DNA synthesis. Dev Biol 36:225–235, 1974

11. Hauschka SD: Clonal analysis of vertebrate myogenesis. II. Environmental influences upon human muscle differentiation. Dev Biol 37:329–344, 1974

12. Slater CR: Control of myogenesis in vitro by chick embryo extract. Dev Biol 50:264–284, 1976

13. Emerson CP: Control of myosin synthesis during myoblast differentiation. In *Pathogenesis of Human Muscular Dystrophies*. Edited by Rowland LP. Excerpta Medica, Amsterdam, 1977, pp 799–809

14. Nadal-Ginard B: Commitment, fusion and biochemical differentiation of a myogenic cell line in the absence of DNA synthesis. Cell 15:855–864, 1978

15. Bonner PH, Hauschka SD: Clonal analysis of vertebrate myogenesis. I. Early developmental events in the chick limb. Dev Biol 37:317–328, 1974

16. Hauschka SD: Clonal analysis of vertebrate myogenesis. III. Developmental changes in the muscle-colony-forming cells of the human fetal limb. Dev Biol 37:345–368, 1974

17. White NK, Bonner PH, Nelson DR, et al: Clonal analysis of vertebrate myogenesis. IV. Medium-dependent classification of colony-forming cells. Dev Biol 44:346–361, 1975

18. Hauschka SD, Haney C, Angello JC, et al: Clonal studies of muscle development: analogies between human and chicken cells *in vitro* and their possible relevance to muscle diseases. In *Pathogenesis of Human Muscular Dystrophies*. Edited by Rowland LP. Excerpta Medica, Amsterdam, 1977, pp 835–856

19. Bonner PH: Clonal analysis of vertebrate myogenesis. V. Nerve-muscle interaction in chick limb bud chorio-allantoic membrane grafts. Dev Biol 47:222–227, 1975

20. Bonner PH: Nerve-dependent changes in clonable myoblast populations. Dev Biol 66:207–219, 1978

21. Womble MD, Bonner PH: Developmental fate of a distinct class of chick myoblasts after transplantation of cloned cells into quail embryos. J Embryol Exp Morphol (in press)

22. White NK, Hauschka SD: Muscle development *in vitro*: a new conditioned medium effect on colony differentiation. Exp Cell Res 67:479–482, 1971

23. Hauschka SD, White NK: Studies on myogenesis in vitro. I. temporal changes in the proportion of muscle-colony-forming cells during the early stages of limb development. II. myoblast-collagen interaction: molecular specificity required. In *Research in Muscle Development and the Muscle Spindle*. Edited by Banker GQ, Przybylski RJ, Van Der Meulen JP, Victor M. Excerpta Medica, Amsterdam, 1972, pp 53–71

24. Linkhart TA, Hauschka SD: Clonal analysis of vertebrate myogenesis. VI. Acetylcholinesterase and acetylcholine receptor in myogenic and non-myogenic clones from chick embryo leg cells. Dev Biol 69:529–548, 1978

25. Hauschka SD, Haney C: Use of living tissue sections for analysis of positional information during development (abstract). J Cell Biol 79:24, 1978

26. Rutz R, Haney C, Hauschka SD: A proximo-distal gradient of muscle colony-forming cells in chick embryo leg buds (abstract). J Cell Biol 83:45, 1979

27. Gospodarowicz D: Localization of a fibroblast growth factor and its effect alone and with hydrocortisone on 3T3 cell growth. Nature 249:123–127, 1974

28. Gowpodarowicz D: Purification of a fibroblast growth factor from bovine pituitary. J Biol Chem 250:2515–2520, 1975

29. Hauschka SD, Clegg CH, Linkhart TA, et al: Mouse myogenesis: karyotypic, morphological, proliferative, and biochemical analysis of permanent clonal cell lines and their subclonal variants (abstract). J Cell Biol 75:383, 1977

30. Quastler H, Sherman FG: Cell population kinetics in the intestinal epithelium of the mouse. Exp Cell Res 17:420–438, 1959

31. Stockdale R, Okazaki K, Nameroff M, et al: 5-Bromodeoxyuridine: effect on myogenesis in vitro. Science 146:533–535, 1964

32. Coleman JR, Coleman AW, Hartline EJH: A clonal study of the reversible inhibition of muscle differentiation by the halogenated thymidine analog 5-Bromodeoxyuridine. Dev Biol 19:527–548, 1969

33. Bischoff R, Holtzer H: Inhibition of myoblast fusion after one round of DNA synthesis in 5-bromodeoxyuridine. J Cell Biol 44:134–150, 1970

34. Rutter WJ, Pictet RL, Morris PW: Toward molecular mechanisms of developmental processes. Annu Rev Biochem 42:601–646, 1973

35. Merrill GF, Witter EB, Hauschka SD: Differentiation of thymidine kinase deficient mouse myoblasts in the presence of 5'-bromodeoxyuridine. Exp Cell Res 129:191–199, 1980

36. Merrill GF, Clegg CH, Linkhart TA, et al: Bromodeoxyuridine inhibits the commitment decision of mouse myoblasts to terminally differentiate. Paper presented at 2nd International Congress on Cell Biology, 1980 (abstr)

DISCUSSION

Dr. Barry Wilson: Is it possible that there is a temperature-sensitive stage for the mitogen or for commitment that could help you catch hold of what might be going?

Dr. Stephen Hauschka: There does not seem to be a natural temperature-sensitive step in commitment. We are trying to derive temperature-sensitive mutants that will not commit even when mitogens are withdrawn.

Dr. James Florini: I have some data that seem almost in direct disagreement with your results. We find just the opposite with somatomedins, which stimulate proliferation, differentiation, and fusion. Insulin, which is used in cull cultures at very high concentrations (and apparently acts as a somatomedin analogue) does the same thing. It is possible that the difference might be explained by Gospodarowicz's suggestions about the effects of fibroblast growth factor (FGF) on cells at low density. We grow our cells at high density, whereas you grow yours at substantially lower density. Gospodarowicz has been suggesting that FGF causes a change in the substratum, which is necessary to allow the cells to proliferate. Maybe we see different things because we are dealing with cultures of very different densities. It is also quite possible that mouse cells differ from rat cells, and we are using different mitogens. It is not possible to say that all mitogens have this effect. Somatomedins are very potent mitogens for the rat muscle cells, and they stimulate rather than prevent differentiation.

Dr. Stephen Hauschka: That is certainly correct. The mouse cells respond only to FGF, and not to other mitogens such as multiple stimulation activity (MSA). With human cells and rat cells, the situation may be different. I think we are both right, and what it indicates is that we just do not know very much yet about how mitogens regulate cell growth.

Dr. James Florini: I agree with both points. We are both right, and we do not know very much about these regulatory processes.

Dr. Stephen Hauschka: We could both be wrong, but let's be optimistic.

Dr. Joav Prives: Dr. Hauschka, consistent with your hypothesis, have you ever seen clones of "revertants" that ignore the presence of FGF in the medium and undergo fusion and terminal differentiation? Have you seen myoblasts that fail to differentiate when mitogens are withdrawn?

Dr. Stephen Hauschka: To answer your first question, so far, we have seen no clones that fuse in the presence of FGF. To answer your second question, we have isolated numerous variants from FGF-responsive myoblasts that fail to fuse in mitogen-depleted medium. Interestingly, these cells appear to have acquired responsiveness to epidermal growth factor (EGF), whereas their parents lack the capacity to respond to EGF even though they have EGF receptors. In addition, these same cells retain their responsiveness to FGF.

Dr. Wilfried Mommaerts: Comparing the present with the immediate past, i.e., an hour and a half ago or so, I now learn that different characteristics and different genes are switched on independently, not in coordination. You did not emphasize this, but your facts seem to show it.

Dr. Stephen Hauschka: No, I think our data are too incomplete to say that the creatine kinase is really being switched on independently of the acetylcholine receptor and myosin. Our data are not complete enough yet to look at coordinated versus sequential switching on of different genes.

Dr. Wilfried Mommaerts: In adult nerve crosses, different characteristics are reprogrammed at very different rates. Certain components can change over within a few weeks. By contrast, it takes about 2 years to make slow myosin fast in the ordinary nerve cross in the cat, even though the lifetimes of those proteins are a matter of days or weeks.

Dr. Helen Blau: Did you fuse your interspecific hybrids with polyethylene glycol?

Dr. Stephen Hauschka: Yes.

Dr. Helen Blau: Will mouse and human muscle cells fuse spontaneously, as chick and rat will?

Dr. Stephen Hauschka: Yes. We can make hybrid myotubes between mouse and human.

Dr. Helen Blau: When you fuse the cells with polyethylene glycol, is the problem due to differences in cell cycle time? Is that why they continue to proliferate instead of differentiating?

Dr. Stephen Hauschka: That is what we guessed. When you fuse cells with polyethylene glycol, you have to have very high concentrations of the cells. We worry that the mitogens might be depleted so rapidly that the mouse partner is commiting during the polyethylene glycol fusion process. The hybrid cells then simply fail to proliferate.

Dr. Sergio Pena: Those of us who work with cultured skin fibroblasts in Duchenne muscular dystrophy (DMD) would like very much to have cultured fibroblasts from a woman who is a double heterozygote for glucose-6-phosphate dehydrogenase and DMD. If anyone has such a person in their clinic, please contact me or any of the other fibroblast workers. We will make sure that these fibroblasts go to the New Jersey or the Montreal repository and that they are available to everyone. That would allow cloning, and would make controlled biochemical studies much easier. One question: as a non-expert in myoblast cultures looking at the development of myogenic rat and mouse lines, I can imagine that a lot of effort has been put in trying to develop myogenic human lines. Why they have not been developed, and what are the main problems?

Dr. Stephen Hauschka: It is thought that mouse cells have the capacity to transform spontaneously, perhaps because they carry endogenous viruses. The human cells simply do not have that capacity when grown under the same culture conditions. We may have to transform them with viruses or chemical carcinogens. Cells transformed in this way retain their ability to differentiate.

69

Muscle Cell Culture: Future Goals for Facilitating the Investigation of Human Muscle Disease

Stephen D. Hauschka, PhD

The rapid accumulation of knowledge concerning molecular aspects of normal skeletal muscle development and function is in sharp contrast to the slow progress being made toward understanding the chemical etiology of most muscle diseases. With all the efforts expended, it seems embarrassing that the molecular basis of a genetically sex-linked disease such as Duchenne muscular dystrophy (DMD) still eludes us.

If one assumes—and this is not a trivial assumption—that the molecular lesions responsible for various muscle diseases will be expressed in cell culture, the etablishment of normal and diseased human muscle cell lines could play a major role in determining the causes of these diseases (1–3). Most important, availability of such cells should also facilitate rational chemotherapeutic approaches to a disease once its molecular basis has been disclosed. The challenge, of course, is that techniques for establishing pure muscle cell lines are still in their infancy. The aim of this chapter is to extrapolate from our present capabilities to optimal situations suggested by recent advances in other cell culture systems. What is feasible at present, and what should we strive for in the future?

MUSCLE CELL CULTURE TECHNIQUES

Culture Medium

Procedures for culturing human muscle cells have been adopted rather directly from those used with avian and rodent myoblasts (4–7). Because human myoblasts appear to grow and differentiate reasonably well under these conditions, little effort toward perfecting them has seemed necessary. However, as human muscle cultures begin replacing animal culture models for both applied and basic experiments, one might question whether the formulation of media with components such as fetal calf serum, horse serum, and chick embryo extract is always consistent with rational experimental design. Cogent arguments for devising an optimal, fully defined culture medium for human muscle cells certainly could be made. Not only would a defined medium lessen the ambiguity due to unidentified constituents, but would also facilitate repeating experiments in different laboratories.

Perfecting an optimal medium is no simple task, but recent reports concerning requirements for trace minerals (8, 9), hormones, and growth factors (10–12) should point the way toward initial improvements. Media approaching fully defined components have been reported for rat myoblasts (13), and analogous media show promise in the mouse myoblast system (Linkhart TA, Merrill GF: unpublished observations).

Muscle Fiber Maintenance

A second aspect requiring improvement is that of muscle fiber maintenance. With the exception of certain organ culture systems in which fully differentiated muscle fibers appear to be maintained for months (14, 15), muscle fibers seldom persist for more than 1 or 2 weeks in vitro. This may be due to an inherent dependence on innervation, because in vivo fibers also degenerate when denervated (16) or when formed in the absence of nerves (17). If innervation is required, the obvious goal is to determine the molecular nature of this interaction (18). In a practical sense, this would permit incorporating the purified trophic factor into culture media.

Because the major pathologic lesion in diseases such as Duchenne muscular dystrophy (DMD) is fiber degeneration, it seems self-evident that long-term maintenance of normal muscle fibers is a prerequisite to obtaining an in vitro model for DMD. The very fact that reproducible differences between normal and human DMD muscle cultures or between control and animal muscular dystrophy cultures have not been reported suggests that the lesions may simply be superseded by rapid onset of an artificial fiber degeneration in all cultures. Solving this problem seems crucial if in vitro models are to be maximally useful in understanding and treating muscle diseases.

Frozen Tissue and Cell Banks

Because diseased and control human muscle tissue are infrequently obtained, it is essential that such material be preserved in a viable state whenever it becomes available. Even though procedures for establishing pure, long-lived, myogenic cell lines require further development, the basic goal here is to stockpile rare tissue samples so that they will be available for study as in vitro techniques are improved. Permanent frozen collections of such tissue will permit repeating experiments, exchange between different investigators, and concurrent analysis of multiple cases of the same disease. Frozen collections should be particularly useful in the instance of tissue obtained from therapeutic abortions at risk for DMD. Because the molecular basis of DMD is not known, comparative analysis specimens from 8 to 10 cases at risk of DMD together with specimens from a series of age-matched control subjects might well disclose a reproducible molecular difference.

Procedures for freezing and long-term storage of cell and tissue samples are already well established (19). We have adapted these techniques to human muscle cultures as well as to fetal and adult tissue samples (see *Appendix* for protocol) and have accumulated an extensive collection representing most developmental stages, as well as tissue from fetuses at risk for DMD. Samples from this collection have been distributed to numerous investigators and are available to anyone requesting them. With these methods, cell cultures have been routinely established from tissue stored for more than 3 years in liquid nitrogen. No noticeable deterioration in cell viability has occurred during this interval.

Amniocytes from Fetuses

As amniocentesis becomes a more prevalent adjunct to genetic counseling, parents with known familial histories of DMD are faced with the difficult question of whether to terminate male fetuses by therapeutic abortion. For many persons the difficulty of this decision would be lessened if amniocytes could provide a direct positive diagnosis of DMD. This would circumvent the present 50% probability of aborting an unaffected male fetus. The possibility that amniocytes might be used for diagnosing DMD in utero seems strengthened by reports of cell surface and cytoskeletal differences in the lymphocytes of proven DMD carriers (see chapters 60 and 61 of this volume).

Clearly, amniocytes from male fetuses at risk for DMD are a valuable resource that should be preserved for analysis of differences attributable to the DMD allele. Because the cytogenetics laboratories that provide sex determinations from amniocytes would not normally save such cells, it seems particularly important that genetic counselors and physicians involved with a potential DMD diagnosis take special care to assure that the remaining amniocytes be frozen for further study. This can be accomplished with standard cell culture procedures and use of the freezing protocol described in the Appendix. Amniocytes are capable of many cell culture doublings, so large numbers can readily be generated for biochemical studies.

As is perhaps typical of other cytogenetics laboratories, the University of Washington facility receives only 1 to 2 requests per year to provide sex determinations from amniocytes of fetuses at risk for DMD. At this rate, it would take years for any single laboratory to acquire a sufficient number of male amniocyte samples to carry out meaningful comparative studies. Throughout the country, however, dozens of cases are handled. In the interest of facilitating comparative studies of amniocytes, it thus seems worthwhile to designate several laboratories as central repositories for frozen amniocyte samples. This would permit ready access to samples from multiple cases as well as assure that potentially valuable samples were not inadvertently lost.

HUMAN MYOBLAST CELL LINES

The goal here is to obtain large numbers of muscle cells that maintain their capacity to differentiate. Achievement of the goal is frustrated by 3 problems: muscle tissue contains numerous cell types; myoblasts have a finite proliferative life span; and serially propagated human myoblasts may lose their ability to differentiate during prolonged cell culture. These problems are not insurmountable, but optimal solutions are not yet available.

The problem of cell type heterogeneity seems best approached by applying subclonal culture techniques. With this procedure, low-density primary cultures are established (7) and single muscle colonies (identified by the presence of multinucleated myotubes) are picked and further expanded. When carefully applied, the use of subclonal techniques assures pure populations of myogenic cells. However, the extensive cell replication required in cultures derived from single cells exacerbates the effects of problems due to a limited proliferative life span and to the instability of muscle differentiation during prolonged cultivation.

In our experience, myogenic cells derived from early human limb buds (day 36 fetus) are capable of 80 to 100 cell doublings. Myoblasts derived from later developmental stages have correspondingly decreased proliferative capacities; for example, those from 3- to 4-month fetuses (the age at which pregnancies at risk for DMD are usually terminated) have the capacity for 40 to 60 doublings, whereas myoblasts from adults are capable of about 30 replications before undergoing proliferative senescence. Less is known concerning the proliferative capacity of myoblasts from diseased muscle tissue. In the 129 dy/dy mouse muscular dystrophy model, most myoblasts exhibit limited proliferative capacity compared to those from age-matched controls (20). By analogy to human DMD (21), we believe this is attributable to the myoblast satellite cell population of dy/dy mice having been stimulated to undergo many additional rounds of replication during repeated cycles of muscle fiber degeneration. Judging from word-of-mouth reports, myoblast replication from DMD biopsies is also extremely limited, but it is not known when the decrease in proliferative potential first occurs.

Theoretically, about 10^9, 10^{12}, and 10^{15} cells could be generated from single myoblasts capable of 30, 40, and 50 doublings, respectively. In practice, the actual cell yield is considerably lower due to the fact that only 30% to 50% of the myoblasts survive each passaging step. Cell yields would also be reduced if myoblasts were permitted to commit to terminal differentiation due to mitogen depletion from the growth medium (22, 23, and chapter 61 of this volume). Expansion of myoblast clones to high cell numbers thus requires scrupulous attention to culture feeding schedules and the wherewithal to invest in huge volumes of medium, numbers of Petri plates, and technician time. As a conservative estimate, it would require 33 cell doublings (approximately 4 weeks' culture time), 1,000 100-mm Petri dishes, and 65 L of growth medium to expand a single human myoblast to 10^9 cells. Clearly, this is no small undertaking; experiments requiring more than about 10^7 pure myogenic cells are impractical.

Although this example might seem to suggest that myoblasts with the capacity for more than about 30 cell doublings would never be required, this would not be the case if one wished to apply somatic genetic analyses or DNA transformation techniques to human myoblasts. Here, for example, a *single* selection step involving a mutation or transformation frequency of 10^{-5} to 10^{-6} would require approximately 20 doublings simply to reexpand the selected cell to 10^6 cells. For such experiments, it seems evident that myoblasts capable of extensive cell proliferation will be required.

As mentioned previously, myoblasts derived from very early human limb bud stages appear to be capable of 80 to 100 doublings; such cells could theoretically be used as a starting source for genetic experiments. The major problem is that during prolonged propagation human myoblasts appear to lose their capacity for muscle differentiation (Hauschka SD, Ose M, Witter E: unpublished data). Little is known concerning the factors governing this loss. Similar behavior, however, has been observed in rat, mouse, and chicken myogenic cells, so it could be related to a normal developmental option in the muscle cell lineage. The most striking aspect of the phenomenon is its apparent randomness. Some clones may exhibit normal muscle differentiation, whereas adjacent colonies derived from the same parental clone exhibit none. Attempts to select for stable sublines by serially passaging colonies that maintain their capacity for differentiation have been unsuccessful. Although the capacity for muscle colony differentiation can be maintained essentially to the point of proliferative senesence (80 to 100 doublings and 8 subclonal passages), sister clones at each passage become differentiation defective. Until such developmental "instability" is understood and methods for circumventing it are devised, this phenomenon will remain a major obstacle to experiments requiring long-term muscle cell propagation.

Cell Lines from DMD Carriers

Although the major emphasis of DMD research is directed toward affected males, clonal cell lines derived from proved female carriers should actually provide the most homogeneous genetic background against which to search for a primary molecular lesion. Because of X-chromosome inactivation, clones from the same carrier will differ only with respect to X-linked alleles, whereas any autosomal allelic differences will be expressed identically by all colonies. From each DMD carrier, one clone type should express alleles from the unaffected X-chromosome and could serve as the normal control; the other clone type should express alleles from the DMD-carrying X-chromosome and could serve as the disease model.

This approach should greatly simplify the task of correlating putative molecular differences, e.g., by 2-dimensional electrophoretic gel patterns of cell proteins, with effects attributable to the DMD allele. In fact, if a proved female carrier were known to be heterozygous for a second X-linked gene (e.g., that for glucose-6-phosphate dehydrogenase) and expression of these alleles was measured in her male offspring, it would be possible to use this marker as an indication of which carrier-derived clones contained the DMD X-chromosome.

Because development of clonal lines of DMD carrier cells requires initiating cultures from single cells, it is important that such cells have as great a proliferative life span as possible. In this regard, clonal cultures derived from DMD carrier muscle biopsy specimens may not suffice, because the proliferative life span of adult myoblasts is inherently low as a result of their age; in carriers, proliferative life span may be reduced even further by additional rounds of in vivo proliferation. Tissue from a female fetus with potential DMD carrier status would be preferable. Alternatively, and assuming that nonskeletal muscle cells also express the DMD lesion, a more accessible source of carrier cells with a high proliferative life span might be umbilical cord tissue. Umbilical cord cells grow well and are capable of many cell doublings.

Parenthetically, umbilical cord and foreskin tissue, are also readily available cell sources from full-term males at risk of DMD. If the donor child is later diagnosed as having DMD, these tissus would provide an excellent source of highly proliferative cells without the necessity of obtaining further biopsy specimens from the child. Physicians involved with such cases should make special efforts to assure that umbilical and foreskin samples are saved for future study. These tissues may be frozen as described in the Appendix.

Application of recent somatic genetic techniques to human muscle cell cultures offers many possibilities for future research. Two of the most likely are: (a) construction of permanent mouse-human myoblast hybrids that retain selected human chromosomes (e.g., a human X-chromosome carrying either the normal or DMD allele); (b) attempts to counteract deleterious effects of the DMD allele by insertion of additional copies of the normal allele into DMD myoblasts.

Mouse-Human Myoblast Hybrids

Mouse-human myoblast hybrids could serve several useful purposes. Because permanent diploid mouse myoblast cell lines are available for use in hybridizations (20, 24), it seems likely that the hybrids might also proliferate indefinitely. Such behavior would negate the limited proliferative life span problem of human cells. Because mouse myoblasts exhibit a lower tendency to produce differentiation-defective progeny than do human myoblasts, mouse-human hybrids might prove similarly stable.

Mouse-human myoblast hybrids could also be used for mapping human muscle-specific genes (25–27). For example, human chromosome 17 should be selectively retained by mouse thymidine kinase–deficient (TK$^-$)-human hybrids grown in hypoxanthine, aminopterin, thymidine (HAT) medium: human chromosome 17 would provide TK to replace the missing mouse enzyme and thus would allow the hybrid cells to circumvent the aminopterin toxicity of HAT; other human chromosomes would be eliminated. If the muscle form of human creatine kinase (mCK) were then detected in differentiating hybrid cells, the gene for mCK could be tentatively assigned to human chromosome 17. A major difficulty with mapping human muscle-specific genes is the near molecular identity of many contractile proteins. Until high-resolution biochemical or immunologic procedures for distinguishing mouse and human contractile proteins are developed, only a few muscle-specific proteins can be mapped.

A related application of mouse-human hybrids would be selection of permanent hybrid cells that retained either the normal or DMD-carrying human X-chromosome. As in the example of TK$^-$, such hybrids should be achievable by using hypoxanthine guanine phosphoribosyltransferase-deficient (HPRT$^-$) mouse myoblasts and selecting for hybrids in HAT medium containing ouabain.

The human X-chromosome would supply HPRT to replace the missing mouse enzyme. The hybrid cells could utilize hypoxanthine and grow in HAT; nonhybrid human cells would be killed by oubain. Production of hybrids containing normal and DMD-carrying human X-chromosomes would then permit molecular comparison of the 2 sets of X-chromosome gene products against a common background of mouse gene products, the goal being to recognize the aberrant DMD gene product. It would be particularly interesting to determine whether the human DMD gene product functioned in the predominantly mouse myoblast environment. If so, such cells could become a useful in vitro model for DMD.

While these goals and applications seem reasonable, they may be difficult to achieve. Using the TK$^-$ and HPRT$^-$ mouse myoblast lines developed in our laboratory, we find that mouse-mouse and mouse-human hybridizations are routinely successful. However, in no case have we succeeded in producing mouse myoblast–human myoblast hybrids. For unexplained reasons, this combination is refractory, although mouse myoblast–human fibroblast, mouse fibroblast–human myoblast, and mouse myoblast (TK$^-$)–mouse myoblast (HPRT$^-$) combinations are viable (Merrill GF: unpublished observations). If this problem cannot be overcome, the applications described could still be approached with mouse myoblast–human fibroblast hybrids, but because this combination abolishes (at least temporarily) the capacity for muscle differentiation in the hybrid, the resulting cell could prove much less useful. For example, the same HAT selection scheme could be used to retain a DMD-carrying X-chromosome in mouse myoblast–human DMD fibroblast hybrids, but if these cells failed to differentiate, analysis of DMD gene function in a muscle cell environment would be precluded.

Insertion of Normal Gene Copies

Altough the molecular basis of DMD is unknown, the disease is presumably due to production of a defective gene product that either fails to integrate properly into a structural complex of the cell or fails to catalyze or regulate the synthesis of a secondary gene product. In either case, if functional copies of the normal allele were inserted into DMD myoblasts, products from these copies might counteract deleterious effects due to DMD allele products.

To some extent, the retarded degeneration of muscle fibers in DMD carrier females may argue for just such counteraction. Assuming random X-chromosome inactivation during early embryogenesis, most muscle fibers should contain mixtures of nuclei expressing either the normal or DMD allele. Presumably, the few rare fibers in which all nuclei express the normal allele are unaffected by DMD and never degenerate, whereas fibers with increasing proportions of nuclei expressing the DMD allele are increasingly prone to degeneration. The question, of course, is what proportion of nuclei expressing the normal allele is required to counteract those expressing the DMD allele? Because the extent of muscle fiber degeneration in carriers appears to be less than that in DMD males, and because statistically most carrier fibers should contain about 50% nuclei expressing each allele, it seems possible that the normal allele can overcome at least a 50% deficit due to the aberrant DMD product. If this were so, then addition of chromosomal material containing a functional normal allele to male DMD cells might override the DMD lesion.

Without having identified the DMD gene product and without having an in vitro DMD model, gene "replacement therapy" is difficult to design and test; in theory, one might envision a protocol similar to the following. Fetal DMD myoblasts capable of extensive proliferation would be mutagenized, and HPRT$^-$ cells would be selected (28). The X-chromosome of these mutants would thus carry 2 markers: DMD and HPRT$^-$. Similarly, TK$^-$ mutants would be selected from a line of normal fetal myoblasts (24). Hybridization of the 2 mutants and selection in HAT should yield tetraploid cells with 1 normal and 1 DMD-carrying X-chromosome. Assuming that such hybrids maintained their capacity for differentiation, as is true for the analogous (HPRT$^-$)-(TK$^-$) mouse myoblast hybrids, the critical issue would be whether the normal X-chromosome could counteract the deleterious effects of the DMD allele. Determining this would require either an in vitro or molecular assay for the DMD lesion; unfortunately, neither assay has been developed.

If these assays were developed, and if the DMD lesion were counteracted, more sophisticated types of in vitro therapy involving cotransformation with cloned regions of the X-chromosome or with pure copies of the normal DMD allele could be envisioned (29, 30). Cotransformation with pure gene copies seems particularly promising, because this procedure yields cotransformed cells with as many as 50 integrated copies of the transforming gene fragments.

Until an in vitro model for DMD is available, until the molecular nature of DMD is understood, and until the normal DMD gene is purified, further compounding of paper speculations and future goals seems presumptuous. What is important to realize is that the solution to the DMD puzzle will be multifaceted. Key molecular experiments await perfection of stable myogenic cell lines that exhibit the DMD lesion. Cell culture techniques thus have the potential for playing a major role in solving the problem.

ACKNOWLEDGMENTS

Without constant interaction with my lively and critical coworkers, Jeff Chamberlain, Chris Clegg, Claire Hainey, Bob Lim, Christy Lin, Tom Linkhart, Gary Merrill, Marshe Ose, Rick Rutz, and Liz Witter, this work would have been impossible. To all of them, and to my typist Laura Glenn, many thanks.

This research was supported by grants from the National Institute of Health and by the Muscular Dystrophy Association, Inc.

APPENDIX: PROTOCOL FOR FREEZING MUSCLE TISSUE AND CELL CULTURE SAMPLES

Tissue Dissection and Freezing

1. Carry out all operations using sterile techniques. Glassware and instruments should not be contaminated by residual detergents, cleaning solutions, or laboratory chemicals.

2. Place the tissue samples in a Petri dish containing sufficient chilled culture medium to cover the specimen. (Any standard medium, such as minimal essential medium with 15% serum of any type, will suffice.) If sterility of the specimen is questionable, rinse it as often as is practical with chilled physiologic saline, and then return it to culture medium. Thumb-sized pieces of muscle or fetal limbs can be stored at 4° C in culture medium for several days with little or no loss of cell viability, but it appears preferable to carry out a rough preliminary dissection if storage for more than 1 day is necessary.

3. Cut the muscle into pieces not exceeding 2 × 2 × 5 mm in size. Remove obvious connective tissue fascia, tendons, nerves, and blood vessels, but it is not necessary to attempt meticulous removal of contaminating tissues.

4. Aspirate the culture medium and add chilled complete medium containing 7.5% dimethyl sulfoxide (DMSO) (92.5 ml of medium plus 7.5 ml of 100% DMSO). Add a volume equivalent to approximately 3 times the residual medium-tissue volume after aspiration.

5. Stir the tissue pieces around in the DMSO-medium and allow 15 minutes for equilibration. Store on ice.

6. Aspirate, add more DMSO-medium as above, stir, and allow another 15 minutes for equilibration.

7. Aspirate, and add more DMSO-medium as above. Further equilibration is not necessary.

8. Transfer tissue pieces to prelabeled freezing vials. For 2-ml "Nunc" vials, add 1 to 1.5 ml of tissue plus DMSO-medium; as much as half the settled volume may be tissue. Use a Pasteur pipette with the tip broken off (diameter of orifice, ~3 mm) for convenient transfer.

9. Screw caps on tightly.

10. Cell freezing protocols call for slow cooling. The remainder of this procedure works, but probably is not as reliable as use of a controlled freezing apparatus. Wrap each vial in 2 Kleenex tissues and place vials (2 to 3 per depression) in a cardboard egg carton.

11. Close the carton and place it in a freezer at −70 to −90° C.

12. Twenty-four hours later, transfer vials to a container of liquid nitrogen. If liquid nitrogen storage is not available, the tissue can be maintained at −70 to −90° C for several years with no apparent loss of viability.

Thawing and Establishing Cell Cultures

1. Remove the vial from the freezer and immediately immerse the lower two-thirds in a water bath at 37° C.

2. As soon as thawing is complete (usually, approximately 2 minutes) uncap the vial and decant the contents into a small Petri dish.

3. Aspirate the DMSO-medium and rinse twice in physiologic saline.

4. Mince the tissue into small pieces with scissors and dissociate with collagenase or trypsin according to usual protocols (e.g., see Hauschka S: Dev Biol 37:329–368, 1974 for dissociation and culture procedures.)

Note that the cell yield from frozen tissue samples obtained from fetal specimens much older than 100 days of development is extremely difficult to assess because of the large amount of fiber debris. In addition, muscle satellite cells may still be attached to short muscle fiber fragments. For these reasons, it appears best simply to subdivide the entire cell and fiber suspension among several large Petri dishes. If attached flattened cells are visible within the first day, residual fiber debris may be aspirated and the culture can be refed and grown several days before passaging. If no attached cells are visible within the first day, the cultures should not be aspirated; rather, they should be left undisturbed and unfed for another 5 to 7 days until fibers and associated satellite cells have had time to attach and spread on the dish surface. The cultures can then be fed and passaged as usual.

Freezing Muscle Cell Culture

1. Dissociate monolayer cultures as usual; resuspend cells in chilled complete growth medium and obtain a cell count.
2. Adjust the cell density to twice that of the final density desired with chilled medium. (We have encountered no problems with final densities ranging from 1×10^5 to 5×10^6 cells/ml.)
3. Add an equal volume of chilled complete growth medium containing 15% DMSO (85 ml of medium plus 15 ml of 100% DMSO).
4. Mix by gentle pipetting and add 1 to 1.5 ml of cell suspension per 2-ml freezing vial.
5. Cap vials tightly and freeze as described above for tissue pieces.

Thawing and Establishing Cultures from Frozen Cells

1. Remove vial from freezer and thaw immediately as described for tissue pieces.
2. Resuspend cells by gentle Pasteur pipetting.
3. Plate cells directly onto dishes containing preequilibrated growth medium. Cells may be diluted in growth medium by gentle pipetting if small cell inocula are required.
4. If the entire thawed sample is placed in a single 100-mm culture dish, it is probably best to aspirate medium and unattached cells 4 to 6 hours after plating and refeed. If smaller volumes of thawed cells are plated, early refeeding is not necessary. As a general rule, we plate thawed human cells at densities of 3×10^4 to 3×10^5 cells/100-mm dish, and grow them 2 to 4 days before subcultivation for experiments.

REFERENCES

1. Askanas V, Engel WK: Diseased human muscle in tissue culture: a new approach to the pathogenesis of human neuromuscular disorders. In *Pathogenesis of the Human Muscular Dystrophies*. Edited by Rowland LP. Excerpta Medica, Amsterdam, 1977, pp 856–871

2. Askanas V: Regeneration of diseased human muscle in vitro as a tool to study the pathogenesis of human neuromuscular disorders. In *Muscle Regeneration*. Edited by Mauro A. Raven Press, New York, 1979, pp 297–304

3. Hauschka SD: Application of clonal assay methods to the analysis of tissue development and diseased states. In *Regulation of Cell Proliferation and Differentiation*. Edited by Nichols WW, Murphy DG. Plenum Press, New York, 1976, pp 143–164

4. Konigsberg IR: Clonal analysis of myogenesis. Science 140:1273–1284, 1963

5. Yaffe D: Retention of differentiation potentialities during prolonged cultivation of myogenic cells. Proc Natl Acad Sci USA 61:477–483, 1968

6. Hauschka SD: Cultivation of muscle tissue. In *Growth Nutrition, and Metabolism of Cells in Culture*, vol II. Edited by Rothblat GH, Cristofalo VJ. Academic Press, New York, 1972, pp 67–130

7. Hauschka SD: Clonal analysis of vertebrate myogenesis. II. Environmental influences upon human muscle differentiation. Dev Biol 37:329–344, 1974

8. McKeehan WL, Hamilton WG, Ham RG: Selenium is an essential trace nutrient for growth of WI-38 diploid human fibroblasts. Proc Natl Acad Sci USA 73:2023–2027, 1976

9. Ham RG, McKeehan WL: Development of improved media and culture conditions for clonal growth of normal diploid cells. In Vitro 14:11–22, 1978

10. Gospodarowicz D, Moran JS: Growth factors in mammalian cell culture. Annu Rev Biochem 45:531–558, 1976

11. Sato G, Reid L: Replacement of serum in cell culture by hormones. Biochemistry and mode of action of hormones. II. Int Rev Biochem 20:219–251, 1978

12. Sato G, Ross R (ed): *Hormones and Cell Culture,* vol A and B. Cold Spring Harbor Laboratory, 1979, pp 1–982

13. Florini JR, Roberts SB: A serum-free medium for the growth of muscle cells in culture. In Vitro 15:983–992, 1979

14. Peterson ER, Crain SM: Regeneration and innervation in cultures of adult mammalian skeletal muscle coupled with fetal rodent spinal cord. Exp Neurol 36:136–159, 1972

15. Peterson ER, Crain SM: Factors involved in muscle atrophy after surgical denervation of long-term cultures of cord-innervated fibers. In *Muscle Regeneration*. Edited by Mauro A. Raven Press, New York, 1979, pp 305–309

16. Gutmann E: Neurotrophic relations. Annu Rev Physiol 38:177–216, 1976

17. Eastlick HL: Studies on transplanted embryonic limbs of the chick. I. The development of muscle in nerveless and innervated grafts. J Exp Zool 93:27–49, 1943

18. Oh TH, Markelonis GJ: Neurotrophic effects of a protein fraction isolated from peripheral nerves on skeletal muscle in culture. In *Muscle Regeneration*. Edited by Mauro A. Raven Press, New York, 1979, pp 417–427

19. Shannon JE, Macy ML: Freezing, storage, and recovery of cell stocks. In *Tissue Culture: Methods and Applications*. Edited by Kruse PF Jr, Patterson MK Jr. Academic Press, New York, 1973, pp 712–718

20. Hauschka SD, Linkhart TA, Clegg C, Merrill G: Clonal studies of human and mouse muscle. In *Muscle Regeneration*. Edited by Mauro A. Raven Press, New York, 1979, pp 311–322

21. Wakayama Y, Schotland DL: Muscle satellite populations in Duchenne Dystrophy. In *Muscle Regeneration*: Edited by Mauro A. Raven Press, New York, 1979, pp 121–129

22. Linkhart TA, Clegg CH, Hauschka SD: Control of mouse myoblast commitment to terminal differentiation by mitogens. Supramolec Struct (in press)

23. Zalin RJ, Linkhart TA, Hauschka SD: The synchronous differentiation of fetal human myoblasts cultured in vitro at high density. Exp Cell Res (in press).

24. Merrill GF, Witter EB, Hauschka SD: Differentiation of thymidine kinase deficient mouse myoblasts in the presence of 5′-bromodeoxyuridine. Exp Cell Res 129:191–199, 1980

25. Weiss MC, Green H: Human-mouse hybrid cell lines containing partial complements of human chromosomes and functioning human genes. Proc Natl Acad Sci USA 78:1104–1111, 1967

26. Ruddle FH, Chapman VM, Ricciuti F, et al: Linkage relationships of seventeen human gene loci as determined by man-mouse somatic cell hybrids. Nature [New Biol] 232:69–73, 1971

27. Ruddle FH, Creagan RP: Parasexual approaches to the genetics of man. Annu Rev Genet 9:407–486, 1975

28. Littlefield JW: Selection of hybrids from matings of fibroblasts in vitro and their presumed recombinants. Science 145:709–810, 1964

29. Wolf SF, Mareni CE, Migeon BR: Isolation and characterization of cloned DNA sequences that hybridize to the human X chromosome. Cell 21:95–102, 1980

30. Wigler M, Sweet R, Sim GK, et al: Transformation of mammalian cells with genes from prokaryotes and eukaryotes. Cell 16:777–785, 1979

Index

Page references to topics in figures or tables are in *italics*.